P9-DFF-244

Statistical Record
OF Health &
Medicine

Charity Anne Dorgan, Editor

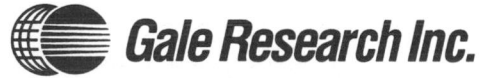
Gale Research Inc.

An International Thomson Publishing Company

I⊤P

NEW YORK • LONDON • BONN • BOSTON • DETROIT • MADRID
MELBOURNE • MEXICO CITY • PARIS • SINGAPORE • TOKYO
TORONTO • WASHINGTON • ALBANY NY • BELMONT CA • CINCINNATI OH

Charity Anne Dorgan, *Editor*

Editorial Code & Data Inc. Staff

Helen S. Fisher, Marlita A. Reddy, and Susan M. Turner, *Contributing Editors*
Karyn Dunford and Robert S. Lazich, *Associate Editors*
Kenneth J. Muth, *Manager, Technical Operations*
Gary Alampi, *Programmer/analyst*

Gale Research Inc. Staff

Karen Boyden, *Coordinating Editor*
Sheila Dow and Jacqueline L. Longe, *Associate Editors*
Mary Beth Trimper, *Production Director*
Mary Kelley, *Production Associate*
Cynthia Baldwin, *Product Design Manager*
Barbara J. Yarrow, *Graphic Services Supervisor*
C. J. Jonik, *Desktop Publisher*

While every effort has been made to ensure the reliability of the information presented in this publication, Gale Research Inc. does not guarantee the accuracy of the data contained herein. Gale accepts no payment for listing; and inclusion in the publication of any organization, agency, institution, publication, service, or individual does not imply endorsement by the editors or publisher. Errors brought to the attention of the publisher and verified to the satisfaction of the publisher will be corrected in future editions.

This publication is a creative work fully protected by all applicable copyright laws, as well as by misappropriation, trade secret, unfair competition, and other applicable laws. The authors and editors of this work have added value to the underlying factual material herein through one or more of the following: unique and original selection, coordination, expression, arrangement, and classification of the information.

All rights to this publication will be vigorously defended.

Copyright © 1995
Gale Research Inc.
835 Penobscot Building
Detroit, MI 48226-4094

All rights reserved including the right of reproduction in whole or in part in any form.

∞™ The paper used in this publication meets the minimum requirements of American National Standard for Information Sciences—Permanence Paper for Printed Library Materials, ANSI Z39.48-1984.

✪ This book is printed on recycled paper that meets Environmental Protection Agency standards.

ISBN 0-8103-9745-5
ISSN 1078-6961
10 9 8 7 6 5 4 3 2 1

Printed in the United States of America
Published simultaneously in the United Kingdom
by Gale Research International Limited
(An affiliated company of Gale Research Inc.)

I(T)P™ Gale Research Inc., an International Thomson Publishing Company.
ITP logo is a trademark under license.

TABLE OF CONTENTS

CHAPTER 6 - HEALTH EXPENDITURES AND FUNDING continued:

Features of This Edition

Statistical Record of Health and Medicine (SRHM) is a comprehensive compilation of national, state, and municipal health and medical statistics drawn from government, academic, association, trade, technical, and media sources. *SRHM* provides broad subject coverage of the field with data on contemporary health-related issues and concerns. Highlights of this edition include:

- More than 960 statistical tables.
- Approximately 380 sources.
- National, state, and local data.
- Comparative statistics from selected foreign countries.
- Summary indicator tables.
- Explanations of health and medical acronyms and abbreviations.
- Annotated source listings.
- Comprehensive keyword index, with extensive cross-references.

Locate Hard-to-Find Data Easily and Quickly

Locating timely and accurate statistical data on health-related matters can be troublesome. Often consumers of professional journals and trade periodicals discard their personal copies only to find that they need to reference a chart or graph from last month's or last year's issue—if indeed the consumer can recall the correct issue in which to locate the material. Libraries (particularly small or specialized ones) cannot purchase every source or retain unlimited back issues of material owing to budget and space constraints, so relevant statistical tables may not be available among the holdings. Frequently charts, graphs, and tables are omitted from online versions of material. *SRHM*, however, provides substantial and detailed coverage of statistics related to major areas of health and medicine. Here are statistics useful to a variety of individuals; for example,

- The student preparing a report or speech.
- The health care practitioner compiling a patient information brochure or journal article.
- The job seeker identifying employment possibilities throughout the United States.
- The consumer of medical services comparing costs of treatments or procedures.

SRHM tables are arranged conveniently by subject for quick access. Related tables are located easily through the Keyword Index and its many cross-references.

Universal Coverage

SRHM covers the health arena comprehensively. Topics include long-standing concerns such as leading causes of death, occupational health and safety, the Consumer Price Index for medical care, trends and projections regarding Social Security's future, and medical malpractice premium rates. In addition, *SRHM* presents a wide range of data on contemporary issues, notably assisted suicide, relative risk of contracting AIDS, domestic violence, and health care reform proposals. Therefore, parents looking for information about their kindergartners' chicken pox or a health care administrator benchmarking cost savings at hospitals with and without quality programs will both find the appropriate statistics easily.

Introduction

"A wise man should consider that health is the greatest of human blessings, and learn how by his own thought to derive benefit from his illnesses." —Hippocrates

In 1990, life expectancy in the United States was 75.4 years. According to the National Center for Health Statistics, the average American will enjoy good health for 64 of those years—about 85 percent of his or her life ("Healthy People 2000 Review." *Health United States, 1992.* Hyattsville, MD: Public Health Service, 1993). The remaining 11.4 years will be spent suffering from any number of diseases, injuries, or disabilities.

Statistical Record of Health and Medicine (SRHM) is a comprehensive compilation of national, state, and municipal health and medical statistics profiling health in the United States, particularly those conditions and concerns causing the average American to sacrifice 15 percent of his or her life to ill health. Data in *SRHM* are drawn from more than 380 government, academic, association, trade, technical, and media sources, thus providing broad subject coverage of health and medical fields. *SRHM* provides statistics on:

- The health status and lifestyle of Americans;
- Specific health care and medical establishments such as hospitals and nursing homes;
- Occupational health and safety;
- Insurance;
- Health care costs and expenditures of consumers, governments, and businesses;
- Health care programs, including Medicaid and Medicare;
- Health care industries, including companies, products, and market trends;
- Medical professions and occupations;
- The medical establishment—from the physician in solo private practice to the largest hospital chains;
- Political issues, opinions and attitudes, and the laws related to health care and medicine; and
- International rankings and comparisons.

This edition also features summary indicator tables, a comprehensive keyword index, annotated source listings, and explanations of acronyms and abbreviations.

Scope and Coverage

Subjects Covered. *SRHM* provides a comprehensive overview of the health arena. Chapters include:

Health Status of Americans. Approximately 150 tables cover health measures, determinants, and conditions in the United States. Topics include aging; children; death; dental health; disabilities and handicaps; diseases and illnesses; environmental health; injuries and accidents; institutionalized populations; life expectancy; men; mental health; pregnancy and childbirth; and women.

Health Care Establishment. This chapter features close to 100 tables profiling health care providers, establishments, treatments, practices, and procedures. Topics include blood banks; health care practitioners; drugs and medicine; home health care; hospitals; immunization and vaccinations; long-term care; medical devices; outpatient services; preventative medicine; surgical and diagnostic procedures; transplants; and treatment options and alternatives.

Lifestyles and Health. Nearly 85 tables show health habits of Americans as well as contemporary health issues and trends. Topics include addiction and recovery; exercise and fitness; insurance coverage; nutrition; poverty; sex; smoking and tobacco; stress; and violence and trauma.

Health in the Workplace. This chapter presents more than 50 tables on occupational health and safety. Topics include health-related costs to businesses; employee benefits; retiree benefits; disabilities; employee injuries and fatalities; lost work time and sick days; wellness promotion programs; and workers' compensation.

Health Expenditures and Funding. Approximately 100 tables cover spending on health care by individuals and governments. Topics include consumer spending; federal government spending; state government spending, local government spending, and trends and projections.

Health Care Programs. The more than 65 tables in this chapter reflect financial, administrative, and delivery programs providing health care to Americans. Topics include Medicaid; Medicare; Social Security; social welfare; and veterans.

Health Care Industries. This chapter features more than 110 tables with varied data on health-related industries, including major players, markets, products and services, and trends. Topics include health services such as kidney dialysis centers and medical equipment rental; hospitals; insurance carriers; laboratories and research firms; medical technology; nursing and personal care facilities; offices and clinics of practitioners; pharmaceutical manufacturers; and retail and wholesale trades.

Medical Professions. Here are in excess of 95 tables presenting occupational data about careers, jobs, and earnings. Topics include associations; education; employment; and salaries and wages.

Medical Establishment. This chapter covers organizations and issues relevant to the medical community through 75 tables. Topics include advertising; computers; construction; food service; grants and contracts; investment and ownership; labor; libraries and information services; licensing; medical practice management; medical publishing; medical research; medical technology; medical waste; philanthropy; and total quality management.

Politics, Opinion, and Law. Close to 60 tables profile ethical, legal, political, and social issues related to health care. Topics include attitudes and opinions on medical costs, privacy, and medical research, among other subjects; elections (campaigns, lobbyists, and like concerns); health care reform; legislation and litigation; and malpractice and abuse.

International Comparisons. Approximately 60 tables compare and rank health care performance of other nations with that of the United States. Topics include costs; death; disease; drugs and medicine; equipment and facilities; grants and contracts; homicide; insurance; life expectancy; medical administration; medical personnel; patient care; politics; research and technology; suicide; and treatments and procedures.

Geographic Area Covered. *SRHM* covers health and medicine in the United States. Depending on the table, data presented may reflect the national, state, or local level. Chapter 12 profiles health care on a worldwide basis. Tables in this chapter offer comparisons and rankings of foreign countries in the subject areas profiled for the United States elsewhere in this edition. Nations selected usually are similar to the United States in economic development.

Period Covered. Most of the material in *SRHM* dates from 1990 or later. If the only data available pre-dated 1990 (1987 Economic Census data, for instance), then that material was included to ensure comprehensive coverage of the field. Some of the tables also present earlier data for historical purposes; for example, to illustrate changes—growth or decline—over time. Whenever possible, projections have been provided to indicate trends and forecasts. In any case, the most recent data available at the time of compilation have been included in this edition.

Sources

Thousands of health-related statistics are produced by a variety of reliable sources each year. Data were selected for inclusion in *SRHM* on the basis of their timeliness, interest or value to researchers and the general public, and their ability to contribute to the comprehensive coverage of the field.

Much of the statistical material included in *SRHM* comes from the U.S. federal government or from state and other government levels under federal mandate. Many of the tables were drawn from statistical services or special reports of major federal departments; for example, the Department of Health and Human Services, the body that administers programs and collects statistics on health and medicine in the United States. Statistics from departments of Commerce, Labor, Education, and Justice frequently are cited, as is material from Congressional hearings.

SRHM also features data from media sources, including newspapers, business periodicals, trade magazines, professional journals, and association publications. These media often rely on the government or other sources for the information they provide. Nevertheless, presentation of material in current literature is indicative of issues, anxieties, and aspirations occupying the American consciousness. In addition, *SRHM* offers statistics collected by associations, special surveys and studies, opinion polls, and election statistics.

Acknowledgments

Many people and organizations contributed data, suggestions, permission, and advice in the compilation of *SRHM*. The editorial staff thanks them all for their help and guidance. Special thanks are due to the AAFRC Trust for Philanthropy, the Conference Board, the Foundation Center, Health Insurance Association of America, Medical Group Management Association, and Medical Library Association.

Comments and Suggestions

Although every effort has been made to ensure the accuracy and timeliness of the data in *SRHM*, errors and omissions may occur. Notification of changes or additions deemed appropriate by users of this edition are appreciated. Comments and suggestions for the improvement of *SRHM* are welcome. Please contact:

Statistical Record of Health and Medicine
Gale Research Inc.
835 Penobscot Building
Detroit, MI 48226-4094
Phone: (313)961-2242
Toll-free: 800-347-GALE
Fax: (313)961-6815

How to Use This Book

Statistical Record of Health and Medicine (SRHM) is organized into 12 chapters, the first of which contains summary indicators. (See the Table of Contents or the Introduction on the preceding pages for a list of chapters.) Each chapter begins with notes that explain its contents and reference related material elsewhere in *SRHM*. To facilitate browsing through 960 *SRHM* tables, the chapter titles also appear in the upper right- or upper left-hand corners of pages.

SRHM chapters are subdivided by alphabetically arranged topics. Topic notations are placed above the first table in subject groupings for easy identification. The topic is shown again in italic type below each subsequent table's reference number.

Organization of Tables

Tables are arranged alphabetically by title within each topic grouping. In addition, each table is numbered sequentially, beginning with the first table in the first chapter. Hence, data may be accessed through table reference numbers or alphabetically by topic and table title.

Tables appear in the Sources list by table number. Tables can be accessed by reference number or by page number using the Table of Contents or the Keyword Index.

Some tables display graphic presentations such as bar graphs and pie charts. If the table has more than one column of data, the number of the column represented by the graphic is identified. Complete tabular data follow each graphic.

A selection of material in *SRHM* is of a textual nature. Nevertheless, these entries contain predominantly statistical data. Occasionally, such entries offer explanatory material.

Special Features

Abbreviations and Acronyms. This list shows all the abbreviations, acronyms, and initialisms that appear in tables throughout *SRHM*. While explanations and translations of abbreviations will be found within the text of tables, a general listing is provided here for the convenience of *SRHM* users. Abbreviations and acronyms are listed in alphabetic order, with explanations following.

Summary Indicators. A brief introductory chapter provides quick access to some of the more conventional material included in the body of *SRHM*. These graphic summaries contain data extracted from one or more tables located elsewhere in the text to offer a convenient overview of health issues such as causes of death or political clout of the medical establishment.

Sources. An appendix lists all the sources cited in tables included in *SRHM*. Sources are arranged alphabetically by author name or title as appropriate. In the case of periodicals, dates of issues consulted are shown. The list provides table references, showing all data citing a particular source.

Keyword Index. This index allows users to access all subjects, issues, diseases, medical specialties, industries, companies, programs, insurance carriers, associations, schools, educational programs, occupations, personal names, and locations cited in the tables of *SRHM*. Each citation is followed by table and page reference numbers. Page references do not necessarily identify the page on which a table begins. In the cases where tables span two or more pages, references point to the page on which the index term appears—which may be the second or subsequent page of a table. Frequent cross-references have been added to index citations to facilitate the location of related topics and tables.

Sample Table

The following sample table shows elements commonly included in *SRHM* tables. Each numbered paragraph corresponds to the numbered item in the sample.

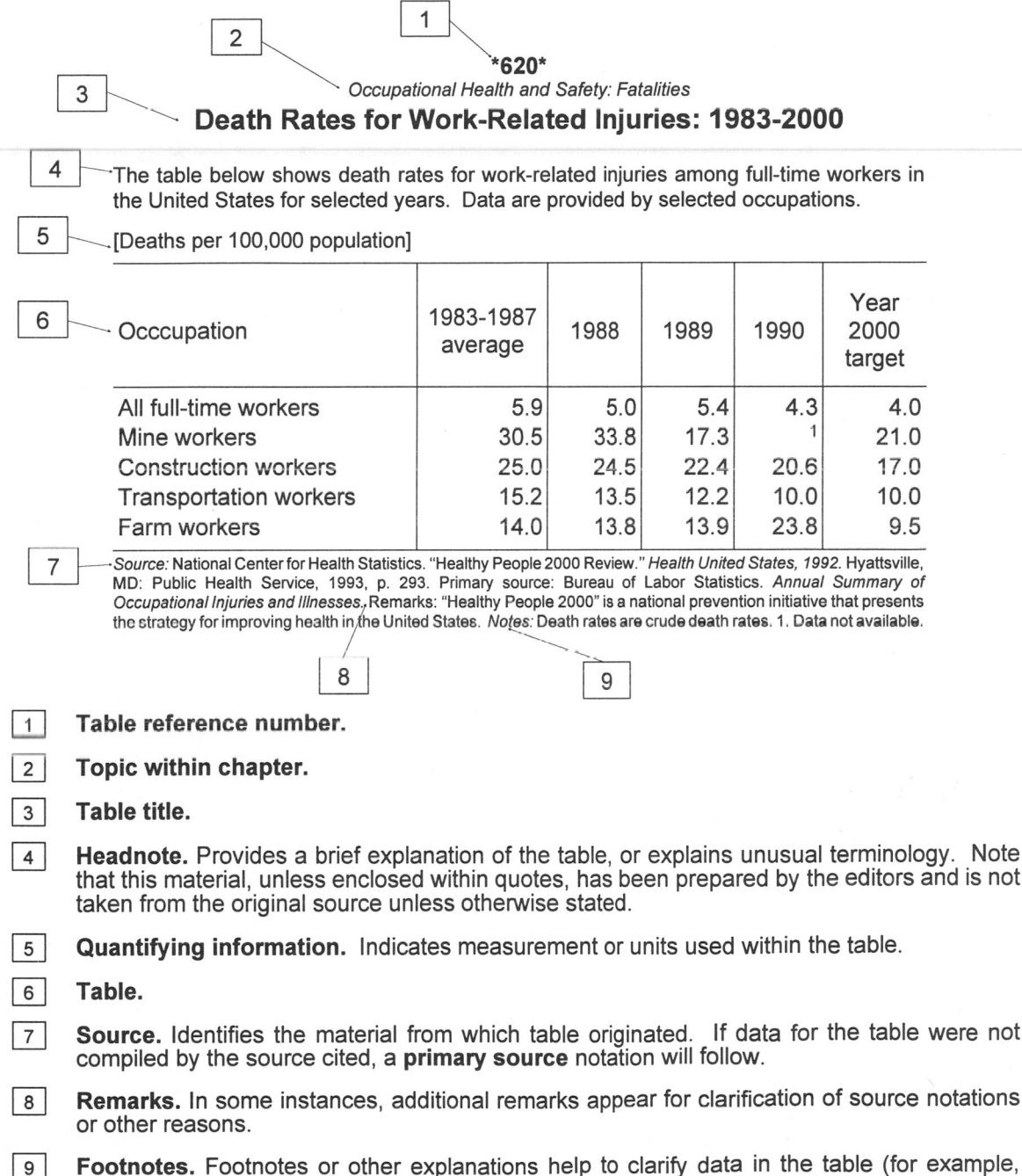

1

2

3

620

Occupational Health and Safety: Fatalities

Death Rates for Work-Related Injuries: 1983-2000

4 The table below shows death rates for work-related injuries among full-time workers in the United States for selected years. Data are provided by selected occupations.

5 [Deaths per 100,000 population]

6

Occcupation	1983-1987 average	1988	1989	1990	Year 2000 target
All full-time workers	5.9	5.0	5.4	4.3	4.0
Mine workers	30.5	33.8	17.3	[1]	21.0
Construction workers	25.0	24.5	22.4	20.6	17.0
Transportation workers	15.2	13.5	12.2	10.0	10.0
Farm workers	14.0	13.8	13.9	23.8	9.5

7 *Source:* National Center for Health Statistics. "Healthy People 2000 Review." *Health United States, 1992.* Hyattsville, MD: Public Health Service, 1993, p. 293. Primary source: Bureau of Labor Statistics. *Annual Summary of Occupational Injuries and Illnesses.* Remarks: "Healthy People 2000" is a national prevention initiative that presents the strategy for improving health in the United States. *Notes:* Death rates are crude death rates. 1. Data not available.

8   **9**

1 **Table reference number.**

2 **Topic within chapter.**

3 **Table title.**

4 **Headnote.** Provides a brief explanation of the table, or explains unusual terminology. Note that this material, unless enclosed within quotes, has been prepared by the editors and is not taken from the original source unless otherwise stated.

5 **Quantifying information.** Indicates measurement or units used within the table.

6 **Table.**

7 **Source.** Identifies the material from which table originated. If data for the table were not compiled by the source cited, a **primary source** notation will follow.

8 **Remarks.** In some instances, additional remarks appear for clarification of source notations or other reasons.

9 **Footnotes.** Footnotes or other explanations help to clarify data in the table (for example, missing information or special criteria for reported information) or to explain and clarify as in the case of translating acronyms and abbreviations.

Abbreviations and Acronyms

Abbreviations and acronyms used in tables or notes are explained within the context of the data presented. The listing below includes all abbreviations, acronyms, and initialisms used in the *Statistical Record of Health and Medicine,* together with their full translations or meanings. One abbreviation may represent multiple items or organizations. Where more than one use is possible, all explanations of the term are provided. Abbreviations and acronyms in this list appear in alphabetic order.

AAMC	Association of American Medical Colleges	**AR**	Arkansas
AAHSLD	Association of Academic Health Sciences Library Directors	**ASHA**	American Speech-Language-Hearing Association
AAP	American Academy of Pediatrics	**ATV**	All-terrain vehicle
ADA	American Dental Association	**AZ**	Arizona
ADA	American Dietetic Association	**BA**	Bachelor of Arts
ADA	Americans With Disabilities Act	**BAC**	Blood alcohol content
ADL	Activities of daily living	**BATF**	Bureau of Alcohol, Tobacco, and Firearms
AFDC	Aid to Families With Dependent Children	**BLS**	Bureau of Labor Statistics
AHCA	American Health Care Association	**BPH**	Benign prostatic hypertrophy
AHIMA	American Health Information Management Association	**BS**	Bachelor of Science
AIDS	Acquired immunodeficiency syndrome	**BSN**	Bachelor of Science in Nursing
AK	Alaska	**CA**	California
AL	Alabama	**CAD**	Computer-assisted ...
ALHHS	Archivists and Librarians in the Health Sciences (formerly Association of Librarians in the History of Health Sciences)	**CAM**	Computer-assist... manufacture
		CAT	Computerized ...omography
		CBO	Congressi... get Office
		CC	Child an...are ...inical
ALS	Amyotrophic lateral sclerosis	**CCC-A**	Certifi...e—Audiology
AMA	American Medical Association		C...
AMHL	Association of Mental Health Librarians		
APA	American Psychological Association		

CCC-SLP	Certificate of Clinical Competence—Speech-Language Pathology
CDC	Centers for Disease Control
CE	Consumer Expenditure Survey
CEO	Chief executive officer
CFOI	Census of Fatal Occupational Injuries
CHAMPUS	Civilian Health and Medical Program of the Uniformed Services
CI	Cumulative incidence
CIA	Clinical Investigator Awards
cm	Centimeter
CMSA	Consolidated Metropolitan Statistical Area
CO	Colorado
COBRA	Consolidated Omnibus Reconciliation Act
COPD	Chronic obstructive pulmonary disease
COTH	Council of Teaching Hospitals
CPI	Consumer Price Index
CPR	Cardiopulmonary resuscitation
CPS	Current Population Survey
CQI	Continuous quality improvement
CRS	Congenital rubella syndrome
CSA	Community Services Administration
CT	Connecticut
DC	District of Columbia
DE	Delaware
DFTERN	fund for full-time equivalent registered nurses
DHHS	U.S. Department of Health and Human Services
DI	Disability insurance
dl	deciliter
DO	Doctor of osteopathy

DOS	Disk operating system
DPT	Diphtheria, pertussis, and tetanus
DRG	Diagnosis-related groups
EAP	Employee Assistance Program
EEDC	Equal Employment Opportunity Commission
EEG	Electroencephalograph
EEO	Equal Employment Opportunity
EKG	Electrocardiograph
ESA	Economics and Statistics Administration
ESRD	End-stage renal disease
FADHPS	Financial Aid for Disadvantage Health Professions Students
FARS	Fatal Accident Reporting System
FAS	Financial accounting standard
FCoA	Federal Council on the Aging
FDA	U.S. Food and Drug Administration
FL	Florida
FMG	Foreign medical graduates
FMI	Food Marketing Institute
FNS	Food and Nutrition Service
FSMB	Federal State Medical Board
FTE	Full-time equivalent
g	gram(s)
GA	Georgia
GAO	U.S. General Accounting Office
GDP	Gross Domestic Product
GF	Government finances
GNP	Gross National Product
GOP	Grand Old Party; Republican Party
HCFA	Health Care Financing Administration
HCV	Hepatitis C virus
HEAL	Health Education Assistance Loan

HHANES	Hispanic Health and Nutrition Examination Survey
HI	Hawaii
HI	Hospital Insurance
HIV	Human immunodeficiency virus
HMO	Health maintenance organization
HR	Human Resources
IA	Iowa
IADL	Instrumental activities for daily living
IAQ	Indoor air quality
ID	Idaho
IL	Illinois
IMG	International medical graduates
IN	Indiana
IPA	Independent Practice Association
IPEDS	Integrated Postsecondary Education Data System
IRA	Individual retirement account
IUD	Intrauterine device
IVDA	Intravenous drug abuse
JAMA	Journal of the American Medical Association
JAVMA	Journal of American Veterinary Medicine Association
JTPA	Job Training Partnership Act
KS	Kansas
KY	Kentucky
LA	Louisiana
LCME	Liaison Committee on Medical Education
LIHEAP	Low-Income Home Energy Assistance Program
LPN	Licensed practical nurse
LSC	Life Safety Code
LSD	Lysergic acid diethylamide
LTC	Long-term care

MA	Massachusetts
MA	Master of Arts
MAA	Medical Assistance for the Aged
MD	Doctor of Medicine
MD	Maryland
ME	Maine
MERIT	Method to Extend Research in Time
MeSH	Medical subject headings
MI	Michigan
MLA	Medical Library Association
MLA-MHLS	Medical Library Association-Mental Health Librarians Section
MMR	Measles-mumps-rubella
MN	Minnesota
MO	Missouri
MRI	Magnetic resonance imager or imaging
MS	Master of Science
MS	Mississippi
MSA	Metropolitan Statistical Area
MSHA	Mine Safety and Health Administration
MT	Montana
NA	Not available; not applicable
NC	North Carolina
NCHS	National Center for Health Statistics
ND	North Dakota
NE	Nebraska
NEISS	National Electronic Injury Surveillance System
NETS	Network of Employers for Traffic Safety
NH	New Hampshire
NHA	National Health Accounts
NHLBI	National Heart, Lung, and Blood Institute
NIA	National Institute on Aging
NIH	National Institutes for Health

NIJ	National Institute of Justice
NJ	New Jersey
NM	New Mexico
no.	Number
NSLP	National School Lunch Program
NV	Nevada
NY	New York
OASDHI	Old-Age, Survivors, and Disability Health Insurance
OASDI	Old-Age, Survivors, and Disability Insurance
OASI	Old-Age, Survivors Insurance
OB	Obstetrics; obstetrician
OECD	Organization for Economic Cooperation and Development
OH	Ohio
OHD	Other health doctorates
OK	Oklahoma
OR	Oregon
OSHA	Occupational Safety and Health Administration
PA	Pennsylvania
PAA	Pulmonary Academic Awards
PAC	Political action committee
PBGC	Pension Benefit Guaranty Corporation
PCAA	Preventive Cardiology Academic Awards
PCP	Phencyclidine
PhD	Doctor of Philosophy
PHS	Public Health Service
POS	Point-of-service plan
PPO	Preferred provider organization
PPA	Physician Scientist Awards
PPS	Prospective Payment System
PR	Puerto Rico

PRK	Photorefractive keratectomy
R&D	Research and development
RCA	Research Career Awards
RN	Registered nurse
RPG	Research Project Grant
RR	Relative risk
SB	School Breakfast
SBIR	Small Business Innovation Research
SBS	Sick building syndrome
SC	South Carolina
SCOR	Specialized Centers for Research
SD	South Dakota
SES	Socioeconomic status
SF	School Funding
SGLI	Servicemen's Group Life Insurance
SMA	State Mental Health Agency
SMI	Supplemental Medical Insurance
SNF	Skilled-nursing facility
SOA	Survey on Aging
SPF	Sun protection factor
SPVDAA	Systemic Pulmonary and Vascular Disease Academic Awards
SSA	Social Security Administration
SSI	Supplemental Security Income
STD	Sexually transmitted disease
TB	Tuberculosis
TMAA	Transfusion Medicine Academic Awards
TN	Tennessee
TQM	Total quality management
TX	Texas
UCLA	University of California, Los Angeles
UN	United Nations
UR	Utilization review

USC	University of Southern California
UT	Utah
VA	U.S. Department of Veterans Affairs
VA	U.S. Veterans Administration
VA	Virginia
VI	Virgin Islands
VMLS/MLA	Veterinary Medical Libraries Section/Medical Library Association
VN	Vocational nurse

VT	Vermont
WA	Washington
WHO	World Health Organization
WI	Wisconsin
WIC	Special Supplemental Food Program for Women, Infants, and Children
WV	West Virginia
WY	Wyoming

Statistical Record
OF Health &
Medicine

Chapter 1
SUMMARY INDICATORS

The 8 tables in this chapter provide an overview of the material included in *Statistical Record of Health and Medicine,* highlighting major aspects of the health field. Each table was compiled from data included elsewhere in *SRHM.* Locations of full data are indicated in the Table column. Listed numbers in this column show table (not page) reference numbers.

★ 1 ★

Death as a Measurement of Health

Segment of population	Leading cause of death	Deaths from leading cause	Denomination	Date	Table
Fetal	Not reported	29,345	Number	1990	0140
Infants	Congenital anomalies	8,239	Number	1990	0141
Children					
1-4 year olds	Accidents	2,566	Number	1990	0022
5-14 year olds	Accidents	3,650	Number	1990	0022
Teens	Accidents	16,241	In thousands	1990	0023
Women	Heart disease	359,270	Number	1990	0154
Men	Heart disease	720,050	Number	1990	0119
Older Americans					
55-59 year olds	Malignant neoplasms	352.7	Per 100,000	-	0014
60-64 year olds	Malignant neoplasms	538.7	Per 100,000	-	0014
65-69 year olds	Heart disease	820.4	Per 100,000	-	0014
70-74 year olds	Heart disease	1,323.4	Per 100,000	-	0014
75-79 year olds	Heart disease	2,098.1	Per 100,000	-	0014
80-84 year olds	Heart disease	3,526.1	Per 100,000	-	0014
85 year olds or older	Heart disease	7,178.7	Per 100,000	-	0014

Source: Data are drawn from tables elsewhere in *Statistical Record of Health and Medicine.*

★ 2 ★

Health Care Industry Receipts

Industry	Amount	Denomination	Percent	Date	Table
Health services					
Medical doctors' offices	$122,470	Million	46.9	1991	0650
Hospitals	$31,523	Million	12.1	1991	0586
Dentists' offices	$29,731	Million	11.4	1991	0648
Nursing and personal care facilities	$28,848	Million	11.0	1991	0636
General medical and surgical hospitals	$24,518	Million	9.4	1991	0582
Skilled nursing care facilities	$23,623	Million	9.0	1991	0641
Medical and dental laboratories	$10,527	Million	4.0	1991	0610
Medical laboratories	$8,849	Million	3.4	1991	0612
Home health care services	$7,381	Million	2.8	1991	0567
Specialty outpatient facilties	$6,426	Million	2.5	1991	0577
Psychiatric hospitals	$5,436	Million	2.1	1991	0590
Chiropractors' offices	$4,986	Million	1.9	1991	0646
Optometrists' offices	$4,430	Million	1.7	1991	0654
Intermediate care facilities	$3,338	Million	1.3	1991	0631
Osteopaths' offices	$2,599	Million	.99	1991	0652
Podiatrists' offices	$1,826	Million	.70	1991	0658
Dental laboratories	$1,678	Million	.64	1991	0607
Specialty hospitals, except psychiatric	$1,569	Million	.60	1991	0594
Kidney dialysis centers	$1,505	Million	.58	1991	0572
Business services					
Medical equipment rental and leasing	$2,424	Million	.86	1991	0575

Source: Data are drawn from tables elsewhere in *Statistical Record of Health and Medicine.*

★ 3 ★

Health Expenditures

Source of spending	Amount	Denomination	Percent distribution	Date	Table
Households	$247.0	Billion	33.9	1991	0411
Businesses	$205.4	Billion	28.2	1991	0342
Federal government	$133.8	Billion	18.4	1991	0418
State and local governments	$120.7	Billion	16.6	1991	0476

Source: Data are drawn from tables elsewhere in *Statistical Record of Health and Medicine.*

★ 4 ★

Health Habits and Living Conditions

People who:	Value	Denomination	Date	Table
Used alcohol in the past year	138,238	In thousands	1991	0258
Used cigarettes in the past year	65,119	In thousands	1991	0319
Used cocaine in the past year	2,594	In thousands	1991	0262
Exercise or play sports regularly	40.7	Percent	1990	0281
Are 20 percent or more above desirable body weights	27.5	Percent	1990	0304
Lack health insurance	37	Million	1991	0287
Live in poverty	33,585	In thousands	1990	0310

Source: Data are drawn from tables elsewhere in *Statistical Record of Health and Medicine.*

★ 5 ★

Health-Related Social Welfare Programs

Programs	Value	Denomination	Date	Table
Medicaid				
Recipients	28,280	In thousands	1991	0495
Payments	$77,048	Million	1991	0495
Medicare				
Enrollment	34,870	In thousands	1991	0506
Payments	$118,546	Million	1991	0506
Public aid				
Aid to Families With Dependent Children				
Recipients	4,708	In thousands	1991	0547
Payments	$390	Average monthly	1991	0547
General assistance cases				
Recipients	1,106	In thousands	1991	0547
Old-age assistance				
Recipients	17	In thousands	1991	0547
Payments	$55	Average monthly	1991	0547
Supplemental Social Insurance				
Recipients	5,118	In thousands	1991	0547
Payments	$321	Average monthly	1991	0547
Social Security				
Beneficiaries	40,568	In thousands	1991	0522
Payments (annual)	268,098	In thousands	1991	0521
Veterans compensation				
Enrollment	3,428	In thousands	1992	0558
Payment	$4,712	Average annual	1992	0558

Source: Data are drawn from tables elsewhere in *Statistical Record of Health and Medicine.*

★6★

Health Services Utilization

Health service	Amount	Denomination	Date	Table
Alternative therapies	19	Visits/year	1990	0254
Doctors' office visits	669,689	Number	1991	0166
Home health care				
Skilled nursing	8.56	Visits/episode	-	0191
Home health aide	7.63	Visits/episode	-	0191
Physical therapy	12.83	Visits/episode	-	0191
Occupational/speech therapy or social work	1.21	Visits/episode	-	0191
Hospitals				
Inpatient care	302	Days	1991	0232
Outpatient care	388	Visits	1991	0232
House calls				
Family practitioners making one or more house calls	65	Percent	1992-1993	0163
General practitioners making one or more house calls	43	Percent	1992-1993	0163

Source: Data are drawn from tables elsewhere in *Statistical Record of Health and Medicine.*

★7★

Medical Salaries

Occupation	Salary	Date	Table
Radiologist	$240,000	1992	0765
Anesthesiologist	$220,000	1992	0765
Surgeon	$207,000	1992	0765
Obstetrician/gynecologist	$190,000	1992	0765
Pathologist	$170,000	1992	0765
Physician	$170,000	1991	0764
Hospital chief of medical affairs	$159,300	1993	0754
Internist	$130,000	1992	0765
Psychiatrist	$120,000	1992	0765
Pediatrician	$112,000	1992	0765
Family practitioner	$100,000	1992	0765
Hospital's chief financial officer	$97,700	1993	0754
Nurse anesthetist	$68,312	1992	0757
Clinical psychologist	$58,240	1990	0747
Hospital's head of marketing	$57,500	1993	0754
Head nurse	$47,911	1992	0757
Clinical nurse specialist	$45,974	1992	0757
Nurse practitioner	$45,012	1992	0757
Physical therapist	$43,281	1990	0747
Staff nurse	$35,982	1992	0757
Pharmacist	$35,200	1990	0760

[Continued]

★ 7 ★

Medical Salaries
[Continued]

Occupation	Salary	Date	Table
Occupational therapist	$35,000	1990	0747
Audiologist	$32,000	1990	0747
Speech-language pathologist	$30,000	1990	0747
Paramedic	$27,320	1991	0748
Emergency medical technician	$23,108	1991	0748
Veterinary technician in small animal practice	$16,600	1991	0749

Source: Data are drawn from tables elsewhere in *Statistical Record of Health and Medicine.*

★ 8 ★

Political Action Committee Contributions

Group	Contributions	Denomination	Percent	Date	Table
Health professionals	$35.5	Million	47.1	1981-1992	0872
Insurance industry	$23.8	Million	31.7	1981-1992	0872
American Medical Association	$14.9	Million	19.9	1981-1992	0871
Pharmaceutical Industry	$10.3	Million	13.7	1981-1992	0872
Hospitals	$7.3	Million	9.7	1981-1992	0872
National Association of Life Underwriters	$6.7	Million	8.9	1981-1992	0871
American Dental Association	$5.3	Million	7.1	1981-1992	0871
American Academy of Ophthalmology	$2.6	Million	3.5	1981-1992	0871
American Hospital Association	$2.2	Million	2.9	1981-1992	0871
American Family Corporation	$2.1	Million	2.8	1981-1992	0871
American Optometric Association	$1.7	Million	2.3	1981-1992	0871

Source: Data are drawn from tables elsewhere in *Statistical Record of Health and Medicine.*

Chapter 2
HEALTH STATUS OF AMERICANS

In *The Book of Answers,* Barbara Berliner reports the value of a human body as more than $171,000—about $169,000 worth of chemicals and $1,200 in blood (New York, New York: Prentice Hall, 1990, p. 102). It is no wonder, then, that people go to great lengths to take care of their bodies, which are ever threatened by a variety of health risks. The tables in this chapter show the effects of diseases, disabilities, and illnesses on specific populations—for example, Older Americans, children, or prisoners—as well as American men and women in general. Specifically, tables profile acute and chronic conditions, notifiable diseases (such as tuberculosis and other highly contagious illnesses), and the leading causes of death. Data also cover health measures and determinants such as life expectancy, birth and death rates, fertility, infant mortality, and prenatal care. Dental and environmental health subjects are covered as well, but the chapter excludes animal health topics since these fall outside of the scope of *Statistical Record of Health and Medicine.* Animal health occupations, however, are included in the chapter on Medical Professions.

Aging

★ 9 ★

Accidents and Older Americans

People over age 65 comprise about 12 percent of the population and suffer 27 percent of all accidental deaths. The National Safety Council reports that each year about 27,000 persons over age 65 die from accidental injuries and thousands of others are severely injured—frequently in mishaps involving motor vehicles. The table below ranks motor vehicles as a cause of accidental death for older Americans.

AGE GROUP	RANK AS A CAUSE OF ACCIDENTAL DEATH
65-74 year olds	Most common cause
Older people in general	Second most common cause

Source: U.S. Department of Health and Human Services. Public Health Service. National Institute on Aging. *Bound for Good Health: A Collection of Age Pages.* Bethesda, MD: National Institute on Aging, c. 1991, n.p.

★ 10 ★

Aging

AIDS and Older Americans

As many as 10 percent of all AIDS cases reported have involved people aged 50 and over. The older population also receives the highest rate of blood transfusions during routine medical care. As a result, the second most common cause of AIDS in people over age 50 (after homosexual and bisexual activity) has been exposure to contaminated blood transfusions received before 1985 when the public blood supply was not being screened for the virus.

Source: U.S. Department of Health and Human Services. Public Health Service. National Institute on Aging. *Bound for Good Health: A Collection of Age Pages.* Bethesda, MD: National Institute on Aging, c. 1991, n.p.

★ 11 ★

Aging

Hearing Impairment in Older Americans

More than 10 million older people in the United States are hearing impaired. The table below shows the percent of older Americans suffering from some degree of hearing loss.

Age group	Percent suffering from hearing loss
65-74 years old	30
75-79 years old	50

Source: U.S. Department of Health and Human Services. Public Health Service. National Institute on Aging. *Bound for Good Health: A Collection of Age Pages.* Bethesda, MD: National Institute on Aging, c. 1991, n.p.

★ 12 ★

Aging

High Blood Pressure and Older Americans

As many as 58 million Americans may have high blood pressure. About 40 percent of whites and more than 50 percent of blacks age 65 and older suffer some form of the disease.

Source: U.S. Department of Health and Human Services. Public Health Service. National Institute on Aging. *Bound for Good Health: A Collection of Age Pages.* Bethesda, MD: National Institute on Aging, c. 1991, n.p.

★ 13 ★

Aging

Hospital Stays of Older Americans for Selected Illnesses

[Discharges from nonfederal short-stay hospitals]

Age and first-listed diagnosis	Average length of stay in days	
	1981	1987
55-59 years		
Heart disease	8.1	5.9
Malignant neoplasms	10.5	9.3
Cerebrovascular disease	9.6	11.7
Inguinal hernia	4.8	2.1
Fractures[1]	8.3	7.4
Hyperplasia of prostate	6.4	4.5
60-64 years		
Heart disease	8.3	6.2
Malignant neoplasms	10.3	8.8
Cerebrovascular disease	11.7	8.9
Hyperplasia of prostate	7.2	4.8
Inguinal hernia	4.8	2.2
Pneumonia[2]	10.8	8.4
65-69 years		
Heart disease	9.3	7.0
Malignant neoplasms	12.8	9.1
Cerebrovascular disease	11.2	8.9
Hyperplasia of prostate	8.5	5.0
Pneumonia[2]	9.9	9.6
Inguinal hernia	5.4	2.6
70-74 years		
Heart disease	9.8	7.2
Malignant neoplasms	12.5	8.5
Cerebrovascular disease	10.9	9.1
Hyperplasia of prostate	8.9	5.3
Pneumonia[2]	12.1	10.0
Inguinal hernia	6.1	3.5
75-79 years		
Heart disease	10.1	7.9
Malignant neoplasms	12.9	9.8
Cerebrovascular disease	14.7	9.4
Pneumonia[2]	11.9	9.9
Hyperplasia of prostate	8.9	5.7
Fractures[1]	16.5	11.7

[Continued]

★ 13 ★

Hospital Stays of Older Americans for Selected Illnesses
[Continued]

Age and first-listed diagnosis	Average length of stay in days	
	1981	1987
80-84 years		
Heart disease	10.3	7.4
Malignant neoplasms	12.7	10.5
Cerebrovascular disease	12.9	9.7
Pneumonia[2]	12.7	10.0
Hyperplasia of prostate	10.3	6.2
Fractures[1]	23.4	13.0
65 years and over		
Heart disease	9.9	7.3
Malignant neoplasms	12.8	9.3
Cerebrovascular disease	12.2	9.1
Pneumonia[2]	11.7	9.8
Hyperplasia of prostate	9.3	5.7
Fractures[1]	16.0	12.0
75 years and over		
Heart disease	10.3	7.6
Malignant neoplasms	12.9	10.1
Cerebrovascular disease	13.4	9.3
Pneumonia[2]	12.1	9.9
Hyperplasia of prostate	10.4	6.3
Fractures[1]	18.2	12.5
85 years and over		
Heart disease	10.7	7.1
Pneumonia[2]	11.9	9.6
Malignant neoplasms	13.4	10.0
Cerebrovascular disease	11.6	8.6
Fractures[1]	15.9	12.9
Hyperplasia of prostate	14.6	8.2

Source: Van Nostrand, J. F., S. E. Furner, and R. Suzman, eds. *Health Data on Older Americans: United States, 1992.* Vital and Health Statistics, Series 3: Analytic and Epidemiological Studies, no. 27. DHHS publication no. (PHS) 93-1411. Hyattsville, MD: U.S. Department of Health and Human Services, Public Health Service, Centers for Disease Control and Prevention, National Center for Health Statistics, 1993, pp. 128-129. Primary source: National Center for Health Statistics: Data from the National Hospital Discharge Survey. *Notes:* 1. All sites. 2. All forms.

★ 14 ★

Aging

Leading Causes of Death for Older Americans

Data are based on the National Vital Statistics System.

Age and cause of death	Rank	Number of deaths per 100,000 resident population
55-59 years		
All causes		978.8
Malignant neoplasms[1]	1	352.7
Heart disease	2	318.9
Cerebrovascular diseases	3	39.4
Accidents[2]	4	32.5
Chronic obstructive pulmonary disease[3]	5	31.3
Chronic liver disease and cirrhosis	6	29.5
Diabetes mellitus	7	19.8
Suicide	8	17.0
Pneumonia and influenza	9	13.4
Septicemia	10	6.8
60-64 years		
All causes		1,539.1
Malignant neoplasms[1]	1	538.7
Heart disease	2	532.5
Cerebrovascular diseases	3	67.0
Chronic obstructive pulmonary disease[3]	4	63.4
Accidents[3]	5	37.1
Chronic liver disease and cirrhosis	6	35.0
Diabetes mellitus	7	32.4
Pneumonia and influenza	8	24.0
Suicide	9	17.0
Nephritis, nephrotic syndrome, and nephrosis	10	12.7
65-69 years		
All causes		2,263.0
Heart disease	1	820.4
Malignant neoplasms[1]	2	736.2
Cerebrovascular diseases	3	116.3
Chronic obstructive pulmonary disease[3]	4	113.6
Diabetes mellitus	5	48.3
Accidents[2]	6	41.4
Pneumonia and influenza	7	41.0
Chronic liver disease and cirrhosis	8	36.9
Nephritis, nephrotic syndrome, and nephrosis	9	20.0
Septicemia	10	17.8
70-74 years		
All causes		3,797.7
Heart disease	1	1,323.4
Malignant neoplasms[1]	2	986.6

[Continued]

★ 14 ★

Leading Causes of Death for Older Americans
[Continued]

Age and cause of death	Rank	Number of deaths per 100,000 resident population
Cerebrovascular diseases	3	224.4
Chronic obstructive pulmonary disease[3]	4	194.1
Pneumonia and influenza	5	80.8
Diabetes mellitus	6	73.1
Accidents[2]	7	58.6
Chronic liver disease and cirrhosis	8	37.7
Nephritis, nephrotic syndrome, and nephrosis	9	35.4
Septicemia	10	28.6
75-79 years		
All causes		5,206.1
Heart disease	1	2,098.1
Malignant neoplasms[1]	2	1,188.4
Cerebrovascular diseases	3	422.0
Chronic obstructive pulmonary disease[3]	4	271.2
Pneumonia and influenza	5	172.7
Diabetes mellitus	6	103.9
Accidents[2]	7	86.5
Nephritis, nephrotic syndrome, and nephrosis	8	62.0
Septicemia	9	50.3
Atherosclerosis	10	49.3
80-84 years		
All causes		8,230.0
Heart disease	1	3,526.1
Malignant neoplasms[1]	2	1,450.3
Cerebrovascular diseases	3	823.7
Pneumonia and influenza	4	358.3
Chronic obstructive pulmonary disease[3]	5	333.7
Diabetes mellitus	6	151.7
Accidents[2]	7	139.0
Atherosclerosis	8	116.9
Nephritis, nephrotic syndrome, and nephrosis	9	108.1
Septicemia	10	88.3
85 years and over		
All causes		15,398.9
Heart disease	1	7,178.7
Cerebrovascular diseases	2	1,762.8
Malignant neoplasms[1]	3	1,612.0
Pneumonia and influenza	4	1,032.1
Atherosclerosis	5	432.6
Chronic obstructive pulmonary disease[3]	6	362.9

[Continued]

★ 14 ★

Leading Causes of Death for Older Americans
[Continued]

Age and cause of death	Rank	Number of deaths per 100,000 resident population
Accidents[2]	7	252.2
Nephritis, nephrotic syndrome, and nephrosis	8	216.4
Diabetes mellitus	9	213.9
Septicemia	10	181.9

Source: Van Nostrand, J. F., S. E. Furner, and R. Suzman, eds. *Health Data on Older Americans: United States, 1992.* Vital and Health Statistics, Series 3: Analytic and Epidemiological Studies, no. 27. DHHS publication no. (PHS) 93-1411. Hyattsville, MD: U.S. Department of Health and Human Services, Public Health Service, Centers for Disease Control and Prevention, National Center for Health Statistics, 1993, pp. 91-92. Primary source: National Center for Health Statistics. *Vital Statistics of the United States.* Vol. II, *Mortality.* Part A. Washington, DC: Public Health Service, 1986. *Notes:* 1. Includes neoplasms of lymphatic and hematopoietic tissues. 2. Includes adverse effects of accidents. 3. Includes allied conditions.

★ 15 ★
Aging

Most Frequent Diagnoses of Older Americans by Office-Based Physicians

Data are based on reporting by a sample of office-based physicians.

Age and frequent all-listed diagnoses[1]	Rank	Number of mentions per 1,000 visits	Rank Male	Rank Female
55-59 years				
Essential hypertension	1	143	1	1
Diabetes mellitus	2	61	2	2
Chronic ischemic heart disease	3	28	3	17
Neurotic disorders	4	26	9	4
Disorders of refraction and accommodation	5	26	6	5
Osteoarthritis and allied disorders	6	25	4	9
Arthropathies, other and unspecified	7	19	10	11
Obesity	8	16	27	10
Bronchitis	9	16	16	13
Acute upper respiratory infections	10	16	47	6
60-64 years				
Essential hypertension	1	159	1	1
Diabetes mellitus	2	83	2	2
Chronic ischemic heart disease	3	46	3	3
Osteoarthritis	4	28	5	5

[Continued]

★ 15 ★

Most Frequent Diagnoses of Older Americans by Office-Based Physicians
[Continued]

Age and frequent all-listed diagnoses[1]	Rank	Number of mentions per 1,000 visits	Rank	
			Male	Female
Disorders of refraction and accommodation	5	26	8	4
Arthropathies	6	21	10	9
Chronic airway obstruction, not elsewhere classified	7	19	4	38
Neurotic disorders	8	19	19	7
Angina pectoris	9	19	6	22
Cardiac dysrhythmias	10	17	16	11
65-69 years				
Essential hypertension	1	157	1	1
Diabetes mellitus	2	78	2	2
Chronic ischemic heart disease	3	47	3	5
Osteoarthritis and allied disorders	4	43	10	3
Cataract	5	30	8	4
Cardiac dysrhythmias	6	26	5	6
Angina pectoris	7	24	6	11
Chronic airway obstruction, not elsewhere classified	8	23	4	17
Arthropathies, other and unspecified	9	23	9	9
Disorders of refraction and accommodation	10	22	11	8
70-74 years				
Essential hypertension	1	145	1	1
Diabetes mellitus	2	81	2	2
Chronic ischemic heart disease	3	53	3	4
Cataract	4	48	5	3
Osteoarthritis and allied disorders	5	35	8	5
Cardiac dysrhythmias	6	27	6	10
Chronic airway obstruction, not elsewhere classified	7	24	4	12
Heart failure	8	25	9	8
Arthropathies	9	24	18	6
Glaucoma	10	24	14	7
75-79 years				
Essential hypertension	1	170	1	1
Diabetes mellitus	2	91	2	2
Chronic ischemic heart disease	3	67	3	4
Cataract	4	61	5	3
Osteoarthritis and allied disorders	5	48	7	5

[Continued]

★ 15 ★

Most Frequent Diagnoses of Older Americans by Office-Based Physicians

[Continued]

Age and frequent all-listed diagnoses[1]	Rank	Number of mentions per 1,000 visits	Rank	
			Male	Female
Heart failure	6	37	6	7
Cardiac dysrhythmias	7	34	4	9
Glaucoma	8	32	8	6
Arthropathies, other and unspecified	9	27	12	8
Neurotic disorders	10	21	15	11
80-84 years				
Essential hypertension	1	133	1	1
Cataract	2	74	5	2
Chronic ischemic heart disease	3	72	2	3
Diabetes mellitus	4	56	8	4
Heart failure	5	54	3	6
Osteoarthritis and allied disorders	6	54	6	5
Glaucoma	7	32	9	7
Cardiac dysrhythmias	8	30	7	11
Other eye disorders	9	27	14	8
Chronic airway obstruction, not elsewhere classified	10	27	4	26
85 years and over				
Essential hypertension	1	122	4	1
Chronic ischemic heart disease	2	77	1	3
Cataract	3	74	3	2
Heart failure	4	66	2	4
Diabetes mellitus	5	44	5	5
Osteoarthritis and allied disorders	6	37	9	6
Glaucoma	7	35	8	8
Cardiac dysrhythmias	8	33[2]	6	12
Other disorders of urethra and urinary tract	9	31[2]	16	9
Other skin cancer	10	31[2]	7	11

Source: Van Nostrand, J. F., S. E. Furner, and R. Suzman, eds. *Health Data on Older Americans: United States, 1992.* Vital and Health Statistics, Series 3: Analytic and Epidemiological Studies, no. 27. DHHS publication no. (PHS) 93-1411. Hyattsville, MD: U.S. Department of Health and Human Services, Public Health Service, Centers for Disease Control and Prevention, National Center for Health Statistics, 1993, pp. 125-126. Primary source: National Center for Health Statistics: Data from the National Ambulatory Medical Care Survey. *Notes:* 1. "All-listed" means listed as first, second, or third diagnosis. 2. Figure does not meet the standard for reliability or precision.

★ 16 ★

Aging

Number of People Older Than Age 65 With Selected Chronic Health Problems and Living Alone: 1990-2020

From the source: "As the older population increases during the twenty-first century, the number of people with chronic health problems who live alone is expected to increase."

[Number in millions]

Condition	1990	2005	2020
Arthritis	5.2	6.1	8.2
Hearing/vision	4.8	5.8	7.6
Hypertension	4.4	5.1	6.8

Source: Aging America: Trends and Projections. 1991 ed. Prepared by the U.S. Senate Special Committee on Aging, the American Association of Retired Persons, the Federal Council on the Aging, and the U.S. Administration on Aging. DHHS Publication No. (FCoA) 91-28001. Washington, DC: U.S. Department of Health and Human Services (DHHS), 1991, p. 227. Primary source: Lewin/ICF estimates based on data from the *Supplement on Aging* (1984) and the Brookings/ICF Long-Term Care Financing Model (1990).

★ 17 ★

Aging

Probable Alzheimer's Disease for Persons Older Than Age 65

It is estimated that 10 percent of all persons over 65 years old have Alzheimer's disease. It is much more prevalent in persons older than 85, with almost half of that group estimated to have the disease to some degree. These data exclude persons in nursing homes or other institutions.

Age group	Percent
65 +	10.0
65 to 74	3.0
75 to 84	19.0
85 +	47.0

Source: Aging America: Trends and Projections. 1991 ed. Prepared by the U.S. Senate Special Committee on Aging, the American Association of Retired Persons, the Federal Council on the Aging, and the U.S. Administration on Aging. DHHS Publication No. (FCoA) 91-28001. Washington, DC: U.S. Department of Health and Human Services (DHHS), 1991, p. 116. Primary source: Evans, Dennis A., and others. "Prevalence of Alzheimer's Disease in a Community Population of Older Persons." *Journal of the American Medical Association* 262, no. 18, 10 November 1989.

★ 18 ★

Aging

Proportion of Poor People Over Age 65 Who Have Selected Chronic Health Problems and Live Alone: 1990

[Numbers in percent]

Condition	Poor	Non-poor
Arthritis	65.0	54.0
Hearing/vision	60.0	50.0
Hypertension	55.0	45.0

Source: Aging America: Trends and Projections. 1991 ed. Prepared by the U.S. Senate Special Committee on Aging, the American Association of Retired Persons, the Federal Council on the Aging, and the U.S. Administration on Aging. DHHS Publication No. (FCoA) 91-28001. Washington, DC: U.S. Department of Health and Human Services (DHHS), 1991, p. 226. Primary source: Lewin/ICF estimates based on data from the 1984 *Supplement on Aging* and the Brookings/ICF Long-Term Care Financing Model (1990).

★ 19 ★

Aging

Urinary Incontinence in Older Americans

At least 1 in 10 persons age 65 or older suffers from incontinence.... Incontinence is not an inevitable result of aging. It is caused by specific changes in body function that often result from diseases or use of medications.... [It] may be brought on by an illness accompanied by fatigue, confusion, or hospital admission.

Source: U.S. Department of Health and Human Services. Public Health Service. National Institute on Aging. *Bound for Good Health: A Collection of Age Pages.* Bethesda, MD: National Institute on Aging, c. 1991, n.p.

Children's Health

★ 20 ★

Chicken Pox

"Chicken pox affects 90 to 95 percent of Americans by the end of adolescence ... and another 2.5 percent over the age of 20. More than 60 percent of the cases occur in children aged 5 to 9."

Source: Rosenthal, Elisabeth. "Doctors Weigh the Cost of a Chicken Pox Vaccine." *New York Times,* 7 July 1993, late edition (final), p. A1. Primary source: Centers for Disease Control.

★ 21 ★

Children's Health

Child Abuse: 1985-1993

A report by the National Committee for the Prevention of Child Abuse indicated that 2,989,000 child abuse cases had been reported. Of that number, 34 percent had been verified. The table below shows the child abuse report rate per 1,000 children since 1985.

Year	Report rate
1985	30
1986	33
1987	34
1988	35
1989	38
1990	40
1991	42
1992	45
1993	45

Source: "Child Abuse: Growing Problem in the USA." *USA TODAY,* 7 April 1994, final edition, p. 8A.

★ 22 ★

Children's Health

Death in Childhood – Ages 1 Through 14: 1990

Table shows the leading causes of death for children ages 1 through 14 years old. Excludes deaths of nonresidents of the United States. Deaths classified according to ninth revision of *International Classification of Diseases.*

Ages	1-4 year olds			5-14 year olds		
	Total	Male	Female	Total	Male	Female
All causes	6,931	3,969	2,962	8,436	5,127	3,309
Accidents	2,566	1,574	992	3,650	2,418	1,232
Malignant neoplasms[1]	513	280	233	1,094	621	473
Congenital anomalies	896	473	423	468	245	223
Homicide and legal intervention	378	208	170	512	299	213
Heart disease	282	141	141	308	169	139
Pneumonia and influenza	171	88	83	134	71	63

Source: 1993 Statistical Abstract of the United States on CD-ROM [machine-readable datafiles]. CD-ABSTR-93. Washington, DC: U.S. Department of Commerce, Economics and Statistics Administration, Bureau of the Census, Data User Services Division, 1993. Primary source: U.S. National Center for Health Statistics. *Vital Statistics of the United States* (annual); and unpublished data. *Note:* 1. Cancer.

★ 23 ★
Children's Health

Death in Childhood – Teens: 1990

```
Accidents - 16,241

Homicide - 7,354

Suicide - 4,859

        Cancer - 1,819

     Heart disease - 917

    HIV/AIDS - 541

    Birth defects - 491

  Stroke - 234

  Pneumonia/flu - 231

  Lung disease - 178
```

Ranking and number of deaths as reported in 1990 for Americans ages 15 to 24.

[In thousands]

Disease or condition	Number of deaths
Accidents	16,241
Homicide	7,354
Suicide	4,859
Cancer	1,819
Heart disease	917
HIV/AIDS	541
Birth defects[1]	491
Stroke	234
Pneumonia/flu	231
Lung disease	178

Source: "Top 10 Teen Killers." *Current Health 2* 20, no. 1 (September 1993), p. 8. *Notes:* 1. Birth defects are conditions present at birth that may or may not be life threatening. Examples include abnormalities of such vital organs as the heart, kidneys, liver, and brain. In the majority of cases, children born with defects serious enough to threaten their lives die in infancy. In a few instances, however, they grow to young adulthood before dying.

★ 24 ★

Children's Health

Health Behaviors of Children

Table shows the responses of 301 children, ages 12-18, and 300 parents when asked if they (or their children in the case of parents) engage in certain health behaviors.

[In percentages]

Behavior	Children (n=301)		Parents (n=300)	
	You	Other kids	Your child	Other kids
Threats				
Sunbathe to tan	52	87	45	79
Drink alcohol	34	81	21	75
Smoke cigarettes	22	83	14	74
Use illegal drugs	10	66	5	64
Chew tobacco	3	46	3	33
Benefits				
Exercise	93	85	94	79
Eat nutritiously	83	75	93	82
Drive safely[1]	82	70	88	87
Wear a safety belt	82	64	87	74
Get enough sleep	66	56	74	64

Source: "Children Don't Expect a Healthy Future." *Nurse Practitioner* (July/August 1993), p. 4.
Notes: 1. Among those age 16 and older (n=72 children) and among those parents with children age 16 and older (n=63).

★ 25 ★

Children's Health

Hearing-Impaired Children

According to child hearing experts, 3 years old is the average age for identifying deaf or severely hearing-impaired children in the United States. A panel of experts assembled by the National Institutes of Health recommended that all infants be tested in the first 3 months of life by an otocoustic emission test, costing an average of $25.

Source: Leary, Warren. "U.S. Panel Backs Testing All Babies to Uncover Hearing Losses Early." *New York Times,* 10 March 1993, p. C12.

★ 26 ★

Children's Health

Lead Exposure and Children

According to the findings of Australian and Boston studies, the mental development of children from middle-class families is just as likely to be damaged from lead exposure (mainly from house paint) as that of children from poor families. An average deficit of 8 I.Q. points was discovered when children's average lifetime blood lead concentrations rose from 10 to 35 micrograms per deciliter. In the Australian study, an average of 10 micrograms per deciliter of lead exposure was linked to significant I.Q. deficits in 10-year-olds.

Source: Brody, Jane E. "Study Documents Lead-Exposure Damage in Middle-Class Children." *New York Times,* 29 October 1992, p. A20.

★ 27 ★

Children's Health

Measles, With Complications: 1991

The figures indicate the proportion of reported measles cases with complications for 1991. Data are provided by age group.

Condition	Total		Age groups					
			Under 5		5-19		20 or older	
	Number	Percent	Number	Percent	Number	Percent	Number	Percent
Otitis media	1,308	14	1,105	23	138	5	65	3
Diarrhea	1,194	12	740	16	212	7	242	13
Pneumonia	815	8	502	11	97	3	216	11
Encephalitis	13	0.1	3	0.1	3	0.1	7	0.4
Hospitalization	2,549	26	1,525	32	343	11	681	36

Source: U.S. Department of Health and Human Services. Public Health Service. Centers for Disease Control and Prevention. "Measles Surveillance—United States, 1991." *CDC Surveillance Summaries. Morbidity and Mortality Weekly Report* 41, no. SS-6, 20 November 1992, p. 8.

★ 28 ★

Children's Health

Mumps

Mumps is a paramyxovirus infection known to cause male infertility, acquired deafness in children, pancreatitis, diabetes, fatal myocarditis, and abortions.

Characteristics of mumps	Frequency or duration
Epidemics	2-3 years
Incubation period	16-18 days
Symptoms in those affected	60-70%
Adults with viral antibodies[1]	80-90%

Source: Peltola, Heikki. "Mumps Vaccination and Meningitis." *Lancet* 341, no. 88511, 17 April 1993, p. 994. *Note:* 1. Unless living in isolated communities.

Death

★ 29 ★

Central Death Rate Projections: 1985-2080

Data are provided by age, sex, and alternative. Includes the populations of Puerto Rico, Guam, American Samoa, the Virgin Islands, and U.S. citizens living abroad. The central death rate is defined as "the ratio of the number of deaths during the year for persons at the tabulated age to the midyear population at that age." Alternatives in the table below are "based on three different sets of assumptions about future net immigration, birth rates, and death rates.... Alternative I is designated as optimistic because among the three projections the assumptions selected produce the most favorable financial effect for the OASDI program. Conversely, the assumptions chosen for Alternative III, designated pessimistic, produce the most unfavorable financial effect."

[Per hundred thousand]

Alternative, sex, and age group	Calendar year										
	1985	1990	2000	2010	2020	2030	2040	2050	2060	2070	2080
Alternative I: Male:											
0	1,177.6	1,042.1	890.7	834.4	795.5	759.5	726.2	695.4	666.8	640.4	615.8
1-4	56.8	53.0	48.1	46.1	44.9	43.9	42.9	41.9	41.0	40.1	39.3
5-9	31.3	28.3	24.4	23.3	22.8	22.4	22.0	21.7	21.3	21.0	20.6
10-14	35.2	32.4	28.4	27.2	26.7	26.2	25.8	25.3	24.9	24.4	24.0
15-19	116.4	110.5	102.1	98.3	96.4	94.6	92.8	91.0	89.3	87.6	86.0
20-24	163.6	156.1	145.1	140.0	137.2	134.6	132.0	129.5	127.0	124.7	122.3
25-29	172.5	168.0	161.4	157.3	154.3	151.5	148.7	146.0	143.3	140.8	138.3
30-34	185.6	177.3	165.3	159.7	156.7	153.8	151.0	148.2	145.6	143.0	140.5
35-39	236.5	219.6	196.2	187.7	183.8	180.1	176.5	173.0	169.7	166.5	163.4
40-44	348.1	321.2	284.1	270.9	264.9	259.1	253.6	248.4	243.3	238.4	233.8
45-49	509.0	473.1	423.7	404.9	395.5	386.7	378.2	370.2	362.5	355.1	348.1

[Continued]

★ 29 ★

Central Death Rate Projections: 1985-2080
[Continued]

Alternative, sex, and age group	Calendar year										
	1985	1990	2000	2010	2020	2030	2040	2050	2060	2070	2080
50-54	844.7	796.2	730.7	704.6	688.7	673.5	659.1	645.4	632.3	619.8	608.0
55-59	1,316.2	1,238.8	1,134.0	1,092.9	1,068.3	1,045.0	1,022.8	1,001.7	981.6	962.5	944.4
60-64	2,078.4	1,965.1	1,831.3	1,750.8	1,710.6	1,672.5	1,636.3	1,601.9	1,569.2	1,538.2	1,508.6
65-69	3,186.6	3,081.1	2,953.8	2,872.9	2,806.5	2,743.5	2,683.7	2,626.9	2,572.9	2,521.6	2,472.9
70-74	4,792.8	4,674.9	4,550.5	4,437.7	4,330.8	4,229.4	4,133.2	4,041.9	3,955.3	3,873.1	3,795.0
75-79	7,308.7	7,172.3	7,057.8	6,895.1	6,720.3	6,554.6	6,397.6	6,248.7	6,107.5	5,973.6	5,846.5
80-84	10,935.3	10,761.4	10,666.1	10,416.8	10,135.6	9,869.1	9,616.6	9,377.3	9,150.4	8,935.3	8,731.3
85-89	15,749.1	15,506.5	15,402.8	15,024.7	14,594.9	14,187.7	13,802.0	13,436.5	13,090.1	12,761.8	12,450.3
90-94	22,547.1	22,142.2	21,867.5	21,261.9	20,605.5	19,984.0	19,395.6	18,838.3	18,310.4	17,810.1	17,335.9
Alternative II:											
Male:											
0	1,177.6	955.9	714.1	644.5	593.7	549.0	509.7	474.9	444.1	416.7	392.3
1-4	56.8	50.3	41.3	38.4	36.7	35.1	33.7	32.3	31.1	29.9	28.8
5-9	31.3	26.5	19.9	18.6	17.9	17.4	16.8	16.3	15.8	15.3	14.8
10-14	35.2	30.6	24.0	22.4	21.6	20.9	20.3	19.6	19.0	18.4	17.9
15-19	116.4	106.8	91.9	86.7	84.0	81.4	78.9	76.5	74.2	72.0	69.8
20-24	163.6	151.3	131.8	124.6	120.7	117.1	113.5	110.1	106.8	103.6	100.5
25-29	172.5	165.1	153.2	146.8	142.3	138.0	133.8	129.8	125.9	122.1	118.5
30-34	185.6	172.0	150.9	142.9	138.4	134.1	130.0	126.1	122.2	118.6	115.0
35-39	236.5	209.0	169.3	158.3	152.8	147.7	142.7	138.0	133.5	129.2	125.1
40-44	348.1	304.4	242.1	225.3	216.9	209.0	201.5	194.4	187.5	181.1	174.9
45-49	509.0	450.8	368.0	343.8	330.5	317.9	306.1	294.8	284.1	274.0	264.3
50-54	844.7	763.7	648.9	613.3	589.6	567.3	546.1	526.0	506.9	488.9	471.7
55-59	1,316.2	1,188.8	1,009.5	954.5	917.5	882.6	849.6	818.3	788.6	760.5	733.8
60-64	2,078.4	1,887.9	1,618.8	1,532.1	1,471.8	1,414.9	1,361.1	1,310.3	1,262.2	1,216.5	1,173.3
65-69	3,180.0	2,900.5	2,680.3	2,551.5	2,449.7	2,353.8	2,263.2	2,177.6	2,096.7	2,020.1	1,947.5
70-74	4,792.8	4,532.9	4,155.2	3,965.0	3,803.0	3,650.4	3,506.5	3,370.8	3,242.6	3,121.5	3,006.9
75-79	7,308.7	6,960.9	6,461.3	6,177.6	5,917.8	5,673.5	5,443.6	5,227.0	5,022.9	4,830.3	4,648.4
80-84	10,935.3	10,419.9	9,699.7	9,264.7	8,860.3	8,480.8	8,124.3	7,789.1	7,473.7	7,176.6	6,896.6
85-89	15,749.1	14,995.6	13,961.2	13,316.9	12,714.6	12,150.1	11,620.6	11,123.5	10,656.4	10,217.2	9,803.8
90-94	22,547.1	21,433.4	19,867.4	18,878.2	17,978.1	17,136.1	16,347.8	15,609.3	14,916.7	14,266.7	13,656.2
Alternative III:											
Male:											
0	1,177.6	877.8	593.9	525.4	473.6	429.2	391.1	358.1	329.5	304.4	282.4
1-4	56.8	47.7	35.6	31.8	29.4	27.2	25.3	23.5	21.9	20.4	19.0
5-9	31.3	24.7	16.4	14.6	13.6	12.7	11.8	11.1	10.3	9.7	9.1
10-14	35.2	28.9	20.2	18.1	16.8	15.7	14.7	13.7	12.8	12.0	11.2
15-19	116.4	103.2	82.8	75.4	70.7	66.4	62.3	58.5	55.0	51.7	48.6
20-24	163.6	146.6	119.9	109.4	102.7	96.5	90.7	85.2	80.1	75.3	70.8
25-29	172.5	162.3	145.8	135.5	127.3	119.7	112.5	105.8	99.6	93.7	88.2
30-34	185.6	166.9	138.2	126.3	118.5	111.1	104.3	98.0	92.0	86.5	81.3
35-39	236.5	199.0	146.7	131.5	122.4	114.0	106.3	99.2	92.6	86.6	80.9
40-44	348.1	288.5	207.3	184.0	169.6	156.6	144.7	133.8	123.9	114.8	106.5
45-49	509.0	429.6	322.5	287.8	262.5	239.7	219.1	200.5	183.6	168.4	154.6
50-54	844.7	732.9	580.1	519.9	471.8	428.6	389.7	354.6	323.1	294.7	269.0
55-59	1,316.2	1,141.3	905.4	810.7	733.5	664.2	602.0	546.2	496.0	450.8	410.2
60-64	2,078.4	1,814.6	1,454.6	1,302.8	1,178.1	1,066.3	966.0	876.0	795.1	722.4	657.0
65-69	3,186.6	2,883.8	2,436.7	2,194.7	1,988.9	1,804.2	1,638.3	1,489.2	1,355.1	1,134.4	1,125.7

[Continued]

★ 29 ★

Central Death Rate Projections: 1985-2080
[Continued]

Alternative, sex, and age group	Calendar year										
	1985	1990	2000	2010	2020	2030	2040	2050	2060	2070	2080
70-74	4,792.8	4,396.1	3,798.6	3,438.3	3,123.6	2,840.8	2,586.5	2,357.5	2,151.4	1,965.5	1,797.9
75-79	7,308.7	6,757.2	5,922.5	5,392.9	4,915.1	4,484.8	4,097.1	3,747.6	3,432.2	3,147.2	2,889.7
80-84	10,935.5	10,091.0	8,833.9	8,060.1	7,365.4	6,738.9	6,173.4	5,662.7	5,200.9	4,783.0	4,404.4
85-89	15,749.1	14,504.1	12,679.2	11,589.3	10,613.2	9,731.5	8,934.5	8,213.3	7,560.2	6,968.0	6,430.5
90-94	22,547.1	20,751.7	18,096.4	16,522.4	15,139.5	13,889.7	12,759.1	11,735.3	10,807.3	9,965.3	9,200.6
Alternative I: **Female:**											
0	927.0	763.5	575.3	516.3	473.3	435.5	402.4	373.1	347.3	324.4	304.1
1-4	45.1	39.3	31.4	29.0	27.5	26.1	24.9	23.7	22.6	21.6	20.6
5-9	23.0	19.6	14.9	13.8	13.2	12.7	12.2	11.7	11.2	10.8	10.4
10-14	21.4	18.8	15.0	13.9	13.3	12.8	12.3	11.8	11.3	10.9	10.4
15-19	43.0	39.5	34.4	32.4	31.1	29.9	28.7	27.6	26.5	25.5	24.5
20-24	51.4	47.6	42.3	40.1	38.5	37.0	35.6	34.2	32.8	31.6	30.4
25-29	60.2	54.4	46.2	43.4	41.7	40.1	38.6	37.1	35.7	34.3	33.1
30-34	72.1	61.9	48.2	44.8	43.1	41.5	39.9	38.5	37.1	35.7	34.4
35-39	107.5	90.3	67.9	62.8	60.4	58.1	55.9	53.8	51.8	49.9	48.1
40-44	175.7	150.6	116.5	107.9	103.6	99.5	95.7	92.0	88.6	85.2	82.1
45-49	281.8	248.6	200.8	186.6	179.1	172.0	165.3	158.9	152.8	147.0	141.5
50-54	465.8	426.5	368.4	347.2	333.3	320.1	307.6	295.8	284.5	273.8	263.5
55-59	713.2	663.8	592.8	564.7	542.1	520.6	500.2	480.9	462.4	444.9	428.2
60-64	1,146.3	1,090.1	1,014.2	973.3	933.2	895.3	859.3	825.2	792.9	762.1	732.9
65-69	1,700.4	1,640.3	1,568.4	1,510.5	1,446.3	1,385.7	1,328.2	1,273.9	1,222.4	1,173.6	1,127.3
70-74	2,610.8	2,457.8	2,259.4	2,158.2	2,060.7	1,968.9	1,882.4	1,800.9	1,723.9	1,651.1	1,582.3
75-79	4,057.2	3,729.8	3,285.1	3,103.4	2,951.7	2,809.7	2,676.5	2,551.5	2,434.1	2,323.8	2,219.9
80-84	6,644.2	6,060.2	5,241.0	4,906.9	4,647.1	4,405.0	4,179.0	3,967.9	3,770.5	3,585.8	3,412.7
85-89	11,545.8	10,592.4	9,218.3	8,596.0	8,116.3	7,670.7	7,256.1	6,869.9	6,509.8	6,173.8	5,860.0
90-94	18,288.9	17,052.4	15,203.3	14,172.1	13,346.3	12,580.7	11,869.6	11,208.4	10,593.3	10,020.4	9,486.4
Alternative II: **Female:**											
0	927.0	827.5	712.3	666.4	634.2	604.3	576.8	551.2	527.6	505.6	485.4
1-4	45.1	41.7	37.4	35.8	34.8	34.0	33.2	32.4	31.6	30.9	30.3
5-9	23.0	20.9	18.1	17.3	17.0	16.7	16.4	16.1	15.8	15.6	15.4
10-14	21.4	19.8	17.6	16.9	16.5	16.2	16.0	15.7	15.4	15.2	14.9
15-19	43.0	40.9	37.9	36.7	36.0	35.3	34.7	34.0	33.4	32.9	32.3
20-24	51.4	49.0	45.9	44.6	43.8	43.0	42.2	41.4	40.7	40.0	39.3
25-29	60.2	56.6	51.8	50.0	49.1	48.3	47.4	46.6	45.8	45.1	44.4
30-34	72.1	65.8	57.5	55.1	54.2	53.4	52.6	51.8	51.1	50.3	49.6
35-39	107.5	96.8	83.0	79.4	78.2	77.0	75.9	74.8	73.8	72.8	71.9
40-44	175.7	160.1	139.6	133.6	131.4	129.4	127.5	125.6	123.9	122.2	120.6
45-49	281.8	261.3	233.2	223.9	220.2	216.7	213.5	210.3	207.4	204.5	201.9
50-54	465.8	261.3	233.2	223.9	220.2	216.7	213.5	210.3	207.4	204.5	201.9
55-59	713.2	684.0	644.7	628.6	618.2	608.4	599.0	590.1	581.6	573.6	565.9
60-64	1,146.3	1,123.2	1,104.5	1,087.3	1,068.0	1,049.7	1,032.3	1,015.7	1,000.0	985.1	970.9
65-69	1,700.4	1,694.7	1,723.7	1,704.8	1,671.8	1,640.5	1,610.7	1,582.5	1,555.6	1,530.2	1,505.9
70-74	2,610.8	2,551.0	2,510.0	2,459.9	2,403.3	2,349.7	2,298.8	2,250.5	2,204.8	2,161.4	2,120.2
75-79	4,057.2	3,884.3	3,682.2	3,565.8	3,467.0	3,373.6	3,285.2	3,201.5	3,122.2	3,047.2	2,976.1
80-84	6,644.2	6,320.2	5,913.5	5,679.2	5,497.0	5,325.0	5,162.5	5,008.9	4,863.6	4,726.2	4,596.2
85-89	11,545.8	11,029.6	10,382.5	9,946.2	9,598.7	9,271.1	8,961.7	8,669.3	8,393.1	8,132.0	7,885.2

[Continued]

★ 29 ★

Central Death Rate Projections: 1985-2080
[Continued]

Alternative, sex, and age group	Calendar year										
	1985	1990	2000	2010	2020	2030	2040	2050	2060	2070	2080
90-94	18,288.9	17,673.7	16,939.1	16,249.2	15,644.9	15,075.2	14,537.2	14,029.0	13,548.9	13,095.2	12,666.3
Alternative III: Female											
0	927.0	705.0	479.6	420.2	376.1	338.5	306.4	278.9	255.1	234.4	216.4
1-4	45.1	37.0	26.5	23.4	21.3	19.5	17.8	16.4	15.0	13.8	12.8
5-9	23.0	18.3	12.3	10.8	9.9	9.1	8.4	7.7	7.1	6.6	6.1
10-14	21.4	17.8	12.9	11.3	10.4	9.5	8.7	8.0	7.4	6.8	6.3
15-19	43.0	38.3	31.4	28.3	26.1	24.0	22.1	20.4	18.8	17.3	16.0
20-24	51.4	46.2	39.3	36.0	33.1	30.4	28.0	25.8	23.8	22.0	20.3
25-29	60.2	52.3	41.6	37.3	34.2	31.4	28.9	26.6	24.5	22.6	20.9
30-34	72.1	58.3	40.6	35.5	32.3	29.4	26.9	24.6	22.5	20.6	18.9
35-39	107.5	84.2	55.7	47.9	43.1	38.8	34.9	31.6	28.6	25.9	23.5
40-44	175.7	141.6	97.3	83.6	74.6	66.7	59.7	53.6	48.2	43.4	39.2
45-49	281.8	236.5	173.2	149.3	132.8	118.3	105.6	94.4	84.6	75.9	68.3
50-54	465.8	412.0	334.6	294.9	261.2	231.7	206.0	183.4	163.6	146.2	131.0
55-59	713.2	644.6	546.0	483.7	428.5	380.2	338.0	301.0	268.6	240.2	215.2
60-64	1,146.3	1,058.3	930.8	832.4	741.0	660.9	590.6	528.8	474.4	426.5	384.2
65-69	1,700.4	1,587.9	1,424.1	1,282.5	1,146.8	1,027.4	922.3	829.5	747.6	675.2	611.0
70-74	2,610.8	2,368.8	2,037.8	1,832.6	1,644.7	1,478.8	1,332.2	1,202.6	1,087.7	985.7	895.1
75-79	4,057.2	3,582.9	2,949.1	2,645.8	2,384.8	2,153.6	1,948.6	1,766.4	1,604.3	1,459.8	1,330.9
80-84	6,644.2	5,821.8	4,676.8	4,180.5	3,776.0	3,416.8	3,097.2	2,812.6	2,558.7	2,331.7	2,128.7
85-89	11,545.8	10,174.8	8,232.7	7,355.4	6,659.0	6,039.2	5,486.4	4,992.6	4,550.8	4,155.0	3,799.0
90-94	18,288.9	16,455.4	13,697.0	12,255.8	11,106.3	10,081.2	9,165.1	8,345.2	7,610.4	6,950.8	6,357.9

Source: U.S. Department of Health and Human Services. Social Security Administration (SSA). Office of the Actuary. "Social Security Area Population Projections." Prepared by Alice H. Wade. *Social Security Bulletin* 51, No. 2 (February 1988), pp. 14-15. *Note:* OASDI stands for Old Age, Survivors, and Disability Insurance.

★ 30 ★
Death

Death Rates, by Age, Sex, and Race: 1970-1991

Number of deaths per 100,000 population in specified group. Excludes deaths of nonresidents of the United States (except as noted) and fetal deaths. The standard population for this table is the total population of the United States enumerated in 1940.

Sex, year, and race	All ages[1]	Under 1 year	1-4 years	5-14 years	15-24 years	25-34 years	35-44 years	45-54 years	55-64 years	65-74 years	75-84 years	85 years and over
Male[2]												
1970	1,090	2,410	93	51	189	215	403	959	2,283	4,874	10,010	17,822
1980	977	1,429	73	37	172	196	299	767	1,815	4,105	8,817	18,801
1985	949	1,220	59	32	139	180	279	672	1,711	3,856	8,502	18,614
1986	945	1,174	58	32	149	195	289	656	1,670	3,787	8,360	18,351
1987	939	1,150	58	32	143	195	292	648	1,649	3,717	8,241	18,212
1988	945	1,145	57	31	147	200	302	633	1,635	3,682	8,237	18,711
1989	926	1,133	55	31	142	204	308	622	1,596	3,558	7,957	18,019
1990	918	1,083	52	29	147	204	310	610	1,553	3,492	7,889	18,057
1991[3]	909	1,007	49	29	161	201	311	598	1,504	3,307	7,663	17,151

[Continued]

★ 30 ★

Death Rates, by Age, Sex, and Race: 1970-1991
[Continued]

Sex, year, and race	All ages[1]	Under 1 year	1-4 years	5-14 years	15-24 years	25-34 years	35-44 years	45-54 years	55-64 years	65-74 years	75-84 years	85 years and over
White:												
1970	1,087	2,113	84	48	171	177	344	883	2,203	4,810	10,099	18,552
1980	983	1,230	66	35	167	171	257	699	1,729	4,036	8,830	19,097
1985	964	1,057	53	30	134	159	243	612	1,626	3,771	8,486	18,980
1988	958	964	52	29	136	173	260	569	1,547	3,588	8,197	19,021
1989	937	941	48	28	129	177	263	556	1,504	3,455	7,913	18,242
1990	931	896	46	26	131	176	268	549	1,467	3,398	7,845	18,268
1991[3]	924	846	43	26	143	172	269	541	1,431	3,246	7,689	17,620
Black:												
1970	1,187	4,299	151	67	321	560	957	1,778	3,257	5,803	9,455	12,222
1980	1,034	2,587	111	47	209	407	690	1,480	2,873	5,131	9,232	16,099
1985	989	2,220	90	42	174	352	630	1,293	2,780	5,172	9,262	15,774
1988	1,026	2,190	92	44	222	417	707	1,297	2,713	5,148	9,455	16,643
1989	1,027	2,172	90	44	235	426	718	1,312	2,700	5,130	9,163	16,752
1990	1,008	2,112	86	41	252	431	700	1,261	2,618	4,946	9,130	16,955
1991[3]	962	1,899	82	44	277	414	707	1,203	2,323	4,286	8,359	14,325
Female[2]												
1970	808	1,864	75	32	68	102	231	517	1,099	2,580	6,678	15,518
1980	785	1,142	55	24	58	76	159	413	934	2,145	5,440	14,747
1985	809	951	45	21	50	69	139	375	926	2,097	5,162	14,554
1986	812	923	46	20	52	72	140	368	914	2,096	5,088	14,494
1987	817	919	46	19	51	75	139	364	909	2,069	5,045	14,514
1988	831	921	46	21	52	75	140	355	916	2,064	5,091	14,851
1989	819	917	46	21	51	76	139	345	894	2,020	4,967	14,395
1990	812	856	41	19	49	74	138	343	879	1,991	4,883	14,274
1991[3]	802	791	45	19	52	74	136	326	855	1,972	4,862	13,328
White:												
1970	813	1,615	66	30	62	84	193	463	1,015	2,471	6,699	15,980
1980	806	963	49	23	56	65	138	373	876	2,067	5,402	14,980
1985	840	799	40	20	48	59	122	342	869	2,027	5,112	14,745
1988	865	754	41	19	49	63	120	320	859	1,996	5,040	15,019
1989	852	740	39	19	48	63	119	311	838	1,949	4,911	14,526
1990	847	690	36	18	46	62	117	309	823	1,924	4,839	14,401
1991[3]	838	645	37	17	48	63	115	296	807	1,915	4,842	13,553
Black:												
1970	829	3,369	129	44	112	231	533	1,044	1,986	3,861	6,692	10,707
1980	733	2,124	84	31	71	150	324	768	1,561	3,057	6,212	12,367
1985	734	1,821	71	29	60	138	277	668	1,533	2,968	6,078	12,703
1988	765	1,834	71	31	69	158	305	655	1,513	2,948	5,991	13,461
1989	763	1,840	73	29	68	161	299	641	1,478	2,936	5,930	13,509

[Continued]

★ 30 ★

Death Rates, by Age, Sex, and Race: 1970-1991
[Continued]

Sex, year, and race	All ages[1]	Under 1 year	1-4 years	5-14 years	15-24 years	25-34 years	35-44 years	45-54 years	55-64 years	65-74 years	75-84 years	85 years and over
1990	748	1,736	68	28	69	160	299	639	1,453	2,866	5,688	13,310
1991[3]	721	1,546	80	28	77	147	298	587	1,328	2,750	5,762	11,856

Source: 1993 Statistical Abstract of the United States on CD-ROM [machine-readable datafiles]. CD-ABSTR-93. Washington, DC: U.S. Department of Commerce, Economics and Statistics Administration, Bureau of the Census, Data User Services Division, 1993. Primary source: U.S. National Center for Health Statistics. Vital Statistics of the United States (annual); Monthly Vital Statistics Report; and unpublished data. Notes: 1. Includes unknown age. 2. Includes other races not shown separately. 3. Preliminary. Includes deaths of nonresidents. Based on a 10-percent sample of deaths.

★ 31 ★
Death

Leading Causes of Death: 1990

Table shows the number and rank for top causes of death in the United States in 1990. Data include all races and are based on the National Vital Statistics System.

Cause	1990	
	Number	Rank
All causes	2,148,463	-
Heart disease	720,058	1
Malignant neoplasms[1]	505,322	2
Cerebrovascular disease	144,088	3
Injuries (unintentional)	91,983	4
Chronic obstructive pulmonary disease	86,679	5
Pneumonia and influenza	79,513	6
Diabetes mellitus	47,664	7
Suicide	30,906	8
Chronic liver disease and cirrhosis	25,815	9
HIV infection	25,188	10
Homicide and legal intervention	24,932	11
Nephritis, nephrotic syndrome, and nephrosis	20,764	12
Septicemia	19,169	13
Atherosclerosis	18,047	14

Source: U.S. Department of Health and Human Services. Public Health Service. Centers for Disease Control and Prevention. National Center for Health Statistics. Health, United States, 1992. Hyattsville, MD: Public Health Service, 1993, pp. 49-51. Primary source: Centers for Disease Control and Prevention. National Center for Health Statistics. Vital Statistics of the United States. Vol. II: Mortality, Part A. Washington, DC: U.S. Government Printing Office; data computed by the Division of Analysis from data compiled by the Division of Vital Statistics. Notes: The code numbers for the cause of death are based on the International Classification of Diseases, 9th revision. Categories for the coding and classification of human immunodeficiency virus (HIV) infection were introduced in the United States beginning with mortality data for 1987. The number of HIV infection deaths based on the National Vital Statistics System differs from the number of deaths among Acquired Immunodeficiency Syndrome (AIDS) cases reported to the Centers for Disease Control (CDC) AIDS Surveillance System. 1. Cancer.

★ 32 ★

Death

Leading Causes of Death, by State: 1990

Deaths per 100,000 resident population enumerated as of April 1. By place of residence. Excludes nonresidents of the United States. Causes of death classified according to ninth revision of *International Classification of Diseases.*

Division and state	Total[1]	Heart disease	Cancer	Cerebro-vascular diseases	Accidents & adverse effects	Chronic obstructive pulmonary diseases[2]	Pneumonia, flu	Diabetes mellitus	Suicide	Chronic liver diseases & cirrhosis	Athero-sclerosis
United States	863.8	289.5	203.2	57.9	37.0	34.9	32.0	19.2	12.4	10.4	7.3
New England	867.4	293.0	217.6	54.0	28.1	34.2	35.4	19.0	10.2	10.5	7.1
Maine	904.5	301.1	227.4	58.6	33.6	45.8	32.9	19.9	12.6	8.9	9.5
New Hampshire	765.2	251.7	191.3	50.6	29.4	34.3	24.7	17.9	13.4	9.9	8.0
Vermont	816.5	253.4	201.9	53.5	34.5	39.3	36.3	19.2	14.9	10.5	5.0
Massachusetts	883.9	295.1	223.5	54.9	25.6	33.0	38.5	20.4	8.8	11.2	6.9
Rhode Island	954.3	342.5	241.9	55.5	27.9	36.0	28.7	22.1	12.7	10.1	11.2
Connecticut	839.9	291.9	207.4	51.7	29.0	30.5	36.1	15.5	9.1	10.0	5.1
Middle Atlantic	960.8	347.8	229.2	54.4	30.0	33.2	36.5	21.3	9.5	11.2	5.8
New York	939.0	353.7	213.5	48.7	28.1	31.6	41.2	15.8	8.6	11.5	5.5
New Jersey	910.5	306.1	232.0	51.4	27.1	29.8	31.4	26.8	7.3	11.8	5.8
Pennsylvania	1,026.4	366.1	251.2	65.0	34.7	37.9	32.9	26.1	12.2	10.4	6.4
East North Central	887.6	307.5	211.4	59.5	34.6	35.1	31.8	22.1	11.3	10.2	8.1
Ohio	911.0	319.6	221.0	58.1	33.9	39.0	28.8	25.3	11.0	9.1	8.1
Indiana	894.1	306.1	210.3	66.7	37.1	38.0	30.0	21.8	13.1	7.5	10.4
Illinois	901.1	308.8	213.8	58.7	34.9	33.1	34.8	19.8	10.1	11.8	6.8
Michigan	847.1	297.2	198.5	55.0	34.0	32.4	30.9	21.7	11.5	12.1	8.7
Wisconsin	873.6	298.7	210.5	64.7	33.8	32.8	35.4	21.9	12.7	8.1	7.8
West North Central	912.2	312.4	208.6	68.2	38.2	39.3	38.5	18.9	12.9	7.2	10.4
Minnesota	794.9	246.3	185.6	64.8	33.5	32.8	33.4	15.7	12.5	6.7	8.2
Iowa	968.2	345.2	218.8	73.5	37.7	42.6	44.0	20.7	12.1	6.7	15.2
Missouri	984.5	348.3	226.8	67.3	42.4	41.5	39.8	21.3	13.8	8.2	8.2
North Dakota	888.9	305.1	209.6	66.7	36.5	34.9	30.7	24.7	11.4	8.1	15.8
South Dakota	908.9	334.8	196.1	73.0	47.0	38.9	36.5	17.2	13.1	7.2	8.2
Nebraska	935.7	319.3	209.0	68.0	36.5	47.0	43.3	16.2	13.9	5.9	14.2
Kansas	899.2	309.5	203.3	68.9	37.6	38.9	38.1	18.4	12.0	6.9	9.9
South Atlantic	900.0	294.4	215.4	61.6	40.2	34.9	27.7	20.2	13.7	10.7	6.6
Delaware	865.2	284.3	225.3	48.6	36.5	33.6	24.9	28.8	12.0	11.0	4.8
Maryland	803.4	248.9	205.6	46.6	29.7	29.4	24.8	21.1	10.2	8.4	4.4
District of Columbia	1,205.0	310.9	254.9	61.6	32.8	25.9	34.4	32.3	6.1	31.6	9.4
Virginia	776.0	248.9	187.9	56.9	35.5	29.2	27.9	14.4	12.9	8.0	5.8
West Virginia	1,080.9	395.8	245.8	65.9	47.1	50.9	39.7	27.2	12.2	10.0	8.6
North Carolina	864.7	280.1	199.6	67.3	44.0	30.9	29.3	19.8	14.0	10.9	5.0
South Carolina	852.2	267.7	194.8	69.5	47.8	29.9	23.4	20.8	12.4	10.3	4.7
Georgia	799.8	252.2	170.3	59.0	44.4	29.5	27.7	15.5	13.6	8.7	6.6
Florida	1,038.7	354.3	261.7	65.7	40.0	43.9	27.0	22.9	16.1	13.1	8.7
East South Central	961.4	326.1	216.8	70.7	51.6	38.3	33.9	19.9	13.2	9.7	7.0
Kentucky	951.8	322.4	228.6	65.9	45.9	42.2	36.7	21.7	14.9	8.6	6.2
Tennessee	949.6	317.8	215.1	73.6	47.6	38.2	34.8	18.7	13.4	10.5	8.3
Alabama	974.6	319.1	214.3	71.7	57.5	37.5	30.3	21.5	12.7	10.7	7.0
Mississippi	976.5	358.3	206.9	70.6	58.0	34.2	33.8	17.1	11.2	8.2	5.5
West South Central	816.7	265.3	186.1	56.6	40.5	31.7	28.2	21.6	12.9	9.1	7.3
Arkansas	1,048.7	339.9	242.6	88.3	50.4	42.2	38.5	22.0	12.5	8.7	6.9
Louisiana	890.3	294.4	206.0	56.8	45.7	29.0	24.0	28.8	13.2	8.6	7.6
Oklahoma	965.7	345.9	211.6	69.8	42.9	42.6	41.0	16.1	12.5	7.9	12.0
Texas	738.7	232.9	168.6	49.8	37.5	29.0	25.4	20.7	13.0	9.4	6.5
Mountain	710.3	210.3	162.1	44.3	41.8	39.0	27.8	15.4	18.5	10.3	6.9
Montana	858.6	247.7	202.9	61.7	49.8	48.7	29.8	19.4	20.9	10.6	8.4
Idaho	740.2	219.7	172.6	54.4	47.4	37.7	31.0	17.0	19.1	5.1	6.8
Wyoming	706.1	214.3	161.2	46.5	44.8	44.1	27.8	14.6	17.9	8.6	5.5
Colorado	655.1	186.5	149.8	40.2	34.2	39.5	28.4	12.3	16.8	9.0	8.3
New Mexico	701.3	198.2	149.5	36.6	52.7	35.2	23.0	21.1	18.7	15.3	7.3
Arizona	785.5	240.3	186.5	47.3	44.4	43.5	32.3	15.1	18.7	11.7	7.0
Utah	533.5	159.0	102.4	39.2	32.7	20.8	23.2	16.7	15.3	6.1	4.5
Nevada	775.3	238.3	187.0	42.7	42.7	47.9	21.7	12.7	24.5	14.1	5.3
Pacific	729.8	227.2	169.1	53.0	35.3	33.7	31.7	12.4	12.9	12.0	7.3
Washington	762.1	230.9	185.0	56.0	36.7	39.9	28.9	15.8	13.9	8.5	9.0
Oregon	884.3	267.4	212.9	66.2	40.2	45.1	34.6	16.7	15.8	9.4	11.2
California	720.3	227.0	164.6	52.0	34.2	32.4	32.6	11.3	12.5	13.1	6.9

[Continued]

★ 32 ★

Leading Causes of Death, by State: 1990

[Continued]

Division and state	Total[1]	Heart disease	Cancer	Cerebro-vascular diseases	Accidents & adverse effects	Chronic obstructive pulmonary diseases[2]	Pneumonia, flu	Diabetes mellitus	Suicide	Chronic liver diseases & cirrhosis	Athero-sclerosis
Alaska	397.8	80.7	85.4	18.7	71.4	16.4	8.7	9.3	12.7	8.4	2.4
Hawaii	612.0	186.6	149.3	47.8	29.0	19.6	26.2	15.2	11.3	6.8	2.1

Source: 1993 Statistical Abstract of the United States on CD-ROM [machine-readable datafiles]. CD-ABSTR-93. Washington, DC: U.S. Department of Commerce, Economics and Statistics Administration, Bureau of the Census, Data User Services Division, 1993. Primary source: U.S. National Center for Health Statistics. *Monthly Vital Statistics Report;* and unpublished data. *Notes:* 1. Includes other causes not shown separately. 2. Includes allied conditions.

Dental Health

★ 33 ★

Alcohol Content of Mouthwash

Figures show the alcohol content of selected national brands of mouthwash.

[In percentages]

Mouthwash brand	Alcohol content
Listerine	26.9
Scope	18.9
Clear Choice	0
Rembrandt	0

Source: "The Bite Is Back." *Chemical Marketing Reporter* 244, no. 6, 9 August 1993, p. SR30.

★ 34 ★
Dental Health

Complete Loss of Permanent Teeth: 1990

Data reflect the percent of persons 18 years of age and older who have lost all their permanent teeth. Data are provided by sex, age, and selected characteristics for 1990.

Characteristic	Both sexes 18 years and over	Male					Female				
		Total	18-29 years	30-44 years	45-64 years	65 years and over	Total	18-29 years	30-44 years	45-64 years	65 years and over
All persons[1]	10.6	9.6	1.4	3.0	14.4	30.9	11.5	1.7	3.4	15.0	33.7
Education level											
Less than 12 years	23.6	21.0	1.4[2]	5.3	26.9	42.4	25.9	1.3[2]	7.9	27.5	46.9
12 years	9.8	8.9	1.3	3.2	16.1	28.8	10.5	2.0	3.4	14.6	30.0
More than 12 years	4.5	4.6	1.5	2.4	6.3	17.0	4.4	1.6	2.3	6.8	14.9
13-15 years	5.4	5.6	1.3	2.7	9.0	25.6	5.3	1.4	2.5	8.9	18.4
16 years or more	3.6	3.7	1.8[2]	2.1	4.6	10.8	3.4	2.0[2]	2.0	4.7	9.9
Income											
Less than $10,000	20.3	16.6	1.0[2]	4.1[2]	30.1	46.5	22.3	1.7[2]	4.8	28.6	48.0
$10,000-$19,999	15.9	15.4	0.6[2]	3.4	20.6	41.6	16.3	2.1	4.9	20.6	36.8
$20,000-$34,999	9.1	9.0	2.3	3.3	15.1	26.5	9.2	2.3	3.5	16.8	23.4
$35,000-$49,999	6.3	7.0	1.1[2]	3.5	15.9	16.8	5.6	1.5[2]	3.9	9.9	15.2
$50,000 or more	4.6	4.6	1.6[2]	2.0	7.4	13.6	4.6	1.5[2]	2.3	7.3	16.7
Race											
White	10.8	9.9	1.4	2.8	14.7	31.4	11.7	1.6	3.5	15.2	32.7
Black	9.3	7.6	1.3[2]	3.6	11.9	29.3	10.6	2.9	2.8	13.5	41.5
Hispanic origin											
Hispanic	4.9	4.4	1.1[2]	1.7[2]	10.2	21.8	5.3	1.6[2]	2.0[2]	6.7	33.1
Non-Hispanic	11.0	10.0	1.4	3.1	14.7	31.2	12.0	1.8	3.5	15.5	33.8
Geographic region											
Northeast	10.8	9.7	2.2	2.0	15.8	29.4	11.7	2.1	2.5	14.0	33.3
Midwest	11.5	10.7	1.4	3.6	16.1	34.5	12.3	1.7	3.7	16.8	35.3
South	11.0	10.0	0.7[2]	3.2	15.8	31.8	11.9	1.5	3.8	15.0	35.4
West	8.4	7.3	1.9	3.2	9.0	26.1	9.4	1.7	3.2	13.7	28.9
Marital status											
Currently married	9.9	10.7	1.5	3.2	14.4	29.4	9.1	2.0	3.4	13.2	28.6
Formerly married	21.1	15.1	2.6[2]	2.5	15.7	36.7	23.5	1.5[2]	3.5	20.2	38.7
Never married	3.3	3.1	1.3	2.7	10.6	35.5	3.4	1.5	2.7	13.9	19.1
Employment status											
Currently employed	5.8	5.7	1.5	2.9	12.2	21.7	6.0	1.7	3.4	12.3	25.5
Unemployed	5.0	5.8	1.1[2]	2.6[2]	18.0	24.4[2]	4.0	1.5[2]	2.6[2]	9.4[2]	24.4[2]
Not in labor force	20.9	23.5	0.9[2]	5.7	23.2	33.0	19.6	1.9	3.4	19.2	34.8

Source: U.S. Department of Health and Human Services. Public Health Service. Centers for Disease Control and Prevention. National Center for Health Statistics. *Health Promotion and Disease Prevention: United States, 1990.* Vital and Health Statistics, Series 10, no. 185. Hyattsville, MD: U.S. Department of Health and Human Services, Public Health Service, Centers for Disease Control and Prevention, National Center for Health Statistics, n.d., p. 56. *Notes:* Data are based on household interviews of the civilian noninstitutionalized population. The survey design, general qualifications, and information on the reliability of the estimates are given in Appendix 1 in the original source. Denominator for each cell excludes unknowns. 1. Includes persons with unknown sociodemographic characteristics. 2. Figure does not meet standard of reliability or precision (more than 30-percent relative standard error in numerator of percent or rate).

★ 35 ★

Dental Health

Cost of Fillings

Type of filling	Average Cost	Average Lifespan (yrs.)
Amalgam	$51	10-20
Composite	64	3-10
Gold	361	20 or more
Ceramic	404	10

Source: "How Dental Fillings Compare." *Consumer Reports* 56 (May 1991), p. 319.

★ 36 ★

Dental Health

Dental Hygiene Habits

Ninety percent of Americans understand that regular dental visits promote healthy teeth and gums. The table below reflects dental hygiene habits of Americans.

Habits	Percent
Brush teeth daily	<50
Brush teeth after each meal	25
Change toothbrush every 3 months	17
Avoid visiting dentist	7

Source: "Brushing Up on Dental Hygiene." *Washington Post,* 11 August 1992, final edition, p. Z5.

★ 37 ★

Dental Health

Dental Visits: 1990

Table below indicates the percent of persons 18 years of age and older who have visited the dentist at least once in the past 12 months. Data are provided by sex, age, and selected characteristics for 1990.

Characteristic	Both sexes 18 years and over	Male					Female				
		Total	18-29 years	30-44 years	45-64 years	65 years and over	Total	18-29 years	30-44 years	45-64 years	65 years and over
All persons[1]	62.5	59.0	57.9	62.9	60.5	48.7	65.7	67.4	74.0	64.9	50.2
Education level											
Less than 12 years	40.4	38.3	45.2	39.5	39.3	30.6	42.2	51.8	52.7	40.7	33.0
12 years	61.3	55.9	55.1	59.0	53.9	53.6	65.5	65.4	70.7	65.5	55.7

[Continued]

★ 37 ★

Dental Visits: 1990
[Continued]

Characteristic	Both sexes 18 years and over	Male					Female				
		Total	18-29 years	30-44 years	45-64 years	65 years and over	Total	18-29 years	30-44 years	45-64 years	65 years and over
More than 12 years	75.3	71.4	66.7	70.9	77.3	69.4	79.3	75.8	81.8	81.2	74.7
13-15 years	71.5	66.3	66.4	65.8	70.0	58.9	76.1	75.5	78.4	75.9	71.1
16 years or more	79.2	75.9	67.2	74.8	81.9	77.1	83.1	76.3	85.2	86.5	79.8
Income											
Less than $10,000	44.5	40.3	58.5	35.2	30.2	19.3	46.8	60.7	50.7	41.7	34.2
$10,000-$19,999	49.1	43.5	48.5	47.7	37.5	37.8	53.6	60.6	57.8	50.7	45.6
$20,000-$34,999	63.2	58.1	58.1	58.7	58.5	55.9	68.0	69.3	71.9	63.6	64.1
$35,000-$49,999	72.5	67.3	62.3	71.3	63.0	74.0	78.1	74.4	82.1	75.0	76.8
$50,000 or more	78.2	74.6	67.5	74.2	77.9	79.2	82.1	78.8	84.5	81.9	76.5
Race											
White	64.1	60.8	59.6	64.8	62.6	50.5	67.2	68.9	75.4	66.6	52.2
Black	51.8	46.0	51.4	48.9	42.5	29.2	56.4	59.1	66.4	53.2	31.1
Hispanic origin											
Hispanic	54.0	47.7	44.3	50.5	53.6	32.1	59.3	55.5	65.8	62.0	42.1
Non-Hispanic	63.3	59.9	59.6	64.0	61.0	49.2	66.3	69.2	74.8	65.1	50.5
Geographic region											
Northeast	66.6	63.9	63.2	70.3	62.5	52.3	69.0	73.1	77.7	68.0	52.6
Midwest	65.0	61.0	59.6	66.0	62.9	48.8	68.7	73.4	75.6	68.4	50.8
South	57.3	53.0	54.4	56.4	52.7	43.4	61.2	62.9	69.7	60.1	45.9
West	64.2	61.5	56.9	62.6	68.2	54.6	66.7	63.3	75.4	65.8	54.9
Marital status											
Currently married	64.4	59.8	53.4	64.4	62.0	51.2	69.0	65.1	75.6	67.8	57.1
Formerly married	53.8	52.5	55.1	59.7	53.2	39.9	54.4	61.0	68.6	57.3	44.4
Never married	63.8	59.1	61.0	56.9	54.9	38.6	69.5	71.2	69.8	60.6	58.5
Employment status											
Currently employed	66.8	62.3	58.0	64.6	63.7	57.3	72.3	70.7	76.7	68.6	60.4
Unemployed	56.9	48.2	49.8	48.0	46.5	38.5[2]	66.4	67.1	64.5	69.9	57.7[2]
Not in labor force	54.2	49.3	60.7	43.5	49.0	46.9	56.6	59.5	66.9	59.2	49.0

Source: U.S. Department of Health and Human Services. Public Health Service. Centers for Disease Control and Prevention. National Center for Health Statistics. *Health Promotion and Disease Prevention: United States, 1990.* Vital and Health Statistics, Series 10, no. 185. Hyattsville, MD: U.S. Department of Health and Human Services, Public Health Service, Centers for Disease Control and Prevention, National Center for Health Statistics, n.d., p. 55. *Notes:* Data are based on household interviews of the civilian noninstitutionalized population. The survey design, general qualifications, and information on the reliability of the estimates are given in Appendix 1 in the original source. Denominator for each cell excludes unknowns. 1. Includes persons with unknown sociodemographic characteristics. 2. Figure does not meet standard of reliability or precision (more than 30-percent relative standard error in numerator of percent or rate).

Disabilities and Handicaps

★ 38 ★

Adults With Special Health Conditions

Table reflects the members of the adult population who reported having a physical, mental, or other health condition in the National Adult Literacy Survey.

[In percentages]

Condition	Adult population affected
Physical, mental, or health condition	12
Visual difficulty	7
Hearing difficulty	7
Learning disability	3
Mental or emotional condition	2
Mental retardation	0[1]
Speech disability	1
Physical disability	9
Long-term illness	8
Other health impairment	6

Source: Kirsch, Irwin S., Ann Jungeblut, Lynn Jenkins, and Andrew Kolstad. *Adult Literacy in America: A First Look at the Results of the National Adult Literacy Survey.* Prepared by Educational Testing Service under contract with National Center for Education Statistics. Washington, DC: U.S. Department of Education, Office of Educational Research and Improvement, September 1990, sec. 1, p. 43. Primary source: U.S. Department of Education. National Center for Education Statistics. National Adult Literacy Survey (1992). *Note:* 1. Percentages below .5 are rounded to 0.

★ 39 ★
Disabilities and Handicaps

Limitation of Activity Caused by Chronic Conditions: 1985 and 1990

Data are based on household interviews of a sample of the civilian noninstitutionalized population.

[Percent of population]

Characteristic	Total with limitation of activity		Limited but not in major activity		Limited in amount or kind of major activity		Unable to carry on major activity	
	1985	1990	1985	1990	1985	1990	1985	1990
Total[1,2]	13.4	12.9	4.2	4.1	5.5	5.0	3.7	3.9
Under 15 years	4.8	4.7	1.2	1.2	3.1	3.1	0.4	0.4
Under 5 years	2.2	2.2	0.6	0.6	1.1	1.0	0.5	0.6
5-14 years	6.2	6.1	1.6	1.6	4.2	4.1	0.4	0.4
15-44 years	8.3	8.5	2.7	2.6	3.6	3.5	1.9	2.4

[Continued]

★ 39 ★

Limitation of Activity Caused by Chronic Conditions: 1985 and 1990
[Continued]

Characteristic	Total with limitation of activity		Limited but not in major activity		Limited in amount or kind of major activity		Unable to carry on major activity	
	1985	1990	1985	1990	1985	1990	1985	1990
45-64 years	23.4	21.8	5.9	5.7	8.8	7.5	8.7	8.6
65 years and over	39.6	37.5	15.5	15.4	13.8	11.9	10.4	10.2
65-74 years	36.7	33.7	14.0	13.2	11.5	9.9	11.2	10.6
75 years and over	44.3	43.3	17.9	18.8	17.3	14.9	9.1	9.6

Source: National Economic, Social, and Environmental Data Bank: The Federal Connection [CD-ROM]. Prepared by U.S. Department of Commerce, Economics and Statistics Administration. Washington, DC: U.S. Department of Commerce, Economics and Statistics Administration, Office of Business Analysis, November 1992. Primary source: National Center for Health Statistics, Division of Health Interview Statistics, data from the National Health Interview Survey. Notes: 1. Age adjusted. 2. Includes all other races not shown separately and unknown family income.

★ 40 ★

Disabilities and Handicaps

Percent Distribution of Persons With Daily Activity Limitations Due to Illness: 1991

Characteristic	All persons	With no activity limitation	With activity limitation	With limitation in major activity	Unable to carry on major activity	Limited in amount or kind of major activity	Limited, but not in major activity
All persons[1]	100.0	85.7	14.3	9.6	4.3	5.4	4.6
Age							
Under 18 years	100.0	94.2	5.8	4.2	0.5	3.7	1.6
18-44 years	100.0	90.8	9.2	6.4	2.8	3.5	2.9
45-64 years	100.0	77.8	22.2	16.3	8.7	7.6	5.9
65 years and over	100.0	62.1	37.9	22.3	10.6	11.7	15.6
65-69 years	100.0	65.2	34.8	26.9	15.2	11.7	7.9
70 years and over	100.0	60.6	39.4	20.1	8.4	11.7	19.2
Sex and age							
Male							
All ages	100.0	86.1	13.9	9.6	4.7	5.0	4.2
Under 18 years	100.0	93.2	6.8	5.0	0.5	4.5	1.8
18-44 years	100.0	90.6	9.4	6.9	3.3	3.5	2.5
45-64 years	100.0	78.5	21.5	16.9	10.2	6.6	4.6
65-69 years	100.0	64.3	35.7	29.4	18.8	10.5	6.3
70 years and over	100.0	62.0	38.0	15.5	7.4	8.2	22.4
Female							
All ages	100.0	85.4	14.6	9.6	3.9	5.7	5.0
Under 18 years	100.0	95.3	4.7	3.3	0.5	2.9	1.4
18-44 years	100.0	91.0	9.0	5.9	2.3	3.5	3.2

[Continued]

★ 40 ★

Percent Distribution of Persons With Daily Activity Limitations Due to Illness: 1991

[Continued]

Characteristic	All persons	With no activity limitation	With activity limitation	With limitation in major activity	Unable to carry on major activity	Limited in amount or kind of major activity	Limited, but not in major activity
45-64 years	100.0	77.2	22.8	15.8	7.3	8.6	7.0
65-69 years	100.0	65.9	34.1	24.9	12.2	12.7	9.2
70 years and over	100.0	59.7	40.3	23.2	9.1	14.1	17.1
Race and age							
White							
All ages	100.0	85.5	14.5	9.6	4.1	5.4	4.9
Under 18 years	100.0	94.3	5.7	4.1	0.5	3.6	1.6
18-44 years	100.0	90.6	9.4	6.3	2.7	3.6	3.1
45-64 years	100.0	78.3	21.7	15.7	8.0	7.7	6.0
65-69 years	100.0	65.8	34.2	26.4	14.5	11.9	7.8
70 years and over	100.0	61.2	38.9	19.4	8.0	11.4	19.5
Black							
All ages	100.0	85.6	14.4	11.0	5.5	5.5	3.4
Under 18 years	100.0	93.2	6.8	5.2	0.5	4.7	1.6
18-44 years	100.0	90.7	9.3	7.3	4.0	3.3	2.0
45-64 years	100.0	71.7	28.3	23.2	15.1	8.2	5.0
65-69 years	100.0	57.6	42.4	33.0	22.0	11.0	9.4
70 years and over	100.0	54.0	46.0	28.6	12.9	15.7	17.4
Family income and age							
Under $10,000							
All ages	100.0	73.4	26.6	19.6	10.1	9.6	7.0
Under 18 years	100.0	89.9	10.1	7.7	0.9	6.8	2.4
18-44 years	100.0	83.0	17.0	13.0	7.5	5.6	4.0
45-64 years	100.0	42.2	57.8	48.9	33.6	15.3	8.8
65-69 years	100.0	47.9	52.1	43.7	26.7	17.0	8.5
70 years and over	100.0	51.4	48.6	27.2	9.0	18.1	21.5
$10,000-$19,999							
All ages	100.0	80.2	19.8	13.7	6.4	7.3	6.1
Under 18 years	100.0	92.8	7.2	5.7	0.7	4.9	1.6
18-44 years	100.0	87.6	12.4	9.1	4.3	4.8	3.3
45-64 years	100.0	64.3	35.7	29.1	17.0	12.1	6.7
65-69 years	100.0	60.6	39.4	31.0	18.3	12.6	8.4
70 years and over	100.0	61.3	38.7	17.9	6.8	11.1	20.8
$20,000-$34,999							
All ages	100.0	87.5	12.5	8.2	3.3	5.0	4.2
Under 18 years	100.0	94.7	5.4	3.9	0.4	3.5	1.4
18-44 years	100.0	91.1	8.9	6.0	2.3	3.7	2.9
45-64 years	100.0	79.1	20.9	15.1	7.1	8.0	5.8
65-69 years	100.0	69.4	30.6	22.9	11.5	11.5	7.7
70 years and over	100.0	66.8	33.2	14.9	6.7	8.2	18.4

[Continued]

★ 40 ★

Percent Distribution of Persons With Daily Activity Limitations Due to Illness: 1991
[Continued]

Characteristic	All persons	With no activity limitation	With activity limitation	With limitation in major activity	Unable to carry on major activity	Limited in amount or kind of major activity	Limited, but not in major activity
$35,000 or more							
All ages	100.0	91.3	8.7	5.4	1.8	3.6	3.3
Under 18 years	100.0	95.3	4.7	3.2	0.4	2.8	1.5
18-44 years	100.0	93.4	6.6	4.0	1.3	2.7	2.6
45-64 years	100.0	86.2	13.8	8.6	3.1	5.5	5.2
65-69 years	100.0	77.7	22.3	16.3	7.7	8.6	6.0
70 years and over	100.0	66.7	33.3	16.7	9.2	7.4	16.7
Geographic region							
Northeast	100.0	87.4	12.6	8.5	3.9	4.5	4.1
Midwest	100.0	85.5	14.5	9.7	3.7	6.0	4.7
South	100.0	84.5	15.5	10.8	5.0	5.8	4.7
West	100.0	86.4	13.6	8.8	4.0	4.7	4.9
Place of residence							
MSA[2]	100.0	86.4	13.6	9.2	4.0	5.1	4.4
Central city	100.0	85.3	14.7	10.1	4.6	5.4	4.6
Not central city	100.0	87.2	12.8	8.6	3.6	5.0	4.3
Not MSA[2]	100.0	83.2	16.8	11.2	5.1	6.1	5.6

Source: U.S. Department of Health and Human Services. Public Health Service. Centers for Disease Control and Prevention. National Center for Health Statistics. *Current Estimates From the National Health Interview Survey, 1991.* Vital and Health Statistics, Series 10: Data From the National Health Survey, no. 184. DHHS publication no. (PHS) 93-1512. Hyattsville, MD: U.S. Department of Health and Human Services, Public Health Service, Centers for Disease Control and Prevention, National Center for Health Statistics, December 1992, pp. 106-107. *Notes:* Data are based on household interviews of the civilian noninstitutionalized population. The survey design, general qualifications, and information on the reliability of the estimates are given in Appendix 1 of the original source. 1. Includes other races and unknown family income. 2. MSA is metropolitan statistical area.

★ 41 ★

Disabilities and Handicaps

Restrictions of Persons With Daily Activity Limitations Due to Illness:1991

Data indicate number of days individuals are restricted due to acute and chronic conditions.

Characteristic	Type of restriction					
	Number of days per person			Number of days in thousands		
	All types	Bed disability	Work or school loss[1]	All types	Bed disability	Work or school loss[1]
All persons[2]	16.1	6.5	5.4	3,996,402	1,612,545	887,025
Age						
Under 5 years	10.9	4.6	...	211,935	89,829	...
5-17 years	9.4	4.1	5.1	432,499	190,601	236,887

[Continued]

★ 41 ★

Restrictions of Persons With Daily Activity Limitations Due to Illness:1991
[Continued]

Characteristic	Type of restriction					
	Number of days per person			Number of days in thousands		
	All types	Bed disability	Work or school loss[1]	All types	Bed disability	Work or school loss[1]
18 years and over	18.3	7.3	5.6	3,351,968	1,332,115	650,138
18-24 years	10.2	4.4	4.6	252,184	108,503	74,386
25-44 years	13.4	5.0	5.5	1,088,353	403,591	356,682
45-64 years	20.8	7.9	6.2	981,232	373,470	199,438
65 years and over	34.0	14.7	5.1	1,030,200	446,552	19,633
Sex and age						
Male						
All ages	14.1	5.4	4.9	1,700,766	656,879	426,423
Under 5 years	11.9	5.1	...	118,007	50,449	...
5-17 years	8.7	3.8	4.8	205,082	90,167	113,756
18 years and over	15.8	5.9	4.9	1,377,677	516,262	312,667
18-24 years	8.7	3.6	3.7	105,233	42,979	31,538
25-44 years	11.6	3.8	4.6	461,909	151,030	165,449
45-64 years	18.4	6.6	5.9	415,772	148,881	103,286
65 years and over	31.2	13.7	5.5	394,764	173,371	12,394
Female						
All ages	17.9	7.5	6.1	2,295,636	955,666	460,602
Under 5 years	9.9	4.2	...	93,928	39,380	...
5-17 years	10.1	4.5	5.5	227,417	100,433	123,131
18 years and over	20.6	8.5	6.3	1,974,291	815,853	337,471
18-24 years	11.7	5.2	5.6	146,951	65,524	42,848
25-44 years	15.2	6.1	6.5	626,444	252,560	191,233
45-64 years	23.0	9.2	6.6	565,460	224,589	96,152
65 years and over	36.0	15.5	4.5	635,436	273,180	7,239
Race and age						
White						
All ages	16.1	6.3	5.5	3,343,859	1,312,883	749,485
Under 5 years	11.3	4.4	...	174,861	68,552	...
5-17 years	9.9	4.3	5.4	367,708	161,238	198,564
18 years and over	18.0	7.0	5.5	2,801,290	1,083,093	550,921
18-24 years	10.6	4.4	4.7	210,125	87,118	64,263
25-44 years	13.1	4.6	5.4	892,799	312,415	295,665
45-64 years	20.0	7.3	6.2	813,604	297,957	172,923
65 years and over	32.5	14.2	5.2	884,761	385,603	18,070
Black						
All ages	17.5	8.0	5.9	540,052	245,659	114,366
Under 5 years	9.6	5.5	...	29,477	16,987	...
5-17 years	7.5	3.4	4.4	54,446	24,366	31,543
18 years and over	22.2	9.9	6.8	456,130	204,305	82,823
18-24 years	9.9	5.3	5.1	34,623	18,523	8,985
25-44 years	16.7	7.7	7.2	160,662	73,983	51,870
45-64 years	28.5	12.1	6.9	138,736	58,927	20,495

[Continued]

★ 41 ★

Restrictions of Persons With Daily Activity Limitations Due to Illness:1991

[Continued]

| Characteristic | Type of restriction | | | | | |
| | Number of days per person | | | Number of days in thousands | | |
	All types	Bed disability	Work or school loss[1]	All types	Bed disability	Work or school loss[1]
65 years and over	47.6	20.6	4.8[4]	122,108	52,871	1,473
Family income and age						
Less than $10,000						
All ages	29.8	12.3	7.6	711,369	294,523	75,753
Under 5 years	12.7	4.9	...	29,310	11,364	...
5-17 years	12.3	5.7	6.9	55,308	25,768	30,934
18 years and over	36.7	15.1	8.3	626,751	257,391	44,819
18-24 years	13.3	5.7	5.4	57,185	24,457	10,541
25-44 years	28.6	12.1	9.9	143,450	60,792	22,033
45-64 years	60.1	23.5	11.4	182,901	71,640	10,522
65 years and over	51.6	21.3	5.9[4]	243,214	100,502	1,723
$10,000-$19,999						
All ages	20.8	8.5	6.6	789,232	323,823	136,032
Under 5 years	13.1	5.9	...	41,794	18,847	...
5-17 years	10.0	4.6	5.9	68,868	31,986	40,419
18 years and over	24.3	9.8	6.9	678,570	272,990	95,614
18-24 years	10.1	3.4	4.9	42,323	14,189	13,582
25-44 years	17.9	7.2	6.7	186,203	74,507	49,213
45-64 years	33.6	13.6	9.8	192,836	77,960	29,274
65 years and over	34.1	14.1	5.0[4]	257,208	106,335	3,544
$20,000-$34,999						
All ages	13.6	5.1	5.9	724,301	269,109	218,005
Under 5 years	10.1	3.7	...	45,354	16,364	...
5-17 years	8.7	3.9	4.9	88,206	39,178	49,696
18 years and over	15.3	5.5	6.3	590,741	213,567	168,309
18-24 years	10.1	4.4	4.9	48,437	21,368	17,327
25-44 years	12.8	4.2	6.2	244,489	81,014	98,636
45-64 years	18.4	7.1	7.2	163,997	62,766	44,778
65 years and over	23.3	8.4	8.7	133,817	48,419	7,568
$35,000 or more						
All ages	11.0	4.2	4.7	983,186	374,261	323,596
Under 5 years	10.7	5.0	...	70,852	32,903	...
5-17 years	9.2	3.8	4.8	161,234	65,982	83,809
18 years and over	11.5	4.2	4.6	751,100	275,376	239,787
18-24 years	8.8	4.0	4.3	61,308	27,434	22,708
25-44 years	10.2	3.5	4.5	346,424	120,035	133,695
45-64 years	12.9	4.3	5.1	253,547	83,751	79,456
65 years and over	20.4	10.0	4.0[3]	89,821	44,157	3,927
Geographic region						
Northeast	13.1	5.1	5.2	658,053	258,366	170,312
Midwest	15.2	5.5	5.5	906,997	329,830	220,107
South	18.2	8.0	5.5	1,529,302	675,048	300,949

[Continued]

★ 41 ★

Restrictions of Persons With Daily Activity Limitations Due to Illness:1991

[Continued]

Characteristic	Type of restriction					
	Number of days per person			Number of days in thousands		
	All types	Bed disability	Work or school loss[1]	All types	Bed disability	Work or school loss[1]
West	16.5	6.4	5.5	902,050	349,301	195,657
Place of residence						
MSA[4]	15.9	6.4	5.4	3,081,071	1,240,553	699,539
Central city	17.6	7.4	5.6	1,350,397	564,930	271,482
Not central city	14.7	5.7	5.3	1,730,674	675,623	428,058
Not MSA[4]	16.7	6.8	5.4	915,331	371,992	187,486

Source: U.S. Department of Health and Human Services. Public Health Service. Centers for Disease Control and Prevention. National Center for Health Statistics. Current Estimates From the National Health Interview Survey, 1991. Vital and Health Statistics, Series 10: Data From the National Health Survey, no. 184. DHHS publication no. (PHS) 93-1512. Hyattsville, MD: U.S. Department of Health and Human Services, Public Health Service, Centers for Disease Control and Disease Prevention, National Center for Health Statistics, December 1992, pp. 110-111. Notes: Data are based on household interviews of the civilian noninstitutionalized population. The survey design, general qualifications, and information on the reliability of the estimates are given in Appendix 1 of the original source. Three dots (...) means the category is not applicable. 1. Sum of school-loss days for children 5-17 years of age and work-loss days for currently employed persons 18 years of age and over. School-loss days are shown for the age group 5-17 years; work-loss days are shown for the age group 18 years and over and each older age group. 2. Includes other races and unknown family income. 3. Figure does not meet standard of reliability or precision. 4. MSA is metropolitan statistical area.

★ 42 ★

Disabilities and Handicaps

Special Education Students, by Race/Ethnicity

[In percentages]

Disability classifications	Race/ethnicity		
	Black	Hispanic	White
Retarded	26	18	11
Learning-disabled	43	55	51
Emotionally disturbed	8	4	8
Speech-impaired	23	23	30

Source: "A Breakdown by Race." U.S. News & World Report, 13 December 1993, p. 54. Primary source: U.S. Department of Education. Office of Civil Rights. 1990 Survey of Schools.

Diseases and Illnesses: Acute Conditions

★ 43 ★

Acute Conditions Per 100 Persons: 1991

Table below reflects the number of acute conditions per 100 persons per year.

Type of acute condition	All ages	Under 5 years	5-17 years	18-24 years	25-44 years	45 years and over		
						Total	45-64 years	65 years and over
All acute conditions	191.8	390.7	270.2	194.6	164.0	123.5	128.4	115.7
Infective and parasitic diseases	18.5	45.9	38.4	14.0	12.5	7.6	9.3	5.1
Common childhood diseases	1.8	10.6	4.7	0.3[1]	0.2[1]	0.1[1]	0.2[1]	-[1]
Intestinal virus, unspecified	4.0	8.5	8.4	3.1[1]	3.6	1.0[1]	1.3[1]	0.5[1]
Viral infections, unspecified	6.1	15.3	10.0	5.3	4.3	3.8	4.8	2.3[1]
Other	6.5	11.5	15.3	5.4	4.4	2.7	3.0	2.2[1]
Respiratory conditions	100.6	183.5	150.1	106.3	88.0	61.8	68.9	50.7
Common cold	28.6	67.2	38.7	34.1	22.9	17.2	17.4	17.0
Other acute upper respiratory infections	11.7	23.0	21.9	8.0	9.5	6.5	7.9	4.3
Influenza	52.1	68.1	78.6	58.1	51.1	31.5	38.2	20.9
Acute bronchitis	4.5	12.0	6.7	3.8	2.9	3.1	3.0	3.3
Pneumonia	1.7	6.5	1.4[1]	1.0[1]	0.8[1]	1.8	0.9[1]	3.3
Other respiratory conditions	2.0	6.8	2.8	1.3[1]	0.8[1]	1.7	1.5[1]	2.0[1]
Digestive system conditions	6.6	10.1	9.1	5.3	5.7	5.6	4.8	6.9
Dental conditions	1.4	3.3[1]	1.2[1]	0.8[1]	1.7	0.9[1]	1.2[1]	0.4[1]
Indigestion, nausea, and vomiting	2.9	2.0[1]	6.1	3.2[1]	2.5	1.4	1.0[1]	2.0[1]
Other digestive conditions	2.4	4.8	1.8	1.3[1]	1.5	3.3	2.5	4.5
Injuries	24.0	23.2	29.6	32.2	23.6	18.7	18.3	19.3
Fractures and dislocations	3.0	1.0[1]	5.0	3.7	2.8	2.3	2.0	2.7
Sprains and strains	5.4	1.1[1]	5.9	7.3	7.2	3.8	3.7	3.9
Open wounds and lacerations	4.7	6.1	6.9	7.6	4.5	2.4	2.9	1.5[1]
Contusions and superficial injuries	4.7	6.1	5.4	7.4	3.3	4.6	4.3	5.1
Other current injuries	6.1	8.9	6.3	6.1	5.8	5.7	5.4	6.0
Selected other acute conditions	30.1	105.0	34.3	25.0	23.9	17.1	15.6	19.2
Eye conditions	1.2	3.0[1]	1.0[1]	0.8[1]	0.7[1]	1.4	0.9[1]	2.2[1]
Acute ear infections	10.3	70.7	14.3	2.7[1]	3.9	1.9	2.5	1.0[1]
Other ear conditions	1.7	6.4	2.9	0.2[1]	1.3	0.8[1]	0.8[1]	0.8[1]
Acute urinary conditions	3.5	2.7[1]	1.7[1]	4.2	4.2	3.7	3.1	4.8
Disorders of menstruation	0.6	...	0.7[1]	1.5[1]	0.7[1]	0.2[1]	0.3[1]	-[1]
Other disorders of female genital tract	1.1	0.3[1]	-[1]	1.8[1]	1.8	1.1	1.0[1]	1.2[1]
Delivery and other conditions of pregnancy and puerperium	1.6	...	0.2[1]	6.5	2.5	-[1]	-[1]	...
Skin conditions	1.9	5.2	2.6	1.6[1]	1.0	1.8	0.9[1]	3.2
Acute musculoskeletal conditions	4.0	1.3[1]	2.7	3.2[1]	4.9	4.8	5.7	3.4
Headaches, excluding migraine	1.3	-[1]	2.9	1.2[1]	1.4	0.7[1]	0.3[1]	1.1[1]

[Continued]

★ 43 ★

Acute Conditions Per 100 Persons: 1991
[Continued]

Type of acute condition	All ages	Under 5 years	5-17 years	18-24 years	25-44 years	45 years and over		
						Total	45-64 years	65 years and over
Fever, unspecified	2.9	15.4	5.3	1.3[1]	1.3	0.7[1]	0.1[1]	1.5[1]
All other acute conditions	11.9	23.1	8.6	11.7	10.3	12.7	11.5	14.6

Source: U.S. Department of Health and Human Services. Public Health Service. Centers for Disease Control and Prevention. National Center for Health Statistics. *Current Estimates From the National Health Interview Survey, 1991*. Vital and Health Statistics, Series 10: Data From the National Health Survey, no. 184. DHHS publication no. (PHS) 93-1512. Hyattsville, MD: U.S. Department of Health and Human Services, Public Health Service, Centers for Disease Control and Prevention, National Center for Health Statistics, December 1992, p. 13. *Notes:* Data are based on household interviews of the civilian noninstitutionalized population. The survey design, general qualifications, and information on the reliability of the estimates are given in Appendix 1 in the original source. Excluded from these estimates are conditions involving neither medical attention nor activity restriction. A dash (-) represents zero. Three dots (...) indicate that the category is not applicable. 1. Figure does not meet standards of reliability or precision.

★ 44 ★

Diseases and Illnesses: Acute Conditions

Bed Days Associated With Acute Conditions: 1991

Data reflect the number of bed days due to acute conditions per 100 persons per year.

Type of acute condition	All ages	Under 5 years	5-17 years	18-24 years	25-44 years	45 years and over		
						Total	45-64 years	65 years and over
All acute conditions	313.6	420.7	334.2	324.1	280.6	305.7	269.6	361.8
Infective and parasitic diseases	27.6	75.9	54.3	28.0	15.4	12.4	11.0[1]	14.5[1]
Common childhood diseases	4.0	21.8[1]	10.6[1]	0.7[1]	0.3[1]	0.4[1]	0.6[1]	-[1]
Intestinal virus, unspecified	5.4	18.1[1]	11.8[1]	3.2[1]	3.7[1]	0.8[1]	0.6[1]	1.1[1]
Viral infections, unspecified	0.8	29.2[1]	14.2	7.8[1]	5.4[1]	7.5	7.5[1]	7.7[1]
Other	8.5	6.8[1]	17.8	16.2[1]	5.9[1]	3.7[1]	2.3[1]	5.8[1]
Respiratory conditions	166.4	227.0	219.1	156.3	140.9	149.7	141.8	161.9
Common cold	24.8	54.1	31.6	32.3	19.1	17.0	16.7	17.4[1]
Other acute upper respiratory infections	12.7	14.2[1]	25.0	10.2[1]	10.4	8.3	7.7[1]	9.2[1]
Influenza	100.3	114.7	137.7	95.1	93.2	83.7	94.8	66.4
Acute bronchitis	9.4	19.5[1]	10.7[1]	9.8[1]	7.9	7.4	10.1[1]	3.4[1]
Pneumonia	14.0	14.3[1]	7.9[1]	6.9[1]	8.1	26.0	9.5[1]	51.6
Other respiratory conditions	5.1	10.2[1]	6.2[1]	2.0[1]	2.2[1]	7.3[1]	3.1[1]	13.8[1]
Digestive system conditions	13.6	9.4[1]	10.0[1]	11.5[1]	12.5	18.8	14.8	24.9
Dental conditions	2.6	4.9[1]	2.7[1]	3.5[1]	2.7[1]	1.6[1]	1.9[1]	1.3[1]
Indigestion, nausea, and vomiting	2.9	3.0[1]	5.5[1]	3.6[1]	1.3[1]	2.7[1]	1.5[1]	4.6[1]
Other digestive conditions	8.1	1.41[1]	1.7[1]	4.4[1]	8.5	14.4	11.5[1]	19.0
Injuries	39.2	8.0[1]	14.8	58.0	41.8	52.8	43.5	67.4
Fractures and dislocations	10.7	1.2[1]	3.4[1]	14.0[1]	8.1	19.1	12.5	29.2
Sprains and strains	8.3	-[1]	2.8[1]	8.4[1]	15.9	5.8[1]	7.0[1]	3.8[1]
Open wounds and lacerations	3.8	1.4[1]	3.7[1]	7.6[1]	5.1[1]	1.7[1]	0.8[1]	3.1[1]
Contusions and superficial injuries	5.1	0.3[1]	1.4[1]	10.5[1]	3.6[1]	8.5	10.1[1]	5.9[1]

[Continued]

★ 44 ★

Bed Days Associated With Acute Conditions: 1991
[Continued]

Type of acute condition	All ages	Under 5 years	5-17 years	18-24 years	25-44 years	45 years and over		
						Total	45-64 years	65 years and over
Other current injuries	11.3	5.1[1]	3.5[1]	17.5[1]	9.1	17.8	13.0	25.3
Selected other acute conditions	45.8	82.0	28.8	49.4	54.1	37.2	31.3	46.3
Eye conditions	0.2[1]	1.8[1]	-[1]	0.7[1]	-[1]	-[1]	-[1]	-[1]
Acute ear infections	9.5	56.6	12.0[1]	2.6[1]	5.2[1]	2.8[1]	2.4[1]	3.3[1]
Other ear conditions	1.0[1]	3.9[1]	2.1[1]	-[1]	0.6[1]	0.2[1]	0.3[1]	-[1]
Acute urinary conditions	4.7	1.1[1]	3.4[1]	2.7[1]	4.6[1]	7.2[1]	6.1[1]	9.0[1]
Disorders of menstruation	1.0[1]	...	0.3[1]	0.5[1]	2.6[1]	0.2[1]	0.3[1]	-[1]
Other disorders of female genital tract	1.3[1]	-[1]	-[1]	1.8[1]	2.5[1]	1.1[1]	0.7[1]	1.6[1]
Delivery and other conditions of pregnancy and puerperium	9.8	...	-[1]	32.8	20.0	-[1]	-[1]	...
Skin conditions	3.4	4.9[1]	2.8[1]	0.8[1]	1.9[1]	5.6[1]	4.1[1]	8.0[1]
Acute musculoskeletal conditions	8.1	-[1]	1.0[1]	2.7[1]	11.3	12.8	14.1	10.6[1]
Headaches, excluding migraines	1.9[1]	-[1]	1.9[1]	2.6[1]	1.7[1]	2.4[1]	2.0[1]	3.0[1]
Fever, unspecified	5.0	13.6[1]	5.2[1]	2.2[1]	3.6[1]	4.9[1]	1.2[1]	10.7[1]
All other acute conditions	20.9	18.5[1]	7.2[1]	21.0[1]	16.0	34.9	27.2	46.8

Source: U.S. Department of Health and Human Services. Public Health Service. Centers for Disease Control and Prevention. National Center for Health Statistics. *Current Estimates From the National Health Interview Survey, 1991.* Vital and Health Statistics, Series 10: Data From the National Health Survey, no. 184. DHHS publication no. (PHS) 93-1512. Hyattsville, MD: U.S. Department of Health and Human Services, Public Health Service, Centers for Disease Control and Prevention, National Center for Health Statistics, December 1992, p. 43. *Notes:* Data are based on household interviews of the civilian noninstitutionalized population. The survey design, general qualifications, and information on the reliability of the estimates are given in Appendix 1 in the original source. Excluded from these estimates are conditions involving neither medical attention nor activity restriction. A dash (-) represents zero. Three dots (...) indicate that the category is not applicable. 1. Figure does not meet standards of reliability or precision.

★ 45 ★

Diseases and Illnesses: Acute Conditions

Deaths From Pneumonia and Influenza, by Age: 1990

Excludes deaths of nonresidents of the United States. Deaths classified according to ninth revision of *International Classification of Diseases.*

Ages	Number of deaths			Death rate per 100,000 population		
	Total	Male	Female	Total	Male	Female
All ages[1] [2]	79,513	36,898	42,615	32.0	30.4	33.4
1 to 4 years old	171	88	83	1.2	1.2	1.1
5 to 14 years old	134	71	63	0.4	0.4	0.4
65 years old and older	70,485	31,256	39,229	226.8	250.2	211.1

Source: 1993 Statistical Abstract of the United States on CD-ROM [machine-readable datafiles]. CD-ABSTR-93. Washington, DC: U.S. Department of Commerce, Economics and Statistics Administration, Bureau of the Census, Data User Services Division, 1993. Primary source: U.S. National Center for Health Statistics. *Vital Statistics of the United States* (annual); and unpublished data. *Notes:* Pneumonia is not a leading cause of death among persons 15 to 64 years old. 1. Includes those deaths with age not stated. 2. Pneumonia only.

★ 46 ★

Diseases and Illnesses: Acute Conditions

Medical Attention for Acute Conditions: 1991

Table indicates percent of acute conditions that received medical attention.

Type of acute condition	All ages	Under 5 years	5-17 years	18-24 years	25-44 years	45 years and over		
						Total	45-64 years	65 years and over
All acute conditions	63.0	82.2	55.1	56.8	58.0	68.0	64.0	75.0
Infective and parasitic diseases	65.4	80.0	63.9	58.4	57.8	64.8	62.5	71.5
Common childhood diseases	70.5	81.4	58.2	100.0[1]	100.0[1]	58.0[1]	58.0[1]	-[1]
Intestinal virus, unspecified	36.3	69.7	27.2	24.2[1]	33.7	32.3[1]	31.9[1]	33.7[1]
Viral infections, unspecified	54.1	76.6	50.0	47.2[1]	44.8	52.1	51.7	53.3[1]
Other	92.4	90.8	94.9	86.7	89.0	95.1	92.9	100.0[1]
Respiratory conditions	46.6	74.4	41.2	35.6	39.0	50.8	47.2	58.6
Common cold	38.9	72.1	28.0	26.9	30.4	40.6	30.5	56.7
Other acute upper respiratory infections	76.6	92.6	67.5	60.4	79.6	82.1	79.0	91.1
Influenza	37.1	62.5	34.2	32.3	31.0	41.2	41.3	40.9
Acute bronchitis	90.3	93.0	86.2	93.9	88.5	93.3	92.5	94.5
Pneumonia	92.3	100.0	100.0[1]	32.9[1]	100.0[1]	88.4	100.0[1]	83.7
Other respiratory conditions	89.5	96.3	79.6	84.2[1]	83.8[1]	96.4	100.0[1]	92.1[1]
Digestive system conditions	66.3	74.5	45.6	87.4	62.2	80.7	78.7	82.9
Dental conditions	64.4	51.4[1]	67.3[1]	100.0[1]	71.0	50.8[1]	50.0[1]	54.6[1]
Indigestion, nausea, and vomiting	44.4	50.8[1]	29.0	78.9[1]	40.7	64.1[1]	71.0[1]	58.8[1]
Other digestive conditions	94.0	100.0	87.1[1]	100.0[1]	88.5	95.9	95.6	96.2
Injuries	88.3	93.5	89.7	90.9	86.3	86.5	89.3	82.3
Fractures and dislocations	99.2	100.0[1]	100.0	93.6	100.0	100.0	100.0	100.0
Sprains and strains	80.4	100.0[1]	79.9	81.2	78.0	83.7	91.1	72.9
Open wounds and lacerations	95.2	96.1	94.7	100.0	94.5	91.8	100.0	67.5[1]
Contusions and superficial injuries	87.5	88.4	88.2	97.1	85.8	83.0	83.4	82.4
Other current injuries	85.1	93.8	86.3	81.9	83.7	83.6	83.1	84.4
Selected other acute conditions	87.4	92.3	75.9	87.9	88.6	91.5	87.1	97.1
Eye conditions	98.3	91.7[1]	100.0[1]	100.0[1]	100.0[1]	100.0	100.0[1]	100.0[1]
Acute ear infections	98.4	99.1	97.8	100.0[1]	98.4	94.3	92.9	100.0[1]
Other ear conditions	87.6	88.5	82.0	100.0[1]	90.4	91.7[1]	86.5[1]	100.0[1]
Acute urinary conditions	98.7	100.0[1]	100.0[1]	100.0	97.0	99.6	99.2	100.0
Disorders of menstruation	63.7	...	37.4[1]	46.7[1]	89.6[1]	68.9[1]	68.9[1]	-[1]
Other disorders of female genital tract	100.0	100.0[1]	-[1]	100.0[1]	100.0	100.0	100.0[1]	100.0[1]
Delivery and other conditions of pregnancy and puerperium	98.7	...	100.0[1]	100.0	97.9	-[1]	-[1]	...
Skin conditions	97.8	100.0	91.2	100.0[1]	100.0	100.0	100.0[1]	100.0
Acute musculoskeletal conditions	81.8	100.0[1]	85.0	70.9[1]	79.8	83.9	79.7	94.8
Headaches, excluding migraine	47.4	-[1]	25.9[1]	82.9[1]	64.9[1]	44.6[1]	-[1]	66.2[1]

[Continued]

★ 46 ★

Medical Attention for Acute Conditions: 1991
[Continued]

Type of acute condition	All ages	Under 5 years	5-17 years	18-24 years	25-44 years	45 years and over		
						Total	45-64 years	65 years and over
Fever, unspecified	43.2	57.9	21.5[1]	15.4[1]	38.6[1]	90.0[1]	-[1]	100.0[1]
All other acute conditions	83.5	94.3	66.6	74.1	82.4	89.2	88.3	90.3

Source: U.S. Department of Health and Human Services. Public Health Service. Centers for Disease Control and Prevention. National Center for Health Statistics. Current Estimates From the National Health Interview Survey, 1991. Vital and Health Statistics, Series 10: Data From the National Health Survey, no. 184. DHHS publication no. (PHS) 93-1512. Hyattsville, MD: U.S. Department of Health and Human Services, Public Health Service, Centers for Disease Control and Prevention, National Center for Health Statistics, December 1992, p. 25. Notes: Data are based on household interviews of the civilian noninstitutionalized population. The survey design, general qualifications, and information on the reliability of the estimates are given in Appendix 1 in the original source. Excluded from these estimates are conditions involving neither medical attention nor activity restriction. A dash (-) represents zero. Three dots (...) indicate that the category is not applicable. 1. Figure does not meet standards of reliability or precision.

★ 47 ★

Diseases and Illnesses: Acute Conditions

Restricted Activity Associated With Acute Conditions: 1991

Data reflect the number of days of restricted activity due to acute conditions per 100 persons per year.

Type of acute condition	All ages	Under 5 years	5-17 years	18-24 years	25-44 years	45 years and over		
						Total	45-64 years	65 years and over
All acute conditions	733.3	996.1	720.5	712.4	682.9	734.7	643.1	877.4
Infectious and parasitic diseases	62.2	155.9	124.2	56.3	35.2	32.0	29.8	35.5
Common childhood diseases	11.0	51.6	28.9	8.8[1]	1.7[1]	0.4[1]	0.7[1]	-[1]
Intestinal virus, unspecified	9.9	23.6[1]	19.5	9.6[1]	7.8	3.0[1]	2.4[1]	3.9[1]
Viral infections, unspecified	20.4	56.5	30.6	14.6[1]	11.9	16.1	16.9	14.9[1]
Other	21.0	24.1[1]	45.3	23.3	13.8	12.5	9.7[1]	16.7[1]
Respiratory conditions	341.6	526.3	407.2	297.7	285.8	328.7	309.4	358.7
Common cold	70.8	150.7	77.5	82.0	54.5	60.3	51.9	73.4
Other acute upper respiratory infections	31.5	50.8	49.4	18.2[1]	28.0	23.8	23.9	23.7
Influenza	184.5	236.9	235.2	169.1	166.2	165.1	181.6	139.3
Acute bronchitis	22.5	51.4	24.0	15.7[1]	17.0	22.3	25.1	18.1[1]
Pneumonia	23.0	24.1[1]	10.8[1]	10.6[1]	15.3	42.2	18.9	78.5
Other respiratory conditions	9.3	12.5[1]	10.3[1]	2.2[1]	4.8[1]	14.9	8.1[1]	25.6
Digestive system conditions	27.3	24.8[1]	18.5	19.7[1]	25.9	37.0	25.0	55.5
Dental conditions	5.6	13.3[1]	4.8[1]	5.5[1]	5.7[1]	4.0[1]	4.4[1]	3.4[1]
Indigestion, nausea, and vomiting	5.3	5.4[1]	9.6[1]	7.2[1]	3.4[1]	4.0[1]	1.9[1]	7.3[1]
Other digestive conditions	16.4	6.1[1]	4.1[1]	7.0[1]	16.8	28.9	18.7	44.8
Injuries	135.6	33.9	75.7	157.2	155.8	168.7	143.9	207.4
Fractures and dislocations	38.9	9.2[1]	27.4	44.8	30.9	59.6	40.8	88.7
Sprains and strains	37.3	-[1]	13.4	47.6	60.7	33.1	33.4	32.5
Open wounds and lacerations	11.1	7.3[1]	10.9[1]	19.9[1]	13.1	7.2[1]	7.6[1]	6.7[1]
Contusions and superficial injuries	18.5	2.6[1]	7.6[1]	13.5[1]	16.6	32.7	31.0	35.2

[Continued]

★ 47 ★

Restricted Activity Associated With Acute Conditions: 1991
[Continued]

Type of acute condition	All ages	Under 5 years	5-17 years	18-24 years	25-44 years	45 years and over		
						Total	45-64 years	65 years and over
Other current injuries	29.8	14.7[1]	16.4	31.3	34.4	36.2	31.0	44.4
Selected other acute conditions	116.3	210.6	74.2	125.2	133.2	97.2	82.4	120.1
Eye conditions	1.8[1]	4.6[1]	0.3[1]	4.5[1]	0.1[1]	3.0[1]	1.7[1]	4.9[1]
Acute ear infections	24.1	155.7	33.9	6.7[1]	9.4	6.1[1]	3.7[1]	9.9[1]
Other ear conditions	1.9[1]	7.9[1]	3.6[1]	-[1]	0.9[1]	0.9[1]	1.0[1]	0.6[1]
Acute urinary conditions	9.9	3.2[1]	4.3[1]	6.0[1]	10.3	15.7	13.4	19.3
Disorders of menstruation	1.7[1]	...	2.5[1]	1.4[1]	3.2[1]	0.2[1]	0.3[1]	-[1]
Other disorders of female genital tract	4.9	-[1]	-[1]	9.5[1]	8.0	4.4[1]	2.5[1]	7.5[1]
Delivery and other conditions of pregnancy and puerperium	25.1	...	1.7[1]	80.0	51.7	-[1]	-[1]	...
Skin conditions	5.6	6.5[1]	5.0[1]	1.5[1]	2.1[1]	10.8	7.5[1]	15.9[1]
Acute musculoskeletal conditions	28.1	2.5[1]	6.1[1]	5.4[1]	37.8	44.8	48.0	39.9
Headaches, excluding migraine	5.2	-[1]	7.6[1]	4.9[1]	5.2[1]	5.1[1]	3.3[1]	8.0[1]
Fever, unspecified	8.0	30.1	9.3[1]	5.3[1]	4.6[1]	6.2[1]	1.2[1]	13.9[1]
All other acute conditions	50.4	44.6	20.6	56.2	47.0	71.2	52.5	100.3

Source: U.S. Department of Health and Human Services. Public Health Service. Centers for Disease Control and Prevention. National Center for Health Statistics. *Current Estimates From the National Health Interview Survey, 1991.* Vital and Health Statistics, Series 10: Data From the National Health Survey, no. 184. DHHS publication no. (PHS) 93-1512. Hyattsville, MD: U.S. Department of Health and Human Services, Public Health Service, Centers for Disease Control and Prevention, National Center for Health Statistics, December 1992, p. 31, *Notes:* Data are based on household interviews of the civilian noninstitutionalized population. The survey design, general qualifications, and information on the reliability of the estimates are given in Appendix 1 in the original source. Excluded from these estimates are conditions involving neither medical attention nor activity restriction. A dash (-) represents zero. Three dots (...) indicate that the category is not applicable. 1. Figure does not meet standards of reliability or precision.

Diseases and Illnesses: AIDS

★ 48 ★

AIDS Averages

Occurrences	Number	Frequency
New HIV infections	1	each 54 seconds
Deaths from AIDS	1	each 9 minutes
New AIDS cases reported	267	each day
College students infected with AIDS	1	per 1,000

Source: Kramer, Larry. "We Have Lost the War Against AIDS." *USA TODAY* (magazine; May 1992), p. 72.

★ 49 ★

Diseases and Illnesses: AIDS

AIDS Life Expectancy

According to the federal Centers for Disease Control and Prevention, the average life expectancy for adults who contract AIDS is 18 months to 2 years after diagnosis.

Source: Freudenheim, Milt. "Insurers Accused of Discrimination in AIDS Coverage." *New York Times,* 1 June 1993, p. D2.

★ 50 ★

Diseases and Illnesses: AIDS

Cost of AIDS

Each year in the United States treatment of AIDS costs an average of $100,000 per patient. Treatment includes multiple hospitalizations with intensive care and outpatient expenses for drugs and services.

Source: "Experts See a Long Battle." *Christian Science Monitor,* 31 July 1992, n.p.

★ 51 ★

Diseases and Illnesses: AIDS

Deaths From HIV Infection, by Age: 1990

Excludes deaths of nonresidents of the United States. Deaths classified according to ninth revision of *International Classification of Diseases.*

Ages	Number of deaths			Death rate per 100,000 population		
	Total	Male	Female	Total	Male	Female
All ages[1]	25,188	22,386	2,802	10.1	18.5	2.2
15 to 24 years old	541	412	129	1.5	2.2	0.7
25 to 44 years old	18,748	16,717	2,031	23.3	41.7	5.0

Source: 1993 Statistical Abstract of the United States on CD-ROM [machine-readable datafiles]. CD-ABSTR-93. Washington, DC: U.S. Department of Commerce, Economics and Statistics Administration, Bureau of the Census, Data User Services Division, 1993. Primary source: U.S. National Center for Health Statistics. *Vital Statistics of the United States* (annual); and unpublished data. *Notes:* "HIV" stands for Human Immunodeficiency Virus. HIV infection is not a leading cause of death among persons aged 1 to 14 or 45 and older. 1. Includes those deaths with age not stated.

★ 52 ★

Diseases and Illnesses: AIDS

Relative Risks of Contracting AIDS

The table below reflects the cumulative incidence (CI) and relative risk (RR) of contracting AIDS. Cumulative incidence indicates AIDS cases reported from June 1, 1981, to January 18, 1988, per million population. Data are shown by racial/ethnic group, exposure category, and geographic region.

Exposure category and region	Hispanic		White		Black		Other	
	CI	RR	CI	RR	CI	RR	CI	RR
Exclusively homosexual men without IVDA[1]								
Northeast	1,242.2	3.3 (3.0, 3.6)	376.8	1.0	893.2	2.4 (2.2, 2.6)	152.5	0.4 (0.3, 0.6)
Midwest	180.6	2.0 (1.5, 2.7)	88.9	1.0	217.7	2.4 (2.1, 2.8)	34.6	0.4 (0.2, 0.9)
South	390.4	1.5 (1.4, 1.7)	255.2	1.0	248.8	1.0 (0.9, 1.1)	35.2	0.1 (0.1, 0.3)
West	400.8	0.6 (0.6, 0.7)	657.5	1.0	747.2	1.1 (1.0, 1.3)	126.3	0.2 (0.2, 0.2)
Bisexual men with IVDA								
Northeast	283.0	5.7 (4.7, 7.0)	49.3	1.0	341.4	6.9 (6.0, 8.0)	37.3	0.8 (0.3, 1.7)
Midwest	57.9	2.7 (1.6, 4.6)	21.5	1.0	114.1	5.3 (4.3, 6.7)	11.5	0.5 (0.1, 2.4)
South	65.4	1.5 (1.1, 2.0)	43.4	1.0	115.9	2.7 (2.3, 3.1)	8.8	0.2 (0.0, 0.9)
West	100.4	1.2 (1.0, 1.4)	86.6	1.0	245.3	2.8 (2.3, 3.5)	33.7	0.4 (0.3, 0.6)
Heterosexual adults with IVDA								
Northeast	1,128.8	30.7 (27.9, 33.7)	36.8	1.0	951.3	25.9 (23.7, 28.2)	15.0	0.4 (0.2, 1.0)
Midwest	47.8	22.6 (13.8, 37.0)	2.1	1.0	43.5	20.6 (14.6, 29.0)	3.8	1.8 (0.3, 11.2)
South	20.0	3.4 (2.3, 4.8)	6.0	1.0	92.4	15.4 (12.9, 18.5)	2.8	0.5 (0.1, 3.0)
West	23.6	3.2 (2.4, 4.5)	7.3	1.0	82.5	11.3 (8.5, 15.2)	2.3	0.3 (0.1, 1.0)
Adults with undetermined means of acquiring HIV infection								
Northeast	91.6	16.7 (12.6, 22.0)	5.5	1.0	78.7	14.3 (11.2, 18.3)	13.3	2.4 (1.0, 6.1)
Midwest	10.8	5.8 (2.3, 14.3)	1.9	1.0	9.1	4.9 (2.9, 8.3)	1.9	1.0 (0.1, 13.4)
South	15.8	3.5 (2.4, 5.3)	4.5	1.0	24.7	5.5 (4.3, 7.1)	7.1	1.6 (0.5, 5.1)
West	15.2	2.5 (1.7, 3.7)	6.0	1.0	45.5	7.6 (5.3, 10.9)	2.3	0.4 (0.1, 1.2)
All AIDS patients (including children)								
Northeast	1,538.8	7.0 (6.7, 7.4)	218.4	1.0	1,445.9	6.6 (6.3, 6.9)	100.0	0.5 (0.3, 0.6)
Midwest	138.6	2.6 (2.1, 3.2)	53.1	1.0	171.8	3.2 (2.9, 3.6)	28.1	0.5 (0.3, 0.9)
South	206.3	1.4 (1.3, 1.6)	143.9	1.0	286.7	2.0 (1.9, 2.1)	31.4	0.2 (0.1, 0.3)
West	227.5	0.6 (0.6, 0.7)	351.0	1.0	560.9	1.6 (1.5, 1.7)	71.5	0.2 (0.2, 0.2)

Source: U.S. Department of Health and Human Services. Public Health Service. Health Resources and Services Administration. *Health Status of Minorities and Low-Income Groups.* 3rd ed. Washington, DC: U.S. Government Printing Office, n.d., p. 207. Primary source: Selik, Richard M., Kenneth G. Castro, and Marguerite Pappaioanou. "Racial/Ethnic Differences in the Risk of AIDS in the United States." *American Journal of Public Health* 78, no. 12 (1988), p. 1542; table 16. *Notes:* Reference group for relative risk was non-Hispanic whites (99% confidence interval around RR in parentheses). 1. History of intravenous drug abuse (IVDA).

Diseases and Illnesses: Cancer

★ 53 ★

Cancer, by Site: 1994

Figures show the estimated deaths, new cases, and 5-year survival rates in the United States for selected cancers. Data are for 1994.

Cancer	Deaths	New cases	5-year survival rate (%)
Lung	153,000	172,000	13
Colon/rectum	56,000	149,000	58
Breast (female)	46,000	182,000	79
Prostate	38,000	200,000	77
Pancreas	25,900	27,000	3
Lymphoma	22,750	52,900	78[1]
			52[2]
Leukemia	19,100	28,600	38
Ovary	13,600	24,000	39
Kidney	11,300	27,600	55
Bladder	10,600	51,200	79
Uterus	10,500	46,000	67[3]
			83[4]
Oral	7,925	29,600	53
Skin melanoma	6,900	32,000	84

Source: "The Big Killers." Time, 25 April 1994, p. 60. Notes: 1. Hodgkin's. 2. Non-Hodgkin's. 3. Cervical. 4. Endometrial.

★ 54 ★

Diseases and Illnesses: Cancer

Causes of Cancer

The table below presents the conditions or factors from which death due to cancer have been attributed.

[In percentages]

Condition or factor	Percent
Diet	35
Tobacco	30
Other	13
Infections	10
Workplace	4
Alcohol	3

[Continued]

★ 54 ★

Causes of Cancer
[Continued]

Condition or factor	Percent
Radiation	3
Pollution	2

Source: "The War's Toll." *Detroit Free Press,* 3 July 1994, p. F1. Primary sources: American Cancer Society; National Cancer Institute. *Notes:* Inherited genetic flaws make 1 person in 10 more susceptible to genetic damage from external factors.

★ 55 ★

Diseases and Illnesses: Cancer

Deaths From Malignant Neoplasms, by Age: 1990

Excludes deaths of nonresidents of the United States. Deaths classified according to ninth revision of *International Classification of Diseases.*

Ages	Number of deaths			Death rate per 100,000 population		
	Total	Male	Female	Total	Male	Female
All ages[1]	505,322	268,283	237,039	203.2	221.3	186.0
1 to 4 years old	513	280	233	3.5	3.7	3.2
5 to 14 years old	1,094	621	473	3.1	3.5	2.8
15 to 24 years old	1,819	1,078	741	4.9	5.7	4.1
25 to 44 years old	21,650	9,835	11,815	26.9	24.5	29.2
45 to 64 years old	134,742	72,933	61,809	291.8	328.7	257.7
65 years old and older	345,387	183,473	161,914	1,111.3	1,468.6	871.2

Source: 1993 Statistical Abstract of the United States on CD-ROM [machine-readable datafiles]. CD-ABSTR-93. Washington, DC: U.S. Department of Commerce, Economics and Statistics Administration, Bureau of the Census, Data User Services Division, 1993. Primary source: U.S. National Center for Health Statistics. *Vital Statistics of the United States* (annual); and unpublished data. *Note:* 1. Includes those deaths with age not stated.

★ 56 ★

Diseases and Illnesses: Cancer

Deaths Per 100,000 From Lung Cancer by Age 75

The table shows estimates of deaths from lung cancer, by age 75, for smokers, non-smokers, and smokers who quit. Estimates assume that smokers began at age 18.

[Deaths in number per 100,000 people]

	Men		Women	
	Deaths from lung cancer	Risk[1] (%)	Deaths from lung cancer	Risk[1] (%)
Never smoked	37.5	3.0	22.0	4.0
Quit at age				
30-39	87.5	7.0	55.0	10.0
40-49	150.0	12.0	82.5	15.0
50-54	237.5	19.0	126.5	23.0
55-59	337.5	27.0	170.5	31.0
60-64	562.5	45.0	269.5	49.0
Current smokers	1,250.0	100.0	550.0	100.0

Source: "Cancer Risk Lingers After Smokers Quit." *New York Times,* 21 March 1993, late edition (final), sec. 1, p. 31. Primary source: Based on studies conducted at the University of Michigan and published in the *Journal of the National Cancer Institute. Note:* 1. Percentages of risk compare nonsmokers to current smokers.

★ 57 ★

Diseases and Illnesses: Cancer

Melanoma Survival Time

Victims of advanced melanoma, a fatal skin cancer, who receive standard treatments have an average survival time of 7.3 months. A new vaccine under testing has given more than half of those receiving it a survival time of 23 months.

Source: Angier, Natalie. "Early Data Finds Promise in New Cancer Therapy." *New York Times,* 31 July 1992, p. A10.

Diseases and Illnesses: Cerebrovascular Disease

★ 58 ★

Deaths From Cerebrovascular Disease, by Age: 1990

Excludes deaths of nonresidents of the United States. Deaths classified according to ninth revision of *International Classification of Diseases.*

Ages	Number of deaths			Death rate per 100,000 population		
	Total	Male	Female	Total	Male	Female
All ages[1]	144,088	56,697	87,391	57.9	46.8	68.6
45 to 64 years old	14,814	7,916	6,898	32.1	35.7	28.8
65 years old and older	125,409	46,785	78,624	403.5	374.5	423.0

Source: 1993 Statistical Abstract of the United States on CD-ROM [machine-readable datafiles]. CD-ABSTR-93. Washington, DC: U.S. Department of Commerce, Economics and Statistics Administration, Bureau of the Census, Data User Services Division, 1993. Primary source: U.S. National Center for Health Statistics. *Vital Statistics of the United States* (annual); and unpublished data. *Notes:* Cerebrovascular disease (stroke) is not a leading cause of death among persons 1 to 44 years old. 1. Includes those deaths with age not stated.

★ 59 ★

Diseases and Illnesses: Cerebrovascular Disease

Types of Strokes

Figures show the types of strokes and their frequency.

[In percentages]

Type of stroke	Occurrence
Thrombotic[1]	60
Embolic[1]	20
Hemorrhagic[2]	20

Source: "The Three Types of Stroke." *FDA Consumer* (June 1994), p. 23. *Notes:* 1. Affects mostly older persons. 2. Affects mostly younger persons.

Diseases and Illnesses: Chronic Conditions

★ 60 ★

Chronic Conditions Per 1,000 Persons: 1991

Type of chronic condition	All ages	Under 45 years			45-64 years	65 years and over		
		Total	Under 18 years	18-44 years		Total	65-74 years	75 years and over
Selected skin and musculoskeletal conditions								
Arthritis	125.2	29.8	1.6[1]	47.3	240.8	484.8	425.6	575.2
Gout, including gouty arthritis	8.6	2.5	-[1]	4.0	17.7	29.1	27.3	31.9
Intervertebral disc disorders	20.0	12.1	0.2[1]	19.4	43.8	27.6	31.1	22.3
Bone spur or tendinitis, unspecified	9.9	5.1	0.6[1]	8.0	21.4	18.7	19.3	17.8
Disorders of bone or cartilage	6.7	3.1	1.7[1]	3.9	10.4	21.3	19.4	24.2
Trouble with bunions	10.7	5.6	1.5[1]	8.1	17.3	29.6	24.0	38.4
Bursitis, unclassified	18.1	8.9	0.5[1]	14.1	41.1	34.0	39.9	24.9
Sebaceous skin cyst	4.7	4.4	1.6[1]	6.1	5.6	4.8[1]	6.6[1]	2.2[1]
Trouble with acne	20.4	28.0	26.5	28.8	4.9	1.6[1]	2.0[1]	1.0[1]
Psoriasis	9.4	7.1	2.6	10.0	15.4	12.8	11.5	14.7
Dermatitis	36.1	36.8	31.5	40.1	36.9	30.8	34.8	24.8
Trouble with dry (itching) skin, unclassified	19.8	16.0	11.5	18.8	23.2	36.2	24.4	54.4
Trouble with ingrown nails	23.8	17.9	7.8	24.2	26.6	52.2	50.2	55.4
Trouble with corns and calluses	19.4	10.7	0.7[1]	16.9	33.2	47.0	40.5	56.9
Impairments								
Visual impairment	32.1	19.6	5.4	28.4	47.5	79.2	56.8	113.3
Color blindness	9.9	8.4	2.7	11.9	13.1	12.9	12.0	14.3
Cataracts	26.5	2.3	1.4[1]	2.9	20.2	173.0	127.6	242.3
Glaucoma	10.4	1.7	0.4[1]	2.5	11.9	57.0	46.0	74.0
Hearing impairment	91.2	36.8	16.1	49.7	141.3	320.5	266.2	403.6
Tinnitus	26.1	9.5	1.7[1]	14.3	50.2	82.4	95.3	62.6
Speech impairment	11.2	11.7	16.7	8.6	10.0	10.3	6.1[1]	16.6
Absence of extremities (excludes tips of fingers or toes only)	5.9	2.9	0.9[1]	4.2	9.8	16.9	16.1	18.0
Paralysis of extremities, complete or partial	5.0	2.9	2.4[1]	3.2	7.1	14.0	8.3[1]	22.8
Deformity or orthopedic impairment	115.5	93.8	25.2	136.4	154.4	177.5	167.1	193.3
Back	71.2	59.0	9.1	89.9	99.3	96.2	95.8	96.7
Upper extremities	13.9	9.1	1.4[1]	13.9	22.1	28.2	30.0	25.4
Lower extremities	43.8	34.6	15.5	46.5	57.9	73.5	68.3	81.5
Selected digestive conditions								
Ulcers	15.0	9.7	1.1[1]	15.1	26.2	27.0	24.4	31.0
Hernia of abdominal cavity	19.7	7.0	2.9	9.5	40.6	58.9	55.0	64.8

[Continued]

★ 60 ★

Chronic Conditions Per 1,000 Persons: 1991
[Continued]

Type of chronic condition	All ages	Under 45 years			45-64 years	65 years and over		
		Total	Under 18 years	18-44 years		Total	65-74 years	75 years and over
Gastritis or duodenitis	11.8	7.9	1.6[1]	11.9	20.2	20.6	21.9	18.5
Frequent indigestion	23.0	16.4	2.2[1]	25.3	34.9	41.7	39.1	45.5
Enteritis or colitis	8.9	5.9	1.8[1]	8.5	11.7	21.5	17.5	27.8
Spastic colon	6.8	5.6	-[1]	9.0	11.1	7.5	9.8	3.9[1]
Diverticula of intestines	7.4	0.9[1]	-[1]	1.4[1]	12.2	36.7	39.8	31.9
Frequent constipation	18.5	11.1	6.2	14.1	19.1	59.7	41.4	87.7
Selected conditions of the genitourinary, nervous, endocrine, metabolic, and blood and blood-forming systems								
Goiter or other disorders of the thyroid	14.8	6.3	0.8[1]	9.6	28.3	41.7	45.8	35.4
Diabetes	29.0	8.8	1.1[1]	13.6	57.4	99.3	103.8	92.6
Anemias	14.3	12.5	6.8	16.0	13.2	26.1	22.5	31.5
Epilepsy	5.8	5.8	6.3	5.5	5.4	6.0	5.7[1]	6.3[1]
Migraine headaches	38.4	39.1	12.6	55.5	47.2	20.6	19.6	22.3
Neuralgia or neuritis, unspecified	1.8	0.7[1]	-[1]	1.1[1]	3.2[1]	5.8	5.7[1]	6.0[1]
Kidney trouble	12.6	9.2	3.1	12.9	17.3	25.1	23.4	27.6
Bladder disorders	15.2	10.6	4.6	14.3	15.6	40.4	30.6	55.5
Diseases of prostate	7.2	0.9[1]	-[1]	1.5[1]	12.3	35.0	38.8	29.2
Diseases of female genital organs	19.5	19.9	3.1	30.4	24.4	9.7	13.4	4.0[1]
Selected circulatory conditions								
Rheumatic fever with or without heart disease	8.8	6.4	0.6[1]	9.9	15.1	13.0	13.9	11.6[1]
Heart disease	82.6	30.8	18.5	38.4	134.1	295.2	256.4	354.3
Ischemic heart disease	29.6	1.8	0.2[1]	2.8	61.1	138.3	127.2	155.3
Heart rhythm disorders	33.5	22.9	14.6	28.1	42.4	79.3	65.9	99.7
Tachycardia or rapid heart	8.4	3.3	1.6[1]	4.4	15.3	26.8	24.1	30.9
Heart murmurs	18.2	17.5	11.9	21.0	18.8	20.8	19.3	23.1
Other and unspecified heart rhythm disorders	6.9	2.1	1.1[1]	2.8	8.3	31.7	22.5	45.6
Other selected diseases of heart, excluding hypertension	19.4	6.1	3.8	7.5	30.5	77.7	63.4	99.5
High blood pressure (hypertension)	111.8	29.3	1.9[1]	46.3	244.0	372.2	376.6	365.5
Cerebrovascular disease	11.5	1.1	0.7[1]	1.4[1]	16.1	63.0	58.2	70.4
Hardening of the arteries	7.5	0.4[1]	-[1]	0.6[1]	11.1	42.7	36.4	52.1
Varicose veins of lower extremities	31.9	16.1	0.4[1]	25.9	58.7	79.5	90.4	62.8
Hemorrhoids	37.4	23.6	0.3[1]	38.0	68.1	67.5	75.7	55.0
Selected respiratory conditions								
Chronic bronchitis	50.5	49.2	53.1	46.7	53.9	52.5	56.2	46.7

[Continued]

★ 60 ★

Chronic Conditions Per 1,000 Persons: 1991

[Continued]

Type of chronic condition	All ages	Under 45 years			45-64 years	65 years and over		
		Total	Under 18 years	18-44 years		Total	65-74 years	75 years and over
Asthma	47.2	50.7	62.5	43.4	40.7	37.2	38.0	35.9
Hay fever or allergic rhinitis without asthma	97.5	99.2	64.6	120.6	107.1	72.9	79.4	62.9
Chronic sinusitis	129.3	116.0	59.6	151.0	171.1	139.5	156.4	113.7
Deviated nasal septum	6.1	6.0	1.6[1]	8.7	7.6	4.2[1]	4.5[1]	3.7[1]
Chronic disease of tonsils or adenoids	11.1	15.3	24.0	10.0	1.1[1]	2.8[1]	3.6[1]	1.8[1]
Emphysema	6.6	0.4[1]	-[1]	0.6[1]	12.8	32.4	32.7	31.9

Source: U.S. Department of Health and Human Services. Public Health Service. Centers for Disease Control and Prevention. National Center for Health Statistics. *Current Estimates From the National Health Interview Survey, 1991.* Vital and Health Statistics, Series 10: Data From the National Health Survey, no. 184. DHHS publication no. (PHS) 93-1512. Hyattsville, MD: U.S. Department of Health and Human Services, Public Health Service, Centers for Disease Control and Prevention, National Center for Health Statistics, December 1992, p. 82. *Notes:* Data are based on household interviews of the civilian noninstitutionalized population. The survey design, general qualifications, and information are given in Appendix 1 of the original source. A dash (-) represents zero. 1. Figure does not meet standard of reliability or precision.

★ 61 ★

Diseases and Illnesses: Chronic Conditions

Deaths From Chronic Liver Disease and Cirrhosis, by Age: 1990

Excludes deaths of nonresidents of the United States. Deaths classified according to ninth revision of *International Classification of Diseases.*

Ages	Number of deaths			Death rate per 100,000 population		
	Total	Male	Female	Total	Male	Female
All ages[1]	25,815	16,627	9,188	10.4	13.7	7.2
45 to 64 years old	10,806	7,515	3,291	23.4	33.9	13.7

Source: 1993 Statistical Abstract of the United States on CD-ROM [machine-readable datafiles]. CD-ABSTR-93. Washington, DC: U.S. Department of Commerce, Economics and Statistics Administration, Bureau of the Census, Data User Services Division, 1993. Primary source: U.S. National Center for Health Statistics. *Vital Statistics of the United States* (annual); and unpublished data. *Notes:* Chronic liver disease and cirrhosis are not leading causes of death among persons aged 1 through 44 or 65 and older. 1. Includes those deaths with age not stated.

★ 62 ★

Diseases and Illnesses: Chronic Conditions

Deaths From Chronic Obstructive Pulmonary Disease, by Age: 1990

Excludes deaths of nonresidents of the United States. Deaths classified according to ninth revision of *International Classification of Diseases.*

Ages	Number of deaths			Death rate per 100,000 population		
	Total	Male	Female	Total	Male	Female
All ages[1]	86,679	49,416	37,263	34.9	40.8	29.2
45 to 64 years old	12,605	6,985	5,620	27.3	31.5	23.4
65 years old and older	72,755	41,712	31,043	234.1	333.9	167.0

Source: *1993 Statistical Abstract of the United States on CD-ROM* [machine-readable datafiles]. CD-ABSTR-93. Washington, DC: U.S. Department of Commerce, Economics and Statistics Administration, Bureau of the Census, Data User Services Division, 1993. Primary source: U.S. National Center for Health Statistics. *Vital Statistics of the United States* (annual); and unpublished data. *Notes:* Chronic obstructive pulmonary disease is not a leading cause of death among persons 1 to 44 years old. 1. Includes those deaths with age not stated.

Diseases and Illnesses: Diabetes

★ 63 ★

Deaths From Diabetes, by Age: 1990

Excludes deaths of nonresidents of the United States. Deaths classified according to ninth revision of *International Classification of Diseases.*

Ages	Number of deaths			Death rate per 100,000 population		
	Total	Male	Female	Total	Male	Female
All ages[1]	47,664	20,266	27,398	19.2	16.7	21.5
45 to 64 years old	9,803	4,983	4,820	21.2	22.5	20.1
65 years old and older	35,523	13,926	21,597	114.3	111.5	116.2

Source: *1993 Statistical Abstract of the United States on CD-ROM* [machine-readable datafiles]. CD-ABSTR-93. Washington, DC: U.S. Department of Commerce, Economics and Statistics Administration, Bureau of the Census, Data User Services Division, 1993. Primary source: U.S. National Center for Health Statistics. *Vital Statistics of the United States* (annual); and unpublished data. *Notes:* Diabetes is not a leading cause of death among persons 1 to 44 years old. 1. Includes those deaths with age not stated.

★ 64 ★

Diseases and Illnesses: Diabetes

Diabetes Prevalence Among Selected Groups

U.S. population group[1]	Percent rate	Rate relative to whites
American Indian[2]	9.1	1.5
Black	10.2	1.6
Cuban	9.3	1.5
Mexican American	13.0	2.1
Pima Indian[3]	43.4	7.0
Puerto Rican	13.4	2.2
White	6.2	1.0

Source: U.S. General Accounting Office. *Diabetes: Status of the Disease Among American Indians, Blacks and Hispanics.* Washington, DC: U.S. General Accounting Office, 1992, p. 4. Primary sources: Hispanic Health and Nutrition Examination Survey, 1982-1984 (HHANES); National Health and Nutrition Examination Survey, 1976-1980 (NHANES II); Indian Health Service, 1991; Knowler, W.C., and others. "Diabetes Mellitus in the Pima Indians: Incidence, Risk Factors and Pathogenesis." *Diabetes/Metabolism Reviews* 6, no. 1 (1990), pp. 1-27. *Notes:* 1. Rates for whites, Cubans, blacks, Mexican Americans, and Puerto Ricans are based on previously diagnosed and undiagnosed cases of diabetes. Undiagnosed cases were detected by administering an oral glucose test to a subsample of the study population. Rates for American Indians and Pima Indians are based on previously diagnosed cases of diabetes. It is likely that there are fewer undiagnosed cases of diabetes in American Indians than other racial groups because of the numerous community education programs and free health care services that are available to American Indians. Thus, it is reasonable to compare the rates, although it is likely that the total prevalence of diabetes in American Indians and Pima Indians is indicated in the table. 2. The rate of American Indians is based on persons 15 years of age or older, 1990 (age-adjusted to the 1980 U.S. population). It is likely that the prevalence rate of American Indians 20 to 74 years of age would be higher than the rate for persons 15 years of age and older because increasing age is a risk factor for diabetes. 3. The rate for Pima Indians is based on persons 25-64 years of age, 1981-88. The rates are not age-adjusted. The Pima Indians, who have the highest recorded prevalence rate of diabetes in the world, have been studied for over 25 years.

★ 65 ★

Diseases and Illnesses: Diabetes

Projects and Funding for Diabetes Research by the U.S. Government: 1991

Type of research and population group	Projects		Funding	
	Number	%	($000)	%
Human (total)[1]				
Hispanic	4	2.0	1,671	5.0
American Indian	46	28.0	7,458	21.0
Black	15	9.0	4,145	11.0
Multiracial[2]	19	12.0	5,965	17.0
White	77	47.0	16,728	46.0
Total	163	100.0	36,089	100.0
Prevention/Behavioral				
Hispanic	0	0.0	70[3]	2.0

[Continued]

★ 65 ★

Projects and Funding for Diabetes Research by the U.S. Government: 1991
[Continued]

Type of research and population group	Projects		Funding	
	Number	%	($000)	%
American Indian	5	36.0	358	8.0
Black	5	36.0	2,048	47.0
Multiracial[2]	1	7.0	258	7.0
White	3	21.0	1,600	37.0
Total	14	100.0	4,361	100.0
Clinical[1]				
Hispanic	1	<1.0	293	1.0
American Indian	35	28.0	6,042	25.0
Black	6	5.0	1,095	4.0
Multiracial[2]	12	10.0	2,559	11.0
White	69	55.0	14,246	58.0
Total	125	100.0	24,357	100.0
Epidemiologic				
Hispanic	3	13.0	1,308	18.0
American Indian	6	26.0	1,050	15.0
Black	4	17.0	1,002	14.0
Multiracial	6	26.0	3,121	44.0
White	4	17.0	666	9.0
Total	23	100.0	7,155	100.0

Source: U.S. General Accounting Office. *Diabetes: Status of the Disease Among American Indians, Blacks and Hispanics.* Washington, DC: U.S. General Accounting Office, 1992, p. 13. Primary source: National Institute of Diabetes and Digestive and Kidney Diseases, 1991 *Notes:* 1. Totals for human and clinical research categories include 2 projects ($122,000) that were targeted to another population group, the human research for whites includes another type of project ($216,000). 2. Involved only non-white populations. 3. The amount from 2 multiracial projects that targeted Hispanics.

★ 66 ★

Diseases and Illnesses: Diabetes

Type II Diabetes, by Age

Data show percent of all adults who will contract Type II diabetes. The largest percentage includes persons older than 75. Fourteen million people are afflicted with diabetes.

Age of occurrence	Percent of adults afflicted
20-44	2.0
45-64	6.0
65-75	9.0
75 and older	18.0

Source: "Adult Onset of Diabetes." *USA TODAY,* 30 November 1992, final edition, p. D1. Primary source: American Diabetes Association and *USA TODAY* research.

Diseases and Illnesses: Heart Disease

★ 67 ★

Cardiovascular Disease

According to the American Heart Association, on average, every 34 seconds an American dies from heart and blood vessel diseases, accounting for nearly 1 million deaths per year. Cardiovascular diseases are the leading cause of death in America, killing more people than cancer or AIDS.

Source: "Away From Politics." *International Herald Tribune,* 19 January 1993, p. 3.

★ 68 ★

Diseases and Illnesses: Heart Disease

Cardiovascular Disease Risk Factors: 1990

Table presents percent of survey participants responding affirmatively to cardiovascular disease risk factors. Data provided by demographic characteristics.

Characteristic	Exercise or play sports regularly		Consider self overweight		High blood pressure cured or under control		Doctor-diagnosed high cholesterol		A lot or a moderate amount of stress	
	Men	Women	Men	Women	Men	Women	Men	Women	Men	Women
Total	43.6	37.4	35.8	52.1	86.3	88.6	30.9	31.3	60.8	67.5
Age										
18-24	59.8	44.8	17.5	40.6	81.7	79.2	11.3	17.3	60.5	68.9
25-44	45.5	40.0	36.1	52.9	83.0	89.3	26.8	20.3	69.8	75.3
45-64	35.2	34.4	46.2	62.6	88.1	88.7	38.8	40.2	60.7	69.3
65 and older	36.5	28.7	33.3	43.3	91.0	89.9	31.3	41.2	32.7	45.5
Race										
White	43.7	38.8	37.0	52.6	87.1	89.2	31.0	31.5	62.6	69.3
Black	41.6	27.6	28.2	51.2	84.3	86.2	29.2	30.3	50.6	57.8
Other	46.1	35.9	24.9	38.0	72.1	82.1	31.6	26.8	49.2	53.4
Education										
Less than 4 years of high school	28.9	22.6	29.5	50.5	81.5	85.6	33.8	39.8	44.6	54.0
4 years of high school	39.8	34.2	35.2	54.9	86.3	89.2	30.8	32.9	58.3	67.4
1-3 years of college	49.8	46.7	37.4	51.4	87.3	91.3	29.7	27.1	67.7	73.7
4 or more years of college	57.5	52.7	40.4	47.8	90.5	90.2	30.2	25.0	72.7	76.1
Income										
Under $10,000	39.7	28.7	24.9	47.1	86.7	86.6	28.6	37.3	55.4	60.9
$10,000-$19,999	35.0	29.7	31.4	52.4	87.3	88.5	29.6	35.9	52.7	65.3
$20,000-$34,999	42.3	38.3	35.4	54.5	84.6	87.6	31.3	31.1	59.6	69.5
$35,000-$49,999	47.0	48.3	38.4	58.3	86.4	92.3	31.7	27.5	66.5	73.7
$50,000 or more	53.7	26.9	42.8	29.5	89.5	92.4	30.8	26.6	72.3	75.9

Source: Metropolitan Life Insurance Company. "Selected Behaviors and Perceptions Among U.S. Adults in 1990." *Statistical Bulletin* 74, no. 4 (October-December 1993), p. 6. *Statistical Bulletin* is a publication of Metropolitan Life Insurance Company. Primary sources: National Center for Health Statistics. 1990 Health Promotion and Disease Prevention supplemental survey to National Health Interview Survey; reported estimates, analyses, and computations by the Health and Safety Education Division of MetLife. *Note:* Percentages do not add because only positive responses are listed.

★ 69 ★

Diseases and Illnesses: Heart Disease

Deaths From Heart Disease, by Age: 1990

Excludes deaths of nonresidents of the United States. Deaths classified according to ninth revision of *International Classification of Diseases.*

Ages	Number of deaths			Death rate per 100,000 population		
	Total	Male	Female	Total	Male	Female
All ages[1]	720,058	360,788	359,270	289.5	297.6	281.8
1 to 4 years old	282	141	141	1.9	1.9	1.9
5 to 14 years old	308	169	139	0.9	0.9	0.8
15 to 24 years old	917	588	329	2.5	3.1	1.8
25 to 44 years old	15,045	11,121	3,924	18.7	27.8	9.7
45 to 64 years old	107,750	75,871	31,879	233.4	342.0	132.9
65 years old and older	594,858	272,397	322,461	1,914.0	2,180.4	1,735.0

Source: 1993 *Statistical Abstract of the United States on CD-ROM* [machine-readable datafiles]. CD-ABSTR-93. Washington, DC: U.S. Department of Commerce, Economics and Statistics Administration, Bureau of the Census, Data User Services Division, 1993. Primary source: U.S. National Center for Health Statistics. *Vital Statistics of the United States* (annual); and unpublished data. *Note:* 1. Includes those deaths with age not stated.

★ 70 ★

Diseases and Illnesses: Heart Disease

Persons Reporting High Blood Pressure

Table reflects the percent of persons 18 years of age and older who have been told at least twice that they have high blood pressure. Data are provided by sex, age, and selected characteristics for 1990.

Characteristic	Both sexes 18 years and over	Male					Female				
		Total	18-29 years	30-44 years	45-64 years	65 years and over	Total	18-29 years	30-44 years	45-64 years	65 years and over
All persons[1]	16.3	15.3	4.1	9.8	24.6	32.0	17.2	4.0	8.1	25.2	39.7
Education level											
Less than 12 years	24.5	20.8	5.0	11.0	29.8	31.6	27.8	4.6	14.5	33.8	42.4
12 years	15.7	14.2	3.3	9.9	24.7	31.7	16.9	4.3	7.7	25.5	39.6
More than 12 years	12.6	13.7	4.5	9.6	21.7	32.7	11.5	3.3	6.8	18.5	35.1
13-15 years	12.8	14.0	4.5	11.5	23.7	37.1	11.7	3.4	8.2	18.9	33.3
16 years or more	12.4	13.3	4.4	8.1	20.5	29.5	11.2	3.1	5.5	18.2	37.5
Income											
Less than $10,000	22.3	15.8	3.1	12.3	29.3	32.1	25.8	4.2	15.1	40.3	44.7
$10,000-$19,999	19.4	18.0	5.3	10.9	31.8	30.1	20.6	5.3	7.1	30.6	39.0
$20,000-$34,999	15.5	15.1	3.8	9.8	25.2	33.8	15.8	4.0	9.8	24.4	38.1
$35,000-$49,999	12.8	13.7	4.7	9.9	21.7	38.3	11.8	3.3	7.3	22.0	32.9
$50,000 or more	13.1	14.6	3.9	9.3	22.5	34.5	11.4	4.0	5.7	18.3	39.5
Race											
White	15.9	15.1	4.0	9.4	23.3	31.5	16.7	3.9	7.1	23.3	39.2
Black	21.3	20.0	5.5	14.2	38.6	38.6	22.3	4.5	15.0	41.2	47.2
Hispanic origin											
Hispanic	10.1	7.5	1.7[2]	5.6	17.8	21.2	12.3	2.9	8.7	23.9	41.1
Non-Hispanic	16.8	16.0	4.4	10.2	25.0	32.4	17.6	4.1	8.0	25.2	39.5
Geographic region											
Northeast	16.3	16.1	4.0	11.2	26.9	29.1	16.4	3.3	6.5	22.9	37.3
Midwest	16.9	15.8	4.3	11.4	22.9	33.5	17.9	4.1	7.7	25.6	43.0
South	17.6	15.9	4.2	9.1	26.7	33.1	19.1	4.9	10.5	28.2	40.6
West	13.5	13.3	3.7	7.9	21.1	30.8	13.7	2.9	6.1	21.6	36.1
Marital status											
Currently married	16.4	17.4	5.1	9.8	24.6	32.3	15.3	4.2	7.5	23.9	37.0
Formerly married	26.7	20.4	7.9[2]	11.0	25.0	31.8	29.3	6.2	10.4	28.9	42.5
Never married	6.6	6.2	3.2	9.1	21.9	27.0	7.1	3.3	8.5	23.8	29.7
Employment status											
Currently employed	11.2	11.8	4.0	9.5	21.1	30.0	10.6	3.6	7.6	20.0	33.7
Unemployed	10.3	11.2	6.7	9.9	21.9	13.3[2]	9.3	1.8[2]	8.2	25.3	29.5[2]
Not in labor force	27.3	28.2	3.3	16.0	40.1	32.6	26.9	5.1	9.5	32.6	40.4

Source: U.S. Department of Health and Human Services. Public Health Service. Centers for Disease Control and Prevention. National Center for Health Statistics. *Health Promotion and Disease Prevention: United States, 1990.* Vital and Health Statistics, Series 10, no. 185. Hyattsville, MD: U.S. Department of Health and Human Services, Public Health Service, Centers for Disease Control and Prevention, National Center for Health Statistics, n.d., p. 33. *Notes:* Data are based on household interviews of the civilian noninstitutionalized population. The survey design, general qualifications, and information on the reliability of the estimates are given in Appendix 1 in the original source. Denominator for each cell excludes unknowns. 1. Includes persons with unknown sociodemographic characteristics. 2. Figure does not meet standard of reliability or precision (more than 30-percent relative standard error in numerator of percent or rate).

Diseases and Illnesses: Notifiable Diseases

★ 71 ★

Notifiable Diseases: 1992

Summary of reported cases in the United States during 1992.

Disease	Cases
AIDS	45,472
Amebiasis	2,942
Anthrax	1
Aseptic meningitis	12,223
Botulism[1]	91
Foodborne	21
Infant	66
Brucellosis	105
Chancroid	1,886
Cholera	103
Diphtheria	4
Encephalitis[2]	774
Indeterminate[2]	NA
Postinfectious[2]	129
Gonorrhea	501,409
Granuloma inguinale	6
Haemophilus influenzae	1,412
Hansen disease	172
Hepatitis A	23,112
Hepatitis B	16,126
Hepatitis non-A, non-B[3]	6,010
Hepatitis, unspecified	884
Legionellosis[4]	1,339
Leptospirosis	54
Lyme disease	9,895
Lymphogranuloma venereum	302
Malaria	1,087
Measles (rubeola)	2,237
Meningococcal infections	2,134
Mumps	2,572
Murine typhus fever	28
Pertussis[5]	4,083
Plague	13
Poliomyelitis[6]	4
Psittacosis	92
Rabies (animal)	8,589
Rabies (human)	1
Rheumatic fever (acute)	75
Rocky Mountain spotted fever	502
Rubella[7]	160
Rubella (congenital syndrome)	11
Salmonellosis[8]	40,912
Shigellosis	23,931

[Continued]

★ 71 ★

Notifiable Diseases: 1992

[Continued]

Disease	Cases
Smallpox	9
Syphilis[10]	33,973
Total, all stages	112,581
Tetanus	45
Toxic-shock syndrome	244
Trichinosis	41
Tuberculosis	26,673
Tularemia	159
Typhoid fever	414
Varicella[11]	158,364
Yellow fever	12

Source: U.S. Department of Health and Human Services. Public Health Service. Centers for Disease Control and Prevention. "Summary of Notifiable Diseases: United States, 1992." *Morbidity and Mortality Weekly Report* 41, no. 55, 24 September 1993, p. 67 *Notes:* 1. Total, including wound and unspecified. 2. Primary. Data reflect change in categories for tabulating encephalitis reports that were recorded by date of report to state health departments. 3. The number of cases of non-A, non-B hepatitis is misleading because in some states reported cases included persons positive for antibody to hepatitis C virus (anti-HCV) identified in routine screening programs who did not have acute hepatitis. 4. Data are recorded by date of report to state health departments. 5. Whooping cough. 6. Paralytic. Annual case reports from state health departments; numbers may not reflect changes based on retrospective case evaluations or late reports. 7. German measles. 8. Excluding typhoid fever. 9. Last documented case occurred in 1949. 10. Primary and secondary. 11. Chicken pox. 12. Last indigenous case reported in 1911; last imported case reported in 1924.

Environmental Health

★ 72 ★

Radiation Exposure and Sources

Source of radiation	Dose to humans[1]	Percent
Natural radon	200	55
From inside human body	39	11
Medical x-rays	39	11
Rocks and soil	28	8
Cosmic radiation	27	8
Nuclear medicine	14	4
Consumer products	10	3
Other	-	<1

[Continued]

★ 72 ★

Radiation Exposure and Sources

[Continued]

Source of radiation	Dose to humans[1]	Percent
Occupational fallout Nuclear energy		

Source: Fox, Michael R. "Radiation and Risk: Hanford Workers' Health and the Decline of Scientific Debate." *21st Century Science and Technology* (fall 1993), p. 37. Primary source: National Council on Radiation Protection and Measures. *Note:* 1, Millirem.

★ 73 ★

Environmental Health

Sick Building Syndrome

The table below reflects the frequency of complaints associated with Sick Building Syndrome (SBS). Data are provided by area of the United States.

[In percentages]

Symptoms	West Coast (6 cities)	Midwest (5 cities)	Central (5 cities)	South (4 cities)	East Coast (5 cities)
Tiredness	38	41	36	40	41
Listlessness	16	14	15	16	19
Headaches	30	36	36	36	38
Watery or itchy eyes	19	18	22	22	22
Dry eyes	19	24	17	17	20
Itchy or runny nose	20	16	18	18	15
Dry throat	16	23	19	21	29
Flu	26	19	21	10	16
No complaints	42	35	34	36	34

Source: "Mind Over IAQ? Scientists Reseach Mental Aspects of Poor Indoor Air." *Facilities Design and Management* (February 1993), p. 21. *Note:* "IAQ" stands for "indoor air quality."

Injuries and Accidents

★ 74 ★

Accidental Death Costs

[Cost in billion dollars]

Type of accident	Cost
Motor vehicle	96.1
Work	63.3
Home	22.0
Public	13.9
All	177.2

Source: National Safety Council. *Accident Facts, 1992.* Itasca, IL: National Safety Council, Safety & Health News Center, 1992, p. 25.

★ 75 ★

Injuries and Accidents

Accidental Deaths, by Type of Accident: 1991

Type of accident	Rate[1]	Average number of deaths		
		Per hour	Per day	Per week
Motor vehicle				
Deaths	5 minutes	5	119	840
Injuries	4 seconds	180	4,400	30,800
Work				
Deaths	53 minutes	1	190	190
Injuries	19 seconds	190	32,700	32,700
Workers-off-the-job				
Deaths	16 minutes	4	640	640
Injuries	13 seconds	290	48,100	48,100
Home				
Deaths	26 minutes	2	390	390
Injuries	10 seconds	350	59,600	59,600
Public nonmotor vehicle				
Deaths	29 minutes	2	350	350
Injuries	14 seconds	260	44,200	44,200
All				
Deaths	5 minutes	10	1,690	1,690
Injuries	4 seconds	980	165,400	165,400

Source: National Safety Council. *Accident Facts, 1992.* Itasca, IL: National Safety Council, Safety & Health News Center, 1992, p. 25. *Note:* 1. Reflects frequency; for example, 1 death every 5 minutes.

★ 76 ★

Injuries and Accidents

Alcohol Involvement for Drivers in Fatal Crashes: 1982 and 1991

Intoxication rates decreased between 1982 and 1991 for drivers of all ages involved in fatal crashes. The decrease was most significant for drivers 65 years of age and older, dropping from 9.9 percent in 1982 to 6.2 percent in 1991.

Drivers involved in fatal crashes	1982		1991		Change in percentage, 1982-1991
	Number of drivers	Percentage with BAC 0.10 g/dl or greater[1]	Number of drivers	Percentage with BAC 0.10 g/dl or greater[1]	
Total	56,029	30.0	54,323	23.9	-20.0
Drivers by age group (years)					
16-20	9,858	31.1	7,989	20.1	-35.0
21-24	9,018	40.0	6,738	33.7	-16.0
25-34	14,787	35.1	14,131	32.3	-8.0
35-44	7,984	27.9	9,475	25.2	-10.0
45-64	8,921	20.7	9,140	15.7	-24.0
Over 64	3,894	9.9	5,459	6.2	-37.0
Drivers by sex					
Male	44,370	32.4	40,680	26.9	-17.0
Female	10,675	18.9	12,806	13.6	-28.0
Drivers by vehicle type					
Passenger cars	34,121	30.6	31,045	23.4	-24.0
Light trucks	11,199	34.7	14,602	28.3	-18.0
Large trucks	4,582	4.3	4,285	2.0	-53.0
Motorcycles	4,490	40.5	2,019	38.6	-5.0

Source: U.S. Department of Transportation. National Highway Traffic Safety Administration. National Center for Statistics and Analysis. *1991 Alcohol Fatal Crash Facts.* Washington, DC: National Center for Statistics and Analysis, Research and Development, c. 1991, p. 5. *Notes:* Numbers shown for groups of drivers do not add to the total number of drivers due to unknown or other data not included. 1. BAC stands for blood alcohol content and is measured in grams (g) per deciliter (dl).

★ 77 ★

Injuries and Accidents

Alcohol Involvement for Nonoccupants Killed in Fatal Crashes: 1982 and 1991

Nonoccupant fatalities	1982		1991		Change in percentage, 1982-1991
	Number of nonoccupant fatalities	Percentage with BAC 0.10 g/dl or greater[2]	Number of nonoccupant fatalities	Percentage with BAC 0.10 g/dl or greater[2]	
Pedestrian fatalities by age group (years)					
16-20	721	47.0	366	34.0	-28.0
21-24	671	53.1	363	50.8	-4.0
25-34	1,109	53.2	986	56.4	+6.0
35-44	779	48.5	812	51.0	+5.0
45-64	1,264	40.7	1,051	36.0	-12.0
Over 64	1,449	13.8	1,288	9.8	-29.0
Total[1]	7,331	33.8	5,797	31.8	-6.0
Pedalcyclist fatalities					
Total	883	14.3	841	17.5	+22.0

Source: U.S. Department of Transportation. National Highway Traffic Safety Administration. National Center for Statistics and Analysis. *1991 Alcohol Fatal Crash Facts*. Washington, DC: National Center for Statistics and Analysis, Research and Development, c. 1991, p. 6. *Notes:* 1. Includes pedestrians under 16 years old and pedestrians of unknown age. 2. BAC stands for blood alcohol content and is measured in grams (g) per deciliter (dl).

★ 78 ★

Injuries and Accidents

Deaths From Bee Stings

An average of 18 to 20 people die from allergic reactions to bee stings every year in the United States.

Source: El-Makkakh, Rif S., and others. "Abuzz Over Bee Keeping." *Science Teacher* 58 (September 1991), pp. 26-31.

★ 79 ★

Injuries and Accidents

Deaths From Hair Dryers

Since January 1991, hair dryers have been made with a safety plug that automatically shuts off if they fall into water. Dryers made before that time may be deadly if they come in contact with water. An average of 17 people a year, most of them children under 10, died from electrocution by hair dryers before the safety feature was added.

Source: "In the Stores." *Consumer Reports* 57 (August 1992), p. 532.

★ 80 ★

Injuries and Accidents

Deaths From Lawn Mowers

The Consumer Product Safety Commission reported an average of 75 deaths annually due to lawn mower accidents in the United States. Accidents most often involved persons over the age of 65 or under the age of 5. In addition, each year there are approximately 55,000 injuries involving lawn mowers.

Source: Wellness Letter 9, no. 10 (July 1993), p. 1. The *Wellness Letter* is a publication of the School of Public Health at the University of California at Berkeley.

★ 81 ★

Injuries and Accidents

Deaths From Toys

Toy	Deaths
Tricycles and riding toys	
Rode into pool or pond	5
Hit by motor vehicle	2
Fell from toy	1
Balloons	
Choking	6
Balls	
Choking	5
Marbles	
Choking	1

[Continued]

★ 81 ★

Deaths From Toys
[Continued]

Toy	Deaths
Toy chests	
Lid closed on head or neck	2
Other	
Choked on toy dart	2
Fell from toy rocking boat	1
Strangled on string of toy car	1
Strangled on loop of crib toy	1
Strangled on plastic jump rope	1
Trapped in toy baseketball net	1
Suffocated under play tent	1

Source: "Toy-related Deaths." *Time,* 13 December 1993, p. 24. Primary source: Consumer Product Safety Commission (January 1992-September 1993).

★ 82 ★

Injuries and Accidents

Motor Vehicle Traffic Fatalities, by Age Group: 1991

Age (years)	Percent of total traffic fatalities
Under 1	0.4
1-4	11.5
5-9	24.2
10-14	25.6
15-19	42.5
20-24	34.2
25-29	22.5
30-34	14.2
35-39	9.6
40-44	6.0
45-54	2.9
55-64	1.2
Over 64	0.4

Source: U.S. Department of Transportation. National Highway Traffic Safety Administration. National Center for Statistics and Analysis. *1991 Traffic Fatality Facts.* Washington, DC: National Center for Statistics and Analysis, Research and Development, c. 1991, p. 1.

★ 83 ★

Injuries and Accidents

Pedalcyclist Fatalities: 1991

Data below indicate fatalities and fatality rates for pedalcyclists. Data are provided by age and sex for 1991.

[Rate per million population]

Age (years)	Male			Female			Total		
	Fatalities	Population (000)	Fatality rate	Fatalities	Population (000)	Fatality rate	Fatalities	Population (000)	Fatality rate
<5	14	9,836	1.42	3	9,386	0.32	17	19,222	0.88
5-9	80	9,337	8.57	21	8,900	2.36	101	18,237	5.54
10-15	153	10,741	14.24	36	10,223	3.52	189	20,964	9.02
16-20	55	9,231	5.96	7	8,760	0.80	62	17,992	3.45
21-24	47	7,688	6.11	11	7,427	1.48	58	15,114	3.84
25-34	117	21,427	5.46	15	21,450	0.70	132	42,877	3.08
35-44	82	19,432	4.22	15	19,840	0.76	97	39,272	2.47
45-54	69	12,563	5.49	4	13,177	0.30	73	25,739	2.84
55-64	45	9,932	4.53	4	11,073	0.36	49	21,005	2.33
65-69	15	4,491	3.34	1	5,546	0.18	16	10,037	1.59
70-79	24	6,013	3.99	3	8,509	0.35	24	14,521	1.86
80+	11	2,287	4.81	1	4,908	0.20	12	7,195	1.67
Unknown	8			0			8		
Total	720	122,979	5.85	121	129,198	0.94	841	252,177	3.33

Source: U.S. Department of Transportation. National Highway Traffic Safety Administration. National Center for Statistics and Analysis. *1991 Pedalcyclist Fatal Crash Facts.* Washington, DC: National Center for Statistics and Analysis, Research and Development, c. 1991, p. 3. Primary source: Population—Bureau of the Census.

★ 84 ★

Injuries and Accidents

Pedestrian Fatalities and Fatality Rates, by Age and Sex: 1991

The data below show that persons younger than age 16 and persons older than age 70 constituted about one-third of all pedestrian fatalities in 1991.

Age (years)	Male			Female			Total		
	Fatalities	Population (000)	Fatality rate[1]	Fatalities	Population (000)	Fatality rate[1]	Fatalities	Population (000)	Fatality rate[1]
<5	144	9,836	1.46	100	9,386	1.07	244	19,222	1.27
5-9	216	9,337	2.31	101	8,900	1.13	317	18,237	1.74
10-15	191	10,741	1.78	104	10,223	1.02	295	20,964	1.41
16-20	251	9,231	2.72	115	8,760	1.31	366	17,992	2.03
21-24	277	7,688	3.60	85	7,427	1.14	363	15,114	2.40
25-34	752	21,427	3.51	234	21,450	1.09	986	42,877	2.30
35-44	613	19,432	3.15	199	19,840	1.00	812	39,272	2.07
45-54	397	12,563	3.16	150	13,177	1.14	547	25,739	2.13
55-64	368	9,932	3.71	136	11,073	1.23	504	21,005	2.40
65-69	148	4,491	3.30	99	5,546	1.79	247	10,037	2.46
70-79	301	6,013	5.01	255	8,509	3.00	556	14,521	3.83

[Continued]

★ 84 ★

Pedestrian Fatalities and Fatality Rates, by Age and Sex: 1991

[Continued]

Age (years)	Male			Female			Total		
	Fatalities	Population (000)	Fatality rate[1]	Fatalities	Population (000)	Fatality rate[1]	Fatalities	Population (000)	Fatality rate[1]
80+	266	2,287	11.63	219	4,908	4.46	485	7,195	6.74
Unknown	59			15			75[2]		
Total	3,983	122,979	3.24	1,812	129,198	1.40	5,797[2]	252,177	2.30

Source: U.S. Department of Transportation. National Highway Traffic Safety Administration. National Center for Statistics and Analysis. *1991 Traffic Fatality Facts.* Washington, DC: National Center for Statistics and Analysis, Research and Development, c. 1991, p. 4. Primary source: Population—Bureau of the Census. *Notes:* 1. Rate per 100,000 population. 2. Includes two fatalities of unknown sex.

★ 85 ★

Injuries and Accidents

Product-Related Injuries: General Household Appliances

Product	Number of cases	Ages					
		All ages	00-04	05-14	15-24	25-64	65+
Cooking ranges, ovens, etc.	627	19.5	67.4	16.4	18.7	14.1	16.7
Irons, clothes steamers[1]	290	7.0	60.3	6.0	4.2	1.6	1.4
Misc. household appliances	400	12.4	27.0	9.2	12.7	10.7	14.1
Refrigerators, freezers	451	14.2	19.9	8.0	14.8	15.5	11.5
Washers & dryers	260	8.6	18.8	4.9	9.3	8.3	7.1

Source: *NEISS Data Highlights* 14 (January-December 1990). These data are compiled by the National Electronic Injury Surveillance System (NEISS). *Note:* 1. Not toys.

★ 86 ★

Injuries and Accidents

Product-Related Injuries: Heating, Cooling, and Ventilating Equipment

Product	Number of cases	Ages					
		All ages	00-04	05-14	15-24	25-64	65+
Air conditioners	156	4.9	5.5	5.1	4.1	5.5	2.7
Chimneys, fireplaces	214	7.6	68.9	4.7	1.4	2.1	4.1
Fans (except stove exhaust fans)	239	7.7	17.0	6.7	8.2	6.7	7.1
Heating stoves & space heaters	410	13.4	87.4	14.9	6.1	6.2	5.0
Pipes, heating & plumbing	324	9.4	10.6	18.0	11.4	7.1	5.8
Radiators, all	321	7.6	50.1	9.1	3.5	3.0	4.2
Other	160	5.2	10.3	2.9	5.9	5.4	3.0

Source: *NEISS Data Highlights* 14 (January-December 1990). These data are compiled by the National Electronic Injury Surveillance System (NEISS).

★ 87 ★
Injuries and Accidents

Product-Related Injuries: Home Communication, Entertainment, and Hobby

Product	Number of cases	Estimated Ages					
		All ages	00-04	05-14	15-24	25-64	65+
Miscellaneous hobby equipment	188	5.8	15.8	9.8	10.3	3.0	1.0
Pet supplies, equipment	283	8.9	14.9	11.8	10.4	7.0	8.2
Sound recording & reproducing equipment	601	17.8	54.8	14.9	22.2	10.9	21.5
Television sets, stands	532	15.2	81.4	16.7	13.0	6.4	11.9
Other	18	.5	2.8	-	.2	.5	.4

Source: NEISS Data Highlights 14 (January-December 1990). These data are compiled by the National Electronic Injury Surveillance System (NEISS).

★ 88 ★
Injuries and Accidents

Product-Related Injuries: Home Furnishings and Accessories

Product	Number of cases	Ages					
		All ages	00-04	05-14	15-24	25-64	65+
Bathtub & shower structures	1,945	59.8	165.1	37.8	44.5	44.7	100.8
Beds, mattresses, pillows	4,960	141.6	663.8	188.1	72.6	49.6	230.7
Carpets and rugs	1,212	37.4	76.0	26.5	22.9	22.3	104.8
Chairs, sofas & sofa beds	4,910	148.5	653.9	157.5	83.7	71.0	226.4
Desks, cabinets, shelves, racks	2,811	83.1	291.3	119.4	68.2	49.3	72.1
Electric fixtures, lamps & equip.	660	20.0	44.9	26.1	22.6	15.2	15.1
Ladders, stools	2,174	68.8	63.1	29.0	38.1	80.9	104.8
Mirrors & mirror glass	306	8.7	16.9	9.7	18.1	5.8	3.0
Misc. household covers and fabrics	227	6.8	10.9	3.3	4.8	6.4	12.4
Other misc. furniture & accessories	645	19.0	38.4	10.5	15.9	21.0	12.7
Sinks & toilets	721	22.6	52.5	16.2	15.1	14.0	55.7
Tables, all types	4,331	127.3	798.9	139.0	71.5	48.9	94.6
Other	349	11.3	38.1	14.0	7.6	7.2	13.1

Source: NEISS Data Highlights 14 (January-December 1990). These data are compiled by the National Electronic Injury Surveillance System (NEISS).

★ 89 ★

Injuries and Accidents

Product-Related Injuries: Home Maintenance Equipment

Product	Number of cases	Ages					
		All ages	00-04	05-14	14-24	25-64	65+
Cleaning equipment, noncaustic/detergent	333	9.8	17.2	10.8	8.5	8.5	11.0
Cleaning agents (except soaps)	582	16.3	92.8	6.6	15.1	10.8	4.8
Drain, oven cleaners, caustics	138	4.1	14.9	1.9	4.8	3.3	2.9
Miscellaneous household chemicals	250	7.5	23.8	9.1	8.9	5.4	2.6
Paints, solvents, lubricants	278	8.7	20.5	5.1	9.5	8.6	5.3
Other	163	4.3	24.4	1.5	2.8	2.6	4.3

Source: NEISS Data Highlights 14 (January-December 1990). These data are compiled by the National Electronic Injury Surveillance System (NEISS).

★ 90 ★

Injuries and Accidents

Product-Related Injuries: Home Structures and Construction Materials

Product	Number of cases	Ages					
		All ages	00-04	05-14	15-24	25-64	65+
Cabinets or door hardware	298	8.8	32.3	12.7	7.8	4.7	8.5
Ceilings, walls, panels (interior)	3,199	88.3	182.4	156.8	150.3	48.0	44.3
Counters and counter tops	397	11.9	69.1	10.9	6.8	6.1	8.5
Fences	1,623	48.6	62.1	122.9	65.4	28.7	17.7
Glass doors, windows and panels	3,062	91.4	132.1	119.1	185.4	63.8	36.2
Handrails, railings and banisters	614	17.0	37.9	27.5	18.7	11.2	13.8
Miscellaneous construction materials	1,074	36.9	29.2	49.8	43.0	35.9	24.2
Nails, carpet tacks, etc.	3,312	102.1	105.2	204.1	126.0	84.4	28.4
Non-glass doors and panels	5,079	138.9	396.2	231.5	162.6	81.2	86.3
Outside attached structures & materials	164	5.3	6.9	6.0	5.3	5.2	4.1
Porches, open side floors, etc.	1,439	47.9	105.3	63.9	39.9	38.2	44.7
Stairs, ramps, landings, floors	23,828	688.3	1,433.4	599.8	657.8	484.4	1,205.7
Windows, door sills, frames	674	20.9	68.9	22.3	22.1	11.4	27.7
Other	259	9.1	11.3	9.0	6.3	9.1	11.0

Source: NEISS Data Highlights 14 (January-December 1990). These data are compiled by the National Electronic Injury Surveillance System (NEISS).

★ 91 ★

Injuries and Accidents

Product-Related Injuries: Home Workshop Equipment

Product	Number of cases	Ages					
		All ages	00-04	05-14	14-24	25-64	65+
Batteries, all types	162	5.0	13.4	5.4	7.1	3.9	1.2
Hoists, lifts, jacks, etc.	167	5.7	2.1	1.5	9.5	7.3	1.3
Miscellaneous workshop equipment	479	15.9	12.6	20.8	21.4	15.0	9.7
Power home tools, exc. saws	353	12.0	1.7	1.7	13.3	16.8	8.6
Power home workshop saws, all	1,127	37.7	5.4	8.8	36.3	45.7	58.9
Welding, soldering, cutting tools	229	7.8	1.0	-	15.8	10.4	.4
Wires, cords, not specified	175	5.8	3.6	7.4	6.3	5.6	5.8
Workshop manual tools	1,455	47.5	23.6	27.5	64.2	57.9	21.7
Other	184	6.1	14.3	4.8	7.6	5.7	2.8

Source: NEISS Data Highlights 14 (January-December 1990). These data are compiled by the National Electronic Injury Surveillance System (NEISS).

★ 92 ★

Injuries and Accidents

Product-Related Injuries: Household Packaging and Containers

Product	Number of cases	Ages					
		All ages	00-04	05-14	15-24	25-64	65+
Cans, other containers	3,082	87.1	184.9	98.7	107.2	74.5	42.9
Glass bottles & jars	991	30.4	56.7	49.5	53.0	20.8	4.9
Paper/cardboard/plastic products	547	17.1	31.8	24.4	17.1	13.8	13.6

Source: NEISS Data Highlights 14 (January-December 1990). These data are compiled by the National Electronic Injury Surveillance System (NEISS).

★ 93 ★

Injuries and Accidents

Product-Related Injuries: Housewares

Product	Number of cases	Ages					
		All ages	00-04	05-14	15-24	25-64	65+
Cookware, pots and pans	443	13.3	27.8	13.6	15.9	11.4	8.4
Cutlery, knives, unpowered	5,872	179.5	76.6	170.0	293.6	190.5	70.8
Drinking glasses	1,796	53.5	53.8	47.8	101.3	50.6	14.3
Miscellaneous housewares	787	23.0	45.6	28.3	25.4	18.4	19.2
Scissors	360	10.8	21.6	25.3	11.4	6.6	4.4

[Continued]

★ 93 ★

Product-Related Injuries: Housewares
[Continued]

Product	Number of cases	Ages					
		All ages	00-04	05-14	15-24	25-64	65+
Small kitchen appliances	566	17.5	26.3	10.4	21.9	18.3	11.8
Tableware and accessories	1,492	44.8	63.0	38.4	69.9	43.9	14.6
Other	118	3.9	4.8	8.3	2.6	3.4	1.7

Source: NEISS Data Highlights 14 (January-December 1990). These data are compiled by the National Electronic Injury Surveillance System (NEISS).

★ 94 ★

Injuries and Accidents

Product-Related Injuries: Miscellaneous

Product	Number of cases	Ages					
		All ages	00-04	05-14	15-24	25-64	65+
Dollies, carts	548	16.5	109.6	14.6	6.6	7.0	12.9
Elevators, other lifts	231	5.8	10.2	4.2	4.9	4.2	13.0
Fireworks and flares	178	5.1	3.9	12.8	8.9	3.2	-
Gasoline and diesel fuels	237	8.2	21.8	7.4	13.0	6.3	3.0
Miscellaneous	1,520	45.6	79.8	124.5	71.3	18.1	17.3
Other	187	5.7	19.5	7.2	8.0	3.4	2.2

Source: NEISS Data Highlights 14 (January-December 1990). These data are compiled by the National Electronic Injury Surveillance System (NEISS).

★ 95 ★

Injuries and Accidents

Product-Related Injuries: Personal Care Items

Product	Number of cases	Ages					
		All ages	00-04	05-14	15-24	25-64	65+
Cigarettes, lighters & fuel	264	7.8	38.7	6.4	8.1	5.1	1.5
Clothing, all	1,509	47.7	59.9	70.5	48.5	37.0	57.2
Grooming devices	406	11.6	63.7	10.6	17.2	5.1	1.3
Holders for personal items	232	6.8	12.7	10.2	3.7	5.6	8.0
Jewelry	762	19.7	88.4	35.4	20.6	8.8	3.9
Paper money & coins	482	11.9	105.3	25.0	1.5	.3	.5
Pencils, pens, other desk supplies	691	18.6	36.3	71.4	16.0	5.7	3.7
Razors, shavers, razor blades	683	18.8	20.1	14.4	35.6	17.3	9.0

[Continued]

★ 95 ★

Product-Related Injuries: Personal Care Items

[Continued]

Product	Number of cases	Ages					
		All ages	00-04	05-14	15-24	25-64	65+
Sewing equipment	427	11.9	20.2	18.4	16.6	8.8	7.0
Other	178	5.6	6.8	4.8	13.4	4.3	1.7

Source: *NEISS Data Highlights* 14 (January-December 1990). These data are compiled by the National Electronic Injury Surveillance System (NEISS).

★ 96 ★

Injuries and Accidents

Product-Related Injuries: Sports and Recreational Equipment

Data show product-related injuries that were treated in hospital emergency departments in the United States and territories.

Product	Number of cases	Estimated number of cases per 100,000 population Ages					
		All ages	00-04	05-14	15-24	25-64	65+
ATVs, mopeds, minibikes, etc.	1,359	50.0	14.5	103.2	129.0	27.9	7.2
Barbecue grills, stoves, equipment	185	6.2	23.4	7.5	3.5	4.9	2.5
Baseball	5,463	174.0	42.6	400.1	358.4	119.2	1.8
Basketball	8,641	257.5	9.9	469.1	885.2	114.9	2.4
Beach, picnic, camping equipment	243	8.1	21.6	17.7	5.1	5.4	3.3
Bicycles & accessories	7,739	233.3	266.5	949.9	256.5	75.3	20.2
Bowling	295	9.1	5.9	8.2	17.3	8.2	5.5
Cheerleading	156	5.0	-	13.5	20.7	-	-
Dancing	549	17.0	5.7	22.5	45.4	11.5	6.4
Exercise equipment	1,055	31.7	45.5	38.5	73.8	21.5	7.1
Fishing	798	27.9	16.5	50.6	30.9	25.4	16.0
Football	5,390	166.6	5.0	466.7	567.2	31.1	.5
Golf	504	16.6	9.8	31.3	13.5	13.9	19.3
Gymnastics & equipment	580	17.8	4.0	88.3	28.1	1.7	.2
Hockey, all kinds	646	19.7	2.7	38.7	68.4	7.5	.1
Horseback riding	876	29.9	7.2	41.8	48.5	30.8	3.9
Ice & roller skating	1,628	52.0	13.8	217.5	53.0	23.7	2.1
Lacrosse, rugby, misc. ball games	1,493	43.3	15.3	147.3	92.9	14.7	.4
Martial arts	354	10.2	.2	14.8	23.3	9.1	-
Nonpowder guns, BBs and pellets	321	9.7	8.1	40.3	15.8	2.0	.3
Playground equipment	3,316	101.7	402.8	465.8	19.3	4.9	2.2
Skateboards	1,085	33.1	14.6	155.8	59.0	2.5	.3
Snowskiing	1,228						
Soccer	1,795	56.2	2.0	167.3	160.7	16.6	.2
Swimming, pools, equipment	1,416	45.4	63.7	129.6	66.8	23.1	5.2
Tennis, badminton, squash	752	22.8	4.3	20.1	48.7	22.1	9.4
Toboggans, sleds, snow discs, etc.	315	11.5	9.8	44.8	15.2	4.1	.4
Track & field activities, equipment	853	23.9	-	41.9	61.8	16.7	2.6
Trampolines	350	13.1	16.1	66.1	11.6	1.6	-
Volleyball	1,510	50.5	-	63.7	142.6	39.5	1.0
Water skiing, tubing, surfing	336	12.1	1.1	6.2	31.1	12.6	.5

[Continued]

★ 96 ★

Product-Related Injuries: Sports and Recreational Equipment
[Continued]

Product	Number of cases	Estimated number of cases per 100,000 population Ages					
		All ages	00-04	05-14	15-24	25-64	65+
Wrestling	584	19.7	1.2	47.1	79.6	2.2	-
Other	575	19.7	16.1	32.9	40.7	14.6	2.6

Source: NEISS Data Highlights 14 (January-December 1990). These data are compiled by the National Electronic Injury Surveillance System (NEISS).

★ 97 ★

Injuries and Accidents

Product-Related Injuries: Yard and Garden Equipment

Product	Number of cases	Ages					
		All ages	00-04	05-14	15-24	25-64	65+
Chain saws	424	15.8	1.0	2.9	16.1	22.8	10.4
Hand garden tools	415	14.2	17.2	24.2	11.0	12.3	12.7
Hatchets & axes	190	6.9	1.4	7.9	8.1	7.5	5.4
Lawn and garden care equipment	599	19.9	20.8	21.9	14.9	18.0	31.0
Lawn mowers, all types	897	31.1	13.6	19.1	24.1	37.9	36.0
Other power lawn equipment	255	9.2	4.2	5.2	8.9	11.5	8.2
Trimmers, small power garden tools	160	5.5	1.3	1.6	4.3	7.1	7.4
Other	118	4.0	6.0	9.7	2.6	2.6	4.2

Source: NEISS Data Highlights 14 (January-December 1990). These data are compiled by the National Electronic Injury Surveillance System (NEISS).

Institutionalized Populations: Emergency Shelters

★ 98 ★

Abused Women in Shelters: 1990

Data are provided by type of institution and by state.

[As of April 1]

Region, division, and state	Population in shelters for abused women[1]
United States	11,768
Northeast	2,170
New England	556
Maine	43
New Hampshire	27
Vermont	29
Massachusetts	269
Rhode Island	33
Connecticut	155
Middle Atlantic	1,614
New York	756
New Jersey	255
Pennsylvania	603
Midwest	2,764
East North Central	2,075
Ohio	496
Indiana	279
Illinois	536
Michigan	506
Wisconsin	258
West North Central	689
Minnesota	230
Iowa	164
Missouri	117
North Dakota	36
South Dakota	41
Nebraska	41
Kansas	60
South	3,975
South Atlantic	1,792
Delaware	36
Maryland	199
District of Columbia	49
Virginia	185
West Virginia	128
North Carolina	315
South Carolina	87

[Continued]

★ 98 ★

Abused Women in Shelters: 1990
[Continued]

Region, division, and state	Population in shelters for abused women[1]
Georgia	192
Florida	601
East South Central	672
Kentucky	190
Tennessee	230
Alabama	127
Mississippi	125
West South Central	1,511
Arkansas	105
Louisiana	244
Oklahoma	113
Texas	1,049
West	2,859
Mountain	824
Montana	49
Idaho	78
Wyoming	45
Colorado	167
New Mexico	108
Arizona	279
Utah	49
Nevada	49
Pacific	2,035
Washington	297
Oregon	251
California	1,257
Alaska	157
Hawaii	73

Source: 1993 Statistical Abstract of the United States on CD-ROM [machine-readable datafiles]. CD-ABSTR-93. Washington, DC: U.S. Department of Commerce, Economics and Statistics Administration, Bureau of the Census, Data User Services Division, 1993. Primary source: U.S. Bureau of the Census. 1990 Census of Population. General Population Characteristics (CP-1). Notes: 1. Results reported from the enumeration of emergency shelters and visible in street locations are not (and were never intended to be) a count of the total population of homeless persons at the national, state, or local level. The data do not represent a complete count of the homeless population. Counts of persons in these two locations represent one of the Bureau's efforts to include homeless persons in the 1990 census.

★ 99 ★

Institutionalized Populations: Emergency Shelters

Homeless Population in Institutions: 1990

Data are provided by type of institution and by state.

[As of April 1]

Region, division, and state	Population in:	
	Emergency shelters for homeless persons[1]	Visible street locations[1]
United States	190,406	49,734
Northeast	62,247	14,653
New England	12,454	970
Maine	462	7
New Hampshire	404	8
Vermont	261	16
Massachusetts	6,476	674
Rhode Island	502	44
Connecticut	4,349	221
Middle Atlantic	49,793	13,683
New York	33,228	10,732
New Jersey	7,725	1,639
Pennsylvania	8,840	1,312
Midwest	30,009	3,324
East North Central	21,423	2,544
Ohio	4,773	188
Indiana	2,530	268
Illinois	8,017	1,755
Michigan	4,290	262
Wisconsin	1,813	71
West North Central	8,586	780
Minnesota	2,483	138
Iowa	1,153	148
Missouri	2,393	215
North Dakota	315	30
South Dakota	437	71
Nebraska	805	20
Kansas	1,000	158
South	46,382	7,975
South Atlantic	27,052	5,025
Delaware	349	19
Maryland	2,706	523
District of Columbia	4,731	131
Virginia	2,842	319
West Virginia	579	33
North Carolina	2,952	259
South Carolina	1,060	102
Georgia	4,122	450
Florida	7,711	3,189
East South Central	5,733	922

[Continued]

★ 99 ★

Homeless Population in Institutions: 1990
[Continued]

Region, division, and state	Population in:	
	Emergency shelters for homeless persons[1]	Visible street locations[1]
Kentucky	1,474	118
Tennessee	2,094	357
Alabama	1,657	364
Mississippi	508	83
West South Central	13,597	2,028
Arkansas	594	62
Louisiana	1,803	184
Oklahoma	2,335	340
Texas	8,865	1,442
West	51,768	23,782
Mountain	9,807	3,215
Montana	494	17
Idaho	539	19
Wyoming	228	13
Colorado	2,721	393
New Mexico	775	164
Arizona	3,014	1,897
Utah	974	276
Nevada	1,062	436
Pacific	41,961	20,567
Washington	4,862	772
Oregon	3,505	564
California	32,063	18,081
Alaska	604	79
Hawaii	927	1,071

Source: *1993 Statistical Abstract of the United States on CD-ROM* [machine-readable datafiles]. CD-ABSTR-93. Washington, DC: U.S. Department of Commerce, Economics and Statistics Administration, Bureau of the Census, Data User Services Division, 1993. Primary source: U.S. Bureau of the Census. *1990 Census of Population.* General Population Characteristics (CP-1). *Notes:* 1. Results reported from the enumeration of emergency shelters and visible in street locations are not (and were never intended to be) a count of the total population of homeless persons at the national, state, or local level. The data do not represent a complete count of the homeless population. Counts of persons in these two locations represent one of the Bureau's efforts to include homeless persons in the 1990 census.

Institutionalized Populations: Mental Health Facilities

★ 100 ★

Facilities and Residents of Facilities for Persons With Mental Retardation: 1990

For year ending June 30. Persons with mental retardation refers to those who have been so designated by state governments in the process of placing them into residential facilities.

Item	State operated facilities[1] 1990[2]	Private facilities[3] 1990
Number of facilities[4]	1,321	41,547
Residents beginning of year	94,675	(NA)
Admissions[5]	5,568	(NA)
Deaths in institutions	1,143	(NA)
Live releases[6]	7,679	(NA)
Residents end of year	91,640	188,902
Rate per 100,000 population[7]	34.7	76.0
Average daily residents	92,729	(NA)
Maintenance expenditures per day per average daily resident (dollars)[8]	196	(NA)

Source: 1993 Statistical Abstract of the United States on CD-ROM [machine-readable datafiles]. CD ABSTR-93. Washington, DC: U.S. Department of Commerce, Economics and Statistics Administration, Bureau of the Census, Data User Services Division, 1993. Primary source: For state-operated facilities: 1990, MN, White, Prouty, Lakin & Blake. Report No. 36; Private facilities: 1990, MN, Lakin, White, Blake, and Prouty. Report No. 38. Notes: "NA" stands for "not available." 1. Data as submitted by many state agencies; figures reflect some estimates Resident patients at the end of a year do not equal the number at the beginning of a succeeding year. Includes estimates for underreporting. 2. Includes data for 108 facilities operated as mental hospitals or other facilities and which have residents with mental retardation. The average daily number of residents with mental retardation in these facilities was 1,487 in 1990. 3. A privately operated living quarter which provides 24-hour, 7-days-a-week responsibility for room, board, and supervision of mentally retarded persons. Excludes single-family homes providing services to a relative; and nursing homes, boarding homes, and foster homes not formally licensed or contracted as mental retardation service providers. 4. Beginning 1985, reflects the development of a large number of community-based, state-operated facilities which were developed in the early 1980's. 5. Includes readmissions and excludes transfers. Excludes people entering newly opened facilities. 6. Total live releases. 7. Based on Bureau of the Census estimated civilian population as of July 1. Estimates reflect revisions based on 1990 Census of Population. 8. Reporting facilities only; includes salaries and wages, purchased provisions, fuel, light, water, etc.

★ 101 ★

Institutionalized Populations: Mental Health Facilities

Mental Health Inpatients and Facilities: 1990

Facilities, beds and inpatients as of year end; other data are for calendar year or fiscal year ending in a month other than December since facilities are permitted to report on either a calendar or fiscal year basis. Excludes private psychiatric office practice and psychiatric service modes of all types in hospitals or outpatient clinics of federal agencies other than U.S. Department of Veterans Affairs. Excludes data from Puerto Rico, Virgin Islands, Guam, and other territories.

| Facility | Number of facilities | Inpatient beds | | Inpatients | | Average daily inpatients | Inpatient care episodes[2] (1,000) | Expenditures | | Patient care staff[4] (1,000) |
		Total (1,000)	Rate[1]	Total (1,000)	Rate[1]			Total (million dollars)	Per capita[3] (dollars)	
Total	5,205	280.7	113.5	231.7	93.8	253.6	2,303.7	28,953	118.0	421.8
Mental hospitals: State and county	266	98.6	39.8	90.2	36.5	89.8	365.2	7,678	31.0	112.6
Private[5]	1,038	79.1	32.0	61.8	25.0	83.8	565.3	8,804	36.0	104.4
General hospitals[6]	1,545	52.5	21.2	37.6	15.2	37.9	983.1	4,604	19.0	71.1
Veterans Administration[7]	130	21.7	8.8	17.2	7.0	17.3	215.5	1,381	6.0	24.3
Free-standing psychiatric outpatient clinics[8]	741	(X)	(X)	(X)	(X)	(X)	(X)	678	3.0	10.3
Other[9]	1,485	28.8	11.7	24.9	10.1	24.8	174.6	5,808	23.0	99.1

Source: *1993 Statistical Abstract of the United States on CD-ROM* [machine-readable datafiles]. CD-ABSTR-93. Washington, DC: U.S. Department of Commerce, Economics and Statistics Administration, Bureau of the Census, Data User Services Division, 1993. Primary source: U.S. Substance Abuse and Mental Health Services Administration. Center for Mental Health Services. Unpublished data. *Notes:* "X" represents "not applicable." 1. Rate per 100,000 population. Based on Bureau of Census estimated civilian population as of July 1. 2. "Inpatient care episodes" is defined as the number of residents in inpatient facilities at the beginning of the year plus the total additions to inpatient facilities during the year. 3. Based on Bureau of the Census estimated civilian population as of July 1. 4. Full-time equivalent. 5. Includes residential treatment centers for emotionally disturbed children. 6. Nonfederal hospitals with separate psychiatric services. 7. Includes U.S. Department of Veterans Affairs (VA) neuropsychiatric hospitals, VA general hospitals with separate psychiatric settings and VA freestanding psychiatric outpatient clinics. 8. Includes mental health facilities which provide only psychiatric outpatient services. 9. Includes other multiservice mental health facilities with two or more settings, which are not elsewhere classified, as well as freestanding partial care facilities which only provide psychiatric partial care services. Number of facilities, expenditures, and staff data also include freestanding psychiatric partial care facilities.

Institutionalized Populations: Military

★ 102 ★

Military Mortality Experience of Enlisted Personnel

Mortality rates are shown for persons covered by Servicemen's Group Life Insurance (SGLI), which, by law, provides insurance to members on active duty in the uniformed services listed in this table. Data shown for three calendar years, 1989-1991.

[Annual death rate per 1,000]

Age group	Total	Accidental	No. of deaths
Total, all Services			
17-19	0.78	0.70	450
20-24	0.82	0.74	1,700
25-29	0.55	0.46	717
30-34	0.58	0.40	483
35-39	0.58	0.34	318

[Continued]

★ 102 ★

Military Mortality Experience of Enlisted Personnel
[Continued]

Age group	Total	Accidental	No. of deaths
40-44	0.90	0.35	199
45-49	1.36	0.47	64
50 and over	7.09	1.15	43
Total, all ages	0.71	0.56	3,974
Army			
17-19	0.77	0.67	163
20-24	0.90	0.82	668
25-29	0.65	0.53	286
30-34	0.64	0.42	183
35-39	0.71	0.42	132
40-44	0.97	0.41	73
45-49	1.34	0.33	24
50 and over	10.85	1.61	27
Total, all ages	0.79	0.62	1,556
Navy			
17-19	0.85	0.78	162
20-24	0.84	0.75	535
25-29	0.56	0.46	207
30-34	0.60	0.43	140
35-39	0.53	0.30	80
40-44	1.04	0.36	64
45-49	1.33	0.28	19
50 and over	2.89	0.03	7
Total, all ages	0.73	0.58	1,214
Air Force			
17-19	0.52	0.43	44
20-24	0.48	0.44	207
25-29	0.39	0.34	150
30-34	0.52	0.35	130
35-39	0.49	0.29	91
40-44	0.67	0.23	49
45-49	1.54	0.81	19
50 and over	10.59	1.18	9
Total, all ages	0.49	0.37	699
Marine Corps			
17-19	0.90	0.86	81
20-24	1.06	0.97	290
25-29	0.71	0.60	74
30-34	0.53	0.43	30
35-39	0.49	0.30	15
40-44	1.18	0.63	13
45-49	0.83	0.83	2

[Continued]

★ 102 ★

Military Mortality Experience of Enlisted Personnel
[Continued]

Age group	Total	Accidental	No. of deaths
50 and over	0.00	0.00	0
Total, all ages	0.89	0.79	505

Source: U.S. Department of Veterans Affairs. Veterans Benefits Administration. Regional Office and Insurance Center. *Servicemen's and Veterans' Group Life Insurance Programs: Twenty-seventh Annual Report, Year Ending June 30, 1992.* Supervised by the Secretary of Veterans Affairs. Philadelphia, PA: Veterans Benefits Administration, c. 1992, pp. 14-15. *Note:* All exposure and deaths for post-separation period excluded.

★ 103 ★

Institutionalized Populations: Military

Military Mortality Experience of Officers and Warrant Officers

Mortality rates are shown for persons covered by Servicemen's Group Life Insurance (SGLI), which, by law, provides insurance to members on active duty in the uniformed services listed in this table. Data shown for three calendar years, 1989-1991.

[Annual death rate per 1,000 population]

Age group	Total	Accidental	No. of deaths
Total, all services			
17-19	0.00	0.00	0
20-24	0.80	0.68	69
25-29	0.72	0.67	169
30-34	0.52	0.43	110
35-39	0.51	0.38	95
40-44	0.56	0.34	85
45-49	0.93	0.24	55
50 and over	1.76	0.39	36
Total, all ages	0.65	0.47	619
Army			
17-19	0.00	0.00	0
20-24	0.80	0.70	24
25-29	0.66	0.57	51
30-34	0.44	0.32	33
35-39	0.46	0.36	29
40-44	0.75	0.43	38
45-49	1.28	0.35	26
50 and over	1.83	0.39	14
Total, all ages	0.66	0.44	215
Navy			
17-19	0.00	0.00	0
20-24	1.08	0.81	28
25-29	0.86	0.81	52
30-34	0.66	0.48	32
35-39	0.49	0.36	22

[Continued]

★ 103 ★

Military Mortality Experience of Officers and Warrant Officers
[Continued]

Age group	Total	Accidental	No. of deaths
40-44	0.53	0.39	19
45-49	0.85	0.13	13
50 and over	2.55	0.48	16
Total, all ages	0.77	0.54	182
Air Force			
17-19	0.00	0.00	0
20-24	0.48	0.48	11
25-29	0.48	0.47	38
30-34	0.47	0.45	35
35-39	0.57	0.39	37
40-44	0.43	0.23	24
45-49	0.67	0.19	14
50 and over	0.86	0.17	5
Total, all ages	0.51	0.38	164
Marine Corps			
17-19	0.00	0.00	0
20-24	0.84	0.84	6
25-29	1.58	1.52	28
30-34	0.68	0.68	10
35-39	0.58	0.50	7
40-44	0.46	0.23	4
45-49	0.73	0.36	2
50 and over	1.36	1.36	1
Total, all ages	0.91	0.83	58

Source: U.S. Department of Veterans Affairs. Veterans Benefits Administration. Regional Office and Insurance Center. *Servicemen's and Veterans' Group Life Insurance Programs: Twenty-seventh Annual Report, Year Ending June 30, 1992.* Supervised by the Secretary of Veterans Affairs. Philadelphia, PA: Veterans Benefits Administration, c. 1992, pp. 12-13. *Note:* All exposure and deaths for post-separation period excluded.

★ 104 ★

Institutionalized Populations: Military

Military Mortality Experience of Service Personnel

Mortality rates are shown for persons covered by Servicemen's Group Life Insurance (SGLI), which, by law, provides insurance to members on active duty in the uniformed services listed in this table. Data shown for three calendar years, 1989-1991.

[Annual death rate per 1,000 population]

Age group	Total	Accidental	No. of deaths
Total, all services			
17-19	0.79	0.71	457
20-24	0.82	0.73	1,790
25-29	0.58	0.50	906

[Continued]

★ 104 ★

Military Mortality Experience of Service Personnel
[Continued]

Age group	Total	Accidental	No. of deaths
30-34	0.56	0.40	601
35-39	0.56	0.35	421
40-44	0.76	0.34	291
45-49	1.10	0.34	123
50 and over	2.88	0.60	86
Total, all ages	2.88	0.60	86
Army			
17-19	0.77	0.67	163
20-24	0.90	0.81	692
25-29	0.65	0.54	337
30-34	0.60	0.40	216
35-39	0.65	0.41	161
40-44	0.88	0.42	111
45-49	1.31	0.34	50
50 and over	4.04	0.69	41
Total, all ages	0.77	0.60	1,771
Navy			
17-19	0.85	0.78	162
20-24	0.85	0.75	563
25-29	0.60	0.51	259
30-34	0.61	0.44	172
35-39	0.52	0.31	102
40-44	0.85	0.37	83
45-49	1.08	0.20	32
50 and over	2.65	0.58	23
Total, all ages	0.74	0.58	1,396
Coast Guard			
17-19	1.21	1.21	7
20-24	0.72	0.66	21
25-29	0.65	0.62	20
30-34	0.30	0.21	7
35-39	0.41	0.41	6
40-44	0.62	0.25	5
45-49	1.16	0.39	3
50 and over	3.31	0.00	3
Total, all ages	0.63	0.51	72
Public Health and National Oceanic and Atmospheric Administration			
17-19	0.00	0.00	0
20-24	0.00	0.00	0
25-29	0.00	0.00	0
30-34	0.35	0.00	1
35-39	0.49	0.25	2
40-44	0.44	0.22	2
45-49	0.32	0.32	1
50 and over	1.65	1.24	4

[Continued]

★ 104 ★

Military Mortality Experience of Service Personnel
[Continued]

Age group	Total	Accidental	No. of deaths
Total, all ages	0.54	0.32	10
Air Force			
17-19	0.52	0.43	44
20-24	0.48	0.44	218
25-29	0.41	0.36	188
30-34	0.51	0.37	165
35-39	0.51	0.32	128
40-44	0.57	0.23	73
45-49	0.99	0.42	33
50 and over	2.10	0.30	14
Total, all ages	0.49	0.37	863
Marine Corps			
17-19	0.90	0.86	81
20-24	1.05	0.96	296
25-29	0.83	0.74	102
30-34	0.56	0.48	40
35-39	0.52	0.35	22
40-44	0.86	0.45	17
45-49	0.78	0.58	4
50 and over	0.95	0.95	1
Total, all ages	0.89	0.79	563

Source: U.S. Department of Veterans Affairs. Veterans Benefits Administration. Regional Office and Insurance Center. *Servicemen's and Veterans' Group Life Insurance Programs: Twenty-seventh Annual Report, Year Ending June 30, 1992.* Supervised by the Secretary of Veterans Affairs. Philadelphia, PA: Veterans Benefits Administration, c. 1992, pp. 10-11. *Note:* All exposure and deaths for post-separation period excluded.

★ 105 ★

Institutionalized Populations: Military

Population in Military Quarters: 1990

Data are provided by type of institution and by state.

[As of April 1]

Region, division, and state	In military quarters
United States	589,700
Northeast	47,252
New England	20,349
Maine	5,153
New Hampshire	923
Vermont	0
Massachusetts	4,439
Rhode Island	2,851
Connecticut	6,983

[Continued]

★ 105 ★

Population in Military Quarters: 1990
[Continued]

Region, division, and state	In military quarters
Middle Atlantic	26,903
New York	12,875
New Jersey	10,102
Pennsylvania	3,926
Midwest	40,203
East North Central	19,261
Ohio	449
Indiana	883
Illinois	16,091
Michigan	1,693
Wisconsin	145
West North Central	20,942
Minnesota	24
Iowa	57
Missouri	6,424
North Dakota	2,245
South Dakota	1,051
Nebraska	1,104
Kansas	10,037
South	312,915
South Atlantic	213,816
Delaware	1,164
Maryland	10,426
District of Columbia	2,181
Virginia	51,869
West Virginia	32
North Carolina	58,378
South Carolina	30,166
Georgia	30,261
Florida	29,339
East South Central	38,432
Kentucky	15,228
Tennessee	11,126
Alabama	6,085
Mississippi	5,993
West South Central	60,667
Arkansas	1,814
Louisiana	10,851
Oklahoma	8,712
Texas	39,290
West	189,330
Mountain	27,269
Montana	1,000
Idaho	740
Wyoming	832

[Continued]

★ 105 ★

Population in Military Quarters: 1990
[Continued]

Region, division, and state	In military quarters
Colorado	12,895
New Mexico	3,088
Arizona	6,071
Utah	1,046
Nevada	1,597
Pacific	162,061
Washington	18,491
Oregon	122
California	115,334
Alaska	8,807
Hawaii	19,307

Source: 1993 Statistical Abstract of the United States on CD-ROM [machine-readable datafiles]. CD-ABSTR-93. Washington, DC: U.S. Department of Commerce, Economics and Statistics Administration, Bureau of the Census, Data User Services Division, 1993. Primary source: U.S. Bureau of the Census. 1990 Census of Population. General Population Characteristics (CP-1).

Institutionalized Populations: Nursing Homes

★ 106 ★

Mobility Impairments in Nursing Home Residents Over Age 75

From the source: "As with home-dwelling frail older persons ... physical disabilities are the sole or primary cause of many persons' nursing home needs."

Impairment	Number impaired	Percent of residents
Chairfast	464,000	42.0
Walk with assistance	301,000	27.0
Walk independently	260,000	24.0
Bedfast	79,000	7.0

Source: U.S. Department of Health and Human Services. Public Health Service. National Institute on Aging. Physical Frailty: A Reducible Barrier to Independence for Older Americans. Report to Congress. NIH Publication No. 91-397. Bethesda, MD: Department of Health and Human Services, Public Health Service, National Institutes of Health (NIH), September 1991, pp. 5-6.

★ 107 ★

Institutionalized Populations: Nursing Homes

Nursing Home Concerns of Families

Category	What troubled them[1] (N=51)	How many see this as their top concern (N=21)
Admission process	8 (15.7%)	5 (23.8%)
Elder leaving own home	3	2
Elder resisting admission	3	2
Selecting a nursing home	2	1
Care provided by staff	16 (31.4%)	5 (23.8%)
Inadequate environment	3	0
Inadequate care	12	5
Use of restraints	1	0
Feelings of family members	7 (13.7%)	3 (14.3%)
Guilt	4	2
Fear that placement will be permanent	3	1
Feelings of residents	15 (29.4%)	6 (28.6%)
Depression	4	0
Loneliness	6	4
Loss of independence	3	1
Unhappiness	2	1
Financing nursing home care	5 (9.8%)	2 (9.5%)

Source: Sorrels, Valarie L. "Nursing Home Fears." *Geriatric Nursing* (September-October 1991), p. 237. *Note:* 1. Family members listed more than one concern.

★ 108 ★

Institutionalized Populations: Nursing Homes

Nursing Home Population: 1980 and 1990

Data are provided by region, division, and state.

Region, division, and state	Number			Percent change 1980 to 1990	Percentage of population in 1990
	1980	1990	Change 1980 to 1990		
United States	1,426,371	1,772,032	345,661	24.2	0.7
Northeast	327,319	399,329	72,010	22.0	0.8
New England	106,344	119,646	13,302	12.5	0.9
Middle Atlantic	220,975	279,683	58,708	26.6	0.7

[Continued]

★ 108 ★

Nursing Home Population: 1980 and 1990
[Continued]

Region, division, and state	Number			Percent change 1980 to 1990	Percentage of population in 1990
	1980	1990	Change 1980 to 1990		
Midwest	472,568	544,650	72,082	15.3	0.9
East North Central	296,088	346,243	50,155	16.9	0.8
West North Central	176,480	198,407	21,927	12.4	1.1
South	396,554	558,382	161,828	40.8	0.7
South Atlantic	163,080	270,930	107,850	66.1	0.6
East South Central	77,060	102,900	25,840	33.5	0.7
West South Central	156,414	184,552	28,138	18.0	0.7
West	229,930	269,671	39,741	17.3	0.5
Mountain	47,139	65,842	18,703	39.7	0.5
Pacific	182,791	203,829	21,038	11.5	0.5
New England	106,344	119,646	13,302	12.5	0.9
Maine	9,570	9,855	285	3.0	0.8
Vermont	4,354	4,809	455	10.5	0.9
New Hampshire	6,673	8,202	1,529	22.9	0.7
Massachusetts	49,728	55,662	5,934	11.9	0.9
Rhode Island	8,146	10,156	2,010	24.7	1.0
Connecticut	27,873	30,962	3,089	11.1	0.9
Middle Atlantic	220,975	279,683	58,708	26.6	0.7
New York	114,276	126,175	11,899	10.4	0.7
New Jersey	34,414	47,054	12,640	36.7	0.6
Pennsylvania	72,285	106,454	34,169	47.3	0.9
East North Central	296,088	346,243	50,155	16.9	0.8
Ohio	71,479	93,769	22,290	31.2	0.9
Indiana	40,112	50,845	10,733	26.8	0.9
Illinois	80,410	93,662	13,252	16.5	0.8
Michigan	55,805	57,622	1,817	3.3	0.6
Wisconsin	48,282	50,345	2,063	4.3	1.0
West North Central	176,480	198,407	21,927	12.4	1.1
Minnesota	44,553	47,051	2,498	5.6	1.1
Iowa	36,217	36,455	238	0.7	1.3
Missouri	37,942	52,060	14,118	37.2	1.0
North Dakota	7,486	8,159	673	9.0	1.3
South Dakota	8,087	9,356	1,269	15.7	1.3
Nebraska	17,650	19,171	1,521	8.6	1.2
Kansas	24,545	26,155	1,610	6.6	1.1
South Atlantic	163,080	270,930	107,850	66.1	0.6
Delaware	2,771	4,596	1,825	65.9	0.7
Maryland	19,821	26,884	7,063	35.6	0.6

[Continued]

★ 108 ★

Nursing Home Population: 1980 and 1990
[Continued]

Region, division, and state	Number			Percent change 1980 to 1990	Percentage of population in 1990
	1980	1990	Change 1980 to 1990		
District of Columbia	2,866	7,008	4,142	144.5	1.2
Virginia	24,323	37,762	13,439	55.3	0.6
West Virginia	6,355	12,591	6,236	98.1	0.7
North Carolina	29,596	47,014	17,418	58.9	0.7
South Carolina	11,666	18,228	6,562	56.2	0.5
Georgia	29,376	36,549	7,173	24.4	0.6
Florida	36,306	80,298	43,992	121.2	0.6
East South Central	77,060	102,900	25,840	33.5	0.7
Kentucky	23,591	27,874	4,283	18.2	0.8
Tennessee	22,014	35,192	13,178	59.9	0.7
Alabama	18,702	24,031	5,329	28.5	0.6
Mississippi	12,753	15,803	3,050	23.9	0.6
West South Central	156,414	184,552	28,138	18.0	0.7
Arkansas	18,631	21,809	3,178	17.1	0.9
Louisiana	22,776	32,072	9,296	40.8	0.8
Oklahoma	25,732	29,666	3,934	15.3	0.9
Texas	89,275	101,005	11,730	13.1	0.6
Mountain	47,139	65,842	18,703	39.7	0.5
Montana	5,479	7,764	2,285	41.7	1.0
Idaho	5,084	6,318	1,234	24.3	0.6
Wyoming	2,198	2,679	481	21.9	0.6
Colorado	16,109	18,506	2,397	14.9	0.6
New Mexico	2,585	6,276	3,691	142.8	0.4
Arizona	8,424	14,472	6,048	71.8	0.4
Utah	4,921	6,222	1,301	26.4	0.4
Nevada	2,339	3,605	1,266	54.1	0.3
Pacific	182,791	203,829	21,038	11.5	0.5
Washington	27,970	32,840	4,870	17.4	0.7
Oregon	16,052	18,200	2,148	13.4	0.6
California	134,756	148,362	13,606	10.1	0.5
Alaska	854	1,202	348	40.7	0.2
Hawaii	3,159	3,225	66	2.1	0.3

Source: U.S. Department of Commerce. Economics and Statistics Administration. Bureau of the Census. *Sixty-five Plus in America.* Prepared by Cynthia M. Taeuber. Washington, DC: U.S. Government Printing Office, 1992, pp. 6-11, 6-12. Primary source: U.S. Bureau of the Census. 1980 data from 1980 Census of Population, *Persons in Institutions and Other Group Quarters* (PC80-2-4D); 1990 data from 1990 Census of Population and Housing, Summary Tape File 1A.

★ 109 ★

Institutionalized Populations: Nursing Homes

Nursing Home Residents With Selected Cognitive Disabilities and Type of Therapy Received

Data are based on personal interviews of the nursing home staff most knowledgeable about the residents sampled.

["-" indicates quantity of zero]

Age and therapy received in past month[1]	Total	No cognitive disabilities	Cognitive disabi- lities[2]	Organic brain syndromes	Alzheimer's disease	Schizophrenia and other psychoses	Depressive disorders	Anxiety disorders	Alcohol and drug abuse	Mental retardation
					Number					
Total[3]	1,464,500	476,500	988,000	677,800	77,500	189,100	213,100	212,000	58,200	81,400
All ages										
					Percent					
Total	100.0	100.0	100.0	100.0	100.0	100.0	100.0	100.0	100.0	100.0
No therapy	70.0	70.7	69.8	72.7	72.0	64.5	63.6	65.5	47.3	63.1
Mental health evaluation or treatment	6.2	3.2	7.6	4.7	5.2[5]	18.5	11.6	9.8	9.5	12.4
Social services by social worker	11.3	9.9	11.9	11.2	10.7	11.6	14.7	12.6	8.8	19.7
Other[4]	23.4	26.1	22.1	20.9	22.6	21.2	26.3	24.6	16.2	28.5
65 years and over										
No therapy	63.2	65.7	62.1	69.9	68.0	49.7	55.5	58.0	49.3	29.9
Mental health evaluation or treatment	4.2	2.6	4.9	4.1	5.2[5]	9.0	8.5	6.2	7.4[5]	4.2[5]
Social services by social worker	9.6	9.0	9.9	10.5	10.3	8.1	12.9	9.4	6.4[3]	8.0
Other[4]	19.9	22.8	18.6	19.6	21.2	15.3	22.6	19.9	16.0	11.6
75 years and over										
No therapy	53.6	57.1	52.0	61.3	52.3	34.8	44.1	48.0	31.4	14.5
Mental health evaluation or treatment	3.1	2.2	3.5	3.3	4.1[5]	4.7	5.4	3.8	2.1[5]	2.7[5]
Social services by social worker	8.0	8.1	8.1	9.2	8.0	5.1	9.2	7.3	2.4[5]	3.9
Other[4]	16.4	19.2	15.0	17.0	14.8	10.0	17.6	15.9	9.1[5]	4.1[5]
85 years and over										
No therapy	29.7	31.6	28.8	35.8	19.5	16.2	21.1	22.3	10.8	4.9[5]
Mental health evaluation or treatment	1.5	1.3	1.7	1.9	2.3[5]	2.2[5]	2.4[5]	1.5[5]	0.4[5]	-
Social services by social worker	4.6	5.2	4.3	5.3	6.2[5]	2.8[5]	3.7	4.6	0.5[5]	0.2[5]
Other[4]	8.6	10.2	7.9	9.7	8.4	5.2	7.8	8.5	1.7[5]	0.6[5]

Source: Van Nostrand, J. F., S. E. Furner, and R. Suzman, eds. *Health Data on Older Americans: United States, 1992.* Vital and Health Statistics, Series 3: Analytic and Epidemiological Studies, no. 27. DHHS publication no. (PHS) 93-1411. Hyattsville, MD: U.S. Department of Health and Human Services, Public Health Service, Centers for Disease Control and Prevention, National Center for Health Statistics, 1993, p. 174. Primary source: National Center for Health Statistics data from the National Nursing Home Survey. *Notes:* Column percents may add to more than 100 because a person may have received several types of therapy. 1. Therapy received either inside or outside the nursing home. 2. Includes residents with all types of cognitive disabilities. Residents with multiple disabilities are counted only once in the total. 3. Residents with more than one type of therapy are counted only once. 4. Includes physical, occupational, recreational, and speech or hearing therapy. 5. Figure does not meet standard of reliability or precision.

★ 110 ★

Institutionalized Populations: Nursing Homes

Nursing Home Residents With Selected Cognitive Disabilities Who Need Help With Instrumental Activities of Daily Living (IADL)

Data are based on personal interviews of the nursing home staff most knowledgeable about the residents sampled.

["-" indicates quantity of zero]

Age and IADLs for which help of another person is required	Total	No cognitive disabilities	Cognitive disabi- lities[1]	Organic brain syndromes	Alzheimer's disease	Schizophrenia and other psychoses
			Number			
All ages	1,489,600	485,300	1,004,300	685,400	78,700	194,300
			Percent			
Number:						
None	15.3	25.7	10.2	5.5	3.2[3]	18.6
1-2	14.9	19.9	12.5	9.3	5.6[3]	13.9
3-4	69.9	54.5	77.3	85.2	91.2	67.5
Type:						
Care of personal possessions	73.4	59.3	80.3	87.8	93.1	68.7
Handling money	75.3	61.3	82.1	87.7	94.0	75.6
Securing personal items[2]	76.2	63.9	82.2	89.0	93.7	71.9
Using the telephone	62.7	49.6	69.0	77.1	84.2	58.2
65 years and over						
Number:						
None	12.3	23.0	7.1	4.6	3.0[3]	9.4
1-2	12.6	18.7	9.7	8.5	5.5[5]	8.1
3-4	63.4	50.4	69.6	82.1	85.1	54.9
Type:						
Care of personal possessions	66.4	54.6	72.1	84.3	86.7	55.5
Handling money	67.6	57.1	72.7	84.1	88.3	58.1
Securing personal items[2]	69.0	59.5	73.6	85.4	87.4	57.6
Using the telephone	57.1	45.8	62.6	74.1	78.9	48.6
75 years and over						
Number:						
None	9.7	19.4	5.0	3.7	2.2[3]	4.0
1-2	10.4	16.2	7.6	7.4	3.7[3]	5.1
3-4	54.1	43.8	59.0	72.4	66.5	40.2

[Continued]

★ 110 ★

Nursing Home Residents With Selected Cognitive Disabilities Who Need Help With Instrumental Activities of Daily Living (IADL)

[Continued]

Age and IADLs for which help of another person is required	Total	No cognitive disabilities	Cognitive disabi- lities[1]	Organic brain syndromes	Alzheimer's disease	Schizophrenia and other psychoses
Type:						
Care of personal possessions	56.5	47.7	60.7	74.2	67.3	40.3
Handling money	57.6	49.8	61.3	74.1	67.5	42.4
Securing personal items[2]	58.8	51.6	62.3	75.5	69.0	41.9
Using the telephone	48.8	39.7	53.2	65.0	60.0	36.3
85 years and over						
Number:						
None	4.4	9.4	2.0	1.6	1.4[3]	1.2[3]
1-2	5.5	9.4	3.5	3.7	0.7[3]	2.0[3]
3-4	30.7	24.8	33.5	43.2	28.4	19.8
Type:						
Care of personal possessions	31.7	27.2	33.9	43.6	27.6	19.7
Handling money	32.4	28.3	34.4	43.9	28.2	20.4
Securing personal items[2]	33.3	29.5	35.2	44.9	29.0	20.7
Using the telephone	27.4	22.5	29.7	38.3	25.4	17.4

Source: Van Nostrand, J. F., S. E. Furner, and R. Suzman, eds. *Health Data on Older Americans: United States, 1992.* Vital and Health Statistics, Series 0: Analytic and Epidemiological Studies, no. 27. DHHS publication no. (PHS) 93-1411. Hyattsville, MD: U.S. Department of Health and Human Services, Public Health Service, Centers for Disease Control and Prevention, National Center for Health Statistics, 1993, pp. 171-172. Primary source: National Center for Health Statistics data from the National Nursing Home Survey. *Notes:* Column percents may not add to 100 because of rounding. 1. Includes residents with all types of cognitive disabilities. Residents with multiple disabilities are counted only once in the total. 2. Securing personal items means shopping for items such as newspapers, toilet articles, and snack foods. 3. Figure does not meet standard of reliability or precision.

Institutionalized Populations: Prisons

★ 111 ★

AIDS Among Correctional Facility Inmates: 1992-1993

Regional distribution of AIDS cases among total inmate population of state and city/county jail sytems from November 1992 through March 1993. The federal prison system is excluded.

Region	State prison systems (n=50)		City/county jail systems (n=31)	
	Total AIDS cases	Percent	Total AIDS cases	Percent
New England[1]	429	5	104	3
Middle Atlantic[2]	4,041	50	1,207	40
East North Central[3]	365	5	157	5
West North Central[4]	83	1	8	0.3
South Atlantic[5]	1,596	20	148	5
East South Central[6]	159	2	29	1
West South Central[7]	346	4	74	2
Mountain[8]	289	4	43	1
Pacific[9]	764	9	1,270	42
Total[10]	8,072	100	3,040	99

Source: Hammett, Theodore M., Lynne Harrold, Michael Gross, and Joel Epstein. *1992 Update: HIV/ AIDS in Correctional Facilities—Issues and Options.* Issues and Practices in Criminal Justice Series. Washington, DC: U.S. Department of Justice, Office of Justice Programs, National Institute of Justice, January 1994, p. 17. Primary source: National Institute of Justice (NIJ)/ Centers for Disease Control (CDC) questionnaire responses. *Notes:* The regional distributions used in this table are standard geographic divisions and are not based on number of AIDS cases. The figures in this table represent the minimum number of correctional AIDS cases to date since the National Institute of Justice (NIJ) survey does not include every U.S. jail system. Recent tightening of case identification and recording may partially explain the large increases in correctional AIDS cases in certain regions since last year. 1. Maine, New Hampshire, Vermont, Massachusetts, Rhode Island, and Connecticut. 2. New York, New Jersey, and Pennsylvania. 3. Ohio, Indiana, Michigan, and Wisconsin. 4. Minnesota, Iowa, Missouri, North Dakota, South Dakota, Nebraska, and Kansas. 5. Delaware, Maryland, District of Columbia, Virginia, West Virginia, North Carolina, South Carolina, Georgia, and Florida. 6. Kentucky, Tennessee, Alabama, and Mississippi. 7. Arkansas, Louisiana, Oklahoma, and Texas. 8. Montana, Idaho, Wyoming, Colorado, New Mexico, Arizona, Utah, and Nevada. 9. Washington, Oregon, California, Alaska, and Hawaii. 10. Due to rounding.

★ 112 ★

Institutionalized Populations: Prisons

Older Male Inmates With Illnesses

Illness	Value
Injuries	76.7
Arthritis	45.4
Hypertension	39.7
Venereal disease	21.6
Ulcers	21.0
Prostate disorders	20.2
Myocardial infarction	19.0
Emphysema	18.5
Diabetes	11.2
Asthma	9.2
Stroke	7.8
Cancer	6.9
Cirrhosis or liver disease	4.2

Chart shows data from column 3.

The table below shows the older male inmates with lifetime histories of specific, physician-diagnosed illnesses as reported by the inmates themselves.

[In percentages]

Illness	Age 50-59 (n=82)	Older than 59 (n=37)	Overall (n=119)
Arthritis	40.2	56.8	45.4
Hypertension	36.7	45.9	39.7
Venereal disease[1]	21.5	21.6	21.6
Ulcers[2]	18.3	27.0	21.0
Prostate disorders	17.1	27.0	20.2
Myocardial infarction	17.7	21.6	19.0
Emphysema	14.6	27.0	18.5
Diabetes	10.1	13.5	11.2
Asthma	8.5	10.8	9.2
Stroke	3.8	16.2	7.8
Cancer	6.3	8.1	6.9
Cirrhosis or liver disease	4.9	2.7	4.2
Injuries[3]	78.5	73.0	76.7

Source: Colsher, Patricia L., Robert B. Wallace, Paul L. Loeffelholz, and Marilyn Sales. "Health Status of Older Male Prisoners: A Comprehensive Survey." *American Journal of Public Health* 82, no. 6 (June 1992), p. 882. *Notes:* 1. Any. 2. Stomach or intestinal. 3. Requiring medical care.

★ 113 ★

Institutionalized Populations: Prisons

Population in Correctional Facilities: 1990

Data are provided by type of institution and by state.

[As of April 1]

Region, division, and state	Population in correctional institutions
United States	1,115,111
Northeast	195,275
New England	33,227
Maine	2,311
New Hampshire	1,991
Vermont	807
Massachusetts	15,471
Rhode Island	2,645
Connecticut	10,002
Middle Atlantic	162,048
New York	90,025
New Jersey	29,093
Pennsylvania	42,930
Midwest	211,192
East North Central	157,275
Ohio	41,618
Indiana	21,726
Illinois	37,334
Michigan	42,849
Wisconsin	13,748
West North Central	53,917
Minnesota	9,969
Iowa	5,630
Missouri	19,975
North Dakota	831
South Dakota	2,543
Nebraska	3,662
Kansas	11,307
South	439,250
South Atlantic	231,369
Delaware	3,347
Maryland	27,025
District of Columbia	4,035
Virginia	33,553
West Virginia	4,439
North Carolina	24,857
South Carolina	18,351
Georgia	40,803
Florida	74,959
East South Central	63,082
Kentucky	13,948
Tennessee	21,335
Alabama	19,226

[Continued]

★ 113 ★

Population in Correctional Facilities: 1990

[Continued]

Region, division, and state	Population in correctional institutions
Mississippi	8,573
West South Central	144,799
Arkansas	8,642
Louisiana	26,792
Oklahoma	15,108
Texas	94,257
West	269,394
Mountain	60,762
Montana	2,174
Idaho	2,871
Wyoming	1,556
Colorado	13,446
New Mexico	5,385
Arizona	22,636
Utah	4,252
Nevada	8,442
Pacific	208,632
Washington	14,569
Oregon	10,912
California	178,199
Alaska	2,630
Hawaii	2,322

Source: 1993 Statistical Abstract of the United States on CD-ROM [machine-readable datafiles]. CD-ABSTR-93. Washington, DC: U.S. Department of Commerce, Economics and Statistics Administration, Bureau of the Census, Data User Services Division, 1993. Primary source: U.S. Bureau of the Census. 1990 Census of Population. General Population Characteristics (CP-1).

★ 114 ★

Institutionalized Populations: Prisons

Positive Drug Tests in Correctional Facilities: 1989-1990

Figures reflect the prison inmates testing positive for illegal drugs from July 1, 1989, through June 30, 1990. Data include results of drug testing at 807 facilities.

[In percentages]

Type of facility	Drugs				
	Amphetamines	Cocaine	Heroin	Marijuana	Meth-amphetamines
General adult population confinement	0.7	1.4	0.9	5.1	1.5
Boot camp	0.7	1.7	1.9	5.2	1.1
Reception/diagnosis and classification	1.4	1.1	1.6	4.2	0.5
Medical treatment/hospitalization confinement	0.4	2.0	0.9	5.8	5.1
Alcohol/drug treatment confinement	1.8	3.0	1.6	7.6	1.2

[Continued]

★ 114 ★

Positive Drug Tests in Correctional Facilities: 1989-1990

[Continued]

Type of facility	Drugs				
	Amphetamines	Cocaine	Heroin	Marijuana	Meth-amphetamines
Youthful offenders	0.1	1.5	0.5	2.1	0.0
Work release/pre-release	1.0	7.0	1.8	6.9	1.0
Returned to custody	2.7	3.5	2.9	9.1	6.2
Other	0.6	4.3	0.6	4.8	0.3

Source: Harlow, Caroline Wolf. *Drug Enforcement and Treatment in Prisons, 1990.* Bureau of Justice Statistics Special Report. Washington, DC: U.S. Bureau of Justice, Office of Justice Programs, Bureau of Justice Statistics, July 1992, p. 9.

★ 115 ★

Institutionalized Populations: Prisons

Prison Stays of the Mentally Ill and Homeless in the United States

According to the findings of recent studies summarized by Dr. Ron Jemelka and his associates at the University of Washington, on a typical day an average of 250,000—or a quarter of a million—mentally ill persons with serious disorders such as schizophrenia and manic depression are homeless, living in public shelters, or in prison. More than 30,000 will be jailed, although there will be no charges against them. They merely must wait in prison until space is available in a state psychiatric hospital.

Source: Torrey, E. Fuller. "The Mental Health Mess." *National Review* 44, 28 December 1992, pp. 22-23.

Life Expectancy

★ 116 ★

Life Expectancy at 65 Years of Age: 1900-1990

The table below shows life expectancy at age 65 according to race and sex for selected years. Data are based on the National Vital Statistics System.

Specified age and year	All races			White			Black		
	Both sexes	Sex		Both sexes	Sex		Both sexes	Sex	
		Male	Female		Male	Female		Male	Female
1900-1902[1,2]	11.9	11.5	12.2	-	11.5	12.2	-	10.4	11.4
1950[2]	13.9	12.8	15	-	12.8	15.1	13.9	12.9	14.9
1960[2]	14.3	12.8	15.8	14.4	12.9	15.9	13.9	12.7	15.1
1970	15.2	13.1	17	15.2	13.1	17.1	14.2	12.5	15.7
1975	16.1	13.8	18.1	16.1	13.8	18.2	15	13.1	16.7
1980	16.4	14.1	18.3	16.5	14.2	18.4	15.1	13	16.8
1981	16.7	14.3	18.6	16.7	14.4	18.7	15.5	13.4	17.3
1982	16.8	14.5	18.7	16.9	14.5	18.8	15.7	13.5	17.5
1983	16.7	14.5	18.6	16.8	14.5	18.7	15.5	13.4	17.3
1984	16.8	14.6	18.6	16.9	14.6	18.7	15.5	13.5	17.2
1985	16.7	14.6	18.6	16.8	14.6	18.7	15.3	13.3	17
1986	16.8	14.7	18.6	16.9	14.8	18.7	15.4	13.4	17
1987	16.9	14.8	18.7	17	14.9	18.8	15.4	13.5	17.1
1988	16.9	14.9	18.6	17	14.9	18.7	15.4	13.4	16.9
1989	17.2	15.2	18.8	17.3	15.2	19	15.5	13.6	17
Provisional data:									
1988[2]	16.9	14.8	18.6	17	14.9	18.7	15.5	13.6	17.1
1989[2]	17.2	15.2	18.8	17.3	15.2	18.9	15.8	13.8	17.4
1990[2]	17.3	15.3	19	17.3	15.3	19	16.1	14.2	17.6

Source: National Economic, Social, and Environmental Data Bank: The Federal Connection [CD-ROM]. Prepared by U.S. Department of Commerce, Economics and Statistics Administration. Washington, DC: U.S. Department of Commerce, Economics and Statistics Administration, Office of Business Analysis, November 1992. Primary sources: 1) U.S. Bureau of the Census. *U.S. Life Tables 1890, 1901, 1910, and 1901-1910.* Prepared by J. W. Glover. Washington, DC: U.S. Government Printing Office, 1921. 2) National Center for Health Statistics. *Vital Statistics Rates in the United States, 1940-1960.* Prepared by R. D. Grove and A. M. Hetzel. DHEW Pub. No. (PHS) 1677. Washington, DC: U.S. Government Printing Office, 1968. 3) *Annual Summary of Births, Marriages, Divorces, and Deaths, United States, 1988.* Monthly Vital Statistics Report, vol. 37, no. 13. DHHS Pub. No. (PHS) 89-1120. Hyattsville, MD: Public Health Service, 26 July 1989. 4) *Annual Summary of Births, Marriages, Divorces, and Deaths, United States, 1989.* Monthly Vital Statistics Report. Hyattsville, MD: Public Health Service, 1991. 4) *Annual Summary of Births, Marriages, Divorces, and Deaths, United States, 1990.* Monthly Vital Statistics Report, vol. 39, no. 13. DHHS Pub. No. (PHS) 91-1120. Hyattsville, MD: Public Health Service, 1991. 5) Unpublished data from the Division of Vital Statistics. 6) Data computed by the Office of Research and Methodology from data compiled by the Division of Vital Statistics. *Notes:* A dash (-) indicates that data were not given in the original source. 1. Death registration area only. The death registration area increased from 10 States and the District of Columbia in 1900 to the coterminous United States in 1933. 2. Includes deaths of nonresidents of the United States.

★117★

Life Expectancy

Life Expectancy of Right-Handers vs. Left-Handers

According to a study by psychologists Diane Halpern and Stanley Coren, published in the *New England Journal of Medicine,* right-handed people live longer than the left-handed: an average of 75 years for those who are right-handed, compared to 66 for left-handed people. Right-handed men lived an average of 10 years longer than left-handed men; while right-handed women lived an average of 5 years longer than left-handed women. Those who are left-handed are 6 times more likely to die in accidents; 4 times more likely to do so while driving.

Source: "Lifestyle—Health: The Right Stuff for a Longer Life." *Newsweek* 117, 15 April 1991, p. 58.

★118★

Life Expectancy

Projected Life Expectancy at Birth and Age 65: 1990-2050

Data are provided by sex.

[In years]

Year	At birth			At age 65		
	Men	Women	Difference	Men	Women	Difference
1990	72.1	79.0	6.9	15.0	19.4	4.4
2000	73.5	80.4	6.9	15.7	20.3	4.6
2010	74.4	81.3	6.9	16.2	21.0	4.8
2020	74.9	81.8	6.9	16.6	21.4	4.8
2030	75.4	82.3	6.9	17.0	21.8	4.8
2040	75.9	82.8	6.9	17.3	22.3	5.0
2050	76.4	83.3	6.9	17.7	22.7	5.0

Source: Aging America: Trends and Projections. 1991 ed. Prepared by the U.S. Senate Special Committee on Aging, the American Association of Retired Persons, the Federal Council on the Aging, and the U.S. Administration on Aging. DHHS Publication No. (FCoA) 91-28001. Washington, DC: U.S. Department of Health and Human Services (DHHS), 1991, p. 23. Primary source: U.S. Bureau of the Census. "Projections of the Population of the United States, by Age, Sex, and Race: 1988 to 2080." Prepared by Gregory Spencer. *Current Population Reports* Series P-25, no. 1018, January 1989.

Men's Health

★119★

Causes of Death for Males: 1990

The table below shows the number of deaths from leading causes for men in the United States. Data are provided by race for 1990.

Cause	All races	White	Black	American Indian	Asian or Pacific Islander
All causes	2,148,463	950,812	145,359	4,877	12,211
Heart disease	720,058	319,362	37,038	1,106	3,238
Cerebrovascular disease	144,088	48,024	7,653	164	853
Malignant neoplasms[1]	505,322	232,608	31,995	629	3,021
Chronic obstructive pulmonary disease	86,679	45,234	3,628	141	412
Pneumonia and influenza	79,513	32,101	4,161	170	462
Chronic liver disease and cirrhosis	25,815	13,889	2,393	184	160
Diabetes mellitus	47,664	16,817	3,049	152	244
Nephritis, nephrotic syndrome, and nephrosis	20,764	8,021	1,806	58	119
Septicemia	19,169	6,786	1,624	50	79
Atherosclerosis	18,047	6,232	563	17	47
HIV infection	25,188	16,106	6,097	33	149
Injuries (unintentional)	91,983	51,348	8,756	883	935
Suicide	30,906	22,448	1,737	214	318
Homicide and legal intervention	24,932	9,147	9,981	177	289

Source: U.S. Department of Health and Human Services. Public Health Service. Centers for Disease Control and Prevention. National Center for Health Statistics. *Health, United States, 1992.* Hyattsville, MD: Public Health Service, 1993, pp. 49-51. Primary source: Centers for Disease Control and Prevention. National Center for Health Statistics. *Vital Statistics of the United States.* Vol. II: *Mortality, Part A.* Washington, DC: U.S. Government Printing Office; data computed by the Division of Analysis from data compiled by the Division of Vital Statistics. *Notes:* The code numbers for the cause of death are based on the *International Classification of Diseases,* 9th revision. Categories for the coding and classification of human immunodeficiency virus (HIV) infection were introduced in the United States beginning with mortality data for 1987. The number of HIV infection deaths based on the National Vital Statistics System differs from the number of deaths among Acquired Immunodeficiency Syndrome (AIDS) cases reported to the Centers for Disease Control (CDC) AIDS Surveillance System. 1. Cancer.

★ 120 ★

Men's Health

Death Rates of Men From Selected Cancers: 1990

Data reflect death rates per 100,000 Americans.

Cancer	Death rate
Lung	76
Prostate	26
Stomach	7

Source: "The War's Toll." *Detroit Free Press,* 3 July 1994, p. F1.

★ 121 ★

Men's Health

Life Expectancy and Good Health for Men

A 35-year-old man who reduces his cholesterol level from 250 to 200 adds 1 year to his life expectancy. Reducing his weight by 30 percent to the ideal level adds an additional year, and eliminating behaviors that promote heart disease would extend his life expectancy by 3.1 years.

Action	Amount added to life expectancy
Controlling blood pressure	12 months
Quitting smoking	10 months
Cholesterol under 200	8 months
Controlling weight	7 months

Source: Scan/Info 3 (May 1991), p. 19. *Scan/Info* is a publication of the Los Angeles Public Library, State of California. Primary sources: *San Francisco Chronicle,* 26 April 1991, p. A30; *Circulation* (April 1991).

★ 122 ★

Men's Health

Prostate Cancer in Older Men

Prostate cancer is one of the most common forms of cancer among American men. About 80 percent of all cases are found in men over 65.

Source: U.S. Department of Health and Human Services. Public Health Service. National Institute on Aging. *Bound for Good Health: A Collection of Age Pages.* Bethesda, MD: National Institute on Aging, c. 1991, n.p.

★ 123 ★

Men's Health

Prostate Enlargement in Older Men

Benign prostatic hypertrophy (BPH) is an enlargement of the prostate. This condition is common in older men; more than half of men in their 60s and as many as 90 percent of men in their 70s and 80s have some symptoms of BPH.

Source: U.S. Department of Health and Human Services. Public Health Service. National Institute on Aging. *Bound for Good Health: A Collection of Age Pages.* Bethesda, MD: National Institute on Aging, c. 1991, n.p.

★ 124 ★

Men's Health

Prostate Surgery

The table shows the average expenditures for prostate surgery and treatment.

[In dollars]

Procedure/condition	Cost
Prostate operation	8,000-12,000
Benign prostate enlargement	3-4 billion[1]

Source: "The Prostate Puzzle." *Consumer Reports* 57 (July 1993), p. 459. *Note:* 1. Annual spending.

★ 125 ★

Men's Health

Sperm Count

Average sperm concentrations have fallen to 66 million spermatozoa per milliliter in 1990, according to a study reported in the *British Medical Journal.* On average, the sperm count of contemporary men is about half of that of their grandfathers' generation.

Source: "Human Sperm Count Study Shows World-Wide Decline." *Wall Street Journal,* 11 September 1992, p. B13.

Mental Health: Cost

★ 126 ★

Cost of Psychotherapy, by State

Data indicate average charge per psychotherapy session for each state.

State	Charge
Alabama	$62-$74
Alaska	$88-$100
Arizona	$88-$100
Arkansas	$62-$74
California	$88-$100
Colorado	$75-$87
Connecticut	$75-$87
Delaware	$62-$74
Florida	$88-$100
Georgia	$62-$74
Hawaii	$62-$74
Idaho	$62-$74
Illinois	$88-$100
Indiana	$75-$87
Iowa	$62-$74
Kansas	$62-$74
Kentucky	$62-$74
Louisiana	$75-$87
Maine	$62-$74
Maryland	$88-$100
Massachusetts	$75-$87
Michigan	$62-$74
Minnesota	$62-$74
Mississippi	$62-$74
Missouri	$62-$74
Montana	$62-$74
Nebraska	$62-$74
Nevada	$88-$100
New Hampshire	$88-$100
New Jersey	$88-$100
New Mexico	$88-$100
New York	$88-$100
North Carolina	$75-$87
North Dakota	$62-$74
Ohio	$75-$87
Oklahoma	$62-$74
Oregon	$75-$87
Pennsylvania	$75-$87
Rhode Island	$75-$87
South Carolina	$62-$74
South Dakota	$75-$87
Tennessee	$75-$87
Texas	$88-$100

[Continued]

★ 126 ★

Cost of Psychotherapy, by State
[Continued]

State	Charge
Utah	$75-$87
Vermont	$62-$74
Virginia	$75-$87
Washington	$62-$74
West Virginia	$62-$74
Wisconsin	$75-$87
Wyoming	$62-$74

Source: "Price Tag: Psychotherapy." *New York Times,* 4 February 1993, late edition (final), sec. C, p. 2. Primary sources: American Psychiatric Association; American Psychoanalytic Association; Mutual of Omaha Company; *Medical Economics;* Bureau of Labor Statistics; Peter Gay, *Freud: A Life for Our Time.*

★ 127 ★

Mental Health: Cost

Cost of Psychotherapy Visits: 1991

The table below reflects average fees charged by mental health professionals for a 45- or 50-minute therapy session. Data are for 1991.

Type of therapy	Average cost per visit
Group	$50 per person
Family	150 per family
Individual	100 per person

Source: "Price Tag: Psychotherapy." *New York Times,* 4 February 1993, late edition (final), sec. C, p. 2. Primary sources: American Psychiatric Association; American Psychoanalytic Association; Mutual of Omaha Company; *Medical Economics;* Bureau of Labor Statistics; Peter Gay, *Freud: A Life for Our Time.*

★ 128 ★

Mental Health: Cost

State Mental Health Agency Per Capita Expenditures: 1990

The table below presents mental health care expenditures per capita for each state. Agencies covered include state mental hospitals, other hospitals, community-based programs, and state mental health support activities for the 1990 fiscal year.

State	State mental health agency
Alabama	38.35
Alaska	72.24
Arizona	27.27
Arkansas	25.92
California	42.32
Colorado	33.55
Connecticut	72.81
Delaware	54.88
District of Columbia	267.86
Florida	37.49
Georgia	50.98
Hawaii	37.58
Idaho	20.37
Illinois	34.43
Indiana	47.05
Iowa	17.07
Kansas	35.41
Kentucky	23.24
Louisiana	28.44
Maine	67.29
Maryland	61.28
Massachusetts	83.91
Michigan	73.73
Minnesota	53.67
Mississippi	33.71
Missouri	35.47
Montana	28.42
Nebraska	29.07
Nevada	33.47
New Hampshire	63.37
New Jersey	57.16
New Mexico	22.88
New York	118.34
North Carolina	45.66
North Dakota	40.24
Ohio	40.93
Oklahoma	35.92
Oregon	40.68
Pennsylvania	56.85
Rhode Island	50.37
South Carolina	51.12
South Dakota	25.34

[Continued]

★ 128 ★

State Mental Health Agency Per Capita Expenditures: 1990

[Continued]

State	State mental health agency
Tennessee	28.84
Texas	22.72
Utah	20.57
Vermont	53.77
Virginia	44.54
Washington	42.96
West Virginia	23.72
Wisconsin	36.62
Wyoming	34.62

Primary source: Center for Mental Health Services and National Institute of Mental Health. *Mental Health, United States, 1992.* Edited by R. W. Manderscheid and M. A. Sonnenschein. DHHS Publication No. (SMA) 92-1942. Washington, DC: U.S. Government Printing Office, 1992, p. 188.

Mental Health: Disorders

★ 129 ★

Depression: 1990

Approximately 11 million Americans suffered from depression and other affective disorders in 1990. More than $12 billion was spent on their treatment, including inpatient care and drugs. In total, depression costs close to $44 billion dollars annually when lost work time and lost productivity are included in the calculations.

Source: "Depression Affects Millions." *Business and Health* 12, no. 4. (Supplement A, 1994), p. 4.

★ 130 ★

Mental Health: Disorders

Mental Disorders Among American Adults

Table provides the estimated number of persons affected by selected mental disorders.

Disorder	Number affected
Schizophrenic disorders	1,749,000
Mood disorders	15,143,000
Bipolar disorders	1,908,000
Depression[1]	7,950,000
Dysthymia	8,586,000
Anxiety disorders	20,034,000
Phobic disorders	17,331,000
Panic disorders	2,067,000
Obsessive-compulsive disorders	3,339,000
Antisocial personality disorders	2,385,000
Any mental disorder	35,139,000
Any mental/substance abuse disorders	44,679,000

Source: U.S. Congress. Office of Technology Assessment. *Psychiatric Disabilities, Employment, and the Americans With Disabilities Act.* OTA-BP- BBS-124. Washington, DC: U.S. Government Printing Office, March 1994, p. 51. Primary source: Regier, D. A., W. E. Narrow, D. S. Rae, and others. "The de Facto U.S. Mental and Addictive Disorders Service System: Epidemiologic Catchment Area Prospective 1-Year Prevalence Rates of Disorders and Services." *Archives of General Psychiatry* 50 (1993), pp. 85- 94. *Note:* 1. Major.

Mental Health: Treatment

★ 131 ★

Seeking Help for Personal or Emotional Problems

Table indicates the percent of persons 18 years of age and older who have sought help for a personal or emotional problem in the past year. Data are provided by sex, age, and selected characteristics for 1990.

Characteristic	Both sexes 18 years and over	Male					Female				
		Total	18-29 years	30-44 years	45-64 years	65 years and over	Total	18-29 years	30-44 years	45-64 years	65 years and over
All persons[1]	12.5	8.6	9.6	10.7	7.8	3.1	16.0	18.5	21.5	13.3	6.8
Educational level											
Less than 12 years	8.5	5.5	8.8	6.7	5.0	2.3	11.3	14.7	18.1	11.1	6.3
12 years	11.3	7.5	8.2	9.4	6.6	2.7	14.2	17.0	18.7	11.2	6.6
More than 12 years	15.6	10.9	11.4	12.5	10.3	4.5	20.6	21.5	24.6	17.8	8.3
13-15 years	14.9	10.4	10.1	12.0	10.1	4.6	19.0	20.8	22.8	15.9	6.8
16 years or more	16.4	11.4	13.5	12.8	10.4	4.5	22.5	22.9	26.4	19.8	10.3

[Continued]

★ 131 ★

Seeking Help for Personal or Emotional Problems
[Continued]

Characteristic	Both sexes 18 years and over	Male					Female				
		Total	18-29 years	30-44 years	45-64 years	65 years and over	Total	18-29 years	30-44 years	45-64 years	65 years and over
Income											
Less than $10,000	14.6	11.8	12.6	16.6	15.9	2.8[2]	16.1	18.3	25.7	21.3	6.1
$10,000-$19,999	12.5	8.3	10.8	11.7	6.7	2.8	16.0	18.8	23.8	14.6	7.5
$20,000-$34,999	12.0	8.0	9.1	10.2	6.5	2.6	16.0	18.7	21.6	11.7	4.8
$35,000-$49,999	13.2	9.3	8.3	10.9	8.5	5.2[2]	17.5	17.7	21.4	13.3	7.9
$50,000 or more	14.0	9.1	9.6	10.4	8.5	3.7[2]	19.3	22.6	22.2	15.0	10.6
Race											
White	12.8	8.7	10.1	10.9	8.1	3.0	16.6	20.0	22.4	13.5	6.9
Black	10.2	7.0	6.6	9.0	6.2	3.9[2]	12.7	11.5	17.2	11.8	6.0
Hispanic origin											
Hispanic	10.3	6.2	7.4	6.0	6.3	-[2]	13.9	12.8	16.8	12.6	9.1[2]
Non-Hispanic	12.6	8.7	9.8	11.1	7.9	3.2	16.2	19.3	21.9	13.4	6.7
Geographic region											
Northeast	11.5	8.4	8.5	11.8	6.9	2.8	14.2	18.5	20.3	10.7	5.1
Midwest	13.3	9.0	10.6	10.4	8.4	3.8	17.3	19.9	23.2	14.5	7.1
South	11.2	7.2	8.1	9.1	6.2	3.1	14.7	15.7	19.8	12.6	7.6
West	14.6	10.4	11.5	12.5	10.5	2.5[2]	18.5	21.7	23.2	16.0	7.0
Marital status											
Currently married	10.7	7.0	8.4	8.7	6.6	2.5	14.5	16.5	18.1	11.4	7.1
Formerly married	17.3	14.8	20.6	20.1	14.3	5.8	18.4	29.1	37.0	19.3	6.9
Never married	14.2	10.7	9.8	14.3	11.8	3.2[2]	18.5	19.1	22.6	11.4	3.3[2]
Employment status											
Currently employed	13.1	8.8	9.4	9.9	7.2	2.8[2]	18.2	19.2	21.7	13.3	6.4
Unemployed	15.9	11.7	12.6	12.2	10.3[2]	2.6[2]	20.4	20.0	26.6	11.9[2]	2.6[2]
Not in labor force	10.8	7.3	9.5	22.0	10.2	3.1	12.6	16.6	20.1	13.4	6.9

Source: U.S. Department of Health and Human Services. Public Health Service. Centers for Disease Control and Prevention. National Center for Health Statistics. *Health Promotion and Disease Prevention: United States, 1990.* Vital and Health Statistics, Series 10, no. 185. Hyattsville, MD: U.S. Department of Health and Human Services, Public Health Service, Centers for Disease Control and Prevention, National Center for Health Statistics, n.d., p. 39. *Notes:* Data are based on household interviews of the civilian noninstitutionalized population. The survey design, general qualifications, and information on the reliability of the estimates are given in Appendix 1 in the original source. Denominator for each cell excludes unknowns. 1. Includes persons with unknown sociodemographic characteristics. 2. Figure does not meet standard of reliability or precision (more than 30-percent relative standard error in numerator of percent or rate).

★ 132 ★

Mental Health: Treatment

Treatment of Mental Illness

Figures below show the 6-month success rates for treatment of selected mental illnesses.

[In percentages]

Disorder	Success rate
Panic disorders	80
Bipolar disorders	80
Depression[1]	65
Schizophrenia	60
Obsessive-compulsive disorders	60

Source: "At a Glance: Snapshots of the Workplace Health Industry." *Workplace Health* (January 1994), p. 15. Primary sources: National Institute of Mental Health; *Business and Health. Note:* 1. Major.

Pregnancy and Childbirth: Abortion

★ 133 ★

Abortion Rates in Selected States

Table below shows the states with the highest and lowest abortion rates in 1992. Data are for women aged 15-44.

[Per 1,000]

State or area	Rate
Highest rates	
Washington, District of Columbia	138.4
New York	46.2
Hawaii	46.0
Nevada	44.2
California	42.1
Lowest rates	
Utah	9.3
West Virginia	7.7
Idaho	7.2
South Dakota	6.8
Wyoming	4.3

Source: "Fewest Abortions Since '79." *USA TODAY,* 16 June 1994, p. 4A. Primary source: Alan Guttmacher Institute.

★ 134 ★

Pregnancy and Childbirth: Abortion

Teen Abortion Distribution by Race/Ethnicity: 1991

Percentages are shown for states without parental consent laws.

Race/ethnicity	Abortion distribution
White, non-Hispanic	55
Black, non-Hispanic	30
Hispanic	12
Asian/other	3

Source: Hall, Mimi. "Study Zeros in on Pregnant Teens, Parents: Both Sides Say New Report Is a Validation of Positions." *USA TODAY,* 20 October 1992, final edition, p. 10A. Primary source: Survey by the Alan Guttmacher Institute, 1991.

Pregnancy and Childbirth: Births

★ 135 ★

Live Births, by State: 1990-1991

Number and rate of registered births. Excludes births to nonresidents of the United States, except as noted. By race of child, except as indicated.

Division and state	Number (1,000)						Ratio per 1,000 population[3]					
	1990					1991 preliminary[3]	1990					1991 preliminary[3]
	All races[1]	White	Black	Hispanic origin[2]			All races[1]	White	Black	Hispanic origin[2]		
				Total	Mexican					Total	Mexican	
United States	4,158.2	3,225.3	724.6	595.1	385.6	4,111.0	16.7	15.5	23.8	26.7	28.7	16.2
New England	201.2	175.3	19.0	15.5	0.6	189.5	15.2	14.6	30.3	27.2	20.1	14.3
Maine	17.4	16.9	0.2	0.1	(Z)	16.6	14.1	14.0	31.7	18.6	13.0	13.2
New Hampshire	17.6	17.1	0.2	(NA)	(NA)	16.1	15.8	15.7	25.6	(NA)	(NA)	13.9
Vermont	8.3	8.2	(Z)	(Z)	(Z)	7.7	14.7	14.7	19.5	8.2	9.7	13.2
Massachusetts	92.7	78.3	10.2	8.4	0.3	86.3	15.4	14.5	34.1	29.3	22.5	14.5
Rhode Island	15.2	13.1	1.3	1.6	0.1	14.6	15.1	14.3	34.5	34.1	35.7	14.5
Connecticut	50.1	41.8	7.0	5.3	0.2	48.3	15.2	14.6	25.6	25.0	20.1	14.8
Middle Atlantic	591.8	450.1	118.7	75.7	5.1	578.8	15.7	15.0	23.8	23.8	34.9	15.2
New York	297.6	216.8	66.3	53.1	3.8	292.4	16.5	16.2	23.2	24.0	41.0	16.2
New Jersey	122.3	92.6	24.5	17.0	0.9	117.8	15.8	15.1	23.6	22.9	30.4	15.1
Pennsylvania	172.0	140.7	27.9	5.6	0.4	168.6	14.5	13.4	25.6	24.3	16.5	13.9
East North Central	675.5	536.7	123.5	34.7	23.8	662.4	16.1	15.0	25.6	24.1	25.2	15.5
Ohio	166.9	137.1	27.7	2.4	1.0	158.6	15.4	14.4	24.0	17.4	17.5	14.4
Indiana	86.2	74.6	10.3	1.9	1.4	84.7	15.6	14.9	23.8	18.8	20.3	14.9
Illinois	195.8	144.8	45.2	24.2	17.7	194.0	17.1	16.2	26.7	26.8	28.3	16.5
Michigan	153.7	117.5	32.9	4.3	2.6	153.4	16.5	15.2	25.5	21.5	18.5	16.4
Wisconsin	72.9	62.7	7.5	1.9	1.2	71.7	14.9	13.9	30.7	20.0	21.3	14.5
West North Central	270.3	235.4	24.1	5.6	4.1	262.4	15.3	14.5	26.9	19.5	19.8	14.5
Minnesota	68.0	61.0	3.1	1.1	0.8	67.0	15.5	14.8	32.7	19.5	22.5	15.1
Iowa	39.4	37.4	1.3	0.6	0.4	36.0	14.2	13.9	26.6	19.1	15.5	12.6
Missouri	79.3	63.8	14.1	1.0	0.7	78.0	15.5	14.2	25.7	15.7	19.0	15.0

[Continued]

Live Births, by State: 1990-1991
[Continued]

Division and state	Number (1,000)						Ratio per 1,000 population[3]					
	1990					1991 preliminary[3]	1990					1991 preliminary[3]
	All races[1]	White	Black	Hispanic origin[2]			All races[1]	White	Black	Hispanic origin[2]		
				Total	Mexican					Total	Mexican	
North Dakota	9.3	8.2	0.1	0.1	0.1	9.1	14.5	13.6	33.8	26.4	26.1	14.0
South Dakota	11.0	9.0	0.1	0.1	0.1	11.0	15.8	14.1	41.4	21.5	20.9	15.4
Nebraska	24.4	22.1	1.6	0.8	0.5	23.9	15.4	14.9	27.0	21.7	17.4	14.7
Kansas	39.0	34.0	3.8	2.0	1.6	37.3	15.7	15.3	26.8	20.9	21.0	14.6
South Atlantic	700.3	476.1	207.2	39.4	8.9	689.1	16.1	14.3	23.2	18.5	28.3	15.5
Delaware	11.1	8.2	2.7	0.3	0.1	11.2	16.7	15.4	23.8	20.4	27.2	16.0
Maryland	80.2	51.0	26.0	2.5	0.5	84.5	16.8	15.0	21.9	20.2	29.7	17.5
District of Columbia	11.9	1.7	9.2	0.9	(Z)	10.0	19.5	9.7	22.9	27.2	14.8	17.0
Virginia	99.4	71.1	24.7	3.5	0.6	96.6	16.1	14.8	21.3	21.6	19.1	15.4
West Virginia	22.6	21.5	1.0	0.1	(Z)	22.2	12.6	12.4	17.1	8.6	8.5	12.2
North Carolina	104.5	69.8	31.7	1.8	1.0	102.4	15.8	13.9	21.7	22.9	30.2	15.2
South Carolina	58.6	35.2	22.7	0.6	0.3	57.7	16.8	14.6	21.8	18.7	24.1	16.0
Georgia	112.7	69.7	41.3	2.3	1.3	110.0	17.4	15.1	23.6	20.8	26.7	16.6
Florida	199.3	147.9	48.1	27.6	5.0	194.5	15.4	13.8	27.3	17.5	31.0	14.6
East South Central	236.4	167.5	66.3	1.2	0.6	232.1	15.6	13.9	22.3	12.4	15.9	14.9
Kentucky	54.4	48.5	5.4	0.3	0.2	54.9	14.8	14.3	20.4	12.5	20.5	14.7
Tennessee	75.0	56.0	18.0	0.4	0.2	73.1	15.4	13.8	23.2	13.6	16.6	14.5
Alabama	63.5	40.8	22.0	0.3	0.2	60.5	15.7	13.7	21.6	14.0	16.8	14.6
Mississippi	43.6	22.2	20.9	0.1	(Z)	43.5	16.9	13.6	22.8	7.3	7.0	16.6
West South Central	472.7	366.1	90.2	117.2	103.5	482.0	17.7	18.2	22.9	25.8	25.9	17.7
Arkansas	36.5	27.2	8.7	0.4	0.2	34.6	15.5	14.0	23.2	20.8	19.7	14.2
Louisiana	72.2	40.7	30.0	0.9	0.2	74.6	17.1	14.3	23.1	10.1	8.6	17.2
Oklahoma	47.6	35.6	5.5	(NA)	(NA)	47.3	15.1	13.8	23.7	(NA)	(NA)	14.7
Texas	316.4	262.6	45.9	115.8	103.0	325.6	18.6	20.6	22.7	26.7	26.5	18.8
Mountain	242.8	212.4	10.2	48.7	31.8	243.4	17.8	18.1	27.2	24.4	22.1	17.5
Montana	11.6	9.7	0.1	0.3	0.1	11.5	14.5	13.1	31.5	24.0	17.3	14.3
Idaho	16.4	15.8	0.1	1.4	1.2	17.2	16.3	16.6	27.3	27.1	27.7	16.6
Wyoming	7.0	6.5	0.1	0.5	0.3	6.8	15.4	15.2	29.7	19.8	17.2	14.6
Colorado	53.5	48.1	3.4	9.3	4.7	54.0	16.2	16.6	25.5	21.9	16.5	16.1
New Mexico	27.4	22.2	0.8	12.2	2.8	28.2	18.1	19.3	25.8	21.1	8.6	18.0
Arizona	69.0	58.1	3.2	19.7	18.9	67.7	18.8	19.6	28.7	28.6	30.7	18.3
Utah	36.3	33.9	0.4	2.0	1.2	35.1	21.1	21.0	33.3	24.1	21.8	20.1
Nevada	21.6	18.1	2.2	3.3	2.5	23.0	18.0	17.9	27.4	26.2	29.1	18.8
Pacific	767.2	605.7	65.3	257.0	207.2	755.5	19.6	21.4	26.6	31.7	32.5	18.8
Washington	79.3	68.2	4.1	5.7	3.9	75.7	16.3	15.8	27.7	26.6	24.8	15.2
Oregon	42.9	38.9	1.3	3.0	2.6	42.8	15.1	14.7	27.3	26.4	30.9	14.6
California	612.6	486.3	58.2	245.6	200.1	605.7	20.6	23.7	26.4	31.9	32.7	19.8
Alaska	11.9	7.6	0.7	0.3	0.2	11.2	21.6	18.3	31.9	18.4	21.5	21.1
Hawaii	20.5	4.7	1.0	2.4	0.3	20.0	18.5	12.7	35.3	29.9	24.2	17.5

Source: *1993 Statistical Abstract of the United States on CD-ROM* [machine-readable datafiles]. CD-ABSTR-93. Washington, DC: U.S. Department of Commerce, Economics and Statistics Administration, Bureau of the Census, Data User Services Division, 1993. Primary source: U.S. National Center for Health Statistics. *Vital Statistics of the United States* (annual); *Monthly Vital Statistics Report. Notes:* "NA" represents "not available." "Z" represents less than 50. 1. Includes other races not shown separately. 2. Persons of Hispanic origin may be of any race. Births by Hispanic origin of mother. 3. Includes births to nonresidents. Provisional. 4. Based on resident population enumerated as of April 1 for 1990 and estimated as of July 1 for 1991.

★ 136 ★

Pregnancy and Childbirth: Births

Low Birth Weight and Births to Teenage Mothers and to Unmarried Women, by State: 1980 and 1990

Represents registered births. Excludes births to nonresidents of the United States. Based on 100 percent of births in all states and the District of Columbia.

Division and state	Births with low birth weight (percent of total)[1]		Births to teenage mothers (percent of total)		Births to unmarried women (percent of total)	
	1980	1990	1980	1990	1980	1990
United States	6.8	7.0	15.6	12.8	18.4	28.0
New England	6.2	5.9	11.6	8.4	15.5	24.2
Maine	6.5	5.1	15.3	10.8	13.9	22.6
New Hampshire	5.4	4.9	10.7	7.2	11.0	16.9
Vermont	5.9	5.3	13.0	8.5	13.7	20.1
Massachusetts	6.1	5.9	10.7	8.0	15.7	24.7
Rhode Island	6.3	6.2	12.3	10.5	15.7	26.3
Connecticut	6.7	6.6	11.4	8.2	17.9[2]	26.6[2]
Middle Atlantic	7.1	7.3	12.6	9.5	21.3	29.9
New York	7.4	7.6	11.8	9.1	23.8[2]	33.0[2]
New Jersey	7.2	7.0	12.3	8.4	21.1	24.3
Pennsylvania	6.5	7.1	13.9	10.9	17.7	28.6
East North Central	6.7	7.1	15.2	13.2	18.0	28.3
Ohio	6.8	7.1	15.7	13.8	17.8[2]	28.9
Indiana	6.3	6.6	17.3	14.5	15.5	26.2
Illinois	7.2	7.6	15.7	13.1	22.5	31.7
Michigan	6.9	7.6	14.0	13.5	16.2[2]	26.2[2]
Wisconsin	5.4	5.9	12.3	10.2	13.9	24.2
West North Central	5.7	5.9	13.5	11.1	13.1	23.2
Minnesota	5.1	5.1	10.4	8.0	11.4	20.9
Iowa	5.0	5.4	12.5	10.2	10.3	21.0
Missouri	6.6	7.1	16.9	14.4	17.6	28.6
North Dakota	4.9	5.5	10.9	8.6	9.2	18.4
South Dakota	5.1	5.1	13.5	10.8	13.4	22.9
Nebraska	5.6	5.3	12.1	9.8	11.6	20.7
Kansas	5.8	6.2	15.0	12.3	12.3	21.5
South Atlantic	8.0	7.9	18.3	14.4	22.2	30.9
Delaware	7.7	7.6	16.7	11.9	24.2	29.0
Maryland	8.2	7.8	14.8	10.5	25.2[2]	29.6
District of Columbia	12.8	15.1	20.7	17.8	56.5	64.9
Virginia	7.5	7.2	15.5	11.7	19.2	26.0
West Virginia	6.7	7.1	20.1	17.8	13.1	25.4
North Carolina	7.9	8.0	19.2	16.2	19.0	29.4
South Carolina	8.6	8.7	19.8	17.1	23.0	32.7
Georgia	8.6	8.7	20.7	16.7	23.2	32.8
Florida	7.6	7.4	18.2	13.9	23.0	31.7
East South Central	7.8	8.2	21.0	18.4	20.9	30.6
Kentucky	6.8	7.1	21.1	17.5	15.1	23.6
Tennessee	8.0	8.2	19.9	17.6	19.9	30.2
Alabama	7.9	8.4	20.6	18.2	22.2	30.1
Mississippi	8.7	9.6	23.2	21.3	28.0	40.5
West South Central	7.3	7.3	19.1	16.3	15.8	22.2

[Continued]

★ 136 ★

Low Birth Weight and Births to Teenage Mothers and to Unmarried Women, by State: 1980 and 1990
[Continued]

Division and state	Births with low birth weight (percent of total)[1]		Births to teenage mothers (percent of total)		Births to unmarried women (percent of total)	
	1980	1990	1980	1990	1980	1990
Arkansas	7.6	8.2	21.6	19.7	20.5	29.4
Louisiana	8.6	9.2	20.1	17.6	23.4	36.8
Oklahoma	6.8	6.6	19.6	16.2	14.0	25.2
Texas	6.9	6.9	18.3	15.6	13.3[2]	17.5[2]
Mountain	6.6	6.8	14.3	12.8	12.7	25.1
Montana	5.6	6.2	12.4	11.5	12.5[2]	23.7
Idaho	5.3	5.7	13.1	12.3	7.9	16.7
Wyoming	7.3	7.4	15.5	13.6	8.2	19.8
Colorado	8.2	8.0	13.3	11.3	13.0	21.2
New Mexico	7.6	7.4	18.2	16.3	16.1	35.4
Arizona	6.2	6.4	16.5	14.2	18.7	32.7
Utah	5.2	5.7	11.0	10.3	6.2	13.5
Nevada	6.6	7.2	15.4	12.6	13.5[2]	25.4[2]
Pacific	5.8	5.7	13.6	11.5	19.6	30.2
Washington	5.1	5.3	12.5	10.8	13.6	23.7
Oregon	4.9	5.0	13.3	12.0	14.8	25.7
California	5.9	5.8	13.9	11.6	21.4[2]	31.6[2]
Alaska	5.4	4.8	11.8	9.7	15.1	26.2
Hawaii	7.1	7.1	11.5	10.5	17.6	24.8

Source: 1993 Statistical Abstract of the United States on CD-ROM [machine-readable datafiles]. CD-ABSTR-93. Washington, DC: U.S. Department of Commerce, Economics and Statistics Administration, Bureau of the Census, Data User Services Division, 1993. Primary source: U.S. National Center for Health Statistics. Vital Statistics of the United States. (annual); Monthly Vital Statistics Report. Notes: 1. Less than 2,500 grams (5 pounds, 8 ounces). 2. Marital status of mother is inferred.

★ 137 ★

Pregnancy and Childbirth: Births

Premature Infants' Survival and Quality of Life

A Johns Hopkins University study found the odds favorable for suvival without major birth defects for premature infants born at 25 weeks of gestation. Figures below compare survival prospects of premature infants 6 months after birth by week of gestation at birth.

Weeks of gestation	Percent surviving 6 months	Percent without severe abnormalities
22	0	NA
23	15	2
24	56	21
25	79	69

Source: "Lines Drawn for Survival of Preemies." *St. Louis Post-Dispatch,* 25 November 1993, p. 14A. *Note:* "NA" represents "not applicable."

Pregnancy and Childbirth: Contraception and Fertility

★ 138 ★

Contraceptive Use: 1992

Figures show the percent distribution for contraceptive use by women ages 15 to 44 who are at risk of unintended pregnancy. Data provided according to marital status for 1992.

Contraceptives and contraceptive users	Total	Married	Unmarried
All users	94	97	92
Nonusers	6	3	8
Pill	39	28	52
Sterilization	31	48	11
Female	19	27	10
Male	12	21	1
Condom	25	19	33
Withdrawal	8	6	11
Rhythm	4	5	4
Diaphragm	4	4	4
Sponge	3	3	3
Suppository	3	1	3
Douche	3	1	4
IUD	1	1	1
Foam	1	1	1

[Continued]

★ 138 ★

Contraceptive Use: 1992
[Continued]

Contraceptives and contraceptive users	Total	Married	Unmarried
Cream/jelly	1	1	1
Implant	1	1	1
Cervical cap	1	1	1

Source: Forrest, Jacqueline Darroch, and Richard R. Fordyce. "Women's Contraceptive Attitudes and Use in 1992." *Family Planning Perspectives* 25, no. 4 (July/August 1993), p. 178. *Notes:* Sum of the proportions using each method exceeds the total proportion of users because some respondents used more than 1 method. 1. Less than 0.5 percent. 2. Intrauterine device.

★ 139 ★

Pregnancy and Childbirth: Contraception and Fertility

Projected Fertility Rates, by Race and Age Group

The total fertility rate is the number of births that 1,000 women would have in their lifetime if, at each year of age, they experienced the birth rates occurring in the specified year. Birth rates represent live births per 1,000 women in age group indicated. Projections are based on middle fertility assumptions.

	1992	2000	2010
All races[1]			
Total fertility rate	2,054	2,073	2,092
Birth rates:			
10 to 14 years old	1.4	1.4	1.5
15 to 19 years old	57.3	57.4	58.7
20 to 24 years old	118.0	119.3	120.0
25 to 29 years old	120.0	120.9	121.0
30 to 34 years old	79.2	80.1	80.5
35 to 39 years old	29.6	30.2	31.0
40 to 44 years old	4.9	5.1	5.4
45 to 49 years old	0.2	0.3	0.3
White			
Total fertility rate	1,953	1,969	1,981
Birth rates:			
10 to 14 years old	0.6	0.6	0.7
15 to 19 years old	46.7	47.3	48.5
20 to 24 years old	109.8	111.2	112.1
25 to 29 years old	119.8	120.2	120.0
30 to 34 years old	79.7	79.9	79.9
35 to 39 years old	29.1	29.5	29.9
40 to 44 years old	4.7	4.7	5.0
45 to 49 years old	0.2	0.2	0.2
Black			
Total fertility rate	2,468	2,461	2,459
Birth rates:			
10 to 14 years old	5.3	5.3	5.2

[Continued]

★ 139 ★

Projected Fertility Rates, by Race and Age Group
[Continued]

	1992	2000	2010
15 to 19 years old	113.7	113.0	112.7
20 to 24 years old	161.6	161.0	160.8
25 to 29 years old	113.8	113.6	113.6
30 to 34 years old	66.6	66.6	66.6
35 to 39 years old	27.2	27.2	27.3
40 to 44 years old	5.2	5.2	5.3
45 to 49 years old	0.3	0.3	0.3
Asian and Pacific Islander			
Total fertility rate	2,335	2,323	2,271
Birth rates:			
10 to 14 years old	0.6	0.6	0.6
15 to 19 years old	28.3	28.0	27.2
20 to 24 years old	95.8	95.1	93.1
25 to 29 years old	152.2	151.6	149.1
30 to 34 years old	123.8	123.2	120.7
35 to 39 years old	53.6	53.4	52.2
40 to 44 years old	11.3	11.3	11.0
45 to 49 years old	1.3	1.3	1.2
American Indian, Eskimo, Aleut			
Total fertility rate	2,874	2,864	2,855
Birth rates:			
10 to 14 years old	1.9	1.9	1.9
15 to 19 years old	105.9	105.2	105.5
20 to 24 years old	210.5	209.7	209.0
25 to 29 years old	142.1	141.6	141.1
30 to 34 years old	76.2	76.1	75.8
35 to 39 years old	31.2	31.2	31.1
40 to 44 years old	6.7	6.7	6.8
45 to 49 years old	0.4	0.4	0.4
Hispanic[2]			
Total fertility rate	2,655	2,648	2,588
Birth rates:			
10 to 14 years old	2.3	2.3	2.2
15 to 19 years old	86.3	86.1	84.1
20 to 24 years old	163.2	162.8	159.1
25 to 29 years old	139.1	138.8	135.6
30 to 34 years old	88.6	88.4	86.4
35 to 39 years old	41.3	41.2	40.2
40 to 44 years old	9.7	9.7	9.5
45 to 49 years old	0.6	0.6	0.6

Source: 1993 Statistical Abstract of the United States on CD-ROM [machine-readable datafiles]. CD-ABSTR-93. Washington, DC: U.S. Department of Commerce, Economics and Statistics Administration, Bureau of the Census, Data User Services Division, 1993. Primary source: U.S. Bureau of the Census. Current Population Reports. P25-1092; and unpublished data. Notes: 1. Includes other races not shown separately. 2. Persons of Hispanic origin may be of any race.

Pregnancy and Childbirth: Infant Mortality

★ 140 ★

Fetal and Infant Deaths, Number and Percent Distribution: 1960-1990

State requirements for reporting of fetal deaths vary. Most states require reporting of fetal deaths of gestations of 20 weeks or more. There is substantial evidence that not all fetal deaths for which reporting is required are reported.

Year	Number						Percent distribution					
	Total	Fetal deaths		Infant deaths			Total	Fetal deaths		Infant deaths		
				Neonatal		Post-				Neonatal		Post-
		Early[1]	Late[2]	Early[3]	Late[4]	neonatal		Early[1]	Late[2]	Early[3]	Late[4]	neonatal
1960	179,353	16,496	51,984	71,125	8,608	31,140	100.0	9.2	29.0	39.7	4.8	17.4
1970	127,628	17,170	35,791	50,821	5,458	18,388	100.0	13.5	28.0	39.8	4.3	14.4
1975	84,321	8,995	24,801	31,396	5,020	14,109	100.0	10.7	29.4	37.2	6.0	16.7
1980	78,879	10754	22,599	25,492	5,126	14,908	100.0	13.6	28.7	32.3	6.5	18.9
1981	75,901	11126	21,470	24,384	4,737	14,184	100.0	14.7	28.3	32.1	6.2	18.7
1982	75,095	11,028	21,666	23,706	4,629	14,066	100.0	14.7	28.9	31.6	6.2	18.7
1983	71,379	10,933	19,819	22,315	4,192	14,120	100.0	15.3	27.8	31.3	5.9	19.8
1984	69,679	10,963	19,136	21,566	4,125	13,889	100.0	15.7	27.5	31.0	5.9	19.9
1985	69,691	10,958	18,703	21,865	4,314	13,851	100.0	15.7	26.8	31.4	6.2	19.9
1986	67,863	11,100	17,872	21,053	4,159	13,679	100.0	16.4	26.3	31.0	6.1	20.2
1987	67,757	11,656	17,693	20,471	4,156	13,781	100.0	17.2	26.1	30.2	6.1	20.3
1988	68,352	11,833	17,609	20,471	4,219	14,220	100.0	17.3	25.8	29.9	6.2	20.8
1989	70,124	12,397	18,072	20,796	4,372	14,487	100.0	17.7	25.8	29.7	6.2	20.7
1990	67,696	12,554	16,791	20,020	4,289	14,042	100.0	18.5	24.8	29.6	6.3	20.7

Source: *1993 Statistical Abstract of the United States on CD-ROM* [machine-readable datafiles]. CD-ABSTR-93. Washington, DC: U.S. Department of Commerce, Economics and Statistics Administration, Bureau of the Census, Data User Services Division, 1993. Primary source: U.S. National Center for Health Statistics. *Vital Statistics of the United States* (annual). *Notes:* 1. 20-27 weeks gestation. 2. 28 weeks or more gestation. 3. Less than 7 days. 4. 7-27 days. 5. 28 days-11 months.

★ 141 ★

Pregnancy and Childbirth: Infant Mortality

Infant Deaths and Infant Mortality Rates, by Cause of Death: 1980 and 1990

Excludes deaths of nonresidents of the United States. Deaths classified according to ninth revision of *International Classification of Diseases*.

Cause of death	Number		Percent distribution		Infant mortality rate[1]	
	1980	1990	1980	1990	1980	1990
Total	45,526	38,351	100	100	12.6	9.2
Congenital anomalies	9,220	8,239	20	21	2.6	2.0
Sudden infant death syndrome	5,510	5,417	12	14	1.5	1.3
Respiratory distress syndrome	4,989	2,850	11	7	1.4	0.7
Disorders relating to short gestation and unspecified low birth weight	3,648	4,013	8	10	1.0	1.0

[Continued]

★ 141 ★

Infant Deaths and Infant Mortality Rates, by Cause of Death: 1980 and 1990

[Continued]

Cause of death	Number		Percent distribution		Infant mortality rate[1]	
	1980	1990	1980	1990	1980	1990
Newborn affected by maternal complications of pregnancy	1,572	1,655	4	4	0.4	0.4
Intrauterine hypoxia and birth asphyxia	1,497	762	3	2	0.4	0.2
Infections specific to the perinatal period	971	875	2	2	0.3	0.2
Accidents and adverse effects	1,166	930	3	2	0.3	0.2
Newborn affected by complications of placenta, cord, and membranes	985	975	2	3	0.3	0.2
Pneumonia and influenza	1,012	634	2	2	0.3	0.2
All other causes	14,956	12,001	33	31	4.1	2.9

Source: 1993 Statistical Abstract of the United States on CD-ROM [machine-readable datafiles]. CD-ABSTR-93. Washington, DC: U.S. Department of Commerce, Economics and Statistics Administration, Bureau of the Census, Data User Services Division, 1993. Primary source: U.S. National Center for Health Statistics. *Vital Statistics of the United States* (annual); *Monthly Vital Statistics Report. Note:* 1. Deaths of infants under 1 year old per 1,000 live births.

Pregnancy and Childbirth: Labor and Delivery

★ 142 ★

Births, by Practitioner: 1990 and 1991

Doctors - 94.8
Midwives - 4.4

Chart shows data from column 2.

Table shows percentage of deliveries by doctors and midwives for 1990 and 1991.

Practitioner	1990	1991
Doctors	95.3	94.8
Midwives	3.9	4.4

Source: "More Midwives." *Detroit News,* 25 April 1994, p. 3C. Primary source: National Center for Health Statistics.

★ 143 ★

Pregnancy and Childbirth: Labor and Delivery

Cesarean Section Deliveries, by Age of Mother: 1970-1991

Based on data collected from the National Hospital Discharge Survey, a sample survey of hospital records of patients discharged in year shown; subject to sampling variability. Beginning 1988, comparisons with data for earlier years should be made with caution as estimates of change may reflect improvements in the 1988 design rather than true changes in hospital use.

Age of mother	1970	1975	1980	1985	1990	1991
Number of cesarean deliveries (1,000)	195	328	619	877	945	933
Rate: Mothers, all ages[1]	5.5	10.4	16.5	22.7	23.5	23.5
Under 20 years	3.9	8.4	14.5	16.1	16.6	18.2
20 to 24 years	4.9	9.0	15.8	21.2	21.0	21.0
25 to 29 years	5.9	11.1	16.7	22.9	23.3	24.3
30 to 34 years	7.5	13.6	18.0	26.6	27.8	26.7
35 years and over	8.3	15.0	20.6	30.7	31.4	28.4

Source: 1993 Statistical Abstract of the United States on CD-ROM [machine-readable datafiles]. CD-ABSTR-93. Washington, DC: U.S. Department of Commerce, Economics and Statistics Administration, Bureau of the Census, Data User Services Division, 1993. Primary source: U.S. National Center for Health Statistics. Unpublished data. *Notes:* 1. Cesarean rates are the number of cesarean deliveries per 100 total deliveries for specified category.

★ 144 ★

Pregnancy and Childbirth: Labor and Delivery

Childbirth Costs

Data below reflect the average total cost of maternity care, doctor's fees, and hospital charges.

	1986	1991
Normal delivery		
Midwest	$2,460	$4,541
United States	2,550	4,720
Caesarean		
Midwest	4,220	7,334
United States	4,270	7,826

Source: "Costs of Having a Baby." *USA TODAY,* 21 March 1993, p. 15A. Primary source: Health Insurance Association of America. *Source Book of Health Insurance Data, 1992.*

★ 145 ★

Pregnancy and Childbirth: Labor and Delivery

Conceptions, Abortions, and Maternal Mortality

According to the World Health Organization, an average of 910,000 conceptions occur each day, of which 150,000 end in abortion. Worldwide, 1 woman dies each minute because of complications during pregnancy or childbirth.

Source: "U.N. Agency on Sex: Pitfalls and Promise." *New York Times,* 25 June 1992, p. A12.

★ 146 ★

Pregnancy and Childbirth: Labor and Delivery

Tuesdays and Birthdays

According to the National Center for Health Statistics (NCHS), more babies are born on Tuesdays than any other day. In 1988, for example, an average of 11,700 babies were born on Tuesdays—9 percent more than the daily average for that year. Similarly, more babies are born in September than any other month. In 1990, there were an average of 12,100 babies born every day in September, compared with a daily average of 11,400 for the entire year.

Source: Waldrop, Judith. "Seasons: The Birthday Boost." *American Demographics* 13 (September 1991), p. 4.

Pregnancy and Childbirth: Prenatal Care

★ 147 ★

Barriers to Prenatal Care

Figures show the percentage of women who cited barriers to prenatal care.

Barrier	Inadequate care	Adequate care
Financial		
Difficulty with insurance	54.5[1]	16.0
Difficulty paying for care	69.7[1]	22.1
Organizational		
Difficulty with appointments	24.6[1]	6.5

[Continued]

★ 147 ★

Barriers to Prenatal Care
[Continued]

Barrier	Inadequate care	Adequate care
Difficulty getting off work or school	5.9	4.9
Difficulty arranging for child care	16.1	11.1
Transportation problems	42.4[1]	21.5
Long waits in provider's office	31.6	31.7
Don't know where to obtain care	37.0[1]	14.6
Personal		
Care poorly valued or understood	25.0[1]	3.7
Didn't know was pregnant	33.2[1]	16.7
Ambivalence or fear about pregnancy	46.0[1]	19.5
Alcohol or drug use	8.1[1]	2.0
Excessive physical or psychological stress	35.3[1]	7.7

Source: Harvey, S. Marie, and Kathy S. Faber. "Obstacles to Prenatal Care Following Implementation of a Community-Based Program to Reduce Financial Barriers." *Family Planning Perspective* 25, no. 1 (January/February 1993), p. 34. *Note:* 1. $p < 001$.

Women's Health

★ 148 ★

AIDS and Women Worldwide

According to a study done by the United Nations, an average of 3,000 women contract the AIDS virus and 500 die every day worldwide. Seventy percent of these women are between the ages of 15 and 25.

Source: "UN Says AIDS Hits Younger Women Harder." *Detroit Free Press,* 29 July 1993, p. 2A.

★ 149 ★
Women's Health

Breast Cancer Cases, by Age: 1992

Nearly half (47.6 percent) of all breast cancer cases in 1992 occurred among women aged 60 or above, yet older women are less likely to have had a mammogram than their younger counterparts.

Age range	Number of cases	Percent of total
40-44	13,100	7.3
45-49	15,800	8.8
50-54	14,900	8.3
55-59	15,800	8.8
60-64	20,700	11.5
65-69	23,800	13.2
70-74	22,000	12.2
75-79	19,300	10.7
Percent who have had mammograms		
50-64	-	34.0
65-74	-	29.0
75-84	-	22.0
85+	-	13.0

Source: Springfield News-Leader, 20 March 1993, p. 4A. Primary source: American Cancer Society; National Cancer Institute. *Note:* A dash (-) stands for not reported by original source.

★ 150 ★
Women's Health

Breast Self-Examinations

Data below show the percent of women 18 years of age and older who know how to do breast self-examination. Data also indicate the percent of those who know how to do breast self-examination and who do the procedure at least 12 times a year. Data are provided by age and selected characteristics for 1990.

Characteristic	Knew breast self-examination					Did breast self-examination				
	Total	18-29 years	30-44 years	45-64 years	65 years and over	Total	18-29 years	30-44 years	45-64 years	65 years and over
All women[1]	88.1	84.9	92.7	90.6	80.5	43.1	36.6	43.6	47.1	45.4
Education level										
Less than 12 years	76.9	75.6	81.3	81.6	71.9	43.9	35.3	41.8	48.8	45.8
12 years	89.7	84.4	93.0	92.9	85.8	43.6	36.7	45.2	46.6	45.2
More than 12 years	92.8	89.5	95.4	94.1	88.6	42.2	36.8	42.7	46.5	45.2
13-15 years	91.7	88.3	95.0	92.4	89.9	43.1	38.5	45.1	44.4	46.6
16 years or more	94.0	91.7	95.7	95.8	86.8	41.3	33.7	40.4	48.6	43.1

[Continued]

★ 150 ★

Breast Self-Examinations
[Continued]

Characteristic	Knew breast self-examination					Did breast self-examination				
	Total	18-29 years	30-44 years	45-64 years	65 years and over	Total	18-29 years	30-44 years	45-64 years	65 years and over
Income										
Less than $10,000	80.0	81.0	84.8	79.6	76.4	42.2	36.2	40.5	49.0	45.9
$10,000-$19,999	85.3	82.2	90.9	87.2	82.1	43.0	39.4	41.5	47.0	44.6
$20,000-$34,999	90.6	86.8	93.2	93.8	86.2	42.3	33.9	44.0	47.2	45.3
$35,000-$49,999	93.3	89.2	95.7	94.1	89.2	43.1	39.9	43.0	47.4	38.7
$50,000 or more	92.5	87.1	94.9	94.0	83.2	41.5	31.3	42.6	44.4	48.2
Race										
White	88.8	85.6	93.5	91.2	81.9	42.3	35.6	42.7	46.1	44.3
Black	86.0	84.8	92.4	88.4	68.3	50.9	43.1	51.3	55.6	61.8
Hispanic origin										
Hispanic	74.7	70.4	77.9	78.0	71.7	44.1	37.7	46.2	47.1	53.6
Non-Hispanic	89.2	87.0	94.2	91.5	80.8	43.1	36.5	43.4	47.1	45.1
Geographic region										
Northeast	86.5	83.2	92.6	89.1	77.4	42.0	35.3	43.7	44.9	42.4
Midwest	90.5	88.0	94.9	92.5	83.3	41.3	33.0	43.1	44.1	44.9
South	89.2	88.3	94.3	90.9	79.3	46.0	39.8	47.0	49.0	49.3
West	84.8	77.2	88.0	89.3	83.1	41.6	36.2	38.6	50.2	42.6
Marital status										
Currently married	90.6	87.8	93.1	92.0	83.8	44.5	39.2	43.6	47.7	48.6
Formerly married	84.8	87.0	92.5	88.5	78.3	43.8	37.3	44.1	45.7	43.4
Never married	82.8	81.3	90.2	80.6	77.4	36.4	33.4	43.1	44.4	37.6
Employment status										
Currently employed	91.3	87.0	94.3	92.1	86.0	42.9	36.3	44.1	47.3	48.1
Unemployed	90.2	87.0	94.0	90.1	91.0	40.7	37.3	43.2	43.0	41.2[2]
Not in labor force	83.4	79.5	87.7	88.6	79.8	43.8	37.3	42.1	47.1	45.0

Source: U.S. Department of Health and Human Services. Public Health Service. Centers for Disease Control and Prevention. National Center for Health Statistics. *Health Promotion and Disease Prevention: United States, 1990.* Vital and Health Statistics, Series 10, no. 185. Hyattsville, MD: U.S. Department of Health and Human Services, Public Health Service, Centers for Disease Control and Prevention, National Center for Health Statistics, n.d., p. 31. *Notes:* Data are based on household interviews of the civilian noninstitutionalized population. The survey design, general qualifications, and information on the reliability of the estimates are given in Appendix 1 in the original source. Denominator for each cell excludes unknowns. 1. Includes women with unknown sociodemographic characteristics. 2. Figure does not meet standard of reliability or precision (more than 30-percent relative standard error in numerator of percent or rate).

★ 151 ★

Women's Health

Death Rates of Women From Selected Cancers: 1990

Data reflect death rates per 100,000 Americans.

Cancer	Death rate
Lung	32
Breast	28
Uterine	7

Source: "The War's Toll." *Detroit Free Press,* 3 July 1994, p. F1.

★ 152 ★

Women's Health

Frequency of Osteoporosis in Older Women

Osteoporosis affects 1 in 4 women over age 60 and is a major cause of fractures in the spine, hip, and wrist. White women are affected most often, particularly those who have a family history of osteoporosis or who have had their ovaries removed at early ages. Women with fair skin or small frames also are susceptible. Men are much less likely than women to contract osteoporosis because of their denser bone structure, among other factors.

Source: U.S. Department of Health and Human Services. Public Health Service. National Institute on Aging. *Bound for Good Health: A Collection of Age Pages.* Bethesda, MD: National Institute on Aging, c. 1991, n.p.

★ 153 ★

Women's Health

Hysterectomies

Cost for a hysterectomy varies. The table below provides the average cost for the surgery in selected cities.

[In dollars]

City	Cost
New York, New York	4,165
Atlanta, Georgia	1,885

Source: The Universal Almanac, 1992. Kansas City, MO: Andrews and McMeel, 1991, p. 262. Primary source: Health Insurance Association of America.

★ 154 ★

Women's Health

Leading Causes of Death for Women: 1990

Figures represent the numbers of women who died from leading killers—
heart disease, cancer, and strokes—in 1990.

Cause of death	Number
Heart disease	359,270
Cancer	237,039
Lung cancer	51,436
Breast cancer	43,391
Stroke	87,391

Source: Painter, Kim. "'Don't Worry About Women' Was Lesson." *USA TODAY,* 10 February 1993, p. 1A. Primary source: National Center for Health Statistics.

★ 155 ★

Women's Health

Life Expectancy and Good Health for Women

Eliminating behaviors that promote heart disease extends the average life
expectancy of a woman by 3.3 years.

Action	Amount added to life expectancy
Cholesterol under 200	10 months
Quitting smoking	8 months
Controlling blood pressure	5 months
Controlling weight	5 months

Source: Scan/Info 3 (May 1991), p. 19. *Scan/Info* is a publication of the Los Angeles Public Library, State of California. Primary sources: *San Francisco Chronicle,* 26 April 1991, p. A30; *Circulation* (April 1991).

★ 156 ★

Women's Health

Pap Smear Testing

According to a study by Marianne C. Fahs and her colleagues at Mount Sinai Medical Center and Memorial Sloan-Kettering Cancer Center in New York, pap smear testing every 3 years for women over 65 years of age would help reduce death from cervical cancer by 73 percent and cost an average of $2,254 per life saved each year.

Source: Winslow, Ron. "Pap Smears for Some Women Over 65 Are Cost-Effective, Study Says." *Wall Street Journal,* 15 September 1992, p. B6.

★ 157 ★

Women's Health

Screening for Ovarian Cancer

Dr. Marilyn Schapira, a researcher at the Medical College of Wisconsin in Milwaukee, and her colleagues found that mass screening for ovarian cancer would add only hours to women's lives. In fact, only 8 hours would be added to the average life expectancy of a 40-year-old woman.

Source: Levy, Doug. "Mass Ovarian Cancer Testing Impractical." *USA TODAY*, 1 June 1993, p. D1.

★ 158 ★

Women's Health

Women Who Have Had Mammograms

Table indicates the percent of women 35 years of age and older who have ever had a mammogram. Data are provided by age and selected characteristics for 1990.

Characteristic	Total 35 years and over	35-39 years	40-49 years	50-59 years	60-69 years	70 years and over
All women[1]	57.7	39.5	64.3	67.9	61.7	50.1
Education level						
Less than 12 years	44.9	29.9	45.4	51.3	49.9	41.3
12 years	59.0	37.6	63.3	69.1	62.7	54.7
More than 12 years	65.5	43.0	71.3	78.8	74.3	63.4
13-15 years	63.2	40.2	69.0	76.3	72.3	60.6
16 years or more	67.9	45.7	73.4	81.5	76.6	67.4
Income						
Less than $10,000	40.9	28.1	43.2	44.5	43.2	41.3
$10,000-$19,999	50.3	26.7	49.1	55.1	57.0	51.6
$20,000-$34,999	58.9	37.8	63.1	68.1	64.6	56.8
$35,000-$49,999	62.9	43.0	66.9	76.2	72.0	58.7
$50,000 or more	71.4	47.4	76.8	82.2	77.2	64.9
Race						
White	58.9	40.9	65.6	69.2	63.5	50.2
Black	51.3	35.7	56.3	61.9	49.1	49.2
Hispanic origin						
Hispanic	49.4	35.5	50.2	58.3	55.8	48.6
Non-Hispanic	58.2	39.8	65.4	68.5	62.0	50.1
Geographic region						
Northeast	58.4	41.4	60.4	70.7	63.5	51.0
Midwest	57.7	40.8	67.0	66.5	61.2	47.9

[Continued]

★ 158 ★

Women Who Have Had Mammograms
[Continued]

Characteristic	Total 35 years and over	35-39 years	40-49 years	50-59 years	60-69 years	70 years and over
South	55.4	40.5	63.0	65.0	56.9	46.4
West	61.1	34.6	67.2	71.4	69.9	59.3
Marital status						
Currently married	61.5	40.8	66.6	71.0	64.0	59.9
Formerly married	51.7	35.3	60.3	60.5	57.7	44.8
Never married	47.4	36.4	48.4	55.1	59.5	47.7
Employment status						
Currently employed	60.5	40.5	65.8	70.3	65.2	57.1
Unemployed	52.9	34.6	54.8	63.0	72.0	60.0[2]
Not in labor force	55.1	36.6	60.6	64.2	60.2	49.6

Source: U.S. Department of Health and Human Services. Public Health Service. Centers for Disease Control and Prevention. National Center for Health Statistics. *Health Promotion and Disease Prevention: United States, 1990.* Vital and Health Statistics, Series 10, no. 185. Hyattsville, MD: U.S. Department of Health and Human Services, Public Health Service, Centers for Disease Control and Prevention, National Center for Health Statistics, n.d., p. 58. *Notes:* Data are based on household interviews of the civilian noninstitutionalized population. The survey design, general qualifications, and information on the reliability of the estimates are given in Appendix 1 in the original source. Denominator for each cell excludes unknowns. 1. Includes women with unknown sociodemographic characteristics. 2. Figure does not meet standard of reliability or precision (more than 30-percent relative standard error in numerator of percent or rate).

Chapter 3
HEALTH CARE ESTABLISHMENT

This chapter features close to 100 tables profiling the role of services and care providers in ensuring the health and well-being of Americans. Covered agencies include doctors' offices, home health care services, hospitals, and long-term care facilities. Tables convey the availability, frequency, and costs associated with specific treatments, practices, and procedures. Tables emphasize trends in health care—for example, visits to alternative therapists and the growth of outpatient services. Data also are provided for consumer-interest topics such as blood bank recalls, hospital overcharges, and performance of inappropriate or unnecessary procedures. Leading providers in selected medical specialities—as well as the cost of common procedures by specialists—will be found in this chapter. Additional information regarding medical specialties has been included in the chapter on Medical Professions.

Blood Banks

★ 159 ★

Blood Bank Errors and Accidents: 1990-1994

The table below indicates the number of reports received by the U.S. Food and Drug Administration (FDA) regarding errors and accidents in the testing, processing, or distributing of donated blood. According to the source, the FDA received 29,586 reports from January 1990 through April 1994.

Problem	Number reported
Storage and shipping	2,506
Inadequate testing for blood type	2,025
Inadequate testing for hepatitis	621
Incorrect product released[1]	621
Donor called back to report hepatitis-related illness	581
Donor later reported history of exchanging sex for drugs or money	433
Donor later reported having sex with an intravenous drug user	433
Donor later reported having had sex with a man who had sex with another man	322
Inadequate testing for HIV	151
Inadequate testing for syphilis	112

[Continued]

★ 159 ★

Blood Bank Errors and Accidents: 1990-1994
[Continued]

Problem	Number of
Donor later reported that a sexual partner tested HIV positive	109
Blood accepted from donor with high risk of AIDS	50
Blood accepted from donor with high risk of hepatitis	36

Source: Newman, Richard J., Doug Podolsky, and Penny Loeb. "Bad Blood." *U.S. News & World Report* 116, no. 25, 27 June 1994, p. 68. *Note:* 1. For example, wrong blood type or plasma instead of platelets.

★ 160 ★

Blood Banks

Blood Centers With Frequent Recall Notices: 1989-1994

The table below presents information about blood centers that received 10 or more recall notices from the U.S. Food and Drug Administration because of failures to meet safety standards. Data were accumulated from October 1989 through March 1994.

Blood bank	Number of recalls	Units recalled
Red Cross (Baltimore, Maryland)	19	149
BloodCare (Dallas, Texas)	15	3,928
Red Cross (St. Paul, Minnesota)	15	95
Red Cross (Charlotte, North Carolina)	14	214
Central Indiana Regional Blood Center (Indianapolis, Indiana)	13	60
Red Cross (Portland, Oregon)	12	124
Red Cross (Peoria, Illinois)	11	62
LifeSource Blood Services (Glenview, Illinois)	11	343
Red Cross (Dedham, Massachusetts)	11	91
Belle Bonfils Memorial Blood Center (Denver, Colorado)	10	15,955
Red Cross (St. Louis, Missouri)	10	20

Source: Newman, Richard J., Doug Podolsky, and Penny Loeb. "Bad Blood." *U.S. News & World Report* 116, no. 25, 27 June 1994, p. 68.

Contact With Health Care Providers

★ 161 ★

General Medical Examinations

Data show the number and percent of U.S. office visits in which general medical examination was the patient's primary reason for seeing the doctor. The median number of diagnostic services per visit also are provided.

	Race[1]		Ethnicity[1]	
	White	Black and other non-white races	Non-Hispanic	Hispanic
Number	27,730,449	3,090,515	29,532,939	1,288,025
Percent	4.8	4.8	5.0	3.2
Median number of diagnostic services	3	3	3	3

Source: U.S. Department of Health and Human Services. Public Health Service. Health Resources and Services Administration. Health Status of Minorities and Low-Income Groups, 3rd ed. Washington, DC: U.S. Government Printing Office, n.d., p. 49. Ethnic classification of the patient was based on the physician's knowledge or judgment. Note: 1. Race and ethnicity are not mutually exclusive classifications.

★ 162 ★

Contact With Health Care Providers

House Call Charges

Figures indicate the fees of physicians for providing primary care in a home setting.

[In dollars]

Charges	Mean	Range	Median
Charge for house call	59.98	18.00-220.00	50.00
Charge required to make house calls financially feasible	112.66	10.00-600.00	100.00

Source: Stevens, Larry. "House Calls; Financial Aspects for Physicians." American Medical News 36, no. 33, 6 September 1993, p. 20. Primary source: American Medical Association, Department of Geriatric Health. Note: Based on a 45- to 60-minute visit.

★ 163 ★

Contact With Health Care Providers

House Calls

Figures indicate the availability of physicians for providing primary care in a home setting.

[In percentages]

Medical specialty	Number of house calls	
	1 or more	24 or more
Family practice	65	14
Internal medicine	43	8

Source: Stevens, Larry. "House Calls; Financial Aspects for Physicians." *American Medical News* 36, no. 33, 6 September 1993, p. 20. Primary source: American Medical Association, Department of Geriatric Health.

★ 164 ★

Contact With Health Care Providers

Interval Since Last Physician Contact: 1991

The table below shows the percent distribution and number of persons contacting physicians at specified intervals.

Characteristic	Interval since last contact									
	Percent distribution[1]					Number in thousands[1]				
	All intervals[2]	Less than 1 year	1 year to less than 2 years	2 years to less than 5 years	5 years or more	All intervals[3]	Less than 1 year	1 year to less than 2 years	2 years to less than 5 years	5 years or more
All persons[4]	100.0	78.5	9.9	8.1	3.5	248,713	191,945	24,138	19,881	8,439
Age										
Under 5 years	100.0	94.4	4.5	1.0	0.1[5]	19,379	17,963	852	192	28
5-17 years	100.0	78.0	12.9	7.3	1.7	46,142	35,316	5,832	3,321	778
18-24 years	100.0	73.6	12.7	10.4	3.4	24,641	17,733	3,053	2,500	814
25-44 years	100.0	73.4	11.3	10.7	4.6	81,098	58,515	9,008	8,512	3,648
45-64 years	100.0	78.0	8.7	8.6	4.7	47,162	36,212	4,031	3,985	2,189
65-74 years	100.0	78.0	8.7	8.6	4.7	47,162	36,212	4,031	3,985	2,189
75 years and over	100.0	89.8	4.0	3.7	2.5	11,991	10,634	479	440	293
Sex and age										
Male										
All ages	100.0	73.0	11.4	10.7	4.9	120,724	86,437	13,448	12,658	5,795
Under 18 years	100.0	82.7	10.5	5.5	1.4	33,535	27,201	3,446	1,808	448
18-44 years	100.0	63.8	14.1	15.3	6.8	51,912	32,325	7,163	7,764	3,424
45-64 years	100.0	72.9	10.0	10.7	6.3	22,626	16,220	2,226	2,388	1,412
65 years and over	100.0	85.4	4.9	5.6	4.1	12,652	10,692	613	699	511
Female										
All ages	100.0	83.7	8.5	5.7	2.1	127,988	105,508	10,690	7,223	2,645
Under 18 years	100.0	83.1	10.3	5.4	1.1	31,986	26,079	3,239	1,706	359
18-44 years	100.0	82.7	9.2	6.1	2.0	53,827	43,923	4,897	3,249	1,038
45-64 years	100.0	82.7	7.5	6.6	3.2	24,536	19,992	1,805	1,597	777
65 years and over	100.0	89.1	4.3	3.9	2.7	17,640	15,514	748	672	471

[Continued]

★ 164 ★

Interval Since Last Physician Contact: 1991
[Continued]

Characteristic	Interval since last contact									
	Percent distribution[1]					Number in thousands[1]				
	All intervals[2]	Less than 1 year	1 year to less than 2 years	2 years to less than 5 years	5 years or more	All intervals[3]	Less than 1 year	1 year to less than 2 years	2 years to less than 5 years	5 years or more
Race and age										
White										
All ages	100.0	79.0	9.6	8.1	3.4	208,202	161,835	19,640	16,505	6,918
Under 18 years	100.0	83.8	9.8	5.3	1.1	52,593	43,348	5,062	2,716	577
18-44 years	100.0	73.9	11.4	10.6	4.2	87,785	63,769	9,797	9,127	3,617
45-64 years	100.0	77.9	8.8	8.6	4.7	40,628	31,167	3,524	3,454	1,868
65 years and over	100.0	87.6	4.7	4.5	3.2	27,197	23,551	1,257	1,209	856
Black										
All ages	100.0	77.6	11.4	7.8	3.2	30,896	23,433	3,441	2,343	966
Under 18 years	100.0	78.7	13.4	6.3	1.7	10,321	7,899	1,343	634	166
18-44 years	100.0	73.6	12.7	9.7	4.1	13,151	9,452	1,630	1,240	521
45-64 years	100.0	81.1	8.1	7.0	3.8	4,861	3,868	387	333	182
65 years and over	100.0	87.6	3.2	5.3	3.9	2,563	2,213	81	135	98
Family income and age										
Under $10,000										
All ages	100.0	80.0	8.2	7.6	4.1	23,892	18,847	1,942	1,802	968
Under 18 years	100.0	81.9	9.7	6.0	2.3	6,823	5,472	651	404	152
18-44 years	100.0	75.9	9.4	9.8	5.0	9,313	6,988	867	898	457
45-64 years	100.0	78.4	7.4	7.7	6.5	3,044	2,355	222	230	194
65 years and over	100.0	86.4	4.3	5.8	3.5	4,712	4,032	202	270	165
$10,000-$19,999										
All ages	100.0	77.0	9.5	9.0	4.5	37,984	28,806	3,544	3,383	1,689
Under 18 years	100.0	78.6	11.8	7.6	2.2	10,092	7,743	1,144	753	212
18-44 years	100.0	70.6	11.2	12.2	6.0	14,600	10,152	1,609	1,754	863
45-64 years	100.0	77.6	7.6	9.3	5.5	5,742	4,414	433	531	310
65 years and over	100.0	86.6	4.8	4.6	4.1	7,549	6,498	357	345	305
$20,000-$34,999										
All ages	100.0	77.2	10.5	8.8	3.5	53,182	40,596	5,499	4,648	1,830
Under 18 years	100.0	81.4	11.6	6.1	0.9	14,610	11,705	1,670	882	128
18-44 years	100.0	72.1	12.0	11.5	4.5	23,917	17,035	2,825	2,717	1,062
45-64 years	100.0	76.6	8.8	9.1	5.5	8,900	6,774	775	804	487
65 years and over	100.0	89.0	4.0	4.3	2.7	5,755	5,081	230	245	153
$35,000 or more										
All ages	100.0	80.9	9.4	7.2	2.5	89,200	71,217	8,312	6,326	2,198
Under 18 years	100.0	87.4	8.4	3.7	0.5	24,142	20,849	2,014	872	128
18-44 years	100.0	76.6	10.9	9.4	3.1	41,023	30,948	4,416	3,790	1,273
45-64 years	100.0	79.9	8.8	7.7	3.6	19,641	15,520	1,702	1,496	694
65 years and over	100.0	89.6	4.1	3.9	2.4	4,395	3,899	180	168	103
Geographic region										
Northeast	100.0	81.2	8.8	7.1	2.9	50,300	40,317	4,387	3,519	1,447
Midwest	100.0	79.5	9.6	7.9	3.0	59,735	46,871	5,657	4,666	1,766
South	100.0	76.8	11.0	8.7	3.5	84,008	63,138	9,009	7,162	2,918
West	100.0	77.7	9.5	8.5	4.3	54,670	41,620	5,086	4,534	2,308
Place of residence										
MSA[6]	100.0	79.0	9.7	7.9	3.4	194,020	150,879	18,558	14,996	6,448
Central city	100.0	79.1	9.7	7.7	3.4	76,512	59,574	7,324	5,828	2,554

[Continued]

★ 164 ★

Interval Since Last Physician Contact: 1991
[Continued]

Characteristic	Interval since last contact									
	Percent distribution[1]					Number in thousands[1]				
	All intervals[2]	Less than 1 year	1 year to less than 2 years	2 years to less than 5 years	5 years or more	All intervals[3]	Less than 1 year	1 year to less than 2 years	2 years to less than 5 years	5 years or more
Not central city	100.0	79.0	9.7	7.9	3.4	117,508	91,305	11,234	9,168	3,894
Not MSA[6]	100.0	76.7	10.4	9.1	3.7	54,693	41,066	5,580	4,885	1,991

Source: U.S. Department of Health and Human Services. Public Health Service. Centers for Disease Control and Prevention. National Center for Health Statistics. Current Estimates From the National Health Interview Survey, 1991. Vital and Health Statistics, Series 10: Data From the National Health Survey, no. 184. DHHS publication no. (PHS) 93-1512. Hyattsville, MD: U.S. Department of Health and Human Services, Public Health Service, Centers for Disease Control and Prevention, National Center for Health Statistics, December 1992, pp. 116-117. Notes: Data are based on household interviews of the civilian noninstitutionalized population. The survey design, general qualifications, and information on the reliability of the estimates are given in Appendix 1 in the original source. 1. Includes physician contacts while an overnight patient in a hospital. 2. Excludes unknown interval. 3. Includes unknown interval. 4. Includes other races and unknown family income. 5. Figure does not meet standard of reliability or precision. 6. MSA is metropolitan statistical area.

★ 165 ★

Contact With Health Care Providers

Obstetric and Gynecology Care Fees

Table reflects the median fees charged by obstetricians and gynecologists for selected treatments and procedures.

[In dollars]

Procedure or treatment	Cost
Complete OB care, cesarean section	2,400.00
Hysterectomy (total, abdominal)	2,197.00
Complete OB care, routine vaginal delivery	2,000.00
Laparoscopy with fulguration of oviducts	1,000.00
Dilation and curettage for abortion[1]	600.00
Dilation and evacuation for abortion	600.00
Dilation and curettage (diagnostic)[1]	572.00

Source: "The Range of Fees for OBG Services." Medical Economics, 11 October 1993, pp. 122-123. Notes: "OB" stands for obstetric. 1. In hospital.

★ 166 ★

Contact With Health Care Providers

Office Visits: 1991

The table below shows the number and percent of office visits. Data provided by patient's reason for the visit.

[Number of visits in thousands]

Primary reason for office visit	Number	Percent
All visits	669,689	100.0
Symptom module	385,861	57.6
General symptoms	44,230	6.6
Symptoms referable to:		
Psychological/mental disorders	18,291	2.7
Nervous system[1]	21,066	3.1
Cardiovascular/lymphatic system	3,417	0.5
Eyes and ears	43,589	6.5
Respiratory system	76,764	11.5
Digestive system	27,074	4.0
Genitourinary system	31,265	4.7
Skin, hair, and nails	43,809	6.5
Musculoskeletal system	76,356	11.4
Disease module	64,926	9.7
Diagnostic, screening, and preventive module	101,002	15.1
Treatment module	65,333	9.8
Injuries and adverse effects module	20,462	3.1
Test results module	6,832	1.0
Administrative module	7,122	1.1
Other[2]	18,150	2.7

Source: Schappert, S.M. *National Ambulatory Medical Care Survey: 1991 Summary.* Advance data from Vital and Health Statistics. No. 230. Hyattsville, MD: National Center for Health Statistics, 1993, p. 7. *Notes:* 1. Excludes sense organs. 2. Includes problems and complaints not elsewhere classified, entries of "none," blanks, and illegible entries.

★ 167 ★

Contact With Health Care Providers

Pediatricians' Fees

Table reflects the median fees charged by pediatricians for selected treatments and procedures.

[In dollars]

Procedure or treatment	Cost
Circumcision of newborn[1]	100.00
History and examination of normal newborn	120.00
MMR virus vaccine (live)	40.00
DPT immunization	25.00

Source: "Pediatricians' Latest Charges." *Medical Economics,* 11 October 1993, p. 121. *Notes:* "MMR" stands for "measles-mumps-rubella." "DPT" stands for "diphtheria, pertussis, and tetanus." 1. Clamp procedure.

★ 168 ★

Contact With Health Care Providers

Physicians' Fee Increases: 1983-1993

Table reflects increases in fees for physicians' services.

[In percentages]

Year	Increases
1983	7.5
1984	6.0
1985	6.9
1986	7.8
1987	6.3
1988	7.5
1989	7.2
1990	7.4
1991	6.1
1992	6.3
1993 (projected)	6.3

Source: "Physicians' Fees and the Cost of Living." *Medical Economics,* 11 October 1993, p. 108. Primary source: Bureau of Labor Statistics. *Notes:* Projections are based on first 8 months. All other figures are based on the Consumer Price Index for December of each year.

★ 169 ★

Contact With Health Care Providers

Physicians' Services Expenditures: 1960-1991

The table below presents expenditures for physicians' services and percent distribution according to source of funds for selected years. Data were compiled by the Health Care Financing Administration.

[In percentages, except as noted]

Year	Total (in billion dollars)	Out-of-pocket payments	Private health insurance	Other private funds	Government Total[1]	Government Medicaid	Government Medicare
1960	5.3	62.7	30.2	0.1	7.1	-	-
1965	8.2	60.6	32.5	0.1	6.8	-	-
1970	13.6	42.8	35.2	0.1	21.9	4.6	11.8
1975	23.3	32.8	39.3	0.1	27.9	7.1	14.6
1980	41.9	26.9	42.9	0.1	30.2	5.1	19.0
1984	67.1	23.4	45.2	0.0	31.4	3.8	21.6
1985	74.0	21.8	45.6	0.0	32.6	3.9	22.5
1986	82.1	20.8	45.7	0.0	33.5	3.9	23.1
1987	93.0	20.4	45.8	0.0	33.8	3.8	23.3
1988	105.1	19.9	46.7	0.0	33.4	3.6	23.0
1989	116.1	19.4	46.4	0.0	34.1	3.7	23.6
1990	128.8	18.7	47.1	0.0	34.2	4.1	23.1
1991	142.0	18.1	47.0	0.0	34.8	4.9	23.1

Source: U.S. Department of Health and Human Services. Public Health Service. Centers for Disease Control and Prevention. National Center for Health Statistics. *Health, United States, 1992.* Hyattsville, MD: Public Health Service, 1993, p. 172. Primary source: Health Care Financing Administration. Office of National Health Statistics. Office of the Actuary. "National Health Expenditures: 1991." *Health Care Financing Review* 14, no. 2 (winter 1992). *Notes:* 1. Includes other government expenditures for these health care services; for example, care funded by the U.S. Department of Veterans Affairs and state and locally financed subsidies to hospitals.

★ 170 ★

Contact With Health Care Providers

Place of Physician Contact: 1991

The table below presents the number of persons contacting physicians each year. The number of contacts also is shown.

Characteristic	Number per person per year[1] All places[2]	Telephone	Office	Hospital	Other	Number in thousands[1] All places[2]	Telephone	Office	Hospital	Other
All persons[3]	5.8	0.7	3.3	0.8	0.9	1,430,509	163,637	829,934	198,054	228,952
Age										
Under 5 years	7.1	1.2	4.3	1.0	0.6	137,908	22,583	83,920	18,526	12,169
5-17 years	3.4	0.4	2.1	0.5	0.4	157,649	17,459	94,878	24,341	20,005
18-24 years	3.9	0.5	2.0	0.6	0.8	96,236	11,184	49,804	15,836	18,887
25-44 years	5.1	0.6	3.0	0.7	0.7	410,158	50,975	242,241	55,063	59,013
45-64 years	6.6	0.7	3.8	1.0	1.0	312,248	35,184	180,743	48,348	46,131
65-74 years	9.2	0.8	5.6	1.2	1.5	168,621	15,291	102,129	21,619	28,007

[Continued]

★ 170 ★

Place of Physician Contact: 1991
[Continued]

Characteristic	Number per person per year[1]					Number in thousands[1]				
	All places[2]	Telephone	Office	Hospital	Other	All places[2]	Telephone	Office	Hospital	Other
75 years and over	12.3	0.9	6.4	1.2	3.7	147,688	10,960	76,220	14,320	44,740
Sex and age										
Male										
All ages	4.9	0.5	2.8	0.8	0.8	588,739	61,951	338,654	92,918	91,002
Under 18 years	4.7	0.6	2.8	0.7	0.5	156,371	21,035	94,595	23,878	15,759
18-44 years	3.4	0.4	1.9	0.5	0.7	178,733	18,754	96,647	27,421	34,351
45-64 years	5.8	0.6	3.4	1.1	0.7	131,513	12,791	77,013	24,473	16,523
65 years and over	9.7	0.7	5.6	1.4	1.9	122,122	9,370	70,399	17,146	24,369
Female										
All ages	6.6	0.8	3.8	0.8	1.1	841,771	101,686	491,280	105,136	137,949
Under 18 years	4.4	0.6	2.6	0.6	0.5	139,186	19,008	84,202	18,990	16,415
18-44 years	6.1	0.8	3.6	0.8	0.8	327,662	43,405	195,398	43,477	43,548
45-64 years	7.4	0.9	4.2	1.0	1.2	180,735	22,392	103,730	23,875	29,608
65 years and over	11.0	1.0	6.1	1.1	2.7	194,187	16,882	107,950	18,793	48,378
Race and age										
White										
All ages	6.0	0.7	3.5	0.8	0.9	1,243,100	149,106	733,957	1259,040	192,510
Under 18 years	4.8	0.7	3.0	0.6	0.5	252,755	35,842	157,547	31,988	25,892
18-44 years	5.0	0.6	2.9	0.6	0.7	436,147	56,517	254,422	57,003	65,238
45-64 years	6.6	0.8	3.9	0.9	0.9	268,848	31,746	159,286	38,408	37,954
65 years and over	10.5	0.9	6.0	1.2	2.3	285,350	25,002	162,702	31,642	63,427
Black										
All ages	4.9	0.3	2.5	1.0	1.0	152,111	10,574	77,814	30,954	31,584
Under 18 years	3.2	0.3	1.6	0.8	0.5	32,924	2,908	16,728	8,137	4,963
18-44 years	4.3	0.3	2.3	0.8	0.8	56,169	3,716	30,832	10,618	10,628
45-64 years	7.5	0.6	3.0	1.8	1.4	36,262	2,755	17,533	8,626	7,024
65 years and over	10.4	0.5[4]	5.0	1.4	3.5	26,755	1,195	12,722	3,572	8,969
Family income and age										
Under $10,000										
All ages	7.6	0.8	3.5	1.4	1.9	181,066	18,281	83,195	33,905	44,678
Under 18 years	5.1	0.4	2.4	1.3	0.9	34,542	2,540	16,704	8,865	6,213
18-44 years	6.1	0.7	2.6	1.1	1.7	56,442	6,126	24,446	9,825	15,810
45-64 years	12.0	1.7	5.2	2.8	2.3	36,443	5,191	15,699	8,486	7,031
65 years and over	11.4	0.9	5.6	1.4	3.3	53,639	4,425	26,346	6,729	15,624
$10,000-$19,999										
All ages	6.0	0.6	3.3	1.0	1.0	227,466	24,678	127,017	37,778	36,872
Under 18 years	4.0	0.5	2.2	0.7	0.6	40,398	4,737	22,138	7,331	6,067
18-44 years	4.7	0.6	2.5	0.9	0.7	69,198	9,121	36,320	13,339	10,135
45-64 years	8.0	0.7	4.6	1.4	1.3	46,142	4,245	26,193	8,125	7,186
65 years and over	9.5	0.9	5.6	1.2	1.8	71,728	6,574	42,366	8,983	13,484
$20,000-$34,999										
All ages	5.6	0.7	3.3	0.8	0.8	296,359	34,870	174,292	41,094	44,685
Under 18 years	4.2	0.6	2.6	0.6	0.5	61,787	9,030	37,771	8,087	6,644
18-44 years	4.8	0.6	2.7	0.7	0.7	115,225	14,102	65,704	17,622	17,415
45-64 years	6.5	0.8	3.9	1.0	0.9	58,175	6,699	34,308	8,767	8,171
65 years and over	10.6	0.9	6.3	1.1	2.2	61,172	5,038	36,509	6,618	12,455

[Continued]

★ 170 ★

Place of Physician Contact: 1991
[Continued]

Characteristic	Number per person per year[1]					Number in thousands[1]				
	All places[2]	Telephone	Office	Hospital	Other	All places[2]	Telephone	Office	Hospital	Other
$35,000 or more										
All ages	5.5	0.8	3.5	0.6	0.7	494,419	67,068	307,852	56,998	58,354
Under 18 years	5.2	0.8	3.4	0.5	0.4	125,521	20,319	82,375	13,092	8,796
18-44 years	5.0	0.7	3.1	0.5	0.6	205,179	28,774	125,927	21,850	26,554
45-64 years	6.1	0.7	3.7	0.9	0.8	119,552	13,425	73,321	16,810	15,152
65 years and over	10.0	1.0	6.0	1.2	1.8	44,166	4,549	26,229	5,245	7,852
Geographic region										
Northeast	5.5	0.6	3.3	0.8	0.8	277,763	28,379	167,707	40,610	39,835
Midwest	5.9	0.7	3.3	0.8	1.0	352,515	44,529	198,112	48,131	59,782
South	5.7	0.6	3.4	0.7	0.9	480,527	53,862	287,059	59,601	75,698
West	5.8	0.7	3.2	0.9	1.0	319,704	36,866	177,057	49,712	53,638
Place of residence										
MSA[5]	5.9	0.7	3.4	0.8	1.0	1,137,796	136,211	654,468	154,110	185,153
Central city	6.0	0.7	3.3	0.9	1.1	460,637	50,393	251,054	70,591	85,528
Not central city	5.8	0.7	3.4	0.7	0.8	677,160	85,819	403,414	83,519	99,626
Not MSA[5]	5.4	0.5	3.2	0.8	0.8	292,713	27,425	175,467	43,944	43,798

Source: U.S. Department of Health and Human Services. Public Health Service. Centers for Disease Control and Prevention. National Center for Health Statistics. *Current Estimates From the National Health Interview Survey, 1991.* Vital and Health Statistics, Series 10: Data From the National Health Survey, no. 184. DHHS publication no. (PHS) 93-1512. Hyattsville, MD: U.S. Department of Health and Human Services, Public Health Service, Centers for Disease Control and Prevention, National Center for Health Statistics, December 1992, pp. 114-115. *Notes:* Data are based on household interviews of the civilian noninstitutionalized population. The survey design, general qualifications, and information on the reliability of the estimates are given in Appendix 1 in the original source. 1. Does not include physician contacts while an overnight patient in a hospital. 2. Includes unknown place of contact. 3. Includes other races and unknown family income. 4. Figure does not meet standard of reliability or precision. 5. MSA is metropolitan statistical area.

★ 171 ★

Contact With Health Care Providers

Telemedicine Costs

Telemedicine is home-based, health-care video conferencing. According to the source, telemedicine involves "using high speed transmissions (which could include satellite or microwave), robotized cameras, built-in microphones and speakers, TV screens, and a translation device called a codec [to make] telemedicine ... an interactive experience controlled by both the patient and doctor. Not only do they see and talk to each other in real time, but they zoom in, zoom out, focus on an entire room or on one person by using a computer keyboard, pen-based stylus or joystick." Use of telemedicine is growing primarily in rural communities.

[In dollars]

Item	Cost
Telemedicine equipment	9,000-50,000
Pay-per-hour charges	20

Source: Miller, Roy. "The New Housecall; Telemedicine Puts a Different Image on Seeing the Doctor." *Dallas Morning News,* 20 December 1993, home final edition, p. 3C.

★ 172 ★

Contact With Health Care Providers

Unnecessary Patient Care

Figures show all unneccessary care performed in selected cities.

City	Admits[1] (1,000)	Days (1,000)	Projected unnecessary (%)
Atlanta, Georgia	92	465	60
Baltimore, Maryland	94	527	65
Birmingham, Alabama	99	537	66
Boston, Massachusetts	90	531	65
Chicago, Illinois	91	504	63
Cincinnati, Ohio	85	438	58
Cleveland, Ohio	85	450	59
Dallas, Texas	84	443	58
Denver, Colorado	87	439	58
Des Molnes, Iowa	85	493	63
Detroit, Michigan	84	487	62
Hartford, Connecticut	84	498	63
Honolulu, Hawaii	70	391	53
Houston, Texas	86	502	63
Indianapolis, Indiana	86	486	62
Kansas City, Missouri	83	443	58
Las Vegas, Nevada	75	391	53
Little Rock, Arkansas	86	490	62
Los Angeles, California	83	426	57
Louisville, Kentucky	90	501	63
Memphis, Tennessee	93	565	67
Miami, Florida	88	500	63
Milwaukee, Wisconsin	93	432	57
Minneapolis-St. Paul, Minnesota	68	333	45
New Orleans, Louisiana	92	565	67
New York, New York	77	600	69
Newark, New Jersey	72	512	64
Norfolk, Virginia	81	436	58
Oklahoma City, Oklahoma	78	424	57
Philadelphia, Pennsylvania	86	542	66
Phoenix, Arizona	77	348	47
Pittsburgh, Pennsylvania	93	546	66
Portland, Oregon	75	322	43
Salt Lake City, Utah	80	407	55
San Diego, California	77	358	49
San Francisco, California	86	423	57
Seattle, Washington	73	325	43
St. Louis, Missouri	88	502	63
Tampa, Florida	82	425	57
Washington, District of Columbia	79	459	60

Source: "Appropriateness and the Effect of Guidelines." *Business and Health* 12, no. 3 (Special Report on Guidelines, 1994), p. 4. Primary source: *M&R Health Cost Guidelines, 1993.* Seattle, WA: Milliman & Robertson, Inc., c. 1993. *Notes:* 1. All acute patient care performed at medical, surgical, mental health, chemical dependency, obstetric, and skilled nursing facilities.

Drugs and Medicine

★ 173 ★

Arthritis Medicines

Research conducted by the Food and Drug Administration indicates that the medicines taken most by people over age 45 are those used to relieve the discomfort of arthritis. There are more than 100 forms of arthritis—with osteoarthritis, rheumatoid arthritis, and gout being the most common. For example, according to the Arthritis Foundation, more than 9 million Americans over 65 have some symptoms of osteoarthritis.

Source: U.S. Department of Health and Human Services. Public Health Service. National Institute on Aging. *Bound for Good Health: A Collection of Age Pages.* Bethesda, MD: National Institute on Aging, c. 1991, n.p.

★ 174 ★

Drugs and Medicine

Cost of Drug Development

A new drug takes an average of 12 years and $230 million to develop. For every successful drug that reaches the pharmacy, 10,000 compounds are rejected.

Source: "Penicillin From a Screen." *Newsweek* 120, 14 September 1992, p. 58.

★ 175 ★

Drugs and Medicine

Cost of Drugs

Table reflects the effect of inflation on drug prices. Rate of inflation was current at time of source's publication.

[In dollars]

Year	Cost of drug	Percent increase
1980	20.00	-
1991	53.76	268
1995	77.06	365
2000	120.88	604

Source: Pryor, David. "Communism Collapses ... But Nothing Changes the Pharmaceutical Industry's Skyrocketing Pricing Practices." *Congressional Record,* 10 September 1991, pS.12618.

★ 176 ★

Drugs and Medicine

Frequency of Price Increases and Percentage Increases for Ansaid

The table below reflects the intervals of price changes. Data are provided in price per pill.

[In dollars]

Date	Ansaid 100 mg price increase	Ansaid 50 mg price increase
01-01-89	0.8000	0.5125
09-17-89	0.8480	0.5433
03-05-90	0.9659	0.6188
01-11-91	1.0576	0.6775
01-03-92	1.0999	0.7046
Percent increase	37.49	37.48

Source: U.S. Senate Special Committee on Aging. *The Effects of Escalating Drug Costs on the Elderly: Hearing Before the Special Committee on Aging.* 102d Cong., 2nd sess., 22 April 1992. Serial no. 102-21. Washington, DC: U.S. Government Printing Office, 1992, p. 54.

★ 177 ★

Drugs and Medicine

Frequency of Price Increases and Percentage Increases for Axid

The table below reflects the intervals of price changes. Data are provided in price per pill.

[In dollars]

Date	Axid 300 mg price increase
05-01-88	1.8257
04-27-89	1.9353
04-10-90	2.0707
03-14-91	2.3813
01-03-92	2.5720
Percent increase	40.88

Source: U.S. Senate Special Committee on Aging. *The Effects of Escalating Drug Costs on the Elderly: Hearing Before the Special Committee on Aging.* 102d Cong., 2nd sess., 22 April 1992. Serial no. 102-21. Washington, DC: U.S. Government Printing Office, 1992, p. 55.

★ 178 ★

Drugs and Medicine

Frequency of Price Increases and Percentage Increases for Ceclor

The table below reflects the intervals of price changes. Data are provided in price per pill.

[In dollars]

Date	Ceclor 250 mg caps price increase
09-01-88	1.2783
04-01-89	1.3933
12-01-89	1.4908
10-15-90	1.6101
05-25-91	1.7550
03-15-92	1.8322
Percent increase	31.50

Source: U.S. Senate Special Committee on Aging. *The Effects of Escalating Drug Costs on the Elderly: Hearing Before the Special Committee on Aging.* 102d Cong., 2nd sess., 22 April 1992. Serial no. 102-21. Washington, DC: U.S. Government Printing Office, 1992, p. 56.

★ 179 ★

Drugs and Medicine

Frequency of Price Increases and Percentage Increases for Ceftin

The table below reflects the intervals of price changes. Data are provided in price per pill.

[In dollars]

Date	Ceftin 250 mg price increase	Ceftin 500 mg price increase
07-10-88	2.0150	3.7090
08-01-89	2.1960	4.1067
01-05-90	2.3495	4.3940
10-09-90	2.5375	4.7455
08-29-91	2.7666	5.1728
03-06-92	2.8885	5.4020
Percent increase	43.35	45.65

Source: U.S. Senate Special Committee on Aging. *The Effects of Escalating Drug Costs on the Elderly: Hearing Before the Special Committee on Aging.* 102d Cong., 2nd sess., 22 April 1992. Serial no. 102-21. Washington, DC: U.S. Government Printing Office, 1992, p. 55.

★ 180 ★

Drugs and Medicine

Frequency of Price Increases and Percentage Increases for Premarin

The table below reflects the intervals of price changes. Data are provided in price per pill.

[In dollars]

Date	Premarin 1.2 mg price increase	Premarin .626 mg price increase
04-01-89	0.2935	0.2143
07-28-89	0.3521	0.2574
03-16-90	0.3853	0.2816
09-01-90	0.42155	0.3081
03-15-91	0.4528	0.3309
02-24-92	0.4726	0.3454
Percent increase	61.02	61.18

Source: U.S. Senate Special Committee on Aging. *The Effects of Escalating Drug Costs on the Elderly: Hearing Before the Special Committee on Aging.* 102d Cong., 2nd sess., 22 April 1992. Serial no. 102-21. Washington, DC: U.S. Government Printing Office, 1992, p. 55.

★ 181 ★

Drugs and Medicine

Frequency of Price Increases and Percentage Increases for Prozac

The table below reflects the intervals of price changes. Data are provided in price per pill.

[In dollars]

Date	Prozac 20 mg price increase
01-04-88	1.3201
01-13-89	1.4389
09-28-89	1.5684
08-30-90	1.6782
05-09-91	1.8292
01-10-92	1.9298
Percent increase	46.19

Source: U.S. Senate Special Committee on Aging. *The Effects of Escalating Drug Costs on the Elderly: Hearing Before the Special Committee on Aging.* 102d Cong., 2nd sess., 22 April 1992. Serial no. 102-21. Washington, DC: U.S. Government Printing Office, 1992, p. 54.

★ 182 ★

Drugs and Medicine

Frequency of Price Increases and Percentage Increases for Ventolin

The table below reflects the intervals of price changes. Data are provided in price per pill.

[In dollars]

Date	Ventolin refill price increase per pill, tablet, etc.
12-18-88	0.7865
07-03-89	0.8953
07-02-90	0.9712
01-24-91	1.0106
06-29-91	1.0559
03-06-92	1.1036
Percent increase	40.32

Source: U.S. Senate Special Committee on Aging. *The Effects of Escalating Drug Costs on the Elderly: Hearing Before the Special Committee on Aging.* 102d Cong., 2nd sess., 22 April 1992. Serial no. 102-21. Washington, DC: U.S. Government Printing Office, 1992, p. 54.

★ 183 ★

Drugs and Medicine

Frequency of Price Increases and Percentage Increases for Xanax

The table below reflects the intervals of price changes. Data are provided in price per pill.

[In dollars]

Date	Xanax 0.5 mg price increase
04-01-88	0.3914
04-01-89	0.4461
07-17-89	0.4774
03-05-90	0.5438
01-11-91	0.5976
01-03-92	0.8490
Percent increase	65.82

Source: U.S. Senate Special Committee on Aging. *The Effects of Escalating Drug Costs on the Elderly: Hearing Before the Special Committee on Aging.* 102d Cong., 2nd sess., 22 April 1992. Serial no. 102-21. Washington, DC: U.S. Government Printing Office, 1992, p. 56.

★ 184 ★

Drugs and Medicine

Mixing Drugs

Older Americans comprise 12-13 percent of the population, but consume 25-30 percent of all medications, including heavy use of over-the-counter drugs. As a group, older people tend to have more long-term illnesses, such as arthritis, diabetes, high blood pressure, and heart disease. They also run the greatest risk of adverse drug interactions since—with advancing age—comes major changes in the body's ability to absorb and dispose of drugs and alcohol.

Source: U.S. Department of Health and Human Services. Public Health Service. National Institute on Aging. *Bound for Good Health: A Collection of Age Pages.* Bethesda, MD: National Institute on Aging, c. 1991, n.p.

★ 185 ★

Drugs and Medicine

rDNA Product Sales Worldwide

World sales of recombinant DNA (rDNA) pharmaceuticals were $4.420 billion in 1992 and are expected to be $7.130 billion in 1997. Data shown are distributed by type in millions of dollars and in percent for 1997.

Type	1992 ($ mil.)	1997 ($ mil.)	1997 share
Erythropoeitin	1,225	1,845	26.9
Human insulin	625	1,035	15.1
Alpha-interferon	565	1,020	14.9
G-CSF	405	870	12.7
Human growth hormone	575	660	9.6
Factor VIII	235	445	6.5
GM-CSF	70	305	4.4
Centoxin/E5 MAbs	75	220	3.2
Orthoclone OKT3	90	160	2.3
T-PA	230	120	1.8
Interleukin-2	20	50	0.7
CD4	-	45	0.7
Gamma-interferon	25	45	0.7
Beta-interferon	20	35	0.5
Hepatitis B Vacc. 50	105	-	0.0

Source: Bio/Technology, 11 March 1993, p. S37. Primary source: Robin Rodgers and Decision Resources, Inc.

Home Health Care

★ 186 ★

Cost Comparison of Inpatient and Inpatient/Home Treatment of Chronic Obstructive Pulmonary Disease Patients

From the source: "The results of the cost-identification analysis, detailed in the table, indicate that the reduction of inpatient stay of chronic obstructive pulmonary disease (COPD) patients in inpatient/home treatment saves approximately $450 per patient in health care resources. When quality of life is factored into the analysis, the cost savings attributed to inpatient/home therapy increases to $520 per patient. Thus, less intensive inpatient treatment of COPD is both cheaper and more cost-effective than the longer inpatient strategies."

[In dollars]

Cost component	Inpatient treatment strategy 1[1]	Inpatient/home treatment strategy 2[2]
Hospital inpatient costs	3,497.68	3,019.91
Physician inpatient costs	+ 50.19	none
Outpatient hospital and physician costs	none	+ 4.92
Personnel	none	+ 16.05
Home medical equipment, supplies and services	none	+ 28.06
Total	3,547.87	3,097.75
Quality of life adjustment	+ 73.13	none
Adjusted total	3,621.00	3,097.75

Source: U.S. Senate Committee on Aging. *Medicare Fraud and Abuse: A Neglected Emergency? Hearing Before the Special Committee on Aging.* 102d Cong., 1st sess., 2 October 1991. Serial no. 102-13. Washington, DC: U.S. Government Printing Office, 1992, p. 232. *Notes:* A plus value in a column reflects an incremental cost. Total costs are used for comparison only and do not reflect total cost of an episode. 1. Strategy #1: Inpatient treatment for COPD—The patient requires inpatient treatment for 7.5 days and then is released to the home setting for follow-up treatment. All patients will require home medical equipment. 2. Strategy #2: Shorter inpatient stay with more intensive home treatment—The patient receives only 6.1 days of inpatient therapy before being released to treatment in the home setting.

★ 187 ★

Home Health Care

Cost Comparison of Inpatient and Inpatient/Home Treatment of Hip Fractures

Inpatient/home treatment saves $2,016.19 per episode and $2,337.88 per quality-adjusted episode.

[In dollars]

Cost component	Inpatient treatment	Inpatient/home treatment
Hospital inpatient costs	6,500.21	4,383.83
Physician inpatient costs	+ 207.93	none
Outpatient hospital and physician costs	none	+ 93.49
Personnel	none	+ 165.57
Home medical equipment, supplies and services	none	+ 49.16
Total	6,708.14	4,692.05
Quality of life adjustment	+ 321.79	none
Adjusted total	7,029.93	4,692.05

Source: U.S. Senate Committee on Aging. *Medicare Fraud and Abuse: A Neglected Emergency? Hearing Before the Special Committee on Aging.* 102d Cong., 1st sess., 2 October 1991. Serial no. 102-13. Washington, DC: U.S. Government Printing Office, 1992, p. 225. *Notes:* A plus in one column reflects an incremental cost. Total costs are used for comparison only and do not reflect total cost of an episode.

★ 188 ★

Home Health Care

Cost Effectiveness of Home Care

The table below indicates the savings to society per quality-adjusted episode. From the source: "The pressure on providers to reduce length of inpatient stay as well as the development of locally managed home medical equipment services that allow for more care in the home are largely responsible for these savings. Physicians are increasingly aware of the availability of home medical equipment and home health care services and factor these choices into their practice decisions. Full realization of the potential of home health care services and home medical equipment services can achieve significant cost savings as well as improve patient satisfaction."

Type of patient	Savings per episode ($)	Prevalence (per year)	Annual savings ($)
Hip fracture	2,300	250,000	575,000,000
Amyotrophic Lateral Sclerosis with pneumonia (ALS)	300	1,533	459,900
Chronic Obstructive Pulmonary Disease (COPD)	520	93,184	48,455,680

Source: U.S. Senate Committee on Aging. *Medicare Fraud and Abuse: A Neglected Emergency? Hearing Before the Special Committee on Aging.* 102d Cong., 1st sess., 2 October 1991. Serial no. 102-13. Washington, DC: U.S. Government Printing Office, 1992, pp. 217, 233. Primary source: Lewin/ICF.

★ 189 ★

Home Health Care

Home Health Agency Visits for Chronic Obstructive Pulmonary Disease Patients

From the source: "The number of home health visits to patients and the cost of a home health visit are provided in the table below. Estimates for charge per visit are 1987 charges inflated to 1990 dollars at a rate of 5.5 percent per year. Assuming the length of an episode is 3 months, the charge per day can be calculated by dividing the total charges by the total days. The charge for an additional 1.4 days of home health visits totals $18.88. When 85 percent of charges is used as a proxy for costs, the total cost attributable to combination therapy is $16.05."

	Visits	Charge/visit ($)	Total charge ($)
Skilled nursing	10.61	74	785.14
Home health aide	5.24	55	288.20
Physical therapy	1.19	75	89.25
Occupational therapy; speech therapy; social work	0.72	83	51.12
Total			1,213.71

Source: U.S. Senate Committee on Aging. *Medicare Fraud and Abuse: A Neglected Emergency? Hearing Before the Special Committee on Aging.* 102d Cong., 1st sess., 2 October 1991. Serial no. 102-13. Washington, DC: U.S. Government Printing Office, 1992, p. 231. Primary source: Branch, L., H. Goldberg, V. Chen, and others. "Medicare Home Health Clients: Who Are They and What Services Do They Receive During an Episode of Care?" *Health Care Financing Review* (April 1990). *Note:* Chronic obstructive pulmonary disease often is referred to as COPD.

★ 190 ★

Home Health Care

Home Health Agency Visits for Pneumonia Patients Per Episode

Type of home visit	Pre-prospective payment system visits	Post-prospective payment system visits
Skilled nursing	0.160	0.455
Home health aide	0.068	0.288

Source: U.S. Senate Committee on Aging. *Medicare Fraud and Abuse: A Neglected Emergency? Hearing Before the Special Committee on Aging.* 102d Cong., 1st sess., 2 October 1991. Serial no. 102-13. Washington, DC: U.S. Government Printing Office, 1992, p. 227. Primary source: Abt Associates Inc. "Episodes of Hospitalization and PPS—Working Paper" (21 September 1988).

★ 191 ★

Home Health Care

Home Health Agency Visits Per Patient Episode

From the source: "A recent paper reports home health utilization by Medicare patients for specific diagnoses. Estimates of per visit charges are based on 1987 allowed charges inflated to 1990 dollars at a rate of 5.5 percent per year. Length of therapy for the inpatient strategy is assumed to be 9 weeks; while patients receiving inpatient and home therapy incur an additional 5.8 days of services at a charge of $194.79. When 85 percent of charges are used as a proxy for costs, the total cost attributable to combination therapy is $165.57."

	Visits	Charge/visit ($)	Total charge
Skilled nursing	8.56	74	633.44
Home health aide	7.63	55	419.65
Physical therapy	12.83	75	962.25
Occupational therapy; speech therapy; social work	1.21	83	100.43
Total			2,115.77

Source: U.S. Senate Committee on Aging. *Medicare Fraud and Abuse: A Neglected Emergency? Hearing Before the Special Committee on Aging.* 102d Cong., 1st sess., 2 October 1991. Serial no. 102-13. Washington, DC: U.S. Government Printing Office, 1992, p. 224. Primary source: Branch, L., H. Goldberg, V. Chen, and others. "Medicare Home Health Clients: Who Are They and What Services Do They Receive During an Episode of Care?" *Health Care Financing Review* (April 1990).

★ 192 ★

Home Health Care

Home Health Care: 1990

Home health care environment	The numbers
People requiring home health care	5 million
Total number of providers	11,000
Medicare certified	5,700
Hospitals	1,780
Total spending on home health care[1]	$7 billion
Medicare	$4 billion
Annual growth rate	20%
Cost comparison	
Skilled nursing care at home	$750/month
Skilled nursing care in an institution	$2,000/month

Source: U.S. Department of Commerce. *U.S. Industrial Outlook '92: Business Forecasts for 350 Industries.* Washington, DC: U.S. Government Printing Office, 1992, p. 43-3. *Note:* 1. Excludes home health care products.

★ 193 ★

Home Health Care

Home Health Care Expenditures, by Source: 1990

Total expenditures equal $6.9 billion.

Source	Percent
Medicare	42.0
Medicaid	32.0
Out-of-pocket	12.0
Private insurance	7.0
Other	7.0

Source: U.S. Department of Labor. Pension and Welfare Benefits Administration. *Trends in Health Benefits.* Washington, DC: U.S. Government Printing Office, 1993, p. 224. Primary source: Health Care Financing Administration, Office of the Actuary, 1992.

Hospitals

★ 194 ★

Hospital Care Expenditures: 1960-1991

Data below indicate expenditures for hospital care and the percent distribution according to source of funds for selected years. Data were compiled by the Health Care Financing Administration.

[In percentages, except as noted]

Year	Total (in billion dollars)	Out-of-pocket payments	Private health insurance	Other private funds	Government Total[1]	Government Medicaid	Government Medicare
1960	9.3	20.7	35.6	1.2	42.5	-	-
1965	14.0	19.6	40.9	1.9	37.6	-	-
1970	27.9	9.0	34.4	3.2	53.4	8.1	18.8
1975	52.4	8.4	34.4	2.8	54.5	8.8	21.9
1980	102.4	5.2	36.6	4.9	53.3	9.4	25.8
1984	157.5	5.1	36.1	4.6	54.1	9.1	28.8
1985	168.3	5.2	35.4	4.9	54.4	9.2	28.9
1986	179.8	4.8	35.5	5.0	54.7	9.2	28.2
1987	194.2	4.5	35.7	5.0	54.8	9.5	27.7
1988	212.0	4.9	36.0	5.3	53.9	9.4	27.1
1989	232.4	4.7	36.3	5.4	53.7	9.8	26.9
1990	258.1	4.0	36.6	5.4	54.0	11.2	26.1
1991	288.6	3.4	35.2	5.1	56.3	15.0	25.4

Source: U.S. Department of Health and Human Services. Public Health Service. Centers for Disease Control and Prevention. National Center for Health Statistics. *Health, United States, 1992.* Hyattsville, MD: Public Health Service, 1993, p. 172. Primary source: Health Care Financing Administration. Office of National Health Statistics. Office of the Actuary. "National Health Expenditures: 1991." *Health Care Financing Review* 14, no. 2 (winter 1992). *Notes:* 1. Includes other government expenditures for these health care services; for example, care funded by the U.S. Department of Veterans Affairs and state and locally financed subsidies to hospitals.

★ 195 ★

Hospitals

Hospital Overcharges

The General Accounting Office estimates that 99 percent of hospital bills contain overcharges. A study done by a private insurer estimates that the average hospital bill contains unnecessary charges of $1,400.

Source: Rosenthal, Elisabeth. "Confusion and Error Are Rife in Hospital Billing Practices." *New York Times,* 27 January 1993, p. C16. **Remarks:** Source includes a discussion of common errors in hospital billing practices.

★ 196 ★
Hospitals

Rural Hospitals

The average charge at rural hospitals is $850 per day. Urban hospitals, which offer a wide array of specialties, charge $1,350 a day.

Source: Smothers, Ronald. "150 Miles Away, the Doctor Is Examining Your Tonsils." *New York Times,* 16 September 1992, p. C14.

★ 197 ★
Hospitals

Top Ten Cardiology Departments at U.S. Hospitals and Health Care Facilities

The table below ranks hospitals according to a mathematical model. Rank is based on each hospital's overall score.

Hospital	Overall score	Reputational score	Mortality rate	COTH member	Residents to beds	Technology score	R.N.'s to beds	Board-certified M.D.'s to beds	Inpatient operations to beds
Mayo Clinic (Rochester, Minnesota)	100.0	32.5%	0.64	Yes	0.37	8	0.73	1.49	21.5
Cleveland Clinic (Cleveland, Ohio)	95.6	32.7%	0.76	Yes	0.59	9	1.47	0.38	19.9
Massachusetts General Hospital (Boston, Massachusetts)	68.9	19.8%	0.77	Yes	0.47	9	1.14	0.66	17.5
Stanford University Medical Center (Stanford, California)	56.0	15.5%	0.95	Yes	0.79	8	0.86	1.81	13.9
Duke University Medical Center (Durham, North Carolina)	54.8	14.1%	0.86	Yes	0.43	9	1.60	0.66	15.3
Bringham and Women's Hospital (Boston, Massachusetts)	54.2	11.7%	0.75	Yes	0.64	8	0.79	1.24	20.0
Emory University Hospital (Atlanta, Georgia)	51.1	12.5%	0.84	Yes	0.31	7	1.28	0.68	17.2
Johns Hopkins Hospital (Baltimore, Maryland)	47.4	8.9%	0.78	Yes	0.45	9	1.43	0.66	15.5
University of California San Francisco Medical Center (San Francisco, California)	45.5	6.8%	0.76	Yes	0.32	8	1.82	1.55	18.3
Texas Heart Institute/St. Luke's Episcopal Hospital (Houston, Texas)	43.4	12.7%	1.16	Yes	0.19	8	1.36	0.62	19.3

Source: "The 16 Specialties: From AIDS to Urology, 114 Hospitals That Offer Top Care." *U.S. News & World Report,* 18 July 1994, pp. 74, 77. *Notes:* "Reputational score" is the percentage of doctors surveyed who named the hospital. "Mortality rate" is the ratio of actual to expected deaths (lower is better). "COTH member" indicates member of Council of Teaching Hospitals. "Residents to beds" is the ratio of interns and residents to beds. "Technology score" is a specialty-specific index from 0 to 9. "R.N.'s to beds" is the ratio of registered nurses to beds. "Board-certified M.D.'s to beds" is the ratio of doctors certified in a specialty to the number of beds. "Inpatient operations to beds" is the ratio of annual inpatient operations to beds.

★ 198 ★
Hospitals

Top Ten Endocrinology Departments at U.S. Hospitals and Health Care Facilities

The table below ranks hospitals according to a mathematical model. Rank is based on each hospital's overall score.

Hospital	Overall score	Reputational score	Mortality rate	COTH member	Residents to beds	Technology score	R.N.'s to beds	Board-certified M.D.'s to beds
Mayo Clinic (Rochester, Minnesota)	100.0	42.5%	0.64	Yes	0.37	8	0.73	1.49
Massachusetts General Hospital (Boston, Massachusetts)	84.3	35.8%	0.77	Yes	0.47	11	1.14	0.66
University of California San Francisco Medical Center (San Francisco, California)	49.4	12.8%	0.76	Yes	0.32	10	1.82	1.55
UCLA Medical Center (Los Angeles, California)[1]	43.7	9.7%	0.77	Yes	0.71	11	1.20	0.82
University of Washington Medical Center (Seattle, Washington)	43.1	7.7%	0.73	Yes	0.30	10	2.06	1.90
Barnes Hospital (St. Louis, Missouri)	42.6	9.9%	0.76	Yes	0.47	11	0.81	0.90
Johns Hopkins Hospital (Baltimore, Maryland)	42.4	9.6%	0.78	Yes	0.45	11	1.43	0.66
University of Chicago Hospitals (Chicago, Illinois)	41.5	10.9%	0.91	Yes	0.75	11	1.38	0.73

[Continued]

★ 198 ★

Top Ten Endocrinology Departments at U.S. Hospitals and Health Care Facilities

[Continued]

Hospital	Overall score	Reputational score	Mortality rate	COTH member	Residents to beds	Technology score	R.N.'s to beds	Board-certified M.D.'s to beds
Deaconess Hospital (Boston, Massachusetts)	41.2	6.3%	0.69	Yes	0.63	10	1.33	0.93
University of Michigan Medical Center (Ann Arbor, Michigan)	40.3	10.2%	0.85	Yes	0.41	10	1.29	0.66

Source: "The 16 Specialties: From AIDS to Urology, 114 Hospitals That Offer Top Care." *U.S. News & World Report,* 18 July 1994, pp. 74, 78. *Notes:* "Reputational score" is the percentage of doctors surveyed who named the hospital. "Mortality rate" is the ratio of actual to expected deaths (lower is better). "COTH member" indicates member of Council of Teaching Hospitals. "Residents to beds" is the ratio of interns and residents to beds. "Technology score" is a specialty-specific index from 0 to 11. "R.N.'s to beds" is the ratio of registered nurses to beds. "Board-certified M.D.'s to beds" is the ratio of doctors certified in a specialty to the number of beds. "NA" indicates "not available." 1. UCLA stands for University of California, Los Angeles.

★ 199 ★

Hospitals

Top Ten Gastroenterology Departments at U.S. Hospitals and Health Care Facilities

The table below ranks hospitals according to a mathematical model. Rank is based on each hospital's overall score.

Hospital	Overall score	Reputational score	Mortality rate	COTH member	Residents to beds	Technology score	R.N.'s to beds	Board-certified M.D.'s to beds	Inpatient operations to beds
Mayo Clinic (Rochester, Minnesota)	100.0	39.7%	0.64	Yes	0.37	8	0.73	1.49	21.5
Johns Hopkins Hospital (Baltimore, Maryland)	67.7	23.7%	0.78	Yes	0.45	11	1.43	0.66	15.5
Massachusetts General Hospital (Boston, Massachusetts)	60.8	19.4%	0.77	Yes	0.47	11	1.14	0.66	17.5
Cleveland Clinic (Cleveland, Ohio)	55.5	15.5%	0.76	Yes	0.59	10	1.47	0.38	19.9
UCLA Medical Center (Los Angeles, California) [1]	53.5	14.3%	0.77	Yes	0.71	11	1.20	0.82	14.6
Duke University Medical Center (Durham, North Carolina)	51.6	15.7%	0.86	Yes	0.43	11	1.60	0.66	15.3
University of California San Francisco Medical Center (San Francisco, California)	49.3	11.2%	0.76	Yes	0.32	10	1.82	1.55	18.3
Mount Sinai Medical Center (New York, New York)	47.8	11.8%	0.79	Yes	0.50	9	1.50	1.11	12.3
Brigham and Women's Hospital (Boston, Massachusetts)	42.0	7.5%	0.75	Yes	0.64	10	0.79	1.24	20.0
University of Chicago Hospitals (Chicago, Illinois)	41.0	10.0%	0.91	Yes	0.75	10	1.38	0.73	17.3

Source: "The 16 Specialties: From AIDS to Urology, 114 Hospitals That Offer Top Care." *U.S. News & World Report,* 18 July 1994, pp. 74, 79. *Notes:* "Reputational score" is the percentage of doctors surveyed who named the hospital. "Mortality rate" is the ratio of actual to expected deaths (lower is better). "COTH member" indicates member of Council of Teaching Hospitals. "Residents to beds" is the ratio of interns and residents to beds. "Technology score" is a specialty-specific index from 0 to 11. "R.N.'s to beds" is the ratio of registered nurses to beds. "Board-certified M.D.'s to beds" is the ratio of doctors certified in a specialty to the number of beds. "Inpatient operations to beds" is the ratio of annual inpatient operations to beds. 1. UCLA stands for University of California, Los Angeles.

★ 200 ★

Hospitals

Top Ten Geriatrics Departments at U.S. Hospitals and Health Care Facilities

The table below ranks hospitals according to a mathematical model. Rank is based on each hospital's overall score.

Hospital	Overall score	Reputational score	Mortality rate	COTH member	Service mix	Residents to beds	Technology score	R.N.'s to beds	Geriatric services	Discharge planning	Board-certified M.D.'s to beds
UCLA Medical Center (Los Angeles, California) [1]	100.0	21.4%	0.77	Yes	7	0.71	12	1.20	4	2	0.82
Mount Sinai Medical Center (New York, New York)	92.7	19.1%	0.79	Yes	9	0.50	10	1.50	6	2	1.11
Duke University Medical Center (Durham, North Carolina)	80.4	16.4%	0.86	Yes	7	0.43	13	1.60	3	2	0.66
Beth Israel Hospital (Boston, Massachusetts)	75.4	12.4%	0.75	Yes	9	0.54	11	1.93	3	2	2.08

[Continued]

★ 200 ★

Top Ten Geriatrics Departments at U.S. Hospitals and Health Care Facilities
[Continued]

Hospital	Overall score	Reputational score	Mortality rate	COTH member	Service mix	Residents to beds	Technology score	R.N.'s to beds	Geriatric services	Discharge planning	Board-certified M.D.'s to beds
Johns Hopkins Hospital (Baltimore, Maryland)	73.2	13.1%	0.78	Yes	8	0.45	12	1.43	1	2	0.66
Massachusetts General Hospital (Boston, Massachusetts)	69.8	11.7%	0.77	Yes	8	0.47	13	1.14	4	2	0.66
University of Michigan Medical Center (Ann Arbor, Michigan)	58.1	8.7%	0.85	Yes	9	0.41	12	1.29	8	2	0.66
University of Washington Medical Center (Seattle, Washington)	55.6	6.0%	0.73	Yes	7	0.30	11	2.06	4	2	1.90
Mayo Clinic (Rochester, Minnesota)	55.3	5.2%	0.64	Yes	5	0.37	9	0.73	5	2	1.49
New York University Medical Center (New York, New York)	50.3	3.4%	0.62	Yes	3	0.20	11	1.15	0	2	1.25

Source: "The 16 Specialties: From AIDS to Urology, 114 Hospitals That Offer Top Care." *U.S. News & World Report,* 18 July 1994, pp. 74, 80. *Notes:* "Reputational score" is the percentage of doctors surveyed who named the hospital. "Mortality rate" is the ratio of actual to expected deaths (lower is better). "COTH member" indicates member of Council of Teaching Hospitals. "Service mix" indicates breadth of community services from 0 to 16. "Residents to beds" is the ratio of interns and residents to beds. "Technology score" is a specialty-specific index from 0 to 13. "R.N.'s to beds" is the ratio of registered nurses to beds. "Geriatric services" indicates number of geriatric services available, from 0 to 9. "Discharge planning" indicates number of postdischarge services available, from 0 to 2. "Board-certified M.D.'s to beds" is the ratio of doctors certified in a specialty to the number of beds. 1. UCLA stands for University of California, Los Angeles.

★ 201 ★

Hospitals

Top Ten Gynecology Departments at U.S. Hospitals and Health Care Facilities

The table below ranks hospitals according to a mathematical model. Rank is based on each hospital's overall score.

Hospital	Overall score	Reputational score	Mortality rate	Residents to beds	Technology score	R.N.'s to beds	Board-certified M.D.'s to beds	Inpatient operations to beds
Johns Hopkins Hospital (Baltimore, Maryland)	100.0	19.2%	0.78	0.45	9	1.43	0.66	15.5
Mayo Clinic (Rochester, Minnesota)	96.9	18.7%	0.64	0.37	5	0.73	1.49	21.5
University of Texas M.D. Anderson Cancer Center (Houston, Texas)	81.3	15.3%	0.78	0.10	8	1.88	0.61	12.4
Brigham and Women's Hospital (Boston, Massachusetts)	71.5	12.6%	0.75	0.64	8	0.79	1.24	20.0
Massachusetts General Hospital (Boston, Masschusetts)	59.8	10.3%	0.77	0.47	9	1.14	0.66	17.5
Duke University Medical Center (Durham, North Carolina)	53.7	8.6%	0.86	0.43	9	1.60	0.66	15.3
Memorial Sloan-Kettering Cancer Center, (New York, New York)	52.8	9.0%	0.67	0.32	6	1.37	0.55	17.9
Los Angeles County-USC Medical Center (Los Angeles, California)[1]	45.7	7.7%	0.99	0.00	6	1.30	0.27	28.7
University of Chicago Hospitals (Chicago, Illinois)	41.0	5.4%	0.91	0.75	9	1.38	0.73	17.3
UCLA Medical Center (Los Angeles, California)[2]	40.1	5.5%	0.77	0.71	9	1.20	0.82	14.6

Source: "The 16 Specialties: From AIDS to Urology, 114 Hospitals That Offer Top Care." *U.S. News & World Report,* 18 July 1994, pp. 74, 82. *Notes:* "Reputational score" is the percentage of doctors surveyed who named the hospital. "Mortality rate" is the ratio of actual to expected deaths (lower is better). "Residents to beds" is the ratio of interns and residents to beds. "Technology score" is a specialty-specific index from 0 to 9. "R.N.'s to beds" is the ratio of registered nurses to beds. "Board-certified M.D.'s to beds" is the ratio of doctors certified in a specialty to the number of beds. "Inpatient operations to beds" is the ratio of annual inpatient operations to beds. 1. USC stands for University of Southern California. 2. UCLA stands for University of California, Los Angeles.

★ 202 ★
Hospitals

Top Ten Hospitals and Health Care Facilities for AIDS Treatment

The table below ranks hospitals according to a mathematical model. Rank is based on each hospital's overall score.

Hospital	Overall score	Reputational score	Mortality rate	COTH member	Residents to beds	Technology score	Discharge planning	R.N.'s to beds	Board-certified M.D.'s to beds
San Francisco General Hospital Medical Center (San Francisco, California)	100.0	40.1%	1.24	No	0.55	6	2	1.52	0.40
Johns Hopkins Hospital (Baltimore, Maryland)	71.9	20.3%	0.78	Yes	0.45	9	2	1.43	0.66
Massachusetts General Hospital (Boston, Massachusetts)	62.0	15.6%	0.77	Yes	0.47	9	2	1.14	0.66
University of California San Francisco Medical Center (San Francisco, California)	55.9	12.0%	0.76	Yes	0.32	8	2	1.82	1.55
Memorial Sloan-Kettering Cancer Center (New York, New York)	50.0	8.4%	0.67	Yes	0.32	5	2	1.37	0.55
UCLA Medical Center (Los Angeles, California)[1]	46.7	9.1%	0.77	yes	0.71	9	2	1.20	0.82
New York University Medical Center (New York, New York)	46.3	5.3%	0.62	Yes	0.20	6	2	1.15	1.25
University of Miami Hospital and Clinics (Miami, Florida)	45.9	9.0%	0.79	Yes	0.30	6	2	1.42	0.27
New York Hospital-Cornell Medical Center (New York, New York)	45.2	7.0%	0.72	Yes	0.38	8	2	1.00	0.99
Mayo Clinic (Rochester, Minnesota)	38.3	2.3%	0.64	Yes	0.37	5	2	0.73	1.49

Source: "The 16 Specialties: From AIDS to Urology, 114 Hospitals That Offer Top Care." *U.S. News & World Report,* 18 July 1994, pp. 74-75. *Notes:* "Reputational score" is the percentage of doctors surveyed who named the hospital. "Mortality rate" is the ratio of actual to expected deaths (lower is better). "COTH member" indicates member of Council of Teaching Hospitals. "Residents to beds" is the ratio of interns and residents to beds. "Technology score" is a specialty-specific index from 0 to 9. "Discharge planning" indicates number of postdischarge services available, from 0 to 2. "R.N.'s to beds" is the ratio of registered nurses to beds. "Board-certified M.D.'s to beds" is the ratio of doctors certified in a specialty to the number of beds. 1. UCLA stands for University of California, Los Angeles.

★ 203 ★
Hospitals

Top Ten Hospitals and Health Care Facilities for Cancer Treatment

The table below ranks hospitals according to a mathematical model. Rank is based on each hospital's overall score.

Hospital	Overall score	Reputational score	Mortality rate	COTH member	Residents to beds	Technology score	R.N.'s to beds	Board-certified M.D.'s to beds	Inpatient operations to beds
Memorial Sloan-Kettering Cancer Center (New York, New York)	100.0	50.4%	0.67	Yes	0.32	8	1.37	0.55	17.9
University of Texas M.D. Anderson Cancer Center (Houston, Texas)	81.5	40.9%	0.78	Yes	0.10	10	1.88	0.61	12.4
Dana-Farber Cancer Institute (Boston, Massachusetts)	57.1	27.3%	0.88	No	0.63	2	1.58	2.17	0.0
Mayo Clinic (Rochester, Minnesota)	56.9	16.4%	0.64	Yes	0.37	7	0.73	1.49	21.5
Roswell Park Cancer Institute (Buffalo, New York)	50.6	7.4%	0.65	No	0.37	8	2.58	0.49	37.7
Fred Hutchinson Cancer Research Center (Seattle, Washington)	50.2	10.4%	0.50	No	0.00	1	0.95	1.13	6.8
Johns Hopkins Hospital (Baltimore, Maryland)	49.7	15.7%	0.78	Yes	0.45	10	1.43	0.66	15.5
University of Washington Medical Center (Seattle, Washington)	43.4	8.8%	0.73	Yes	0.30	8	2.06	1.90	14.8
Stanford University Medical Center (Stanford, California)	38.5	10.3%	0.95	YEs	0.79	9	0.88	1.81	13.9
Duke University Medical Center (Durham, North Carolina)	36.6	7.6%	0.86	Yes	0.43	11	1.60	0.66	15.3

Source: "The 16 Specialties: From AIDS to Urology, 114 Hospitals That Offer Top Care." *U.S. News & World Report,* 18 July 1994, pp. 74, 76. *Notes:* "Reputational score" is the percentage of doctors surveyed who named the hospital. "Mortality rate" is the ratio of actual to expected deaths (lower is better). "COTH member" indicates member of Council of Teaching Hospitals. "Residents to beds" is the ratio of interns and residents to beds. "Technology score" is a specialty-specific index from 0 to 11. "R.N.'s to beds" is the ratio of registered nurses to beds. "Board-certified M.D.'s to beds" is the ratio of doctors certified in a specialty to the number of beds. "Inpatient operations to beds" is the ratio of annual inpatient operations to beds.

★ 204 ★

Hospitals

Top Ten Neurology Departments at U.S. Hospitals and Health Care Facilities

The table below ranks hospitals according to a mathematical model. Rank is based on each hospital's overall score.

Hospital	Overall score	Reputational score	Mortality rate	COTH member	Residents to beds	Technology score	R.N.'s to beds	Board-certified M.D.'s to beds
Mayo Clinic (Rochester, Minnesota)	100.0	35.9%	0.64	Yes	0.37	6	0.73	1.49
Massachusetts General Hospital (Boston, Massachusetts)	83.8	30.1%	0.77	Yes	0.47	9	1.14	0.66
Johns Hopkins Hospital (Baltimore, Maryland)	78.0	26.8%	0.78	Yes	0.45	9	1.43	0.66
Columbia-Presbyterian Medical Center (New York, New York)	67.5	21.8%	0.78	Yes	0.31	9	1.05	0.81
University of California San Francisco Medical Center (San Francisco, California)	66.7	19.3%	0.76	Yes	0.32	8	1.82	1.55
New York Hospital-Cornell Medical Center (New York, New York)	53.4	12.7%	0.72	Yes	0.38	7	1.00	0.99
Cleveland Clinic (Cleveland, Ohio)	47.7	9.2%	0.76	Yes	0.59	9	1.47	0.38
Barnes Hospital (St. Louis, Missouri)	46.8	9.8%	0.76	Yes	0.47	9	0.81	0.90
Hospital of the University of Pennsylvania (Philadelphia, Pennsylvania)	44.3	8.6%	0.84	Yes	0.73	9	1.33	0.94
UCLA Medical Center (Los Angeles, California)[1]	40.2	5.2%	0.77	Yes	0.71	9	1.20	0.82

Source: "The 16 Specialties: From AIDS to Urology, 114 Hospitals That Offer Top Care." *U.S. News & World Report,* 18 July 1994, pp. 74, 83. *Notes:* "Reputational score" is the percentage of doctors surveyed who named the hospital. "Mortality rate" is the ratio of actual to expected deaths (lower is better). "COTH member" indicates member of Council of Teaching Hospitals. "Residents to beds" is the ratio of interns and residents to beds. "Technology score" is a specialty-specific index from 0 to 9. "R.N.'s to beds" is the ratio of registered nurses to beds. "Board-certified M.D.'s to beds" is the ratio of doctors certified in a specialty to the number of beds. 1. UCLA stands for University of California, Los Angeles.

★ 205 ★

Hospitals

Top Ten Ophthalmology Departments at U.S. Hospitals and Health Care Facilities

The table below ranks hospitals according to reputational scores from physician surveys of the previous 3 years.

Hospital	Reputational score	Board-certified M.D.'s to beds	Technology score	Inpatient operations to beds	COTH member
University of Miami/Bascom Palmer Eye Institute (Miami, Florida)	40.0%	2.13	2	37.8	No
Johns Hopkins Hospital/Wilmer Eye Institute (Baltimore, Maryland)	37.7%	0.66	17	15.5	Yes
Wills Eye Hospital (Philadelphia, Pennsylvania)	35.4%	1.10	3	44.5	No
Massachusetts Eye and Ear Infirmary (Boston, Massachusetts)	29.8%	0.39	3	78.4	No
UCLA Medical Center/Jules Stein Eye Institute (Los Angeles, California)	22.3%	0.82	17	14.6	Yes
University of Iowa Hospitals and Clinics (Iowa City, Iowa)	16.1%	0.54	18	25.5	Yes
Doheny Eye Hospital (Los Angeles, California)	8.7%	1.08	0	31.3	No
Barnes Hospital (St. Louis, Missouri)	7.3%	0.90	17	11.1	Yes
Duke University Medical Center (Durham, North Carolina)	5.0%	0.66	19	15.3	Yes
University of California San Francisco Medical Center (San Francisco, California)	4.6%	1.55	17	18.3	Yes

Source: "The 16 Specialties: From AIDS to Urology, 114 Hospitals That Offer Top Care." *U.S. News & World Report,* 18 July 1994, pp. 74, 88. *Notes:* "Reputational score" is the percentage of doctors surveyed who named the hospital. "Board-certified M.D.'s to beds" is the ratio of doctors certified in a specialty to the number of beds. "Technology score" is an index from 0 to 19. "Inpatient operations to beds" is the ratio of annual inpatient operations to beds. "COTH member" indicates member of Council Teaching Hospitals. 1. UCLA stands for University of California, Los Angeles.

★ 206 ★

Hospitals

Top Ten Orthopedics Departments at U.S. Hospitals and Health Care Facilities

The table below ranks hospitals according to a mathematical model. Rank is based on each hospital's overall score.

Hospital	Overall score	Reputational score	Mortality rate	COTH member	Residents to beds	Technology score	R.N.'s to beds	Board-certified M.D.'s to beds	Inpatient operations to beds
Hospital for Special Surgery (New York, New York)	100.0	28.5%	0.16	Yes	0.18	4	0.78	0.77	27.8
Mayo Clinic (Rochester, Minnesota)	57.9	28.6%	0.64	Yes	0.37	4	0.73	1.49	21.5
Massachusetts General Hospital (Boston, Massachusetts)	42.5	19.2%	0.77	Yes	0.47	5	1.14	0.66	17.5
Johns Hopkins Hospital (Baltimore, Maryland)	26.4	7.6%	0.78	Yes	0.45	5	1.43	0.66	15.5
Duke University Medical Center, (Durham, North Carolina)	25.1	7.4%	0.86	Yes	0.43	5	1.60	0.66	15.3
University of Washington Medical Center (Seattle, Washington)	25.0	5.3%	0.73	Yes	0.30	4	2.06	1.90	14.8
Cleveland Clinic (Cleveland, Ohio)	23.9	5.3%	0.76	Yes	0.59	5	1.47	0.38	19.9
UCLA Medical Center (Los Angeles, California)[1]	22.7	4.6%	0.77	Yes	0.71	5	1.20	0.82	14.6
University of Iowa Hospitals and Clinics (Iowa, City, Iowa)	22.2	5.2%	0.92	Yes	0.78	5	1.34	0.54	25.5
University of Tennessee Medical Center (Memphis, Tennessee)	21.7	5.5%	0.77	No	0.24	2	0.72	2.28	14.6

Source: "The 16 Specialties: From AIDS to Urology, 114 Hospitals That Offer Top Care." *U.S. News & World Report,* 18 July 1994, pp. 74, 84. *Notes:* "Reputational score" is the percentage of doctors surveyed who named the hospital. "Mortality rate" is the ratio of actual to expected deaths (lower is better). "COTH member" indicates member of Council of Teaching Hospitals. "Residents to beds" is the ratio of interns and residents to beds. "Technology score" is a specialty-specific index from 0 to 5. "R.N.'s to beds" is the ratio of registered nurses to beds. "Board-certified M.D.'s to beds" is the ratio of doctors certified in a specialty to the number of beds. "Inpatient operations to beds" is the ratio of annual inpatient operations to beds. 1. UCLA stands for University of California, Los Angeles.

★ 207 ★

Hospitals

Top Ten Otolaryngology Departments at U.S. Hospitals and Health Care Facilities

The table below ranks hospitals according to a mathematical model. Rank is based on each hospital's overall score.

Hospital	Overall score	Reputational score	Mortality rate	COTH member	Residents to beds	Technology score	R.N.'s to beds	Board-certified M.D.'s to beds	Inpatient operations to beds
Massachusetts Eye and Ear Infirmary (Boston, Massachusetts)	100.0	16.0%	0.35	No	0.46	2	2.18	0.39	78.4
Johns Hopkins Hospital (Baltimore, Maryland)	84.7	21.4%	0.78	Yes	0.45	9	1.43	0.66	15.5
New York Eye and Ear Infirmary (New York, New York)	83.1	3.3%	0.24	No	0.30	2	0.84	4.54	52.2
University of Iowa Hospitals and Clinics (Iowa City, Iowa)	79.9	20.4%	0.92	Yes	0.78	9	1.34	0.54	25.5
Manhattan Eye, Ear and Throat Hospital (New York, New York)	75.0	4.4%	0.28	No	0.43	1	0.53	4.21	95.9
Mayo Clinic (Rochester, Minnesota)	59.5	11.0%	0.65	Yes	0.37	6	0.73	1.49	21.5
UCLA Medical Center, (Los Angeles, California)[1]	54.1	9.6%	0.77	Yes	0.71	9	1.20	0.82	14.6
University of Michigan Medical Center (Ann Arbor, Michigan)	50.6	9.7%	0.85	Yes	0.41	8	1.29	0.66	16.8
Barnes Hospital (St. Louis, Missouri)	48.8	8.2%	0.76	Yes	0.47	9	0.81	0.90	11.1
University of Texas M.D. Anderson Cancer Center (Houston, Texas)	48.7	8.4%	0.78	Yes	0.10	9	1.88	0.81	12.4

Source: "The 16 Specialties: From AIDS to Urology, 114 Hospitals That Offer Top Care." *U.S. News & World Report,* 18 July 1994, pp. 74, 85. *Notes:* "Reputational score" is the percentage of doctors surveyed who named the hospital. "Mortality rate" is the ratio of actual to expected deaths (lower is better). "COTH member" indicates member of Council of Teaching Hospitals. "Residents to beds" is the ratio of interns and residents to beds. "Technology score" is a specialty-specific index from 0 to 9. "R.N.'s to beds" is the ratio of registered nurses to beds. "Board-certified M.D.'s to beds" is the ratio of doctors certified in a specialty to the number of beds. "Inpatient operations to beds" is the ratio of annual inpatient operations to beds. 1. UCLA stands for University of California, Los Angeles.

★ 208 ★

Hospitals

Top Ten Pediatrics Departments at U.S. Hospitals and Health Care Facilities

The table below ranks hospitals according to reputational scores from physician surveys of the previous 3 years.

Hospital	Reputational score	Board-certified M.D.'s to beds	Technology score	R.N.'s to beds	COTH member
Children's Hospital (Boston, Massachusetts)	36.1%	1.25	10	1.60	Yes
Children's Hospital of Philadelphia (Philadelphia, Pennsylvania)	26.5%	1.13	10	1.89	Yes
Johns Hopkins Hospital (Baltimore, Maryland)	21.0%	0.66	17	1.43	Yes
University Hospitals of Cleveland/Rainbow Babies and Children's Hospital (Cleveland, Ohio)	10.3%	1.26	18	1.73	Yes
Children's Hospital Los Angeles (Los Angeles, California)	9.8%	0.62	0	1.45	No
Children's Hospital of Pittsburgh (Pittsburgh, Pennsylvania)	8.1%	1.96	4	2.06	Yes
Children's National Medical Center (Washington, D.C.)	7.6%	1.02	8	1.82	Yes
Children's Hospital Medical Center (Cincinnati, Ohio)	6.9%	2.10	8	2.18	Yes
Children's Hospital (Denver, Colorado)	6.6%	1.38	8	1.74	No
Children's Memorial Hospital (Chicago, Illinois)	6.3%	0.95	9	1.99	Yes

Source: "The 16 Specialties: From AIDS to Urology, 114 Hospitals That Offer Top Care." *U.S. News & World Report,* 18 July 1994, pp. 74, 88. *Notes:* "Reputational score" is the percentage of doctors surveyed who named the hospital. "Board-certified M.D.'s to beds" is the ratio of doctors certified in a specialty to the number of beds. "Technology score" is an index from 0 to 19. "R.N.'s to beds" is the ratio of registered nurses to beds. "COTH member" indicates member of Council Teaching Hospitals.

★ 209 ★

Hospitals

Top Ten Psychiatry Departments at U.S. Hospitals and Health Care Facilities

The table below ranks hospitals according to reputational scores from physician surveys of the previous 3 years.

Hospital	Reputational score	Board-certified M.D.'s to beds	Discharge planning	R.N.'s to beds	COTH member	Technology score	R.N.'s to L.P.N's
McLean Hospital (Belmont, Massachusetts)	14.2%	0.48	2	0.66	No	3	5.0
Menninger Clinic (Topeka, Kansas)	14.0%	0.19	2	0.48	No	0	2
Johns Hopkins Hospital (Baltimore, Maryland)	9.1%	0.66	2	1.43	Yes	17	42.9
New York Hospital–Cornell Medical Center (New York, New York)	9.0%	0.99	2	1.00	Yes	16	30.5
UCLA Medical Center (Los Angeles, California)[1]	6.3%	0.51	2	0.52	No	0	4.7
Sheppard and Enoch Pratt (Baltimore, Maryland)	8.0%	0.08	2	0.28	No	0	2
Massachusetts General Hospital (Boston, Massachusetts)	7.7%	0.66	2	1.14	Yes	19	27.9
Institute of Living (Hartford, Connecticut)	6.1%	0.16	2	0.45	No	0	2
Columbia-Presbyterian Medical Center (New York, New York)	5.0%	0.81	2	1.05	Yes	16	23.5
Mayo Clinic (Rochester, Minnesota)	4.0%	0.93	2	0.86	Yes	13	5.3

Source: "The 16 Specialties: From AIDS to Urology, 114 Hospitals That Offer Top Care." *U.S. News & World Report,* 18 July 1994, pp. 74, 89. *Notes:* "Reputational score" is the percentage of doctors surveyed who named the hospital. "Board-certified M.D.'s to beds" is the ratio of doctors certified in a specialty to the number of beds. "Discharge planning" indicates number of post-discharge services available, from 0 to 2. "R.N.'s to beds" is the ratio of registered nurses to beds. "COTH member" indicates member of Council of Teaching Hospitals. "Technology score" is an index from 0 to 19. "R.N.'s to L.P.N.'s" is the ratio of registered nurses to licensed practical nurses. 1. UCLA stands for University of California, Los Angeles. 2. Not available.

★ 210 ★

Hospitals

Top Ten Rehabilitation Departments at U.S. Hospitals and Health Care Facilities

The table below ranks hospitals according to reputational scores from physician surveys of the previous 3 years.

Hospital	Reputational score	Board-certified M.D.'s to beds	Discharge planning	R.N.'s to beds	Geriatric services	Technology score
Rehabilitation Institute of Chicago (Chicago, Illinois)	34.7%	0.14	1	0.52	1	1
University of Washington Medical Center (Seattle, Washington)	24.9%	1.90	2	2.06	4	15
Craig Hospital (Englewood, Colorado)	17.0%	0.11	2	0.41	0	1
Institute for Rehabilitation and Research (Houston, Texas)	15.2%	0.34	1	0.35	0	1
New York University Medical Center/Rusk Institute for Rehabilitation Medicine (New York, New York)	14.5%	1.25	2	1.15	0	13
Mayo Clinic (Rochester, Minnesota)	12.8%	0.93	2	0.86	5	13
Los Angles County-Rancho Los Angeles Medical Center (Downey, California)	10.4%	0.15	2	1.01	5	5
Ohio State University Medical Center (Columbus, Ohio)	8.1%	0.68	2	1.11	5	11
Thomas Jefferson University Hospital (Philadelphia, Pennsylvania)	7.3%	1.12	2	1.44	3	16
Baylor University Medical Center (Dallas, Texas)	7.0%	0.40	2	1.38	3	14

Source: "The 16 Specialties: From AIDS to Urology, 114 Hospitals That Offer Top Care." *U.S. News & World Report,* 18 July 1994, pp. 74, 89. *Notes:* "Reputational score" is the percentage of doctors surveyed who named the hospital. "Board-certified M.D.'s to beds" is the ratio of doctors certified in a specialty to the number of beds. "Discharge planning" indicates number of post-discharge services available, from 0 to 2. "R.N.'s to beds" is the ratio of registered nurses to beds. "Geriatric services" indicates number of geriatric services available, from 0 to 9. "Technology score" is an index from 0 to 19.

★ 211 ★

Hospitals

Top Ten Rheumatology Departments at U.S. Hospitals and Health Care Facilities

The table below ranks hospitals according to a mathematical model. Rank is based on each hospital's overall score.

Hospital	Overall score	Reputational score	Mortality rate	COTH member	Residents to beds	Technology score	R.N.'s to beds	Board-certified M.D.'s to beds
Hospital for Special Surgery (New York, New York)	100.0	17.6%	0.10	Yes	0.18	4	0.76	0.77
Mayo Clinic (Rochester, Minnesota)	70.6	31.2%	0.64	Yes	0.37	4	0.73	1.49
Brigham and Women's Hospital (Boston, Massachusetts)	47.3	17.5%	0.75	Yes	0.64	4	0.78	1.24
UCLA Medical Center (Los Angeles, California) [1]	43.3	14.8%	0.77	Yes	0.71	5	1.20	0.82
Johns Hopkins Hospital (Baltimore, Maryland)	42.9	14.9%	0.78	Yes	0.45	5	1.43	0.66
Massachusetts General Hospital (Boston, Massachusetts)	38.7	12.5%	0.77	Yes	0.47	5	1.14	0.66
University of Alabama Hospital at Birmingham (Birmingham, Alabama)	34.0	12.3%	1.03	Yes	0.46	4	0.92	0.60
Duke University Medical Center (Durham, North Carolina)	33.8	10.0%	0.86	Yes	0.43	5	1.60	0.66
Cleveland Clinic (Cleveland, Ohio)	33.6	8.7%	0.76	Yes	0.59	5	1.47	0.38
New York University Medical Center (New York, New York)	31.1	5.8%	0.62	Yes	0.20	4	1.15	1.25

Source: "The 16 Specialties: From AIDS to Urology, 114 Hospitals That Offer Top Care." *U.S. News & World Report,* 18 July 1994, pp. 74, 86. *Notes:* "Reputational score" is the percentage of doctors surveyed who named the hospital. "Mortality rate" is the ratio of actual to expected deaths (lower is better). "COTH member" indicates member of Council of Teaching Hospitals. "Residents to beds" is the ratio of interns and residents to beds. "Technology score" is a specialty-specific index from 0 to 5. "R.N.'s to beds" is the ratio of registered nurses to beds. "Board-certified M.D.'s to beds" is the ratio of doctors certified in a specialty to the number of beds. 1. UCLA stands for University of California, Los Angeles.

★ 212 ★

Hospitals

Top Ten Urology Departments at U.S. Hospitals and Health Care Facilities

The table below ranks hospitals according to a mathematical model. Rank is based on each hospital's overall score.

Hospital	Overall score	Reputational score	Mortality rate	COTH member	Residents to beds	Technology score	R.N.'s to beds	Board-certified M.D.'s to beds	Inpatient operations to beds
Mayo Clinic (Rochester, Minnesota)	100.0	30.5%	0.64	Yes	0.37	8	0.73	1.49	21.5
Johns Hopkins Hospital (Baltimore, Maryland)	95.6	31.5%	0.78	Yes	0.45	11	1.43	0.66	15.5
Cleveland Clinic (Cleveland, Ohio)	73.5	19.9%	0.76	Yes	0.59	10	1.47	0.38	19.9
UCLA Medical Center (Los Angeles, California)[1]	65.5	16.2%	0.77	Yes	0.71	11	1.20	0.82	14.6
Memorial Sloan-Kettering Cancer Center (New York, New York)	58.2	10.8%	0.67	Yes	0.32	8	1.37	0.55	17.9
Stanford University Medical Center (Stanford, California)	55.9	14.3%	0.95	Yes	0.79	11	0.86	1.81	13.9
Barnes Hospital (St. Louis, Missouri)	54.7	11.7%	0.76	Yes	0.47	11	0.81	0.90	11.1
University of Texas M.D. Anderson Cancer Center (Houston, Texas)	49.9	9.8%	0.78	Yes	0.10	10	1.88	0.61	12.4
Massachusetts General Hospital (Boston, Massachusetts)	47.2	7.8%	0.77	Yes	0.47	11	1.14	0.66	17.5
Duke University Medical Center (Durham, North Carolina)	44.5	8.0%	0.86	Yes	0.43	11	1.60	0.66	15.3

Source: "The 16 Specialties: From AIDS to Urology, 114 Hospitals That Offer Top Care." *U.S. News & World Report,* 18 July 1994, pp. 74, 87. *Notes:* "Reputational score" is the percentage of doctors surveyed who named the hospital. "Mortality rate" is the ratio of actual to expected deaths (lower is better). "COTH member" indicates member of Council of Teaching Hospitals. "Residents to beds" is the ratio of interns and residents to beds. "Technology score" is a specialty-specific index from 0 to 11. "R.N.'s to beds" is the ratio of registered nurses to beds. "Board-certified M.D.'s to beds" is the ratio of doctors certified in a specialty to the number of beds. "Inpatient operations to beds" is the ratio of an annual inpatient operations to beds. 1. UCLA stands for University of California, Los Angeles.

Immunization and Vaccinations

★ 213 ★

Cost of Immunization

The table below indicates the average cost to doctors for drugs used in the immunization of children.

Disease	Cost
Diphtheria/tetanus/pertussis	$49.85
Oral polio	39.64
Measles/mumps/rubella	50.58
Hemophilus influenza	58.20
Hepatitis B	32.12
Total	230.39

Source: "Kids, Shots, and Drug Research: Let's Get Some Answers." *Business Week* 23, 15 February 1992, p. 38. Primary source: Children's Defense Fund, Centers for Disease Control.

★214★

Immunization and Vaccinations

Reported Cases of Diseases Preventable by Childhood Vaccination: 1993-1994

Table shows the number of reported cases of diseases preventable by routine childhood vaccination. Data for 1993 are final, but data for 1994 are provisional.

Disease	Number of cases January 1994	Total cases		Number of cases among children under age 5[1]	
		1993	1994	1993	1994
Congenital rubella syndrome (CRS)	0	1	0	0	0
Diphtheria	0	0	0	0	0
Haemophilus influenzae[2]	73	95	73	39	26
Hepatitis B[3]	636	733	636	6	19
Measles	4	14	4	7	1
Mumps	65	106	65	21	7
Pertussis	198	222	198	108	117
Poliomyelitis paralytic[4]	-	-	-	-	-
Rubella	3	11	3	4	0
Tetanus	1	1	1	0	0

Source: U.S. Department of Health and Human Services. Public Health Service. Centers for Disease Control and Prevention. "Notices to Readers." *Morbidity and Mortality Weekly Report* 43, no. 8, 4 March 1994, p. 151. *Notes:* 1. For 1993 and 1994, age data were available for 85 percent or more cases, except for 1994 age data for pertussis, which were available at 76 percent. 2. Invasive disease; *haemophilus influenzae* serotype is not routinely reported to the National Notifiable Diseases Surveillance System. 3. Because most hepatitis B virus infections among infants and children under age 5 are asymptomatic (although likely to become chronic), acute disease surveillance does not reflect the incidence of this problem in this age group or the effectiveness of hepatitis B vaccination of infants. 4. No cases of suspected poliomyelitis have been reported in 1994; 3 cases of suspected poliomyelitis were reported in 1993. Four of the 5 suspected cases with onset in 1992 were confirmed; the confirmed cases were vaccine associated.

Long-term Care: Insurance

★ 215 ★

Average Annual Premiums for Long-term Care Insurance Policies: 1990

[In dollars]

Initial age of purchaser	Individual policy without inflation adjustment[1]	Individual policy with inflation adjustment[1]	Employer-based plans[2]
30			125
40			176
50	483	658	328
65	1,135	1,395	1,108
79	3,841	4,194	4,438

Source: U.S. Department of Labor. Pension and Welfare Benefits Administration. *Trends in Health Benefits.* Washington, DC: U.S. Government Printing Office, 1993, p. 221. Primary source: Van Gelder, Susan, and Diane Johnson "Long-term Care Insurance: A Market Update." *HIAA* (January 1991), tables 5 and 7. *Notes:* 1. Generally, for a plan providing $80 per day for nursing home care, a 20-day deductible and 4 years of coverage. 2. Generally, for a plan providing $80 per day for nursing care, a 90-day deductible and 4 years of coverage.

★ 216 ★

Long-term Care: Insurance

Expected Role of Private Long-term Care Insurance

Table below indicates the total, projected long-term care (LTC) expenditures and the percent of expenditures covered by private insurance.

[Expenditures in billions of 1989 dollars]

	Total expenditures	Percent of expenditures
1990	46.0	2.0
2005	75.9	4.0
2020	132.6	6.6

Source: Aging America: Trends and Projections. 1991 ed. Prepared by the U.S. Senate Special Committee on Aging, the American Association of Retired Persons, the Federal Council on the Aging, and the U.S. Administration on Aging. DHHS Publication No. (FCoA) 91-28001. Washington, DC: U.S. Department of Health and Human Services (DHHS), 1991, p. 175. Primary source: Brookings/ICF Long-Term Care Financing Model, unpublished data (1990).

★ 217 ★

Long-term Care: Insurance

Long-term Care Insurance Sales: 1987-1991

The table below presents the number of long-term care policies sold for each type of purchaser; for example, individuals, groups, or employers.

Year	Individual	Group association	Employer sponsored	Other	Total
1987	637,795	112,744	0	0	786,539
1988	917,701	186,589	20,406	2,797	1,127,493
1989	1,249,611	263,112	51,568	11,103	1,575,394
1990	1,428,533	315,495	133,078	22,810	1,928,415

Source: U.S. Department of Labor. Pension and Welfare Benefits Administration. *Trends in Health Benefits.* Washington, DC: U.S. Government Printing Office, 1993, p. 222. Primary source: Health Insurance Association of America. Unpublished data.

★ 218 ★

Long-term Care: Insurance

Purchasers of Long-term Care Insurance: 1988-1990

Table reflects average age of purchasers of long-term care insurance. Data are provided by type of purchaser.

Year	Individual	Group association	Employer (median)
1988	70	70	40
1989	72	70	43
1990	72	69	43

Source: U.S. Department of Labor. Pension and Welfare Benefits Administration. *Trends in Health Benefits.* Washington, DC: U.S. Government Printing Office, 1993, p. 222. Primary source: Health Insurance Association of American. Unpublished data.

Long-term Care: Nursing Homes

★ 219 ★

Nursing Home Costs

In 1990, the average cost of nursing home care was $31,000 per year, or $86 per day—double the cost in 1980. Prices ranged from $60,000 in large cities to $20,000 in rural areas.

Source: Wilson, Virginia. "Policies for Old-Age Care" *Newsweek* 120, 20 April 1992, p. 61.

★ 220 ★

Long-term Care: Nursing Homes

Nursing Home Expenditures: 1960-1991

The data below reflect expenditures for nursing home care and the percent distribution according to source of funds for selected years. Data were compiled by the Health Care Financing Administration.

[In percentages, except as noted]

Year	Total (in billion dollars)	Out-of-pocket payments	Private health insurance	Other private funds	Government		
					Total[1]	Medicaid	Medicare
1960	1.0	80.0	0.0	6.4	13.6	-	-
1965	1.7	64.5	0.1	5.8	29.5	-	-
1970	4.9	48.2	0.3	4.9	46.6	28.0	5.0
1975	9.9	42.1	0.7	4.8	52.3	47.5	2.9
1980	20.0	43.3	0.9	3.1	52.7	48.6	2.1
1984	31.2	47.8	1.1	2.1	48.9	44.9	1.8
1985	34.1	48.6	1.0	1.9	48.5	44.6	1.7
1986	36.7	49.1	1.0	1.9	48.0	44.1	1.6
1987	39.7	47.9	1.0	1.9	49.2	45.2	1.6
1988	42.8	48.1	1.1	1.9	48.9	44.4	2.2
1989	47.5	44.2	1.1	1.9	52.7	43.4	7.2
1990	53.3	45.3	1.1	1.9	51.7	45.1	4.5
1991	59.9	43.1	1.1	1.9	53.9	47.4	4.4

Source: U.S. Department of Health and Human Services. Public Health Service. Centers for Disease Control and Prevention. National Center for Health Statistics. *Health, United States, 1992.* Hyattsville, MD: Public Health Service, 1993, p. 172. Primary source: Health Care Financing Administration. Office of National Health Statistics. Office of the Actuary. "National Health Expenditures: 1991." *Health Care Financing Review* 14, no. 2 (winter 1992). *Notes:* 1. Includes other government expenditures for these health care services; for example, care funded by the U.S. Department of Veterans Affairs and state and locally financed subsidies to hospitals.

★ 221 ★

Long-term Care: Nursing Homes

Nursing Home Expenditures, by Source: 1990

Total expenditures equal $53.1 billion.

Source	Percent
Out-of-pocket	45.0
Medicaid	45.0
Medicare	5.0
Private insurance	1.0
Other	4.0

Source: U.S. Department of Labor. Pension and Welfare Benefits Administration. *Trends in Health Benefits.* Washington, DC: U.S. Government Printing Office, 1993, p. 223. Primary source: Health Care Financing Administration, Office of the Actuary, 1992.

★ 222 ★

Long-term Care: Nursing Homes

Projected Nursing Home Expenditures for Persons Over Age 65: 1990, 2005, and 2020

Data are provided by source of payment.

[Numbers in billions of 1989 dollars]

Source of payment	1990	2005	2020
Medicare	1.1	1.8	3.2
Medicaid	15.7	27.0	45.0
Out-of-pocket	20.8	35.2	64.4
Total	37.6	64.0	112.6

Source: Aging America: Trends and Projections. 1991 ed. Prepared by the U.S. Senate Special Committee on Aging, the American Association of Retired Persons, the Federal Council on the Aging, and the U.S. Administration on Aging. DHHS Publication No. (FCoA) 91-28001. Washington, DC: U.S. Department of Health and Human Services (DHHS), 1991, p. 172. Primary source: Brookings/ICF Long Term-Care Financing Model, unpublished data (1990).

★ 223 ★

Long-term Care: Nursing Homes

Sources of Payment for Nursing Home Residents

Data are based on reporting by a sample of nursing homes.

["-" indicates quantity of zero]

Primary source of payment	Both sexes				Male				Female			
	55-64 years	65-74 years	75-84 years	85 years and over	55-64 years	65-74 years	75-84 years	85 years and over	55-64 years	65-74 years	75-84 years	85 years and over
All sources												
Number of residents (in thousands)	88	209	502	604	43	79	140	114	45	130	362	490
Average monthly charge	1,358	1,367	1,471	1,492	1,415	1,330	1,457	1,510	1,304	1,389	1,476	1,487
Own income or family support												
Number of residents (in thousands)	27	71	229	272	14	27	63	62	12	44	167	210
Average monthly charge	1,118	1,425	1,450	1,513	1,258	1,349	1,455	1,535	953	1,472	1,448	1,506
Medicare												
Number of residents (in thousands)	1^2	5^2	10	5^2	1^2	2^2	3^2	1^2	-	3^2	7	4^2
Average monthly charge	3,507	1,748	2,360	1,966	3,507	1,903	2,676	2,289	-	1,614	2,220	1,901
Medicaid												
Skilled nursing facility benefit:												
Number of residents (in thousands)	17	31	82	110	7	0	22	17	11	22	60	93
Average monthly charge	1,981	1,846	1,904	1,839	1,963	1,810	1,889	1,912	1,992	1,860	1,909	1,826
Intermediate care facility benefit:												
Number of residents (in thousands)	30	78	159	192	12	28	42	28	18	49	117	165
Average monthly charge	1,291	1,229	1,295	1,303	1,400	1,248	1,244	1,283	1,222	1,218	1,314	1,306
Other government assistance or welfare												
Number of residents (in thousands)	6^2	14	12	11	4^2	5^2	5^2	2^2	3^2	9	6^2	9
Average monthly charge	710	770	908	1,185	641	797	1,058	1,042	801	758	789	1,217
All other sources[1]												
Number of residents (in thousands)	7	10	10	13	6^2	8	5^2	4^2	1^2	3^2	6^2	9
Average monthly charge	1,414	1,136	997	957	1,460	1,126	1,044	1,078	1,209	1,166	957	897

Source: Van Nostrand, J. F., S. E. Furner, and R. Suzman, eds. *Health Data on Older Americans: United States, 1992.* Vital and Health Statistics, Series 3: Analytic and Epidemiological Studies, no. 27. DHHS publication no. (PHS) 93-1411. Hyattsville, MD: U.S. Department of Health and Human Services, Public Health Service, Centers for Disease Control and Prevention, National Center for Health Statistics, 1993, p. 221. Primary source: National Center for Health Statistics data from the National Hospital Discharge Survey. *Notes:* 1. Includes religious organizations, Veterans' Administration contracts, initial payment-life care funds, and unknown. 2. Figure does not meet standard of reliability or precision.

Medical Devices

★ 224 ★

Axillary Thermometers

Adhesive-strip axillary thermometers are being marketed as alternatives to traditional glass rectal and oral or electric thermometers. They are considered more comfortable for treating children, jaw surgery, and other patients. Though only used 10 percent of the time, adhesive-strip axillary thermometers can be easier—no hands needed—and quicker than traditional ones. Figures below indicate the time needed for results for each type of thermometer.

[In minutes]

Thermometer	Time for results
Adhesive-strip axillary thermometer	3
Electric thermometer	5
Glass axillary thermometer	8-15

Source: "PyMaH Promoting Ease of Use With New Axillary Thermometer." *Health Industry Today* 56, no. 10 (October 1993), p. 16. *Note:* Adhesive-strip thermometers cost approximately $0.08 each.

★ 225 ★

Medical Devices

High-Tech Dental Instruments

New equipment is under development to speed procedures and lessen pain associated with dental treatments. Developments include computer imaging and intraoral video cameras to illustrate the condition of a patient's mouth or to preview corrective and cosmetic dental work. Much of the technology has been slow in making its way to dentists' offices, though, owing to high costs. The table below reflects the estimated costs of selected new dental technology.

Equipment	Technology	Cost
Cerec system[1]	CAD/CAM	$57,000[4]
Sopha system[2]	CAD/CAD	$70,000
Lasers[3]	-	$30,000

Source: Crichton, Ginger Munsch. "The Latest High-Tech Instruments Will Make Your Visits With the Dentist Speedier—and More Comfortable." *Dallas Morning News,* 19 April 1993, home final edition, p. 3C. *Notes:* CAD/CAM stands for computer-assisted design/computer-assisted manufacture. 1. Cerec system manufactures veneers, inlays, and onlays. 2. Sopha system manufactures crowns. 3. Lasers are used for "soft tissue" procedures such as removing gum tissue. 4. $1,100/month to lease.

★ 226 ★

Medical Devices

Home Medical Equipment, Supplies, and Services: 1990

The table below indicates prices for the purchase or rental of medical equipment and supplies. Data are provided per episode.

Home medical equipment	Rental/ purchase	Fee/price[1] ($)
Hospital bed, manual	Rental	192.53
Walker - wheeled	Rental	49.77
Drop-arm commode	Rental	67.84
Toilet safety rails	Purchase	41.40
Transfer bath bench	Purchase	98.58
Total cost (9 weeks)		450.12

Source: U.S. Senate Committee on Aging. *Medicare Fraud and Abuse: A Neglected Emergency? Hearing Before the Special Committee on Aging.* 102d Cong., 1st sess., 2 October 1991. Serial no. 102-13. Washington, DC: U.S. Government Printing Office, 1992, p. 224. *Note:* 1. 9 weeks.

★ 227 ★

Medical Devices

Home Medical Equipment, Supplies, and Services Used by Amyotrophic Lateral Sclerosis Patients

Table displays the monthly costs associated with home medical equipment, supplies, and services ($940.88) for the care and treatment of patients with Amyotrophic lateral sclerosis (ALS; or Lou Gehrig's disease). The costs associated with 1.3 days of equipment are $40.21.

[Amount in 1990 dollars]

Home medical equipment	Cost/month
Oxygen - portable	322.84
Oxygen - stationary	275.51
Hospital bed - electric	195.73
Bed trapeze	40.57
Walker	22.12
Bedside commode	30.15
Flotation mattress	46.18
Toilet safety rails	2.30
Bathtub/shower chair	5.48
Total costs per month	940.88

Source: U.S. Senate Committee on Aging. *Medicare Fraud and Abuse: A Neglected Emergency? Hearing Before the Special Committee on Aging.* 102d Cong., 1st sess., 2 October 1991. Serial no. 102-13. Washington, DC: U.S. Government Printing Office, 1992, p. 228. Primary source: Lewin/ICF.

★ 228 ★

Medical Devices

Home Medical Equipment, Supplies, and Services Used by Chronic Obstructive Pulmonary Disease Patients

It is assumed that all chronic obstructive pulmonary disease (COPD) patients will require home medical equipment services upon discharge from the hospital. It is further assumed that inpatient/home treatment patients will require an additional 1.4 days of home medical equipment costs.

Home medical equipment	Cost/month ($)
Oxygen - stationary and portable	322.84
Ventolin and aerosol inhaler	21.47
Walker - wheeled	22.12
Hospital bed - electric	195.73
Bedside commode	30.15
Overbed table	17.40
Monthly total	609.71

Source: U.S. Senate Committee on Aging. *Medicare Fraud and Abuse: A Neglected Emergency? Hearing Before the Special Committee on Aging.* 102d Cong., 1st sess., 2 October 1991. Serial no. 102-13. Washington, DC: U.S. Government Printing Office, 1992, p. 231. Primary source: Lewin/ICF.

★ 229 ★

Medical Devices

Implant Use: 1992-1993

Figures represent the number of medical procedures by specialty that required the use of biomaterials during a one-year period (1992-1993).

Specialty	Number of procedures
Urology	2.65 million
Cardiology and thoracic surgery	2.27 million
Ophthalmology	1.58 million
Orthopedics	617,000[1]
Reconstructive surgery	208,410
Neurology	75,000

Source: Feder, Barnaby J. "Implant Industry Is Facing Cutback by Top Suppliers." *New York Times,* 25 April 1994, late edition, p. A1. Primary source: Health Industry Manufacturers Association. *Note:* 1. Data from 1991.

★ 230 ★

Medical Devices

Latex Gloves

Latex gloves are used by health care providers to protect themselves and patients from the spread of disease. A study compared the use and leakage of gloves from surgical intensive care and AIDS units. Data below reflect the total number of gloves used and the number that leaked.

Variables	Totals		Gloves that leaked	
	Percent	n/N	Percent	n/N
Duration of use				
1-2 minutes	68	1,962/2,900	10	188/1,1962
3-5 minutes	32	938/2,900	55	512/938
Secretion contact				
None	45	1,300/2,900	23	301/1,300
Blood	18	530/2,900	31	164/530
Urine or feces	37	1,070/2,900	22	235/1,070
Contact level				
Direct[1]	64	1,862/2,900	35	648/1,862
Indirect[2]	36	1,038/2,900	29	297/1,038

Source: Korniewicz, Denise M., Marie Kirwin, Kay Cresci, and others. "In-use Comparison of Latex Gloves in Two High-Risk Units: Surgical Intensive Care and Acquired Immunodificiency Syndrome." *Heart & Lung* 21, no. 1 (January 1992), p. 83. *Notes:* 1. Touches patient and equipment. 2. Does not touch patient; equipment only.

★ 231 ★

Medical Devices

Magnetic Resonance Imaging

Introduced in 1984, magnetic resonance imaging (MRI) is an example of high-tech medicine. Twenty years ago doctors would drill holes in a patient's skull, inject dye, then x-ray to determine if a brain tumor was present. Today the patient simply would be scanned by one of the 3,600 MRI machines in the United States. The data below reflect the growth and proportion of MRI in America.

Magnetic resonance imaging equipment	Percent
Increase since introduction	20
MRIs in United States compared to rest of world	50[1]

Source: Zaldivar, R. A. "High-Tech Love Affair; Lust for Latest Technology Breaking Health Care's Back." *Phoenix Gazette,* 30 July 1993, final edition, p. A2. *Note:* 1. Approximation.

Outpatient Services

★ 232 ★

Inpatient vs. Outpatient Care: 1981 and 1991

Table below compares hospital size, occupancy, and patient visits for in-patient and outpatient care during 1981 and 1991.

[In millions]

	1981	1991
Beds	1.36	1.20
In-patient days	007	302
Outpatient visits	265	388

Source: "Hospitals Seeing More Outpatients." *Food Management* (July 1993), p. 52. Primary source: American Hospital Association.

★ 233 ★

Outpatient Services

Market Share of Outpatient Surgery

Laparoscopy - 75	
Arthroscopy - 74	
Tonsillectomy/adenoidectomy - 72	
Myringotomy/tubes - 66	
Cataract surgery - 61	
Nasal surgery - 60	
Repair wounds, superficial - 53	
Foot procedures - 41	
	Excision of benign skin lesions - 13
	Incision and drainage of cysts - 7

Chart shows data from column 2.

Approximately 155 million outpatient procedures are performed annually in hospitals. The table below shows the market share of hospitals and non-hospital care providers for selected outpatient procedures.

[In percentages]

	Number performed	Place	
		Hospitals	Non-hopital settings
Arthroscopy	1.1 million	74	26
Cataract surgery	1.6 million	61	39
Excision of benign skin lesions	7.3 million	13	87
Foot procedures	1.7 million	41	59
Incision and drainage of cysts	6.7 million	7	93
Laparoscopy[1]	634,000	75	25
Myringotomy/tubes	1.1 million	66	34
Nasal surgery	1.1 million	60	40
Repair wounds, superficial	2.6 million	53	47
Tonsillectomy/adenoidectomy	715,000	72	28

Source: "Outpatient Procedures: New Data Show Services Likely to Shift to Non-hospital Settings." *Hospitals and Health Networks,* 20 July 1993, p. 52. *Note:* 1. Surgical.

Preventive Medicine

★ 234 ★

Blood Pressure Checks

The table below reflects the percent of Americans 18 years of age and older who had their blood pressures checked in the past year. Data are provided by sex, age, and selected characteristics for 1990.

Characteristic	Both sexes 18 years and over	Male					Female				
		Total	18-29 years	30-44 years	45-64 years	65 years and over	Total	18-29 years	30-44 years	45-64 years	65 years and over
All persons[1]	87.0	82.7	77.6	80.6	85.8	90.9	90.8	92.1	89.9	90.0	91.7
Education level											
Less than 12 years	85.4	81.2	73.2	74.0	83.3	89.8	88.9	89.7	84.2	87.5	91.8
12 years	86.5	82.2	77.8	80.0	85.3	92.1	89.9	91.3	88.5	89.1	91.9
More than 12 years	88.2	83.9	79.3	82.5	87.4	91.4	92.7	93.7	92.4	92.7	91.1
13-15 years	87.6	82.6	79.5	81.4	85.7	92.0	92.0	93.6	90.8	91.9	91.5
16 years or more	88.8	85.0	79.1	83.3	88.5	91.0	93.4	93.9	93.9	93.4	90.6
income											
Less than $10,000	86.2	79.8	78.0	73.9	82.4	86.2	89.5	91.1	83.4	89.6	91.5
$10,000-$19,999	85.5	80.8	73.9	76.5	82.6	91.2	89.2	90.9	85.6	87.0	92.7
$20,000-$34,999	86.1	81.6	77.0	79.1	84.5	91.9	90.4	92.4	89.7	90.1	88.8
$35,000-$49,999	87.3	83.9	78.2	82.6	88.3	94.5	91.0	92.5	91.0	89.9	90.0
$50,000 or more	88.7	85.1	81.2	84.0	87.0	91.8	92.6	94.0	92.6	91.6	93.2
Race											
White	86.9	82.9	78.0	80.3	85.8	91.2	90.6	92.0	89.8	89.6	91.4
Black	89.2	84.7	81.6	84.3	87.5	89.0	92.6	93.1	90.9	93.3	94.4
Hispanic origin											
Hispanic	81.8	73.3	68.9	72.1	78.7	85.7	88.3	88.2	88.6	86.3	92.7
Non-Hispanic	87.4	83.4	78.5	81.3	86.1	91.1	90.9	92.6	90.0	90.1	91.6
Geographic region											
Northeast	88.7	85.5	81.2	84.7	87.5	90.7	91.4	92.5	91.3	90.8	91.3
Midwest	87.2	83.2	78.8	80.8	85.3	92.3	90.8	92.2	90.1	89.7	91.7
South	87.1	82.3	76.7	80.5	86.1	89.5	91.2	92.7	90.0	90.5	92.2
West	84.9	80.2	74.5	76.6	84.3	92.0	89.2	90.4	88.2	88.3	90.9
Marital status											
Currently married	87.6	84.4	77.7	81.9	86.7	91.8	90.7	92.1	90.1	90.3	91.1
Formerly married	88.3	81.6	81.8	76.8	82.3	88.0	90.9	92.9	89.4	89.4	92.4
Never married	83.6	77.4	77.4	76.1	78.1	87.3	90.9	92.0	89.0	87.0	88.3
Employment status											
Currently employed	85.8	81.3	77.7	80.2	85.5	89.6	90.9	91.8	90.2	91.0	90.6

[Continued]

★ 234 ★

Blood Pressure Checks
[Continued]

Characteristic	Both sexes 18 years and over	Male					Female				
		Total	18-29 years	30-44 years	45-64 years	65 years and over	Total	18-29 years	30-44 years	45-64 years	65 years and over
Unemployed	84.9	79.3	76.5	83.4	79.8	68.9[2]	90.7	92.6	88.2	90.6	94.7
Not in labor force	89.7	88.1	77.9	85.1	87.7	91.4	90.5	92.5	89.0	88.4	91.8

Source: U.S. Department of Health and Human Services. Public Health Service. Centers for Disease Control and Prevention. National Center for Health Statistics. *Health Promotion and Disease Prevention: United States, 1990.* Vital and Health Statistics, Series 10, no. 185. Hyattsville, MD: U.S. Department of Health and Human Services, Public Health Service, Centers for Disease Control and Prevention, National Center for Health Statistics, n.d., p. 32. *Notes:* Data are based on household interviews of the civilian noninstitutionalized population. The survey design, general qualifications, and information on the reliability of the estimates are given in Appendix 1 in the original source. Denominator for each cell excludes unknowns. 1. Includes persons with unknown sociodemographic characteristics. 2. Figure does not meet standard of reliability or precision (more than 30-percent relative standard error in numerator of percent or rate).

★ 235 ★

Preventive Medicine

Cholesterol Checks

The table below indicates the percent of persons 18 years of age and older who had their blood cholesterol levels checked. Data are provided by sex, age, and selected characteristics for 1990.

Characteristic	Both sexes 18 years and over	Male					Female				
		Total	18-29 years	30-44 years	45-64 years	65 years and over	Total	18-29 years	30-44 years	45-64 years	65 years and over
All persons[1]	52.7	49.9	24.5	48.2	65.9	71.4	55.3	32.2	53.2	69.4	70.5
Education level											
Less than 12 years	44.6	40.7	13.3	28.2	50.2	62.8	48.1	21.0	36.2	57.0	62.4
12 years	48.7	43.1	20.2	39.1	62.2	72.3	53.2	28.0	48.0	69.5	73.9
More than 12 years	60.8	60.0	34.2	59.1	77.1	82.8	61.5	40.8	61.7	77.8	80.6
13-15 years	54.0	51.5	29.7	52.1	72.6	77.9	56.2	35.9	57.1	74.1	79.0
16 years or more	67.7	67.6	42.0	64.5	80.1	86.4	67.9	49.6	66.1	81.5	82.7
Income											
Less than $10,000	40.8	32.3	21.0	26.4	44.9	49.0	45.4	24.0	35.9	58.5	64.5
$10,000-$19,999	46.0	40.8	18.3	32.0	51.4	68.9	50.3	27.4	39.9	61.9	72.3
$20,000-$34,999	50.6	46.8	26.3	43.0	59.0	77.2	54.4	34.6	51.5	70.0	72.4
$35,000-$49,999	55.7	52.7	22.9	53.3	70.2	84.9	58.9	38.3	58.5	73.3	79.1
$50,000 or more	65.3	65.0	34.1	64.7	77.7	87.4	65.5	41.4	65.1	77.7	78.9
Race											
White	54.7	52.4	25.8	50.6	67.9	73.2	56.8	33.2	54.6	70.1	71.5
Black	42.1	35.4	19.7	34.7	51.3	49.8	47.4	28.1	46.2	66.0	61.1
Hispanic origin											
Hispanic	37.5	30.0	14.7	31.6	47.9	57.2	43.9	27.7	45.0	63.9	62.2
Non-Hispanic	54.0	51.5	25.6	49.7	66.9	71.9	56.3	32.9	54.0	69.8	70.8
Geographic region											
Northeast	52.5	50.3	23.5	49.7	66.3	69.0	54.4	34.6	50.5	66.3	67.0

[Continued]

★ 235 ★

Cholesterol Checks
[Continued]

Characteristic	Both sexes 18 years and over	Male					Female				
		Total	18-29 years	30-44 years	45-64 years	65 years and over	Total	18-29 years	30-44 years	45-64 years	65 years and over
Midwest	54.7	52.2	26.8	50.5	67.1	75.0	57.0	32.7	54.4	72.0	72.8
South	51.8	48.1	24.7	46.2	63.5	67.3	55.1	32.1	54.3	68.5	69.6
West	52.2	49.9	22.4	47.3	67.6	76.8	54.4	29.6	52.7	71.0	73.3
Marital status											
Currently married	56.8	56.5	27.1	50.5	68.2	74.9	57.2	32.9	53.7	70.8	74.6
Formerly married	58.3	50.5	30.5	43.8	55.3	60.0	61.5	31.6	52.3	66.6	67.5
Never married	33.2	28.5	22.3	39.2	52.1	53.8	39.0	31.4	51.1	60.5	68.2
Employment status											
Currently employed	51.0	48.0	25.6	49.2	66.3	73.8	54.5	35.4	55.1	72.2	74.8
Unemployed	39.1	33.6	16.7	38.8	56.3	53.8[2]	45.1	30.8	48.5	65.5	83.3[2]
Not in labor force	57.7	59.0	20.8	37.0	65.3	71.0	57.1	24.6	47.9	65.4	69.9

Source: U.S. Department of Health and Human Services. Public Health Service. Centers for Disease Control and Prevention. National Center for Health Statistics. *Health Promotion and Disease Prevention: United States, 1990.* Vital and Health Statistics, Series 10, no. 185. Hyattsville, MD: U.S. Department of Health and Human Services, Public Health Service, Centers for Disease Control and Prevention, National Center for Health Statistics, n.d., p. 36. *Notes:* Data are based on household interviews of the civilian noninstitutionalized population. The survey design, general qualifications, and information on the reliability of the estimates are given in Appendix 1 in the original source. Denominator for each cell excludes unknowns. 1. Includes persons with unknown sociodemographic characteristics. 2. Figure does not meet standard of reliability or precision (more than 30-percent relative standard error in numerator of percent or rate).

★ 236 ★

Preventive Medicine

Cost of Preventive Practices

Data indicate the median costs of a year of life saved by selected interventions.

[In dollars]

Intervention	Cost
Childhood immunizations	<0
Prenatal care	<0
Flu shots	600
Water chlorination	4,000
Pneumonia vaccination	12,000
Breast cancer screening	17,000
Construction safety rules	38,000
Home radon control	141,000
Asbestos controls	1.9 million
Radiation controls	27.4 million

Source: Stipp, David. "Prevention May Be Costlier Than a Cure." *Wall Street Journal,* 6 July 1994, p. B1. Harvard Lifesaving Study.

★ 237 ★

Preventive Medicine

Preventable Medical Conditions

The table below reflects preventable medical conditions, including the number of those affected or cases reported, deaths per year for each, and the cost of treatment.

Condition	Number per year	Deaths per year	Cost per patient ($)
Heart disease	7 million affected	500,000	30,000.00[1]
Cancer	1 million new cases	510,000	29,000.00[2]
Stroke	600,000 strokes	150,000	22,000.00
Injuries	2.3 million hospitalized[3]	142,500	570,000.00[4]
HIV	1-1.5 million infected[5]	Not reported	75,000.00[6]
Alcoholism	18.5 million persons	105,000	250,000.00[7]
Drug abuse[8]		Not reported	63,000.00[9]
Cocaine	1.3 million persons		
Intravenous drugs	900,000 persons		
Heroin	500,00 persons		
Drug-exposed babies	375,000 babies		
Low birth-weight babies	260,000 babies born	23,000	10,000.00[10]

Source: Health Insurance Association of America (HIAA). *Source Book of Health Insurance Data, 1993.* Washington, DC: Health Insurance Association of America, 1994, p. 8. Used with permission of HIAA. *Notes:* 1. 284,000 bypass procedures are performed each year. 2. Lung cancer treatment. 3. 177,000 are spinal cord injuries. 4. Lifetime, quadriplegia. 5. 147,525 AIDS cases (January 1990). 6. Cost reflects lifetime treatment. 7. Cost of liver transplant. 8. Regular users. 9. 5 years. 10. Intensive care.

Surgical and Diagnostic Procedures

★ 238 ★

Diagnostic and Other Nonsurgical Procedures: 1980-1990

Figures below represent the number of procedures and the number per 1,000 population for diagnostic and nonsurgical procedures performed on inpatients discharged from nonfederal short-stay hospitals. Data are provided by sex, age, and procedure. Data are based on a sample of hospital records.

Sex, age, and procedure category	Procedures in thousands				Procedures per 1,000 population			
	1980[1]	1988	1989[2]	1990	1980[1]	1988	1989[2]	1990
MALES								
All ages[2,3,4]	3,386	6,665	7,202	7,378	31.3	55.6	59.3	59.6
Angiocardiography using contrast material	174	749	767	833	1.6	6.4	6.5	6.9
Computerized axial tomography (CAT scan)	152	775	721	736	1.4	6.3	5.8	5.8
Diagnostic ultrasound	114	599	628	667	1.0	5.1	5.2	5.4
Cystoscopy	543	399	356	350	5.1	3.2	2.8	2.7
Radioisotope scan	236	315	287	268	2.1	2.6	2.3	2.1
Arteriography using contrast material	180	246	233	217	1.7	2.0	1.9	1.7
Endoscopy of large intestine without biopsy	228	170	158	148	2.1	1.4	1.2	1.2
Under 15 years[2,4]	217	424	566	546	8.3	15.6	20.5	19.4
Spinal tap	39	84	97	94	1.5	3.1	3.5	3.4
Diagnostic ultrasound	6[5]	51	49	47	0.2[5]	1.9	1.8	1.7
Computerized axial tomography (CAT scan)	17	42	46	41	0.7	1.5	1.7	1.5
Electroencephalogram	5[5]	15	17	17	0.2[5]	0.5	0.6	0.6
Radioisotope scan	8[5]	11	14	11	0.3[5]	0.4	0.5	0.4
Application of cast or splint	21	14	12	10	0.8	0.5	0.4	0.4
Cystoscopy	23	5	5	5	0.9	5	5	5
15-44 years[2,4]	884	1,382	1,477	1,584	17.3	24.4	25.9	27.6
Computerized axial tomography (CAT scan)	37	218	196	216	0.7	3.8	3.4	3.8
Diagnostic ultrasound	25	111	117	118	0.5	2.0	2.0	2.1
Angiocardiography using contrast material	30	89	98	102	0.6	1.6	1.7	1.8
Contrast myelogram	88	79	65	58	1.7	1.4	1.1	1.0
Radioisotope scan	48	62	58	47	0.9	1.1	1.0	0.8
Arthroscopy of knee	94	55	55	43	1.8	1.0	1.0	0.7
Cystoscopy	80	36	37	35	1.6	0.6	0.6	0.6
Endoscopy of large intestine without biopsy	52	25	25	21	1.0	0.4	0.4	0.4
Application of cast or splint	54	27	25	22	1.1	0.5	0.4	0.4
45-64 years[2,4]	1,128	2,038	2,103	2,106	53.4	92.6	94.4	93.5
Angiocardiography using contrast material	106	388	386	428	5.0	17.6	17.3	19.0
Diagnostic ultrasound	41	173	188	184	1.9	7.9	8.5	8.1
Computerized axial tomography (CAT scan)	43	200	179	170	2.0	9.1	8.1	7.5
Radioisotope scan	75	102	88	81	3.5	4.7	3.9	3.6
Cystoscopy	153	93	84	80	7.3	4.2	3.8	3.6
Arteriography using contrast material	76	95	77	65	3.6	4.3	3.4	2.9
Endoscopy of large intestine without biopsy	86	48	36	42	4.0	2.2	1.6	1.9
65 years and over[2,4]	1,158	2,821	3,056	3,143	111.8	228.4	241.8	243.3
Computerized axial tomography (CAT scan)	54	316	299	309	5.2	25.6	23.7	23.9
Angiocardiography using contrast material	35	264	274	297	3.4	21.3	21.7	23.0
Diagnostic ultrasound	42	264	274	319	4.0	21.4	21.7	24.7
Cystoscopy	287	266	232	232	27.7	21.6	18.3	18.0

[Continued]

★ 238 ★

Diagnostic and Other Nonsurgical Procedures: 1980-1990

[Continued]

Sex, age, and procedure category	Procedures in thousands				Procedures per 1,000 population			
	1980[1]	1988	1989[2]	1990	1980[1]	1988	1989[2]	1990
Endoscopy of small intestine without biopsy	35	113	131	123	3.3	9.1	10.4	9.5
Radioisotope scan	105	139	127	129	10.1	11.3	10.1	10.0
Arteriography using contrast material	72	110	117	109	7.0	8.9	9.3	8.4
Endoscopy of large intestine without biopsy	86	94	95	84	8.3	7.6	7.5	6.5
FEMALES								
All ages[2,3,4]	3,532	6,902	9,471	10,077	27.5	47.3	64.7	68.0
Diagnostic ultrasound	204	963	930	941	1.6	6.6	6.3	6.2
Computerized axial tomography (CAT scan)	154	838	798	770	1.2	5.6	5.3	4.9
Angiocardiography using contrast material	84	439	432	510	0.7	3.1	3.0	3.5
Radioisotope scan	289	390	347	335	2.1	2.6	2.3	2.1
Endoscopy of small intestine without biopsy	164	279	291	294	1.3	1.8	1.9	1.9
Endoscopy of large intestine without biopsy	307	238	255	250	2.3	1.5	1.6	1.5
Cystoscopy	324	143	131	135	2.6	1.0	0.9	0.9
Laparoscopy (excluding that for ligation and division of fallopian tubes)	235	133	125	147	1.8	0.9	0.9	1.0
Under 15 years[2,4]	191	356	418	403	7.6	13.8	15.9	15.0
Spinal tap	26	70	75	71	1.0	2.7	2.9	2.7
Computerized axial tomography (CAT scan)	10	39	37	27	0.4	1.5	1.4	1.0
Diagnostic ultrasound	5[5]	45	33	43	0.2[5]	1.7	1.3	1.6
Electroencephalogram	5	19	14	14	5	0.7	0.5	0.5
Angiocardiography using contrast material	5	5	11	6[5]	5	5	0.4	0.2[5]
Application of cast or splint	13	9[5]	7[5]	6[5]	0.5	0.3[5]	0.3[5]	0.2[5]
Radioisotope scan	6[5]	6[5]	6[5]	9[5]	0.2[5]	0.2[5]	0.2[5]	0.3[5]
Cystoscopy	38	5[5]	5	5	1.5	0.2[5]	5	5
15-44 years[2,4]	1,203	1,643	3,850	4,217	22.7	28.3	66.1	72.0
Diagnostic ultrasound	94	365	348	309	1.8	6.3	6.0	5.3
Computerized axial tomography (CAT scan)	36	156	157	144	0.7	2.7	2.7	2.5
Laparoscopy (excluding that for ligation and division of fallopian tubes)	214	124	118	120	4.1	2.1	2.0	2.0
Biliary tract X-ray	60	109	94	102	1.1	1.9	1.6	1.7
Radioisotope scan	49	62	60	58	0.9	1.1	1.0	1.0
Contrast myelogram	66	57	46	36	1.2	1.0	0.8	0.6
Endoscopy of large intestine without biopsy	77	29	41	34	1.5	0.5	0.7	0.6
Cystoscopy	97	44	38	39	1.8	0.8	0.7	0.7
45-64 years[2,4]	1,030	1,711	1,771	1,861	44.2	71.4	73.3	76.3
Diagnostic ultrasound	44	176	190	174	1.9	7.3	7.9	7.1
Computerized axial tomography (CAT scan)	42	188	176	163	1.8	7.8	7.3	6.7
Angiocardiography using contrast material	49	189	173	214	2.1	7.9	7.2	8.8
Radioisotope scan	92	113	99	79	3.9	4.7	4.1	3.2
Biliary tract X-ray	48	63	73	64	2.1	2.6	3.0	2.6
Endoscopy of small intestine without biopsy	55	68	67	71	2.3	2.8	2.8	2.9
Endoscopy of large intestine without biopsy	94	54	58	59	4.0	2.3	2.4	2.4
Cystoscopy	93	33	37	37	4.0	1.4	1.5	1.5
65 years and over[2,4]	1,107	3,192	3,431	3,596	72.1	177.2	187.0	192.6
Computerized axial tomography (CAT scan)	66	455	428	436	4.3	25.3	23.3	23.3
Diagnostic ultrasound	62	377	359	415	4.0	20.9	19.6	22.2
Angiocardiography using contrast material	21	209	220	245	1.4	11.6	12.0	13.1
Radioisotope scan	143	209	182	189	9.3	11.6	9.9	10.1

[Continued]

★ 238 ★

Diagnostic and Other Nonsurgical Procedures: 1980-1990

[Continued]

Sex, age, and procedure category	Procedures in thousands				Procedures per 1,000 population			
	1980[1]	1988	1989[2]	1990	1980[1]	1988	1989[2]	1990
Endoscopy of small intestine without biopsy	55	150	163	168	3.6	8.3	8.9	9.0
Endoscopy of large intestine without biopsy	131	154	155	156	8.5	8.6	8.4	8.4
Cystoscopy	96	61	51	56	6.2	3.4	2.8	3.0

Source: National Economic, Social, and Environmental Data Bank: The Federal Connection [CD-ROM]. Prepared by U.S. Department of Commerce, Economics and Statistics Administration. Washington, DC. U.S. Department of Commerce, Economics and Statistics Administration, Office of Business Analysis, November 1992. Primary source: National Center for Health Statistics, Division of Health Care Statistics. Data from the National Hospital Discharge Survey. *Notes:* Excludes newborn infants. Data do not reflect total use of procedures because procedures for outpatients are not included in the National Hospital Discharge Survey. For example, CAT scans are frequently performed on outpatients. Rates are based on the civilian population. In each sex and age group, data are shown for the 5 most common procedures in 1980 and 1989. Procedure categories are based on the *International Classification of Diseases*, 9th revision, Clinical Modification. For a listing of the code numbers, see Appendix II, table IX, in the primary source. 1. Comparisons of 1980 with later years should be made with caution as estimates of change may reflect improvements in the design (see Appendix I) rather than true changes in hospital use. 2. Beginning in 1989, the definition of some surgical and diagnostic and other nonsurgical procedures was revised, thus causing a discontinuity in the trends for the totals. See Appendix II in the primary source. 3. Rates are age adjusted. 4. Includes nonsurgical procedures not shown. 5. Estimates based on fewer than 30 discharges are not shown; estimates based on 30-59 discharges should be used with caution.

★ 239 ★

Surgical and Diagnostic Procedures

Inappropriate Procedures: 1991 and 1992

Figures show the percentage of inappropriate commonly performed procedures.

[In percentages]

Procedure	Procedures performed inappropriately
Coronary angiography	2.3
Knee arthroscopy	4.0
Laminectomy	8.8
Dilation and curettage	9.4
Ear, nose, and throat procedures	9.6
Carpal tunnel	10.9
Hysterectomy	19.7

Source: "Appropriateness and the Effect of Guidelines." *Business and Health* 12, no. 3 (Special Report on Guidelines, 1994), p. 4. Primary source: Value Health Science Inc. (Santa Monica, California), 1993.

★ 240 ★

Surgical and Diagnostic Procedures

Procedures for Inpatients Discharged From Short-Stay Hospitals: 1990-1991

Excludes newborn infants and discharges from federal hospitals.

Procedure	Number of procedures (1,000)		Rate per 1,000 population[2]	
	1990[1]	1991[1]	1990[1]	1991[1]
Both sexes				
Surgical procedures, total[3][4]	23,051	23,403	92.4	93.4
Procedures to assist delivery[4]	2,491	2,558	10.0	10.2
Cesarean section	945	933	3.8	3.7
Cardiac catheterization	995	1,000	4.0	4.0
Reduction of fracture[5]	609	665	2.4	2.7
Repair of current obstetric laceration	795	795	3.2	3.2
Hysterectomy	591	546	2.4	2.2
Diagnostic and other non-surgical procedures[4][6]	17,455	20,519	70.0	81.9
CAT scan[7]	1,506	1,459	6.0	5.8
Diagnostic ultrasound	1,608	1,592	6.4	6.4
Angiocardiography and arteriography[8]	1,735	1,718	7.0	6.9
Radioisotope scan	603	539	2.4	2.2
Cystoscopy	485	427	1.9	1.7
Male				
Surgical procedures, total[3][4]	8,538	8,692	70.6	71.5
Cardiac catheterization	620	603	5.1	5.0
Prostatectomy	364	363	3.0	3.0
Reduction of fracture[5]	300	337	2.5	2.8
Repair of inguinal hernia	181	155	1.5	1.3
Diagnostic and other non-surgical procedures[4][6]	7,378	8,572	61.0	70.5
Angiocardiography and arteriography[8]	1,051	989	8.7	8.1
CAT scan[7]	736	702	6.1	5.8
Female				
Surgical procedures, total[4][3]	14,513	14,711	113.0	114.0
Procedures to assist delivery[4]	2,491	2,558	19.4	19.8
Cesarean section	945	933	7.4	7.2
Repair of current obstetric laceration	795	795	6.2	6.2
Hysterectomy	591	546	4.6	4.2
Diagnostic and other non-surgical procedures[4][6]	10,077	11,947	78.5	92.6

[Continued]

★ 240 ★

Procedures for Inpatients Discharged From Short-Stay Hospitals: 1990-1991

[Continued]

Procedure	Number of procedures (1,000)		Rate per 1,000 population[2]	
	1990[1]	1991[1]	1990[1]	1991[1]
Diagnostic ultrasound	941	940	7.3	7.3
CAT scan[7]	770	757	6.0	5.9

Source: 1993 Statistical Abstract of the United States on CD-ROM [machine-readable datafiles]. CD ABSTR-93. Washington, DC: U.S. Department of Commerce, Economics and Statistics Administration, Bureau of the Census, Data User Services Division, 1993. Primary source: U.S. National Center for Health Statistics. Vital and Health Statistics. Series 13; and unpublished data. Notes: 1. Comparisons beginning 1988 with data for earlier years should be made with caution as estimates of change may reflect improvements in the design rather than true changes in hospital use. 2. Based on Bureau of the Census estimated civilian population as of July 1. Population estimates do not reflect revised estimates based on the 1990 Census of Population. 3. Includes other types of surgical procedures not shown separately. 4. Beginning in 1989, the definition of some surgical and diagnostic and other non-surgical procedures was revised, causing a discontinuity in the trends for some totals. 5. Excluding skull, nose, and jaw. 6. Includes other non-surgical procedures not shown separately. 7. Computerized axial tomography. 8. Using contrast material.

Surgical and Diagnostic Procedures: Cost

★ 241 ★

Cancer Detection Costs

The overall costs of cancer in the United States in 1990 were estimated to have been $104 billion, or $416 per person. The table below presents some average costs relating to cancer detection.

Procedure	Average cost	Denomination
Mammographic exam	$120	Per person
Pap test	$10	Per lab fee
Fecal-occult blood test	$5	Per test
Sigmoidscopy	$100	Per procedure

Source: Brown, Martin L. "The National Economic Burden of Cancer: An Update." Journal of the National Cancer Institute 82, 5 December 1990, pp. 1811-1814.

★ 242 ★

Surgical and Diagnostic Procedures: Cost

Cardio/thoracic Surgeons' Charges for Selected Procedures

Table reflects the median fees.

[In dollars]

Procedure or treatment	Cost
Coronary artery bypass, with 3 coronary grafts	5,486.00
Replacement of aortic valve, with cardiopulmonary bypass	5,000.00
Insertion of permanent pacemaker with transvenous electrodes[1]	1,550.00

Source: "Cardio/thoracic Surgeons' Latest Fees." *Medical Economics,* 11 October 1993, p. 126. *Note:* 1. Ventricular.

★ 243 ★

Surgical and Diagnostic Procedures: Cost

Gastroenterologists' Charges for Selected Procedures

Table reflects the median fees.

[In dollars]

Procedure or treatment	Cost
Esophagogastroduodenoscopy, diagnostic	427.00
Liver biopsy[1]	250.00
Esophageal dilation[2]	150.00

Source: "What Gastroenterologists Charge for Three Procedures." *Medical Economics,* 11 October 1993, p. 130. *Notes:* 1. Percutaneous needle. 2. By unguided sound or bougie; initial session.

★ 244 ★

Surgical and Diagnostic Procedures: Cost

Knee Replacement Costs

Each year an average of 1 million patients have part or all of the cartilage in their knees removed due to injuries. Sometimes the surgery is extensive, replacing the knee with an artificial joint. In 1992, about 187,000 such operations were performed in the United States at an average cost of $40,000.

Source: "Cartilage Transplants in Knees Show Promise." *Wall Street Journal,* 9 June 1993, p. B1.

★ 245 ★

Surgical and Diagnostic Procedures: Cost

Neurosurgeons' Charges for Selected Procedures

Table reflects the median fees.

[In dollars]

Procedure or treatment	Cost
Craniotomy[1]	3,615.00
Laminectomy, lumbar[2]	3,500.00
Discectomy, anterior[3]	3,275.00
Cranioplasty[4]	2,847.00
Neuroplasty[5]	1,000.00

Source: "Median Fees for Neurosurgeons' Services." *Medical Economics,* 11 October 1993, p. 128. *Notes:* 1. For evacuation of hematoma. 2. More than 2 vertebral segments. 3. Includes osteophytectomy; cervical, single interspace. 4. For skull defect larger than 5 cm diameter. 5. Median nerve at carpal tunnel.

★ 246 ★

Surgical and Diagnostic Procedures: Cost

Orthopedic Surgeons' Charges for Selected Procedures

Table reflects the median fees.

[In dollars]

Procedure or treatment	Cost
Total hip arthroplasty	4,200.00
Total knee arthroplasty	4,142.00
Lumbar arthrodesis	3,461.00
Hip fracture, open treatment	2,392,00
Knee arthroscopy with meniscectomy	1,926.00
Diagnostic knee arthroscopy	844.00
Colles' fracture, closed manipulation	545.00
Arthrocentesis of knee[1]	69.00

Source: "What Orthopedic Surgeons Are Charging." *Medical Economics,* 11 October 1993, p. 125. *Note:* 1. Does not include pre- and post-operative care.

★ 247 ★

Surgical and Diagnostic Procedures: Cost

Plastic Surgeons' Charges for Selected Procedures

Table reflects the median fees.

[In dollars]

Procedure or treatment	Cost
Reduction mammaplasty[2]	4,500.00
Mammaplasty, augmentation, with prosthetic implant[2]	3,000.00
Rhinoplasty, complete	3,000.00
Rhytidectomy, forehead	2,410.00
Suction-assisted lipectomy, trunk	1,750.00
Blepharoplasty, upper eyelid[2]	1,500.00
Excision of benign lesion, except skin tag[1]	144.00

Source: "Big Swing in Plastic Surgeons' Charges." *Medical Economics,* 11 October 1993, pp. 126-127. *Notes:* 1. 0.5 cm or less. 2. Bilateral.

★ 248 ★

Surgical and Diagnostic Procedures: Cost

Surgeons' Charges for Selected Procedures

Table reflects the median fees charged by general surgeons.

[In dollars]

Procedure or treatment	Cost
Subtotal gastrectomy without vagotomy	2,119.00
Laparoscopy (surgical); cholecystectomy	2,000.00
Modified radical mastectomy	1,800.00
Cholecystectomy	1,503.00
Appendectomy	1,000.00
Inguinal hernia repair[1]	974.00
Excision of cyst fibroadenoma from breast tissue[2]	550.00

Source: "General Surgeons' Charges for Seven Procedures." *Medical Economics,* 11 October 1993, p. 124. *Notes:* 1. Age 5 or over. 2. One or more lesions.

★ 249 ★

Surgical and Diagnostic Procedures: Cost

Surgical Procedure Costs in Selected U.S. Cities: 1992

Data reflect charges for selected surgical procedures by geographic area for 1992.

[In dollars]

Place	Excision of breast lesion[1]	Cesarean section	Abdominal hysterectomy	Oophorectomy	Salpingo-oophorectomy	Coronary bypass (triple)	Appendectomy	Cholecytectomy
Atlanta, Georgia	628	2,643	2,253	1,488	1,562	5,733	1,052	2,920
Chicago, Illinois	656	2,539	2,543	1,576	1,570	6,063	1,150	1,899
Dallas, Texas	631	2,253	2,133	1,494	1,579	5,661	1,001	1,802
Denver, Colorado	482	1,505	1,852	1,036	1,095	5,146	932	1,450
Los Angeles, California	802	1,465	2,987	1,821	1,563	7,071	1,430	2,258
New York, New York	1,365	4,994	1,234	2,513	3,099	8,500	1,850	2,980
Philadelphia, Pennsylvania	674	2,587	2,615	1,822	1,996	6,414	1,111	1,685

Source: Health Insurance Association of America (HIAA). *Source Book of Health Insurance Data, 1993.* Washington, DC: Health Insurance Association of America, 1994, p. 73. Used with permission of HIAA. Primary source: Health Insurance Association of America. Prevailing Healthcare Charges System (1992). *Note:* 1. Lumpectomy.

Transplants

★ 250 ★

Organ Donors, by Race/Ethnicity: 1991

Organ	All donors	Donors (%)				
		White	Black	Hispanic	Asian	Other
Total	4,532	80.4	10.2	7.5	0.9	1.0
Kidney	4,272	81.1	9.9	7.1	0.9	1.0
Liver	3,166	80.5	10.0	7.8	0.9	0.8
Pancreas	1,069	83.4	7.9	7.1	1.0	0.6
Heart	2,148	80.3	9.9	8.2	0.8	0.8
Heart/lung	51	81.6	8.2	8.2	2.0	0.0
Lung	345	79.9	11.6	7.3	0.3	0.9
Multiple organ	3,445	80.7	9.8	7.7	0.9	0.9

Source: Richardson, Rod. "Blacks Reluctant to Donate Organs." *Detroit News,* 1 March 1993, p. 2A. Primary source: United Network for Organ Sharing.

★ 251 ★

Transplants

People Waiting for Transplants: 1993

Kidney - 23,586

Heart - 2,840

Liver - 2,644

Lung - 1,081

Pancreas - 998

Heart/lung - 184

Table shows the number of people on the National Organ Transplantation Waiting List as of May 12, 1993.

Organ	Number awaiting transplants
Kidney	23,586
Liver	2,644
Pancreas	998
Heart	2,840
Heart/lung	184
Lung	1,081

Source: Evans, Roger W. "Organ Procurement Expenditures and the Role of Financial Incentives." *Journal of the American Medical Association (JAMA)* 269, no. 24, 23-30 June 1993, p. 3114. Primary source: United Network for Organ Sharing.

Treatment Options and Alternatives

★ 252 ★

Ailments Treated With Alternative Therapies

In 1992, there were 425 million visits to providers of alternative care such as acupuncture or chiropractic. The table below lists the most common ailments treated through unconventional therapies.

[In percentages]

Ailment	Patients visiting alternative therapists
Back problems	36
Anxiety	28
Headache	27
Sprains/strains	22
Insomnia	20
Depression	20

Source: "USA Snapshots." USA TODAY, 6 October 1993, p. 1A. Primary source: New England Journal of Medicine. Survey of 1,539 adults.

★ 253 ★

Treatment Options and Alternatives

Spending on Alternative Medical Treatment: 1990

Figures below represent out-of-pocket expenditures for alternative therapies as compared to expenditures for all hospitalizations. Data for 1990.

[In billion dollars]

Care	Expenditures
Alternative treatments	13.7
All hospitalizations	12.8

Source: "At a Glance: Snapshots of the Workplace Health Industry." Workplace Health (May 1993), p. 15. Primary source: New York Times.

★ 254 ★

Treatment Options and Alternatives

Visits to Alternative Therapists

A 1990 national survey conducted by Dr. David M. Eisenberg of Beth Israel Hospital and Harvard Medical School found that Americans spent $13.7 billion on alternative medicine, such as chiropractic manipulation of the spine, relaxation techniques, spiritual healing, herbal medicine, and homeopathy. Those who relied on alternative therapists averaged 19 visits during the year. The problems that frequently caused people to seek unconventional therapy were backaches, anxiety, allergies, and chronic pain. Those most likely to use alternative treatment are well-educated, middle-income whites between 25 and 49 years of age, living in the western states.

Source: Angier, Natalie. "Unusual Therapy Gains Popularity." *New York Times,* 26 January 1993, p. A12.

Chapter 4
LIFESTYLES AND HEALTH

For years Americans have been hearing: "You are what you eat." In this era of counting fat grams and eating fiber, the adage now more than ever illustrates the effect of personal lifestyle on one's health. Data in this chapter show the positive consequences of good health habits such as exercise and nutrition and the consequences of health risks (substance abuse, smoking, and like behaviors) on the U.S. population. Tables reflecting living conditions—stress, domestic violence, poverty, and lack of health insurance—are presented as well. Issues specific to occupational health—for example, job-related stress—are included in the chapter on Health in the Workplace.

Addiction and Recovery: Alcohol

★ 255 ★

Alcohol Advertisements: 1990-1991

Data below indicate the number of alcohol advertisements on television each hour.

Type of promotion	Type of program				
	Situation comedy	Drama	College sports	Major professional sports	Other professional sports
Beer commercial	0.13	0.23	1.16	2.20	0.43
Wine/wine cooler commercial	0.09	0.06	0.06	0.18	0.16
Stadium sign	-	-	0.00	2.08	1.75
On-site promotion	-	-	0.00	0.00	0.98
Brief sponsorship	-	-	0.26	1.22	0.28
Total	0.22	0.29	1.48	5.68	3.60

Source: "Alcohol Portrayals and Advertising on Television." *Alcohol Health and Research World* 17, no. 1 (1993), p. 63.
Notes: The prime time data are from the fall 1990. The sports data are from the fall 1990 through the summer of 1991.

★ 256 ★
Addiction and Recovery: Alcohol

Alcohol Consumption: 1990

Percent of persons in the United States 18 years of age and older who had consumed an average of 1 ounce or more of ethanol a day (2 or more drinks of beer, wine, or liquor) in the past 2 weeks. Data are provided by sex, age, and selected characteristics.

Characteristic	Both sexes 18 years and over	Male					Female				
		Total	18-29 years	30-44 years	45-64 years	65 years and over	Total	18-29 years	30-44 years	45-64 years	65 years and over
All persons[1]	5.5	9.7	10.3	9.7	9.8	8.5	1.7	1.7	1.6	2.0	1.7
Education level											
Less than 12 years	5.1	9.2	11.1	12.8	9.1	5.4	1.5	1.7[2]	2.9	1.1[2]	1.0
12 years	5.9	11.2	12.2	11.9	10.2	9.1	1.7	1.8	1.5	1.9	1.7
More than 12 years	5.4	8.7	8.2	7.5	9.9	12.0	1.9	1.5	1.5	2.6	3.3
13-15 years	5.5	9.3	8.6	9.6	10.0	8.6	2.1	1.5	1.7	2.8	3.9
16 years or more	5.3	8.2	7.4	5.9	9.8	14.5	1.7	1.5[2]	1.3	2.5	2.4[2]
Income											
Less than $10,000	4.8	10.0	11.3	12.6	9.0	5.8	2.0	2.6	3.5	1.8[2]	0.6[2]
$10,000-$19,999	4.9	8.8	11.4	9.2	8.3	5.7	1.7	1.4[2]	2.4	1.7[2]	1.6
$20,000-$34,999	5.8	10.3	10.8	10.5	10.5	8.3	1.5	1.6	1.2	1.6	1.8[2]
$35,000-$49,999	5.6	9.3	7.6	10.3	8.0	12.8	1.5	0.8[2]	1.3	1.8[2]	3.6[2]
$50,000 or more	6.7	10.7	10.3	8.2	12.5	16.7	2.3	1.1[2]	1.7	3.0	6.6[2]
Race											
White	5.8	10.1	11.0	9.7	10.4	9.0	1.8	1.9	1.6	2.1	1.9
Black	4.3	8.2	8.1	11.8	5.6	3.4[2]	1.2	0.6[2]	2.1	1.2[2]	0.4[2]
Hispanic origin											
Hispanic	4.6	8.8	6.6	9.6	11.9	7.4[2]	1.1	1.7[2]	0.6[2]	0.6[2]	1.3[2]
Non-Hispanic	5.6	9.8	10.8	9.7	9.7	8.5	1.8	1.6	1.8	2.1	1.7
Geographic region											
Northeast	5.4	9.9	10.9	9.9	9.4	8.9	1.6	2.4	1.2	1.3[2]	1.4[2]
Midwest	5.6	10.2	12.4	10.7	8.6	7.8	1.4	0.8[2]	1.9	1.8	1.0[2]
South	5.2	9.0	9.3	9.4	9.1	7.0	1.8	1.8	1.6	2.0	1.8
West	6.1	10.3	9.1	8.9	12.6	11.6	2.2	1.7	1.8	2.7	3.0
Marital status											
Currently married	5.3	8.9	9.6	8.8	9.0	8.7	1.6	1.3	1.4	1.9	2.4
Formerly married	5.3	13.8	15.7	14.8	16.5	8.0	1.8	2.8[2]	2.2	2.2	1.2
Never married	6.6	10.3	10.6	10.6	6.4[2]	6.5[2]	2.1	1.9	2.8	1.9[2]	1.9[2]
Employment status											
Currently employed	6.1	9.6	9.7	9.6	9.6	8.6	1.9	2.0	1.5	2.1	2.5[2]
Unemployed	9.0	15.8	20.6	12.4	11.1[2]	20.5[2]	1.6[2]	0.2[2]	2.4[2]	1.7[2]	9.0[2]
Not in labor force	4.0	9.2	10.2	9.6	10.3	8.4	1.6	1.0[2]	1.9	1.7	1.6

Source: U.S. Department of Health and Human Services. Public Health Service. Centers for Disease Control and Prevention. National Center for Health Statistics. *Health Promotion and Disease Prevention: United States, 1990.* Vital and Health Statistics, Series 10, no. 185. Hyattsville, MD: U.S. Department of Health and Human Services, Public Health Service, Centers for Disease Control and Prevention, National Center for Health Statistics, n.d., p. 50. *Notes:* Data are based on household interviews of the civilian noninstitutionalized population. The survey design, general qualifications, and information on the reliability of the estimates are given in Appendix 1 in the original source. Denominator for each cell excludes unknowns. 1. Includes persons with unknown sociodemographic characteristics. 2. Figure does not meet standard of reliability or precision (more than 30 percent relative standard error in numerator of percent or rate).

★ 257 ★

Addiction and Recovery: Alcohol

Alcohol Treatment Programs: 1991

Data below reflect state-funded client treatment admissions by race/ethnicity and by state or U.S. territory.

[For fiscal year 1991]

State	Hispanic	Native American	White, not of Hispanic origin	Black, not of Hispanic origin	Asian or Pacific Islander	Other	Not reported	Total
Alabama	N/A	N/A	5,443	1,748	N/A	21	0	7,212
Alaska	0	4,828	4,100	141	0	335	70	9,474
Arizona	4,379	4,197	15,998	1,358	70	0	0	26,002
Arkansas	51	49	5,693	1,396	2	0	0	7,191
California	12,570	2,410	81,790	28,450	640	1,140	0	127,000
Colorado	14,696	3,016	33,505	3,400	165	54	0	54,836
Connecticut	1,294	N/A	9,418	3,320	N/A	69	5,435	19,536[1]
Delaware	81	0	2,756	1,250	2	0	24	4,113
District of Columbia	0	0	1,321	3,478	0	98	0	4,897
Florida	3,846	195	47,547	10,376	84	164	1,082	63,294
Georgia	77	22	17,927	8,343	9	49	0	26,427
Guam	3	1	34	0	84	0	0	122
Hawaii	66	119	1,120	55	648	306	14	2,328
Idaho	379	224	3,668	18	6	37	0	4,332
Illinois	2,665	186	28,726	15,720	124	0	0	47,421
Indiana	157	19	11,161	2,417	14	32	5	13,805
Iowa	308	236	16,808	535	35	31	254	18,207
Kansas	725	347	9,037	1,143	26	29	28	11,335
Kentucky	N/A	N/A	12,252	1,017	N/A	48	403	13,720
Louisiana	11	14	6,939	1,273	5	13	0	8,255
Maine	0	446	9,918	70	11	40	0	10,485
Maryland	N/A	N/A	12,264	5,688	N/A	244	6	18,202[2]
Massachusetts	2,373	333	46,942	4,273	127	1,157	0	55,205
Michigan	493	872	32,664	6,426	49	276	132	40,912
Minnesota	1,253	8,519	35,305	3,032	74	88	353	48,624
Mississippi	0	42	4,635	3,412	0	0	0	8,089
Missouri	187	167	18,843	6,595	23	26	39	25,880
Montana	106	1,217	6,389	27	8	17	0	7,764
Nebraska	959	2,932	17,719	1,188	35	46	15	22,894
Nevada	635	693	8,837	1,036	51	116	0	11,368
New Hampshire	43	41	4,792	75	4	0	22	4,977
New Jersey	2,470	60	17,078	10,516	0	106	30	30,260
New Mexico	4,143	2,519	2,646	133	6	0	8	9,455
New York	13,489	1,033	100,036	42,741	0	1,011	2,581	160,891
North Carolina	87	342	19,135	9,506	0	83	77	29,230
North Dakota	8	408	2,485	4	2	6	25	2,938
Ohio	207	20	14,953	5,545	0	43	0	20,768
Oklahoma	259	1,521	9,041	1,173	19	0	0	12,013
Oregon	N/A	N/A	N/A	N/A	N/A	N/A	N/A	N/A
Pennsylvania	756	N/A	28,137	6,138	29	62	N/A	35,122
Puerto Rico	7,816	0	0	0	0	0	0	7,816
Rhode Island	131	6	2,215	260	2	67	6,186	8,867
South Carolina	71	37	17,884	7,444	8	1	2	25,447

[Continued]

★ 257 ★

Alcohol Treatment Programs: 1991

[Continued]

State	Hispanic	Native American	White, not of Hispanic origin	Black, not of Hispanic origin	Asian or Pacific Islander	Other	Not reported	Total
South Dakota	0	1,687	4,671	65	0	65	0	6,488
Tennessee	9	9	4,093	1,121	4	8	0	5,244
Texas	4,066	122	8,113	1,768	25	4	0	14,098
Utah	1,499	2,071	9,411	277	87	27	89	13,461
Vermont	0	0	3,287	0	0	0	116	3,403
Virginia	797	78	29,355	10,064	80	754	807	41,935
Washington	N/A	N/A	N/A	N/A	N/A	N/A	N/A	N/A
West Virginia	5	4	10,775	764	1	0	3	11,549
Wisconsin	1,341	2,598	76,682	3,101	84	0	0	83,806
Wyoming	N/A	N/A	N/A	N/A	N/A	N/A	N/A	N/A
Total	84,511	43,640	873,545	217,880	2,643	6,673	17,806	1,246,698
Percent of total	6.8	3.5	70.0	17.5	.2	.5	1.4	100.0

Source: U.S. Department of Health and Human Services. Public Health Service. National Institutes of Health. National Institute on Alcohol Abuse and Alcoholism. National Institute on Drug Abuse. *State Resource and Services Related to Alcohol and Other Drug Abuse Problems for Fiscal Year 1990.* Rockville, MD: U.S. Department of Health and Human Services. National Institutes of Health. National Institute on Alcohol Abuse and Alcoholism. National Institute on Drug Abuse, n.d., p. 26. State Alcohol and Drug Abuse Profile (SADAP), FY 1990; data are included for "only those programs which received at least some funds administered by the State Alcohol/Drug Agency during the State's Fiscal Year (FY) 1990." *Notes:* N/A indicates information not available. 1. Asian or Pacific Islanders and Native Americans are included under "Other." 2. "Other" includes all categories except White and Black.

★ 258 ★

Addiction and Recovery: Alcohol

Alcohol Use: 1991

[Estimates shown for 1991]

	Ever used				Used in past year				Used in past month			
	Total	Hispanic	White	Black	Total	Hispanic	White	Black	Total	Hispanic	White	Black
Percent rate estimates												
Age												
12-17	46.4	45.9	48.2	40.7	40.3	40.2	41.9	35.2	20.3	22.5	20.4	20.1
18-25	90.2	82.2	93.2	82.5	82.8	72.3	86.8	72.8	63.6	52.8	67.2	56.0
26-34	92.4	85.7	94.4	88.6	80.9	74.4	83.7	72.7	61.7	57.2	63.8	57.1
35+	87.5	81.0	88.9	84.4	65.1	64.4	66.4	56.6	49.5	47.8	50.9	40.3
Sex												
Male	89.0	86.0	90.6	84.2	72.7	75.0	73.6	66.1	58.1	60.2	59.2	52.2
Female	80.7	68.9	83.3	74.7	63.9	54.9	66.8	54.5	44.3	34.9	46.6	36.5
Total	84.7	77.4	86.8	79.0	68.1	64.9	70.1	59.8	50.9	47.5	52.7	43.7
Population estimates (in thousands)												
Age												
12-17	9,339	1,043	6,766	1,265	8,123	911	5,892	1,093	4,092	510	2,866	624
18-25	25,689	2,466	19,161	3,238	23,605	2,170	17,839	2,857	18,130	1,585	13,814	2,196
26-34	35,789	3,321	27,292	4,160	31,320	2,881	24,198	3,414	23,886	2,216	18,456	2,679
35+	101,040	5,697	83,394	9,536	75,190	4,534	62,331	6,400	57,123	3,366	47,760	4,556
Sex												
Male	86,576	6,922	68,662	8,782	70,699	6,032	55,805	6,895	56,493	4,841	44,900	5,450

[Continued]

★ 258 ★

Alcohol Use: 1991
[Continued]

	Ever used				Used in past year				Used in past month			
	Total	Hispanic	White	Black	Total	Hispanic	White	Black	Total	Hispanic	White	Black
Female	85,281	5,603	67,951	9,416	67,539	4,464	54,456	6,869	46,739	2,837	37,996	4,604
Total	171,857	12,525	136,613	18,199	138,238	10,496	110,260	13,764	103,232	7,678	82,896	10,054

Source: U.S. Department of Health and Human Services. Public Health Service. Alcohol, Drug Abuse, and Mental Health Administration. *National Household Survey on Drug Abuse: Population Estimates, 1991.* Rockville, MD: U.S. Department of Health and Human Services. Public Health Service. Alcohol, Drug Abuse, and Mental Health Administration, n.d., pp. 85-87. Primary source: National Institute on Drug Abuse. 1991 National Household Survey on Drug Abuse.

★ 259 ★

Addiction and Recovery: Alcohol

Cost of Alcohol Abuse: 1985 and 1990

The table below indicates the estimated economic costs of alcohol abuse for selected years.

[Amounts in million dollars]

Type of cost	1985[1] Amount	1990[2] Amount	1990[2] Percent distribution
Total	70,338	98,623	100.0
Core costs	58,181	80,763	81.9
Direct costs	6,010	10,512	10.7
Specialty organizations	2,281	3,469	3.5
Short-stay hospitals	3,017	4,589	4.7
Office-based physicians	141	240	0.2
Other professional services	173	329	0.3
Nursing homes	703	1,095	1.1
Support costs	495	790	0.8
Indirect costs	51,371	70,251	71.2
Morbidity	27,388	36,627	37.1
Noninstitutionalized population	27,208	36,404	36.9
Institutionalized population	180	223	0.2
Mortality[3]	23,983	33,624	34.1
Other related costs	10,546	15,771	16.0
Direct costs	7,380	10,436	10.6
Crime	4,251	5,807	5.9
Motor vehicle crashes	2,584	3,876	3.9
Fire destruction	457	633	0.6
Social welfare administration	88	120	0.1
Indirect costs	3,166	5,335	5.4
Victims of crime	465	576	0.6
Incarceration	2,701	4,759	4.8

[Continued]

★ 259 ★

Cost of Alcohol Abuse: 1985 and 1990
[Continued]

Type of cost	1985[1] Amount	1990[2] Amount	1990[2] Percent distribution
Special diseases Fetal alcohol syndrome	1,611	2,089	2.1

Source: Rice, Dorothy P. "The Economic Cost of Alcohol Abuse and Alcohol Dependence: 1990." *Alcohol Health and Research World* 17, no. 1 (1993), p. 11. *Notes:* 1. Rice, D. P., S. Kelman, L. S. Miller, and S. Dunmeyer. *The Economic Costs of Alcohol and Drug Abuse and Mental Illness: 1985.* Report submitted to the U.S. Department of Health and Human Services, Alcohol, Drug Abuse, and Mental Health Administration, Office of Financing and Coverage Policy. DHHS Pub. No. (ADM)90-1694. San Francisco: University of California, Institute for Health and Aging, 1990. 2. Costs for 1990 are based on socioeconomic indexes applied to 1985 estimates. 3. Discounted at 6 percent.

★ 260 ★

Addiction and Recovery: Alcohol

Frequency of Alcohol Use: 1991

[Estimates shown for 1991]

	At least once				12 or more times				Once a week or more			
	Total	Hispanic	White	Black	Total	Hispanic	White	Black	Total	Hispanic	White	Black
Percent rate estimates												
Age												
12-17	40.3	40.2	41.9	35.2	14.4	14.9	14.9	12.6	5.1	7.2	4.9	5.5
18-25	82.8	72.3	86.8	72.8	53.0	41.7	57.1	44.2	24.8	19.8	26.5	23.1
26-34	80.9	74.4	83.7	72.7	51.1	46.5	53.3	46.6	24.1	22.6	24.4	27.3
35+	65.1	64.4	66.4	56.6	39.9	39.9	40.9	34.6	22.1	23.7	22.7	19.8
Sex												
Male	72.7	75.0	73.6	66.1	51.5	52.9	52.6	46.0	29.4	31.3	29.9	28.7
Female	63.9	54.9	66.8	54.5	32.0	23.9	34.0	27.1	13.7	9.7	14.5	12.8
Total	68.1	64.9	70.1	59.8	41.4	38.3	43.0	35.7	21.2	20.4	21.9	20.0
Population estimates (in thousands)												
Age												
12-17	8,123	911	5,892	1,093	2,900	337	2,090	392	1,035	163	691	172
18-25	23,605	2,170	17,839	2,857	15,102	1,253	11,743	1,736	7,063	593	5,448	907
26-34	31,320	2,881	24,198	3,414	19,785	1,802	15,424	2,187	9,323	875	7,052	1,282
35+	75,190	4,534	62,331	6,400	46,102	2,811	38,359	3,907	25,549	1,671	21,333	2,241
Sex												
Male	70,699	6,032	55,805	6,895	50,097	4,259	39,864	4,803	28,549	2,516	22,691	2,995
Female	67,539	4,464	54,456	6,869	33,792	1,944	27,753	3,420	14,421	787	11,833	1,608
Total	138,238	10,496	110,260	13,764	83,889	6,203	67,616	8,223	42,970	3,303	34,524	4,603

Source: U.S. Department of Health and Human Services. Public Health Service. Alcohol, Drug Abuse, and Mental Health Administration. *National Household Survey on Drug Abuse: Population Estimates, 1991.* Rockville, MD: U.S. Department of Health and Human Services. Public Health Service. Alcohol, Drug Abuse, and Mental Health Administration, n.d., pp. 121-123. Primary source: National Institute on Drug Abuse. 1991 National Household Survey on Drug Abuse.

Addiction and Recovery: Drug Abuse

★ 261 ★

Analgesics Use: 1991

[Estimates shown for 1991]

	Ever used				Used in past year				Used in past month			
	Total	Hispanic	White	Black	Total	Hispanic	White	Black	Total	Hispanic	White	Black
Percent rate estimates												
Age												
12-17	4.4	3.6	4.8	3.9	3.3	2.9	3.6	2.6	1.1	1.2	1.0	1.4
18-25	10.2	6.5	11.4	6.8	5.3	4.1	5.9	3.0	1.5	1.5	1.5	1.3
26-34	9.8	4.1	11.1	6.8	3.6	1.5	4.0	3.3	1.0	0.5	1.1	0.9
35 +	4.1	3.0	4.2	3.3	1.3	0.8	1.3	1.8	0.3	0.3	0.2	0.8
Sex												
Male	6.8	4.0	7.4	5.1	2.6	1.6	2.8	2.3	0.6	0.5	0.6	1.1
Female	5.4	4.0	5.6	4.4	2.4	2.1	2.4	2.5	0.8	0.9	0.7	0.9
Total	6.1	4.0	6.5	4.7	2.5	1.9	2.6	2.4	0.7	0.7	0.6	1.0
Population estimates (in thousands)												
Age												
12-17	895	82	677	121	668	65	510	81	217	28	146	43
18-25	2,904	195	2,344	268	1,517	122	1,213	118	428	46	310	51
26-34	3,781	160	3,213	317	1,399	60	1,145	156	397	21	310	42
35 +	4,758	208	3,979	371	1,506	56	1,204	208	361	21	215	88
Sex												
Male	6,652	323	5,644	528	2,555	128	2,134	244	596	40	428	110
Female	5,685	322	4,569	549	2,536	174	1,939	319	807	76	552	114
Total	12,337	645	10,213	1,077	5,090	302	4,072	563	1,403	116	980	224

Source: U.S. Department of Health and Human Services. Public Health Service. Alcohol, Drug Abuse, and Mental Health Administration. *National Household Survey on Drug Abuse: Population Estimates, 1991.* Rockville, MD: U.S. Department of Health and Human Services. Public Health Service. Alcohol, Drug Abuse, and Mental Health Administration, n.d., pp. 79-81. Primary source: National Institute on Drug Abuse. 1991 National Household Survey on Drug Abuse.

★ 262 ★

Addiction and Recovery: Drug Abuse

Cocaine Use: 1991

[Estimates shown for 1991]

Age/sex	Ever used				Used in past year				Used in past month			
	Total	Hispanic	White	Black	Total	Hispanic	White	Black	Total	Hispanic	White	Black
Percent rate estimates												
Age												
12-17	2.4	3.7	2.4	1.7	1.5	3.0	1.4	1.5	0.4	1.3	0.3	0.5
18-25	17.9	15.0	20.3	10.1	7.7	7.1	8.3	6.0	2.0	2.7	1.7	3.1
26-34	25.8	186	27.9	22.2	5.1	4.5	4.9	7.5	1.8	2.0	1.6	2.7
35 +	7.0	7.9	6.6	9.7	1.6	2.3	1.4	2.4	0.5	1.0	0.2	1.3

[Continued]

★ 262 ★

Cocaine Use: 1991
[Continued]

Age/sex	Ever used				Used in past year				Used in past month			
	Total	Hispanic	White	Black	Total	Hispanic	White	Black	Total	Hispanic	White	Black
Sex												
Male	14.4	15.1	14.3	15.7	4.2	5.2	4.0	5.3	1.3	2.0	1.1	2.6
Female	9.2	7.4	9.7	7.6	2.2	2.4	2.0	2..7	0.6	1.2	0.4	1.2
Total	11.7	11.2	12.0	11.3	3.1	3.8	3.0	3.9	0.9	1.6	0.7	1.8
Population estimates												
(in thousands)												
Age												
12-17	491	84	339	54	311	67	193	47	83	30	36	15
18-25	5,099	452	4,170	398	2,194	214	1,702	237	582	81	353	120
26-34	10,001	721	8,064	1,042	1,978	176	1,424	354	703	78	475	127
35+	8,124	557	6,232	1,100	1,900	161	1,346	266	523	69	232	151
Sex												
Male	14,016	1,213	10,871	1,633	4,062	421	2,996	558	1,266	164	808	267
Female	9,698	601	7,935	961	2,321	197	1,669	346	626	94	288	146
Total	23,715	1,814	18,805	2,594	6,383	618	4,665	904	1,892	258	1,096	413

Source: U.S. Department of Health and Human Services. Public Health Service. Alcohol, Drug Abuse, and Mental Health Administration. *National Household Survey on Drug Abuse: Population Estimates, 1991.* Rockville, MD: U.S. Department of Health and Human Services. Public Health Service. Alcohol, Drug Abuse, and Mental Health Administration, n.d., pp. 31-33. Primary source: National Institute on Drug Abuse. 1991 National Household Survey on Drug Abuse.

★ 263 ★

Addiction and Recovery: Drug Abuse

Cocaine Use, Frequency: 1991

Cocaine includes crack.

[Estimates shown for 1991]

	At least once				12 or more times				Once a week or more			
	Total	Hispanic	White	Black	Total	Hispanic	White	Black	Total	Hispanic	White	Black
Percent rate estimates												
Age												
12-17	1.5	3.0	1.4	1.5	0.5	1.2	0.4	0.6	0.3	0.8	0.2	0.6
18-25	7.7	7.1	8.3	6.0	1.9	2.3	1.6	3.2	0.8	1.3	0.6	1.4
26-34	5.1	4.5	4.9	7.5	1.5	1.6	1.3	3.1	0.7	0.9	0.4	1.6
35+	1.6	2.3	1.4	2.4	0.6	1.4	0.4	1.4	0.3	0.4	0.2	0.9
Sex												
Male	4.2	5.2	4.0	5.3	1.2	2.1	1.0	2.2	0.5	0.9	0.3	1.5
Female	2.2	2.4	2.0	2.7	0.7	1.0	0.5	1.7	0.4	0.5	0.3	0.8
Total	3.1	3.8	3.0	3.9	0.9	1.6	0.7	1.9	0.4	0.7	0.3	1.1
Population estimates												
(in thousands)												
Age												
12-17	311	67	193	47	106	26	80	20	69	19	32	18
18-25	2,194	214	1,702	237	536	68	330	126	230	39	133	55
26-34	1,978	176	1,424	354	594	63	368	145	256	33	129	75
35+	1,900	161	1,346	266	638	96	387	155	301	25	174	101

[Continued]

★ 263 ★

Cocaine Use, Frequency: 1991
[Continued]

	At least once				12 or more times				Once a week or more			
	Total	Hispanic	White	Black	Total	Hispanic	White	Black	Total	Hispanic	White	Black
Sex												
Male	4,062	421	2,996	558	1,136	172	724	231	480	72	253	152
Female	2,321	197	1,669	346	739	82	420	214	375	44	215	97
Total	6,383	618	4,665	904	1,874	254	1,144	445	855	116	469	249

Source: U.S. Department of Health and Human Services. Public Health Service. Alcohol, Drug Abuse, and Mental Health Administration. *National Household Survey on Drug Abuse: Population Estimates, 1991.* Rockville, MD: U.S. Department of Health and Human Services. Public Health Service. Alcohol, Drug Abuse, and Mental Health Administration, n.d., pp. 115-117. Primary source: National Institute on Drug Abuse. 1991 National Household Survey on Drug Abuse.

★ 264 ★

Addiction and Recovery: Drug Abuse

Crack Cocaine Users in Neighborhoods

Table shows reported crack cocaine users by race/ethnicity.

Characteristics	Neighborhoods with at least one crack cocaine user[1]	Neighborhoods with no crack cocaine users[2]
All	100	100
Race/ethnicity		
White American	35.9	53.5
Hispanic American	33.1	23.9
African American	28.3	20.6
Other	2.7	2.0

Source: Lillie-Blanton, Marsha, James C. Anthony, and Charles R. Schuster. "Probing the Meaning of Racial/Ethnic Group Comparisons in Crack Cocaine Smoking." *Journal of the American Medical Association (JAMA)* 269, no. 8, 24 February 1993, p. 996. Primary source: National Household Survey on Drug Abuse. *Notes:* 1. Includes 128 neighborhoods and 939 residents. 2. Includes 1,404 neighborhoods and 7,875 residents.

★ 265 ★

Addiction and Recovery: Drug Abuse

Crack Use: 1991

[Estimates shown for 1991]

Age/sex	Ever used				Used in past year				Used in past month			
	Total	Hispanic	White	Black	Total	Hispanic	White	Black	Total	Hispanic	White	Black
Percent rate estimates												
Age												
12-17	0.9	1.3	0.8	1.1	0.4	0.4	0.3	0.9	0.1	0.2	0.1	0.3
18-25	3.7	3.3	3.7	4.7	1.0	0.9	0.8	2.5	0.4	0.5	0.2	1.7
26-34	3.7	3.7	2.8	9.2	0.8	0.7	0.5	3.1	0.4	0.6	0.3	1.3
35+	1.0	1.1	0.8	3.0	0.3	0.6	0.2	0.6	0.2	0.4	0.1	0.3
Sex												
Male	2.6	3.2	2.0	6.3	0.8	0.9	0.5	2.2	0.4	0.6	0.3	1.2
Female	1.3	1.1	1.1	2.6	0.3	0.4	0.2	0.8	0.1	0.2	[1]	0.4
Total	1.9	2.1	1.5	4.3	0.5	0.6	0.3	1.5	0.2	0.4	0.2	0.7
Population estimates												
(in thousands)												
Age												
12-17	179	30	115	33	85	9	48	28	22	4	10	8
18-25	1,068	99	756	185	290	26	164	99	114	16	34	65
26-34	1,430	143	808	432	312	26	133	145	169	22	88	59
35+	1,209	76	740	337	334	43	195	63	174	27	108	39
Sex												
Male	2,552	256	1,549	656	744	72	409	228	393	51	217	125
Female	1,334	92	869	331	277	32	131	106	87	17	[1]	47
Total	3,886	348	2,418	987	1,021	105	540	334	479	68	239	172

Source: U.S. Department of Health and Human Services. Public Health Service. Alcohol, Drug Abuse, and Mental Health Administration. *National Household Survey on Drug Abuse: Population Estimates, 1991.* Rockville, MD: U.S. Department of Health and Human Services. Public Health Service. Alcohol, Drug Abuse, and Mental Health Administration, n.d., pp. 37-39. Primary source: National Institute on Drug Abuse. 1991 National Household Survey on Drug Abuse. *Note:* 1. Low precision; no estimate reported.

★ 266 ★

Addiction and Recovery: Drug Abuse

Hallucinogen Use: 1991

[Estimates shown for 1991]

Age/sex	Ever used				Used in past year				Used in past month			
	Total	Hispanic	White	Black	Total	Hispanic	White	Black	Total	Hispanic	White	Black
Percent rate estimates												
Age												
12-17	3.4	3.5	3.9	1.2	2.1	1.9	2.5	1.0	0.8	0.4	0.9	0.4
18-25	13.2	7.5	15.8	5.4	4.8	2.1	5.9	1.8	1.2	0.6	1.3	1.0
26-34	15.6	9.1	18.0	6.0	1.2	0.8	1.2	0.7	0.2	0.2	0.2	0.3
35+	5.4	5.6	5.7	3.7	0.5	0.3	0.5	0.4	0.1	0.1	0.1	0.1
Sex												
Male	10.3	9.1	11.1	6.2	1.7	0.9	1.9	1.2	0.5	0.2	0.6	0.6
Female	6.4	3.9	7.3	2.4	1.0	1.0	1.2	0.5	0.2	0.3	0.2	0.1

[Continued]

★ 266 ★

Hallucinogen Use: 1991

[Continued]

	Ever used				Used in past year				Used in past month			
	Total	Hispanic	White	Black	Total	Hispanic	White	Black	Total	Hispanic	White	Black
Total	8.2	6.5	9.1	4.1	1.4	1.0	1.5	0.8	0.3	0.3	0.4	0.3
Population estimates												
(in thousands)												
Age												
12-17	679	79	547	36	427	44	348	33	155	10	132	12
18-25	3,751	224	3,251	211	1,361	64	1,208	70	328	19	271	38
26-34	6,028	353	5,218	281	446	30	345	35	88	7	66	14
35+	6,233	396	5,311	421	553	22	487	44	121	9	106	6
Sex												
Male	9,975	731	8,379	649	1,685	75	1,449	122	505	17	424	61
Female	6,717	321	5,948	300	1,102	85	939	59	188	28	151	9
Total	16,692	1,052	14,327	949	2,787	160	2,388	181	693	48	575	70

Source: U.S. Department of Health and Human Services. Public Health Service. Alcohol, Drug Abuse, and Mental Health Administration. *National Household Survey on Drug Abuse; Population Estimates, 1991.* Rockville, MD: U.S. Department of Health and Human Services. Public Health Service. Alcohol, Drug Abuse, and Mental Health Administration, n.d., pp. 49-51. Primary source: National Institute on Drug Abuse. 1991 National Household Survey on Drug Abuse.

★ 267 ★

Addiction and Recovery: Drug Abuse

Illicit Drug Use: 1991

Illicit drugs include marijuana and the nonmedical use of psychotherapeutics, inhalants, cocaine, hallucinogens, and heroin.

[Estimates shown for 1991]

Age/sex	Ever used				Used in past year				Used in past month			
	Total	Hispanic	White	Black	Total	Hispanic	White	Black	Total	Hispanic	White	Black
Percent rate estimates												
Age												
12-17	20.1	17.9	20.6	20.4	14.8	13.3	15.1	15.2	6.8	7.9	6.7	7.1
18-25	54.7	40.3	59.2	46.4	29.2	20.9	31.5	25.6	15.4	11.6	16.0	16.7
26-34	61.8	42.2	65.7	58.0	18.4	13.1	18.3	23.1	8.9	6.2	8.5	13.9
35+	27.6	25.1	27.1	34.1	6.6	7.1	6.2	9.6	3.0	3.8	2.5	5.6
Sex												
Male	41.1	37.4	41.0	47.2	14.8	15.5	14.0	20.0	7.5	7.8	6.9	12.3
Female	33.5	24.7	34.8	32.6	11.1	8.5	11.2	11.9	5.0	5.0	4.7	6.9
Total	37.1	31.0	37.8	39.2	12.8	12.0	12.5	15.8	6.2	6.4	5.8	9.4
Population estimates												
(in thousands)												
Age												
12-17	4,044	406	2,892	635	2,988	302	2,120	474	1,370	178	942	222
18-25	15,593	1,210	12,163	1,820	8,312	629	6,468	1,003	4,392	349	3,294	656
26-34	23,946	1,635	19,004	2,725	7,144	508	5,298	1,083	3,441	241	2,458	651
35+	31,768	1,764	25,458	3,852	7,617	502	5,847	1,089	3,444	268	2,391	629
Sex												
Male	39,927	3,007	31,109	4,920	14,386	1,246	10,618	2,144	7,326	630	5,231	1,285

[Continued]

★ 267 ★

Illicit Drug Use: 1991
[Continued]

Age/sex	Ever used				Used in past year				Used in past month			
	Total	Hispanic	White	Black	Total	Hispanic	White	Black	Total	Hispanic	White	Black
Female	35,424	2,008	28,409	4,113	11,676	694	9,115	1,505	5,320	405	3,855	873
Total	75,351	5,015	59,517	9,033	26,062	1,940	19,733	3,649	12,647	1,035	9,086	2,158

Source: U.S. Department of Health and Human Services. Public Health Service. Alcohol, Drug Abuse, and Mental Health Administration. *National Household Survey on Drug Abuse: Population Estimates, 1991.* Rockville, MD: U.S. Department of Health and Human Services. Public Health Service. Alcohol, Drug Abuse, and Mental Health Administration, n.d., pp. 19-21. Primary source: National Institute on Drug Abuse. 1991 National Household Survey on Drug Abuse.

★ 268 ★

Addiction and Recovery: Drug Abuse

Inhalant Use: 1991

[Estimates shown for 1991]

	Ever used				Used in past year				Used in past month			
	Total	Hispanic	White	Black	Total	Hispanic	White	Black	Total	Hispanic	White	Black
Percent rate estimates												
Age												
12-17	7.0	6.6	7.7	5.1	4.1	4.1	4.5	2.9	1.8	2.9	1.6	1.9
18-25	10.9	6.6	12.8	4.4	3.5	1.4	4.1	1.4	1.5	0.7	1.7	0.9
26-34	9.2	6.3	10.4	4.7	0.9	0.7	0.9	1.4	0.5	0.4	0.5	0.5
35 +	2.7	2.8	2.6	2.9	0.6	0.6	0.6	0.9	0.2	0.2	0.1	0.6
Sex												
Male	7.1	6.3	7.5	4.8	1.7	1.3	1.8	1.4	0.7	0.7	0.7	0.8
Female	4.1	3.4	4.3	3.0	1.1	1.2	1.1	1.3	0.5	0.8	0.4	0.9
Total	5.6	4.9	5.8	3.8	1.4	1.3	1.4	1.3	0.6	0.7	0.5	0.8
Population estimates (in thousands)												
Age												
12-17	1,414	150	1,078	158	820	92	627	90	359	65	229	59
18-25	3,108	198	2,625	173	991	43	853	54	431	22	343	35
26-34	3,574	243	2,994	220	356	29	249	67	182	17	135	24
35 +	3,174	194	2,440	330	709	39	539	98	242	17	118	73
Sex												
Male	6,892	508	5,653	502	1,673	103	1,357	144	701	59	501	78
Female	4,378	278	3,485	379	1,203	101	911	165	512	62	324	114
Total	11,270	786	9,138	881	2,876	203	2,268	309	1,213	121	825	192

Source: U.S. Department of Health and Human Services. Public Health Service. Alcohol, Drug Abuse, and Mental Health Administration. *National Household Survey on Drug Abuse: Population Estimates, 1991.* Rockville, MD: U.S. Department of Health and Human Services. Public Health Service. Alcohol, Drug Abuse, and Mental Health Administration, n.d., pp. 43-45. Primary source: National Institute on Drug Abuse. 1991 National Household Survey on Drug Abuse.

★ 269 ★

Addiction and Recovery: Drug Abuse

Marijuana Use: 1991

[Estimates shown for 1991]

Age/sex	Ever used				Used in past year				Used in past month			
	Total	Hispanic	White	Black	Total	Hispanic	White	Black	Total	Hispanic	White	Black
Percent rate estimates												
Age												
12-17	13.0	12.2	13.2	13.7	10.1	9.4	10.3	10.4	4.3	4.6	4.4	4.5
18-25	50.5	36.2	54.9	43.0	24.6	16.9	26.7	22.0	13.0	9.1	13.7	14.6
26-34	59.5	39.3	63.5	55.1	14.5	9.4	14.3	19.2	7.0	4.2	6.6	11.9
35 +	23.9	21.8	23.4	31.3	4.2	4.7	3.9	6.5	2.1	2.3	1.9	3.5
Sex												
Male	37.9	34.4	37.7	44.4	12.0	12.5	11.3	17.1	6.3	5.9	6.0	10.1
Female	29.2	20.2	30.4	28.7	7.5	5.1	7.6	8.3	3.4	2.8	3.2	4.9
Total	33.4	27.3	34.0	35.8	9.6	8.7	9.4	12.3	4.8	4.3	4.5	7.2
Population estimates												
(in thousands)												
Age												
12-17	2,625	275	1,856	425	2,032	214	1,451	324	874	104	622	139
18-25	14,395	1,086	11,278	1,687	7,002	507	5,493	863	3,714	273	2,819	573
26-34	23,048	1,523	18,360	2,588	5,609	364	4,124	899	2,705	162	1,902	559
35 +	27,621	1,531	21,948	3,541	4,907	331	3,705	737	2,428	163	1,791	396
Sex												
Male	36,833	2,769	28,611	4,631	11,627	1,003	8,541	1,779	6,135	476	4,515	1,054
Female	30,856	1,647	24,831	3,611	7,922	413	6,232	1,043	3,586	228	2,619	614
Total	67,689	4,416	53,442	8,242	19,549	1,416	14,773	2,823	9,721	703	7,134	1,667

Source: U.S. Department of Health and Human Services. Public Health Service. Alcohol, Drug Abuse, and Mental Health Administration. *National Household Survey on Drug Abuse: Population Estimates, 1991.* Rockville, MD: U.S. Department of Health and Human Services. Public Health Service. Alcohol, Drug Abuse, and Mental Health Administration, n.d., pp. 25-27. Primary source: National Institute on Drug Abuse. 1991 National Household Survey on Drug Abuse.

★ 270 ★

Addiction and Recovery: Drug Abuse

Marijuana Use, Frequency: 1991

[Estimates shown for 1991]

Age/sex	At least once				12 or more times				Once a week or more			
	Total	Hispanic	White	Black	Total	Hispanic	White	Black	Total	Hispanic	White	Black
Percent rate estimates												
Age												
12-17	10.1	9.4	10.3	10.4	4.8	4.3	5.0	5.3	2.4	2.5	2.5	2.6
18-25	24.6	16.9	26.7	22.0	11.8	8.0	12.5	13.0	6.8	4.7	6.9	9.1
26-34	14.5	9.4	14.3	19.2	7.1	4.5	6.6	10.8	4.2	3.3	3.6	8.0
35 +	4.2	4.7	3.9	6.5	2.0	2.4	1.9	3.3	1.1	0.6	1.0	2.3
Sex												
Male	12.0	12.5	11.3	17.1	6.4	6.2	6.0	9.9	3.8	3.5	3.5	7.1
Female	7.5	5.1	7.6	8.3	3.0	2.2	2.9	4.1	1.5	1.1	1.4	2.6
Total	9.6	8.7	9.4	12.3	4.6	4.2	4.4	6.7	2.6	2.3	2.4	4.6

[Continued]

★ 270 ★
Marijuana Use, Frequency: 1991
[Continued]

	At least once				12 or more times				Once a week or more			
	Total	Hispanic	White	Black	Total	Hispanic	White	Black	Total	Hispanic	White	Black
Population estimates (in thousands)												
Age												
12-17	2,032	214	1,451	324	975	98	701	164	487	58	347	82
18-25	7,002	507	5,493	863	3,363	239	2,572	510	1,945	141	1,427	356
26-34	5,609	364	4,124	899	2,737	176	1,919	507	1,612	130	1,035	376
35+	4,907	331	3,705	737	2,283	167	1,745	372	1,245	40	950	255
Sex												
Male	11,627	1,003	8,541	1,779	6,224	498	4,578	1,037	3,683	282	2,625	743
Female	7,922	413	6,232	1,043	3,135	182	2,359	516	1,607	87	1,134	326
Total	19,549	1,416	14,773	2,823	9,358	680	6,937	1,553	5,289	368	3,759	1,068

Source: U.S. Department of Health and Human Services. Public Health Service. Alcohol, Drug Abuse, and Mental Health Administration. *National Household Survey on Drug Abuse: Population Estimates, 1991.* Rockville, MD: U.S. Department of Health and Human Services. Public Health Service. Alcohol, Drug Abuse, and Mental Health Administration, n.d., pp. 109-111. Primary source: National Institute on Drug Abuse. 1991 National Household Survey on Drug Abuse.

★ 271 ★
Addiction and Recovery: Drug Abuse

Psychotherapeutics Use: 1991

Psychotherapeutics include sedatives, tranquilizers, stimulants, or analgesics. The nonmedical use of any of these is considered drug abuse.

[Estimates shown for 1991]

	Ever used				Used in past year				Used in past month			
	Total	Hispanic	White	Black	Total	Hispanic	White	Black	Total	Hispanic	White	Black
Percent rate estimates												
Age												
12-17	7.5	5.7	8.2	5.8	5.4	4.1	5.9	4.1	1.9	1.7	1.9	1.8
18-25	18.0	11.3	20.6	10.5	8.7	6.5	9.5	5.8	2.9	2.1	3.2	2.0
26-34	20.0	11.0	22.7	12.7	6.2	2.9	6.8	5.3	2.2	1.3	2.4	1.7
35+	9.6	8.2	10.0	7.1	2.8	2.0	2.8	3.4	0.9	1.0	0.7	1.7
Sex												
Male	13.4	10.5	14.4	9.2	4.5	3.1	4.7	4.2	1.5	1.3	1.4	1.8
Female	11.7	7.7	12.7	8.2	4.6	3.6	4.7	4.4	1.6	1.5	1.5	1.7
Total	12.6	9.1	13.5	8.7	4.5	3.3	4.7	4.3	1.5	1.4	1.4	1.7
Population estimates (in thousands)												
Age												
12-17	1,508	128	1,145	180	1,086	94	824	127	373	38	267	55
18-25	5,117	340	4,237	411	2,471	194	1,955	226	817	64	648	77
26-34	7,767	427	6,566	598	2,402	113	1,977	251	866	51	693	78
35+	11,070	578	9,369	804	3,202	141	2,594	388	1,006	71	663	193
Sex												
Male	13,059	844	10,948	959	4,349	253	3,530	437	1,414	103	1,038	188

[Continued]

★ 271 ★

Psychotherapeutics Use: 1991
[Continued]

	Ever used				Used in past year				Used in past month			
	Total	Hispanic	White	Black	Total	Hispanic	White	Black	Total	Hispanic	White	Black
Female	12,404	630	10,368	1,034	4,812	289	3,820	555	1,647	121	1,234	215
Total	25,463	1,474	21,317	1,993	9,161	542	7,350	992	3,062	224	2,272	403

Source: U.S. Department of Health and Human Services. Public Health Service. Alcohol, Drug Abuse, and Mental Health Administration. *National Household Survey on Drug Abuse: Population Estimates, 1991.* Rockville, MD: U.S. Department of Health and Human Services. Public Health Service. Alcohol, Drug Abuse, and Mental Health Administration, n.d., pp. 55-57. Primary source: National Institute on Drug Abuse. 1991 National Household Survey on Drug Abuse.

★ 272 ★

Addiction and Recovery: Drug Abuse

Sedative Use: 1991

[Estimates shown for 1991]

Age/sex	Ever used				Used in past year				Used in past month			
	Total	Hispanic	White	Black	Total	Hispanic	White	Black	Total	Hispanic	White	Black
Percent rate estimates												
Age												
12-17	2.4	2.2	2.7	1.2	1.3	1.2	1.4	1.0	0.5	0.8	0.6	0.1
18-25	4.3	2.3	5.1	2.4	1.9	1.3	2.2	0.9	0.6	0.5	0.7	0.2
26-34	7.5	3.4	8.6	3.8	1.2	0.8	1.2	1.1	0.4	0.3	0.3	0.3
35 +	3.5	3.3	3.5	3.4	0.7	0.3	0.7	1.3	0.3	[1]	0.3	0.7
Sex												
Male	4.8	4.2	5.0	3.3	1.0	0.9	1.0	1.1	0.4	0.3	0.3	0.5
Female	3.8	1.8	4.2	2.9	1.1	0.6	1.1	1.2	0.4	0.3	0.4	0.4
Total	4.3	3.0	4.6	3.0	1.0	0.7	1.1	1.2	0.4	0.3	0.4	0.5
Population estimates (in thousands)												
Age												
12-17	492	49	378	38	267	26	198	32	102	18	80	4
18-25	1,227	68	1,047	95	547	38	455	37	176	16	140	8
26-34	2,887	133	2,490	179	464	32	357	50	136	13	85	15
35 +	4,077	231	3,330	390	852	24	645	147	342	[1]	258	80
Sex												
Male	4,666	337	3,815	342	973	70	731	112	345	21	253	51
Female	4,017	144	3,430	360	1,157	51	924	154	410	27	309	55
Total	8,684	481	7,245	702	2,130	121	1,655	266	755	48	562	106

Source: U.S. Department of Health and Human Services. Public Health Service. Alcohol, Drug Abuse, and Mental Health Administration. *National Household Survey on Drug Abuse: Population Estimates, 1991.* Rockville, MD: U.S. Department of Health and Human Services. Public Health Service. Alcohol, Drug Abuse, and Mental Health Administration, n.d., pp. 67-69. Primary source: National Institute on Drug Abuse. 1991 National Household Survey on Drug Abuse. *Note:* 1. Low estimates; no estimates reported.

★ 273 ★

Addiction and Recovery: Drug Abuse

Stimulant Use: 1991

[Estimates shown for 1991]

Age/sex	Ever used				Used in past year				Used in past month			
	Total	Hispanic	White	Black	Total	Hispanic	White	Black	Total	Hispanic	White	Black
Percent rate estimates												
Age												
12-17	3.0	2.1	3.5	0.8	1.9	1.4	2.2	0.4	0.5	0.2	0.6	0.1
18-25	9.4	5.1	11.3	3.3	3.4	2.8	3.8	1.9	0.8	0.5	0.9	0.3
26-34	12.2	6.3	14.3	5.0	1.9	0.8	2.2	1.1	0.5	0.3	0.5	0.2
35 +	5.4	4.7	5.8	3.3	0.5	0.3	0.5	0.6	0.1	0.1	0.2	0.1
Sex												
Male	8.2	6.5	9.1	3.3	1.5	1.0	1.6	1.0	0.4	0.4	0.5	0.2
Female	5.9	3.1	6.7	3.3	1.2	1.1	1.2	0.9	0.2	0.1	0.3	0.1
Total	7.0	4.8	7.9	3.3	1.3	1.1	1.4	0.9	0.3	0.3	0.4	0.2
Population estimates (in thousands)												
Age												
12-17	597	47	495	25	389	33	315	12	106	6	83	5
18-25	2,667	152	2,330	128	965	83	777	75	217	16	188	13
26-34	4,738	244	4,130	236	729	33	636	53	179	14	155	11
35 +	6,248	331	5,411	369	625	24	498	70	165	8	143	15
Sex												
Male	7,984	525	6,924	347	1,478	84	1,237	101	415	32	346	26
Female	6,266	249	5,442	411	1,231	89	990	109	253	11	224	16
Total	14,249	775	12,366	758	2,709	172	2,227	210	668	43	570	42

Source: U.S. Department of Health and Human Services. Public Health Service. Alcohol, Drug Abuse, and Mental Health Administration. *National Household Survey on Drug Abuse: Population Estimates, 1991.* Rockville, MD: U.S. Department of Health and Human Services. Public Health Service. Alcohol, Drug Abuse, and Mental Health Administration, n.d., pp. 61-63. Primary source: National Institute on Drug Abuse. 1991 National Household Survey on Drug Abuse.

★ 274 ★

Addiction and Recovery: Drug Abuse

Tranquilizer Use: 1991

[Estimates shown for 1991.]

Age/sex	Ever used				Used in past year				Used in past month			
	Total	Hispanic	White	Black	Total	Hispanic	White	Black	Total	Hispanic	White	Black
Percent rate estimates												
Age												
12-17	2.1	1.0	2.6	1.1	1.3	0.5	1.6	0.6	0.3	0.1	0.4	0.2
18-25	7.5	3.7	8.9	3.9	2.6	1.2	3.1	1.5	0.6	0.2	0.8	0.4
26-34	10.1	5.4	11.5	5.7	2.5	1.2	2.8	1.9	0.8	0.2	0.8	0.6
35 +	4.2	4.2	4.4	2.4	1.2	1.1	1.3	1.0	0.3	0.6	0.3	0.2
Sex												
Male	6.0	5.1	6.5	3.5	1.6	1.1	1.8	1.1	0.4	0.2	0.4	0.1
Female	5.2	2.8	5.9	2.9	1.7	1.0	1.9	1.3	0.5	0.5	0.5	0.5
Total	5.6	3.9	6.2	3.1	1.7	1.0	1.8	1.2	0.4	0.4	0.4	0.3

[Continued]

★ 274 ★

Tranquilizer Use: 1991
[Continued]

Age/sex	Ever used				Used in past year				Used in past month			
	Total	Hispanic	White	Black	Total	Hispanic	White	Black	Total	Hispanic	White	Black
Population estimates (in thousands)												
Age												
12-17	423	22	362	35	259	12	224	17	69	2	59	8
18-25	2,126	112	1,824	153	742	35	630	58	179	6	157	16
26-34	3,900	208	3,336	266	972	46	814	88	294	8	242	28
35 +	4,881	296	4,163	271	1,435	76	1,204	117	347	41	241	28
Sex												
Male	5,007	410	4,913	363	1,590	88	1,343	112	381	18	311	13
Female	5,524	228	4,772	361	1,817	81	1,529	169	508	38	388	67
Total	11,331	637	9,685	724	3,408	170	2,872	281	889	57	698	80

Source: U.S. Department of Health and Human Services. Public Health Service. Alcohol, Drug Abuse, and Mental Health Administration. *National Household Survey on Drug Abuse: Population Estimates, 1991.* Rockville, MD: U.S. Department of Health and Human Services. Public Health Service. Alcohol, Drug Abuse, and Mental Health Administration, n.d., pp. 73-75. Primary source: National Institute on Drug Abuse. 1991 National Household Survey on Drug Abuse.

★ 275 ★

Addiction and Recovery: Drug Abuse

Trends in Drug Use Among High School Seniors: 1975-1991

Data indicates trends in drug use among high school seniors by type of drug and frequency of use.

[- indicates data not collected]

Type of drug and frequency of use	Class of 1975	Class of 1980	Class of 1985	Class of 1986	Class of 1987	Class of 1900	Class of 1909	Class of 1000	Class of 1001
Percent reporting having ever used drugs									
Alcohol	90.4	93.2	92.2	91.3	92.2	92.0	90.7	89.5	88.0
Any illicit drug abuse	55.2	65.4	60.6	57.6	56.6	53.9	50.9	47.9	-
Marijuana only	19.0	26.7	20.9	19.9	20.8	21.4	19.5	18.5	-
Any illicit drug other than marijuana[1]	36.2	38.7	39.7	37.7	35.8	32.5	31.4	29.4	-
Use of selected drugs									
Cocaine	9.0	15.7	17.3	16.9	15.2	12.1	10.3	9.4	7.8
Heroin	2.2	1.1	1.2	1.1	1.2	1.1	1.3	1.3	0.9
LSD	11.3	9.3	7.5	7.2	8.4	7.7	8.3	8.7	8.8
Marijuana/hashish	47.3	60.3	54.2	50.9	50.2	47.2	43.7	40.7	36.7
PCP	-	9.6	4.9	4.8	3.0	2.9	3.9	2.8	2.9
Percent reporting use of drugs in the past 12 months									
Alcohol	84.8	87.9	85.6	84.5	85.7	85.3	82.7	80.6	77.7
Any illicit drug abuse	45.0	53.1	46.3	44.3	41.7	38.5	35.4	32.5	-
Marijuana only	18.8	22.7	18.9	18.4	17.6	17.4	15.4	14.6	-
Any illicit drug other than marijuana[1]	26.2	30.4	27.4	25.9	24.1	21.1	20.0	17.9	-

[Continued]

★ 275 ★

Trends in Drug Use Among High School Seniors: 1975-1991
[Continued]

Type of drug and frequency of use	Class of 1975	Class of 1980	Class of 1985	Class of 1986	Class of 1987	Class of 1988	Class of 1989	Class of 1990	Class of 1991
Use of selected drugs									
Cocaine	5.6	12.3	13.1	12.7	10.3	7.9	6.5	5.3	3.5
Heroin	1.0	0.5	0.6	0.5	0.5	0.5	0.6	0.5	0.4
LSD	7.2	6.5	4.4	4.5	5.2	4.8	4.9	5.4	5.2
Marijuana/hashish	40.0	48.8	40.6	38.8	36.3	33.1	29.6	27.0	23.9
PCP	-	4.4	2.9	2.4	1.3	1.2	2.4	1.2	1.4

Percent reporting use of drugs in the past 30 days

Alcohol	68.2	72.0	65.9	65.3	66.4	63.9	60.0	57.1	54.0
Any illicit drug abuse	30.7	37.2	29.7	27.1	24.7	21.3	19.7	17.2	-
Marijuana only	15.3	18.8	14.8	13.9	13.1	11.3	10.6	9.2	-
Any illicit drug other than marijuana[1]	15.4	18.4	14.9	13.2	11.6	10.0	9.1	8.0	-
Use of selected drugs									
Cocaine	1.9	5.2	6.7	6.2	4.3	3.4	2.8	1.9	1.4
Heroin	0.4	0.2	0.3	0.2	0.2	0.2	0.3	0.2	0.2
LSD	2.3	2.3	1.6	1.7	1.8	1.8	1.8	1.9	1.9
Marijuana/hashish	27.1	33.7	25.7	23.4	21.0	18.0	16.7	14.0	13.8
PCP	-	1.4	1.6	1.3	0.6	0.3	1.4	0.4	0.5

Source: U.S. Department of Education. Office of Educational Research and Improvement. National Center for Education Statistics. *Digest of Education Statistics, 1992.* Washington, DC: U.S. Government Printing Office, 1992, p. 139. Primary source: U.S. Department of Health and Human Services. Alcohol, Drug Abuse, and Mental Health Administration. *Drug Use Among American High School Students and Other Young Adults: National Trends Through 1988* and press release dated January 1992. This table was prepared in May 1992. *Notes:* Source includes data for additional years. A revised questionnaire was used in 1982 and later years to reduce the inappropriate reporting of nonprescription stimulants. This slightly reduced the number of positive responses for some types of drug abuse. 1. Other illicit drugs include any use of hallucinogens, cocaine, heroin, or any other use of opiates, stimulants, sedatives, or tranquilizers not under a doctor's orders.

★ 276 ★

Addiction and Recovery: Drug Abuse

Trends in Reported Drug Use Among 12- to 17-Year-Olds: 1972-1991

Figures reflect the percentage of youths 12 to 17 years old who have reported using drugs during the past 30 days and the past year.

[- indicates data not available.]

Drug	1972	1974	1976	1977	1979	1982	1985	1988	1990	1991

Percentage reporting drug use during past 30 days

Any illicit use	-	-	-	-	17.6	12.7	14.9	9.2	8.1	6.8
Marijuana	7.0	12.0	12.3	16.6	16.7	11.5	12.0	6.4	5.2	4.3
Hallucinogens	1.4	1.3	0.9	1.6	2.2	1.4	1.2	0.8	0.9	0.8
Cocaine	0.6	1.0	1.0	0.8	1.4	1.6	1.5	1.1	0.6	0.4
Heroin	-	-	-	-	-	-	-	0.1	-	0.1

[Continued]

★ 276 ★

Trends in Reported Drug Use Among 12- to 17-Year-Olds: 1972-1991

[Continued]

Drug	1972	1974	1976	1977	1979	1982	1985	1988	1990	1991
Nonmedical use of										
Stimulants	-	1.0	1.2	1.3	1.2	2.6	1.6	1.2	1.0	0.5
Sedatives	-	1.0	-	0.8	1.1	1.3	1.0	0.6	0.9	0.5
Tranquilizers	-	1.0	1.1	0.7	0.6	0.9	0.6	0.2	0.5	0.3
Analgesics	-	-	-	-	0.6	07	1.6	0.9	1.4	1.1
Alcohol	-	34.0	32.4	31.2	37.2	30.2	31.0	25.2	24.5	20.3
Cigarettes	-	25.0	23.4	22.3	12.1	14.7	15.3	11.8	11.6	10.8

Percentage reporting drug use during past year

Drug	1972	1974	1976	1977	1979	1982	1985	1988	1990	1991
Any illicit use	-	-	-	-	26.0	22.0	23.7	16.8	15.9	14.8
Marijuana	-	18.5	18.4	22.3	24.1	20.6	19.7	2.6	11.3	10.1
Hallucinogens	3.6	4.3	2.8	3.1	4.7	3.6	2.7	2.8	2.4	2.1
Cocaine	1.5	2.7	2.3	2.6	4.2	4.1	4.0	2.9	2.2	1.5
Heroin	-	-	-	0.6	-	-	-	0.4	0.6	0.2
Nonmedical use of										
Stimulants	-	3.0	2.2	3.7	2.9	5.6	4.3	2.8	3.0	1.9
Sedatives	-	2.0	1.2	2.0	2.2	3.7	2.9	1.7	2.2	1.3
Tranquilizers	-	2.0	1.8	2.9	2.7	3.3	3.4	1.6	1.5	1.3
Analgesics	-	-	-	-	2.2	3.7	3.8	3.0	4.8	3.3
Alcohol	-	51.0	49.3	47.5	53.6	52.4	51.7	44.6	41.0	40.3
Cigarettes	-	-	-	-	13.3	24.8	25.8	22.8	22.2	20.1

Source: U.S. Department of Education. Office of Educational Research and Improvement. National Center for Education Statistics. *Digest of Education Statistics, 1002.* Washington, DC: U.S. Government Printing Office, 1992, p. 138. Primary source. U.S. Department of Health and Human Services. National Institute on Drug Abuse. *National Household Survey on Drug Abuse.* Various years. This table was prepared in April 1992.

★ 277 ★

Addiction and Recovery: Drug Abuse

Trends in Reported Drug Use Among 18- to 25-Year-Olds: 1972-1991

Figures reflect the percentage of adults 18 to 25 years old who have reported using drugs during the past 30 days and the past year.

[- indicates data not available.]

Drug	1972	1974	1976	1977	1979	1982	1985	1988	1990	1991

Percentage reporting drug use during past 30 days

Drug	1972	1974	1976	1977	1979	1982	1985	1988	1990	1991
Any illicit use	-	-	-	-	37.1	30.4	25.7	17.8	14.9	15.4
Marijuana	27.8	25.2	25.0	27.4	35.4	27.4	21.8	15.5	12.7	13.0
Hallucinogens	-	2.5	1.1	2.0	4.4	1.7	1.9	1.9	0.8	1.2
Cocaine	-	3.1	2.0	3.7	9.3	6.8	7.6	4.5	2.2	2.0

[Continued]

★ 277 ★

Trends in Reported Drug Use Among 18- to 25-Year-Olds: 1972-1991

[Continued]

Drug	1972	1974	1976	1977	1979	1982	1985	1988	1990	1991
Heroin	-	-	-	-	-	-	-	0.1	0.1	0.1
Nonmedical use of										
Stimulants	-	3.7	4.7	2.5	3.5	4.7	3.7	2.4	1.2	0.8
Sedatives	-	1.6	2.3	2.8	2.8	2.6	1.6	0.9	0.7	0.6
Tranquilizers	-	1.2	2.6	2.4	2.1	1.6	1.6	1.0	0.5	0.6
Analgesics	-	-	-	-	1.0	1.0	1.8	1.5	1.2	1.5
Alcohol	-	69.3	69.0	70.0	75.9	70.9	71.4	65.3	63.3	63.6
Cigarettes	-	48.8	49.4	47.3	42.6	39.5	36.8	35.2	31.5	32.2

Percentage reporting drug use during past year

	1972	1974	1976	1977	1979	1982	1985	1988	1990	1991
Any illicit use	-	-	-	-	49.4	43.4	42.6	32.0	28.7	29.2
Marijuana	-	34.2	35.0	38.7	46.9	40.4	36.9	27.9	24.6	24.6
Hallucinogens	-	6.1	6.0	6.4	9.9	6.9	4.0	5.6	3.9	4.8
Cocaine	-	8.1	7.0	10.2	19.6	18.8	16.3	12.1	7.5	7.7
Heroin	-	0.8	0.6	1.2	0.8	-	0.6	0.3	0.5	0.3
Nonmedical use of										
Stimulants	-	8.0	8.8	10.4	10.4	10.8	9.9	6.4	3.4	3.4
Sedatives	-	4.2	5.7	8.2	7.3	8.7	5.0	3.3	2.0	1.9
Tranquilizers	-	4.6	6.2	7.8	7.1	5.9	6.4	4.6	2.4	2.6
Analgesics	-	-	-	-	5.2	4.4	6.6	5.5	4.1	5.3
Alcohol	-	77.1	77.9	79.8	86.6	87.1	87.2	81.7	80.2	82.8
Cigarettes	-	-	-	-	46.7	47.2	44.3	44.7	39.7	41.2

Source: U.S. Department of Education. Office of Educational Research and Improvement. National Center for Education Statistics. *Digest of Education Statistics, 1992.* Washington, DC: U.S. Government Printing Office, 1992, p. 302. Primary source: U.S. Department of Health and Human Services. National Institute on Drug Abuse. *National Household Survey on Drug Abuse.* Various years. This table was prepared in April 1992.

Addiction and Recovery: Substance Abuse

★ 278 ★

Cost of Substance Abuse, by State

This table indicates the charge per substance abuse incident for selected health care providers.

[In dollars]

State	Hospital room and board	Hospital ancillary	Hospital physician
Alabama	5,830	1,390	520
Arizona	6,480	1,800	800
Arkansas	4,490	1,680	450
California	6,390	1,760	750
Colorado	4,880	1,040	380
Connecticut	4,420	1,200	270
Florida	5,600	1,390	770
Georgia	5,560	1,800	890
Illinois	6,150	1,310	540
Indiana	5,510	1,230	410
Iowa	3,110	950	250
Kansas	5,920	1,170	560
Kentucky	5,780	1,090	640
Louisiana	6,410	2,600	840
Maine	4,720	840	170
Maryland	4,470	770	300
Massachusetts	3,450	1,310	460
Michigan	4,070	1,480	250
Minnesota	3,800	670	310
Mississippi	4,060	1,760	540
Missouri	5,670	1,380	560
Montana	5,290	320	210
Nevada	5,240	1,420	660
New Hampshire	6,940	1,010	280
New Jersey	6,300	780	550
New Mexico	6,500	2,630	840
New York	6,330	1,040	360
North Carolina	4,880	1,090	460
Ohio	5,410	940	380
Oklahoma	5,490	1,220	160
Oregon	3,330	710	70
Pennsylvania	5,400	720	210
Rhode Island	5,400	400	70
South Carolina	6,100	1,250	250
Tennessee	5,180	1,330	580
Texas	5,320	3,750	1,080
Utah	5,560	1,890	470
Vermont	7,700	1,020	80
Virginia	6,280	1,220	590

[Continued]

★ 278 ★

Cost of Substance Abuse, by State
[Continued]

State	Hospital room and board	Hospital ancillary	Hospital physician
Washington	4,200	1,360	150
West Virginia	4,590	1,900	1,270
Wisconsin	3,980	960	470

Source: Metropolitan Life Insurance Company. Claims data. Merged and edited by Corporate Health Strategies Inc. Analyses and computations by Metropolitan Life Insurance Company, Safety Education Division. Primary source: *Statistical Bulletin* (October-December 1991). *Note:* States with fewer than 20 cases have been excluded.

★ 279 ★

Addiction and Recovery: Substance Abuse

Cost of Substance Abuse, Per Person

Substance abuse costs $177 billion annually for direct, indirect, and related charges. This translates into an average of $750 for every man, woman, and child in the United States.

Source: U.S. House Committee on Ways and Means. *Impact of Substance Abuse on State and Local Child Welfare Systems: Hearing.* Prepared by Richard L. Jones of the Child Welfare League of America. 30 April 1991. Washington, DC: U.S. Government Printing Office, 1991, n.p.

Exercise and Fitness

★ 280 ★

Exercise and Health

According to RAND Corporation, an average of 21 minutes of life would be gained and an average of 24 cents would be saved in medical and other costs for each additional mile walked or ran by a sedentary person.

Source: Wellness Letter 8, no. 8 (May 1992), p. 1.

★ 281 ★

Exercise and Fitness

Exercise or Sports Play: 1990

The table below indicates the percent of persons in the United States 18 years of age and older who exercised or played sports regularly in 1990. Data provided by sex, age, and selected characteristics.

[In percentages]

Characteristic	Both sexes 18 years and over	Male					Female				
		Total	18-29 years	30-44 years	45-64 years	65 years and over	Total	18-29 years	30-44 years	45-64 years	65 years and over
All persons[1]	40.7	44.0	56.1	44.3	35.6	36.9	37.7	44.2	40.1	34.6	29.1
Educational level											
Less than 12 years	25.9	29.3	45.0	23.2	20.6	29.5	22.8	28.1	21.6	22.0	21.1
12 years	37.0	40.3	51.5	37.3	32.0	37.1	34.4	38.5	34.1	33.4	30.5
More than 12 years	52.1	54.3	66.1	53.9	46.6	47.5	49.8	56.7	49.7	45.1	42.3
13-15 years	48.5	50.3	65.2	46.5	37.5	42.2	47.0	53.9	44.8	42.5	42.2
16 years or more	55.8	57.9	67.6	59.5	52.4	51.4	53.2	61.7	54.4	47.8	42.3
Income											
Less than $10,000	32.9	40.4	61.8	28.8	22.0	26.1	28.9	38.3	27.2	21.4	24.8
$10,000-$19,999	32.3	35.3	47.9	33.3	24.3	30.6	29.9	36.5	30.0	24.8	27.5
$20,000-$34,999	40.5	42.6	56.0	40.3	30.9	41.4	38.5	43.7	39.0	34.9	33.4
$35,000-$49,999	46.1	47.2	57.6	49.6	33.3	47.4	44.8	53.2	44.4	38.8	41.3
$50,000 or more	51.7	54.1	62.7	54.8	49.5	49.6	49.1	57.1	50.7	44.5	37.5
Race											
White	41.5	44.1	55.0	45.0	36.3	37.8	39.1	46.4	42.1	35.7	29.9
Black	34.3	42.2	61.7	39.6	28.3	25.1	27.9	32.2	29.4	25.5	19.1
Hispanic origin											
Hispanic	34.9	38.4	46.7	38.5	24.4	32.1	31.9	35.1	33.4	27.8	21.2
Non-Hispanic	41.2	44.5	57.3	44.7	36.3	37.1	38.3	45.6	40.7	35.2	29.4
Geographic region											
Northeast	37.4	41.8	53.6	43.5	34.1	31.8	33.5	42.8	36.5	31.1	21.9
Midwest	41.5	43.8	55.5	45.4	36.0	33.3	39.3	46.7	40.2	37.3	30.9
South	39.0	42.8	56.7	42.3	32.1	37.6	35.7	42.6	38.4	31.3	27.7
West	45.9	48.3	58.0	46.8	41.8	45.7	43.5	45.4	46.1	41.1	38.5
Marital status											
Currently married	39.4	40.7	49.0	42.7	35.7	38.0	38.0	40.8	40.0	36.2	31.6
Formerly married	34.3	40.4	48.2	48.1	35.9	32.8	31.8	35.6	39.5	31.7	27.5
Never married	51.3	56.3	61.3	49.7	32.3	33.5	45.0	49.2	42.4	25.0	25.0
Employment status											
Currently employed	43.2	45.6	55.7	45.2	37.0	36.0	40.3	46.0	40.5	34.7	32.4

[Continued]

★ 281 ★

Exercise or Sports Play: 1990

[Continued]

Characteristic	Both sexes 18 years and over	Male					Female				
		Total	18-29 years	30-44 years	45-64 years	65 years and over	Total	18-29 years	30-44 years	45-64 years	65 years and over
Unemployed	42.7	43.4	53.5	40.8	28.9	34.6[2]	42.0	46.8	40.6	34.7	34.6[2]
Not in labor force	35.4	38.6	59.7	30.6	30.4	37.1	33.8	39.4	39.0	34.5	28.7

Source: U.S. Department of Health and Human Services. Public Health Service. Centers for Disease Control and Prevention. National Center for Health Statistics. *Health Promotion and Disease Prevention: United States, 1990.* Vital and Health Statistics, Series 10, no. 185. Hyattsville, MD: U.S. Department of Health and Human Services, Public Health Service, Centers for Disease Control and Prevention, National Center for Health Statistics, n.d., p. 40. *Notes:* Data are based on household interviews of the civilian noninstitutionalized population. The survey design, general qualifications, and information on the reliability of the estimates are given in Appendix 1 in the original source. Denominator for each cell excludes unknowns. 1. Includes persons with unknown sociodemographic characteristic. 2. Figure does not meet standard of reliability or precision (more than 30 percent relative standard error in numerator of percent or rate).

★ 282 ★

Exercise and Fitness

Knowledge of the Need for Exercise: 1990

Table below indicates the percent of persons 18 years of age and older who specified that exercise needs to be performed 3 times per week and maintained 20 minutes per session in order to strengthen the heart and lungs. Data provided by sex, age, and selected characteristics.

[In percentages]

Characteristic	Both sexes 18 years and over	Male					Female				
		Total	18-29 years	30-44 years	45-64 years	65 years and over	Total	18-29 years	30-44 years	45-64 years	65 years and over
All persons[1]	5.2	4.9	4.0	6.0	5.3	3.0	5.5	5.2	7.5	5.4	2.8
Education level											
Less than 12 years	2.8	2.4	2.5	3.1	2.0	2.0	3.3	4.6	4.2	3.2	2.1
12 years	4.4	3.3	2.7	4.0	3.8	2.2	5.3	4.8	6.5	5.3	3.6
More than 12 years	7.2	7.3	6.0	8.0	8.4	5.2	7.2	5.8	9.2	7.2	3.0
13-15 years	5.9	6.1	5.0	6.4	7.9	4.9	5.7	4.8	7.2	6.3	2.3[2]
16 years or more	8.6	8.4	7.8	9.2	8.7	5.4	8.9	7.7	11.0	8.1	3.8[2]
Income											
Less than $10,000	3.2	2.5	3.0	3.0[2]	2.1[2]	1.4[2]	3.7	4.2	4.8	4.3	2.2
$10,000-$19,999	3.7	3.2	3.1	3.8	3.1	2.7	4.1	4.2	4.9	4.2	3.3
$20,000-$34,999	5.5	4.5	5.1	5.2	3.3	3.6	6.5	6.7	8.3	5.5	3.7
$35,000-$49,999	6.9	6.4	4.6	7.7	6.2	4.4[2]	7.5	7.0	8.1	7.5	5.2[2]
$50,000 or more	6.9	6.8	3.4	8.0	7.8	4.6[2]	7.1	4.5	9.4	6.2	2.8[2]
Race											
White	5.5	5.2	4.3	6.4	5.6	3.3	5.7	5.4	7.8	5.6	2.9
Black	3.9	3.1	2.9	3.5	4.1	0.5[2]	4.6	4.5	6.2	4.0	2.0[2]
Hispanic origin											
Hispanic	3.4	2.9	2.2[2]	3.5	3.0[2]	3.5	3.9	3.4	4.6	4.7	1.1[2]
Non-Hispanic	5.4	5.0	4.2	6.2	5.5	3.0	5.7	5.4	7.7	5.5	2.9

[Continued]

★ 282 ★

Knowledge of the Need for Exercise: 1990

[Continued]

Characteristic	Both sexes 18 years and over	Male					Female				
		Total	18-29 years	30-44 years	45-64 years	65 years and over	Total	18-29 years	30-44 years	45-64 years	65 years and over
Geographic region											
Northeast	5.2	4.7	4.5	5.3	5.8	2.0^2	5.5	4.6	7.7	5.0	4.0
Midwest	6.0	5.8	4.8	7.9	5.5	3.5	6.2	6.5	8.0	5.4	3.6
South	4.5	3.8	2.6	4.8	4.7	2.3	5.1	5.2	6.9	5.4	1.4
West	5.5	5.5	4.9	6.2	5.6	4.7	5.6	4.1	7.8	5.8	2.9
Marital status											
Currently married	5.8	5.2	5.5	5.9	5.6	3.0	6.3	5.7	8.2	5.5	3.2
Formerly married	4.0	3.9	3.5^2	5.0	3.9	2.3^2	4.1	5.2	5.6	5.1	2.5
Never married	4.5	4.1	3.0	7.2	5.1^2	5.2^2	4.9	4.7	5.8	5.8^2	4.0^2
Employment status											
Currently employed	5.9	5.4	4.3	6.1	5.8	4.0	6.4	5.4	7.8	6.1	2.2^2
Unemployed	4.3	3.6	2.1^2	4.6^2	5.2^2	$-^2$	5.0	3.4^2	7.7	3.5^2	6.4^2
Not In labor force	3.9	3.1	3.1	4.4	3.3	2.8	4.3	5.1	6.7	4.5	2.9

Source: U.S. Department of Health and Human Services. Public Health Service. Centers for Disease Control and Prevention. National Center for Health Statistics. *Health Promotion and Disease Prevention: United States, 1990.* Vital and Health Statistics, Series 10, no. 185. Hyattsville, MD: U.S. Department of Health and Human Services, Public Health Service, Centers for Disease Control and Prevention, National Center for Health Statistics, n.d., p. 45. *Notes:* Data are based on household interviews of the civilian noninstitutionalized population. The survey design, general qualifications, and information on the reliability of the estimates are given in Appendix 1 in the original source. Denominator for each cell excludes unknowns. 1. Includes persons with unknown sociodemographic characteristics. 2. Figure does not meet standard of reliability or precision (more than 30 percent relative standard error in numerator of percent or rate).

★ 283 ★

Exercise and Fitness

Physical Activity at Work: 1990

Table reflects the percent of persons in the United States 18 years of age and older whose job or main daily activity requires at least a moderate amount of physical work. Data provided by sex, age, and selected characteristics.

[In percentages]

Characteristic	Both sexes 18 years and over	Male					Female				
		Total	18-29 years	30-44 years	45-64 years	65 years and over	Total	18-29 years	30-44 years	45-64 years	65 years and over
All persons[1]	39.3	43.6	54.2	47.6	39.1	23.3	35.3	36.5	37.4	37.0	27.5
Education level											
Less than 12 years	44.2	49.1	63.6	65.2	52.3	22.9	39.9	46.1	52.1	46.2	25.7
12 years	46.7	56.5	64.8	65.1	49.8	26.1	38.9	39.9	42.7	38.8	30.3
More than 12 years	29.7	30.4	39.1	31.6	23.8	21..3	28.9	29.2	29.5	28.3	26.6
13-15 years	37.8	44.2	50.0	48.8	36.1	22.0	32.0	30.6	34.7	30.6	29.6
16 years or more	21.4	18.3	20.3	18.5	16.0	20.7	25.2	26.8	24.6	26.0	22.4
Income											
Less than $10,000	35.3	37.1	42.1	50.2	30.9	21.1	34.4	35.8	46.6	39.5	23.8

[Continued]

★ 283 ★

Physical Activity at Work: 1990
[Continued]

Characteristic	Both sexes 18 years and over	Male					Female				
		Total	18-29 years	30-44 years	45-64 years	65 years and over	Total	18-29 years	30-44 years	45-64 years	65 years and over
$10,000-$19,999	46.7	50.2	60.2	64.9	45.8	26.4	43.8	46.6	50.0	45.1	34.5
$20,000-$34,999	45.9	53.2	59.3	59.6	53.1	25.1	38.9	36.3	40.7	43.4	31.8
$35,000-$49,999	41.2	46.1	55.8	45.0	43.9	30.5	35.7	33.0	36.0	39.3	29.2
$50,000 or more	29.5	30.5	49.2	28.4	24.9	18.1	28.4	31.0	28.6	28.1	20.5
Race											
White	38.7	43.2	55.3	46.8	38.2	23.6	34.6	36.1	36.2	36.1	27.8
Black	44.1	48.2	52.7	54.8	44.9	22.8	40.8	40.5	43.8	46.4	24.1
Hispanic origin											
Hispanic	45.0	54.3	53.0	60.6	54.6	23.6	37.1	35.5	40.5	38.7	25.2
Non-Hispanic	38.8	42.7	54.4	46.4	38.2	23.3	35.2	36.7	37.2	37.0	27.6
Geographic region											
Northeast	37.9	41.5	51.0	45.3	35.7	27.0	34.6	36.3	37.8	35.7	26.4
Midwest	41.6	45.3	56.8	48.5	41.2	24.9	38.2	40.2	40.4	39.0	30.8
South	39.4	44.1	56.2	49.0	39.2	20.4	35.2	36.0	37.8	38.3	25.1
West	37.6	42.7	50.9	46.3	39.7	22.8	32.7	33.5	33.1	33.7	29.1
Marital status											
Currently married	40.3	42.8	57.1	47.8	39.6	24.7	37.6	39.7	37.6	37.4	35.1
Formerly married	33.2	39.0	65.5	48.6	37.8	18.1	30.8	35.2	39.7	37.0	21.8
Never married	41.3	48.4	51.6	45.6	34.7	19.5	32.6	33.1	32.5	31.8	27.2
Employment status											
Currently employed	43.7	50.2	59.2	49.3	43.8	37.6	35.9	36.7	34.9	36.6	34.3
Unemployed	41.3	42.6	48.1	42.5	32.1	43.9[2]	39.9	34.5	45.1	43.4	29.0[2]
Not in labor force	29.8	20.6	23.8	20.3	19.3	20.3	34.2	36.3	44.4	37.4	26.8

Source: U.S. Department of Health and Human Services. Public Health Service. Centers for Disease Control and Prevention. National Center for Health Statistics. *Health Promotion and Disease Prevention: United States, 1990.* Vital and Health Statistics, Series 10, no. 185. Hyattsville, MD: U.S. Department of Health and Human Services, Public Health Service, Centers for Disease Control and Prevention, National Center for Health Statistics, n.d., p. 43. *Notes:* Data are based on household interviews of the civilian noninstitutionalized population. The survey design, general qualifications, and information on the reliability of the estimates are given in Appendix 1 in the original source. Denominator for each cell excludes unknowns. 1. Includes persons with unknown sociodemographic characteristics. 2. Figure does not meet standard of reliability or precision (more than 30 percent relative standard error in numerator of percent or rate).

★ 284 ★

Exercise and Fitness

Student Participation in Athletic Extracurricular Activities: 1990

Individual sports - 23.2	
Basketball - 19.9	
Baseball/softball - 15.6	
Football - 15.9	
Other team sport - 14.2	
Soccer - 7.6	
	Cheerleading - 5.9
	Swim team - 3.9

Chart shows data from column 1.

The table below reflects the participation of tenth graders in extracurricular activities of an athletic nature. Data provided by selected student characteristics.

[In percentages]

Extracurricular activities	Total	Sex		Race/ethnicity					Socioeconomic status[1]		
		Male	Female	White	Black	Hispanic	Asian	Native American	Low	Middle	High
Baseball/softball	15.6	19.2	12.1	16.0	13.7	15.7	13.9	19.8	14.0	16.8	15.2
Basketball	19.9	24.3	15.4	18.2	30.9	16.6	22.8	21.8	18.4	20.8	19.8
Cheerleading	5.9	1.7	10.0	5.3	9.9	5.2	3.8	14.6	5.3	6.2	6.2
Football	15.9	28.9	2.9	14.7	22.6	16.0	16.2	14.5	15.5	16.5	15.2
Soccer	7.6	9.1	6.1	7.9	4.0	8.5	10.2	5.9	4.6	6.8	11.6
Swim team	3.9	3.9	3.9	4.1	2.8	3.3	5.2	3.7	2.3	3.3	6.2
Other team sport	14.2	11.1	17.2	14.5	11.3	13.5	19.7	18.0	11.0	14.5	17.1
Individual sports	23.2	27.7	18.7	23.9	21.9	17.9	28.4	20.4	16.7	21.8	31.9

Source: U.S. Department of Education. Office of Educational Research and Improvement. National Center for Education Statistics. *Digest of Education Statistics, 1992.* Washington, DC: U.S. Government Printing Office, 1992, p.136. Primary source: U.S. Department of Education. National Center for Educational Statistics. National Educational Longitudinal Study of 1990: First Followup Survey. This table was prepared in May 1992. *Notes:* 1. Socioeconomic status (SES) was measured by a composite score on parental education and occupations and on family income. The "Low" SES group is the lowest quartile; the "Middle" SES group is the middle two quartiles, and the "High" group is the upper quartile.

★ 285 ★

Exercise and Fitness

Walking for Exercise: 1990

Data reflect percent of persons in the United States 18 years of age and older who walked for exercise in the past 2 weeks. Data provided by sex, age, and selected characteristics.

[In percentages]

Characteristic	Both sexes 18 years and over	Male					Female				
		Total	18-29 years	30-44 years	45-64 years	65 years and over	Total	18-29 years	30-44 years	45-64 years	65 years and over
All persons[1]	45.1	40.9	34.2	38.9	44.5	51.6	48.9	50.7	49.7	49.4	44.3
Education level											
Less than 12 years	38.2	37.3	35.2	29.3	36.3	46.2	39.0	40.8	38.6	40.6	37.0
12 years	43.4	37.8	32.0	34.7	41.8	53.1	47.8	48.8	46.6	48.4	47.5
More than 12 years	50.2	45.0	36.1	43.9	50.7	57.9	55.5	56.5	54.9	57.0	52.1
13-15 years	47.8	41.2	34.0	40.8	46.8	57.1	53.8	54.4	52.1	56.8	51.7
16 years or more	52.6	48.4	39.7	46.2	53.2	58.5	57.6	60.4	57.5	57.3	52.6
Income											
Less than $10,000	45.9	44.3	39.4	49.1	51.0	44.5	46.8	50.6	48.4	44.4	42.9
$10,000-$19,999	42.7	40.3	33.5	36.8	42.1	51.4	44.6	45.3	46.3	42.4	44.2
$20,000-$34,999	44.8	41.4	35.7	38.8	44.2	54.6	48.2	50.5	47.3	49.3	43.8
$35,000-$49,999	46.6	40.6	34.3	40.1	41.7	61.7	53.1	54.6	53.4	50.3	56.6
$50,000 or more	48.6	43.1	34.1	39.7	49.0	57.6	54.6	54.6	54.0	56.5	48.2
Race											
White	45.3	40.8	32.9	38.5	44.8	52.4	49.5	51.3	50.0	50.3	44.9
Black	45.0	42.8	42.5	42.4	43.9	42.6	46.8	48.7	49.5	45.1	38.4
Hispanic origin											
Hispanic	36.9	32.5	29.1	32.2	31.6	60.6	40.5	39.9	42.4	38.5	40.6
Non-Hispanic	45.8	41.5	34.8	39.5	45.2	51.4	49.7	52.2	50.3	50.1	44.4
Geographic region											
Northeast	47.7	44.8	39.2	41.9	48.6	54.9	50.3	51.8	52.5	51.3	43.6
Midwest	46.6	41.5	36.2	40.1	43.6	50.9	51.3	54.1	51.0	51.7	47.2
South	43.5	38.9	32.2	37.1	42.1	50.2	47.5	51.7	48.4	46.1	41.6
West	43.4	39.5	30.9	37.4	45.2	51.7	47.1	44.2	47.7	50.1	46.3
Marital status											
Currently married	45.0	41.3	33.6	37.4	44.2	52.1	48.7	48.7	48.7	50.5	44.0
Formerly married	45.5	43.7	30.4	42.6	43.8	49.6	46.2	45.3	50.4	46.4	44.0
Never married	45.0	38.0	34.7	44.3	50.4	50.9	53.5	53.5	56.2	48.6	50.1
Employment status											
Currently employed	43.3	38.0	33.3	37.7	42.6	45.0	49.6	51.2	49.8	48.2	45.4

[Continued]

★ 285 ★
Walking for Exercise: 1990
[Continued]

Characteristic	Both sexes 18 years and over	Male					Female				
		Total	18-29 years	30-44 years	45-64 years	65 years and over	Total	18-29 years	30-44 years	45-64 years	65 years and over
Unemployed	48.3	44.7	41.1	48.5	45.4	51.3[2]	52.2	52.8	54.2	45.8	59.0[2]
Not in labor force	48.6	50.7	37.5	53.8	53.4	53.2	47.6	49.0	48.6	51.4	44.0

Source: U.S. Department of Health and Human Services. Public Health Service. Centers for Disease Control and Prevention. National Center for Health Statistics. Health Promotion and Disease Prevention: United States, 1990. Vital and Health Statistics, Series 10, no. 185. Hyattsville, MD: U.S. Department of Health and Human Services, Public Health Service, Centers for Disease Control and Prevention, National Center for Health Statistics, n.d., p. 41. Notes: Data are based on household interviews of the civilian noninstitutionalized population. The survey design, general qualifications, and information on the reliability of the estimates are given in Appendix 1 in the original source. Denominator for each cell excludes unknowns. 1. Includes persons with unknown sociodemographic characteristics. 2. Figure does not meet standard of reliability or precision (more than 30 percent relative standard error in numerator of percent or rate).

★ 286 ★
Exercise and Fitness

Weight Loss and Lower Blood Pressure

Weight loss was found to be the most effective way to reduce blood pressure, according to the Trials of Hypertension Prevention—a multicenter study of 2,000 hypertensive people on nondrug therapies—initiated by the National Heart, Lung, and Blood Institute. Typically, a weight loss of 15 pounds over a 6-month time period resulted in a drop of nearly 4 mmHg in diastolic and 2.5 mmHg in systolic blood pressure. After 2 years of a nondrug regime (sodium and alcohol restrictions, exercise, and weight loss), people lowered their diastolic blood pressures by an average of 9 mmHg and their systolic pressures by 11 mmHg

Source: "How to Lower Blood Pressure." Consumer Reports 57 (May 1992), pp. 300-301.

Insurance Coverage

★ 287 ★

Americans Without Health Insurance: 1991

Approximately 37 million people, 17 percent of the population, carried no health insurance in 1991. The table below shows precentages of those without insurance.

	Percentage
Working family head	34.4
Children	26.0
Working dependent	21.6
Unemployed	17.0
Elderly	1.0

Source: Lee, Jessica, and Mimi Hall. "White House Presses Health-Care Plan." *USA TODAY*, 23 February 1993, final edition, p. 4A. Primary source: Employee Benefits Research Institute.

★ 288 ★

Insurance Coverage

Health Insurance Coverage and Poverty: 1991

The table below indicates the number and percent distribution of the population at all income levels and below the poverty level that are covered by some form of health insurance. Data provided by race/ethnicity.

[In thousands]

Age, race, and Hispanic origin	Total	Covered by some form of health insurance all or part of year					Not covered
		Total	Private insurance[1]	Medicaid[1]	Medicare[1]	CHAMPUS, VA or military health plan[1]	
Number							
All income levels							
Hispanic origin[2]	22,068	15,106	10,336	4,577	1,309	521	6,962
White	210,121	183,033	159,596	16,900	28,940	7,855	27,088
Black	31,312	24,850	15,454	8,282	3,248	1,481	6,462
Income below poverty level							
Hispanic origin[2]	6,339	3,773	836	3,022	319	56	2,566
White	23,747	16,333	6,035	9,782	3,307	463	7,414
Black	10,242	7,927	1,513	6,241	1,169	144	2,315
Percent distribution							
All income levels							
Hispanic origin[2]	100.0	68.5	46.8	20.7	5.9	2.4	31.5

[Continued]

★ 288 ★

Health Insurance Coverage and Poverty: 1991
[Continued]

Age, race, and Hispanic origin	Total	Covered by some form of health insurance all or part of year					Not covered
		Total	Private insurance[1]	Medicaid[1]	Medicare[1]	CHAMPUS, VA or military health plan[1]	
White	100.0	87.1	76.0	8.1	13.8	3.7	12.9
Black	100.0	79.4	49.4	26.4	10.4	4.7	20.6
Income below poverty level							
Hispanic origin[2]	100.0	59.5	13.2	47.7	5.0	0.9	40.5
White	100.0	68.8	25.4	41.2	13.9	1.9	31.2
Black	100.0	77.4	14.8	60.9	11.4	1.4	22.6

Source: U.S. Bureau of the Census. *Poverty in the United States: 1991.* Current Population Reports. Series P-60, no. 181. Washington, DC: U.S. Government Printing Office, 1992, p. xviii. *Notes:* VA is an acronym for Veterans Administration. 1. Includes those also covered by other insurance. 2. Persons of Hispanic origin may be of any race.

★ 289 ★

Insurance Coverage

Health Insurance Coverage, by Race/Ethnicity: 1989-1991

Number of uninsured is shown by year for each race/ethnicity.

Year	Hispanics	Whites	Blacks
1989	6.67	19.20	5.84
1990	6.73	20.22	6.09
1991	6.72	20.41	6.51

Source: *Detroit Free Press,* 10 February 1993, p. 10A. Primary source: Harvard Center for National Health Program Studies. Based on U.S. Census data.

★ 290 ★

Insurance Coverage

Income, Poverty, and Health Insurance Coverage: 1990-1992

According to the source, there are increasing numbers of people living below the poverty level, with a growing number also lacking health insurance coverage. For example, the number of uninsured rose by 2 million from 1991 to 1992, bringing the total number of uninsured to 37.4 million. Data below represent the median household income, percent of persons in poverty, and the percent of persons without health insurance coverage for each state. Data provided are for a 3-year average (1990- 1992).

State	Median income ($)	Poverty rate	Without insurance
Alabama	25,348	18.4	17.3
Alaska	41,996	11.1	14.9
Arizona	30,875	14.5	15.8
Arkansas	24,164	18.1	17.6
California	35,195	15.1	19.0
Colorado	32,718	11.6	12.4
Connecticut	42,069	8.0	7.5
Delaware	34,124	7.3	12.7
District of Columbia	30,182	20.0	22.0
Florida	28,058	15.0	18.7
Georgia	28,835	16.9	16.1
Hawaii	40,773	9.9	6.8
Idaho	27,283	14.6	16.4
Illinois	33,161	14.2	11.8
Indiana	28,491	13.5	11.5
Iowa	29,195	10.4	9.0
Kansas	30,913	11.2	11.0
Kentucky	24,882	18.6	13.6
Louisiana	25,197	22.3	20.8
Maine	29,298	13.5	11.1
Maryland	39,021	10.2	12.3
Massachusetts	37,419	10.6	10.1
Michigan	32,522	14.0	9.4
Minnesota	31,740	12.6	8.8
Mississippi	20,769	24.6	19.3
Missouri	28,532	14.6	13.1
Montana	25,756	15.1	12.0
Nebraska	30,039	10.0	8.7
Nevada	33,443	11.9	19.3
New Hampshire	40,188	7.4	10.9
New Jersey	40,687	9.6	11.3
New Mexico	26,792	21.4	21.0
New York	32,639	15.0	12.6
North Carolina	27,920	14.4	14.2
North Dakota	26,965	13.4	7.4
Ohio	31,461	12.4	10.5
Oklahoma	25,922	17.0	19.5
Oregon	31,548	11.3	13.3
Pennsylvania	30,800	11.2	8.8

[Continued]

★ 290 ★

Income, Poverty, and Health Insurance Coverage: 1990-1992

[Continued]

State	Median income ($)	Poverty rate	Without insurance
Rhode Island	32,239	10.0	10.2
South Carolina	28,934	17.2	15.4
South Dakota	26,036	14.0	12.2
Tennessee	24,593	16.5	13.6
Texas	29,050	17.1	21.9
Utah	31,883	10.1	11.5
Vermont	32,081	11.3	10.6
Virginia	37,699	10.1	15.5
Washington	34,509	9.8	10.7
West Virginia	22,636	19.4	15.0
Wisconsin	32,817	10.0	7.9
Wyoming	30,642	10.4	11.9

Source: "Americans Living in Poverty, Lacked Health Insurance." In CENDATA [online service]. Washington, DC: U.S. Bureau of the Census, 1993 [cited 22 November 1993]. No. 5.1. Primary sources: 1) *Money Income of Households, Families, and Persons in the United States: 1992.* Series P60-184. 2) *Poverty in the United States: 1992.* Series P60-185. 3) *Census and You* (November issue).

★ 291 ★

Insurance Coverage

Medical Insurance Costs Per Person: 1992

The table below reflects medical insurance expenditures for 1992.

[In dollars]

Type of coverage	Cost
Medicare, aged	4,050
Medicare, disabled	3,567
Medicaid	3,313
Medigap supplements	1,639
Small group insurance	1,507
Large group insurance	1,495
Individual insurance	1,458

Source: Johnson, Julie. "Government Health Spending Soars." *American Medical News,* 10 May 1993, p. 26. Primary source: Milliman & Robertson, Inc.

★ 292 ★

Insurance Coverage

Sources of Health Insurance Coverage: 1990

Data reflect sources of health insurance coverage for noninstitutionalized Americans under the age of 65.

Source	Percent
Employment-related private	64.1
Uninsured	15.7
Medicaid	9.9
Other private	5.2
CHAMPUS, VA, or military	4.0
Medicare	1.6

Source: U.S. Congress. Office of Technology Assessment. *Does Health Insurance Make a Difference? Background Paper.* OTA-BP-H-99. Washington, DC: U.S. Government Printing Office, September 1992, p. 51. Primary sources: 1) U.S. Congress. Office of Technology Assessment, 1992. Based on Current Population Survey (March 1991). 2) U.S. Department of Commerce. Bureau of the Census. *Poverty in the United States: 1990.* Current Population Reports. Series P-60, no. 175. Washington, DC: U.S. Government Printing Office, 1991.

★ 293 ★

Insurance Coverage

Uninsured, by Race/Ethnicity

Hispanic - 32

Black - 21

White - 11

Data indicate racial and/or ethnic characteristics of the 37 million Americans lacking health insurance coverage.

[In percentages]

Race	Percent
Hispanic	32
Black	21
White	11

Source: McCoy, Frank. "Where Does It Hurt?" *Black Enterprise* (May 1994), p. 18. Primary source: U.S. Department of Health and Human Services.

★ 294 ★

Insurance Coverage

Uninsured Children: 1991

Data reflects percentage of those under 18 years old having no health insurance coverage.

Race/ethnicity	Percent uninsured
All races	12.3
Latino	26.2
Black	14.8
White	11.7

Source: Mide, Susan. "Healing the Hurt of Homeless Kids." *USA TODAY,* 23 November 1992, final edition, p. 13A. Primary source: Centers for Disease Control. Census survey (March 1992).

★ 295 ★

Insurance Coverage

Uninsured Residents in Selected States: 1992

The table below indicates the states with the most and least number of uninsured people.

[In percentages]

States	Percent
With greatest portion of uninsured residents	
Nevada	20.0
Oklahoma	25.8
Louisiana	25.7
Texas	25.7
District of Columbia	25.5
With lowest portion of uninsured residents	
Wisconsin	10.5
North Dakota	10.5
Minnesota	10.0
Connecticut	9.6
Hawaii	8.1

Source: "Currents." *Hospitals & Health Networks,* 20 January 1994, pp. 16-17.

Nutrition

★ 296 ★

Calcium Sources

The table below rates various sources of calcium, with A+ being the best sources and F being the worst.

[In milligrams (mg.)]

Source	Serving	Mg.	Rating
Almonds, toasted and unblanched	1 oz.	80	B+
Brazil nuts	1 oz.	50	B+
Broccoli, chopped and cooked	1/2 cup	36	B+
Buttermilk	1 cup	285	A+
Figs, dried	5 pieces	135	B+
Hazelnuts	1 oz.	55	B+
Kale, chopped and cooked	1/2 cup	47	B+
Kidney beans, cooked	1/2 cup	39	B+
Meat	--	[1]	F
Mozzarella cheese (from skim milk)	1 oz.	183	A+
Mustard greens, chopped and cooked	1/2 cup	52	B+
Pak-choi, shredded and cooked	1/2 cup	79	B+
Pinto beans, cooked	1/2 cup	45	B+
Prunes, dried	5 pieces	21	B+
Salmon, canned (pink with bones)	3 oz.	181	A
Sardines	7 pieces	321	A
Skim milk	1 cup	302	A+
Spinach, cooked	1/2 cup	122	F
Yogurt (from skim milk)	8 oz.	452	A+

Source: Perlmutter, Cathy. *Prevention* 43, no. 11 (November 1991), p. 61. *Note:* 1. Insignificant.

★ 297 ★
Nutrition

Dietary Guidelines

The table below presents dietary guidelines for females, 25- to 50-years old. Data are based on average daily needs and presume moderate levels of activity. Males and teenagers require more calories.

	Amount
Calories	1,800
Cholesterol	300 mg (max.)
Fat	60 g (max.)[1]
Sodium	3,000 mg (max.)

Source: "What the Nutritional Information Means." *Orlando Sentinel Tribune,* 22 November 1992, p. L2. *Note:* 1. Fat intake should be 30 percent less than daily calories.

★ 298 ★
Nutrition

Eating Breakfast: 1990

This table reflects the percent of persons in the United States 18 years of age and older who indicated that they ate breakfast almost everyday in 1990. Data are provided by sex, age, and selected characteristics.

Characteristic	Both sexes 18 years and over	Male					Female				
		Total	18-29 years	30-44 years	45-64 years	65 years and over	Total	18-29 years	30-44 years	45-64 years	65 years and over
All persons[1]	56.4	54.6	45.1	45.1	59.1	86.2	58.0	42.7	49.8	63.5	84.8
Education level											
Less than 12 years	58.6	57.6	48.7	40.3	54.3	84.6	59.5	36.6	37.9	59.1	82.7
12 years	52.6	50.6	43.4	40.1	56.4	85.3	54.2	40.3	42.7	62.1	84.7
More than 12 years	50.0	50.0	47.5	49.7	00.0	00.0	01.0	47.5	50.7	00.0	00.0
13-15 years	53.5	50.6	45.4	43.0	569	88.3	56.1	44.2	51.6	65.7	86.7
16 years or more	64.2	61.9	51.1	54.9	68.2	91.1	67.0	53.6	65.6	70.9	92.1
Income											
Less than $10,000	54.1	51.5	40.9	40.1	52.6	81.4	55.5	37.2	34.0	58.7	82.8
$10,000-$19,999	56.6	56.1	41.3	43.8	56.3	86.0	56.9	39.0	42.4	59.8	84.8
$20,000-$34,999	55.2	54.2	46.7	42.8	59.6	88.5	56.2	43.2	48.9	62.7	87.3
$35,000-$49,999	53.7	51.3	44.8	47.2	54.2	86.3	56.4	49.2	50.8	64.3	87.6
$50,000 or more	57.2	54.1	44.9	45.5	61.9	89.5	60.5	46.6	58.8	66.2	86.5
Race											
White	57.8	55.6	45.5	45.7	59.4	87.4	59.8	43.9	51.6	64.8	85.8
Black	46.9	47.0	41.6	38.3	53.0	75.8	46.7	37.0	38.7	55.0	73.8
Hispanic origin											
Hispanic	52.5	52.7	50.9	47.2	57.5	80.5	52.2	44.1	47.5	63.6	80.4
Non-Hispanic	56.7	54.8	44.4	44.9	59.2	86.4	58.4	42.5	50.0	63.5	84.9

[Continued]

★ 298 ★

Eating Breakfast: 1990
[Continued]

Characteristic	Both sexes 18 years and over	Male					Female				
		Total	18-29 years	30-44 years	45-64 years	65 years and over	Total	18-29 years	30-44 years	45-64 years	65 years and over
Geographic region											
Northeast	59.9	57.8	48.7	47.6	63.5	86.6	61.8	45.6	54.8	65.8	84.9
Midwest	55.9	53.8	41.7	44.1	59.2	87.6	57.9	40.9	48.9	63.7	87.8
South	54.5	53.2	42.4	45.1	56.6	84.6	55.7	41.5	46.2	61.4	83.2
West	56.6	55.1	50.3	43.9	58.7	87.1	58.0	44.1	52.0	64.5	83.4
Marital status											
Currently married	57.8	56.9	45.7	45.1	60.2	87.6	58.6	45.6	51.8	65.0	85.6
Formerly married	61.5	54.0	37.2	43.1	51.2	78.7	64.6	37.0	41.2	59.0	83.7
Never married	46.9	47.7	45.0	46.7	61.3	90.7	45.9	40.1	48.2	64.0	90.9
Employment status											
Currently employed	50.5	49.9	45.2	44.9	58.1	84.4	51.3	41.9	49.2	61.4	78.8
Unemployed	46.3	46.5	43.8	49.4	44.3	71.1[2]	46.1	42.6	46.4	46.0	94.9
Not in labor force	69.4	72.1	45.0	45.9	65.3	86.7	68.1	44.7	52.2	67.4	85.5

Source: U.S. Department of Health and Human Services. Public Health Service. Centers for Disease Control and Prevention. National Center for Health Statistics. *Health Promotion and Disease Prevention: United States, 1990.* Vital and Health Statistics, Series 10, no. 185. Hyattsville, MD: U.S. Department of Health and Human Services, Public Health Service, Centers for Disease Control and Prevention, National Center for Health Statistics, n.d., p. 25. *Notes:* Data are based on household interviews of the civilian noninstitutionalized population. The survey design, general qualifications, and information on the reliability of the estimates are given in Appendix 1 in the original source. Denominator for each cell excludes unknowns. 1. Includes persons with unknown sociodemographic characteristics. 2. Figure does not meet standard of reliability or precision (more than 30 percent relative standard error in numerator of percent or rate).

★ 299 ★

Nutrition

Fat and Meat

The table below presents data on the fat content and calories for various cuts of meat. Data are ranked by fat content.

Meat	Cut	Type	Fat[1]	Calories
Pork	Center loin	roast	8.9	196
Beef	Flank	steak	8.6	176
Beef	Tenderloin	--	8.5	179
Beef	Top loin	steak	8.0	176
Lamb	Loin	chop; roast	7.8	173
Lamb	Sirloin	chop; roast	7.8	173
Beef	Top sirloin	steak; roast	6.1	165
Beef	Tip round	steak; roast	5.9	157
Lamb	Leg	shank	5.7	153
Beef	Top round	steak; roast	4.2	153
Beef	Eye of round	roast	4.2	143
Pork	Tenderloin	--	4.1	141

Source: Moore, Mary Carroll, and Jean Rogers. *Prevention* 43, no. 11 (November 1991), p. 74. *Notes:* Data reflect average values for 3 ounces of cooked meat; 4 ounces, trimmed, before cooking. 1. In grams.

★ 300 ★
Nutrition

Fat Profiles of Meat

The table below presents data on the fat content of various grades of meat. Data are ranked by fat content.

[In grams]

Grade of meat	Profile	Fat per serving[1]
USDA Prime	Fattiest	10.5
USDA Choice	Leaner	9.5
USDA Select	Leanest	7.4

Source: Moore, Mary Carroll, and Jean Rogers. *Prevention* 43, no. 11 (November 1991), p. 80. *Notes:* USDA is the designation for United States Department of Agriculture. 1. Serving based on 3-ounce trimmed and broiled filet minon.

★ 301 ★
Nutrition

Lamb v. Chicken

The data below compare the nutritional content of lamb and chicken.

Meat	Serving	Calories	Fat (g)
Leg of lamb, roasted (with fat trimmed)	3-inch slice	217	8.8
Chicken breast, roasted (with skin)	3.5 oz.	193	7.6

Source: Lane, Charlotte Balcomb. "Lamb Gaining Favor in Central Florida." *Orlando Sontinol,* 31 March 1994, p. H8.

★ 302 ★

Nutrition

Nutritional Value of Chinese Food

The Center for Science in the Public Interest purchased sample dinners from Chinese restaurants in selected U.S. cities. The dinners then were analyzed by independent labs to determine their nutritional value. The table below reflects some of the findings. Data are ranked by percent of calories from fat.

Dish	Cups	Calories	Fat (g)	Percent calories/fat	Percent calories/ saturated fat	Cholesterol (mg)	Sodium (mg)
Soy sauce	1 tbls.	11	0	0	0	0	1,029
Fortune cookie[1]	1	30	0	6	0	0	22
Szechuan shrimp	4	927	19	18	2	336	2,457
Stir-fried vegetables	4	746	19	22	4	0	2,153
Shrimp with garlic sauce	3	945	27	25	4	307	2,951
Chinese chow mein	5	1,005	32	28	9	205	2,446
House fried rice	4	1,484	50	30	6	346	2,682
House lo mein	5	1,059	36	31	6	175	3,460
Hot-and-sour soup	1	112	4	32	8	129	1,088
Orange crispy beef	4	1,766	66	33	6	296	3,135
Beef with broccoli	4	1,175	46	35	7	228	3,146
Sweet-and-sour pork	4	1,613	71	39	7	118	818
Kung Pao chicken	5	1,620	76	42	7	277	2,608
Moo shu pork	4	1,228	64	47	10	465	2,593
Soup noodles[1]	1/2	150	8	48	0	0	300
Egg roll	1 roll	190	11	52	2	7	463
Chow mein noodles[2]	1/2	119	7	53	1	0	99

Source: Gorov, Lynda. "Nutritionists See Little Good Fortune in Chinese Food." *Boston Globe,* 2 September 1993, city edition, p. 1. Primary source: Center for Science in the Public Interest. Related source: "Report Cites Fat, Cholesterol in Some Popular Chinese Dishes." *Louisville Courier-Journal,* 1 September 1993, metro edition, p. 4A. *Notes:* 1. LaChoy. 2. *USDA Handbook* 8.

★ 303 ★

Nutrition

Obese Persons Attempting to Lose Weight: 1990

Data indicate overweight persons 18 years of age and older who were attempting to lose weight in 1990.

Characteristic	Both sexes 18 years and over	Male					Female				
		Total	18-29 years	30-44 years	45-64 years	65 years and over	Total	18-29 years	30-44 years	45-64 years	65 years and over
All persons[1]	53.1	44.7	45.6	45.8	44.7	40.1	61.9	65.0	66.9	63.6	48.8
Education level											
Less than 12 years	46.4	35.7	37.9	33.7	36.4	34.8	54.6	62.9	58.6	57.4	46.4
12 years	53.5	43.0	44.7	41.7	43.9	41.9	63.2	62.6	67.1	66.8	49.0
More than 12 years	57.6	50.9	50.3	52.0	51.0	45.6	67.5	70.7	70.1	66.1	56.2
13-15 years	56.3	46.1	48.0	45.8	45.2	46.4	69.0	71.0	70.0	70.1	58.8
16 years or more	59.0	55.8	54.2	58.7	55.5	45.2	65.2	70.0	70.3	61.5	52.3

[Continued]

★ 303 ★

Obese Persons Attempting to Lose Weight: 1990
[Continued]

Characteristic	Both sexes 18 years and over	Male					Female				
		Total	18-29 years	30-44 years	45-64 years	65 years and over	Total	18-29 years	30-44 years	45-64 years	65 years and over
Income											
Less than $10,000	52.2	44.7	43.3	45.4	53.4	34.1	55.2	57.9	65.6	58.7	43.0
$10,000-$19,999	51.1	41.2	43.9	41.5	36.0	44.3	58.8	67.4	61.0	59.6	50.1
$20,000-$34,999	52.9	42.5	41.9	45.5	42.3	34.5	64.4	67.9	67.1	63.7	55.8
$35,000-$49,999	55.3	49.4	49.0	47.7	51.8	50.8	63.7	62.3	69.6	60.6	40.2
$50,000 or more	58.8	51.2	54.7	49.9	52.4	42.9	72.4	73.8	72.2	74.2	59.7
Race											
White	53.4	44.9	45.9	45.8	45.1	41.0	62.8	67.3	67.4	64.6	50.3
Black	51.6	42.1	41.5	45.9	41.1	33.7	58.2	57.8	63.8	60.4	40.6
Hispanic origin											
Hispanic	53.0	40.5	48.4	40.9	36.3	32.7[2]	63.1	62.0	65.6	65.1	50.0
Non-Hispanic	53.1	45.0	45.4	46.4	45.3	40.4	61.8	65.5	66.9	63.6	48.8
Geographic region											
Northeast	56.0	48.2	50.3	49.7	46.9	44.9	64.2	68.1	68.2	69.1	49.5
Midwest	55.3	45.0	44.3	46.6	44.7	42.5	66.2	72.0	67.8	68.6	56.0
South	48.4	40.4	40.5	42.0	41.9	32.0	56.5	58.4	64.9	55.6	42.6
West	55.8	48.3	53.9	47.9	46.7	47.1	63.6	66.4	68.0	65.1	48.6
Marital status											
Currently married	52.8	44.4	44.5	45.3	44.9	40.7	63.8	61.5	67.7	64.7	52.8
Formerly married	52.8	45.0	47.5[2]	50.4	43.4	39.2	55.5	70.2	65.3	59.6	46.1
Never married	55.4	46.0	47.1	47.0	41.4	34.2[2]	66.2	68.1	64.0	71.1	45.2[2]
Employment status											
Currently employed	52.9	45.1	46.6	45.4	44.1	41.1	64.9	66.4	66.9	63.9	46.0
Unemployed	52.6	46.2	42.1	48.4	49.3	33.3[2]	61.6	75.2	52.5	65.3	25.0[2]
Not in labor force	53.6	42.8	38.3	50.8	46.6	40.0	58.5	61.4	68.7	63.2	49.2

Source: U.S. Department of Health and Human Services. Public Health Service. Centers for Disease Control and Prevention. National Center for Health Statistics. *Health Promotion and Disease Prevention: United States, 1990.* Vital and Health Statistics, Series 10, no. 185. Hyattsville, MD: U.S. Department of Health and Human Services, Public Health Service, Centers for Disease Control and Prevention, National Center for Health Statistics, n.d., p. 29. *Notes:* Data are based on household interviews of the civilian noninstitutionalized population. The survey design, general qualifications, and information on the reliability of the estimates are given in Appendix 1 in the original source. Denominator for each cell excludes unknowns. 1. Includes persons with unknown sociodemographic characteristics. 2. Figure does not meet standard of reliability or precision (more than 30 percent relative standard error in numerator of percent or rate).

★ 304 ★
Nutrition

Obesity: 1990

This table reflects the persons 18 years of age and older who were 20 percent or more above their desirable body weights in 1990.

Characteristic	Both sexes 18 years and over	Male					Female				
		Total	18-29 years	30-44 years	45-64 years	65 years and over	Total	18-29 years	30-44 years	45-64 years	65 years and over
All persons[1]	27.5	29.6	20.1	32.0	37.8	26.3	25.6	15.9	24.7	34.2	28.2
Education level											
Less than 12 years	32.7	30.0	18.8	30.9	42.9	25.4	35.2	21.7	36.4	47.4	33.0
12 years	28.6	31.2	21.3	35.9	37.6	29.5	26.5	17.9	26.4	33.7	27.5
More than 12 years	23.8	28.2	19.3	29.7	35.3	24.1	19.3	11.6	20.6	25.7	20.4
13-15 years	25.5	30.1	19.2	35.2	39.1	25.1	21.5	13.4	25.5	27.5	21.0
16 years or more	22.0	26.5	19.6	25.5	32.9	23.3	16.6	8.4	16.0	23.9	19.7
Income											
Less than $10,000	29.3	24.0	15.7	31.6	36.5	22.3	32.2	20.7	40.2	49.5	30.1
$10,000-$19,999	28.5	27.5	18.8	32.6	37.3	25.6	29.2	19.1	30.5	40.2	29.1
$20,000-$34,999	28.2	30.2	20.1	32.5	40.1	27.5	26.4	16.0	27.3	36.0	27.7
$35,000-$49,999	27.8	31.3	22.9	32.8	39.1	22.8	23.9	13.0	25.1	31.9	22.4
$50,000 or more	24.9	31.0	21.7	31.3	36.6	25.1	18.4	9.1	15.5	26.7	24.7
Race											
White	26.7	29.7	19.8	32.2	37.8	26.3	24.0	14.7	22.7	32.1	26.6
Black	38.0	35.1	26.5	36.6	46.8	29.5	40.4	25.0	41.9	54.2	47.8
Hispanic origin											
Hispanic	27.6	26.7	13.8	33.4	40.0	25.5	28.4	20.3	30.1	39.0	32.3
Non-Hispanic	27.5	29.9	20.9	31.9	37.7	26.3	25.3	15.3	24.1	33.8	28.1
Geographic region											
Northeast	27.2	30.0	21.7	31.5	37.9	26.3	24.8	14.3	22.3	33.7	28.3
Midwest	29.1	31.4	19.4	33.9	40.3	30.8	27.0	15.8	25.4	36.8	31.0
South	28.2	30.3	22.7	33.9	36.1	25.4	26.4	16.7	27.2	34.2	27.7
West	24.7	26.1	15.2	27.2	37.7	21.5	23.3	16.3	22.2	31.3	25.1
Marital status											
Currently married	29.2	33.3	26.7	33.8	39.3	26.4	25.2	15.5	23.5	32.9	28.0
Formerly married	29.1	26.3	17.1	24.8	30.9	25.3	30.2	21.6	26.3	37.3	29.1
Never married	19.8	19.3	15.6	27.3	30.0	26.9	20.4	15.6	32.0	37.9	18.6
Employment status											
Currently employed	27.3	30.5	21.2	32.1	38.2	26.7	23.4	14.3	23.9	32.0	28.8
Unemployed	26.4	29.5	20.9	34.3	37.5	43.4[2]	23.0	14.5	27.2	35.8	10.8[2]
Not in labor force	28.1	26.4	12.6	29.0	36.3	26.0	28.9	20.2	26.8	37.2	28.2

Source: U.S. Department of Health and Human Services. Public Health Service. Centers for Disease Control and Prevention. National Center for Health Statistics. *Health Promotion and Disease Prevention: United States, 1990.* Vital and Health Statistics, Series 10, no. 185. Hyattsville, MD: U.S. Department of Health and Human Services, Public Health Service, Centers for Disease Control and Prevention, National Center for Health Statistics, n.d., p. 27. *Notes:* Data are based on household interviews of the civilian noninstitutionalized population. The survey design, general qualifications, and information on the reliability of the estimates are given in Appendix 1 in the original source. Denominator for each cell excludes unknowns. 1. Includes persons with unknown sociodemographic characteristics. 2. Figure does not meet standard of reliability or precision (more than 30 percent relative standard error in numerator of percent or rate).

★ 305 ★

Nutrition

Popcorn and Fat

Many have held popcorn to be the healthiest snack food; however, the Center for Science in the Public Interest warns that the method of preparing popcorn may jeopardize its nutritional value—movie theatre popcorn in particular. Approximately 70 percent of the movie theatres use coconut oil—an agent that raises blood cholesterol levels—to prepare their popcorn. The result is a snack that—depending on the serving size—may contain the equivalent of four days' worth of saturated fats.

[In grams]

Popcorn preparation method	Total fat	Saturated fat	Trans fat[1]	Calories
Popped in coconut oil, with butter-flavored topping	50	26	3	632
Popped in coconut oil, plain	27	19	none	398
Popped in canola shortening, plain	22	3	1	361
Commercial air-popped, plain[2]	6	1	none	210

Source: "Consumer Group Gives Movie Popcorn Two Thumbs Down." *Detroit News,* 26 April 1994, p. 2A. Primary source: The Center for Science in the Public Interest. *Notes:* Data presumes each serving to be a small bag of popcorn, about 7 cups. 1. Believed to increase cholesterol. 2. Lightly sprayed with soybean oil.

★ 306 ★

Nutrition

Vitamin Sales: 1992-1993

The table reflects vitamin sale growths from 1992 to 1993.

[In percentages]

Vitamin	Percent
Vitamin E	31
Vitamin A-beta carotene	19
Vitamin C	13
Vitamin B	4

Source: "At a Glance: Snapshots of the Workplace Health Industry." *Workplace Health* (July/August 1993), p. 15. Primary Sources: 1) Information Resources, Inc. 2) *Wall Street Journal.*

★ 307 ★

Nutrition

Water and Nutrition

Water is essential for almost every physiological funtion—from maintaining body temperature to transporting nutrients through the circulatory system. Humans are mostly water. The table below indicates just how much water a body contains.

[In percentages]

Body or body part	Percent
Adult	60-70
Baby	90
Brain	90
Blood	85
Muscles	75
Liver	69
Bones	22

Source: Condor, Bob. "Have You Juggled Your 8 Glasses Today?" *Chicago Tribune,* 13 February 1994, Zone C, p. 1.

★ 308 ★

Nutrition

Weight Loss Program Costs

The table below reflects the average cost per pound of weight loss for a 12-week diet program.

Program	Average Cost
HMR	$7.94
Medifast	6.35
Optifast	9.98
United Weight Control	11.56
Diet Center	4.08
Jenny Craig	10.43
Nutrisystems	8.62
Registered Dietitian	6.80
Weight Watchers	1.10
TOPS	0.03
Overeaters Anonymous	0.00

Source: "The Cost of Losing Weight." *New York Times,* 24 November 1992, p. C11. Primary source: *Journal of the American College of Nutrition.*

Poverty

★ 309 ★

Poverty Income Thresholds: 1992

[In dollars]

Poverty income thresholds	Amount
Individual, aged 65 or older	6,729
Couple, householder aged 65 or older	8,489
Family of four	14,343

Source: U.S. Department of Health and Human Services. Social Security Administration (SSA). *Annual Statistical Supplement to the "Social Security Bulletin," 1992.* SSA Publication No. 13-11700. Washington, DC: U.S. Department of Health and Human Services, Social Security Administration, Office of Research and Statistics, 1993, p. 4.

★ 310 ★
Poverty

Poverty Status of Persons, Families, and Children Under 18: 1959-1990

The table below reflects the number of persons, families, and children under 18 years of age below the poverty level. Data are provided by race/ethnicity.

[In thousands]

Year and race/ethnicity	Related All persons	In all families			In families with female householder, no husband present	
		Total	Related Householder	children under 18	Total	children under 18
All races						
1959	39,490	34,562	8,320	17,208	7,014	4,145
1960	39,851	34,925	8,243	17,288	7,247	4,095
1965	33,185	28,358	6,721	14,388	7,524	4,562
1966	28,510	23,809	5,784	12,146	6,861	4,262
1970	25,420	20,330	5,260	10,235	7,503	4,689
1971	25,559	20,405	5,303	10,344	7,797	4,850
1972	24,460	19,577	5,075	10,082	8,114	5,094
1973	22,973	18,299	4,828	9,453	8,178	5,171
1974	23,370	18,817	4,922	9,967	8,462	5,361
1975	25,877	20,789	5,450	10,882	8,846	5,597
1976	24,975	19,632	5,311	10,081	9,029	5,583
1977	24,720	19,505	5,311	10,028	9,205	5,658
1978	24,497	19,062	5,280	9,722	9,269	5,687
1979	26,072	19,964	5,461	9,993	9,400	5,635

[Continued]

★ 310 ★

Poverty Status of Persons, Families, and Children Under 18: 1959-1990
[Continued]

Year and race/ethnicity	Related All persons	In all families			In families with female householder, no husband present	
		Total	Related Householder	children under 18	Total	children under 18
1980	29,272	22,601	6,217	11,114	10,120	5,866
1981	31,822	24,850	6,851	12,068	11,051	6,305
1982	34,398	27,349	7,512	13,139	11,701	6,696
1983	35,303	27,933	7,647	13,427	12,072	6,747
1984	33,700	26,458	7,277	12,929	11,831	6,772
1985	33,064	25,729	7,223	12,483	11,600	6,716
1986	32,370	24,754	7,023	12,257	11,944	6,943
1987	32,221	24,725	7,005	12,275	12,148	7,074
1988	31,745	24,048	6,876	11,935	11,972	6,742
1989[1]	31,528	244,066	6,784	12,001	11,668	6,808
1990	33,585	25,232	7,098	12,715	12,578	7,363
White[2]						
1960	28,309	24,262	6,115	11,229	4,296	2,357
1965	22,496	18,508	4,824	8,595	4,092	2,321
1970	17,484	13,323	3,708	6,138	3,761	2,247
1975	17,770	13,799	3,838	6,748	4,577	2,813
1980	19,699	14,587	4,195	6,817	4,940	2,813
1981	21,553	16,127	4,670	7,429	5,600	3,120
1982	23,517	18,015	5,118	8,282	5,686	3,249
1983	23,984	18,377	5,220	8,534	6,017	3,388
1984	22,955	17,299	4,925	8,086	5,866	3,377
1985	22,860	17,125	4,983	7,838	5,990	3,372
1986	22,183	16,393	4,811	7,714	6,171	3,522
1987	21,195	15,593	4,567	7,398	5,989	3,474
1988	20,715	15,001	4,471	7,095	5,950	3,385
1989[1]	20,785	15,179	4,409	7,164	5,723	3,320
1990	22,326	15,916	4,622	7,696	6,210	3,597
Black[2]						
1959	9,927	9,112	1,860	5,022	2,416	1,475
1966	8,867	8,090	1,620	4,774	3,160	2,107
1970	7,548	6,683	1,481	3,922	3,656	2,383
1975	7,545	6,533	1,513	3,884	4,168	2,724
1980	8,579	7,190	1,826	3,906	4,984	2,944
1981	9,173	7,780	1,972	4,170	5,222	3,051

[Continued]

★ 310 ★

Poverty Status of Persons, Families, and Children Under 18: 1959-1990
[Continued]

Year and race/ethnicity	Related All persons	In all families			In families with female householder, no husband present	
		Total	Related Householder	children under 18	Total	children under 18
1982	9,697	8,355	2,158	4,388	5,698	3,269
1983	9,882	8,376	2,161	4,273	5,736	3,187
1984	9,490	8,104	2,094	4,320	5,666	3,234
1985	8,926	7,504	1,983	4,057	5,342	3,181
1986	8,983	7,401	1,987	4,037	5,473	3,251
1987	9,520	7,848	2,117	4,234	5,789	3,394
1988	9,356	7,650	2,090	4,148	5,601	3,130
1989[1]	9,302	7,704	2,077	4,257	5,530	3,256
1990	9,837	8,160	2,193	4,412	6,005	3,543
Hispanic origin[3]						
1975	2,991	2,755	627	1,619	1,053	694
1980	3,491	3,143	751	1,718	1,319	809
1981	3,713	3,349	792	1,874	1,465	909
1982	4,301	3,865	916	2,117	1,601	990
1983	4,633	4,113	981	2,251	1,670	1,018
1984	4,806	4,192	991	2,317	1,764	1,093
1985	5,236	4,605	1,074	2,512	1,983	1,247
1986	5,117	4,469	1,085	2,413	1,921	1,194
1987	5,422	4,761	1,168	2,606	2,045	1,241
1988	5,357	4,700	1,141	2,576	2,052	1,208
1989[1]	5,430	4,659	1,133	2,496	1,902	1,163
1990	6,006	5,091	1,244	2,750	2,115	1,314

Source: U.S. Department of Education. Office of Educational Research and Improvement. National Center for Education Statistics. *Digest of Education Statistics, 1992.* Washington, DC: U.S. Government Printing Office, 1992, p. 27. Primary source: U.S. Department of Commerce. Bureau of the Census. *Current Population Reports.* Series P-60, no. 175. This table was prepared in January 1992. *Notes:* 1. Revised from previously published data. 2. Includes persons of Hispanic origin. 3. Persons of Hispanic origin may be of any race.

Sex

★ 311 ★

Abstinence: 1994

A survey asked adults and adolescents for their opinions of messages by celebrities espousing abstinence and/or safe sex. Of the adults polled, 78 percent agreed that the abstinence message was "good," and 72 percent indicated that safe sex messages did not "trouble" them. Of the teenagers, 72 percent agreed that the abstinence message was "good," with 85 percent indicating that safe sex messages did not "trouble" them. Overall, 44 percent of the respondents in 1994 reported that teenagers "hear too little" about "saying no to sex," as compared to 54 percent in 1991. The data below reflect the opinions of those surveyed as to when the abstinence message is most effective.

[In percentages]

Reasons to abstain from sex	Adults	Teenagers
Health risks (e.g., AIDS)	51	38
Unplanned pregnancy	26	33
Morality	16	8

Source: McNichol, Tom. "The New Sex Vow: 'I Won't' Until 'I Do.'" *USA WEEKEND,* 25-27 March 1994, p. 5. Primary source: A national poll of 1,004 adults and 252 teenagers conducted by ICR Research in February 1994. *Notes:* Results may not add to 100 percent because answers of "Don't Know" have been eliminated.

★ 312 ★
Sex

Condom Use

The table below reflects students who reported that they had sexual intercourse and used a condom during the three months prior to being surveyed.

Race/ethnicity	Percentage
Black	47.1
White	45.9
Hispanic	38.4

Source: Painter, Kim. "Lifestyles Remain a Major Barrier to Condom Use." *USA TODAY,* 7 July 1992, final edition, p. 4D. Primary source: U.S. Youth Risk Behavior Survey, 1990.

★ 313 ★

Sex

Number of Sexual Partners of Americans: 1992

According to the source, Americans averaged 1.12 sexual partners in 1992. The data below indicate the number of sexual partners reported by Americans.

Number of partners	Percent
One	72
Two	6
Three	2
Four or more	2
None	17

Source: "Sex, Lies, and Statistics." *The Economist,* 23 October 1993, p. 32. Primary source: General Social Survey, 1992-1993.

★ 314 ★

Sex

Sexual Activity

According to the World Health Organization, there are more than 100 million acts of sexual intercourse every day, resulting in 350,000 cases of sexually transmitted diseases.

Source: "U.N. Agency on Sex: Pitfalls and Promise." *New York Times,* 25 June 1992, p. A12.

★ 315 ★

Sex

Sexually Transmitted Diseases: 1992

The data below reflect new cases of sexually transmitted diseases (STDs), which affect 12 million people each year.

Disease	Number
HIV	40,000
Syphilis	120,000
Hepatitis B	200,000
Genital herpes	500,000
Human papillomavirus	1,000,000
Gonorrhea	1,100,000

[Continued]

★ 315 ★

Sexually Transmitted Diseases: 1992

[Continued]

Disease	Number
Trichomoniasis	3,000,000
Chlamydia	4,000,000

Source: Painter, Kim. "U.S. Found Lagging in Fighting STDs." *USA TODAY,* 1 April 1993, p. 8D. Primary sources: The Alan Guttmacher Institute.

★ 316 ★

Sex

Teens, Sex, and Disease: 1994

This table reflects the sexual activity of American teenagers.

[In percentages]

Teenagers	Percent
High school seniors	
Having had sexual intercourse	72
Having had at least 4 partners	19
High school students	
Using condoms	45

Source: Peterson, Karen S. "TV Condom Ads May Reach Teens, Panelists Say." *USA TODAY,* 11 January 1994, p. 3D. Primary source: Centers for Disease Control and Prevention, January 1994.

Smoking and Tobacco Use

★ 317 ★

Cigarette Smoking: 1990

The table below reflects the percent of persons in the United States 18 years of age and older who smoked cigarettes in 1990. Data are provided by sex, age, and selected characteristics.

[In percentages]

Characteristic	Both sexes 18 years and over	Male					Female				
		Total	18-29 years	30-44 years	45-64 years	65 years and over	Total	18-29 years	30-44 years	45-64 years	65 years and over
All persons[1]	25.5	28.4	28.6	33.6	29.3	14.6	22.8	25.3	25.8	24.8	11.5
Education level											
Less than 12 years	31.8	37.3	44.6	54.0	39.4	17.4	27.1	40.9	40.3	29.9	10.9
12 years	29.6	33.5	33.4	40.9	32.3	16.2	26.5	29.8	32.1	25.5	11.9
More than 12 years	18.3	20.0	16.1	23.9	21.5	8.7	16.6	14.5	17.2	20.5	11.8
13-15 years	23.0	26.2	20.4	34.3	27.6	8.9	20.2	17.3	23.5	22.8	13.0
16 years or more	13.5	14.5	8.8	16.0	17.6	8.6	12.3	9.3	11.1	18.2	10.2
Income											
Less than $10,000	31.6	37.3	30.6	59.7	47.0	21.1	28.6	31.9	46.6	33.2	13.2
$10,000-$19,999	29.8	34.1	35.8	44.7	40.7	16.4	26.3	31.9	36.5	26.1	12.2
$20,000-$34,999	26.9	30.3	30.6	37.0	30.5	13.0	23.5	22.3	27.1	26.5	12.1
$35,000-$49,999	23.4	25.5	22.8	28.4	27.4	10.9	21.0	19.7	22.4	22.5	10.2
$50,000 or more	19.3	21.3	20.6	24.1	20.7	10.1	17.2	17.7	16.2	19.0	12.3
Race											
White	25.6	28.0	29.1	33.0	28.7	13.7	23.4	27.1	26.1	25.4	11.5
Black	26.2	32.5	26.7	38.8	36.7	21.5	21.2	17.9	27.2	22.6	11.1
Hispanic origin											
Hispanic	23.0	30.9	28.5	35.9	30.2	19.4	16.3	15.7	18.6	18.1	5.1[2]
Non-Hispanic	25.7	28.2	28.6	33.4	29.3	14.4	23.4	26.7	26.6	25.3	11.7
Geographic region											
Northeast	23.9	26.8	28.0	31.1	26.7	15.0	21.3	25.9	24.6	22.2	10.3
Midwest	27.4	29.4	31.9	33.6	30.2	14.0	25.6	29.4	29.8	27.6	10.1
South	26.5	30.4	29.4	35.9	32.5	16.4	22.9	24.9	25.4	25.7	12.2
West	23.2	25.6	24.1	32.1	25.9	11.6	20.9	20.9	23.2	22.6	13.5
Marital status											
Currently married	24.6	27.1	32.2	31.5	27.0	12.6	22.1	27.6	23.1	21.9	10.5
Formerly married	30.3	41.1	43.9	49.3	44.4	23.8	25.9	44.3	37.9	33.5	12.4
Never married	24.3	26.7	25.4	32.6	28.8	12.7	21.3	20.2	28.0	23.2	8.8[2]
Employment status											
Currently employed	26.9	29.2	28.1	31.8	27.9	16.3	24.2	24.5	24.6	24.5	15.5

[Continued]

★ 317 ★

Cigarette Smoking: 1990
[Continued]

Characteristic	Both sexes 18 years and over	Male					Female				
		Total	18-29 years	30-44 years	45-64 years	65 years and over	Total	18-29 years	30-44 years	45-64 years	65 years and over
Unemployed	38.8	45.8	43.1	53.1	43.5	16.7[2]	31.2	29.8	38.1	25.1	6.4[2]
Not in labor force	21.3	23.3	25.5	51.7	33.3	14.2	20.3	26.5	28.1	25.2	11.0

Source: U.S. Department of Health and Human Services. Public Health Service. Centers for Disease Control and Prevention. National Center for Health Statistics. *Health Promotion and Disease Prevention: United States, 1990.* Vital and Health Statistics, Series 10, no. 185. Hyattsville, MD: U.S. Department of Health and Human Services, Public Health Service, Centers for Disease Control and Prevention, National Center for Health Statistics, n.d., p. 46. *Notes:* Data are based on household interviews of the civilian noninstitutionalized population. The survey design, general qualifications, and information on the reliability of the estimates are given in Appendix 1 in the original source. Denominator for each cell excludes unknowns. 1. Includes persons with unknown sociodemographic characteristics. 2. Figure does not meet standard of reliability or precision (more than 30 percent relative standard error in numerator of percent or rate).

★ 318 ★
Smoking and Tobacco Use

Cigarette Smoking Among High School Students

Data indicate the percent of high school students who reported that they smoked cigarettes frequently. Data shown for each race/ethnicity.

Race/ethnicity	Percent
White	15.4
Hispanics	6.8
Black	3.1

Source: "Which Students Smoke Most?" *USA TODAY,* 15 July 1992, final edition, p. 1D. *Note:* Hispanics may be of any race.

★ 319 ★
Smoking and Tobacco Use

Cigarette Use: 1991

[Estimates shown for 1991]

	Ever used				Used in past year				Used in past month			
	Total	Hispanic	White	Black	Total	Hispanic	White	Black	Total	Hispanic	White	Black
Percent rate estimates												
Age												
12-17	37.9	31.9	41.7	25.6	20.1	16.7	23.2	9.6	10.8	8.7	12.7	4.3
18-25	71.2	58.0	76.5	57.0	41.2	33.0	45.3	28.9	32.2	24.7	35.7	22.0
26-34	76.4	69.2	78.4	74.0	38.0	34.6	38.3	40.8	32.9	28.6	33.2	36.8
35+	78.0	66.3	80.0	75.6	30.0	31.1	29.2	35.7	26.6	27.7	25.8	32.6
Sex												
Male	77.3	70.7	79.7	70.2	34.7	35.8	34.3	36.3	28.7	29.7	28.1	31.5
Female	68.5	50.7	72.2	61.3	29.7	24.8	30.7	28.5	25.5	19.7	26.5	24.8
Total	72.7	60.6	75.8	65.4	32.1	30.3	32.4	32.1	27.0	24.7	27.3	27.9

[Continued]

★ 319 ★

Cigarette Use: 1991
[Continued]

	Ever used				Used in past year				Used in past month			
	Total	Hispanic	White	Black	Total	Hispanic	White	Black	Total	Hispanic	White	Black
Population estimates (in thousands)												
Age												
12-17	7,632	723	5,860	795	4,052	377	3,264	297	2,180	197	1,783	135
18-25	20,299	1,742	15,732	2,237	11,750	992	9,312	1,132	9,167	742	7,345	865
26-34	29,576	2,682	22,668	3,474	14,726	1,340	11,079	1,915	12,736	1,107	9,612	1,727
35+	90,025	4,662	75,056	8,547	34,591	2,188	27,362	4,037	30,721	1,946	24,217	3,688
Sex												
Male	75,131	5,688	60,454	7,327	33,757	2,879	26,021	3,787	27,867	2,393	21,336	3,291
Female	72,400	4,122	58,862	7,726	31,362	2,018	24,996	3,594	26,937	1,599	21,621	3,123
Total	147,531	9,809	119,316	15,053	65,119	4,897	51,017	7,381	54,805	3,993	42,957	6,414

Source: U.S. Department of Health and Human Services. Public Health Service. Alcohol, Drug Abuse, and Mental Health Administration. *National Household Survey on Drug Abuse: Population Estimates, 1991.* Rockville, MD: U.S. Department of Health and Human Services. Public Health Service. Alcohol, Drug Abuse, and Mental Health Administration, n.d., pp. 91-93. Primary source: National Institute on Drug Abuse. 1991 National Household Survey on Drug Abuse.

★ 320 ★

Smoking and Tobacco Use

Smokeless Tobacco Use: 1991

[Estimates shown for 1991]

	Ever used				Used in past year				Used in past month			
	Total	Hispanic	White	Black	Total	Hispanic	White	Black	Total	Hispanic	White	Black
Percent rate estimates												
Age												
12-17	11.8	4.2	14.9	4.0	6.1	2.0	7.9	1.2	3.0	1.1	3.8	0.8
18-25	21.8	9.2	20.4	7.0	8.7	2.7	11.0	2.0	5.8	1.7	7.5	1.2
26-34	16.4	8.9	19.2	7.5	5.0	2.0	5.9	2.3	3.5	0.8	4.3	1.5
35+	11.7	4.7	12.4	12.8	3.4	0.6	3.7	2.9	2.8	0.4	3.0	2.8
Sex												
Male	25.7	11.5	29.1	15.5	9.0	2.7	10.6	3.4	6.4	1.5	7.6	2.6
Female	3.3	1.5	3.2	4.8	0.8	0.3	0.7	1.5	0.6	0.2	0.4	1.5
Total	14.0	6.5	15.7	9.6	4.7	1.5	5.5	2.4	3.4	0.8	3.9	2.0
Population estimates (in thousands)												
Age												
12-17	2,367	94	2,087	126	1,233	45	1,107	36	599	25	536	25
18-25	6,222	277	5,432	297	2,484	80	2,262	77	1,666	50	1,534	47
26-34	6,347	344	5,542	350	1,945	79	1,715	108	1,373	32	1,232	69
35+	13,549	331	11,598	1,442	3,948	45	3,514	329	3,216	29	2,823	313
Sex												
Male	25,013	925	22,036	1,613	8,781	221	8,025	358	6,269	121	5,777	270
Female	3,471	122	2,623	602	830	28	574	191	584	15	348	184
Total	28,484	1,047	24,659	2,215	9,611	248	8,599	550	6,854	136	6,125	454

Source: U.S. Department of Health and Human Services. Public Health Service. Alcohol, Drug Abuse, and Mental Health Administration. *National Household Survey on Drug Abuse: Population Estimates, 1991.* Rockville, MD: U.S. Department of Health and Human Services. Public Health Service. Alcohol, Drug Abuse, and Mental Health Administration, n.d., pp. 97-99. Primary source: National Institute on Drug Abuse. 1991 National Household Survey on Drug Abuse.

★ 321 ★

Smoking and Tobacco Use

Smokers of 25 or More Cigarettes Per Day: 1990

Data indicate percent of smokers in the United States 18 years of age and older who smoked 25 or more cigarettes each day in 1990. Data are provided by sex, age, and selected characteristics.

[In percentages]

Characteristic	Both sexes 18 years and over	Male					Female				
		Total	18-29 years	30-44 years	45-64 years	65 years and over	Total	18-29 years	30-44 years	45-64 years	65 years and over
All persons[1]	22.9	28.5	14.5	31.0	39.0	26.6	16.6	8.8	19.6	21.8	12.0
Education level											
Less than 12 years	22.2	25.1	15.2	31.6	30.8	19.3	18.7	10.6	25.1	24.8	11.5
12 years	23.4	29.6	15.4	33.6	39.2	35.1	17.2	8.7	21.4	21.1	13.7
More than 12 years	22.7	30.1	11.9	27.8	46.5	31.3	13.5	7.1	13.7	20.0	9.0[2]
13-15 years	23.1	30.6	12.3	29.2	53.2	36.3[2]	14.5	8.1	16.0	20.0	12.0[2]
16 years or more	22.0	29.3	10.5[2]	25.5	39.9	27.7[2]	11.6	3.5[2]	8.9	20.0	3.8[2]
Income											
Less than $10,000	17.3	20.9	10.2	30.2	27.4	13.5[2]	14.8	5.0[2]	24.4	17.4	14.8
$10,000-$19,999	22.3	27.2	18.7	26.4	38.2	30.9	17.2	12.0	23.2	21.3	7.8[2]
$20,000-$34,999	22.3	27.2	12.9	29.9	38.7	30.7	16.2	9.5	17.3	22.1	12.6[2]
$35,000-$49,999	25.3	31.2	18.2	31.1	42.0	27.2[2]	17.4	10.6	18.8	21.0	13.5[2]
$50,000 or more	28.1	35.4	9.1[2]	38.6	45.5	34.7[2]	18.3	5.1[2]	19.2	25.3	11.4[2]
Race											
White	25.4	32.1	16.2	35.1	43.6	30.3	18.0	9.4	21.6	23.6	12.8
Black	6.0	7.4	7.7[2]	7.4	6.9[2]	7.2[2]	4.2	3.8[2]	4.7[2]	4.9[2]	-[2]
Hispanic origin											
Hispanic	6.8	8.9	2.9[2]	11.3	13.2[2]	16.9[2]	3.5[2]	2.3[2]	4.1[2]	4.6[2]	-[2]
Non-Hispanic	24.1	30.3	15.9	32.8	40.8	27.1	17.4	9.3	20.6	22.7	12.2
Geographic region											
Northeast	21.3	26.3	14.2	27.7	36.3	26.0	15.9	10.2	16.4	22.3	11.4[2]
Midwest	24.2	30.9	18.4	35.0	39.2	27.0	17.2	8.2	20.9	22.6	12.1[2]
South	23.8	29.2	12.4	33.6	39.1	26.3	17.4	10.0	22.1	20.8	12.1
West	20.8	26.1	13.0	24.1	41.2	27.5	14.7	6.0[2]	16.4	21.7	12.1[2]
Marital status											
Currently married	25.2	31.8	15.8	32.0	40.7	31.4	17.2	10.4	19.3	21.6	8.9[2]
Formerly married	23.7	30.6	28.2	32.9	34.1	16.6	19.2	10.1[2]	22.2	22.7	13.8
Never married	13.5	16.3	12.3	23.1	31.3	19.7[2]	9.4	5.8	15.5	18.2[2]	14.1[2]
Employment status											
Currently employed	24.0	29.0	15.2	30.8	40.4	30.3	16.7	9.8	19.0	21.7	8.3[2]
Unemployed	23.9	28.2	12.6[2]	33.1	47.4	61.5[2]	17.0	8.5[2]	20.1	30.8[2]	-[2]
Not in labor force	19.8	26.3	11.1	31.9	32.4	25.4	16.2	6.7	21.1	21.5	12.6

Source: U.S. Department of Health and Human Services. Public Health Service. Centers for Disease Control and Prevention. National Center for Health Statistics. *Health Promotion and Disease Prevention: United States, 1990.* Vital and Health Statistics, Series 10, no. 185. Hyattsville, MD: U.S. Department of Health and Human Services, Public Health Service, Centers for Disease Control and Prevention, National Center for Health Statistics, n.d., p. 47. *Notes:* Data are based on household interviews of the civilian noninstitutionalized population. The survey design, general qualifications, and information on the reliability of the estimates are given in Appendix 1 in the original source. Denominator for each cell excludes unknowns. 1. Includes persons with unknown sociodemographic characteristics. 2. Figure does not meet standard of reliability or precision (more than 30 percent relative standard error in numerator of percent or rate).

★ 322 ★

Smoking and Tobacco Use

Smokers Who Are Aware of Its Dangers: 1990

This table reflects the percent of smokers in the United States 18 years of age and older who reported being aware that smoking increases the likelihood of heart disease. Data are for 1990 and are provided by sex, age, and selected characteristics.

[In percentages]

Characteristic	Both sexes 18 years and over	Male					Female				
		Total	18-29 years	30-44 years	45-64 years	65 years and over	Total	18-29 years	30-44 years	45-64 years	65 years and over
All persons[1]	88.9	87.5	89.8	90.9	84.1	73.5	90.6	93.0	94.0	87.9	77.9
Education level											
Less than 12 years	81.3	79.4	82.6	84.5	76.7	67.4	83.6	88.5	88.1	78.9	74.7
12 years	90.5	88.5	91.5	90.5	84.3	77.3	92.4	94.5	94.8	90.3	79.0
More than 12 years	93.7	93.4	95.2	94.7	91.3	83.9	94.0	95.2	96.0	93.1	82.2
13-15 years	92.9	92.9	95.5	94.1	89.8	71.8	93.0	94.9	94.8	92.3	77.0
16 years or more	95.0	94.3	94.1	95.6	92.8	93.1	96.0	96.5	98.3	94.0	91.3
Income											
Less than $10,000	83.7	80.8	88.8	80.9	75.7	68.3	85.7	93.2	89.0	77.5	73.0
$10,000-$19,999	87.6	85.9	88.9	88.9	81.9	77.0	89.4	91.1	93.0	88.9	76.6
$20,000-$34,999	91.9	90.1	92.3	91.5	86.8	82.6	94.0	95.5	94.6	92.1	92.8
$35,000-$49,999	91.3	89.7	97.4	93.8	85.8	76.0	93.5	94.8	96.5	89.6	72.9
$50,000 or more	94.0	93.6	95.1	96.5	89.5	88.7	94.4	97.2	98.0	89.2	90.2
Race											
White	90.0	89.0	90.6	92.1	86.3	76.8	91.0	93.4	94.4	88.5	78.9
Black	84.3	81.8	86.3	86.0	77.6	59.2	87.3	89.7	91.4	82.1	72.1
Hispanic origin											
Hispanic	83.8	82.3	77.6	84.9	86.3	79.2[2]	86.0	89.4	89.2	76.9	74.2[2]
Non-Hispanic	89.3	88.0	91.2	91.5	84.1	73.2	90.8	93.3	94.3	88.4	78.0
Geographic region											
Northeast	91.4	91.0	96.4	93.4	85.9	78.3	91.9	92.7	96.7	88.3	82.4
Midwest	91.1	90.4	93.3	93.4	86.8	75.5	91.8	95.8	93.4	89.0	78.8
South	85.9	84.3	84.0	89.1	81.6	70.9	87.8	90.0	91.9	86.3	72.0
West	89.1	86.3	88.6	88.8	83.6	70.1	92.5	95.0	95.8	88.9	82.7
Marital status											
Currently married	89.6	87.6	90.6	90.8	84.2	76.6	92.0	93.1	95.2	89.0	80.0
Formerly married	86.1	85.3	89.7	92.7	82.8	66.5	86.6	94.0	91.2	86.2	76.7
Never married	89.9	88.7	89.0	89.3	87.0	74.6[2]	91.8	92.6	92.8	85.6	76.6[2]
Employment status											
Currently employed	90.6	88.9	89.6	91.4	85.1	74.3	92.9	94.6	94.4	89.7	78.1

[Continued]

★ 322 ★

Smokers Who Are Aware of Its Dangers: 1990

[Continued]

Characteristic	Both sexes 18 years and over	Male					Female				
		Total	18-29 years	30-44 years	45-64 years	65 years and over	Total	18-29 years	30-44 years	45-64 years	65 years and over
Unemployed	90.5	88.7	88.0	94.5	80.1	61.5[2]	93.4	96.6	93.8	82.5	100.0[2]
Not in labor force	84.5	80.9	91.8	84.0	81.1	73.5	86.4	88.6	92.7	85.7	77.8

Source: U.S. Department of Health and Human Services. Public Health Service. Centers for Disease Control and Prevention. National Center for Health Statistics. *Health Promotion and Disease Prevention: United States, 1990.* Vital and Health Statistics, Series 10, no. 185. Hyattsville, MD: U.S. Department of Health and Human Services, Public Health Service, Centers for Disease Control and Prevention, National Center for Health Statistics, n.d., p. 49. *Notes:* Data are based on household interviews of the civilian noninstitutionalized population. The survey design, general qualifications, and information on the reliability of the estimates are given in Appendix 1 in the original source. Denominator for each cell excludes unknowns. 1. Includes persons with unknown sociodemographic characteristics. 2. Figure does not meet standard of reliability or precision (more than 30 percent relative standard error in numerator of percent or rate).

★ 323 ★

Smoking and Tobacco Use

Weight Gain of Smokers Who Quit the Habit

Dr. David F. Williamson, an epidemiologist at the Federal Centers for Disease Control in Atlanta, conducted two surveys of 9,004 people during the 1970s and 1980s. He found the average weight gain for those who quit smoking to be between 6 and 8 pounds over a 5-year period. A weight gain of 30 pounds occured in 1 of 10 people who quit smoking, especially in those who were underweight.

Source: "Modest Weight Gain Found in Those Who Quit Smoking." *New York Times,* 15 March 1991, p. A21.

Stress

★ 324 ★

Laughter and Health

According to Joan Coggin, a cardiologist at Loma Linda University School of Medicine in California, laughter has proven health benefits because it leads to stress reduction and relaxation.

	Laughs per day
Adults	15
Children	400

Source: "Laugh—It's Healthy." *Glamour* (December 1992), p. 33.

★ 325 ★

Stress

Stress Reduction for Healthier Living

Data show percent of survey respondents who reported intentionally reducing stress in the last 5 years in order to live healthier lives.

[In percentages]

Age	Percent[1]
18-39	44.0
40+	56.0

Source: Belden & Russonello Research and Communications. *Health and Longevity: Results of a National Survey Conducted for the Alliance for Aging Research.* Washington, DC: Belden & Russonello, December 1992, p. 17. *Notes:* Data represent the results of a national telephone survey conducted in December 1992. A total of 906 adults responded. Senior Americans (50 years or older) represented 34 percent of the sample. 1. Percentages are weighted.

★ 326 ★

Stress

Stressful Jobs

The table below indicates responses of 1,299 employees reporting on their experiences with stress-related conditions in the preceding week.

[In percentages]

Condition	High-stress job	Low-stress job
Fatigue/exhaustion	65	30
Tight back/shoulder muscles	58	32
Anger	51	30
Insomnia	45	20
Anxiety	45	16
Headaches	44	17

Source: "At a Glance: Snapshots of the Workplace Health Industry." *Workplace Health* (May 1993), p. 15. Primary sources: 1) Northwestern National Life, 1992. 2) *Business and Health.*

Violence and Trauma: Crime

★ 327 ★

Crime Index Offenses: 1992

The table below reflects the percent distribution of crimes for 1992.

Crime	Percent
Larceny/theft	54.8
Burglary	20.6
Motor vehicle theft	11.1
Aggravated assault	7.8
Robbery	4.7
Forcible rape	.8
Murder	> .2

Source: U.S. Department of Justice. Federal Bureau of Investigation. *Crime in the United States, 1992: Uniform Crime Reports.* Washington, DC: U.S. Government Printing Office, 3 October 1993, p. 8.

★ 328 ★

Violence and Trauma: Crime

Regional Violent Crime Rates: 1992

The table below reflects the rate of violent crime by specific regions of the United States.

[Per 100,000 inhabitants]

Region	Crime rate
West	864.0
South	809.6
Northeast	731.5
Midwest	607.2

Source: U.S. Department of Justice. Federal Bureau of Investigation. *Crime in the United States, 1992: Uniform Crime Reports.* Washington, DC: U.S. Government Printing Office, 3 October 1993, p. 9.

Violence and Trauma: Domestic Violence

★ 329 ★

Domestic Homicide Among Females: 1976-1992

The figures below represent episodes of domestic violence ending in the murders of females, ages 18 to 34, in selected years.

Year	Number
1976	732
1980	813
1992	702

Source: Viviano, JoAnne. "State Takes Aim at Spouse Abuse." *Sunday Macomb Daily* (Macomb County, Michigan), 3 July 1994, pp. 1A, 5A. Primary source: Northeastern University College of Criminal Justice.

★ 330 ★

Violence and Trauma: Domestic Violence

Price of Domestic Violence

According to the Women's Center, between 4 and 6 million women are battered annually, or 1 every 5 seconds. The table below reflects contact with health care providers initiated as a result of domestic violence.

Health care provider	Contacts due to domestic violence
Emergency rooms	30,000 visits
Physicians	40,000 visits
Hospitalization	100,000 days

Source: Viviano, JoAnne. "State Takes Aim at Spouse Abuse." *Sunday Macomb Daily* (Macomb County, Michigan), 3 July 1994, p. 1A. Primary source: American Medical Association.

Violence and Trauma: Homicide

★ 331 ★

Murder Circumstances by Family Relationship: 1992

Data below reflect the relationship of the victim to the offender.

Circumstances	Total	Husband	Wife	Mother	Father	Son	Daughter	Brother	Sister	Other family
Total[1]	22,540	383	913	121	169	325	235	167	42	393
Felony-type total	4,887	22	37	4	13	31	27	5	5	44
Suspected felony-type total	280	---	4	1	---	---	---	---	---	---
Other than felony-type total	11,152	323	762	97	140	276	194	146	30	307

Source: U.S. Department of Justice. Federal Bureau of Investigation. *Crime in the United States, 1992: Uniform Crime Reports.* Washington, DC: U.S. Government Printing Office, 3 October 1993, p. 19. *Notes:* 1. Total murder victims for whom supplemental homicide data were received.

★ 332 ★

Violence and Trauma: Homicide

Who Kills

The table below indicates the relationships of victims with their killers.

[In percentages]

Killers	Percent
Of women	
Other acquaintance	29
Spouse	22
Other intimate partner	17
Nonspouse family member	16
Stranger	12
Friend	4
Of men	
Other acquaintance	50
Stranger	21
Nonspouse family member	11
Friend	9
Other intimate partner	5
Spouse	4

Source: Colburn, Don. "When Violence Begins at Home." *Washington Post Health,* 15 March 1994, p. 7. Primary source: U.S. Department of Justice.

Violence and Trauma: Suicide

★ 333 ★

Suicide Rate

Each year an average of 30,000 people commit suicide, or 1 person every 17.1 minutes.

Source: U.S. Department of Health and Human Services. Public Health Service. Centers for Disease Control and Prevention. National Center for Health Statistics. *Health, United States, 1991.* Hyattsville, MD: Public Health Service, 1992, n.p.

★ 334 ★

Violence and Trauma: Suicide

Suicides, by Age

Age	Percentage
24 and under	17
25-44	39
45-64	23
65-84	19
85 and over	2

Source: "Suicide's Victims." *USA TODAY,* 24 February 1993, p. 1A. Primary source: National Center for Health Statistics.

★ 335 ★

Violence and Trauma: Suicide

Suicides in the Military: 1991

An average of 250 active members of the armed services commit suicide each year. The table below presents suicide rates related to military personnel for the year 1991.

[Per 100,000]

	Suicide rate
Males between the ages of 18 and 34 years old[1]	20.0
Army	14.3
Combined branches of armed services	12.6

Source: "18% Rise in Suicides in the Army Is Found Between 1987 and 1991." *New York Times,* 8 September 1992, p. A14. *Note:* 1. The majority of military personnel fall within this group.

Violence and Trauma: War

★ 336 ★

Causes of Fratricide

Coordination - 45
Target misidentification - 26
Inexperience - 19
Unknown - 10

The table below indicates the causes of direct fire fratricides in World War II and the Korean and Vietnam conflicts.

[% = Incidents by category/58 total incidents]

Cause	Percent
Coordination	45
Target misidentification	26
Inexperience	19
Unknown	10

Source: U.S. Congress. Office of Technology Assessment. *Who Goes There: Friend or Foe?* OTA-ISC-537. Washington, DC: U.S. Government Printing Office, June 1993, p. 24. Primary source: U.S. Army.

★ 337 ★

Violence and Trauma: War

Women Veterans and Sexual Trauma: 1990-1992

The table below indicates the number of women veterans treated in vet centers for the aftermaths of sexual trauma.

Women veterans treated	Fiscal year		
	1990	1991	1992[1]
None	58	61	66
1 to 10	58	69	74
11 to 20	0	0	2
Vet centers responding	116	130	142

Source: U.S. Senate Committee on Veterans' Affairs. *Women's Health Progams Act of 1992.* Report to accompany S. 2973. 102d Cong., 2d sess., 17 September 1992. Washington, DC: U.S. Government Printing Office, 1992, p. 58. *Note:* 1. Figures "to date."

Violence and Trauma: Youths

★ 338 ★

Drug and Discipline Problems in Schools: 1990-1991

Figures reflect the percentage of public elementary and secondary school teachers and principals reporting drug and discipline problems in their schools. Teachers and principals rated these problems as "serious" or "moderate." Data are provided by location of school.

[- indicates data not collected]

Problem	Total		Urban		Suburban		Town		Rural	
	Teachers	Principals	Teachers	Principals	Teachers	Principals	Teachers	Principals	Teachers	Principals
Student alcohol use	23	11	16	9	22	7	28	9	29	16
Student drug use	17	6	17	7	18	4	18	6	17	6
Student tobacco use	24	13	21	12	22	10	30	13	25	17
Sale of drugs on school grounds	6	1	8	1	6	2	5	0	4	1
Physical conflicts among students	28	22	37	29	27	26	25	22	18	14
Racial tensions	14	5	20	8	18	5	10	4	6	3
Robbery or theft of items over $10	12	7	15	9	14	6	10	4	8	9
Student absenteeism/class cutting	37	25	44	36	36	24	38	23	28	20
Student possession of weapons	5	3	10	7	3	1	3	2	1	1
Student tardiness	39	34	47	48	41	33	34	30	28	27
Trespassing	9	7	16	13	7	7	5	3	4	5
Vandalism of school property	22	12	30	18	20	10	21	7	16	11
Physical abuse of teachers	3	1	6	5	4	1	2	1	1	1
Teacher absenteeism	-	14	-	20	-	14	-	11	-	12
Teacher alcohol or drug use	-	1	-	2	-	2	-	1	-	2
Verbal abuse of teachers	29	11	41	17	28	10	22	10	21	7

Source: U.S. Department of Education. Office of Educational Research and Improvement. National Center for Education Statistics. *Digest of Education Statistics, 1992.* Washington, DC: U.S. Government Printing Office, 1992, p. 140. Primary source: U.S. Department of Education. National Center for Education Statistics. "Public School Principal Survey on Safe, Disciplined, Drug-Free Schools" and "Teacher Survey on Safe, Disciplined, Drug-Free Schools." This table was prepared in April 1992. *Note:* 1. Less than 0.5 percent.

Chapter 5
HEALTH IN THE WORKPLACE

In one survey of business professionals, respondents identified health care as the foremost human resources issue of the decade. (See the table titled "Most Important Human Resources Issues for the 1990s" in the chapter on Politics, Opinion, and Law.) The tables in this chapter show some of the factors that make health care an important issue in the workplace. Coverage includes such topics as sick days and lost work time due to illness or injury; violence and stress on the job; wellness promotion programs of employers; and continuation of benefits through retirement years. The cost of providing health care coverage to employees also is presented. For information about expenditures for health care by individuals and governments, see the chapter on Health Expenditures and Funding.

Cost to Business

★ 339 ★

Cost Per Hour for Employee Compensation and Benefits: 1987-1990

Data reflect hourly costs to private industry employers for compensation and benefits for their workforces. Data provided as a percentage of total compensation for March 1987, 1988, 1989, and 1990.

Compensation component	March 1987	March 1988	March 1989	March 1990
Total compensation	100.0	100.0	100.0	100.0
Wages and salaries	73.2	72.7	72.7	72.4
Total benefit costs	26.8	27.3	27.3	27.6
Paid leave	6.9	7.0	7.0	6.9
Supplemental pay	2.4	2.4	2.4	2.5
Insurance	5.4	5.6	6.0	6.1
Retirement and savings	3.6	3.3	2.9	3.0

[Continued]

★ 339 ★

Cost Per Hour for Employee Compensation and Benefits: 1987-1990
[Continued]

Compensation component	March 1987	March 1988	March 1989	March 1990
Legally required benefits	8.4	8.8	8.9	9.0
Other benefits	.1	.2	.1	[1]

Source: U.S. Department of Labor. Pension and Welfare Benefits Administration. *Trends in Health Benefits.* Washington, DC: U.S. Government Printing Office, 1993, p. 309. Primary source: U.S. Bureau of Labor Statistics. *Employer Costs for Employee Compensation. Note:* 1. Less than 0.05 percent.

★ 340 ★

Cost to Business

Health Care Benefit Cost Increases: 1993

Data are based on responses to a survey of nearly 2,400 employers. According the survey, in 1993, the average cost of health care benefits was $3,781 per employee.

[In dollars, except as noted]

Region	Average cost	Percent increase[1]
Nationwide average	3,781	8.0
Eastern United States	4,260	10.0
Midwestern United States	4,020	9.4
Southern United States	3,262	6.6
Western United States	3,620	5.3

Source: "Costs of Health-care Benefits Rise in 1993." *Personnel Journal* (June 1994), p. 18. Primary source: Foster Higgins. *Note:* 1. Increase from cost in 1992.

★ 341 ★

Cost to Business

Health Care Costs as a Percentage of Company Earnings

According to an A. Foster Higgins & Co. survey of 1,955 businesses and governments, health care costs consumed 26 percent of the average employer's net earnings. A. Foster Higgins is a benefits consulting firm.

Source: Freudenheim, Milt. "Health Care: A Growing Burden." *New York Times,* 29 January 1991, p. D1. Source also includes average amount businesses pay for health care per employee and percentage change from previous year's costs.

★ 342 ★

Cost to Business

Health Expenditures of U.S. Businesses: 1965-1991

This table profiles the expenditures of businessess for health services and supplies. Where businesses pay dedicated funds into government health programs (e.g., Medicare), costs are assigned to businesses accordingly. Estimates of national health care expenditures by source of funds aim to track government-sponsored health programs over time, and do not delineate the role of business employers in paying for health care. Data also indicate the percent distribution of businesses' health-related expenditures for selected years. Please see corresponding tables on spending by households, federal government, and state and local governments.

Type of payer	1965	1967	1970	1975	1980	1985	1987	1988	1989	1990	1991
	Amount in billion dollars[1]										
Total[1]	38.2	47.9	69.1	124.7	238.9	407.2	476.9	526.2	583.6	652.4	728.6
Private	30.3	35.0	50.1	86.2	162.0	279.0	327.5	362.5	398.3	436.6	474.1
Private business	6.0	8.3	13.7	27.8	64.3	113.5	131.8	151.0	167.0	187.9	205.4
Private employer share of private health insurance premiums	4.9	5.6	9.8	19.9	47.9	83.9	95.0	110.9	122.8	140.2	152.7
Private employer contribution to Medicare hospital insurance trust fund[2]	0.0	1.4	2.1	5.0	10.5	20.3	24.6	26.2	28.1	29.5	32.8
Workers' compensation and temporary disability insurance medical benefits and administration	0.8	1.0	1.4	2.4	5.1	7.8	10.5	12.0	14.1	16.0	17.5
Industrial inplant health services	0.2	0.2	0.3	0.5	0.9	1.4	1.7	1.9	2.1	2.2	2.4
	Percent distribution										
Total	100.0	100.0	100.0	100.0	100.0	100.0	100.0	100.0	100.0	100.0	100.0
Private	79.3	73.2	72.6	69.2	67.8	68.5	68.7	68.9	68.2	66.9	65.1
Private business	15.6	17.3	19.8	22.3	26.9	27.9	27.6	28.7	28.6	28.8	28.2
Private employer share of private health insurance premiums	12.9	11.7	14.2	16.0	20.0	20.6	19.9	21.1	21.0	21.5	21.0
Private employer contribution to Medicare hospital insurance trust fund[2]	0.0	2.9	3.0	4.0	4.4	5.0	5.2	5.0	4.8	4.5	4.5
Workers' compensation and temporary disability insurance medical benefits and administration	2.2	2.2	2.1	2.0	2.1	1.9	2.2	2.3	2.4	2.4	2.4
Industrial inplant health services	0.6	0.5	0.5	0.4	0.4	0.4	0.4	0.4	0.4	0.3	0.3

Source: U.S. Department of Health and Human Services. Public Health Service. Centers for Disease Control and Prevention. National Center for Health Statistics. *Health, United States, 1992.* Hyattsville, MD: Public Health Service, 1993, p. 170. Primary source: Health Care Financing Administration. Office of National Health Statistics. Office of the Actuary. "Business, Households, and Governments—Health Spending 1991." *Health Care Financing Review* 14, no.3 (winter 1993). *Notes:* Data are compiled by the Health Care Financing Administration. 1. Excludes research and construction. 2. Includes one-half of self-employment contribution to Medicare hospital insurance trust fund.

★ 343 ★

Cost to Business

Health Insurance Costs of Employers, by Employee Characteristics: 1994

Figures show the estimated costs of employers for health insurance coverage for male and female employees. Data provided by worker ages.

[In dollars]

Age	Men	Women
18-24 years old	710	900
25-34 years old	1,500	1,780
35-44 years old	2,380	2,410
45-54 years old	3,200	2,580
55-64 years old	3,960	2,300

Source: Stevens, Carol. "Who Will Pay Health Bill for Early Retirees?" *Detroit News,* 27 February 1994, p. 1A. Primary sources: Employee Benefit Research Institute; Lewin-VHI health consultants.

★ 344 ★

Cost to Business

Health Insurance Costs Per Employee: 1992

Data note cost of health insurance per employee by size of company.

Size of company	Average cost per employee
Fewer than 500	$3,500
500-999	3,628
1,000-2,499	3,599
2,500-4,999	3,579
5,000-9,999	3,714
10,000-19,000	3,847
20,000-39,000	4,003
40,000 +	3,775

Source: "Company Health Costs Soar." *USA TODAY,* 27 April 1993, p. 2A. Primary source: Employee Benefit Research Institute; A. Foster Higgins & Co., Inc. **Remarks**: Source also includes average health insurance costs per employee, 1984-1992, and percentage of companies offering health insurance to full-time employees by size of company.

★ 345 ★

Cost to Business

Health Insurance Plan Costs, by Plan Type: 1990-1992

Figures represent the average medical plan cost per employee. Data provided by plan type.

Plan	Cost per employee		
	1990	1991	1992
Traditional indemnity plans	3,161	3,573	4,080
Preferred Provider Organizations	2,952	3,355	3,708
Point-of-Service plans	-	3,291	3,566
Health Maintenance Organizations	2,683	3,046	3,313

Source: "Benefits." *Personnel Journal* (November 1993), p. 48B. Primary source: A. Foster Higgins & Co. Inc.

★ 346 ★

Cost to Business

Medical Plan Costs, by U.S. Region

The data below indicate the annual cost of medical plans per employee in various regions of the United States. Spending of U.S. employers for health insurance for their employees averaged $3,573 per worker in 1991—a 13 percent increase from the previous year.

[In dollars]

Region	Cost
Pacific	3,421
Mountain	3,218
North Central	3,443
South Central	3,236
Middle Atlantic	3,942
South Atlantic	3,495
New England	3,958

Source: Thompson, Roger. "Employers' Costs for Employees Soar; Health Benefits." *Nation's Business* 80, no. 5 (May 1992), p. 62. Primary source: A. Foster Higgins & Company, Inc.

★ 347 ★

Cost to Business

Traditional Medical Plan Coverage Costs Per Employee: 1992

The table below presents the cost per employee for traditional (indemnity plan), health maintenance organization (HMO), and preferred provider organization (PPO) medical coverage in selected U.S. cities.

City	Indemnity plans	HMOs	PPOs
Atlanta, Georgia	3,729	3,311	3,363
Chicago, Illinois	4,245	3,088	3,684
Cleveland, Ohio	4,027	3,727	3,459
Dallas-Fort Worth, Texas	3,917	3,330	3,837
Houston, Texas	3,627	3,575	[1]
Los Angeles, California	4,350	3,189	4,457
Minneapolis-St. Paul, Minnesota	3,347	2,969	3,121
New York, New York	4,852	3,448	3,871
Orange County, California	4,276	3,124	4,315
Philadelphia, Pennsylvania	4,696	3,319	3,708
San Francisco, California	4,531	3,092	4,459
Seattle, Washington	3,554	3,092	3,114

Source: "Indemnity Plan Costs vs. Managed-Care Plan Costs in Selected U.S. Cities, 1992." *Modern Healthcare,* 8 March 1993, p. 12. "Health Care Coverage in the '90s." *Los Angeles Times,* 8 March 1993, p. D2. "Shifting Health Traditions." *Miami Herald,* 2 March 1993, p. C1. Primary source: A. Foster Higgins. *Foster Higgins 1992 Health Care Benefits Survey. Note:* 1. Not reported.

Cost to Business: Cost Control

★ 348 ★

Curbing the Cost of Health Care

The table below illustrates the revised cap on small company payments for health care coverage as a percentage of payroll as proposed in President Clinton's health care legislation.

[Annual wage is in thousands. Firm size is shown in percent.]

Average annual wage	Firm size		
	Less than 25	25-50	50-75
Less than $12	3.5	4.4	5.3
$12-$15	4.4	5.3	6.2
$15-$18	5.3	6.2	7.1
$18-$21	6.2	7.1	7.9

[Continued]

★ 348 ★

Curbing the Cost of Health Care
[Continued]

Average annual wage	Firm size		
	Less than 25	25-50	50-75
$21-$24	7.1	7.9	7.9
More than $24	7.9	7.9	7.9

Source: Carlson, Eugene. "What Small-Business Owners Face Under Health Plan." *Wall Street Journal,* 28 October 1993, p. B2. Primary source: White House.

★ 349 ★

Cost to Business: Cost Control

Effect of Clinton Health Plan on Employer Health Costs

The table below compares the current cost per employee for health care with projected decreases (or increases) from President Clinton's health plan. Data provided by industry.

[In dollars]

Industry	Current costs per worker	Projected decrease (-) or increase (+) in costs
Communications	6,572	-3,502
Utilities	4,871	-2,067
Mining	4,776	-1,728
Manufacturing (durable goods)	3,801	-1,349
Manufacturing (nondurable goods)	3,017	-649
Wholesale trade	2,426	-249
Transportation	2,221	+191
Services	1,480	+697
Construction	1,572	+800
Retail	788	+1,303
Agriculture	394	+1,647
Private households	0	+2,041

Source: Wessel, David. "Health Costs to Fall in Some Industries, Increase in Others, New Analysis Shows." *Wall Street Journal,* 9 February 1994, p. A3. Primary source: Congressional Budget Office. Based on forthcoming paper by Henry Aaron and Barry Bosworth (Brookings Institution). *Notes:* Cost estimates include retirees, but do not reflect subsidies or cost controls in Clinton plan. 1. Includes those who do not receive health insurance.

★ 350 ★
Cost to Business: Cost Control

Employer Savings From Mail Order Drug Purchasing Programs

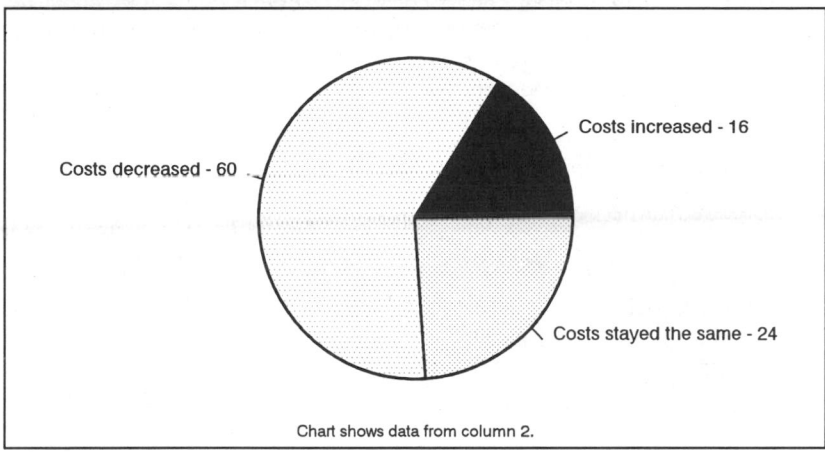

Costs decreased - 60

Costs increased - 16

Costs stayed the same - 24

Chart shows data from column 2.

Approximately 30 percent of employers offer mail order drug purchasing programs. Under these plans, employees may order maintenance medications at discounts, decreasing costs for employers' prescription drug programs. The table below compares the changes in costs to employers with separate card and mail order prescription drug programs.

[In percentages]

Costs	Separate card plan	Separate mail order plan
Costs increased	51	16
Costs stayed the same	21	24
Costs decreased	28	60

Source: "Effect of Drug Programs on Total Drug Costs." *National Underwriter,* 26 April 1993, p. 25. Primary source: Foster Higgins Health Care Benefits Survey, 1992. *Note:* Based on employers implementing separate drug plans in the past 3 years.

★ 351 ★

Cost to Business: Cost Control

Health Care Cost Containment Methods

Financial accounting standard (FAS) 106 requires companies to plan ahead for retiree medical benefit costs. In response to the rule, effective January 1, 1993, companies began taking measures to limit their FAS 106 liability. Figures below represent percentages of companies adopting particular cost containment methods. Data are based on a survey of 780 employers.

Cost containment method	Percent
Increase retiree contributions	48
Increase deductible or copayment	44
Use managed care	38
Tighten eligibility	29
Cap employer contributions	23

Source: "At a Glance: Snapshots of the Workplace Health Industry." *Workplace Health* (March 1993), p. 15. Primary source: William M. Mercer, Inc.

Cost to Business: Taxes

★ 352 ★

Employer Health Insurance Tax Expenditures: 1975-1995

Fiscal year	Exclusion of contributions for medical insurance premiums and medical care (billions of dollars)	Total of tax expenditure items for individuals (billions of dollars)	Net exclusion of medical insurance and care as a percentage of total tax expenditures for individuals (percent)
1975	3.3	70.6	4.7
1976	4.5	72.7	6.2
1977	5.6	87.5	6.4
1978	7.1	92.6	7.7
1979	11.1	112.2	9.9
1980	12.1	139.1	8.7
1981	14.1	179.8	7.8
1982	16.4	198.4	8.3
1983[1]	18.7	239.1	6.4
1984	19.1	248.0	7.7

[Continued]

★ 352 ★

Employer Health Insurance Tax Expenditures: 1975-1995
[Continued]

Fiscal year	Exclusion of contributions for medical insurance premiums and medical care (billions of dollars)	Total of tax expenditure items for individuals (billions of dollars)	Net exclusion of medical insurance and care as a percentage of total tax expenditures for individuals (percent)
1985	21.1	270.3	7.8
1986	23.4	304.6	7.7
1987	24.6	353.4	7.0
1988	24.7	259.1	9.5
1989	26.6	255.4	10.4
1990	29.8	279.9	10.6
1991	33.3	277.6	12.0
1992	38.0	297.0	12.8
1993	42.4	316.4	13.4
1994	46.8	337.1	13.9
1995	49.5	357.0	13.9

Source: U.S. Department of Labor. Pension and Welfare Benefits Administration. *Trends in Health Benefits.* Washington, DC: U.S. Government Printing Office, 1993, p. 96. Primary sources: 1) U.S. House of Representatives Committee on Ways and Means, *Overview of the Federal Tax System,* 1976-1990 editions. 2) U.S. Office of Management and Budget. *Special Analyses, Budget of the United States Government* (annual). *Note:* 1. The methodology for estimating tax expenditures changed in 1983

★ 353 ★

Cost to Business: Taxes

Simulated Effects of Taxing Employee Health Insurance Benefits

Policy	Percentage annual increase in federal personal income tax revenue			
	Aggregate	Average worker in		
		Low-wage industry[1]	Medium-wage industry[2]	High-wage industry[3]
Tax all health insurance contributions	8.3	7.7	6.8	10.8
Tax health insurance contributions above $1,125 per year (1982 dollars)	1.5	0.2	0.6	4.3
Tax all employee benefits	17.6	14.5	13.9	25.9

Source: U.S. Department of Labor. Pension and Welfare Benefits Administration. *Trends in Health Benefits.* Washington, DC: U.S. Government Printing Office, 1993, p. 98. Primary source: Woodbury, Stephen A., and Wei-Jang Huang. *The Tax Treatment of Fringe Benefits.* W.E. Upjohn Institute, 1991. *Notes:* Figures are simulated average annual revenue effects between 1969 and 1982 of policy changes relative to current tax law, based upon econometric estimates of the demand for health insurance and other employee benefits. 1. Average wage between $11,630 and $17,041. 2. Average wage between $17,643 and $22,550. 3. Average wage between $23,103 and $39,498.

Employee Benefits

★ 354 ★

COBRA Coverage: 1987-1991

The Consolidated Onmibus Budget Reconcilliation Act (COBRA) became law in 1985 and ensures the temporary continuation of health plan coverage for former (and certain current) employees, their spouses, and their dependent children. Qualifying individuals may purchase coverage from their former employers at group rates. The table below reflects the characteristics of those obtaining coverage through COBRA, as well the average number of months they were on COBRA, from 1987-1991.

Characteristics	All events	Qualifying events		
		Work related	Disability	Family related
Average number of months on COBRA				
Ages				
All ages	7	7	13	9
18-24 years old	5	4	0	6
25-40 years old	6	5	5	10
41-60 years old	8	7	15	15
61-64 years old	12	12	14	18
65 years old or older	11	10	0	14
Females	7	6	8	9
Males	7	7	17	7
Total	7	7	13	9

Source: U.S. Department of Labor. Pension and Welfare Benefits Administration. *Health Benefits and the Workforce.* Washington, DC: U.S. Government Printing Office, 1992, p. 114. Primary source: 1987-1991 CobraServ.

★ 355 ★

Employee Benefits

Employees Enrolled in Health Care Plans, by Industry: 1992

Data indicate the percent of employees enrolled in various health care plans for selected industries. Data are for 1992.

	Health care plans			
	Conventional plans[1]	HMOs	PPOs	POS plans
Manufacturing	44	17	32	7
Transportation/communication	37	29	24	9
Retail	53	18	24	4
Finance	36	30	29	5
Services	43	23	19	14
State/local governments	45	31	22	3
Health care	35	28	33	3
High tech	39	34	22	6

Source: "Managed Care Facts." *Hospitals,* 5 April 1993, p. 20. Primary source: KPMG Peat Marwick Survey of 1,057 firms (1992). *Notes:* "HMO" stands for health maintenance organization; "PPO" stands for preferred provider organization; "POS" stands for point-of-service plans. 1. Traditional indemnity plans.

★ 356 ★

Employee Benefits

Employees With Employer- or Union-Provided Group Health Plans, by Occupation: 1991

In thousands, except percentages. For wage and salary workers 15 years old and over as of March 1992. Based on *Current Population Survey.*

Occupation	Total	Employees with group health plans	
		Number	Percent
Total	134,023	69,828	52.1
Executive, administrative & managerial occupations	15,814	10,728	67.8
Professional specialty occupations	17,232	11,448	66.4
Technical/related support occupations	4,612	3,104	67.3
Sales workers	16,197	6,865	42.4
Administrative support occupations including clerical	21,199	12,202	57.6
Precision production occupations Craft/repair	14,545	8,183	56.3
Machine operators Assemblers[1]	8,602	5,384	62.6
Transportation/material moving occupations	5,259	3,085	58.7
Handlers, equipment cleaners[2]	5,888	2,276	38.7
Service workers	19,693	5,813	29.5

[Continued]

★ 356 ★

Employees With Employer- or Union-Provided Group Health Plans, by Occupation: 1991

[Continued]

Occupation	Total	Employees with group health plans	
		Number	Percent
Private households	1,098	19	1.7
Other	18,596	5,794	31.2
Farming, forestry & fishing occupations	3,977	662	16.6
Armed Forces	1,005	77	7.6

Source: 1993 Statistical Abstract of the United States on CD-ROM [machine-readable datafiles]. CD-ABSTR-93. Washington, DC: U.S. Department of Commerce, Economics and Statistics Administration, Bureau of the Census, Data User Services Division, 1993. Primary source: U.S. Bureau of the Census. Unpublished data. Notes: 1. Includes inspectors. 2. Includes helpers and laborers.

★ 357 ★

Employee Benefits

Employees With Employer- or Union-Provided Group Health Plans, by Selected Characteristic: 1991

In thousands, except percentages. For wage and salary workers 15 years old and over as of March 1992. Based on *Current Population Survey.*

Occupation	Total	Employees with group health plans	
		Number	Percent
Total	134,023	69,828	52.1
Age			
15 to 24 years	23,028	5,430	23.6
25 to 44 years	70,761	40,638	57.4
45 to 64 years	35,484	21,930	61.8
65 years and over	4,750	1,829	38.5
Work experience			
Full-time	104,537	65,107	62.3
50 weeks or more	80,388	55,938	69.6
27 to 49 weeks	14,492	6,915	47.7
26 weeks or fewer	9,657	2,254	23.3
Part-time	29,486	4,720	16.0
50 weeks or more	12,010	2,686	22.4
27 to 49 weeks	7,078	1,141	16.1
26 weeks or fewer	10,398	893	8.6
Employer size			
Under 25	40,383	10,620	26.3
25 to 99	17,263	8,661	50.2
100 to 499	18,635	11,508	61.8

[Continued]

★ 357 ★

Employees With Employer- or Union-Provided Group Health Plans, by Selected Characteristic: 1991

[Continued]

Occupation	Total	Employees with group health plans	
		Number	Percent
500 to 999	7,320	4,857	66.4
Over 1,000	50,422	34,181	67.8

Source: 1993 Statistical Abstract of the United States on CD-ROM [machine readable datafiles]. CD-ABSTR-93. Washington, DC: U.S. Department of Commerce, Economics and Statistics Administration, Bureau of the Census, Data User Services Division, 1993. Primary source: U.S. Bureau of the Census. Unpublished data.

★ 358 ★

Employee Benefits

Employer-Based Long-term Care Insurance Plans: 1987-1991

The table below reflects the number of long-term care insurance plans sold to employers between 1987 and 1991.

Year	Each year	Cumulative
1987	2	-
1988	5	7
1989	47	54
1990	81	135
1991	51	186

Source: U.S. Department of Labor. Pension and Welfare Benefits Administration. *Trends in Health Benefits*. Washington, DC: U.S. Government Printing Office, 1993, p. 221. Primary source: Health Insurance Association of America. Unpublished data.

★ 359 ★

Employee Benefits

Full-time Employees and Special Medical Care Benefits: 1989 and 1990

The table below shows the percent of full-time participants by type of plan and coverage for selected special medical care benefits; for example, well-baby care or organ transplants. Data are provided by type of employer and type of plan.

Employer and benefit	All plans combined	Plans	
		HMO	non-HMO
Medium and large firms[1]			
Hearing care[2]	26	93	12
Orthoptics[3]	3	[4]	4
Physical examinations (routine)	28	97	14
Organ transplants	26	23	26
Well-baby care	34	95	22
Immunization and innoculation	28	98	14
Small firms[5]			
Hearing care[2]	16	92	4
Orthoptics[3]	1	-	1
Physical examinations (routine)	26	98	15
Organ transplants	28	13	31
Well-baby care	32	97	22
Immunization and innoculation	23	96	12
Dental care (preventive)[6]	2	9	[4]
Vision examinations[7]	12	71	3
State and local governments[8]			
Hearing care[2]	27	84	11
Orthoptics[3]	1	[4]	1
Physical examinations (routine)	36	97	19
Organ transplants	32	20	36
Well-baby care	39	96	23
Immunization and innoculation	33	95	16

[Continued]

★ 359 ★

Full-time Employees and Special Medical Care Benefits: 1989 and 1990
[Continued]

Employer and benefit	All plans combined	Plans HMO	non-HMO
Dental care (preventive)[6]	2	10	4
Vision examinations[7]	19	73	4

Source: U.S. Congress. Office of Technology Assessment. *Does Health Insurance Make a Difference? Background Paper.* OTA-BP-H-99. Washington, DC: U.S. Government Printing Office, September 1992, p. 53. Primary sources: U.S. Department of Labor. Bureau of Labor Statistics. *Employee Benefits in Medium and Large Firms, 1989.* Bulletin 2363. Washington, DC: U.S. Government Printing Office, June 1990; U.S. Department of Labor. Bureau of Labor Statistics. *Employee Benefits in Small Private Establishments, 1990.* Bulletin 2388. Washington, DC: U.S. Government Printing Office, June 1990; U.S. Department of Labor. Bureau of Labor Statistics. *Employee Benefits in State and Local Governments, 1990.* Washington, DC: U.S. Government Printing Office, 1991. *Notes:* "HMO" stands for health maintenance organization. Where applicable, "-" indicates no employees in the category. 1. Data from 1989. Medium and large firms are establishments with 100 workers or more in all private nonfarm industries, excluding (in the 1989 survey) firms in Alaska and Hawaii. According to the Bureau of Labor Statistics (BLS), its survey of these firms provides representative data on 32.4 million full-time employees. 2. Plan provides, as a minimum, coverage for hearing examination expenses. 3. Exercises to improve the function of eye muscles. 4. Less than 0.5 percent. 5. Data for 1990. Small firms are defined as those private nonfarm firms with fewer than 100 workers. According to the Bureau of Labor Statistics (BLS), its survey of these firms provided representative data on 40.8 million full- and part-time employees. Data shown in this table are for full-time employees only. According to the BLS, insurance benefits—sickness and accident insurance, long-term disability insurance, medical care, dental care, and life insurance—were available to one-tenth or fewer part-time workers. No further details were provided on benefits available to part-time workers in the BLS report. 6. Includes plans that provide only examinations and x-rays. 7. Includes plans that provide examinations only. 8. Data for 1990. According to the Bureau of Labor Statistics (BLS), these data represent about 13 million full-time employees in all state and local governments in the 50 states and the District of Columbia. Detailed data for 1.6 million part-time workers were not provided.

★ 360 ★

Employee Benefits

Full-time Employees Participating in Selected Health-Related Benefit Programs: 1991

The table below presents the percentages of full-time employees participating in selected employee benefit programs in medium and private establishments during 1991. Participants are workers covered by a paid time off, insurance, retirement, or capital accumulation plan. Employees subject to a minimum service requirement before they are eligible for benefit coverage are counted as participants even if they have not met the requirement at the time of the survey. If employees are required to pay part of the cost of a benefit, only those who elect the coverage and pay their shares are counted as participants. Benefits for which the employee must pay the full premium are outside the scope of the survey. Only current employees are counted as participants; retirees are excluded.

Benefit programs	All employees	Professional, technical, and related employees	Clerical and sales employees	Production and service employees
Paid:				
Sick leave	67	87	82	48
Maternity leave	2	3	2	1
Paternity leave	1	1	1	1

[Continued]

★ 360 ★

Full-time Employees Participating in Selected Health-Related Benefit Programs: 1991
[Continued]

Benefit programs	All employees	Professional, technical, and related employees	Clerical and sales employees	Production and service employees
Unpaid:				
Maternity leave	37	43	38	33
Paternity leave	26	31	26	23
Sickness and accident insurance	45	32	35	57
Wholly employer financed	33	19	23	46
Partly employer financed	11	13	12	10
Long-term disability insurance	40	61	49	24
Wholly employer financed	31	46	38	20
Partly employer financed	9	15	11	4
Medical care	83	85	81	84
Employee coverage:				
Wholly employer financed	41	38	35	46
Partly employer financed	42	47	46	38
Family coverage:				
Wholly employer financed	26	21	22	31
Partly employer financed	57	64	59	53
Dental care	60	67	60	57
Employee coverage:				
Wholly employer financed	35	36	31	37
Partly employer financed	25	31	29	20
Family coverage:				
Wholly employer financed	26	25	23	29
Partly employer financed	34	42	37	28

Source: U.S. Department of Labor. Bureau of Labor Statistics. *Employee Benefits in Medium and Large Private Establishments, 1991.* Bulletin 2422. Washington, DC: U.S. Government Printing Office, May 1993, p. 5. *Notes:* Because of rounding, sums of individual items may not equal totals. Where applicable, "-" indicates no employees in the category. 1. Less than 0.5 percent.

★ 361 ★

Employee Benefits

Industries That Do Not Offer Health Insurance Coverage

The table below shows the industries that do not offer health insurance coverage to employees.

[In percentages]

Industry	Percent
Retail	43
Services	17
Construction	15
Transportation	6
Wholesale	6
Manufacturing	6
Finance	5

Source: "Health Care Coverage." *San Francisco Examiner,* 28 November 1993, p. E1. Primary source: Lewin-ICF 1991 Retirement Plan Survey.

★ 362 ★

Employee Benefits

Self-Insured Health Benefits

The table below shows the percent of companies that self-fund health insurance benefits for their employees. Data are provided by number of employees.

Number of employees	Percent that self-fund medical indemnity plans
10-49	6
50-199	37
200-499	60
500-999	52
1,000-4,999	69
5,000-9,999	86
10,000-19,999	84
20,000 +	89

Source: Schachner, Michael. "Large Companies Still See Self-Funding as Health Care Cure." *Business Insurance,* 7 February 1994, p. 3. Primary source: A. Foster Higgins & Co. Inc.

★ 363 ★

Employee Benefits

Sources of Employees' Health Insurance, by Company Size

[In percentages]

Employer size	Sources of health insurance				No health insurance
	Own employer	Spouse's employer	Other private[1]	Public source[2]	
Self-employed	22.7	25.8	26.0	4.2	22.9
Fewer than 10 employees	22.1	23.4	15.5	7.9	33.0
10-24 employees	36.7	20.2	10.0	6.9	27.6
25-99 employees	51.7	16.0	7.5	6.4	20.7
100-499 employees	62.8	14.1	5.4	5.6	14.4
500-999 employees	66.5	14.4	5.6	4.7	11.0
1,000 or more employees	69.3	12.4	5.1	6.3	10.0

Source: "Ranks of the Uninsured Increase." *Nation's Business* (May 1994), p. 59. Primary source: Employee Benefit Research Institute. *Notes:* 1. Purchased by individuals. 2. Including Medicare and Medicaid.

★ 364 ★

Employee Benefits

Workers Without Health Insurance

The table below reflects the percentage of working Americans without health insurance coverage. Data are provided by size of employer.

Company size	Uninsured (%)
Self-employed	22
Under 10 employees	32
10-24 employees	25
25-99 employees	21
100-499 employees	13

Source: Thompson, Roger. "Small Firms' Stake in Health Reform." *Nation's Business* 81, no. 11 (November 1993), p. 18. Primary source: Employee Benefit Research Institute.

Employee Benefits: Retirees

★ 365 ★

Cutting Retiree Health Insurance Benefits

Table below presents the percent of companies who have ended or restricted their health care insurance coverage for retired employees. Data are based on a survey of 2,000 companies conducted by the consulting firm of A. Foster Higgins. Survey samples were not necessarily representative of all companies.

Year	Number of companies surveyed	Have ended[1] or plan to end[2] benefits	Have reduced[1] or plan to reduce[2] benefits
1989	1,380	3.0	43.0
1990	1,180	5.0	58.0
1991	1,114	7.0	65.0

Source: Freudenheim, Milt. "Retirees Threatened With Loss of Insurance." *New York Times,* 28 June 1992, sec. 1, pp. 1, 20. Primary source: A. Foster Higgins, a consulting firm. *Notes:* 1. In 1990 or 1991. 2. In 1992 or 1993.

★ 366 ★

Employee Benefits: Retirees

Employer Health Care Plans for Retirees, by Company Size

The table below reflects expectations of employees surveyed in 1993 concerning the availability of employer health care plan coverage for retired private wage-and-salary workers. Data are for currently covered workers aged 46 years or older.

[In percentages, except as noted]

Company size	Number of workers[1] (in thousands)	Coverage available throughout retirement	Coverage available until age 65	No coverage during retirement	Don't know or no response
1-9 employees	250	26	10	28	36
10-24 employees	201	28	8	28	35
25-99 employees	380	27	8	25	40
100-499 employees	413	35	9	26	30
500-999 employees	185	34	8	25	34
1,000 or more employees	1,456	55	7	13	25

Source: "Employer-Provided Health Care Insurance." *New York Times,* 19 June 1994, p. F21. Primary source: Employee Benefits Supplement to the April 1993 *Current Population Survey. Note:* 1. Nationally.

★ 367 ★

Employee Benefits: Retirees

Future Health-Related Spending on Retirees by Selected Major Corporations

The institution of financial accounting standard (FAS) 106 in 1993 required companies to reserve funds for health care coverage of their retirees, to report their health care obligations to retirees, and to forecast future spending increases for retirees in financial statements. The table below shows the amounts set aside for health care spending for retirees by selected large corporations.

[In billion dollars]

Company	Amount
Fortune top 50 companies	115.2
General Motors	35.6
Ford Motor Company	12.7
Chrysler Corporation	7.5
IBM	6.9
DuPont	5.5

Source: "Health Care Write-Down." *American Medical News,* 1 November 1993, p. 30. Primary source: 1992 annual reports.

★ 368 ★

Employee Benefits: Retirees

Retiree Benefit Modifications

A survey of 230 companies revealed that 90 percent of those offering medical benefits to retirees are altering or planning to alter those programs in response to rising costs and changing accounting practices. The table below shows modifications to retiree health benefits.

Status of modifications	Percent
No modifications made or considered	10
Modifications considered	16
Modifications to address:	
New accounting rules	43
Costs	20
New accounting rules and costs	37
Modifications made[1]	74
Modifications to address:	
New accounting rules	25
Costs	22
New accounting rules and costs	53

Source: "By the Numbers: Why Retiree Medical Benefits Are Changing." *Journal of Accountancy* (September 1993), p. 20. Primary source: Buck Consultants. *Notes:* 1. Includes those having made modifications and considering additional changes.

★ 369 ★

Employee Benefits: Retirees

Sources of Health Insurance for Early Retirees

The table below shows the sources of health insurance for workers retiring early.

Source of coverage	Number of retirees covered
Employer coverage	1.7 million
Other[1]	870,000
Uninsured	349,200

Source: Stevens, Carol. "Who Will Pay Health Bill for Early Retirees?" *Detroit News,* 27 February 1994, p. 1A. Primary sources: Employee Benefit Research Institute; Lewin-VHI health consultants. *Notes:* 1. Includes insurance purchased privately and public programs for the poor and disabled.

★ 370 ★

Employee Benefits: Retirees

U.S. Firms Offering Health Care Benefits to Retirees: 1991-1992

[In percentages]

Company size	1992	1991
200-999 employees	37	44
1,000-4,999 employees	52	56
5,000 or more employees	72	72

Source: Rose, Robert L. "Retiree Health Coverage Erodes at Small, Midsize Firms." *Wall Street Journal,* 16 April 1993, p. B2. Primary source: KPMG Peat Marwick survey.

Occupational Health and Safety: Disabilities

★ 371 ★

Americans With Disabilities Act Charges: July 1992-July 1993

Figures below represent percentages of Americans With Disabilities Act (ADA) charges filed with the Equal Employment Opportunity Commission (EEOC) between July 26, 1992, and July 31, 1993. Data reflect complaints for specific, alleged diseases and disorders. In total, 12,962 charges were filed with the EEOC during this time period.

Problem	Percent
Back impairment	18.5
Mental illness	9.8
Retaliation	7.3
Heart impairment	4.3
Neurological disorder	3.7
Diabetes	3.6
Vision impairment	3.3
Hearing impairment	3.3
Arthritis	2.8
Cancer	2.7
All other	40.8

Source: Hansen, Mark. "The ADA's Wide Reach: Little League and Health Insurers Among Those Covered by Act." ABA Journal (December 1993), p. 14. Primary source: Equal Employment Opportunity Commission.

★ 372 ★

Occupational Health and Safety: Disabilities

Men With Work Disabilities Who Are Employed: 1990

Figures show civilian noninstitutionalized persons 16 years and over only.

State	Number	Percent of all persons 16 years old and older
Alabama	41,119	1.3
Alaska	6,582	1.7
Arizona	40,298	1.4
Arkansas	28,233	1.6
California	297,384	1.3
Colorado	42,136	1.7
Connecticut	35,193	1.3

[Continued]

★ 372 ★

Men With Work Disabilities Who Are Employed: 1990
[Continued]

State	Number	Percent of all persons 16 years old and older
Delaware	7,405	1.4
D.C.	5,440	1.1
Florida	146,067	1.4
Georgia	74,119	1.5
Hawaii	11,042	1.3
Idaho	14,545	2.0
Illinois	100,899	1.1
Indiana	59,900	1.4
Iowa	33,463	1.6
Kansas	27,404	1.5
Kentucky	42,144	1.5
Louisiana	40,569	1.3
Maine	18,208	1.9
Maryland	53,612	1.4
Massachusetts	61,299	1.3
Michigan	100,973	1.4
Minnesota	57,947	1.7
Mississippi	26,058	1.4
Missouri	56,894	1.4
Montana	11,093	1.8
Nebraska	19,032	1.6
Nevada	17,527	1.9
New Hampshire	13,517	1.6
New Jersey	68,044	1.1
New Mexico	16,561	1.5
New York	154,144	1.1
North Carolina	76,369	1.5
North Dakota	6,933	1.4
Ohio	121,344	1.5
Oklahoma	42,841	1.8
Oregon	45,704	2.1
Pennsylvania	119,302	1.3
Rhode Island	11,719	1.5
South Carolina	36,550	1.4
South Dakota	8,701	1.7
Tennessee	52,936	1.4
Texas	178,428	1.4
Utah	20,284	1.8
Vermont	7,700	1.8
Virginia	65,791	1.4
Washington	69,591	1.9
West Virginia	19,138	1.4
Wisconsin	53,846	1.4

[Continued]

★ 372 ★

Men With Work Disabilities Who Are Employed: 1990
[Continued]

State	Number	Percent of all persons 16 years old and older
Wyoming	5,487	1.7
U.S. Total	2,671,515	1.4

Source: Census of Population and Housing, 1990: Summary Tape File 3C on CD-ROM [machine-readable datafiles]. Prepared by Bureau of the Census. Washington, DC: The Bureau, 1992.

★ 373 ★
Occupational Health and Safety: Disabilities

Men With Work Disabilities Who Are Prevented From Working: 1990

Figures show civilian noninstitutionalized persons 16 years and over only.

State	Number	Percent of all persons 16 years old and older
Alabama	72,094	2.32
Alaska	3,791	0.96
Arizona	46,431	1.67
Arkansas	46,720	2.60
California	335,049	1.47
Colorado	33,416	1.33
Connecticut	26,551	1.01
Delaware	6,998	1.35
D.C.	8,394	1.67
Florida	172,256	1.66
Georgia	93,470	1.89
Hawaii	10,382	1.21
Idaho	11,051	1.51
Illinois	119,013	1.35
Indiana	64,004	1.51
Iowa	25,860	1.21
Kansas	22,609	1.20
Kentucky	86,015	3.03
Louisiana	83,027	2.66
Maine	18,966	1.99
Maryland	46,585	1.25
Massachusetts	68,746	1.43
Michigan	130,507	1.84
Minnesota	36,484	1.10

[Continued]

★ 373 ★

Men With Work Disabilities Who Are Prevented From Working: 1990

[Continued]

State	Number	Percent of all persons 16 years old and older
Mississippi	52,874	2.77
Missouri	67,806	1.72
Montana	11,610	1.94
Nebraska	13,529	1.13
Nevada	14,323	1.53
New Hampshire	10,542	1.23
New Jersey	69,325	1.13
New Mexico	22,662	2.04
New York	219,816	1.55
North Carolina	93,231	1.79
North Dakota	5,492	1.14
Ohio	156,136	1.87
Oklahoma	46,852	1.95
Oregon	34,902	1.59
Pennsylvania	157,563	1.68
Rhode Island	13,407	1.67
South Carolina	54,138	2.03
South Dakota	6,593	1.28
Tennessee	85,512	2.25
Texas	108,416	1.57
Utah	13,319	1.15
Vermont	6,201	1.43
Virginia	74,397	1.54
Washington	57,222	1.53
West Virginia	50,864	3.62
Wisconsin	49,417	1.32
Wyoming	4,425	1.33
U.S. Total	3,158,993	1.65

Source: Census of Population and Housing, 1990: Summary Tape File 3C on CD-ROM [machine-readable datafiles]. Prepared by Bureau of the Census. Washington, DC: The Bureau, 1992.

★ 374 ★

Occupational Health and Safety: Disabilities

States With the Highest and Lowest Incidence of Work Disability: 1990

[Rate per 1,000 people]

State	Disability rate
States with highest disability rates	
West Virginia	126.2
Kentucky	114.3
Arkansas	111.7
Mississippi	109.8
Louisiana	102.9
Oklahoma	101.6
Maine	101.5
Oregon	100.1
Tennessee	97.3
Montana	97.0
States with lowest disability rates	
Kansas	72.0
Massachusetts	72.0
Nebraska	71.4
Maryland	70.5
North Dakota	69.7
Illinois	68.9
Alaska	66.3
Hawaii	65.9
Connecticut	63.8
New Jersey	61.8

Source: "The State of Affairs in Work Disability." *Small Business Reports* 19, no. 1 (January 1994), p. 35. Primary source: *Morbidity and Mortality Weekly Report.*

★ 375 ★

Occupational Health and Safety: Disabilities

Women With Work Disabilities Who Are Employed: 1990

Figures show civilian noninstitutionalized persons 16 years and over only.

State	Number	Percent of all persons 16 years old or older
Alabama	22,845	0.74
Alaska	3,719	0.95
Arizona	25,401	0.91
Arkansas	16,717	0.93
California	197,300	0.87
Colorado	28,266	1.12
Connecticut	24,126	0.92
Delaware	6,008	1.16
D.C.	5,464	1.09
Florida	89,025	0.86
Georgia	44,464	0.90
Hawaii	7,042	0.82
Idaho	8,515	1.17
Illinois	67,391	0.77
Indiana	40,588	0.96
Iowa	21,092	0.99
Kansas	17,247	0.92
Kentucky	22,692	0.80
Louisiana	22,514	0.72
Maine	11,250	1.18
Maryland	34,907	0.93
Massachusetts	41,822	0.07
Michigan	69,962	0.99
Minnesota	40,557	1.22
Mississippi	14,097	0.74
Missouri	35,686	0.91
Montana	6,569	1.10
Nebraska	11,748	0.98
Nevada	10,068	1.08
New Hampshire	9,426	1.10
New Jersey	46,701	0.76
New Mexico	9,192	0.83
New York	107,710	0.76
North Carolina	48,030	0.92
North Dakota	4,019	0.84
Ohio	80,147	0.96
Oklahoma	24,962	1.04
Oregon	29,964	1.37
Pennsylvania	75,939	0.81
Rhode Island	8,764	1.09
South Carolina	22,418	0.84
South Dakota	5,918	1.14

[Continued]

★ 375 ★

Women With Work Disabilities Who Are Employed: 1990
[Continued]

State	Number	Percent of all persons 16 years old or older
Tennessee	31,723	0.83
Texas	99,925	0.79
Utah	11,405	0.99
Vermont	4,407	1.01
Virginia	40,151	0.83
Washington	43,609	1.17
West Virginia	9,797	0.70
Wisconsin	36,074	0.97
Wyoming	3,163	0.95
U.S. Total	1,700,526	0.89

Source: Census of Population and Housing, 1990: Summary Tape File 3C on CD-ROM [machine-readable datafiles]. Prepared by Bureau of the Census. Washington, DC: The Bureau, 1992.

★ 376 ★

Occupational Health and Safety: Disabilities

Women With Work Disabilities Who Are Prevented From Working: 1990

Figures show civilian noninstitutionalized persons 16 years and over only.

State	Number	Percent of all persons 16 years old or older
Alabama	77,462	2.5
Alaska	4,137	1.1
Arizona	46,886	1.7
Arkansas	47,169	2.6
California	382,270	1.7
Colorado	36,011	1.4
Connecticut	30,159	1.2
Delaware	8,168	1.6
D.C.	10,140	2.0
Florida	170,465	1.6
Georgia	108,241	2.2
Hawaii	9,948	1.2
Idaho	11,288	1.5
Illinois	137,578	1.6
Indiana	71,858	1.7

[Continued]

★ 376 ★

Women With Work Disabilities Who Are Prevented From Working: 1990

[Continued]

State	Number	Percent of all persons 16 years old or older
Iowa	28,292	1.3
Kansas	24,509	1.3
Kentucky	82,849	2.9
Louisiana	82,162	2.6
Maine	18,550	1.9
Maryland	55,632	1.5
Massachusetts	72,617	1.5
Michigan	145,474	2.0
Minnesota	36,575	1.1
Mississippi	57,400	3.0
Missouri	71,376	1.8
Montana	10,361	1.7
Nebraska	14,191	1.2
Nevada	13,809	1.5
New Hampshire	10,643	1.2
New Jersey	83,887	1.4
New Mexico	20,798	1.9
New York	257,918	1.8
North Carolina	108,389	2.1
North Dakota	5,568	1.2
Ohio	171,634	2.1
Oklahoma	49,564	2.1
Oregon	37,552	1.7
Pennsylvania	174,353	1.9
Rhode Island	14,002	1.7
South Carolina	62,238	2.3
South Dakota	6,458	1.2
Tennessee	96,770	2.5
Texas	209,403	1.7
Utah	14,884	1.3
Vermont	6,368	1.5
Virginia	78,175	1.6
Washington	62,814	1.7
West Virginia	43,456	3.1
Wisconsin	50,634	1.4
Wyoming	3,951	1.2
U.S. Total	3,435,036	1.8

Source: Census of Population and Housing, 1990: Summary Tape File 3C on CD-ROM [machine-readable datafiles]. Prepared by Bureau of the Census. Washington, DC: The Bureau, 1992.

Occupational Health and Safety: Fatalities

★ 377 ★

Fatal Work Injuries: 1991

Figures show percent distribution of 3,465 fatal work injuries in 31 states. Data provided by demographic characteristics.

Characteristics	Fatal occupational injuries
Employment status	
Wage and salary workers	81
Self-employed[1]	19
Sex and age	
Men	92
Women	8
Both sexes:	
Under 20 years old	5
20-24 years old	7
25-34 years old	26
35-44 years old	25
45-54 years old	17
55-64 years old	13
65 years old and older	7
Race/Origin	
Asian or Pacific Islander	3
Black	9
Hispanic	9
White	84
Other or unknown	4

Source: U.S. Department of Labor. Bureau of Labor Statistics. *Fatal Workplace Injuries in 1991: A Collection of Data and Analysis.* Report 845. Washington, DC: U.S. Government Printing Office, April 1993, p. 3. Primary source: 31 participating states in the 1991 Census of Fatal Occupational Injuries (CFOI) program. *Notes:* Percentages may not add to total due to rounding. Participating states include Arizona, California, Colorado, Connecticut, Delaware, Georgia, Hawaii, Idaho, Indiana, Iowa, Kansas, Kentucky, Maine, Maryland, Massachusetts, Michigan, Minnesota, Montana, Nebraska, Nevada, New Hampshire, New Jersey, North Carolina, Oklahoma, Oregon, Tennessee, Texas, Utah, Washington, Wisconsin, and Wyoming. 1. May include unpaid family workers, owners of incorporated businesses, or members of partnerships.

★ 378 ★

Occupational Health and Safety: Fatalities

Murder in the Workplace

An employee who murders at his or her workplace stands a 1 in 4 chance of ending the violent episode by committing suicide.

Source: "Just the Facts." *Detroit News,* 12 April 1994, p. 7D. Primary source: *Harper's Magazine.*

★ 379 ★

Occupational Health and Safety: Fatalities

Work-Related Deaths and Death Rates, by Industry: 1992

Industry	Deaths	Death rate[1]
All industries	8,500	7
Agriculture[2]	1,200	37[3]
Mining, quarrying[2]	200	29
Construction	1,300	22
Manufacturing	600	3
Transportation and public utilities	1,200	20
Trade[2]	1,000	4
Services[2]	1,300	3
Government	1,700	9

Source: "Work Accidents." *Traffic Safety* (November/December 1993), p. 21. *Notes:* 1. Deaths per 100,000 workers in each division. 2. Agriculture includes forestry and fishing. Mining and quarrying include oil and gas extraction. Preliminary Mine Safety and Health Administration (MSHA) reports show 97 deaths in coal, metal, and nonmetal mining in 1992. Trade includes wholesale and retail trade. Services include finance, insurance, and real estate. 3. Agriculture rate excludes deaths of persons under 14 years of age. Rates for other industry divisions do not require this adjustment. Deaths of persons under 14 are included in the agriculture death total.

★ 380 ★

Occupational Health and Safety: Fatalities

Worker Fatalities: 1992

Data reflect findings from the first national census of occupational fatalities conducted by the Bureau of Labor Statistics. The survey identified 6,083 worker fatalities in 1992.

[In percentages]

Cause of fatality	Percent
Transportation accident	40
Assaults and violent acts	20
Homicides	17
Suicides	3
Highway accidents	18
Contact with objects	16
Exposure to harmful substances	10
Falls	10
Nonhighway accidents	7
Aircraft accidents	6
Struck by vehicle	6

Source: Laabs, Jennifer J. "Danger at Work: Fatalities and Injuries on the Rise." *Personnel Journal* (February 1994), p. 12.

Occupational Health and Safety: Injuries and Accidents

★ 381 ★

Business Losses Due to Motor Vehicle Accidents

The Network of Employers for Traffic Safety (NETS) found that lost work time due to motor vehicle accidents costs businesses $16.4 billion annually. Workers' compensation for each on-the-job motor vehicle-related fatality averages $110,500. Each injury averages $2,400.

Source: "Safety First." *Business Week* 22, 2 November 1992, p. 37.

★ 382 ★

Occupational Health and Safety: Injuries and Accidents

Employee Injuries: 1992

Figures reflect injuries per 100 full-time workers. Data provided for 1992.

Industry	Injuries	Rank	Incident rate	Rank
Eating and drinking places	387.8	1	8.9	7
Hospitals	341.1	2	11.2	5
Grocery stores	252.8	3	12.3	4
Nursing facilities	224.5	4	18.2	2
Trucking/courier services	191.0	5	13.3	3
Department stores	153.8	6	10.4	6
Motor vehicles/equipment	147.2	7	18.3	1

Source: "... And So Are Some Other Things: Overall Injuries Seem to Be on the Upswing." *Restaurant Business,* 20 January 1994, p. 21. Primary source: U.S. Department of Labor. Bureau of Labor Statistics.

Occupational Health and Safety: Lost Work Time

★ 383 ★

Lost Workdays Due to Injury and Illness

Table shows the lost workdays per 100 full-time workers in selected industries.

Industry	Lost workdays	
	Injury	Illness
Ship and boat building and repairing	337.4	30.5
Logging	274.8	4.7
Iron and steel foundries	184.5	24.9
Railroad equipment	183.0	16.3
Structural clay products	179.5	17.0
Office furniture	131.1	36.5
Millwork[1]	141.9	11.9

Source: "Office Furniture Workers Miss Most Workdays." *Wood and Wood Products* (January 1994), p. 14. Primary source: U.S. Department of Labor. *Note:* 1. Includes cabinetmakers.

★ 384 ★

Occupational Health and Safety: Lost Work Time

Occupational Injury and Illness Cases and Lost Time: 1972-1991

Figures show the occupational injury and illness incidence rates for private industry during 1972 through 1991. The incidence rates represent the number of injuries and illnesses or lost workdays per 100 full-time workers.

Year[1]	Total cases	Lost workday cases	Nonfatal cases without lost workdays	Lost workdays
1972	10.9	3.3	7.6	47.9
1973	11.0	3.4	7.5	53.3
1974	10.4	3.5	6.9	54.6
1975	9.1	3.3	5.8	56.1
1976	9.2	3.5	5.7	60.5
1977	9.3	3.8	5.5	61.6
1978[2]	9.4	4.1	5.3	63.5
1979[2]	9.5	4.3	5.2	67.7
1980	8.7	4.0	4.7	65.2
1981	8.3	3.8	4.5	61.7
1982	7.7	3.5	4.2	58.7
1983[2]	7.6	3.4	4.2	58.5
1984[2]	8.0	3.7	4.3	63.4
1985	7.9	3.6	4.3	64.9
1986	7.9	3.6	4.3	65.8
1987	8.3	3.8	4.4	69.9
1988	8.6	4.0	4.6	76.1
1989	8.6	4.0	4.6	78.7
1990	8.8	4.1	4.7	84.0
1991	8.4	3.9	4.5	86.5

Source: U.S. Department of Labor. Bureau of Labor Statistics. *Occupational Injuries and Illnesses in the United States by Industry, 1991.* Bulletin 2424. Washington, DC: U.S. Government Printing Office, May 1993, p. 1. *Notes:* Data for 1976-1991 exclude farms with fewer than 11 employees. 1. Data for 1972-1975 are based on the *Standard Industrial Classification Manual* (1967 edition); data for 1976-1987 are based on the *Standard Industrial Classification Manual* (1972 edition); and data for 1988-1991 are based on the *Standard Industrial Classification Manual* (1987 edition). 2. In 1978, 1979, 1983, and 1984, small nonfarm employers in low-risk industries were not surveyed. To maintain comparability with the other data, a statistical method was developed to provide estimates for those employers.

★ 385 ★

Occupational Health and Safety: Lost Work Time

Reasons for Lost Work Time

The table below presents the most frequent reasons given for work time lost due to illness. Data include the average number of sick days taken per year for selected illnesses and conditions.

Reason	Days off per year
Flu	76
Sprains	30
Fractures	23
Colds	21

Source: "Hello Boss...." *Detroit Free Press,* 14 March 1993, p. 3A. Primary source: National Center for Health Statistics.

★ 386 ★

Occupational Health and Safety: Lost Work Time

Sick Days, by City

The table below presents the frequency with which employees call in sick. Data are provided by selected cities.

City	Sick days
Atlanta, Georgia	6
Baltimore, Maryland	8
Boston, Massachusetts	6
Chicago, Illinois	6
Cincinnati, Ohio	6
Dallas, Texas	5
Denver, Colorado	4
Detroit, Michigan	4
Houston, Texas	6
Indianapolis, Indiana	6
Los Angeles-Long Beach, California	6
Miami-Hialeah, Florida	4
Minneapolis-St. Paul, Minnesota	5
Newark, New Jersey	5
New Orleans, Louisiana	7
New York, New York	5
Philadelphia, Pennsylvania	4
Phoenix, Arizona	6
Portland, Oregon	5
Riverside-San Bernardino, California	9
San Diego, California	5
San Francisco-Oakland, California	6
Seattle, Washington	4

[Continued]

★ 386 ★

Sick Days, by City
[Continued]

City	Sick days
St. Louis, Missouri	5
Washington, District of Columbia	5

Source: "Something's in the Air." *Small Business Reports* 19, no. 3 (March 1994), p. 64. Primary source: National Center for Health Statistics.

★ 387 ★

Occupational Health and Safety: Lost Work Time

Sick Days: Mondays and Heart Attacks

Results of a Harvard Medical School study identified Monday from 7:00 a.m. until 10:00 a.m. as the time when employed people are at greatest risk of heart attacks. The study suggests that stress associated with returning to work after the weekend make Monday mornings the peak risk period.

Source: "Monday Tops List for Risk." *Detroit News,* 20 July 1994, p. E1.

Wellness Promotion

★ 388 ★

Employees' Health-Related Perks: 1991-1993

The table below reflects the health-enhancing benefits provided by employers during 1991, 1992, and 1993. Data are from a survey of 600 U.S. businesses.

[In percentages]

Benefit	1991	1992	1993
Gym facilities	14	12	10
Sports teams	28	20	24
Stress management programs	N/A	N/A	16
Wellness programs	N/A	21	20

Source: Peters, Shannon. "Employers Provide More Parties, Fewer Gym Facilities in 1993." *Personnel Journal* (May 1994), p. 13. Primary source: Tempforce Inc.

★ 389 ★

Wellness Promotion

Private Work Sites With Fitness/Exercise Facilities: 1992

Table reflects the work sites with 50 or more employees that offer facilities or programs (information or activities) that promote health, exercise, and physical fitness.

[In percentages]

Wellness promotion facility	Percent of work sites offering
Locker room with showers	24
Indoor exercise area	12
Aerobics equipment	10
Strength training equipment	9
Other	41

Source: "How Employers Are Helping Workers Stay Healthy." *Washington Post,* 18 May 1993, final edition, p. Z5. *Note:* 1. For example, counseling, classes, or videos.

★ 390 ★

Wellness Promotion

Workplace Wellness Issues

Data reflect the percentages of organizations with policies or programs dedicated to wellness issues in the workplace.

Issue and program	All organizations	Number of employees				
		100-499	500-999	1,000-2,499	2,500-9,999	10,000 or more
Drugs						
Test employees for drug use (with probable cause)	38	36	48	46	49	50
Test employees for drug use (without probable cause)	11	10	15	16	16	25
Test job applicants for drug use	37	31	54	55	58	62
Have formal policy on substance abuse	86	84	93	92	90	98
Conduct or sponsor training about substance abuse	33	29	47	44	50	60
Have an Employee Assistance Program (EAP)[1]	52	47	65	72	79	88
AIDS						
AIDS antibody testing of employees	1	1	3	1	1	2
AIDS antibody testing of job applicants	1	1	2	0	2	3
Have formal AIDS policy	20	19	29	24	27	26
Have AIDS education program	21	19	34	25	28	28

[Continued]

★ 390 ★

Workplace Wellness Issues
[Continued]

Issue and program	All organizations	Number of employees				
		100-499	500-999	1,000-2,499	2,500-9,999	10,000 or more
Smoking						
Have policy limiting smoking at work	77	76	80	76	79	87
Have policy banning smoking at work	56	57	53	55	49	51
Do not hire smokers	2	1	2	2	2	2

Source: "Social Issues at Work." *Training* (October 1993), p. 55. *Note:* 1. Handles substance abuse problems.

Workers' Compensation

★ 391 ★

Workers' Compensation Benefit Payments: 1987-1990

Table reflects the estimated workers' compensation benefit payment amounts for 1987 through 1990. Data provided by type of benefit.

[In million dollars]

Benefit	1987	1988	1989	1990
Regular program	25,773	29,234	32,837	36,804
Medical and hospitalization	9,794	11,401	13,299	15,067
Compensation	15,979	17,833	19,538	21,737
Disability	15,046	16,956	18,553	20,635
Survivor	933	877	985	1,102
Black lung program	1,545	1,499	1,479	1,434
Medical and hospitalization	118	117	125	120
Compensation	1,426	1,381	1,354	1,314
Disability	698	657	618	577
Survivor	729	725	736	737
Total[1]	27,318	30,733	34,316	38,238
Medical and hospitalization	9,912	11,518	13,424	15,187
Compensation	17,406	19,215	20,892	23,051
Disability	15,775	17,613	19,171	21,212
Survivor	1,631	1,602	1,721	1,839

Source: U.S. House Committee on Ways and Means. *Overview of Entitlement Programs, 1993 Green Book: Background Material and Data Programs Within the Jurisdiction of the Committee on Ways and Means.* 103d Cong., 1st sess., 7 July 1993. Washington, DC: U.S. Government Printing Office, 1993, p. 1706. Primary sources: *Social Security Bulletin* 55, no. 1 (spring 1992); Social Security Adminstration. *Note:* 1. Regular and black lung programs combined.

★ 392 ★
Workers' Compensation

Workers' Compensation Claims: 1990-1992

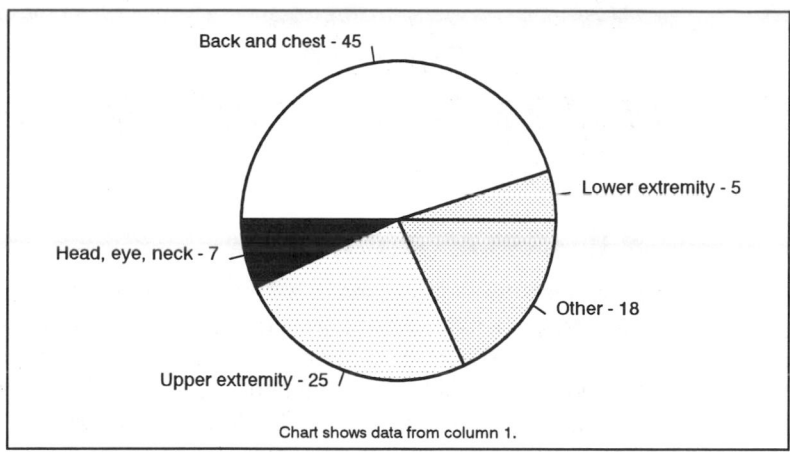

Back and chest - 45

Lower extremity - 5

Head, eye, neck - 7

Other - 18

Upper extremity - 25

Chart shows data from column 1.

Data reflect the cost of workers' compensation claims per body part injured. Data cover April 1990 through May 1992.

Body part	Percent of claims	Cost
Back and chest	45	$211,242
Upper extremity	25	$116,305
Head, eye, neck	7	$33,293
Lower extremity	5	$25,615
Other	18	$86,124

Source: "Workers' Compensation Claims." *Occupational Health and Safety* 62, no. 10 (October 1993), p. 76.

Chapter 6
HEALTH EXPENDITURES AND FUNDING

This chapter presents tables about spending on health and medical care in America. According to the Social Security Administration, "health and medical care expenditures in the United States, including expenditures for medical research and medical facilities construction, were estimated at $751.8 billion for 1991. This amount constituted 13.2 percent of the gross domestic product" (U.S. Department of Health and Human Services. Social Security Administration. "Social Security Programs in the United States, 1993." *Social Security Bulletin* 4, no. 4, 22 December 1993). The private sector was responsible for approximately 56 percent of this spending, while governments accounted for the remaining 44 percent. Tables in this chapter show the sources of health-related spending for consumer and government sectors; for example, an individual's out-of-pocket payments or government financing of programs such as Medicaid. Tables also reflect the use of funds; that is, a family's spending for medical services and supplies or payments to health insurance carriers. The business sector is another major source of health care funding. Tables illustrating spending by businesses are included in Health in the Workplace chapter. Data regarding expenditures for specific social welfare programs—for example, Medicare—also will be found in the chapter on Health Care Programs.

Consumer Spending

★ 393 ★

Aggregate Expenditures for Health Care: 1988-1991

The table below provides a comparison of estimated aggregate expenditures for health care from the Consumer Expenditure (CE) Survey and National Health Accounts (NHA) for 1988 through 1991. From the source: This table "shows a comparison of aggregate out-of-pocket health care expenditures from the Consumer Expenditure Survey and the National Health Accounts. Expenditures by patients in nursing homes, which are not covered in the CE survey, are excluded from the comparison.... As reported in the CE survey, aggregate health care expenditures were $150 billion in 1991, or about 73 percent of the $205 billion estimated from the NHA. Of the CE survey total, $64 billion was spent on health insurance, $34 billion was spent on medical commodities, and $52 billion was spent on medical services. The medical commodities total was 65 percent of the NHA estimate, and the medical services total was 79 percent of the NHA estimate. The ratios for the health insurance estimates are relatively stable from 1988 through 1991. Moderate variations in the ratios for the medical commodities total and the medical services total have occurred over the period" (pp. 12-13).

Expenditure categories	Consumer Expenditure Survey (in billions)				Ratio of CE to NHA			
	1988 ($)	1989 ($)	1990 ($)	1991 ($)	1988	1989	1990	1991
Health care, total	119	132	141	150	0.74	0.75	0.76	0.73
Health insurance premiums[1]	45	51	56	64	.71	.72	.71	.74
Medical care, total[2]	74	81	85	86	.76	.76	.79	.72
Medical commodities, total	28	31	33	34	.66	.69	.66	.65
Drugs and sundries[3]	22	25	26	27	.64	.64	.63	.60
Medical equipment and supplies[3]	5	7	6	7	.80	1.03	.83	.90
Medical services, total	46	50	52	52	.83	.83	.82	.79
Professional services	36	40	45	43	.80	.81	.85	.76
Hospital care	10	10	8	10	.99	.89	.73	.96

Source: U.S. Department of Labor. Bureau of Labor Statistics. *Consumer Expenditure Survey, 1990-1991.* Washington, DC: U.S. Government Printing Office, September 1993, pp. 12. "This bulletin presents detailed information from the Consumer Expenditure Survey for 1990 and 1991. The data shown here are combined, or integrated, from the Diary and Interview components of the survey. Integrated data provide a complete accounting of consumer expenditures and income, which neither component alone is designed to do" (p. iii). Primary source for NHA data: U.S. Department of Health and Human Services. Health Care Financing Administration. "National Health Expenditures, 1991." *Health Care Financing Review* (spring 1993). Estimates have been revised using a rebenchmarking procedure that adjusts the category estimates to proportions from the CE survey. *Notes:* Sums may not equal totals due to rounding. 1. NHA data used to obtain the ratios are derived from NHA out-of-pocket estimates of health insurance data from: Levit, Katherine R., and Cathy A. Cowan. "The Burden of Health Care Costs: Business, Households, and Governments." *Health Care Financing Review* (winter 1990), table 1. 2. Excludes nursing home care and medical equipment repairs. 3. CE categories have been rearranged to match NHA.

★ 394 ★
Consumer Spending

Health Care Expenditures, by Composition of Consumer Unit: 1991

Data below reflect the characteristics of consumers and their average annual health care expenditures for 1991. Data are provided by composition of consumer unit.

["n.a." indicates "not applicable."]

| Item | Total husband and wife consumer units | Husband and wife only | Husband and wife with children |||| Other husband and wife consumer units | One parent, at least one child under 18 | Single person and other consumer units |
			Total husband and wife with children	Oldest child under 6	Oldest child 6 to 17	Oldest child 18 or over			
Number of consumer units (in thousands)	54,017	21,553	28,589	6,267	14,178	8,144	3,875	6,112	37,788
Consumer unit characteristics									
Income before taxes[1] ($)	44,460	40,579	47,303	43,046	47,983	49,638	44,627	20,302	21,255
Income after taxes[1] ($)	40,158	36,098	43,060	39,125	43,446	45,663	40,887	18,884	19,387
Age of reference person	47.3	55.1	41.2	31.5	39.2	52.2	48.7	36.0	49.7
Average number in consumer unit									
Persons	3.2	2.0	3.9	3.5	4.2	3.9	5.0	2.9	1.5
Children under 18	1.0	n.a.	1.6	1.5	2.2	.6	1.6	1.7 [2]	.2
Persons 65 and over	.3	.6	.1	[2]	[2]	.2	.5	[2]	.3
Earners	1.8	1.2	2.0	1.7	1.9	2.6	2.4	1.0	.9
Vehicles	2.6	2.3	2.7	2.2	2.6	3.3	2.8	1.1	1.2
Percent distribution									
Sex of reference person									
Male	88	89	88	91	86	89	86	9	41
Female	12	11	12	9	14	11	14	91	59
Housing tenure									
Homeowner	79	82	77	63	78	86	74	34	46
With mortgage	53	40	63	56	69	58	52	27	20
Without mortgage	26	42	14	7	10	28	22	8	26
Renter	21	18	23	37	22	14	26	66	54
Race of reference person									
Black	7	5	7	6	8	8	16	30	13
White and other	93	95	93	94	92	92	84	70	87
Education of reference person									
Elementary (1-8)	8	11	6	3	4	10	15	5	13
High school (9-12)	44	44	44	41	42	48	47	55	40
College	47 [3]	45 [3]	50 [3]	55 [3]	53 [3]	42 [3]	37	39 [3]	46
Never attended and other							1		1
At least one vehicle owned	96	95	97	96	98	98	93	69	75
Average annual expenditures ($)	37,134	32,937	40,037	36,075	40,839	41,798	39,177	21,653	20,092
Health care	1,963	2,131	1,854	1,614	1,733	2,252	1,825	779	1,095
Health insurance	816	923	740	702	658	913	779	359	475
Medical services	723	696	751	667	739	838	656	273	360
Drugs	315	407	248	184	220	349	291	95	186
Medical supplies	109	104	114	62	116	151	98	52	74

[Continued]

★ 394 ★

Health Care Expenditures, by Composition of Consumer Unit: 1991

[Continued]

Item	Total husband and wife consumer units	Husband and wife only	Husband and wife consumer units				Other husband and wife consumer units	One parent, at least one child under 18	Single person and other consumer units
			Husband and wife with children						
			Total husband and wife with children	Oldest child under 6	Oldest child 6 to 17	Oldest child 18 or over			
Addenda									
Health care	22	25	21	9[4]	15	41	12[4]	3[4]	45

Source: U.S. Department of Labor, Bureau of Labor Statistics. *Consumer Expenditure Survey, 1990-1991.* Washington, DC: U.S. Government Printing Office, September 1993, pp. 30-33. From the source: This table "presents detailed information from the Consumer Expenditure Survey for 1990 and 1991. The data shown here are combined, or integrated, from the Diary and Interview components of the survey. Integrated data provide a complete accounting of consumer expenditures and income, which neither component alone is designed to do" (p. iii). *Notes:* Health insurance expenditures include spending on health maintenance plans (HMOs), Blue Cross/Blue Shield, commercial or other health insurance, Medicare, and Medicare supplemental insurance. Medical services cover hospital rooms and services, physicians' services, services by professionals other than physicians, eye and dental care, lab tests, x-rays, and other medical care, including that provided in retirement communities or convalescent and nursing homes. The drugs category comprises prescription, nonprescription, and over-the-counter (internal and respiratory) medications. Medical supplies include topicals and dressings, antiseptics, bandages, cotton, first aid kits, contraceptives, syringes, ice bags, thermometers, sunlamps, vaporizers, heating pads, medical appliances (such as braces, canes, crutches, walkers, eyeglasses, and hearing aids), and the rental and repair of medical equipment. 1. Components of income and taxes are derived from "complete income reports" only; that is, respondents provided values for major sources of income, such as wages and salaries, self-employment income, and Social Security income. 2. Value less than 0.05. 3. Value less than 0.5. 4. Data are likely to have large sampling errors.

★ 395 ★
Consumer Spending

Health Care Expenditures, by Housing Tenure, Race of Reference Person, and Type of Area: 1991

This table shows consumer characteristics and average annual health care expenditures for 1991. Data are provided by housing tenure, race/ethnicity, and location.

["n.a." indicates "not applicable."]

Item	All consumer units	Housing tenure		Race of reference person		Type of area	
		Homeowner	Renter	White or other	Black	Urban	Rural
Number of consumer units (in thousands)	97,918	61,870	36,048	87,155	10,763	84,497	13,421
Consumer unit characteristics							
Income before taxes[1] ($)	33,901	41,033	22,039	35,311	21,929	34,867	27,540
Income after taxes[1] ($)	30,729	37,009	20,285	31,929	20,544	31,547	25,348
Age of reference person	47.5	51.9	40.1	47.7	46.3	47.1	50.2
Average number in consumer unit							
Persons	2.6	2.7	2.3	2.5	2.8	2.5	2.7
Children under 18	.7	.7	.7	.7	1.0	.7	.7
Persons 65 and over	.3	.4	.2	.3	.2	.3	.4
Earners	1.4	1.5	1.2	1.4	1.3	1.4	1.4
Vehicles	2.0	2.4	1.2	2.1	1.1	1.9	2.5
Percent distribution							
Sex of reference person							
Male	65	72	54	68	46	63	78
Female	35	28	46	32	54	37	22

[Continued]

★ 395 ★

Health Care Expenditures, by Housing Tenure, Race of Reference Person, and Type of Area: 1991
[Continued]

Item	All consumer units	Housing tenure		Race of reference person		Type of area	
		Homeowner	Renter	White or other	Black	Urban	Rural
Housing tenure							
Homeowner	63	100	n.a.	66	41	61	80
With mortgage	39	61	n.a.	40	25	39	38
Without mortgage	25	39	n.a.	26	17	22	41
Renter	37	n.a.	100	34	59	39	20
Race of reference person							
Black	11	7	18	n.a.	100	12	6
White and other	89	93	82	100	n.a.	88	94
Education of reference person							
Elementary (1-8)	10	10	9	9	15	9	16
High school (9-12)	43	43	44	42	53	42	50
College	46	46	46	48	32	48	33
Never attended and other	1	2	1	1	1	2	1
At least one vehicle owned	86	94	73	89	66	85	92
Average annual expenditures ($)	29,614	34,531	21,066	30,794	20,091	30,382	24,785
Health care	1,554	1,927	912	1,640	857	1,525	1,736
Health insurance	656	822	370	688	400	642	746
Medical services	555	679	341	590	272	554	560
Drugs	252	312	147	264	149	239	332
Medical supplies	92	113	54	99	37	91	98
Addenda							
Health care	29	36	19	33	4[3]	28	40

Source: U.S. Department of Labor. Bureau of Labor Statistics. *Consumer Expenditure Survey, 1990-1991.* Washington, DC: U.S. Government Printing Office, September 1993, pp. 38-41. From the source: This table "presents detailed information from the Consumer Expenditure Survey for 1990 and 1991. The data shown here are combined, or integrated, from the Diary and Interview components of the survey. Integrated data provide a complete accounting of consumer expenditures and income, which neither component alone is designed to do" (p. iii). *Notes:* Health insurance expenditures include spending on health maintenance plans (HMOs), Blue Cross/Blue Shield, commercial or other health insurance, Medicare, and Medicare supplemental insurance. Medical services cover hospital rooms and services, physicians' services, services by professionals other than physicians, eye and dental care, lab tests, x-rays, and other medical care, including that provided in retirement communities or convalescent and nursing homes. The drugs category comprises prescription, nonprescription, and over-the-counter (internal and respiratory) medications. Medical supplies include topicals and dressings, antiseptics, bandages, cotton, first aid kits, contraceptives, syringes, ice bags, thermometers, sunlamps, vaporizers, heating pads, medical appliances (such as braces, canes, crutches, walkers, eyeglasses, and hearing aids), and the rental and repair of medical equipment. 1. Components of income and taxes are derived from "complete income reports" only; that is, respondents provided values for major sources of income, such as wages and salaries, self-employment income, and Social Security income. 2. Value less than 0.5. 3. Data are likely to have large sampling errors.

★ 396 ★
Consumer Spending

Health Care Expenditures, by Number of Earners in Consumer Unit: 1991

Data below reflect consumer characteristics and average annual health care expenditures for 1991. Data are provided by number of earners in consumer units.

["n.a." indicates "not applicable."]

Item	All consumer units	Single consumers		Consumer units of two or more persons			
		No earner	One earner	No earner	One earner	Two earners	Three or more earners
Number of consumer units (in thousands)	97,918	10,364	16,802	8,928	19,146	32,766	9,912
Consumer unit characteristics							
Income before taxes[1] ($)	33,901	10,327	22,746	18,556	31,661	46,013	56,122
Income after taxes[1] ($)	30,729	9,947	20,183	17,157	29,053	41,376	51,135
Age of reference person	47.5	70.1	38.2	62.7	47.7	41.2	46.6
Average number in consumer unit							
Persons	2.6	1.0	1.0	2.5	3.0	3.1	4.4
Children under 18	.7	n.a.	n.a.	.5	1.1	.9	1.2
Persons 65 and over	.3	.8	.1	1.2	.3	.1	.1
Earners	1.4	n.a.	1.0	n.a.	1.0	2.0	3.3
Vehicles	2.0	.7	1.2	1.5	2.0	2.4	3.4
Percent distribution							
Sex of reference person							
Male	65	27	55	66	65	79	80
Female	35	73	45	34	35	21	20
Housing tenure							
Homeowner	63	57	33	71	67	71	81
With mortgage	39	7	21	14	40	56	64
Without mortgage	25	50	12	57	27	16	16
Renter	37	43	67	29	33	29	19
Race of reference person							
Black	11	11	10	15	14	8	11
White and other	89	89	90	85	86	92	89
Education of reference person							
Elementary (1-8)	10	27	4	20	11	5	7
High school (9-12)	43	45	32	56	48	42	44
College	46	26	64	23	41	53	48
Never attended and other	1	2	2	1	1	2	1
At least one vehicle owned	86	57	80	77	89	96	97
Average annual expenditures ($)	29,614	12,744	20,499	19,529	29,407	37,581	45,513
Health care	1,554	1,457	741	2,096	1,668	1,670	1,945
Health insurance	656	706	297	1,033	721	663	724
Medical services	555	416	280	483	561	679	806
Drugs	252	286	108	460	281	233	274
Medical supplies	92	50	56	120	104	95	141

[Continued]

★ 396 ★

Health Care Expenditures, by Number of Earners in Consumer Unit: 1991
[Continued]

Item	All consumer units	Single consumers		Consumer units of two or more persons			
		No earner	One earner	No earner	One earner	Two earners	Three or more earners
Addenda Health care	29	119	17	7[3]	19	18	37

Source: U.S. Department of Labor. Bureau of Labor Statistics. *Consumer Expenditure Survey, 1990-1991.* Washington, DC: U.S. Government Printing Office, September 1993, pp. 34-37. From the source: This table "presents detailed information from the Consumer Expenditure Survey for 1990 and 1991. The data shown here are combined, or integrated, from the Diary and Interview components of the survey. Integrated data provide a complete accounting of consumer expenditures and income, which neither component alone is designed to do" (p. iii). *Notes:* Health insurance expenditures include spending on health maintenance plans (HMOs), Blue Cross/Blue Shield, commercial or other health insurance, Medicare, and Medicare supplemental insurance. Medical services cover hospital rooms and services, physicians' services, services by professionals other than physicians, eye and dental care, lab tests, x-rays, and other medical care, including that provided in retirement communities or convalescent and nursing homes. The drugs category comprises prescription, nonprescription, and over-the-counter (internal and respiratory) medications. Medical supplies include topicals and dressings, antiseptics, bandages, cotton, first aid kits, contraceptives, syringes, ice bags, thermometers, sunlamps, vaporizers, heating pads, medical appliances (such as braces, canes, crutches, walkers, eyeglasses, and hearing aids), and the rental and repair of medical equipment. 1. Components of income and taxes are derived from "complete income reports" only; that is, respondents provided values for major sources of income, such as wages and salaries, self-employment income, and Social Security income. 2. Value less than 0.5. 3. Data are likely to have large sampling errors.

★ 397 ★

Consumer Spending

Health Care Expenditures, by Occupation of Reference Person: 1991

Figures represent consumers by specific characteristics and their average annual health care expenditures for 1991. Data are provided by occupations of reference persons.

Item	Self-employed units	Wage and salary earners						Retired workers	All others, including those not reporting
		Total wage and salary earners	Managers and professionals	Technical, sales, and clerical workers	Service workers	Construction workers and mechanics	Operators, fabricators, and laborers		
Number of consumer units (in thousands)	7,056	64,439	21,430	17,045	6,935	6,246	12,782	16,776	9,647
Consumer unit characteristics									
Income before taxes[1] ($)	42,939	39,430	53,812	36,388	22,908	35,872	30,249	18,614	17,412
Income after taxes[1] ($)	39,342	35,548	47,788	32,925	21,317	32,675	27,796	17,235	16,217
Age of reference person	47.7	40.6	41.8	39.6	41.9	39.6	39.7	73.1	49.1
Average number in consumer unit									
Persons	2.8	2.7	2.7	2.5	2.7	3.0	3.0	1.8	2.7
Children under 18	.8	.8	.8	.7	.8	.9	.9	.1	.9
Persons 65 and over	.2	.1	.1	.1	.2	[2]	.1	1.2	.3
Earners	1.9	1.7	1.7	1.7	1.6	1.8	1.8	.3	.5
Vehicles	2.5	2.1	2.2	2.0	1.7	2.5	2.3	1.5	1.3
Percent distribution									
Sex of reference person									
Male	82	71	72	55	55	94	87	55	35
Female	18	29	28	45	45	6	13	45	65
Housing tenure									
Homeowner	78	60	68	55	44	64	61	77	47
With mortgage	49	46	57	42	30	50	43	14	21
Without mortgage	29	14	11	14	14	14	19	63	26
Renter	22	40	32	45	56	36	39	23	53
Race of reference person									
Black	6	10	6	11	21	7	12	9	24

[Continued]

★ 397 ★

Health Care Expenditures, by Occupation of Reference Person: 1991

[Continued]

| Item | Self-employed units | Wage and salary earners | | | | | | Retired workers | All others, including those not reporting |
		Total wage and salary earners	Managers and professionals	Technical, sales, and clerical workers	Service workers	Construction workers and mechanics	Operators, fabricators, and laborers		
White and other	94	90	94	89	79	93	88	91	76
Education of reference person									
Elementary (1-8)	10	5	1	3	10	6	11	25	18
High school (9-12)	41	40	17	39	53	62	64	48	54
College	49	55	82	58	37	32	24	25	25
Never attended and other	3	3	2	3	3	3	1	1	2
At least one vehicle owned	95	91	94	89	79	96	91	77	65
Average annual expenditures ($)	36,072	33,154	42,802	31,383	23,205	29,925	26,455	19,284	18,861
Health care	2,121	1,394	1,659	1,321	1,267	1,285	1,175	2,096	1,260
Health insurance	985	536	647	525	466	469	436	1,092	458
Medical services	761	562	652	527	551	549	470	484	479
Drugs	289	201	229	187	183	185	190	417	274
Medical supplies	87	90	101	81	67	82	80	102	49
Addenda									
Health care	30	20	38	13	8[4]	11[4]	8	45	67

Source: U.S. Department of Labor. Bureau of Labor Statistics. *Consumer Expenditure Survey, 1990-1991.* Washington, DC: U.S. Government Printing Office, September 1993, pp. 46-49. From the source: This table "presents detailed information from the Consumer Expenditure Survey for 1990 and 1991. The data shown here are combined, or integrated, from the Diary and Interview components of the survey. Integrated data provide a complete accounting of consumer expenditures and income, which neither component alone is designed to do" (p. iii). *Notes:* Health insurance expenditures include spending on health maintenance plans (HMOs), Blue Cross/Blue Shield, commercial or other health insurance, Medicare, and Medicare supplemental insurance. Medical services cover hospital rooms and services, physicians' services, services by professionals other than physicians, eye and dental care, lab tests, x-rays, and other medical care, including that provided in retirement communities or convalescent and nursing homes. The drugs category comprises prescription, nonprescription, and over-the-counter (internal and respiratory) medications. Medical supplies include topicals and dressings, antiseptics, bandages, cotton, first aid kits, contraceptives, syringes, ice bags, thermometers, sunlamps, vaporizers, heating pads, medical appliances (such as braces, canes, crutches, walkers, eyeglasses, and hearing aids), and the rental and repair of medical equipment. 1. Components of income and taxes are derived from "complete income reports" only; that is, respondents provided values for major sources of income, such as wages and salaries, self-employment income, and Social Security income. 2. Value less than 0.05. 3. Value less than 0.5. 4. Data are likely to have large sampling errors.

★ 398 ★

Consumer Spending

Health Care Expenditures, by Region of Residence: 1991

Data reflect consumer characteristics and average annual health care expenditures for 1991. Data are provided by region.

| Item | All consumer units | Regions | | | |
		Northeast	Midwest	South	West
Number of consumer units (in thousands)	97,918	20,400	24,813	32,741	19,964
Consumer unit characteristics					
Income before taxes[1] ($)	33,901	36,953	31,535	31,706	37,167
Income after taxes[1] ($)	30,729	33,186	29,124	28,889	33,123
Age of reference person	47.5	48.7	47.1	47.6	46.7

[Continued]

★ 398 ★

Health Care Expenditures, by Region of Residence: 1991
[Continued]

Item	All consumer units	Regions			
		Northeast	Midwest	South	West
Average number in consumer unit					
Persons	2.6	2.5	2.5	2.5	2.7
Children under 18	.7	.6	.7	.7	.8
Persons 65 and over	.3	.3	.3	.3	.3
Earners	1.4	1.3	1.4	1.4	1.4
Vehicles	2.0	1.6	2.1	1.9	2.2
Percent distribution					
Sex of reference person					
Male	65	63	67	65	66
Female	35	37	33	35	34
Housing tenure					
Homeowner	63	61	65	64	61
With mortgage	39	36	37	38	44
Without mortgage	25	26	28	27	17
Renter	37	39	35	36	39
Race of reference person					
Black	11	10	10	16	5
White and other	89	90	90	84	95
Education of reference person					
Elementary (1-8)	10	9	9	13	8
High school (9-12)	43	47	46	42	37
College	46	44	44	44	55
Never attended and other	1	1	2	1	2
At least one vehicle owned	86	79	88	88	90
Average annual expenditures ($)	29,614	31,026	27,675	28,062	33,131
Health care	1,554	1,504	1,482	1,669	1,506
Health insurance	656	669	631	697	607
Medical services	555	528	521	581	580
Drugs	252	223	243	295	221
Medical supplies	92	84	87	96	98

[Continued]

★ 398 ★

Health Care Expenditures, by Region of Residence: 1991
[Continued]

Item	All consumer units	Regions			
		Northeast	Midwest	South	West
Addenda Health care	29	16	50	29	17

Source: U.S. Department of Labor. Bureau of Labor Statistics. *Consumer Expenditure Survey, 1990-1991*. Washington, DC: U.S. Government Printing Office, September 1993, pp. 42-45. From the source: This table "presents detailed information from the Consumer Expenditure Survey for 1990 and 1991. The data shown here are combined, or integrated, from the Diary and Interview components of the survey. Integrated data provide a complete accounting of consumer expenditures and income, which neither component alone is designed to do" (p. iii). *Notes:* Data are presented in four major regions. The Northeast region includes Connecticut, Maine, Massachusetts, New Hampshire, New Jersey, New York, Pennsylvania, Rhode Island, and Vermont. The Midwest region is comprised of Illinois, Indiana, Iowa, Kansas, Michigan, Minnesota, Missouri, Nebraska, North Dakota, Ohio, South Dakota, and Wisconsin. The South includes Alabama, Arkansas, Delaware, District of Columbia, Florida, Georgia, Kentucky, Louisiana, Maryland, Mississippi, North Carolina, Oklahoma, South Carolina, Tennessee, Texas, Virginia, and West Virginia. The West covers Alaska, Arizona, California, Colorado, Hawaii, Idaho, Montana, Nevada, New Mexico, Oregon, Utah, Washington, and Wyoming. Health insurance expenditures include spending on health maintenance plans (HMOs), Blue Cross/Blue Shield, commercial or other health insurance, Medicare, and Medicare supplemental insurance. Medical services cover hospital rooms and services, physicians' services, services by professionals other than physicians, eye and dental care, lab tests, x-rays, and other medical care, including that provided in retirement communities or convalescent and nursing homes. The drugs category comprises prescription, nonprescription, and over-the-counter (internal and respiratory) medications. Medical supplies include topicals and dressings, antiseptics, bandages, cotton, first aid kits, contraceptives, syringes, ice bags, thermometers, sunlamps, vaporizers, heating pads, medical appliances (such as braces, canes, crutches, walkers, eyeglasses, and hearing aids), and the rental and repair of medical equipment. 1. Components of income and taxes are derived from "complete income reporters" only; that is, respondents provided values for major sources of income, such as wages and salaries, self-employment income, and Social Security income. 2. Value less than 0.5.

★ 399 ★

Consumer Spending

Health Care Expenditures, by Size of Consumer Unit: 1991

Data below reflect consumer characteristics and average annual health care expenditures for 1991. Data are provided by size of consumer unit.

["n.a." indicates "not applicable."]

Item	All consumer units	One person	Two or more persons	Two persons	Three persons	Four persons	Five or more persons
Number of consumer units (in thousands)	97,918	27,166	70,752	30,219	16,233	14,036	10,264
Consumer unit characteristics							
Income before taxes[1] ($)	33,901	18,057	40,119	36,955	40,124	46,196	40,985
Income after taxes[1] ($)	30,729	16,318	36,385	33,106	36,696	41,745	38,077
Age of reference person	47.5	50.4	46.4	52.4	44.1	40.1	41.2
Average number in consumer unit							
Persons	2.6	1.0	3.2	2.0	3.0	4.0	5.7
Children under 18	.7	n.a.	1.0	.1	.7	1.7	2.9
Persons 65 and over	.3	.3	.3	.5	.2	.1	.1
Earners	1.4	.6	1.7	1.2	1.8	2.0	2.2
Vehicles	2.0	1.0	2.3	2.1	2.3	2.6	2.7

[Continued]

★ 399 ★

Health Care Expenditures, by Size of Consumer Unit: 1991
[Continued]

Item	All consumer units	One person	Two or more persons	Two persons	Three persons	Four persons	Five or more persons
Percent distribution							
Sex of reference person							
Male	65	45	73	73	70	78	75
Female	35	55	27	27	30	22	25
Housing tenure							
Homeowner	63	42	71	72	69	75	67
With mortgage	39	16	47	37	49	63	54
Without mortgage	25	26	24	35	20	12	14
Renter	37	58	29	28	31	25	33
Race of reference person							
Black	11	11	11	8	13	11	17
White and other	89	89	89	92	87	89	83
Education of reference person							
Elementary (1-8)	10	13	9	10	9	5	11
High school (9-12)	43	37	46	45	47	44	49
College	46	49	45	45	44	51	39
Never attended and other	1	1	2	1	2	2	1
At least one vehicle owned	86	71	92	92	92	94	91
Average annual expenditures ($)	29,614	17,569	34,234	30,648	34,389	38,806	38,269
Health care	1,554	1,014	1,761	1,862	1,759	1,705	1,546
Health insurance	656	453	734	801	763	666	583
Medical services	555	332	640	595	657	712	648
Drugs	252	176	281	349	245	226	210
Medical supplies	92	54	106	117	94	101	104
Addenda							
Health care	29	56	19	22	24	15	9

Source: U.S. Department of Labor. Bureau of Labor Statistics. *Consumer Expenditure Survey, 1990-1991.* Washington, DC: U.S. Government Printing Office, September 1993, pp. 26-29. From the source: This table "presents detailed information from the Consumer Expenditure Survey for 1990 and 1991. The data shown here are combined, or integrated, from the Diary and Interview components of the survey. Integrated data provide a complete accounting of consumer expenditures and income, which neither component alone is designed to do" (p. iii). *Notes:* Health insurance expenditures include spending on health maintenance plans (HMOs), Blue Cross/Blue Shield, commercial or other health insurance, Medicare, and Medicare supplemental insurance. Medical services cover hospital rooms and services, physicians' services, services by professionals other than physicians, eye and dental care, lab tests, x-rays, and other medical care, including that provided in retirement communities or convalescent and nursing homes. The drugs category comprises prescription, nonprescription, and over-the-counter (internal and respiratory) medications. Medical supplies include topicals and dressings, antiseptics, bandages, cotton, first aid kits, contraceptives, syringes, ice bags, thermometers, sunlamps, vaporizers, heating pads, medical appliances (such as braces, canes, crutches, walkers, eyeglasses, and hearing aids), and the rental and repair of medical equipment. 1. Components of income and taxes are derived from "complete income reporters" only; that is, respondents provided values for major sources of income, such as wages and salaries, self-employment income, and Social Security income. 2. Value less than 0.5.

★ 400 ★
Consumer Spending

Health Care Expenditures for Consumer Units, by Age of Reference Person: 1984 and 1991

From the source: This table "shows total expenditures, health care expenditures, and shares of health care expenditures by age of the reference person in 1984 and 1991.... From 1984 to 1991, out-of-pocket health care expenditures increased 48 percent for all consumer units. Much of this increase stems from a sharp rise in health insurance expenditures. Health insurance expenditures increased 77 percent for all consumer units.... During the same period, medical service expenditures by all consumer units increased 22 percent but fell as a share of the total health budget from 43 percent in 1984 to 36 percent in 1991.... Health care expenditures make up a larger portion of the total budget of older consumer units (those age 65 and older) than of younger consumer units. These expenses account for almost 12 percent of total expenditures of those consumer units headed by someone age 65 or older and 2 percent of total expenditures of those consumer units headed by someone under age 25. Older households have less income, lower total expenditures, and more costly health care needs on average than the younger groups. Within the health care budget, the older groups allocate a larger portion to health insurance and prescription drugs and a smaller portion to medical services than do the younger groups. Older households spent close to 50 percent of their total health care dollars on health insurance, whereas the youngest households (those under 25 years old) spent 40 percent. This difference is partially explained by differences in the percent reporting—93 percent of older consumer units reported health insurance expenditures and 19 percent of the youngest consumer units reported health insurance expenditures. Much of this gap is accounted for by Medicare expenditures: 86 percent of older consumer units and none of the youngest consumer units reported Medicare expenditures" (pp. 8-9). Data from 1984 were used for comparison since that year was the first for which integrated data from the current Consumer Expenditure (CE) Survey were available. See Source note below.

[In dollars, unless otherwise noted]

	All consumer units	Age							
		Under 25	25-34	35-44	45-54	55-64	65 and over	65-74	75 and over
Total expenditures									
1984	21,975	13,461	22,294	28,214	28,696	23,401	13,941	15,842	11,122
1991	29,614	16,745	29,280	36,446	38,137	31,945	19,692	22,564	15,782
Health care, total									
1984	1,049	371	746	976	1,245	1,255	1,493	1,485	1,504
1991	1,554	361	1,030	1,488	1,727	1,846	2,257	2,300	2,197
Share of total expenditures (percent)									
1984	4.8	2.8	3.3	3.5	4.3	5.4	10.7	9.4	13.5
1991	5.2	2.2	3.5	4.1	4.5	5.8	11.5	10.2	13.9
Shares of health care budget (percent)									
Health care	100.0	100.0	100.0	100.0	100.0	100.0	100.0	100.0	100.0
Health insurance									
1984	35.3	29.1	33.2	31.0	31.6	36.1	41.6	44.0	37.9
1991	42.2	39.9	40.5	39.2	36.7	40.6	49.2	47.0	52.4
Medical services									
1984	43.3	50.1	48.4	50.5	49.0	42.2	32.8	31.1	35.2
1991	35.7	36.3	40.5	42.3	40.9	36.3	25.7	29.2	20.7
Drugs									
1984	15.9	15.1	13.1	13.7	14.5	17.6	18.6	18.5	19.0
1991	16.2	15.5	13.3	12.2	15.3	18.4	19.7	18.3	21.7

[Continued]

★ 400 ★

Health Care Expenditures for Consumer Units, by Age of Reference Person: 1984 and 1991

[Continued]

	All consumer units	Age							
		Under 25	25-34	35-44	45-54	55-64	65 and over	65-74	75 and over
Medical supplies									
1984	5.5	5.9	5.1	4.8	4.9	4.5	7.0	6.4	7.9
1991	5.9	8.3	5.7	6.3	7.1	4.5	5.4	5.6	5.2

Source: U.S. Department of Labor. Bureau of Labor Statistics. *Consumer Expenditure Survey, 1990-1991*. Washington, DC: U.S. Government Printing Office, September 1993, p. 9. "This bulletin presents detailed information from the Consumer Expenditure Survey for 1990 and 1991. The data shown here are combined, or integrated, from the Diary and Interview components of the survey. Integrated data provide a complete accounting of consumer expenditures and income, which neither component alone is designed to do" (p. iii). *Notes:* Health insurance expenditures include spending on health maintenance plans (HMOs), Blue Cross/Blue Shield, commercial or other health insurance, Medicare, and Medicare supplemental insurance. Medical services cover hospital rooms and services, physicians' services, services by professionals other than physicians, eye and dental care, lab tests, x-rays, and other medical care, including that provided in retirement communities or convalescent and nursing homes. The drugs category comprises prescription, nonprescription, and over-the-counter (internal and respiratory) medications. Medical supplies include topicals and dressings, antiseptics, bandages, cotton, first aid kits, contraceptives, syringes, ice bags, thermometers, sunlamps, vaporizers, heating pads, medical appliances (such as braces, canes, crutches, walkers, eyeglasses, and hearing aids), and the rental and repair of medical equipment.

★ 401 ★

Consumer Spending

Health Care Expenditures for Consumer Units With Reference Persons Aged Under 25: 1990-1991

Figures below show average annual health care expendituires and characterisics of consumer units represented by persons under 25 years old. Data are provided by income before taxes.

Item	Complete reporting of income							
	Total complete reporting	Less than $5,000	$5,000 to $9,999	$10,000 to $14,999	$15,000 to $19,999	$20,000 to $29,999	$30,000 to $39,000	$40,000 and over
Number of consumer units (in thousands)	6,655	1,776	1,491	920	769	874	511	313
Consumer unit characteristics								
Income before taxes[1] ($)	14,202	2,585	7,368	12,276	16,951	24,467	34,040	50,535
Income after taxes[1] ($)	13,381	2,572	7,246	11,721	15,972	22,732	31,627	46,550
Age of reference person	21.5	20.2	21.3	21.9	22.0	22.6	22.4	22.7
Average number in consumer unit								
Persons	1.8	1.2	1.8	1.9	2.0	2.3	2.6	2.6
Children under 18	.4	.1	.6	.5	.5	.5	.5	.3
Persons 65 and over	[2]	[2]	[2]	[2]	[2]	[3]	[3]	[2]
Earners	1.3	1.0	.9	1.2	1.4	1.6	2.0	2.2
Vehicles	1.2	.6	.8	1.3	1.4	1.7	2.2	2.5
Percent distribution								
Sex of reference person								
Male	54	44	46	59	59	65	71	71
Female	46	56	54	41	41	35	29	29

[Continued]

★ 401 ★

Health Care Expenditures for Consumer Units With Reference Persons Aged Under 25: 1990-1991

[Continued]

Item	Complete reporting of income							
	Total complete reporting	Less than $5,000	$5,000 to $9,999	$10,000 to $14,999	$15,000 to $19,999	$20,000 to $29,999	$30,000 to $39,000	$40,000 and over
Housing tenure								
Homeowner	9	2	3	6	14	11	29	31
With mortgage	7	4	1	5	8	11	25	29
Without mortgage	2	1	2	1	5	4	4	2
Renter	91	98	97	94	86	89	71	69
Race of reference person								
Black	10	8	16	9	11	11	3	7
White and other	90	92	84	91	89	89	97	93
Education of reference person								
Elementary (1-8)	2	1	3	3	2	3	1	2
High school (9-12)	41	29	41	44	47	51	55	43
College	56	70	56	53	51	46	45	55
Never attended and other	4	4	4	3	3	3	3	3
At least one vehicle owned	73	54	62	81	88	89	95	95
Average annual expenditures ($)	16,915	9,007	12,647	16,296	18,539	23,360	28,755	36,819
Health care	405	192	202	316	699	675	761	723
Health insurance	129	31	55	86	193	280	318	286
Medical services	175	107	77	126	364	262	297	254
Drugs	64	24	52	70	86	87	99	108
Medical supplies	37	30	18[5]	33	57	46	47[5]	75[5]
Addenda								
Health care	4[5]	1[5]	7[5]	1[5]	5[5]	8[5]	3	1[5]

Source: U.S. Department of Labor. Bureau of Labor Statistics. *Consumer Expenditure Survey, 1990-1991.* Washington, DC: U.S. Government Printing Office, September 1993, pp. 102-105. From the source: This table "presents detailed information from the Consumer Expenditure Survey for 1990 and 1991. The data shown here are combined, or integrated, from the Diary and Interview components of the survey. Integrated data provide a complete accounting of consumer expenditures and income, which neither component alone is designed to do" (p. iii). *Notes:* Health insurance expenditures include spending on health maintenance plans (HMOs), Blue Cross/Blue Shield, commercial or other health insurance, Medicare, and Medicare supplemental insurance. Medical services cover hospital rooms and services, physicians' services, services by professionals other than physicians, eye and dental care, lab tests, x-rays, and other medical care, including that provided in retirement communities or convalescent and nursing homes. The drugs category comprises prescription, nonprescription, and over-the-counter (internal and respiratory) medications. Medical supplies include topicals and dressings, antiseptics, bandages, cotton, first aid kits, contraceptives, syringes, ice bags, thermometers, sunlamps, vaporizers, heating pads, medical appliances (such as braces, canes, crutches, walkers, eyeglasses, and hearing aids), and the rental and repair of medical equipment. 1. Components of income and taxes are derived from "complete income reporters" only; that is, respondents provided values for major sources of income, such as wages and salaries, self-employment income, and Social Security income. 2. Value less than 0.05. 3. No data reported. 4. Value less than 0.5. 5. Data are likely to have large sampling errors.

★ 402 ★

Consumer Spending

Health Care Expenditures for Consumer Units With Reference Persons Ages 25 to 34: 1990-1991

Figures below show average annual health care expenditures and characteristics of consumer units represented by persons between the ages of 25 and 34 years old. Data are provided by income before taxes.

Item	Total complete reporting	Complete reporting of income						
		Less than $5,000	$5,000 to $9,999	$10,000 to $14,999	$15,000 to $19,999	$20,000 to $29,999	$30,000 to $39,000	$40,000 and over
Number of consumer units (in thousands)	18,268	617	1,483	1,747	1,643	3,968	3,282	5,526
Consumer unit characteristics								
Income before taxes[1] ($)	33,160	2,887	7,668	12,489	17,270	24,906	34,240	59,928
Income after taxes[1] ($)	30,101	2,971	7,598	11,976	16,250	23,081	31,135	53,446
Age of reference person	29.8	29.6	29.1	29.4	29.4	29.5	29.9	30.2
Average number in consumer unit								
Persons	2.8	2.5	2.8	2.7	2.5	2.7	2.8	2.9
Children under 18	1.1	1.1	1.4	1.3	1.0	1.0	1.0	1.0
Persons 65 and over	[2]	[3]	[2]	[2]	[2]	[2]	[2]	[2]
Earners	1.5	1.0	.9	1.1	1.3	1.5	1.7	1.9
Vehicles	1.9	1.0	.9	1.4	1.5	1.8	2.2	2.3
Percent distribution								
Sex of reference person								
Male	69	49	37	50	61	70	78	81
Female	31	51	63	50	39	30	22	19
Housing tenure								
Homeowner	45	21	12	19	26	39	54	71
With mortgage	41	12	7	13	21	35	49	67
Without mortgage	5	8	6	6	6	4	5	4
Renter	55	79	88	81	74	61	46	29
Race of reference person								
Black	11	23	33	17	13	10	9	4
White and other	89	77	67	83	87	90	91	96
Education of reference person								
Elementary (1-8)	3	2	10	5	5	2	1	1
High school (9-12)	41	55	53	56	49	46	38	29
College	55	41	36	39	47	52	60	70
Never attended and other	[4]	1	1	[4]	[3]	[3]	[3]	[3]
At least one vehicle owned	90	63	63	84	90	94	96	97
Average annual expenditures ($)	29,681	14,782	13,617	16,646	20,153	24,595	31,430	45,152
Health care	1,029	446	301	558	790	965	1,149	1,481
Health insurance	411	178	93	205	310	417	495	563
Medical services	410	146	114	210	278	358	454	635
Drugs	141	88	74	99	142	137	134	186
Medical supplies	66	34[5]	19	44	61	54	67	98

[Continued]

★ 402 ★

Health Care Expenditures for Consumer Units With Reference Persons Ages 25 to 34: 1990-1991

[Continued]

Item	Complete reporting of income							
	Total complete reporting	Less than $5,000	$5,000 to $9,999	$10,000 to $14,999	$15,000 to $19,999	$20,000 to $29,999	$30,000 to $39,000	$40,000 and over
Addenda								
Health care	8	7[5]	4[5]	7[5]	7[5]	4[5]	11[5]	10

Source: U.S. Department of Labor. Bureau of Labor Statistics. *Consumer Expenditure Survey, 1990-1991.* Washington, DC: U.S. Government Printing Office, September 1993, pp. 106-109. From the source: This table "presents detailed information from the Consumer Expenditure Survey for 1990 and 1991. The data shown here are combined, or integrated, from the Diary and Interview components of the survey. Integrated data provide a complete accounting of consumer expenditures and income, which neither component alone is designed to do" (p. iii). *Notes:* Health insurance expenditures include spending on health maintenance plans (HMOs), Blue Cross/Blue Shield, commercial or other health insurance, Medicare, and Medicare supplemental insurance. Medical services cover hospital rooms and services, physicians' services, services by professionals other than physicians, eye and dental care, lab tests, x-rays, and other medical care, including that provided in retirement communities or convalescent and nursing homes. The drugs category comprises prescription, nonprescription, and over-the-counter (internal and respiratory) medications. Medical supplies include topicals and dressings, antiseptics, bandages, cotton, first aid kits, contraceptives, syringes, ice bags, thermometers, sunlamps, vaporizers, heating pads, medical appliances (such as braces, canes, crutches, walkers, eyeglasses, and hearing aids), and the rental and repair of medical equipment. 1. Components of income and taxes are derived from "complete income reporters" only; that is, respondents provided values for major sources of income, such as wages and salaries, self-employment income, and Social Security income. 2. Value less than 0.05. 3. No data reported. 4. Value less than 0.5. 5. Data are likely to have large sampling errors.

★ 403 ★

Consumer Spending

Health Care Expenditures for Consumer Units With Reference Persons Ages 35 to 44: 1990-1991

Figures below show average annual health care expenditures and characteristics of consumer units represented by persons between 35 and 44 years old. Data are provided by income before taxes.

Item	Complete reporting of income							
	Total complete reporting	Less than $5,000	$5,000 to $9,999	$10,000 to $14,999	$15,000 to $19,999	$20,000 to $29,999	$30,000 to $39,000	$40,000 and over
Number of consumer units (in thousands)	18,299	714	1,081	1,332	1,450	2,936	2,935	7,853
Consumer unit characteristics								
Income before taxes[1] ($)	41,547	1,897	7,834	12,340	17,468	24,851	34,544	68,049
Income after taxes[1] ($)	37,169	1,876	7,700	12,044	16,590	22,661	31,322	60,103
Age of reference person	39.4	38.9	39.2	39.2	39.1	39.4	39.2	39.7
Average number in consumer unit								
Persons	3.3	2.6	3.0	3.1	3.1	3.1	3.2	3.5
Children under 18	1.3	1.1	1.4	1.3	1.3	1.3	1.3	1.4
Persons 65 and over	2	3	2	2	2	2	2	2
Earners	1.8	1.1	1.2	1.3	1.6	1.7	1.8	2.0
Vehicles	2.3	1.3	1.3	1.4	1.7	2.0	2.5	2.8
Percent distribution								
Sex of reference person								
Male	70	46	43	43	58	66	75	83
Female	30	54	57	57	42	34	25	17

[Continued]

★ 403 ★

Health Care Expenditures for Consumer Units With Reference Persons Ages 35 to 44: 1990-1991

[Continued]

Item	Complete reporting of income							
	Total complete reporting	Less than $5,000	$5,000 to $9,999	$10,000 to $14,999	$15,000 to $19,999	$20,000 to $29,999	$30,000 to $39,000	$40,000 and over
Housing tenure								
Homeowner	66	35	39	38	47	53	68	85
With mortgage	57	22	27	26	36	43	57	79
Without mortgage	9	13	12	11	11	9	11	6
Renter	34	65	61	62	53	47	32	15
Race of reference person								
Black	12	27	21	29	13	14	11	5
White and other	88	73	79	71	87	86	89	95
Education of reference person								
Elementary (1-8)	4	12	10	9	10	4	2	2
High school (9-12)	37	44	51	58	51	46	40	25
College	58	43	37	33	39	50	58	73
Never attended and other	4	4	2	4	4	3	4	4
At least one vehicle owned	92	71	70	78	90	91	96	98
Average annual expenditures ($)	37,053	17,858	15,817	18,350	23,950	26,486	33,632	52,167
Health care	1,472	813	624	1,037	1,120	1,262	1,459	1,870
Health insurance	537	290	237	271	326	531	613	658
Medical services	644	385	227	536	366	504	577	871
Drugs	188	110	110	162	188	149	184	225
Medical supplies	104	28[5]	50	68	240	79	85	116
Addenda								
Health care	35	7[5]	6[5]	180[5]	4[5]	17	25	33

Source: U.S. Department of Labor. Bureau of Labor Statistics. *Consumer Expenditure Survey, 1990-1991.* Washington, DC: U.S. Government Printing Office, September 1993, pp. 110-113. From the source: This table "presents detailed information from the Consumer Expenditure Survey for 1990 and 1991. The data shown here are combined, or integrated, from the Diary and Interview components of the survey. Integrated data provide a complete accounting of consumer expenditures and income, which neither component alone is designed to do" (p. iii). *Notes:* Health insurance expenditures include spending on health maintenance plans (HMOs), Blue Cross/Blue Shield, commercial or other health insurance, Medicare, and Medicare supplemental insurance. Medical services cover hospital rooms and services, physicians' services, services by professionals other than physicians, eye and dental care, lab tests, x-rays, and other medical care, including that provided in retirement communities or convalescent and nursing homes. The drugs category comprises prescription, nonprescription, and over-the-counter (internal and respiratory) medications. Medical supplies include topicals and dressings, antiseptics, bandages, cotton, first aid kits, contraceptives, syringes, ice bags, thermometers, sunlamps, vaporizers, heating pads, medical appliances (such as braces, canes, crutches, walkers, eyeglasses, and hearing aids), and the rental and repair of medical equipment. 1. Components of income and taxes are derived from "complete income reporters" only; that is, respondents provided values for major sources of income, such as wages and salaries, self-employment income, and Social Security income. 2. Value less than 0.05. 3. No data reported. 4. Value less than 0.5. 5. Data are likely to have large sampling errors.

★ 404 ★
Consumer Spending

Health Care Expenditures for Consumer Units With Reference Persons Ages 45 to 54: 1990-1991

Figures below show average annual health care expenditures and characteristics of consumer units represented by persons between 45 and 54 years old. Data are provided by income before taxes.

Item	Complete reporting of income							
	Total complete reporting	Less than $5,000	$5,000 to $9,999	$10,000 to $14,999	$15,000 to $19,999	$20,000 to $29,999	$30,000 to $39,000	$40,000 and over
Number of consumer units (in thousands)	12,543	545	833	888	809	1,946	1,634	5,888
Consumer unit characteristics								
Income before taxes[1] ($)	45,945	406	7,400	12,507	17,347	24,950	34,624	74,664
Income after taxes[1] ($)	41,616	52	6,976	12,076	16,186	23,240	31,681	67,141
Age of reference person	49.2	49.4	49.5	49.4	49.4	49.3	49.2	49.1
Average number in consumer unit								
Persons	2.9	2.2	2.3	2.4	2.9	2.7	2.9	3.2
Children under 18	.7	.4	.6	.6	.8	.6	.6	.7
Persons 65 and over	[2]	[2]	[2]	.1[3]	[2]	[2]	.1	[2]
Earners	1.9	1.1	1.1	1.3	1.6	1.8	2.0	2.3
Vehicles	2.6	1.4	1.3	1.4	1.6	2.2	2.6	3.3
Percent distribution								
Sex of reference person								
Male	68	53	39	40	49	62	70	81
Female	32	47	61	60	51	38	30	19
Housing tenure								
Homeowner	74	60	47	46	61	65	76	89
With mortgage	59	39	27	25	44	47	58	76
Without mortgage	16	21	20	21	17	18	19	12
Renter	26	40	53	54	39	35	24	11
Race of reference person								
Black	12	26	23	14	21	16	9	7
White and other	88	74	77	86	79	84	91	93
Education of reference person								
Elementary (1-8)	8	22	14	20	12	8	8	3
High school (9-12)	44	49	59	62	61	55	51	32
College	48	28	26	19	27	36	40	66
Never attended and other	[4]	[5]	1	[4]	[5]	[4]	[4]	[4]
At least one vehicle owned	92	75	70	79	83	95	96	99
Average annual expenditures ($)	39,120	17,426	15,860	18,077	22,480	25,496	32,572	56,227
Health care	1,665	1,074	919	1,381	1,045	1,285	1,619	2,094
Health insurance	593	424	393	294	451	500	617	725
Medical services	701	365	306	838	322	472	574	930
Drugs	252	221	167	204	207	223	301	278
Medical supplies	119	64[3]	53	44	65	91	126	161

[Continued]

★ 404 ★

Health Care Expenditures for Consumer Units With Reference Persons Ages 45 to 54: 1990-1991

[Continued]

Item	Complete reporting of income							
	Total complete reporting	Less than $5,000	$5,000 to $9,999	$10,000 to $14,999	$15,000 to $19,999	$20,000 to $29,999	$30,000 to $39,000	$40,000 and over
Addenda								
Health care	63	73[3]	15[3]	1[3]	17[3]	18[3]	29	109

Source: U.S. Department of Labor. Bureau of Labor Statistics. *Consumer Expenditure Survey, 1990-1991.* Washington, DC: U.S. Government Printing Office, September 1993, pp. 114-117. From the source: This table "presents detailed information from the Consumer Expenditure Survey for 1990 and 1991. The data shown here are combined, or integrated, from the Diary and Interview components of the survey. Integrated data provide a complete accounting of consumer expenditures and income, which neither component alone is designed to do" (p. iii). *Notes:* Health insurance expenditures include spending on health maintenance plans (HMOs), Blue Cross/Blue Shield, commercial or other health insurance, Medicare, and Medicare supplemental insurance. Medical services cover hospital rooms and services, physicians' services, services by professionals other than physicians, eye and dental care, lab tests, x-rays, and other medical care, including that provided in retirement communities or convalescent and nursing homes. The drugs category comprises prescription, nonprescription, and over-the-counter (internal and respiratory) medications. Medical supplies include topicals and dressings, antiseptics, bandages, cotton, first aid kits, contraceptives, syringes, ice bags, thermometers, sunlamps, vaporizers, heating pads, medical appliances (such as braces, canes, crutches, walkers, eyeglasses, and hearing aids), and the rental and repair of medical equipment. 1. Components of income and taxes are derived from "complete income reporters" only; that is, respondents provided values for major sources of income, such as wages and salaries, self-employment income, and Social Security income. 2. Value less than 0.05. 3. Data are likely to have large sampling errors. 4. Value less than 0.5. 5. No data reported.

★ 405 ★
Consumer Spending

Health Care Expenditures for Consumer Units With Reference Persons Ages 55 to 64: 1990-1991

Figures below show average annual health care expenditures and characteristics of consumer units represented by persons between 45 and 54 years old. Data are provided by income before taxes.

Item	Complete reporting of income							
	Total complete reporting	Less than $5,000	$5,000 to $9,999	$10,000 to $14,999	$15,000 to $19,999	$20,000 to $29,999	$30,000 to $39,000	$40,000 and over
Number of consumer units (in thousands)	10,020	599	1,269	1,042	878	1,553	1,201	3,479
Consumer unit characteristics								
Income before taxes[1] ($)	36,832	46	7,586	12,434	17,335	24,881	34,579	72,170
Income after taxes[1] ($)	33,132	-1,894	7,420	11,740	16,543	23,286	31,761	64,000
Age of reference person	59.7	59.9	60.4	60.3	60.4	60.1	59.4	59.0
Average number in consumer unit								
Persons	2.3	1.8	1.9	2.2	2.1	2.2	2.4	2.7
Children under 18	.2	.1[2]	.2	.3	.2	.2	.2	.2
Persons 65 and over	.1	[3]	.1	.1	.1	.1	.1	.1
Earners	1.4	.7	.7	1.0	1.1	1.4	1.7	2.0
Vehicles	2.3	1.2	1.2	2.0	1.8	2.4	2.7	3.0
Percent distribution								
Sex of reference person								
Male	71	43	49	59	66	73	84	83
Female	29	57	51	41	34	27	16	17

[Continued]

★ 405 ★

Health Care Expenditures for Consumer Units With Reference Persons Ages 55 to 64: 1990-1991
[Continued]

Item	Complete reporting of income							
	Total complete reporting	Less than $5,000	$5,000 to $9,999	$10,000 to $14,999	$15,000 to $19,999	$20,000 to $29,999	$30,000 to $39,000	$40,000 and over
Housing tenure								
Homeowner	80	59	57	76	74	80	84	93
With mortgage	40	20	22	26	23	39	45	57
Without mortgage	40	39	36	50	52	41	39	36
Renter	20	41	43	24	26	20	16	7
Race of reference person								
Black	11	18	24	15	13	9	8	5
White and other	89	82	76	85	87	91	92	95
Education of reference person								
Elementary (1-8)	15	22	31	26	19	17	10	4
High school (9-12)	47	55	51	49	61	49	51	37
College	38	19	17	23	20	34	38	59
Never attended and other	4	3	1	1	4	3	5	4
At least one vehicle owned	90	65	68	88	92	94	96	98
Average annual expenditures ($)	31,740	17,276	14,725	19,050	19,902	24,924	32,075	51,202
Health care	1,855	1,316	1,235	1,861	1,674	1,535	1,894	2,357
Health insurance	727	459	507	818	839	600	747	849
Medical services	680	596	382	611	443	531	580	985
Drugs	352	201	300	361	336	324	461	379
Medical supplies	95	59[2]	46	71	56	79	105	143
Addenda								
Health care	26	14[2]	5[2]	23[2]	19[2]	9[2]	31[2]	46

Source: U.S. Department of Labor. Bureau of Labor Statistics. *Consumer Expenditure Survey, 1990-1991.* Washington, DC: U.S. Government Printing Office, September 1993, pp. 118-121. From the source: This table "presents detailed information from the Consumer Expenditure Survey for 1990 and 1991. The data shown here are combined, or integrated, from the Diary and Interview components of the survey. Integrated data provide a complete accounting of consumer expenditures and income, which neither component alone is designed to do" (p. iii). *Notes:* Health insurance expenditures include spending on health maintenance plans (HMOs), Blue Cross/Blue Shield, commercial or other health insurance, Medicare, and Medicare supplemental insurance. Medical services cover hospital rooms and services, physicians' services, services by professionals other than physicians, eye and dental care, lab tests, x-rays, and other medical care, including that provided in retirement communities or convalescent and nursing homes. The drugs category comprises prescription, nonprescription, and over-the-counter (internal and respiratory) medications. Medical supplies include topicals and dressings, antiseptics, bandages, cotton, first aid kits, contraceptives, syringes, ice bags, thermometers, sunlamps, vaporizers, heating pads, medical appliances (such as braces, canes, crutches, walkers, eyeglasses, and hearing aids), and the rental and repair of medical equipment. 1. Components of income and taxes are derived from "complete income reporters" only; that is, respondents provided values for major sources of income, such as wages and salaries, self-employment income, and Social Security income. 2. Data are likely to have large sampling errors. 3. Value less than 0.05. 4. Value less than 0.5. 5. No data reported.

★ 406 ★
Consumer Spending

Health Care Expenditures for Consumer Units With Reference Persons Ages 65 and Over: 1990-1991

Figures below show average annual health care expenditures and characteristics of consumer units represented by persons 65 years old and older. Data are provided by income before taxes.

Item	Complete reporting of income							
	Total complete reporting	Less than $5,000	$5,000 to $9,999	$10,000 to $14,999	$15,000 to $19,999	$20,000 to $29,999	$30,000 to $39,000	$40,000 and over
Number of consumer units (in thousands)	17,937	1,233	5,120	3,463	2,329	2,891	1,340	1,562
Consumer unit characteristics								
Income before taxes[1] ($)	19,427	3,416	7,533	12,377	17,314	24,281	34,275	68,098
Income after taxes[1] ($)	18,113	3,050	7,417	12,116	16,627	22,204	31,661	61,366
Age of reference person	74.2	75.9	75.8	74.7	73.9	72.8	71.4	71.4
Average number in consumer unit								
Persons	1.7	1.3	1.3	1.6	1.9	2.0	2.2	2.5
Children under 18	.1	[2]	[2]	[2]	.1	[2]	.1	.2
Persons 65 and over	1.4	1.1	1.1	1.4	1.5	1.5	1.5	1.5
Earners	.4	.2	.2	.3	.4	.5	.9	1.2
Vehicles	1.5	.7	.9	1.3	1.7	2.0	2.2	2.5
Percent distribution								
Sex of reference person								
Male	53	25	34	51	65	68	75	78
Female	47	75	66	49	35	32	25	22
Housing tenure								
Homeowner	78	59	65	79	82	87	92	92
With mortgage	15	9	7	12	13	19	25	32
Without mortgage	63	50	58	67	69	68	67	60
Renter	22	41	35	21	18	13	8	8
Race of reference person								
Black	9	24	13	7	8	3	4	5
White and other	91	76	87	93	92	97	96	95
Education of reference person								
Elementary (1-8)	26	45	38	24	26	16	10	8
High school (9-12)	47	36	45	51	53	49	46	36
College	26	15	13	23	21	34	43	56
Never attended and other	1	3	3	2	[2]	[3]	[3]	[3]
At least one vehicle owned	78	51	60	79	88	94	96	97
Average annual expenditures ($)	19,541	10,299	11,693	16,768	18,916	23,464	29,364	44,811
Health care	2,240	1,804	1,678	2,027	2,455	2,812	2,739	3,103
Health insurance	1,052	702	802	1,022	1,177	1,282	1,253	1,430
Medical services	619	717	402	414	647	886	837	982
Drugs	470	293	400	477	533	522	537	582
Medical supplies	100	92	75	114	98	121	112	109

[Continued]

★ 406 ★

Health Care Expenditures for Consumer Units With Reference Persons Ages 65 and Over: 1990-1991

[Continued]

Item	Complete reporting of income							
	Total complete reporting	Less than $5,000	$5,000 to $9,999	$10,000 to $14,999	$15,000 to $19,999	$20,000 to $29,999	$30,000 to $39,000	$40,000 and over
Addenda								
Health care	75	460	100	38	15[4]	11[4]	17[4]	27[4]

Source: U.S. Department of Labor. Bureau of Labor Statistics. *Consumer Expenditure Survey, 1990-1991.* Washington, DC: U.S. Government Printing Office, September 1993, pp. 122-125. From the source: This table "presents detailed information from the Consumer Expenditure Survey for 1990 and 1991. The data shown here are combined, or integrated, from the Diary and Interview components of the survey. Integrated data provide a complete accounting of consumer expenditures and income, which neither component alone is designed to do" (p. iii). *Notes:* Health insurance expenditures include spending on health maintenance plans (HMOs), Blue Cross/Blue Shield, commercial or other health insurance, Medicare, and Medicare supplemental insurance. Medical services cover hospital rooms and services, physicians' services, services by professionals other than physicians, eye and dental care, lab tests, x-rays, and other medical care, including that provided in retirement communities or convalescent and nursing homes. The drugs category comprises prescription, nonprescription, and over-the-counter (internal and respiratory) medications. Medical supplies include topicals and dressings, antiseptics, bandages, cotton, first aid kits, contraceptives, syringes, ice bags, thermometers, sunlamps, vaporizers, heating pads, medical appliances (such as braces, canes, crutches, walkers, eyeglasses, and hearing aids), and the rental and repair of medical equipment. 1. Components of income and taxes are derived from "complete income reporters" only; that is, respondents provided values for major sources of income, such as wages and salaries, self-employment income, and Social Security income. 2. Value less than 0.05. 3. Value less than 0.5. 4. Data are likely to have large sampling errors.

★ 407 ★

Consumer Spending

Health Care Expenditures in Selected Midwestern Metropolitan Statistical Areas: 1990-1991

Data below reflect characteristics and the average annual health care expenditures of consumers living in the midwestern United States. Data are provided by metropolitan statistical areas.

Item	All consumer units in the midwest	Chicago	Detroit	Milwaukee	Minneapolis-St. Paul	Cleveland	Cincinnati	St. Louis	Kansas City
Number of consumer units (in thousands)	24,509	3,105	1,847	577	1,108	1,181	743	1,053	691
Consumer unit characteristics									
Income before taxes[1] ($)	30,287	39,230	35,702	31,440	38,571	30,322	33,185	35,814	37,280
Income after taxes[1] ($)	27,868	35,810	33,739	29,676	34,095	28,537	31,612	33,104	35,932
Age of reference person	47.0	47.4	47.0	44.3	45.2	47.6	46.3	47.5	46.6
Average number in consumer unit									
Persons	2.5	2.8	2.5	2.6	2.5	2.4	2.6	2.7	2.8
Children under 18	.7	.8	.6	.7	.7	.6	.7	.7	.8
Persons 65 and over	.3	.2	.3	.3	.2	.3	.3	.3	.3
Earners	1.4	1.5	1.4	1.5	1.6	1.3	1.4	1.5	1.5
Vehicles	2.1	1.6	2.2	2.0	2.4	1.8	2.1	2.0	2.1
Percent distribution									
Sex of reference person									
Male	67	65	71	64	63	60	76	65	68
Female	33	35	29	36	37	40	24	35	32
Housing tenure									
Homeowner	65	61	67	57	65	58	66	69	71
With mortgage	38	41	43	35	52	34	43	43	53
Without mortgage	27	20	25	22	13	23	22	26	17
Renter	35	39	33	43	35	42	34	31	29
Race of reference person									
Black	10	17	16	14	3	15	9	14	10

[Continued]

★ 407 ★

Health Care Expenditures in Selected Midwestern Metropolitan Statistical Areas: 1990-1991

[Continued]

Item	All consumer units in the midwest	Chicago	Detroit	Milwaukee	Minneapolis-St. Paul	Cleveland	Cincinnati	St. Louis	Kansas City
White and other	90	83	84	86	97	85	91	86	90
Education of reference person									
Elementary (1-8)	10	9	6	8	4	9	9	12	4
High school (9-12)	47	47	43	47	42	52	51	42	48
College	43	44	50	45	54	39	40	45	48
Never attended and other	2	2	1	3	2	2	2	1	3
At least one vehicle owned	88	77	91	82	89	84	90	88	90
Average annual expenditures ($)	26,815	32,568	29,732	27,843	34,801	26,960	27,781	27,743	28,189
Health care	1,410	1,439	1,304	1,228	1,438	1,430	1,583	1,416	1,964
Health insurance	591	459	523	553	756	609	729	695	873
Medical services	489	680	526	414	336	491	497	380	773
Drugs	245	220	175	181	217	233	289	260	252
Medical supplies	85	80	80	80	129	97	68	82	66
Addenda									
Health care	49	29[4]	167	32[4]	19[4]	16[4]	24	20	183

Source: U.S. Department of Labor. Bureau of Labor Statistics. *Consumer Expenditure Survey, 1990-1991.* Washington, DC: U.S. Government Printing Office, September 1993, pp. 90-93. From the source: This table "presents detailed information from the Consumer Expenditure Survey for 1990 and 1991. The data shown here are combined, or integrated, from the Diary and Interview components of the survey. Integrated data provide a complete accounting of consumer expenditures and income, which neither component alone is designed to do" (p. iii). *Notes:* Health insurance expenditures include spending on health maintenance plans (HMOs), Blue Cross/Blue Shield, commercial or other health insurance, Medicare, and Medicare supplemental insurance. Medical services cover hospital rooms and services, physicians' services, services by professionals other than physicians, eye and dental care, lab tests, x-rays, and other medical care, including that provided in retirement communities or convalescent and nursing homes. The drugs category comprises prescription, nonprescription, and over-the-counter (internal and respiratory) medications. Medical supplies include topicals and dressings, antiseptics, bandages, cotton, first aid kits, contraceptives, syringes, ice bags, thermometers, sunlamps, vaporizers, heating pads, medical appliances (such as braces, canes, crutches, walkers, eyeglasses, and hearing aids), and the rental and repair of medical equipment. 1. Components of income and taxes are derived from "complete income reporters" only; that is, respondents provided values for major sources of income, such as wages and salaries, self-employment income, and Social Security income. 2. Value less than 0.5. 3. No data reported. 4. Data are likely to have large sampling errors.

★ 408 ★

Consumer Spending

Health Care Expenditures in Selected Northeastern Metropolitan Statistical Areas: 1990-1991

Data below reflect the characteristics and the average annual health care expenditures of consumers living in the northeastern United States. Data are provided by metropolitan statistical areas.

Item	All consumer units in the northeast	New York	Philadelphia	Boston	Pittsburgh	Buffalo
Number of consumer units (in thousands)	20,330	6,552	2,028	1,781	969	553
Consumer unit characteristics						
Income before taxes[1] ($)	36,243	41,448	41,450	42,042	36,499	30,022
Income after taxes[1] ($)	32,809	37,858	36,592	39,053	29,744	29,671
Age of reference person	48.3	49.0	48.5	45.7	49.5	48.5

[Continued]

★ 408 ★

Health Care Expenditures in Selected Northeastern Metropolitan Statistical Areas: 1990-1991

[Continued]

Item	All consumer units in the northeast	New York	Philadelphia	Boston	Pittsburgh	Buffalo
Average number in consumer unit						
Persons	2.5	2.6	2.6	2.5	2.4	2.5
Children under 18	.6	.6	.7	.7	.6	.7
Persons 65 and over	.3	.3	.3	.3	.4	.3
Earners	1.4	1.3	1.4	1.4	1.2	1.3
Vehicles	1.6	1.3	1.5	1.6	1.5	1.5
Percent distribution						
Sex of reference person						
Male	63	57	63	63	64	66
Female	37	43	37	37	36	34
Housing tenure						
Homeowner	60	53	67	58	70	61
With mortgage	35	33	36	41	33	35
Without mortgage	25	20	30	16	37	26
Renter	40	47	33	42	30	39
Race of reference person						
Black	10	16	20	5	7	10
White and other	90	84	80	95	93	90
Education of reference person						
Elementary (1-8)	9	11	6	4	11	10
High school (9-12)	47	45	49	42	50	43
College	44	44	45	53	40	47
Never attended and other	2	2	1	2	3	2
At least one vehicle owned	78	69	79	81	77	80
Average annual expenditures ($)	30,264	34,583	31,795	30,835	28,626	25,119
Health care	1,450	1,533	1,648	1,498	1,290	1,149
Health insurance	611	531	753	735	552	565
Medical services	543	737	594	461	389	365
Drugs	214	196	202	199	265	142
Medical supplies	82	70	98	103	84	76

[Continued]

★ 408 ★

Health Care Expenditures in Selected Northeastern Metropolitan Statistical Areas: 1990-1991

[Continued]

Item	All consumer units in the northeast	New York	Philadelphia	Boston	Pittsburgh	Buffalo
Addenda Health care	32	16	186	16[4]	4[4]	7[4]

Source: U.S. Department of Labor. Bureau of Labor Statistics. *Consumer Expenditure Survey, 1990-1991.* Washington, DC: U.S. Government Printing Office, September 1993, pp. 86-89. From the source: This table "presents detailed information from the Consumer Expenditure Survey for 1990 and 1991. The data shown here are combined, or integrated, from the Diary and Interview components of the survey. Integrated data provide a complete accounting of consumer expenditures and income, which neither component alone is designed to do" (p. iii). *Notes:* Health insurance expenditures include spending on health maintenance plans (HMOs), Blue Cross/Blue Shield, commercial or other health insurance, Medicare, and Medicare supplemental insurance. Medical services cover hospital rooms and services, physicians' services, services by professionals other than physicians, eye and dental care, lab tests, x-rays, and other medical care, including that provided in retirement communities or convalescent and nursing homes. The drugs category comprises prescription, nonprescription, and over-the-counter (internal and respiratory) medications. Medical supplies include topicals and dressings, antiseptics, bandages, cotton, first aid kits, contraceptives, syringes, ice bags, thermometers, sunlamps, vaporizers, heating pads, medical appliances (such as braces, canes, crutches, walkers, eyeglasses, and hearing aids), and the rental and repair of medical equipment. 1. Components of income and taxes are derived from "complete income reporters" only; that is, respondents provided values for major sources of income, such as wages and salaries, self-employment income, and Social Security income. 2. Value less than 0.5. 3. No data reported. 4. Data are likely to have large sampling errors.

★ 409 ★
Consumer Spending

Health Care Expenditures in Selected Southern Metropolitan Statistical Areas: 1990-1991

Data below reflect characteristics and the average annual health care expenditures of consumers living in southern states. Data are provided by metropolitan statistical areas.

Item	All consumer units in the South	Washington, DC	Baltimore	Atlanta	Miami	Dallas-Fort Worth	Houston
Number of consumer units (in thousands)	32,696	1,485	855	1,124	1,338	1,533	1,380
Consumer unit characteristics							
Income before taxes[1] ($)	30,649	46,275	40,367	38,535	33,703	38,804	34,539
Income after taxes[1] ($)	27,883	39,353	35,375	33,803	31,084	34,059	31,195
Age of reference person	47.7	43.6	44.9	44.3	50.6	42.1	45.1
Average number in consumer unit							
Persons	2.5	2.2	2.6	2.7	2.4	2.5	2.6
Children under 18	.7	.5	.7	.7	.5	.7	.7
Persons 65 and over	.3	.2	.2	.2	.5	.2	.2
Earners	1.4	1.5	1.4	1.6	1.3	1.6	1.4
Vehicles	1.9	1.7	1.6	1.9	1.5	1.8	1.9
Percent distribution							
Sex of reference person							
Male	64	57	64	59	61	65	67
Female	36	43	36	41	39	35	33

[Continued]

★ 409 ★

Health Care Expenditures in Selected Southern Metropolitan Statistical Areas: 1990-1991

[Continued]

Item	All consumer units in the South	Washington, DC	Baltimore	Atlanta	Miami	Dallas-Fort Worth	Houston
Housing tenure							
Homeowner	65	58	61	62	58	51	54
With mortgage	38	48	44	46	40	33	32
Without mortgage	27	9	17	16	19	18	22
Renter	35	42	39	38	42	49	46
Race of reference person							
Black	17	25	25	30	19	8	16
White and other	83	75	75	70	81	92	84
Education of reference person							
Elementary (1-8)	13	5	5	10	15	8	11
High school (9-12)	43	31	45	33	37	35	42
College	44	63	50	57	47	56	46
Never attended and other	1	1	2	1	2	1	2
At least one vehicle owned	88	82	85	88	85	93	87
Average annual expenditures ($)	27,543	38,560	33,208	34,163	32,053	33,500	32,298
Health care	1,635	1,962	1,401	1,778	1,686	1,543	1,458
Health insurance	667	687	596	717	765	644	545
Medical services	577	893	562	681	630	548	603
Drugs	296	265	177	269	224	262	224
Medical supplies	95	117	67	110	68	89	85
Addenda							
Health care	30	31	19[3]	15[3]	9[3]	26	42

Source: U.S. Department of Labor. Bureau of Labor Statistics. *Consumer Expenditure Survey, 1990-1991.* Washington, DC: U.S. Government Printing Office, September 1993, pp. 94-97. From the source: This table "presents detailed information from the Consumer Expenditure Survey for 1990 and 1991. The data shown here are combined, or integrated, from the Diary and Interview components of the survey. Integrated data provide a complete accounting of consumer expenditures and income, which neither component alone is designed to do" (p. iii). *Notes:* Health insurance expenditures include spending on health maintenance plans (HMOs), Blue Cross/Blue Shield, commercial or other health insurance, Medicare, and Medicare supplemental insurance. Medical services cover hospital rooms and services, physicians' services, services by professionals other than physicians, eye and dental care, lab tests, x-rays, and other medical care, including that provided in retirement communities or convalescent and nursing homes. The drugs category comprises prescription, nonprescription, and over-the-counter (internal and respiratory) medications. Medical supplies include topicals and dressings, antiseptics, bandages, cotton, first aid kits, contraceptives, syringes, ice bags, thermometers, sunlamps, vaporizers, heating pads, medical appliances (such as braces, canes, crutches, walkers, eyeglasses, and hearing aids), and the rental and repair of medical equipment. 1. Components of income and taxes are derived from "complete income reporters" only; that is, respondents provided values for major sources of income, such as wages and salaries, self-employment income, and Social Security income. 2. Value less than 0.5. 3. Data are likely to have large sampling errors.

★ 410 ★

Consumer Spending

Health Care Expenditures in Selected Western Metropolitan Statistical Areas: 1990-1991

Data below reflect characteristics and average annual health care expenditures of consumers living in western states. Data are provided by metropolitan statistical area.

Item	All consumer units in the west	Los Angeles	San Francisco	San Diego	Portland	Seattle	Honolulu	Anchorage
Number of consumer units (in thousands)	19,908	5,165	2,520	912	668	1,049	242	89
Consumer unit characteristics								
Income before taxes[1] ($)	36,278	39,356	42,215	36,952	36,339	39,921	41,499	50,560
Income after taxes[1] ($)	32,361	35,650	36,748	33,444	32,190	35,103	37,794	44,053
Age of reference person	46.2	46.9	44.6	43.4	45.6	45.3	49.0	41.4
Average number in consumer unit								
Persons	2.7	2.8	2.6	2.4	2.5	2.5	2.8	2.7
Children under 18	.8	.8	.6	.7	.7	.6	.7	.8
Persons 65 and over	.3	.3	.2	.3	.2	.3	.4	.1
Earners	1.4	1.3	1.5	1.3	1.5	1.5	1.5	1.7
Vehicles	2.2	1.9	2.0	1.8	2.3	2.4	1.6	2.6
Percent distribution								
Sex of reference person								
Male	66	64	60	67	64	68	65	69
Female	34	36	40	33	36	32	35	31
Housing tenure								
Homeowner	59	56	58	50	59	61	49	58
With mortgage	43	43	45	35	44	47	38	48
Without mortgage	17	13	13	14	15	14	11	10
Renter	41	44	42	50	41	39	51	42
Race of reference person								
Black	5	8	8	5	1	3	2	5
White and other	95	92	92	95	99	97	98	95
Education of reference person								
Elementary (1-8)	8	13	5	8	3	3	8	4
High school (9-12)	36	34	28	32	35	36	39	38
College	55	52	67	60	61	60	52	58
Never attended and other	2	1	3	3	3	1	1	1
At least one vehicle owned	90	88	87	90	90	89	84	94
Average annual expenditures ($)	32,797	35,673	39,707	32,983	29,228	35,086	36,394	43,991
Health care	1,525	1,485	1,536	1,178	1,318	1,646	1,623	1,730
Health insurance	583	535	656	465	570	509	701	463
Medical services	628	677	582	473	436	811	585	915
Drugs	225	189	198	171	234	239	217	244
Medical supplies	89	85	100	69	78	87	120	108

[Continued]

★ 410 ★

Health Care Expenditures in Selected Western Metropolitan Statistical Areas: 1990-1991

[Continued]

Item	All consumer units in the west	Los Angeles	San Francisco	San Diego	Portland	Seattle	Honolulu	Anchorage
Addenda Health care	39	15	16[4]	16[4]	23	201[4]	129[4]	17[4]

Source: U.S. Department of Labor. Bureau of Labor Statistics. *Consumer Expenditure Survey, 1990-1991.* Washington, DC: U.S. Government Printing Office, September 1993, pp. 98-101. From the source: This table "presents detailed information from the Consumer Expenditure Survey for 1990 and 1991. The data shown here are combined, or integrated, from the Diary and Interview components of the survey. Integrated data provide a complete accounting of consumer expenditures and income, which neither component alone is designed to do" (p. iii). *Notes:* Health insurance expenditures include spending on health maintenance plans (HMOs), Blue Cross/Blue Shield, commercial or other health insurance, Medicare, and Medicare supplemental insurance. Medical services cover hospital rooms and services, physicians' services, services by professionals other than physicians, eye and dental care, lab tests, x-rays, and other medical care, including that provided in retirement communities or convalescent and nursing homes. The drugs category comprises prescription, nonprescription, and over-the-counter (internal and respiratory) medications. Medical supplies include topicals and dressings, antiseptics, bandages, cotton, first aid kits, contraceptives, syringes, ice bags, thermometers, sunlamps, vaporizers, heating pads, medical appliances (such as braces, canes, crutches, walkers, eyeglasses, and hearing aids), and the rental and repair of medical equipment. 1. Components of income and taxes are derived from "complete income reporters" only; that is, respondents provided values for major sources of income, such as wages and salaries, self-employment income, and Social Security income. 2. Value less than 0.5. 3. No data reported. 4. Data are likely to have large sampling errors.

★ 411 ★

Consumer Spending

Health Services and Supplies Expenditures and Percent Distribution of U.S. Households for Selected Years: 1965-1991

This table profiles the health expenditures of households. Where households pay dedicated funds into government health programs (e.g., Medicare), costs are assigned to households accordingly. See corresponding charts on business, federal government, and state and local government spending for profiles of other sources of health care spending.

Type of Payer	1965	1967	1970	1975	1980	1985	1987	1988	1989	1990	1991
	\multicolumn{11}{c}{Amount in billion[1]s ($)}										
Total[1]	38.2	47.9	69.1	124.7	238.9	407.2	476.9	526.2	583.6	652.4	728.6
Private	30.3	35.0	50.1	86.2	162.0	279.0	327.5	362.5	398.3	436.6	474.1
Household (individuals)	23.7	26.0	35.0	55.9	90.8	153.6	181.9	196.1	213.8	228.9	247.0
Employee share of private health insurance premiums and individual policy premiums	4.6	4.9	6.0	9.9	16.6	30.0	37.5	37.7	42.7	46.6	52.2
Employee and self-employment contributions and voluntary premiums paid to Medicare hospital insurance trust fund[2]	0.0	1.6	2.4	5.7	12.0	24.0	29.4	31.2	33.7	35.6	39.9
Premiums paid by individuals to Medicare supplementary medical insurance trust fund	0.0	0.6	1.0	1.7	2.7	5.2	6.1	8.7	11.2	10.2	10.7
Out-of-pocket health spending by individuals	19.0	18.9	25.6	38.5	59.5	94.4	108.8	118.5	126.2	136.5	144.3
Non-patient revenue	0.6	0.8	1.5	2.5	7.0	12.0	13.8	15.4	17.5	19.8	21.7
	\multicolumn{11}{c}{Percent distribution}										
Total	100.0	100.0	100.0	100.0	100.0	100.0	100.0	100.0	100.0	100.0	100.0
Private	79.3	73.2	72.6	69.2	67.8	68.5	68.7	68.9	68.2	66.9	65.1
Household (individuals)	62.0	54.2	50.7	44.8	38.0	37.7	38.1	37.3	36.6	35.1	33.9
Employee share of private health insurance premiums and individual policy premiums	12.2	10.2	8.7	7.9	6.9	7.4	7.9	7.2	7.3	7.1	7.2
Employee and self-employment contributions and voluntary premiums paid to Medicare hospital insurance trust fund[2]	0.0	3.3	3.4	4.6	5.0	5.9	6.2	5.9	5.8	5.5	5.5
Premiums paid by individuals to Medicare supplementary medical insurance trust fund	0.0	1.3	1.4	1.4	1.1	1.3	1.3	1.7	1.9	1.6	1.5

[Continued]

★ 411 ★

Health Services and Supplies Expenditures and Percent Distribution of U.S. Households for Selected Years: 1965-1991
[Continued]

Type of Payer	1965	1967	1970	1975	1980	1985	1987	1988	1989	1990	1991
Out-of-pocket health spending by individuals	49.8	39.5	37.1	30.9	24.9	23.2	22.8	22.5	21.6	20.9	19.8
Non-patient revenue	1.7	1.7	2.2	2.0	2.9	2.9	2.9	2.9	3.0	3.0	3.0

Source: U.S. Department of Health and Human Services. Public Health Service. Centers for Disease Control and Prevention. National Center for Health Statistics. *Health, United States, 1992.* Hyattsville, MD: Public Health Service, 1993, p. 170. Primary source: Health Care Financing Administration. Office of National Health Statistics. Office of the Actuary. "Business, Households, and Governments—Health Spending 1991." *Health Care Financing Review* 14, no.3 (winter 1993). *Notes:* Data are compiled by the Health Care Financing Administration. 1. Excludes research and construction. 2. Includes one-half of self-employment contribution to Medicare hospital insurance trust fund.

★ 412 ★

Consumer Spending

Health Services Expenditures: 1980, 1985, and 1991

Data below reflect average annual expenditures and the percent of consumer units reporting expenditures for selected health services. From the source: "From 1984 to 1991, out-of-pocket health care expenditures increased 48 percent for all consumer units. Much of this increase stems from a sharp rise in health insurance expenditures. Health insurance expenditures increased 77 percent for all consumer units. Health insurance is now the largest portion of the health care budget, rising from 35 percent of total health care in 1984 to 42 percent in 1991. Accounting for the rise in health insurance expenditures is an increase in participation in health plans and a rise in premiums. More consumer units are now self-insuring or are sharing the cost with their employers. Also, more are purchasing supplemental plans. The percent of all consumer units reporting expenditures for health insurance rose from 53 percent in 1984 to 59 percent in 1991. The types of health insurance consumer units are now choosing are also changing. Participation in health maintenance organizations (HMOs) rose from 3 percent in 1984 to 9 percent in 1991 for all consumer units. Participation in supplements to Medicare, dental, and other health insurance rose from 9 percent in 1984 to 12 percent in 1991. However, the percent of consumer units reporting Blue Cross/Blue Shield expenditures fell from 16 percent in 1984 to 13 percent in 1991" (p. 8). Data from 1984 were used for comparison since that year was the first for which integrated data from the current Consumer Expenditure (CE) Survey were available. See Source note below.

Item	1980	1985	1991
Health maintenance plans	8	24	91
Percent reporting	2.1	4.2	9.2
Blue Cross/Blue Shield	84	109	156
Percent reporting	18.5	15.6	13.5
Other commercial health insurance plans	83	147	221
Percent reporting	20.7	22.4	21.8
Medicare	29	49	99
Percent reporting	18.9	19.8	21.2

[Continued]

★ 412 ★

Health Services Expenditures: 1980, 1985, and 1991

[Continued]

Item	1980	1985	1991
Commercial Medicare supplements and other health insurance	21	46	89
Percent reporting	7.1	9.1	12.3

Source: U.S. Department of Labor. Bureau of Labor Statistics. *Consumer Expenditure Survey, 1990-1991.* Washington, DC: U.S. Government Printing Office, September 1993, p. 6. "This bulletin presents detailed information from the Consumer Expenditure Survey for 1990 and 1991. The data shown here are combined, or integrated, from the Diary and Interview components of the survey. Integrated data provide a complete accounting of consumer expenditures and income, which neither component alone is designed to do" (p. iii).

★ 413 ★

Consumer Spending

Hidden Health Care Costs Per Household

Owing to hidden costs, the average expenditure on health care per household is $8,000. These costs include an average of $2,300 spent directly by members of the household; $1,580 in out-of-pocket payments per household to health care providers; $590 in payroll deductions for employee contributions to group insurance; $130 in deduction from Social Security checks as the employee-paid premium for federal supplemental medical insurance; $3,930 per household for higher rates of federal income, Social Security, state income, state sales, and other taxes to support federal, state, and local health efforts. In addition, employers contribute an average of $1,580 per household for health benefits.

Source: "Hidden Factors Boost Annual Cost to $8,000 for Average Household." *Christian Science Monitor,* 18 November 1991, p. 10.

★ 414 ★

Consumer Spending

Revenue Loss From Selected Tax Expenditures for Individuals: 1992

[Millions of dollars]

Provision	Revenue loss
Net exclusion of pension contributions and earnings	51,170
Deductibility of mortgage interest on owner-occupied homes	40,545
Exclusion of contributions for medical insurance premiums and medical care	33,470
Exclusion of Old-Age and Survivors Insurance (Social Security) benefits for retired workers	18,000
Deductibility of charitable contributions	16,800

[Continued]

★414★

Revenue Loss From Selected Tax Expenditures for Individuals: 1992
[Continued]

Provision	Revenue loss
Deferral of capital gains on home sales	13,925
Exclusion of interest on life insurance savings	7,960
Exclusion of Individual Retirement Account contributions and earnings	7,265
Exclusion of untaxed Medicare benefits	6,700
Credit for child and dependent care expenses	4,395
Deductibility of medical expenses	3,170
Earned income credit	2,540
Special Employee Stock Ownership Plan rules	2,055
Exclusion of Keogh contributions and earnings	1,780
Exclusion of employee meals and lodging	780
Exclusion of railroad retirement benefits	310

Source: U.S. Department of Labor. Pension and Welfare Benefits Administration. *Trends in Health Benefits.* Washington, DC: U.S. Government Printing Office, 1993, p. 95. Primary source: U.S. Office of Management and Budget. *The Budget for Fiscal Year, 1992.*

Government Spending: Federal

★415★

Federal Government Health-Related Expenditures: 1970-1971 and 1989-1990

The table below reflects health-related expenditures of the federal government.

Social services and income maintenance expenditures	1970-1971	1980-1981	1988-1989	1989-1990
	In millions ($)			
General expenditures[1]	150,422	422,301	910,438	1,002,224
Public welfare	2,220	22,395	87,580	93,903
Hospitals and health	3,630	11,277	23,404	24,647
Social insurance administration	1,086	2,799	7,165	7,506
	Percentage distribution			
General expenditures[1]	100.0	100.0	100.0	100.0
Public welfare	1.5	5.3	9.6	9.4
Hospitals and health	2.4	2.7	2.6	2.5
Social insurance administration	0.7	0.7	0.8	0.7

Source: U.S. Department of Education. Office of Educational Research and Improvement. National Center for Education Statistics. *Digest of Education Statistics, 1992.* Washington, DC: U.S. Government Printing Office, 1992, p. 37. Primary source: U.S. Department of Commerce. Bureau of the Census. *Government Finances, 1989-1990.* Series GF/90-5. This table was prepared in February 1992. *Note:* 1. Excludes duplicative intergovernmental transactions.

★ 416 ★

Government Spending: Federal

Federal Pension and Health Programs as a Percentage of GNP and the Budget: 1965-2040

From the source: "Rising health care costs, rather than spending for retirement income, account for most of the current increase in public spending on the elderly.... Social Security retirement and disability benefits, which grew from 2.5 percent of gross national product (GNP) in 1965 to 5.2 percent in 1983, are projected to decline to 4.2 percent by 2005, and then increase slightly to 5.7 percent by 2030. Other pension benefits paid from the federal budget are expected to decline from 2 percent of GNP currently to about 1.2 percent of GNP by 2030."

Year	Pension programs as a percent of GNP[1]	Health programs as a percent of GNP[1]	Total as a percent of of GNP[1]	Total as a percent of of budget[2]
1965	4.1	0.3	4.4	24.9
1970	4.7	1.4	6.1	30.0
1975	6.4	2.0	8.4	37.1
1980	6.5	2.3	8.8	38.2
1982	7.1	2.7	9.7	39.6
1984	7.0	2.8	9.8	39.7
1986	6.6	3.0	9.6	39.4
1988	6.4	3.2	9.6	39.4
1990	6.6[3]	3.1[3]	9.7	40.4
1995	6.2	3.7	9.9	41.3
2000	5.8	4.0	9.8	40.8
2005	5.6	4.4	10.0	41.7
2010	6.0	4.7	10.7	44.6
2015	6.0	5.0	11.0	45.8
2020	6.5	5.4	11.9	49.6
2025	7.0	5.9	12.9	53.9
2030	7.1	6.4	13.5	56.3
2035	7.1	7.0	14.1	58.8
2040	7.0	7.5	14.5	60.4

Source: Aging America: Trends and Projections. 1991 ed. Prepared by the U.S. Senate Special Committee on Aging, the American Association of Retired Persons, the Federal Council on the Aging, and the U.S. Administration on Aging. DHHS Publication No. (FCoA) 91-28001. Washington, DC: U.S. Department of Health and Human Services (DHHS), 1991, p. 242. Primary source: Palmer, John L., and Barbara B. Torrey. *Health Care Financing and Pension Programs.* Paper prepared for the Urban Institute Conference on Federal Budget Policy in the 1980s, September 29-30, 1983. *Notes:* 1. Estimates for 1984-1988 are based on Congressional Budget Office (CBO) baseline assumptions, August 1983; forecasts for 1990 and beyond are based on intermediate assumptions of the Social Security and Medicare actuaries. 2. Forecasts for 1990 and beyond are based on the assumption that the budget accounts for 24 percent of GNP. 3. The discontinuity in the estimates of pension and health benefits as a percent of GNP between 1986 and 1990 is due to the Social Security trustees assuming that Old-Age, Survivors, and Disability Insurance (OASDI) will grow at a faster rate in the late 1980s than Congressional Budget Office assumes, and the Health Insurance trustees assuming that Medicare will grow at a slower rate than CBO assumes.

★ 417 ★

Government Spending: Federal

Federal Spending for Health – With Projections – for Selected Years: 1980-1998

From the source: "'Federal health spending' excludes spending for health by the Department of Defense. Spending for discretionary programs in the 1993-1998 period is increased each year to reflect projected inflation, starting from the 1993 appropriated levels. Although the Congressional Budget Office's projections of total federal spending assume compliance with the discretionary spending limits for the 1993-1995 period, the Budget Enforcement Act does not specify programmatic changes to achieve those limits. Thus, it is not possible to adjust projections for individual programs to reflect the overall limits" (p. 76).

["n.a." indicates "not applicable."]

	1980	1985	1990	1991	1992	1993	1994	1995	1996	1997	1998
	In billions of nominal dollars										
Total federal spending	590.9	946.4	1,252.7	1,323.8	1,381.8	1,452.9	1,506.8	1,574.5	1,642.8	1,733.0	1,839.1
Federal health spending											
Medicare[1]	32.1	65.8	98.1	104.5	119.0	134.1	152.3	171.7	192.7	215.3	239.3
Medicaid[2]	14.0	22.7	41.1	52.5	67.8	80.3	91.9	105.0	117.7	131.0	145.9
Veterans Affairs	6.5	9.5	12.1	12.9	14.1	14.9	15.7	16.2	16.7	17.2	18.0
Other[3]	9.2	10.9	16.6	18.7	21.8	24.9	26.2	27.3	28.4	29.7	31.0
Total	61.8	108.9	168.0	188.6	222.7	254.2	286.1	320.2	355.5	393.2	434.2
	As percentage of total federal spending										
Federal health spending	10.5	11.5	13.4	14.2	16.1	17.5	19.0	20.3	21.6	22.7	23.6
	As a percentage of federal spending for health										
Medicare[1]	51.9	60.4	58.4	55.4	53.4	52.7	53.2	53.6	54.2	54.8	55.1
Medicaid[2]	22.7	20.8	24.5	27.8	30.4	31.6	32.1	32.8	33.1	33.3	33.6
Veterans Affairs	10.5	8.7	7.2	6.8	6.3	5.9	5.5	5.1	4.7	4.4	4.1
Other[3]	14.9	10.0	9.9	9.9	9.8	9.8	9.2	8.5	8.0	7.5	7.1
Total	100.0	100.0	100.0	100.0	100.0	100.0	100.0	100.0	100.0	100.0	100.0

Source: U.S. Congress. Congressional Budget Office (CBO). *Trends in Health Spending: An Update.* A CBO Study. Washington, DC: Congressional Budget Office, June 1993, pp. 76-77. Primary source: Congressional Budget Office calculations and projections (January 1993). *Notes:* Details may not add to total because of rounding. 1. Medicare expenditures are calculated net of premium income from enrollees. (The Medicare program was enacted in 1965.) 2. Medicaid spending for 1965 reflects expenditures under the Medical Assistance for the Aged (MAA) program, which was established in 1960. MAA served as the foundation for the Medicaid program, enacted in 1965. 3. Includes federal employee and annuitant health benefits, as well as other health services and research.

★ 418 ★

Government Spending: Federal

Health Services and Supplies Expenditures and Percent Distribution of Federal Government for Selected Years: 1965-1991

This table profiles the health expenditures of the federal government. Where businesses or households pay dedicated funds into government health programs (e.g., Medicare), costs are assigned to businesses and households accordingly. This results in a lower share of expenditures being assigned to the federal government than for tabulations of expenditures by source of funds. Estimates of national expenditures by source of funds aim to track government-sponsored health programs over time and do not delineate the role of business employers in paying for health care. See corresponding charts on business, household, and state and local government spending for profiles of other sources of health care spending.

Type of Payer	1965	1967	1970	1975	1980	1985	1987	1988	1989	1990	1991
						Amount in billion[1]s ($)					
Total[1]	38.2	47.9	69.1	124.7	238.9	407.2	476.9	526.2	583.6	652.4	728.6
Public	7.9	12.8	18.9	38.5	76.8	128.2	149.4	163.7	185.4	215.8	254.5
Federal government	3.4	7.0	10.4	21.3	42.6	68.9	77.0	84.3	96.5	113.7	133.8
Employer contributions to private health insurance	0.2	0.2	0.3	1.2	2.2	4.3	4.8	6.4	8.0	9.1	9.8
Other[2]	3.3	6.8	10.1	20.1	40.3	64.5	72.2	77.9	88.5	104.6	124.0
						Percent distribution					
Total	100.0	100.0	100.0	100.0	100.0	100.0	100.0	100.0	100.0	100.0	100.0
Public	20.7	26.8	27.4	30.8	32.2	31.5	31.3	31.1	31.8	33.1	34.9
Federal government	9.0	14.6	15.0	17.1	17.8	16.9	16.2	16.0	16.5	17.4	18.4
Employer contributions to private health insurance	0.4	0.5	0.4	0.9	0.9	1.1	1.0	1.2	1.4	1.4	1.3
Other[2]	8.6	14.1	14.7	16.1	16.9	15.9	15.1	14.8	15.2	16.0	17.0

Source: U.S. Department of Health and Human Services. Public Health Service. Centers for Disease Control and Prevention. National Center for Health Statistics. *Health, United States, 1992.* Hyattsville, MD: Public Health Service, 1993, pp. 170-171. Primary source: Health Care Financing Administration. Office of National Health Statistics. Office of the Actuary. "Business, Households, and Governments—Health Spending 1991." *Health Care Financing Review* 14, no.3 (winter 1993). *Notes:* Data are compiled by the Health Care Financing Administration. 1. Excludes research and construction. 2. Includes expenditures for federal programs such as Medicaid and Medicare with adjustments for contributions by employers and individuals and for premiums paid to the Medicare insurance trust fund.

Government Spending: Local

★ 419 ★

Local Government Health-Related Finances, by State: 1989-1990

[In thousand dollars]

State	Social services and income maintenance						
	Public welfare	Cash assistance payments	Vendor payments	Other public welfare	Hospitals	Health	Social insurance administration
United States	23,953,290	10,326,473	1,624,948	12,001,869	27,986,606	11,222,965	11,035
Alabama	28,579	510	8,653	19,416	814,126	113,870	-
Alaska	6,627	-	-	6,627	31,190	51,932	-
Arizona	207,201	-	160,082	47,119	239,145	92,817	-

[Continued]

★419★

Local Government Health-Related Finances, by State: 1989-1990
[Continued]

State	Social services and income maintenance				Hospitals	Health	Social insurance administration
	Public welfare	Cash assistance payments	Vendor payments	Other public welfare			
Arkansas	1,730	-	-	1,730	201,671	43,410	-
California	7,912,933	5,679,045	176,417	2,057,471	4,666,377	2,397,737	-
Colorado	412,851	181,298	16,227	215,326	310,946	100,391	-
Connecticut	167,921	45,290	27,192	95,439	20,119	66,540	-
Delaware	717	-	5	712	-	527	-
District of Columbia	672,426	113,150	351,146	208,130	286,312	156,704	11,035
Florida	199,240	3,861	39,623	155,756	1,904,822	306,388	-
Georgia	34,630	-	48	34,582	2,086,115	287,475	-
Hawaii	8,600	-	-	8,600	-	8,411	-
Idaho	22,074	48	7,126	14,900	138,386	23,675	-
Illinois	257,878	210	3,106	254,562	697,182	227,687	-
Indiana	306,565	172,157	17,915	116,493	834,237	70,832	-
Iowa	122,092	1,536	22,283	98,273	343,797	116,246	-
Kansas	26,052	-	1,514	24,538	213,331	87,535	-
Kentucky	19,264	295	3,672	15,297	223,012	118,613	-
Louisiana	39,260	65	16,183	23,012	674,402	41,980	-
Maine	18,086	318	3,448	14,320	33,707	7,018	-
Maryland	37,079	-	4,763	32,316	195	194,982	-
Massachusetts	62,330	1,837	484	60,009	537,682	61,321	-
Michigan	353,406	7,699	53,284	292,423	623,666	856,886	-
Minnesota	1,098,294	479,883	27,003	591,408	584,371	209,410	-
Mississippi	18,268	280	1,016	16,972	683,304	46,964	-
Missouri	71,284	18	1,684	69,582	387,806	126,848	-
Montana	25,155	-	-	25,155	26,535	25,996	-
Nebraska	31,912	339	2,186	29,387	297,307	27,776	-
Nevada	39,304	12	9,370	29,922	189,207	34,601	-
New Hampshire	80,037	4,456	4,197	71,384	732	11,607	-
New Jersey	900,696	479,580	28,354	392,762	261,670	182,824	-
New Mexico	24,137	-	12,941	11,196	94,905	12,388	-
New York	6,850,081	2,726,272	317,968	3,805,841	3,569,790	1,238,615	-
North Carolina	374,722	87,989	21,067	265,666	989,531	560,101	-
North Dakota	28,256	336	2,463	25,457	239	6,694	-
Ohio	1,202,738	232,173	196,297	774,268	557,602	831,672	-
Oklahoma	14,033	-	1,060	12,973	404,681	43,563	-
Oregon	25,747	2	1,173	24,572	115,809	175,440	-
Pennsylvania	878,111	7	832	877,272	78,033	681,061	-
Rhode Island	21,536	17,134	1,487	2,915	-	1,828	-
South Carolina	11,787	-	657	11,130	663,747	53,999	-
South Dakota	10,187	36	4,531	5,620	15,471	6,478	-
Tennessee	80,219	380	6,880	72,959	847,213	107,202	-
Texas	115,607	623	31,433	83,551	2,097,051	503,544	-
Utah	4,755	-	-	4,755	17,984	71,159	-
Vermont	830	-	-	830	9	2,840	-
Virginia	452,423	53,583	31,006	367,834	262,274	232,782	-

[Continued]

★ 419 ★

Local Government Health-Related Finances, by State: 1989-1990
[Continued]

State	Social services and income maintenance						
	Public welfare	Cash assistance payments	Vendor payments	Other public welfare	Hospitals	Health	Social insurance administration
Washington	9,648	272	-	9,376	394,090	188,692	-
West Virginia	1,646	-	-	1,646	129,808	38,985	-
Wisconsin	660,531	35,779	8,172	616,580	286,666	355,708	-
Wyoming	3,805	-	-	3,805	150,351	11,211	-

Source: U.S. Department of Commerce. Economics and Statistics Administration. Bureau of the Census. *Government Finances, 1989-1990: Preliminary Report.* Series GF-90-5P. Washington, DC: U.S. Government Printing Office, September 1991, pp. 1-52. *Note:* Detail may not add to total because of rounding.

★ 420 ★

Government Spending: Local

Local Government Spending on Health Care in Alabama: 1990-1991

Local government spending for social service and income maintenance items is provided below. Data reflect city, urban town, and township government expenditures by function, thus grouping health-related activities (public welfare, hospitals, social insurance, and veterans' services) to provide a comprehensive picture of spending. Totals for these categories are not provided since they are meant only as presentational guidelines. According to the source: "Functions cannot be equated specifically with a single federal or state government program. Instead they represent broader activities of government that have remained virtually unchanged over many years so that as specific programs expand and contract they will remain useful for analytical purposes. Medicaid, for example, is a well-known program that is included in the larger public welfare function, specifically as a medical vendor payment, along with all other social welfare activities" (p. viii).

[Dollar amounts in thousands]

| City | Social service and income maintenance expenditures | | |
	Public welfare	Hospitals	Health
Birmingham	-	-	1,793
Huntsville	380	-	4,025
Mobile	-	-	968
Montgomery	31	385	2,048
Tuscaloosa	-	-	301

Source: U.S. Bureau of the Census. *City Government Finances, 1990-1991.* Series GF/91-4. Washington, DC: U.S. Government Printing Office, 1993, p. 6. "Data in this report pertain to government fiscal years that ended between July 1, 1990, and June 30, 1991.... About three-fourths of all city governments in the nation had a fiscal year ending in either December (42 percent) or June (32 percent). September and April were the next most common months in which city governments ended their fiscal years. Of all townships, three-fifths had fiscal years corresponding directly with the calendar year 1990 (i.e., they ended their fiscal years on December 31, 1990). March, February, and June had the next most common fiscal year ending dates for townships" (p. vi). *Notes:* Detail may not add to total due to rounding. The Public Welfare heading covers the support of and assistance to needy persons contingent upon their need, excluding pensions to former employees and other benefits not contingent upon need. Among the expenditures in this category are: Cash assistance paid directly to needy persons under categorical programs (e.g., Old Age Assistance, Aid to Families With Dependent Children, Aid to the Blind, and Aid to the Disabled) or under any welfare programs; vendor payments made directly to private purveyors for medical care, burial, and other commodities and services provided under welfare programs; and provision and operation by the city of welfare institutions. Hospital data reflects spending for hospital facilities established or operated directly by city and township governments, the provision of health care, and support of other public or private hospitals. The Health category covers outpatient health services other than hospital care, including public health administration; research and education; categorical health programs; treatment and immunization clinics; nursing; environmental health activities (e.g., air and water pollution control); ambulance service provided separately from fire protection services; school health services provided by health agencies; other general public health activities (e.g., mosquito abatement). Health and hospital services provided directly by the city through its own hospitals and health agencies and any payments to other governments for such purposes are classed under those functional headings.

★ 421 ★

Government Spending: Local

Local Government Spending on Health Care in Alaska: 1990-1991

Local government spending for social service and income maintenance items is provided below. Data reflect city, urban town, and township government expenditures by function, thus grouping health-related activities (public welfare, hospitals, social insurance, and veterans' services) to provide a comprehensive picture of spending. Totals for these categories are not provided since they are meant only as presentational guidelines. According to the source: "Functions cannot be equated specifically with a single federal or state government program. Instead they represent broader activities of government that have remained virtually unchanged over many years so that as specific programs expand and contract they will remain useful for analytical purposes. Medicaid, for example, is a well-known program that is included in the larger public welfare function, specifically as a medical vendor payment, along with all other social welfare activities" (p. viii).

[Dollar amounts in thousands]

City	Social service and income maintenance expenditures		
	Public welfare	Hospitals	Health
Anchorage	-	-	29,060

Source: U.S. Bureau of the Census. *City Government Finances, 1990-1991.* Series GF/91-4. Washington, DC: U.S. Government Printing Office, 1993, p. 6. "Data in this report pertain to government fiscal years that ended between July 1, 1990, and June 30, 1991.... About three-fourths of all city governments in the nation had a fiscal year ending in either December (42 percent) or June (32 percent). September and April were the next most common months in which city governments ended their fiscal years. Of all townships, three-fifths had fiscal years corresponding directly with the calendar year 1990 (i.e., they ended their fiscal years on December 31, 1990). March, February, and June had the next most common fiscal year ending dates for townships" (p. vi). *Notes:* Detail may not add to total due to rounding. The Public Welfare heading covers the support of and assistance to needy persons contingent upon their need, excluding pensions to former employees and other benefits not contingent upon need. Among the expenditures in this category are: Cash assistance paid directly to needy persons under categorical programs (e.g., Old Age Assistance, Aid to Families With Dependent Children, Aid to the Blind, and Aid to the Disabled) or under any welfare programs; vendor payments made directly to private purveyors for medical care, burial, and other commodities and services provided under welfare programs; and provision and operation by the city of welfare institutions. Hospital data reflects spending for hospital facilities established or operated directly by city and township governments, the provision of health care, and support of other public or private hospitals. The Health category covers outpatient health services other than hospital care, including public health administration; research and education; categorical health programs; treatment and immunization clinics; nursing; environmental health activities (e.g., air and water pollution control); ambulance service provided separately from fire protection services; school health services provided by health agencies; other general public health activities (e.g., mosquito abatement). Health and hospital services provided directly by the city through its own hospitals and health agencies and any payments to other governments for such purposes are classed under those functional headings.

★ 422 ★

Government Spending: Local

Local Government Spending on Health Care in Arizona: 1990-1991

Local government spending for social service and income maintenance items is provided below. Data reflect city, urban town, and township government expenditures by function, thus grouping health-related activities (public welfare, hospitals, social insurance, and veterans' services) to provide a comprehensive picture of spending. Totals for these categories are not provided since they are meant only as presentational guidelines. According to the source: "Functions cannot be equated specifically with a single federal or state government program. Instead they represent broader activities of government that have remained virtually unchanged over many years so that as specific programs expand and contract they will remain useful for analytical purposes. Medicaid, for example, is a well-known program that is included in the larger public welfare function, specifically as a medical vendor payment, along with all other social welfare activities" (p. viii).

[Dollar amounts in thousands]

City	Social service and income maintenance expenditures		
	Public welfare	Hospitals	Health
Glendale	95	-	-
Mesa	191	-	-
Phoenix	1,531	-	1,716
Tempe	-	-	726
Tucson	2,031	-	897

Source: U.S. Bureau of the Census. *City Government Finances, 1990-1991.* Series GF/91-4. Washington, DC: U.S. Government Printing Office, 1993, p. 6-7. "Data in this report pertain to government fiscal years that ended between July 1, 1990, and June 30, 1991.... About three-fourths of all city governments in the nation had a fiscal year ending in either December (42 percent) or June (32 percent). September and April were the next most common months in which city governments ended their fiscal years. Of all townships, three-fifths had fiscal years corresponding directly with the calendar year 1990 (i.e., they ended their fiscal years on December 31, 1990). March, February, and June had the next most common fiscal year ending dates for townships" (p. vi). *Notes:* Detail may not add to total due to rounding. The Public Welfare heading covers the support of and assistance to needy persons contingent upon their need, excluding pensions to former employees and other benefits not contingent upon need. Among the expenditures in this category are: Cash assistance paid directly to needy persons under categorical programs (e.g., Old Age Assistance, Aid to Families With Dependent Children, Aid to the Blind, and Aid to the Disabled) or under any welfare programs; vendor payments made directly to private purveyors for medical care, burial, and other commodities and services provided under welfare programs; and provision and operation by the city of welfare institutions. Hospital data reflects spending for hospital facilities established or operated directly by city and township governments, the provision of health care, and support of other public or private hospitals. The Health category covers outpatient health services other than hospital care, including public health administration; research and education; categorical health programs; treatment and immunization clinics; nursing; environmental health activities (e.g., air and water pollution control); ambulance service provided separately from fire protection services; school health services provided by health agencies; other general public health activities (e.g., mosquito abatement). Health and hospital services provided directly by the city through its own hospitals and health agencies and any payments to other governments for such purposes are classed under those functional headings.

★ 423 ★

Government Spending: Local

Local Government Spending on Health Care in Arkansas: 1990-1991

Local government spending for social service and income maintenance items is provided below. Data reflect city, urban town, and township government expenditures by function, thus grouping health-related activities (public welfare, hospitals, social insurance, and veterans' services) to provide a comprehensive picture of spending. Totals for these categories are not provided since they are meant only as presentational guidelines. According to the source: "Functions cannot be equated specifically with a single federal or state government program. Instead they represent broader activities of government that have remained virtually unchanged over many years so that as specific programs expand and contract they will remain useful for analytical purposes. Medicaid, for example, is a well-known program that is included in the larger public welfare function, specifically as a medical vendor payment, along with all other social welfare activities" (p. viii).

[Dollar amounts in thousands]

City	Social service and income maintenance expenditures		
	Public welfare	Hospitals	Health
Little Rock	-	-	3,470

Source: U.S. Bureau of the Census, *City Government Finances, 1990-1991*, Series GF/91-4. Washington, DC: U.S. Government Printing Office, 1993, p. 7. "Data in this report pertain to government fiscal years that ended between July 1, 1990, and June 30, 1991.... About three-fourths of all city governments in the nation had a fiscal year ending in either December (42 percent) or June (32 percent). September and April were the next most common months in which city governments ended their fiscal years. Of all townships, three-fifths had fiscal years corresponding directly with the calendar year 1990 (i.e., they ended their fiscal years on December 31, 1990). March, February, and June had the next most common fiscal year ending dates for townships" (p. vi). *Notes:* Detail may not add to total due to rounding. The Public Welfare heading covers the support of and assistance to needy persons contingent upon their need, excluding pensions to former employees and other benefits not contingent upon need. Among the expenditures in this category are: Cash assistance paid directly to needy persons under categorical programs (e.g., Old Age Assistance, Aid to Families With Dependent Children, Aid to the Blind, and Aid to the Disabled) or under any welfare programs; vendor payments made directly to private purveyors for medical care, burial, and other commodities and services provided under welfare programs; and provision and operation by the city of welfare institutions. Hospital data reflects spending for hospital facilities established or operated directly by city and township governments, the provision of health care, and support of other public or private hospitals. The Health category covers outpatient health services other than hospital care, including public health administration; research and education; categorical health programs; treatment and immunization clinics; nursing; environmental health activities (e.g., air and water pollution control); ambulance service provided separately from fire protection services; school health services provided by health agencies; other general public health activities (e.g., mosquito abatement). Health and hospital services provided directly by the city through its own hospitals and health agencies and any payments to other governments for such purposes are classed under those functional headings.

★ 424 ★

Government Spending: Local

Local Government Spending on Health Care in California: 1990-1991

Local government spending for social service and income maintenance items is provided below. Data reflect city, urban town, and township government expenditures by function, thus grouping health-related activities (public welfare, hospitals, social insurance, and veterans' services) to provide a comprehensive picture of spending. Totals for these categories are not provided since they are meant only as presentational guidelines. According to the source: "Functions cannot be equated specifically with a single federal or state government program. Instead they represent broader activities of government that have remained virtually unchanged over many years so that as specific programs expand and contract they will remain useful for analytical purposes. Medicaid, for example, is a well-known program that is included in the larger public welfare function, specifically as a medical vendor payment, along with all other social welfare activities" (p. viii).

[Dollar amounts in thousands]

City	Social service and income maintenance expenditures		
	Public welfare	Hospitals	Health
Alameda	-	-	465
Alhambra	-	-	1,345
Anaheim	-	-	3,526
Berkeley	-	-	15,252
Burbank	-	-	3,170
Carson	-	-	94
Chula Vista	-	-	468
Compton	-	-	1,615
Concord	-	-	602
Corona	-	-	785
Costa Mesa	-	-	3,659
Daly City	-	-	93
Downey	-	-	1,082
El Cajon	-	-	1,419
El Monte	-	-	87
Escondido	-	-	974
Fontana	-	-	208
Fremont	-	-	1,638
Fullerton	-	-	916
Garden Grove	-	-	2,099
Glendale	-	-	825
Hayward	-	-	698
Huntington Beach	-	-	1,358
Inglewood	-	-	2,127
Irvine	-	-	742
Lakewood	-	-	60
Lancaster	-	-	184
Long Beach	-	-	15,340
Los Angeles	-	-	10,560

[Continued]

★ 424 ★

Local Government Spending on Health Care in California: 1990-1991

[Continued]

City	Social service and income maintenance expenditures		
	Public welfare	Hospitals	Health
Modesto	-	-	395
Moreno Valley	-	-	453
Norwalk	-	-	300
Oakland	1,268	-	5
Oceanside	-	-	4,002
Ontario	-	-	3,691
Orange	-	-	2,247
Pasadena	-	-	4,990
Pomona	-	-	694
Richmond	-	-	116
Riverside	-	-	982
Sacramento	-	-	1,899
Salinas	-	-	832
San Bernardino	-	-	689
San Diego	1,604	-	1,473
San Francisco	265,369	296,532	164,571
Santa Ana	-	-	1,173
Santa Barbara	-	-	736
Santa Clarita	-	-	103
Santa Monica	-	-	347
Santa Rosa	-	-	367
Simi Valley	-	-	602
South Gate	-	-	76
Stockton	-	-	581
Sunnyvale	-	-	13
Thousand Oaks	-	-	147
Torrance	-	-	2,919
Vallejo	-	-	358
Visalia	-	-	40
West Covina	-	-	1,113

[Continued]

★ 424 ★

Local Government Spending on Health Care in California: 1990-1991

[Continued]

City	Social service and income maintenance expenditures		
	Public welfare	Hospitals	Health
Westminister	-	-	1,777
Whittier	-	10	77

Source: U.S. Bureau of the Census. *City Government Finances, 1990-1991.* Series GF/91-4. Washington, DC: U.S. Government Printing Office, 1993, p. 7-15. "Data in this report pertain to government fiscal years that ended between July 1, 1990, and June 30, 1991.... About three-fourths of all city governments in the nation had a fiscal year ending in either December (42 percent) or June (32 percent). September and April were the next most common months in which city governments ended their fiscal years. Of all townships, three-fifths had fiscal years corresponding directly with the calendar year 1990 (i.e., they ended their fiscal years on December 31, 1990). March, February, and June had the next most common fiscal year ending dates for townships" (p. vi). *Notes:* Detail may not add to total due to rounding. The Public Welfare heading covers the support of and assistance to needy persons contingent upon their need, excluding pensions to former employees and other benefits not contingent upon need. Among the expenditures in this category are: Cash assistance paid directly to needy persons under categorical programs (e.g., Old Age Assistance, Aid to Families With Dependent Children, Aid to the Blind, and Aid to the Disabled) or under any welfare programs; vendor payments made directly to private purveyors for medical care, burial, and other commodities and services provided under welfare programs; and provision and operation by the city of welfare institutions. Hospital data reflects spending for hospital facilities established or operated directly by city and township governments, the provision of health care, and support of other public or private hospitals. The Health category covers outpatient health services other than hospital care, including public health administration; research and education; categorical health programs; treatment and immunization clinics; nursing; environmental health activities (e.g., air and water pollution control); ambulance service provided separately from fire protection services; school health services provided by health agencies; other general public health activities (e.g., mosquito abatement). Health and hospital services provided directly by the city through its own hospitals and health agencies and any payments to other governments for such purposes are classed under those functional headings.

★ 425 ★

Government Spending: Local

Local Government Spending on Health Care in Colorado: 1990-1991

Local government spending for social service and income maintenance items is provided below. Data reflect city, urban town, and township government expenditures by function, thus grouping health-related activities (public welfare, hospitals, social insurance, and veterans' services) to provide a comprehensive picture of spending. Totals for these categories are not provided since they are meant only as presentational guidelines. According to the source: "Functions cannot be equated specifically with a single federal or state government program. Instead they represent broader activities of government that have remained virtually unchanged over many years so that as specific programs expand and contract they will remain useful for analytical purposes. Medicaid, for example, is a well-known program that is included in the larger public welfare function, specifically as a medical vendor payment, along with all other social welfare activities" (p. viii).

[Dollar amounts in thousands]

City	Social service and income maintenance expenditures		
	Public welfare	Hospitals	Health
Arvada	216	-	-
Aurora	-	-	130
Boulder	2,011	-	-
Colorado Springs	-	89,901	545
Denver	102,851	80,862	44,100
Fort Collins	-	-	10
Lakewood	-	-	490
Pueblo	486	-	-

Source: U.S. Bureau of the Census. *City Government Finances, 1990-1991.* Series GF/91-4. Washington, DC: U.S. Government Printing Office, 1993, p. 16. "Data in this report pertain to government fiscal years that ended between July 1, 1990, and June 30, 1991.... About three-fourths of all city governments in the nation had a fiscal year ending in either December (42 percent) or June (32 percent). September and April were the next most common months in which city governments ended their fiscal years. Of all townships, three-fifths had fiscal years corresponding directly with the calendar year 1990 (i.e., they ended their fiscal years on December 31, 1990). March, February, and June had the next most common fiscal year ending dates for townships" (p. vi). *Notes:* Detail may not add to total due to rounding. The Public Welfare heading covers the support of and assistance to needy persons contingent upon their need, excluding pensions to former employees and other benefits not contingent upon need. Among the expenditures in this category are: Cash assistance paid directly to needy persons under categorical programs (e.g., Old Age Assistance, Aid to Families With Dependent Children, Aid to the Blind, and Aid to the Disabled) or under any welfare programs; vendor payments made directly to private purveyors for medical care, burial, and other commodities and services provided under welfare programs; and provision and operation by the city of welfare institutions. Hospital data reflects spending for hospital facilities established or operated directly by city and township governments, the provision of health care, and support of other public or private hospitals. The Health category covers outpatient health services other than hospital care, including public health administration; research and education; categorical health programs; treatment and immunization clinics; nursing; environmental health activities (e.g., air and water pollution control); ambulance service provided separately from fire protection services; school health services provided by health agencies; other general public health activities (e.g., mosquito abatement). Health and hospital services provided directly by the city through its own hospitals and health agencies and any payments to other governments for such purposes are classed under those functional headings.

★ 426 ★

Government Spending: Local

Local Government Spending on Health Care in Connecticut: 1990-1991

Local government spending for social service and income maintenance items is provided below. Data reflect city, urban town, and township government expenditures by function, thus grouping health-related activities (public welfare, hospitals, social insurance, and veterans' services) to provide a comprehensive picture of spending. Totals for these categories are not provided since they are meant only as presentational guidelines. According to the source: "Functions cannot be equated specifically with a single federal or state government program. Instead they represent broader activities of government that have remained virtually unchanged over many years so that as specific programs expand and contract they will remain useful for analytical purposes. Medicaid, for example, is a well-known program that is included in the larger public welfare function, specifically as a medical vendor payment, along with all other social welfare activities" (p. viii).

[Dollar amounts in thousands]

| City | Social service and income maintenance expenditures | | |
	Public welfare	Hospitals	Health
Bridgeport	24,118	-	6,120
Hartford	44,917	-	6,189
New Britain	3,567	-	3,254
New Haven	25,856	-	2,622
Norwalk	7,510	-	3,330
Stamford	14,350	-	4,857
Waterbury	10,593	-	3,734

Source: U.S. Bureau of the Census. *City Government Finances, 1990-1991.* Series GF/91-4. Washington, DC: U.S. Government Printing Office, 1993, p. 17. "Data in this report pertain to government fiscal years that ended between July 1, 1990, and June 30, 1991.... About three-fourths of all city governments in the nation had a fiscal year ending in either December (42 percent) or June (32 percent). September and April were the next most common months in which city governments ended their fiscal years. Of all townships, three-fifths had fiscal years corresponding directly with the calendar year 1990 (i.e., they ended their fiscal years on December 31, 1990). March, February, and June had the next most common fiscal year ending dates for townships" (p. vi). *Notes:* Detail may not add to total due to rounding. The Public Welfare heading covers the support of and assistance to needy persons contingent upon their need, excluding pensions to former employees and other benefits not contingent upon need. Among the expenditures in this category are: Cash assistance paid directly to needy persons under categorical programs (e.g., Old Age Assistance, Aid to Families With Dependent Children, Aid to the Blind, and Aid to the Disabled) or under any welfare programs; vendor payments made directly to private purveyors for medical care, burial, and other commodities and services provided under welfare programs; and provision and operation by the city of welfare institutions. Hospital data reflects spending for hospital facilities established or operated directly by city and township governments, the provision of health care, and support of other public or private hospitals. The Health category covers outpatient health services other than hospital care, including public health administration; research and education; categorical health programs; treatment and immunization clinics; nursing; environmental health activities (e.g., air and water pollution control); ambulance service provided separately from fire protection services; school health services provided by health agencies; other general public health activities (e.g., mosquito abatement). Health and hospital services provided directly by the city through its own hospitals and health agencies and any payments to other governments for such purposes are classed under those functional headings.

★ 427 ★

Government Spending: Local

Local Government Spending on Health Care in Delaware: 1990-1991

Local government spending for social service and income maintenance items is provided below. Data reflect city, urban town, and township government expenditures by function, thus grouping health-related activities (public welfare, hospitals, social insurance, and veterans' services) to provide a comprehensive picture of spending. Totals for these categories are not provided since they are meant only as presentational guidelines. According to the source: "Functions cannot be equated specifically with a single federal or state government program. Instead they represent broader activities of government that have remained virtually unchanged over many years so that as specific programs expand and contract they will remain useful for analytical purposes. Medicaid, for example, is a well-known program that is included in the larger public welfare function, specifically as a medical vendor payment, along with all other social welfare activities" (p. viii).

[Dollar amounts in thousands]

City	Social service and income maintenance expenditures		
	Public welfare	Hospitals	Health
Wilmington	55	-	-

Source: U.S. Bureau of the Census. *City Government Finances, 1990-1991.* Series GF/91-4. Washington, DC: U.S. Government Printing Office, 1993, p. 17. "Data in this report pertain to government fiscal years that ended between July 1, 1990, and June 30, 1991.... About three-fourths of all city governments in the nation had a fiscal year ending in either December (42 percent) or June (32 percent). September and April were the next most common months in which city governments ended their fiscal years. Of all townships, three-fifths had fiscal years corresponding directly with the calendar year 1990 (i.e., they ended their fiscal years on December 31, 1990). March, February, and June had the next most common fiscal year ending dates for townships" (p. vi). *Notes:* Detail may not add to total due to rounding. The Public Welfare heading covers the support of and assistance to needy persons contingent upon their need, excluding pensions to former employees and other benefits not contingent upon need. Among the expenditures in this category are: Cash assistance paid directly to needy persons under categorical programs (e.g., Old Age Assistance, Aid to Families With Dependent Children, Aid to the Blind, and Aid to the Disabled) or under any welfare programs; vendor payments made directly to private purveyors for medical care, burial, and other commodities and services provided under welfare programs; and provision and operation by the city of welfare institutions. Hospital data reflects spending for hospital facilities established or operated directly by city and township governments, the provision of health care, and support of other public or private hospitals. The Health category covers outpatient health services other than hospital care, including public health administration; research and education; categorical health programs; treatment and immunization clinics; nursing; environmental health activities (e.g., air and water pollution control); ambulance service provided separately from fire protection services; school health services provided by health agencies; other general public health activities (e.g., mosquito abatement). Health and hospital services provided directly by the city through its own hospitals and health agencies and any payments to other governments for such purposes are classed under those functional headings.

★ 428 ★

Government Spending: Local

Local Government Spending on Health Care in District of Columbia: 1990-1991

Local government spending for social service and income maintenance items is provided below. Data reflect city, urban town, and township government expenditures by function, thus grouping health-related activities (public welfare, hospitals, social insurance, and veterans' services) to provide a comprehensive picture of spending. Totals for these categories are not provided since they are meant only as presentational guidelines. According to the source: "Functions cannot be equated specifically with a single federal or state government program. Instead they represent broader activities of government that have remained virtually unchanged over many years so that as specific programs expand and contract they will remain useful for analytical purposes. Medicaid, for example, is a well-known program that is included in the larger public welfare function, specifically as a medical vendor payment, along with all other social welfare activities" (p. viii).

[Dollar amounts in thousands]

| City | Social service and income maintenance expenditures | | | |
	Public welfare	Hospitals	Health	Other
Washington	691,629	357,065	163,988	11,555

Source: U.S. Bureau of the Census. *City Government Finances, 1990-1991.* Series GF/91-4. Washington, DC: U.S. Government Printing Office, 1993, p. 18. "Data in this report pertain to government fiscal years that ended between July 1, 1990, and June 30, 1991.... About three-fourths of all city governments in the nation had a fiscal year ending in either December (42 percent) or June (32 percent). September and April were the next most common months in which city governments ended their fiscal years. Of all townships, three-fifths had fiscal years corresponding directly with the calendar year 1990 (i.e., they ended their fiscal years on December 31, 1990). March, February, and June had the next most common fiscal year ending dates for townships" (p. vi). *Notes:* Detail may not add to total due to rounding. The Public Welfare heading covers the support of and assistance to needy persons contingent upon their need, excluding pensions to former employees and other benefits not contingent upon need. Among the expenditures in this category are: Cash assistance paid directly to needy persons under categorical programs (e.g., Old Age Assistance, Aid to Families With Dependent Children, Aid to the Blind, and Aid to the Disabled) or under any welfare programs; vendor payments made directly to private purveyors for medical care, burial, and other commodities and services provided under welfare programs; and provision and operation by the city of welfare institutions. Hospital data reflects spending for hospital facilities established or operated directly by city and township governments, the provision of health care, and support of other public or private hospitals. The Health category covers outpatient health services other than hospital care, including public health administration; research and education; categorical health programs; treatment and immunization clinics; nursing; environmental health activities (e.g., air and water pollution control); ambulance service provided separately from fire protection services; school health services provided by health agencies; other general public health activities (e.g., mosquito abatement). Health and hospital services provided directly by the city through its own hospitals and health agencies and any payments to other governments for such purposes are classed under those functional headings.

★ 429 ★

Government Spending: Local

Local Government Spending on Health Care in Florida: 1990-1991

Local government spending for social service and income maintenance items is provided below. Data reflect city, urban town, and township government expenditures by function, thus grouping health-related activities (public welfare, hospitals, social insurance, and veterans' services) to provide a comprehensive picture of spending. Totals for these categories are not provided since they are meant only as presentational guidelines. According to the source: "Functions cannot be equated specifically with a single federal or state government program. Instead they represent broader activities of government that have remained virtually unchanged over many years so that as specific programs expand and contract they will remain useful for analytical purposes. Medicaid, for example, is a well-known program that is included in the larger public welfare function, specifically as a medical vendor payment, along with all other social welfare activities" (p. viii).

[Dollar amounts in thousands]

City	Social service and income maintenance expenditures		
	Public welfare	Hospitals	Health
Clearwater	-	-	1,699
Gainesville	17	-	102
Hollywood	197	-	3
Jacksonville	12,788	18,171	12,253
Miami	1,075	-	76
Miami Beach	59	20	5,322
St. Petersburg	-	-	4,117
Tallahassee	223	127	130
Tampa	-	-	3,694

Source. U.S. Bureau of the Census. *City Government Finances, 1990-1991.* Series GF/91-4. Washington, DC: U.S. Government Printing Office, 1993, p. 18-19. "Data in this report pertain to government fiscal years that ended between July 1, 1990, and June 30, 1991.... About three-fourths of all city governments in the nation had a fiscal year ending in either December (42 percent) or June (32 percent). September and April were the next most common months in which city governments ended their fiscal years. Of all townships, three-fifths had fiscal years corresponding directly with the calendar year 1990 (i.e., they ended their fiscal years on December 31, 1990). March, February, and June had the next most common fiscal year ending dates for townships" (p. vi). *Notes:* Detail may not add to total due to rounding. The Public Welfare heading covers the support of and assistance to needy persons contingent upon their need, excluding pensions to former employees and other benefits not contingent upon need. Among the expenditures in this category are: Cash assistance paid directly to needy persons under categorical programs (e.g., Old Age Assistance, Aid to Families With Dependent Children, Aid to the Blind, and Aid to the Disabled) or under any welfare programs; vendor payments made directly to private purveyors for medical care, burial, and other commodities and services provided under welfare programs; and provision and operation by the city of welfare institutions. Hospital data reflects spending for hospital facilities established or operated directly by city and township governments, the provision of health care, and support of other public or private hospitals. The Health category covers outpatient health services other than hospital care, including public health administration; research and education; categorical health programs; treatment and immunization clinics; nursing; environmental health activities (e.g., air and water pollution control); ambulance service provided separately from fire protection services; school health services provided by health agencies; other general public health activities (e.g., mosquito abatement). Health and hospital services provided directly by the city through its own hospitals and health agencies and any payments to other governments for such purposes are classed under those functional headings.

★ 430 ★

Government Spending: Local

Local Government Spending on Health Care in Georgia: 1990-1991

Local government spending for social service and income maintenance items is provided below. Data reflect city, urban town, and township government expenditures by function, thus grouping health-related activities (public welfare, hospitals, social insurance, and veterans' services) to provide a comprehensive picture of spending. Totals for these categories are not provided since they are meant only as presentational guidelines. According to the source: "Functions cannot be equated specifically with a single federal or state government program. Instead they represent broader activities of government that have remained virtually unchanged over many years so that as specific programs expand and contract they will remain useful for analytical purposes. Medicaid, for example, is a well-known program that is included in the larger public welfare function, specifically as a medical vendor payment, along with all other social welfare activities" (p. viii).

[Dollar amounts in thousands]

| City | Social service and income maintenance expenditures | | |
	Public welfare	Hospitals	Health
Atlanta	470	-	-
Columbus	5,657	-	2,760
Savannah	788	-	-

Source: U.S. Bureau of the Census. *City Government Finances, 1990-1991.* Series GF/91-4. Washington, DC: U.S. Government Printing Office, 1993, p. 19-20. "Data in this report pertain to government fiscal years that ended between July 1, 1990, and June 30, 1991.... About three-fourths of all city governments in the nation had a fiscal year ending in either December (42 percent) or June (32 percent). September and April were the next most common months in which city governments ended their fiscal years. Of all townships, three-fifths had fiscal years corresponding directly with the calendar year 1990 (i.e., they ended their fiscal years on December 31, 1990). March, February, and June had the next most common fiscal year ending dates for townships" (p. vi). *Notes:* Detail may not add to total due to rounding. The Public Welfare heading covers the support of and assistance to needy persons contingent upon their need, excluding pensions to former employees and other benefits not contingent upon need. Among the expenditures in this category are: Cash assistance paid directly to needy persons under categorical programs (e.g., Old Age Assistance, Aid to Families With Dependent Children, Aid to the Blind, and Aid to the Disabled) or under any welfare programs; vendor payments made directly to private purveyors for medical care, burial, and other commodities and services provided under welfare programs; and provision and operation by the city of welfare institutions. Hospital data reflects spending for hospital facilities established or operated directly by city and township governments, the provision of health care, and support of other public or private hospitals. The Health category covers outpatient health services other than hospital care, including public health administration; research and education; categorical health programs; treatment and immunization clinics; nursing; environmental health activities (e.g., air and water pollution control); ambulance service provided separately from fire protection services; school health services provided by health agencies; other general public health activities (e.g., mosquito abatement). Health and hospital services provided directly by the city through its own hospitals and health agencies and any payments to other governments for such purposes are classed under those functional headings.

★ 431 ★

Government Spending: Local

Local Government Spending on Health Care in Hawaii: 1990-1991

Local government spending for social service and income maintenance items is provided below. Data reflect city, urban town, and township government expenditures by function, thus grouping health-related activities (public welfare, hospitals, social insurance, and veterans' services) to provide a comprehensive picture of spending. Totals for these categories are not provided since they are meant only as presentational guidelines. According to the source: "Functions cannot be equated specifically with a single federal or state government program. Instead they represent broader activities of government that have remained virtually unchanged over many years so that as specific programs expand and contract they will remain useful for analytical purposes. Medicaid, for example, is a well-known program that is included in the larger public welfare function, specifically as a medical vendor payment, along with all other social welfare activities" (p. viii).

[Dollar amounts in thousands]

City	Social service and income maintenance expenditures		
	Public welfare	Hospitals	Health
Honolulu	-	-	9,647

Source: U.S. Bureau of the Census. *City Government Finances, 1990-1991.* Series GF/91-4. Washington, DC: U.S. Government Printing Office, 1993, p. 20. "Data in this report pertain to government fiscal years that ended between July 1, 1990, and June 30, 1991.... About three-fourths of all city governments in the nation had a fiscal year ending in either December (42 percent) or June (32 percent). September and April were the next most common months in which city governments ended their fiscal years. Of all townships, three-fifths had fiscal years corresponding directly with the calendar year 1990 (i.e., they ended their fiscal years on December 31, 1990). March, February, and June had the next most common fiscal year ending dates for townships" (p. vi). *Notes:* Detail may not add to total due to rounding. The Public Welfare heading covers the support of and assistance to needy persons contingent upon their need, excluding pensions to former employees and other benefits not contingent upon need. Among the expenditures in this category are: Cash assistance paid directly to needy persons under categorical programs (e.g., Old Age Assistance, Aid to Families With Dependent Children, Aid to the Blind, and Aid to the Disabled) or under any welfare programs; vendor payments made directly to private purveyors for medical care, burial, and other commodities and services provided under welfare programs; and provision and operation by the city of welfare institutions. Hospital data reflects spending for hospital facilities established or operated directly by city and township governments, the provision of health care, and support of other public or private hospitals. The Health category covers outpatient health services other than hospital care, including public health administration; research and education; categorical health programs; treatment and immunization clinics; nursing; environmental health activities (e.g., air and water pollution control); ambulance service provided separately from fire protection services; school health services provided by health agencies; other general public health activities (e.g., mosquito abatement). Health and hospital services provided directly by the city through its own hospitals and health agencies and any payments to other governments for such purposes are classed under those functional headings.

★ 432 ★

Government Spending: Local

Local Government Spending on Health Care in Idaho: 1990-1991

Local government spending for social service and income maintenance items is provided below. Data reflect city, urban town, and township government expenditures by function, thus grouping health-related activities (public welfare, hospitals, social insurance, and veterans' services) to provide a comprehensive picture of spending. Totals for these categories are not provided since they are meant only as presentational guidelines. According to the source: "Functions cannot be equated specifically with a single federal or state government program. Instead they represent broader activities of government that have remained virtually unchanged over many years so that as specific programs expand and contract they will remain useful for analytical purposes. Medicaid, for example, is a well-known program that is included in the larger public welfare function, specifically as a medical vendor payment, along with all other social welfare activities" (p. viii).

[Dollar amounts in thousands]

City	Social service and income maintenance expenditures		
	Public welfare	Hospitals	Health
Boise City	-	-	308

Source: U.S. Bureau of the Census. *City Government Finances, 1990-1991.* Series GF/91-4. Washington, DC: U.S. Government Printing Office, 1993, p. 20. "Data in this report pertain to government fiscal years that ended between July 1, 1990, and June 30, 1991.... About three-fourths of all city governments in the nation had a fiscal year ending in either December (42 percent) or June (32 percent). September and April were the next most common months in which city governments ended their fiscal years. Of all townships, three-fifths had fiscal years corresponding directly with the calendar year 1990 (i.e., they ended their fiscal years on December 31, 1990). March, February, and June had the next most common fiscal year ending dates for townships" (p. vi). *Notes:* Detail may not add to total due to rounding. The Public Welfare heading covers the support of and assistance to needy persons contingent upon their need, excluding pensions to former employees and other benefits not contingent upon need. Among the expenditures in this category are: Cash assistance paid directly to needy persons under categorical programs (e.g., Old Age Assistance, Aid to Families With Dependent Children, Aid to the Blind, and Aid to the Disabled) or under any welfare programs; vendor payments made directly to private purveyors for medical care, burial, and other commodities and services provided under welfare programs; and provision and operation by the city of welfare institutions. Hospital data reflects spending for hospital facilities established or operated directly by city and township governments, the provision of health care, and support of other public or private hospitals. The Health category covers outpatient health services other than hospital care, including public health administration; research and education; categorical health programs; treatment and immunization clinics; nursing; environmental health activities (e.g., air and water pollution control); ambulance service provided separately from fire protection services; school health services provided by health agencies; other general public health activities (e.g., mosquito abatement). Health and hospital services provided directly by the city through its own hospitals and health agencies and any payments to other governments for such purposes are classed under those functional headings.

★ 433 ★

Government Spending: Local

Local Government Spending on Health Care in Illinois: 1990-1991

Local government spending for social service and income maintenance items is provided below. Data reflect city, urban town, and township government expenditures by function, thus grouping health-related activities (public welfare, hospitals, social insurance, and veterans' services) to provide a comprehensive picture of spending. Totals for these categories are not provided since they are meant only as presentational guidelines. According to the source: "Functions cannot be equated specifically with a single federal or state government program. Instead they represent broader activities of government that have remained virtually unchanged over many years so that as specific programs expand and contract they will remain useful for analytical purposes. Medicaid, for example, is a well-known program that is included in the larger public welfare function, specifically as a medical vendor payment, along with all other social welfare activities" (p. viii).

[Dollar amounts in thousands]

City	Social service and income maintenance expenditures		
	Public welfare	Hospitals	Health
Arlington Heights	-	-	1,141
Aurora	-	-	231
Chicago	96,545	-	84,623
Peoria	-	-	76
Rockford	3,621	-	40
Springfield	-	-	2,658

Source: U.S. Bureau of the Census. *City Government Finances, 1990-1991.* Series GF/91-4. Washington, DC: U.S. Government Printing Office, 1993, p. 20-21. "Data in this report pertain to government fiscal years that ended between July 1, 1990, and June 30, 1991.... About three-fourths of all city governments in the nation had a fiscal year ending in either December (42 percent) or June (32 percent). September and April were the next most common months in which city governments ended their fiscal years. Of all townships, three-fifths had fiscal years corresponding directly with the calendar year 1990 (i.e., they ended their fiscal years on December 31, 1990). March, February, and June had the next most common fiscal year ending dates for townships" (p. vi). *Notes:* Detail may not add to total due to rounding. The Public Welfare heading covers the support of and assistance to needy persons contingent upon their need, excluding pensions to former employees and other benefits not contingent upon need. Among the expenditures in this category are: Cash assistance paid directly to needy persons under categorical programs (e.g., Old Age Assistance, Aid to Families With Dependent Children, Aid to the Blind, and Aid to the Disabled) or under any welfare programs; vendor payments made directly to private purveyors for medical care, burial, and other commodities and services provided under welfare programs; and provision and operation by the city of welfare institutions. Hospital data reflects spending for hospital facilities established or operated directly by city and township governments, the provision of health care, and support of other public or private hospitals. The Health category covers outpatient health services other than hospital care, including public health administration; research and education; categorical health programs; treatment and immunization clinics; nursing; environmental health activities (e.g., air and water pollution control); ambulance service provided separately from fire protection services; school health services provided by health agencies; other general public health activities (e.g., mosquito abatement). Health and hospital services provided directly by the city through its own hospitals and health agencies and any payments to other governments for such purposes are classed under those functional headings.

★ 434 ★

Government Spending: Local

Local Government Spending on Health Care in Indiana: 1990-1991

Local government spending for social service and income maintenance items is provided below. Data reflect city, urban town, and township government expenditures by function, thus grouping health-related activities (public welfare, hospitals, social insurance, and veterans' services) to provide a comprehensive picture of spending. Totals for these categories are not provided since they are meant only as presentational guidelines. According to the source: "Functions cannot be equated specifically with a single federal or state government program. Instead they represent broader activities of government that have remained virtually unchanged over many years so that as specific programs expand and contract they will remain useful for analytical purposes. Medicaid, for example, is a well-known program that is included in the larger public welfare function, specifically as a medical vendor payment, along with all other social welfare activities" (p. viii).

[Dollar amounts in thousands]

| City | Social service and income maintenance expenditures | | |
	Public welfare	Hospitals	Health
Evansville	-	-	3,067
Fort Wayne	-	-	794
Gary	-	-	4,433
Hammond	-	-	763
Indianapolis	65,984	127,348	28,769
South Bend	-	-	615

Source: U.S. Bureau of the Census. *City Government Finances, 1990-1991.* Series GF/91-4. Washington, DC: U.S. Government Printing Office, 1993, p. 21-22. "Data in this report pertain to government fiscal years that ended between July 1, 1990, and June 30, 1991.... About three-fourths of all city governments in the nation had a fiscal year ending in either December (42 percent) or June (32 percent). September and April were the next most common months in which city governments ended their fiscal years. Of all townships, three-fifths had fiscal years corresponding directly with the calendar year 1990 (i.e., they ended their fiscal years on December 31, 1990). March, February, and June had the next most common fiscal year ending dates for townships" (p. vi). *Notes:* Detail may not add to total due to rounding. The Public Welfare heading covers the support of and assistance to needy persons contingent upon their need, excluding pensions to former employees and other benefits not contingent upon need. Among the expenditures in this category are: Cash assistance paid directly to needy persons under categorical programs (e.g., Old Age Assistance, Aid to Families With Dependent Children, Aid to the Blind, and Aid to the Disabled) or under any welfare programs; vendor payments made directly to private purveyors for medical care, burial, and other commodities and services provided under welfare programs; and provision and operation by the city of welfare institutions. Hospital data reflects spending for hospital facilities established or operated directly by city and township governments, the provision of health care, and support of other public or private hospitals. The Health category covers outpatient health services other than hospital care, including public health administration; research and education; categorical health programs; treatment and immunization clinics; nursing; environmental health activities (e.g., air and water pollution control); ambulance service provided separately from fire protection services; school health services provided by health agencies; other general public health activities (e.g., mosquito abatement). Health and hospital services provided directly by the city through its own hospitals and health agencies and any payments to other governments for such purposes are classed under those functional headings.

★ 435 ★

Government Spending: Local

Local Government Spending on Health Care in Iowa: 1990-1991

Local government spending for social service and income maintenance items is provided below. Data reflect city, urban town, and township government expenditures by function, thus grouping health-related activities (public welfare, hospitals, social insurance, and veterans' services) to provide a comprehensive picture of spending. Totals for these categories are not provided since they are meant only as presentational guidelines. According to the source: "Functions cannot be equated specifically with a single federal or state government program. Instead they represent broader activities of government that have remained virtually unchanged over many years so that as specific programs expand and contract they will remain useful for analytical purposes. Medicaid, for example, is a well-known program that is included in the larger public welfare function, specifically as a medical vendor payment, along with all other social welfare activities" (p. viii).

[Dollar amounts in thousands]

City	Social service and income maintenance expenditures		
	Public welfare	Hospitals	Health
Cedar Rapids	-	-	3,664
Davenport	317	-	1,363
Des Moines	2,859	-	1,696
Sioux City	-	-	153

Source: U.S. Bureau of the Census. *City Government Finances, 1990-1991.* Series GF/91-4. Washington, DC: U.S. Government Printing Office, 1993, p. 22. "Data in this report pertain to government fiscal years that ended between July 1, 1990, and June 30, 1991.... About three-fourths of all city governments in the nation had a fiscal year ending in either December (42 percent) or June (32 percent). September and April were the next most common months in which city governments ended their fiscal years. Of all townships, three-fifths had fiscal years corresponding directly with the calendar year 1990 (i.e., they ended their fiscal years on December 31, 1990). March, February, and June had the next most common fiscal year ending dates for townships" (p. vi). *Notes:* Detail may not add to total due to rounding. The Public Welfare heading covers the support of and assistance to needy persons contingent upon their need, excluding pensions to former employees and other benefits not contingent upon need. Among the expenditures in this category are: Cash assistance paid directly to needy persons under categorical programs (e.g., Old Age Assistance, Aid to Families With Dependent Children, Aid to the Blind, and Aid to the Disabled) or under any welfare programs; vendor payments made directly to private purveyors for medical care, burial, and other commodities and services provided under welfare programs; and provision and operation by the city of welfare institutions. Hospital data reflects spending for hospital facilities established or operated directly by city and township governments, the provision of health care, and support of other public or private hospitals. The Health category covers outpatient health services other than hospital care, including public health administration; research and education; categorical health programs; treatment and immunization clinics; nursing; environmental health activities (e.g., air and water pollution control); ambulance service provided separately from fire protection services; school health services provided by health agencies; other general public health activities (e.g., mosquito abatement). Health and hospital services provided directly by the city through its own hospitals and health agencies and any payments to other governments for such purposes are classed under those functional headings.

★ 436 ★

Government Spending: Local

Local Government Spending on Health Care in Kansas: 1990-1991

Local government spending for social service and income maintenance items is provided below. Data reflect city, urban town, and township government expenditures by function, thus grouping health-related activities (public welfare, hospitals, social insurance, and veterans' services) to provide a comprehensive picture of spending. Totals for these categories are not provided since they are meant only as presentational guidelines. According to the source: "Functions cannot be equated specifically with a single federal or state government program. Instead they represent broader activities of government that have remained virtually unchanged over many years so that as specific programs expand and contract they will remain useful for analytical purposes. Medicaid, for example, is a well-known program that is included in the larger public welfare function, specifically as a medical vendor payment, along with all other social welfare activities" (p. viii).

[Dollar amounts in thousands]

City	Social service and income maintenance expenditures		
	Public welfare	Hospitals	Health
Kansas City	-	-	1,134
Overland Park	671	-	204
Topeka	-	-	6,040
Wichita	-	-	1,413

Source: U.S. Bureau of the Census. *City Government Finances, 1990-1991.* Series GF/91-4. Washington, DC: U.S. Government Printing Office, 1993, p. 23. "Data in this report pertain to government fiscal years that ended between July 1, 1990, and June 30, 1991.... About three-fourths of all city governments in the nation had a fiscal year ending in either December (42 percent) or June (32 percent). September and April were the next most common months in which city governments ended their fiscal years. Of all townships, three-fifths had fiscal years corresponding directly with the calendar year 1990 (i.e., they ended their fiscal years on December 31, 1990). March, February, and June had the next most common fiscal year ending dates for townships" (p. vi). *Notes:* Detail may not add to total due to rounding. The Public Welfare heading covers the support of and assistance to needy persons contingent upon their need, excluding pensions to former employees and other benefits not contingent upon need. Among the expenditures in this category are: Cash assistance paid directly to needy persons under categorical programs (e.g., Old Age Assistance, Aid to Families With Dependent Children, Aid to the Blind, and Aid to the Disabled) or under any welfare programs; vendor payments made directly to private purveyors for medical care, burial, and other commodities and services provided under welfare programs; and provision and operation by the city of welfare institutions. Hospital data reflects spending for hospital facilities established or operated directly by city and township governments, the provision of health care, and support of other public or private hospitals. The Health category covers outpatient health services other than hospital care, including public health administration; research and education; categorical health programs; treatment and immunization clinics; nursing; environmental health activities (e.g., air and water pollution control); ambulance service provided separately from fire protection services; school health services provided by health agencies; other general public health activities (e.g., mosquito abatement). Health and hospital services provided directly by the city through its own hospitals and health agencies and any payments to other governments for such purposes are classed under those functional headings.

★ 437 ★

Government Spending: Local

Local Government Spending on Health Care in Kentucky: 1990-1991

Local government spending for social service and income maintenance items is provided below. Data reflect city, urban town, and township government expenditures by function, thus grouping health-related activities (public welfare, hospitals, social insurance, and veterans' services) to provide a comprehensive picture of spending. Totals for these categories are not provided since they are meant only as presentational guidelines. According to the source: "Functions cannot be equated specifically with a single federal or state government program. Instead they represent broader activities of government that have remained virtually unchanged over many years so that as specific programs expand and contract they will remain useful for analytical purposes. Medicaid, for example, is a well-known program that is included in the larger public welfare function, specifically as a medical vendor payment, along with all other social welfare activities" (p. viii).

[Dollar amounts in thousands]

City	Social service and income maintenance expenditures		
	Public welfare	Hospitals	Health
Lexington-Fayette	6,568	-	11,292
Louisville	10,101	2,841	4,031

Source: U.S. Bureau of the Census. *City Government Finances, 1990-1991.* Series GF/91-4. Washington, DC: U.S. Government Printing Office, 1993, p. 23. "Data in this report pertain to government fiscal years that ended between July 1, 1990, and June 30, 1991.... About three-fourths of all city governments in the nation had a fiscal year ending in either December (42 percent) or June (32 percent). September and April were the next most common months in which city governments ended their fiscal years. Of all townships, three-fifths had fiscal years corresponding directly with the calendar year 1990 (i.e., they ended their fiscal years on December 31, 1990). March, February, and June had the next most common fiscal year ending dates for townships" (p. vi). *Notes:* Detail may not add to total due to rounding. The Public Welfare heading covers the support of and assistance to needy persons contingent upon their need, excluding pensions to former employees and other benefits not contingent upon need. Among the expenditures in this category are: Cash assistance paid directly to needy persons under categorical programs (e.g., Old Age Assistance, Aid to Families With Dependent Children, Aid to the Blind, and Aid to the Disabled) or under any welfare programs; vendor payments made directly to private purveyors for medical care, burial, and other commodities and services provided under welfare programs; and provision and operation by the city of welfare institutions. Hospital data reflects spending for hospital facilities established or operated directly by city and township governments, the provision of health care, and support of other public or private hospitals. The Health category covers outpatient health services other than hospital care, including public health administration; research and education; categorical health programs; treatment and immunization clinics; nursing; environmental health activities (e.g., air and water pollution control); ambulance service provided separately from fire protection services; school health services provided by health agencies; other general public health activities (e.g., mosquito abatement). Health and hospital services provided directly by the city through its own hospitals and health agencies and any payments to other governments for such purposes are classed under those functional headings.

★ 438 ★

Government Spending: Local

Local Government Spending on Health Care in Louisiana: 1990-1991

Local government spending for social service and income maintenance items is provided below. Data reflect city, urban town, and township government expenditures by function, thus grouping health-related activities (public welfare, hospitals, social insurance, and veterans' services) to provide a comprehensive picture of spending. Totals for these categories are not provided since they are meant only as presentational guidelines. According to the source: "Functions cannot be equated specifically with a single federal or state government program. Instead they represent broader activities of government that have remained virtually unchanged over many years so that as specific programs expand and contract they will remain useful for analytical purposes. Medicaid, for example, is a well-known program that is included in the larger public welfare function, specifically as a medical vendor payment, along with all other social welfare activities" (p. viii).

[Dollar amounts in thousands]

City	Social service and income maintenance expenditures		
	Public welfare	Hospitals	Health
Baton Rouge	1,083	22,232	5,746
Kenner	477	-	-
Lafayette	122	-	680
New Orleans	20,112	-	12,569
Terrebonne Parish Consolidated Government	298	49,611	1,065

Source: U.S. Bureau of the Census. *City Government Finances, 1990-1991.* Series GF/91-4. Washington, DC: U.S. Government Printing Office, 1993, p. 23-24. "Data in this report pertain to government fiscal years that ended between July 1, 1990, and June 30, 1991.... About three-fourths of all city governments in the nation had a fiscal year ending in either December (42 percent) or June (32 percent). September and April were the next most common months in which city governments ended their fiscal years. Of all townships, three-fifths had fiscal years corresponding directly with the calendar year 1990 (i.e., they ended their fiscal years on December 31, 1990). March, February, and June had the next most common fiscal year ending dates for townships" (p. vi). *Notes:* Detail may not add to total due to rounding. The Public Welfare heading covers the support of and assistance to needy persons contingent upon their need, excluding pensions to former employees and other benefits not contingent upon need. Among the expenditures in this category are: Cash assistance paid directly to needy persons under categorical programs (e.g., Old Age Assistance, Aid to Families With Dependent Children, Aid to the Blind, and Aid to the Disabled) or under any welfare programs; vendor payments made directly to private purveyors for medical care, burial, and other commodities and services provided under welfare programs; and provision and operation by the city of welfare institutions. Hospital data reflects spending for hospital facilities established or operated directly by city and township governments, the provision of health care, and support of other public or private hospitals. The Health category covers outpatient health services other than hospital care, including public health administration; research and education; categorical health programs; treatment and immunization clinics; nursing; environmental health activities (e.g., air and water pollution control); ambulance service provided separately from fire protection services; school health services provided by health agencies; other general public health activities (e.g., mosquito abatement). Health and hospital services provided directly by the city through its own hospitals and health agencies and any payments to other governments for such purposes are classed under those functional headings.

★ 439 ★

Government Spending: Local

Local Government Spending on Health Care in Maine: 1990-1991

Local government spending for social service and income maintenance items is provided below. Data reflect city, urban town, and township government expenditures by function, thus grouping health-related activities (public welfare, hospitals, social insurance, and veterans' services) to provide a comprehensive picture of spending. Totals for these categories are not provided since they are meant only as presentational guidelines. According to the source: "Functions cannot be equated specifically with a single federal or state government program. Instead they represent broader activities of government that have remained virtually unchanged over many years so that as specific programs expand and contract they will remain useful for analytical purposes. Medicaid, for example, is a well-known program that is included in the larger public welfare function, specifically as a medical vendor payment, along with all other social welfare activities" (p. viii).

[Dollar amounts in thousands]

City	Social service and income maintenance expenditures		
	Public welfare	Hospitals	Health
Portland	7,130	7,187	942

Source: U.S. Bureau of the Census. *City Government Finances, 1990-1991.* Series GF/91-4. Washington, DC: U.S. Government Printing Office, 1993, p. 24. "Data in this report pertain to government fiscal years that ended between July 1, 1990, and June 30, 1991.... About three-fourths of all city governments in the nation had a fiscal year ending in either December (42 percent) or June (32 percent). September and April were the next most common months in which city governments ended their fiscal years. Of all townships, three-fifths had fiscal years corresponding directly with the calendar year 1990 (i.e., they ended their fiscal years on December 31, 1990). March, February, and June had the next most common fiscal year ending dates for townships" (p. vi). *Notes:* Detail may not add to total due to rounding. The Public Welfare heading covers the support of and assistance to needy persons contingent upon their need, excluding pensions to former employees and other benefits not contingent upon need. Among the expenditures in this category are: Cash assistance paid directly to needy persons under categorical programs (e.g., Old Age Assistance, Aid to Families With Dependent Children, Aid to the Blind, and Aid to the Disabled) or under any welfare programs; vendor payments made directly to private purveyors for medical care, burial, and other commodities and services provided under welfare programs; and provision and operation by the city of welfare institutions. Hospital data reflects spending for hospital facilities established or operated directly by city and township governments, the provision of health care, and support of other public or private hospitals. The Health category covers outpatient health services other than hospital care, including public health administration; research and education; categorical health programs; treatment and immunization clinics; nursing; environmental health activities (e.g., air and water pollution control); ambulance service provided separately from fire protection services; school health services provided by health agencies; other general public health activities (e.g., mosquito abatement). Health and hospital services provided directly by the city through its own hospitals and health agencies and any payments to other governments for such purposes are classed under those functional headings.

★ 440 ★

Government Spending: Local

Local Government Spending on Health Care in Maryland: 1990-1991

Local government spending for social service and income maintenance items is provided below. Data reflect city, urban town, and township government expenditures by function, thus grouping health-related activities (public welfare, hospitals, social insurance, and veterans' services) to provide a comprehensive picture of spending. Totals for these categories are not provided since they are meant only as presentational guidelines. According to the source: "Functions cannot be equated specifically with a single federal or state government program. Instead they represent broader activities of government that have remained virtually unchanged over many years so that as specific programs expand and contract they will remain useful for analytical purposes. Medicaid, for example, is a well-known program that is included in the larger public welfare function, specifically as a medical vendor payment, along with all other social welfare activities" (p. viii).

[Dollar amounts in thousands]

City	Social service and income maintenance expenditures		
	Public welfare	Hospitals	Health
Baltimore	1,775	-	55,847

Source: U.S. Bureau of the Census. *City Government Finances, 1990-1991.* Series GF/91-4. Washington, DC: U.S. Government Printing Office, 1993, p. 24. "Data in this report pertain to government fiscal years that ended between July 1, 1990, and June 30, 1991.... About three-fourths of all city governments in the nation had a fiscal year ending in either December (42 percent) or June (32 percent). September and April were the next most common months in which city governments ended their fiscal years. Of all townships, three-fifths had fiscal years corresponding directly with the calendar year 1990 (i.e., they ended their fiscal years on December 31, 1990). March, February, and June had the next most common fiscal year ending dates for townships" (p. vi). *Notes:* Detail may not add to total due to rounding. The Public Welfare heading covers the support of and assistance to needy persons contingent upon their need, excluding pensions to former employees and other benefits not contingent upon need. Among the expenditures in this category are: Cash assistance paid directly to needy persons under categorical programs (e.g., Old Age Assistance, Aid to Families With Dependent Children, Aid to the Blind, and Aid to the Disabled) or under any welfare programs; vendor payments made directly to private purveyors for medical care, burial, and other commodities and services provided under welfare programs; and provision and operation by the city of welfare institutions. Hospital data reflects spending for hospital facilities established or operated directly by city and township governments, the provision of health care, and support of other public or private hospitals. The Health category covers outpatient health services other than hospital care, including public health administration; research and education; categorical health programs; treatment and immunization clinics; nursing; environmental health activities (e.g., air and water pollution control); ambulance service provided separately from fire protection services; school health services provided by health agencies; other general public health activities (e.g., mosquito abatement). Health and hospital services provided directly by the city through its own hospitals and health agencies and any payments to other governments for such purposes are classed under those functional headings.

Government Spending: Local

Local Government Spending on Health Care in Massachusetts: 1990-1991

Local government spending for social service and income maintenance items is provided below. Data reflect city, urban town, and township government expenditures by function, thus grouping health-related activities (public welfare, hospitals, social insurance, and veterans' services) to provide a comprehensive picture of spending. Totals for these categories are not provided since they are meant only as presentational guidelines. According to the source: "Functions cannot be equated specifically with a single federal or state government program. Instead they represent broader activities of government that have remained virtually unchanged over many years so that as specific programs expand and contract they will remain useful for analytical purposes. Medicaid, for example, is a well-known program that is included in the larger public welfare function, specifically as a medical vendor payment, along with all other social welfare activities" (p. viii).

[Dollar amounts in thousands]

City	Social service and income maintenance expenditures		
	Public welfare	Hospitals	Health
Boston	126,648	230,806	322
Brockton	923	-	358
Cambridge	8,653	50,158	792
Fall River	1,101	342	2,339
Lowell	806	-	1,179
Lynn	5,450	-	747
New Bedford	657	-	1,854
Newton	105	-	832
Quincy	404	83,189	429
Somerville	216	-	649

[Continued]

★ 441 ★

Local Government Spending on Health Care in Massachusetts: 1990-1991
[Continued]

City	Social service and income maintenance expenditures		
	Public welfare	Hospitals	Health
Springfield	581	15,362	1,149
Worcester	7,401	7,087	3,538

Source: U.S. Bureau of the Census. *City Government Finances, 1990-1991.* Series GF/91-4. Washington, DC: U.S. Government Printing Office, 1993, p. 24-26. "Data in this report pertain to government fiscal years that ended between July 1, 1990, and June 30, 1991.... About three-fourths of all city governments in the nation had a fiscal year ending in either December (42 percent) or June (32 percent). September and April were the next most common months in which city governments ended their fiscal years. Of all townships, three-fifths had fiscal years corresponding directly with the calendar year 1990 (i.e., they ended their fiscal years on December 31, 1990). March, February, and June had the next most common fiscal year ending dates for townships" (p. vi). *Notes:* Detail may not add to total due to rounding. The Public Welfare heading covers the support of and assistance to needy persons contingent upon their need, excluding pensions to former employees and other benefits not contingent upon need. Among the expenditures in this category are: Cash assistance paid directly to needy persons under categorical programs (e.g., Old Age Assistance, Aid to Families With Dependent Children, Aid to the Blind, and Aid to the Disabled) or under any welfare programs; vendor payments made directly to private purveyors for medical care, burial, and other commodities and services provided under welfare programs; and provision and operation by the city of welfare institutions. Hospital data reflects spending for hospital facilities established or operated directly by city and township governments, the provision of health care, and support of other public or private hospitals. The Health category covers outpatient health services other than hospital care, including public health administration; research and education; categorical health programs; treatment and immunization clinics; nursing; environmental health activities (e.g., air and water pollution control); ambulance service provided separately from fire protection services; school health services provided by health agencies; other general public health activities (e.g., mosquito abatement). Health and hospital services provided directly by the city through its own hospitals and health agencies and any payments to other governments for such purposes are classed under those functional headings.

★ 442 ★

Government Spending: Local

Local Government Spending on Health Care in Michigan: 1990-1991

Local government spending for social service and income maintenance items is provided below. Data reflect city, urban town, and township government expenditures by function, thus grouping health-related activities (public welfare, hospitals, social insurance, and veterans' services) to provide a comprehensive picture of spending. Totals for these categories are not provided since they are meant only as presentational guidelines. According to the source: "Functions cannot be equated specifically with a single federal or state government program. Instead they represent broader activities of government that have remained virtually unchanged over many years so that as specific programs expand and contract they will remain useful for analytical purposes. Medicaid, for example, is a well-known program that is included in the larger public welfare function, specifically as a medical vendor payment, along with all other social welfare activities" (p. viii).

[Dollar amounts in thousands]

City	Social service and income maintenance expenditures		
	Public welfare	Hospitals	Health
Ann Arbor	650	-	-
Dearborn	927	-	226
Detroit	-	67	97,844
Flint	266	173,629	89
Lansing	1,345	-	-
Southfield	334	-	-

Source: U.S. Bureau of the Census. *City Government Finances, 1990-1991.* Series GF/91-4. Washington, DC: U.S. Government Printing Office, 1993, p. 26-27. "Data in this report pertain to government fiscal years that ended between July 1, 1990, and June 30, 1991.... About three-fourths of all city governments in the nation had a fiscal year ending in either December (42 percent) or June (32 percent). September and April were the next most common months in which city governments ended their fiscal years. Of all townships, three-fifths had fiscal years corresponding directly with the calendar year 1990 (i.e., they ended their fiscal years on December 31, 1990). March, February, and June had the next most common fiscal year ending dates for townships" (p. vi). *Notes:* Detail may not add to total due to rounding. The Public Welfare heading covers the support of and assistance to needy persons contingent upon their need, excluding pensions to former employees and other benefits not contingent upon need. Among the expenditures in this category are: Cash assistance paid directly to needy persons under categorical programs (e.g., Old Age Assistance, Aid to Families With Dependent Children, Aid to the Blind, and Aid to the Disabled) or under any welfare programs; vendor payments made directly to private purveyors for medical care, burial, and other commodities and services provided under welfare programs; and provision and operation by the city of welfare institutions. Hospital data reflects spending for hospital facilities established or operated directly by city and township governments, the provision of health care, and support of other public or private hospitals. The Health category covers outpatient health services other than hospital care, including public health administration; research and education; categorical health programs; treatment and immunization clinics; nursing; environmental health activities (e.g., air and water pollution control); ambulance service provided separately from fire protection services; school health services provided by health agencies; other general public health activities (e.g., mosquito abatement). Health and hospital services provided directly by the city through its own hospitals and health agencies and any payments to other governments for such purposes are classed under those functional headings.

★ 443 ★

Government Spending: Local

Local Government Spending on Health Care in Minnesota: 1990-1991

Local government spending for social service and income maintenance items is provided below. Data reflect city, urban town, and township government expenditures by function, thus grouping health-related activities (public welfare, hospitals, social insurance, and veterans' services) to provide a comprehensive picture of spending. Totals for these categories are not provided since they are meant only as presentational guidelines. According to the source: "Functions cannot be equated specifically with a single federal or state government program. Instead they represent broader activities of government that have remained virtually unchanged over many years so that as specific programs expand and contract they will remain useful for analytical purposes. Medicaid, for example, is a well-known program that is included in the larger public welfare function, specifically as a medical vendor payment, along with all other social welfare activities" (p. viii).

[Dollar amounts in thousands]

City	Social service and income maintenance expenditures		
	Public welfare	Hospitals	Health
Bloomington	-	-	2,166
Minneapolis	-	-	10,003
St. Paul	-	-	7,950

Source: U.S. Bureau of the Census. *City Government Finances, 1990-1991.* Series GF/91-4. Washington, DC: U.S. Government Printing Office, 1993, pp. 27-28. "Data in this report pertain to government fiscal years that ended between July 1, 1990, and June 30, 1991.... About three-fourths of all city governments in the nation had a fiscal year ending in either December (42 percent) or June (32 percent). September and April were the next most common months in which city governments ended their fiscal years. Of all townships, three-fifths had fiscal years corresponding directly with the calendar year 1990 (i.e., they ended their fiscal years on December 31, 1990). March, February, and June had the next most common fiscal year ending dates for townships" (p. vi). *Notes:* Detail may not add to total due to rounding. The Public Welfare heading covers the support of and assistance to needy persons contingent upon their need, excluding pensions to former employees and other benefits not contingent upon need. Among the expenditures in this category are: Cash assistance paid directly to needy persons under categorical programs (e.g., Old Age Assistance, Aid to Families With Dependent Children, Aid to the Blind, and Aid to the Disabled) or under any welfare programs; vendor payments made directly to private purveyors for medical care, burial, and other commodities and services provided under welfare programs; and provision and operation by the city of welfare institutions. Hospital data reflects spending for hospital facilities established or operated directly by city and township governments, the provision of health care, and support of other public or private hospitals. The Health category covers outpatient health services other than hospital care, including public health administration; research and education; categorical health programs; treatment and immunization clinics; nursing; environmental health activities (e.g., air and water pollution control); ambulance service provided separately from fire protection services; school health services provided by health agencies; other general public health activities (e.g., mosquito abatement). Health and hospital services provided directly by the city through its own hospitals and health agencies and any payments to other governments for such purposes are classed under those functional headings.

★ 444 ★

Government Spending: Local

Local Government Spending on Health Care in Mississippi: 1990-1991

Local government spending for social service and income maintenance items is provided below. Data reflect city, urban town, and township government expenditures by function, thus grouping health-related activities (public welfare, hospitals, social insurance, and veterans' services) to provide a comprehensive picture of spending. Totals for these categories are not provided since they are meant only as presentational guidelines. According to the source: "Functions cannot be equated specifically with a single federal or state government program. Instead they represent broader activities of government that have remained virtually unchanged over many years so that as specific programs expand and contract they will remain useful for analytical purposes. Medicaid, for example, is a well-known program that is included in the larger public welfare function, specifically as a medical vendor payment, along with all other social welfare activities" (p. viii).

[Dollar amounts in thousands]

City	Social service and income maintenance expenditures		
	Public welfare	Hospitals	Health
Jackson	-	-	-

Source: U.S. Bureau of the Census. *City Government Finances, 1990-1991.* Series GF/91-4. Washington, DC: U.S. Government Printing Office, 1993, p. 28. "Data in this report pertain to government fiscal years that ended between July 1, 1990, and June 30, 1991.... About three-fourths of all city governments in the nation had a fiscal year ending in either December (42 percent) or June (32 percent). September and April were the next most common months in which city governments ended their fiscal years. Of all townships, three-fifths had fiscal years corresponding directly with the calendar year 1990 (i.e., they ended their fiscal years on December 31, 1990). March, February, and June had the next most common fiscal year ending dates for townships" (p. vi). *Notes:* Detail may not add to total due to rounding. The Public Welfare heading covers the support of and assistance to needy persons contingent upon their need, excluding pensions to former employees and other benefits not contingent upon need. Among the expenditures in this category are: Cash assistance paid directly to needy persons under categorical programs (e.g., Old Age Assistance, Aid to Families With Dependent Children, Aid to the Blind, and Aid to the Disabled) or under any welfare programs; vendor payments made directly to private purveyors for medical care, burial, and other commodities and services provided under welfare programs; and provision and operation by the city of welfare institutions. Hospital data reflects spending for hospital facilities established or operated directly by city and township governments, the provision of health care, and support of other public or private hospitals. The Health category covers outpatient health services other than hospital care, including public health administration; research and education; categorical health programs; treatment and immunization clinics; nursing; environmental health activities (e.g., air and water pollution control); ambulance service provided separately from fire protection services; school health services provided by health agencies; other general public health activities (e.g., mosquito abatement). Health and hospital services provided directly by the city through its own hospitals and health agencies and any payments to other governments for such purposes are classed under those functional headings.

★ 445 ★

Government Spending: Local

Local Government Spending on Health Care in Missouri: 1990-1991

Local government spending for social service and income maintenance items is provided below. Data reflect city, urban town, and township government expenditures by function, thus grouping health-related activities (public welfare, hospitals, social insurance, and veterans' services) to provide a comprehensive picture of spending. Totals for these categories are not provided since they are meant only as presentational guidelines. According to the source: "Functions cannot be equated specifically with a single federal or state government program. Instead they represent broader activities of government that have remained virtually unchanged over many years so that as specific programs expand and contract they will remain useful for analytical purposes. Medicaid, for example, is a well-known program that is included in the larger public welfare function, specifically as a medical vendor payment, along with all other social welfare activities" (p. viii).

[Dollar amounts in thousands]

City	Social service and income maintenance expenditures		
	Public welfare	Hospitals	Health
Independence	-	-	1,157
Kansas City	3	27,766	13,657
St. Louis	3,744	18,450	18,129
Springfield	3,951	-	3,109

Source: U.S. Bureau of the Census. *City Government Finances, 1990-1991.* Series GF/91-4. Washington, DC: U.S. Government Printing Office, 1993, p. 28. "Data in this report pertain to government fiscal years that ended between July 1, 1990, and June 30, 1991.... About three-fourths of all city governments in the nation had a fiscal year ending in either December (42 percent) or June (32 percent). September and April were the next most common months in which city governments ended their fiscal years. Of all townships, three-fifths had fiscal years corresponding directly with the calendar year 1990 (i.e., they ended their fiscal years on December 31, 1990). March, February, and June had the next most common fiscal year ending dates for townships" (p. vi). *Notes:* Detail may not add to total due to rounding. The Public Welfare heading covers the support of and assistance to needy persons contingent upon their need, excluding pensions to former employees and other benefits not contingent upon need. Among the expenditures in this category are: Cash assistance paid directly to needy persons under categorical programs (e.g., Old Age Assistance, Aid to Families With Dependent Children, Aid to the Blind, and Aid to the Disabled) or under any welfare programs; vendor payments made directly to private purveyors for medical care, burial, and other commodities and services provided under welfare programs; and provision and operation by the city of welfare institutions. Hospital data reflects spending for hospital facilities established or operated directly by city and township governments, the provision of health care, and support of other public or private hospitals. The Health category covers outpatient health services other than hospital care, including public health administration; research and education; categorical health programs; treatment and immunization clinics; nursing; environmental health activities (e.g., air and water pollution control); ambulance service provided separately from fire protection services; school health services provided by health agencies; other general public health activities (e.g., mosquito abatement). Health and hospital services provided directly by the city through its own hospitals and health agencies and any payments to other governments for such purposes are classed under those functional headings.

★ 446 ★

Government Spending: Local

Local Government Spending on Health Care in Montana: 1990-1991

Local government spending for social service and income maintenance items is provided below. Data reflect city, urban town, and township government expenditures by function, thus grouping health-related activities (public welfare, hospitals, social insurance, and veterans' services) to provide a comprehensive picture of spending. Totals for these categories are not provided since they are meant only as presentational guidelines. According to the source: "Functions cannot be equated specifically with a single federal or state government program. Instead they represent broader activities of government that have remained virtually unchanged over many years so that as specific programs expand and contract they will remain useful for analytical purposes. Medicaid, for example, is a well-known program that is included in the larger public welfare function, specifically as a medical vendor payment, along with all other social welfare activities" (p. viii).

[Dollar amounts in thousands]

| City | Social service and income maintenance expenditures | | |
	Public welfare	Hospitals	Health
Billings	-	-	41

Source: U.S. Bureau of the Census. *City Government Finances, 1990-1991.* Series GF/91-4. Washington, DC: U.S. Government Printing Office, 1993, p. 29. "Data in this report pertain to government fiscal years that ended between July 1, 1990, and June 30, 1991.... About three-fourths of all city governments in the nation had a fiscal year ending in either December (42 percent) or June (32 percent). September and April were the next most common months in which city governments ended their fiscal years. Of all townships, three-fifths had fiscal years corresponding directly with the calendar year 1990 (i.e., they ended their fiscal years on December 31, 1990). March, February, and June had the next most common fiscal year ending dates for townships" (p. vi). *Notes:* Detail may not add to total due to rounding. The Public Welfare heading covers the support of and assistance to needy persons contingent upon their need, excluding pensions to former employees and other benefits not contingent upon need. Among the expenditures in this category are: Cash assistance paid directly to needy persons under categorical programs (e.g., Old Age Assistance, Aid to Families With Dependent Children, Aid to the Blind, and Aid to the Disabled) or under any welfare programs; vendor payments made directly to private purveyors for medical care, burial, and other commodities and services provided under welfare programs; and provision and operation by the city of welfare institutions. Hospital data reflects spending for hospital facilities established or operated directly by city and township governments, the provision of health care, and support of other public or private hospitals. The Health category covers outpatient health services other than hospital care, including public health administration; research and education; categorical health programs; treatment and immunization clinics; nursing; environmental health activities (e.g., air and water pollution control); ambulance service provided separately from fire protection services; school health services provided by health agencies; other general public health activities (e.g., mosquito abatement). Health and hospital services provided directly by the city through its own hospitals and health agencies and any payments to other governments for such purposes are classed under those functional headings.

★ 447 ★

Government Spending: Local

Local Government Spending on Health Care in Nebraska: 1990-1991

Local government spending for social service and income maintenance items is provided below. Data reflect city, urban town, and township government expenditures by function, thus grouping health-related activities (public welfare, hospitals, social insurance, and veterans' services) to provide a comprehensive picture of spending. Totals for these categories are not provided since they are meant only as presentational guidelines. According to the source: "Functions cannot be equated specifically with a single federal or state government program. Instead they represent broader activities of government that have remained virtually unchanged over many years so that as specific programs expand and contract they will remain useful for analytical purposes. Medicaid, for example, is a well-known program that is included in the larger public welfare function, specifically as a medical vendor payment, along with all other social welfare activities" (p. viii).

[Dollar amounts in thousands]

City	Social service and income maintenance expenditures		
	Public welfare	Hospitals	Health
Lincoln	-	44,666	4,065
Omaha	-	-	1,026

Source: U.S. Bureau of the Census. *City Government Finances, 1990-1991.* Series GF/91-4. Washington, DC: U.S. Government Printing Office, 1993, p. 29. "Data in this report pertain to government fiscal years that ended between July 1, 1990, and June 30, 1991.... About three-fourths of all city governments in the nation had a fiscal year ending in either December (42 percent) or June (32 percent). September and April were the next most common months in which city governments ended their fiscal years. Of all townships, three-fifths had fiscal years corresponding directly with the calendar year 1990 (i.e., they ended their fiscal years on December 31, 1990). March, February, and June had the next most common fiscal year ending dates for townships" (p. vi). *Notes:* Detail may not add to total due to rounding. The Public Welfare heading covers the support of and assistance to needy persons contingent upon their need, excluding pensions to former employees and other benefits not contingent upon need. Among the expenditures in this category are: Cash assistance paid directly to needy persons under categorical programs (e.g., Old Age Assistance, Aid to Families With Dependent Children, Aid to the Blind, and Aid to the Disabled) or under any welfare programs; vendor payments made directly to private purveyors for medical care, burial, and other commodities and services provided under welfare programs; and provision and operation by the city of welfare institutions. Hospital data reflects spending for hospital facilities established or operated directly by city and township governments, the provision of health care, and support of other public or private hospitals. The Health category covers outpatient health services other than hospital care, including public health administration; research and education; categorical health programs; treatment and immunization clinics; nursing; environmental health activities (e.g., air and water pollution control); ambulance service provided separately from fire protection services; school health services provided by health agencies; other general public health activities (e.g., mosquito abatement). Health and hospital services provided directly by the city through its own hospitals and health agencies and any payments to other governments for such purposes are classed under those functional headings.

★ 448 ★

Government Spending: Local

Local Government Spending on Health Care in Nevada: 1990-1991

Local government spending for social service and income maintenance items is provided below. Data reflect city, urban town, and township government expenditures by function, thus grouping health-related activities (public welfare, hospitals, social insurance, and veterans' services) to provide a comprehensive picture of spending. Totals for these categories are not provided since they are meant only as presentational guidelines. According to the source: "Functions cannot be equated specifically with a single federal or state government program. Instead they represent broader activities of government that have remained virtually unchanged over many years so that as specific programs expand and contract they will remain useful for analytical purposes. Medicaid, for example, is a well-known program that is included in the larger public welfare function, specifically as a medical vendor payment, along with all other social welfare activities" (p. viii).

[Dollar amounts in thousands]

| City | Social service and income maintenance expenditures | | |
	Public welfare	Hospitals	Health
Las Vegas	391	-	1,584
Reno	-	-	651

Source: U.S. Bureau of the Census. *City Government Finances, 1990-1991.* Series GF/91-4. Washington, DC: U.S. Government Printing Office, 1993, p. 29. "Data in this report pertain to government fiscal years that ended between July 1, 1990, and June 30, 1991.... About three-fourths of all city governments in the nation had a fiscal year ending in either December (42 percent) or June (32 percent). September and April were the next most common months in which city governments ended their fiscal years. Of all townships, three-fifths had fiscal years corresponding directly with the calendar year 1990 (i.e., they ended their fiscal years on December 31, 1990). March, February, and June had the next most common fiscal year ending dates for townships" (p. vi). *Notes:* Detail may not add to total due to rounding. The Public Welfare heading covers the support of and assistance to needy persons contingent upon their need, excluding pensions to former employees and other benefits not contingent upon need. Among the expenditures in this category are: Cash assistance paid directly to needy persons under categorical programs (e.g., Old Age Assistance, Aid to Families With Dependent Children, Aid to the Blind, and Aid to the Disabled) or under any welfare programs; vendor payments made directly to private purveyors for medical care, burial, and other commodities and services provided under welfare programs; and provision and operation by the city of welfare institutions. Hospital data reflects spending for hospital facilities established or operated directly by city and township governments, the provision of health care, and support of other public or private hospitals. The Health category covers outpatient health services other than hospital care, including public health administration; research and education; categorical health programs; treatment and immunization clinics; nursing; environmental health activities (e.g., air and water pollution control); ambulance service provided separately from fire protection services; school health services provided by health agencies; other general public health activities (e.g., mosquito abatement). Health and hospital services provided directly by the city through its own hospitals and health agencies and any payments to other governments for such purposes are classed under those functional headings.

★ 449 ★

Government Spending: Local

Local Government Spending on Health Care in New Hampshire: 1990-1991

Local government spending for social service and income maintenance items is provided below. Data reflect city, urban town, and township government expenditures by function, thus grouping health-related activities (public welfare, hospitals, social insurance, and veterans' services) to provide a comprehensive picture of spending. Totals for these categories are not provided since they are meant only as presentational guidelines. According to the source: "Functions cannot be equated specifically with a single federal or state government program. Instead they represent broader activities of government that have remained virtually unchanged over many years so that as specific programs expand and contract they will remain useful for analytical purposes. Medicaid, for example, is a well-known program that is included in the larger public welfare function, specifically as a medical vendor payment, along with all other social welfare activities" (p. viii).

[Dollar amounts in thousands]

City	Social service and income maintenance expenditures		
	Public welfare	Hospitals	Health
Manchester	1,505	-	1,687
Nashua	316	-	910

Source: U.S. Bureau of the Census. *City Government Finances, 1990-1991.* Series GF/91-4. Washington, DC: U.S. Government Printing Office, 1993, p. 29. "Data in this report pertain to government fiscal years that ended between July 1, 1990, and June 30, 1991.... About three-fourths of all city governments in the nation had a fiscal year ending in either December (42 percent) or June (32 percent). September and April were the next most common months in which city governments ended their fiscal years. Of all townships, three-fifths had fiscal years corresponding directly with the calendar year 1990 (i.e., they ended their fiscal years on December 31, 1990). March, February, and June had the next most common fiscal year ending dates for townships" (p. vi). *Notes:* Detail may not add to total due to rounding. The Public Welfare heading covers the support of and assistance to needy persons contingent upon their need, excluding pensions to former employees and other benefits not contingent upon need. Among the expenditures in this category are: Cash assistance paid directly to needy persons under categorical programs (e.g., Old Age Assistance, Aid to Families With Dependent Children, Aid to the Blind, and Aid to the Disabled) or under any welfare programs; vendor payments made directly to private purveyors for medical care, burial, and other commodities and services provided under welfare programs; and provision and operation by the city of welfare institutions. Hospital data reflects spending for hospital facilities established or operated directly by city and township governments, the provision of health care, and support of other public or private hospitals. The Health category covers outpatient health services other than hospital care, including public health administration; research and education; categorical health programs; treatment and immunization clinics; nursing; environmental health activities (e.g., air and water pollution control); ambulance service provided separately from fire protection services; school health services provided by health agencies; other general public health activities (e.g., mosquito abatement). Health and hospital services provided directly by the city through its own hospitals and health agencies and any payments to other governments for such purposes are classed under those functional headings.

★ 450 ★

Government Spending: Local

Local Government Spending on Health Care in New Jersey: 1990-1991

Local government spending for social service and income maintenance items is provided below. Data reflect city, urban town, and township government expenditures by function, thus grouping health-related activities (public welfare, hospitals, social insurance, and veterans' services) to provide a comprehensive picture of spending. Totals for these categories are not provided since they are meant only as presentational guidelines. According to the source: "Functions cannot be equated specifically with a single federal or state government program. Instead they represent broader activities of government that have remained virtually unchanged over many years so that as specific programs expand and contract they will remain useful for analytical purposes. Medicaid, for example, is a well-known program that is included in the larger public welfare function, specifically as a medical vendor payment, along with all other social welfare activities" (p. viii).

[Dollar amounts in thousands]

City	Social service and income maintenance expenditures		
	Public welfare	Hospitals	Health
Camden	2,694	-	294
Clifton[1]	50	-	638
Dover township (Ocean Co.)	708	-	222
East Orange[1]	3,890	-	3,396
Edison township	372	-	785
Elizabeth	795	-	2,630
Hamilton township (Mercer Co.)	760	-	1,185
Jersey City	6,843	2,917	7,000
Newark	47,303	-	8,497
Paterson	901	-	1,455
Trenton	2,368	-	1,540
Woodbridge township	88	-	778

Source: U.S. Bureau of the Census. *City Government Finances, 1990-1991.* Series GF/91-4. Washington, DC: U.S. Government Printing Office, 1993, p. 30-31. "Data in this report pertain to government fiscal years that ended between July 1, 1990, and June 30, 1991.... About three-fourths of all city governments in the nation had a fiscal year ending in either December (42 percent) or June (32 percent). September and April were the next most common months in which city governments ended their fiscal years. Of all townships, three-fifths had fiscal years corresponding directly with the calendar year 1990 (i.e., they ended their fiscal years on December 31, 1990). March, February, and June had the next most common fiscal year ending dates for townships" (p. vi). *Notes:* Detail may not add to total due to rounding. The Public Welfare heading covers the support of and assistance to needy persons contingent upon their need, excluding pensions to former employees and other benefits not contingent upon need. Among the expenditures in this category are: Cash assistance paid directly to needy persons under categorical programs (e.g., Old Age Assistance, Aid to Families With Dependent Children, Aid to the Blind, and Aid to the Disabled) or under any welfare programs; vendor payments made directly to private purveyors for medical care, burial, and other commodities and services provided under welfare programs; and provision and operation by the city of welfare institutions. Hospital data reflects spending for hospital facilities established or operated directly by city and township governments, the provision of health care, and support of other public or private hospitals. The Health category covers outpatient health services other than hospital care, including public health administration; research and education; categorical health programs; treatment and immunization clinics; nursing; environmental health activities (e.g., air and water pollution control); ambulance service provided separately from fire protection services; school health services provided by health agencies; other general public health activities (e.g., mosquito abatement). Health and hospital services provided directly by the city through its own hospitals and health agencies and any payments to other governments for such purposes are classed under those functional headings. 1. Data are for 1989-1990.

★ 451 ★

Government Spending: Local

Local Government Spending on Health Care in New Mexico: 1990-1991

Local government spending for social service and income maintenance items is provided below. Data reflect city, urban town, and township government expenditures by function, thus grouping health-related activities (public welfare, hospitals, social insurance, and veterans' services) to provide a comprehensive picture of spending. Totals for these categories are not provided since they are meant only as presentational guidelines. According to the source: "Functions cannot be equated specifically with a single federal or state government program. Instead they represent broader activities of government that have remained virtually unchanged over many years so that as specific programs expand and contract they will remain useful for analytical purposes. Medicaid, for example, is a well-known program that is included in the larger public welfare function, specifically as a medical vendor payment, along with all other social welfare activities" (p. viii).

[Dollar amounts in thousands]

City	Social service and income maintenance expenditures		
	Public welfare	Hospitals	Health
Albuquerque	2,522	-	6,456

Source: U.S. Bureau of the Census. *City Government Finances, 1990-1991.* Series GF/91-4. Washington, DC: U.S. Government Printing Office, 1993, p. 31. "Data in this report pertain to government fiscal years that ended between July 1, 1990, and June 30, 1991.... About three-fourths of all city governments in the nation had a fiscal year ending in either December (42 percent) or June (32 percent). September and April were the next most common months in which city governments ended their fiscal years. Of all townships, three-fifths had fiscal years corresponding directly with the calendar year 1990 (i.e., they ended their fiscal years on December 31, 1990). March, February, and June had the next most common fiscal year ending dates for townships" (p. vi). *Notes:* Detail may not add to total due to rounding. The Public Welfare heading covers the support of and assistance to needy persons contingent upon their need, excluding pensions to former employees and other benefits not contingent upon need. Among the expenditures in this category are: Cash assistance paid directly to needy persons under categorical programs (e.g., Old Age Assistance, Aid to Families With Dependent Children, Aid to the Blind, and Aid to the Disabled) or under any welfare programs; vendor payments made directly to private purveyors for medical care, burial, and other commodities and services provided under welfare programs; and provision and operation by the city of welfare institutions. Hospital data reflects spending for hospital facilities established or operated directly by city and township governments, the provision of health care, and support of other public or private hospitals. The Health category covers outpatient health services other than hospital care, including public health administration; research and education; categorical health programs; treatment and immunization clinics; nursing; environmental health activities (e.g., air and water pollution control); ambulance service provided separately from fire protection services; school health services provided by health agencies; other general public health activities (e.g., mosquito abatement). Health and hospital services provided directly by the city through its own hospitals and health agencies and any payments to other governments for such purposes are classed under those functional headings.

★ 452 ★

Government Spending: Local

Local Government Spending on Health Care in New York: 1990-1991

Local government spending for social service and income maintenance items is provided below. Data reflect city, urban town, and township government expenditures by function, thus grouping health-related activities (public welfare, hospitals, social insurance, and veterans' services) to provide a comprehensive picture of spending. Totals for these categories are not provided since they are meant only as presentational guidelines. According to the source: "Functions cannot be equated specifically with a single federal or state government program. Instead they represent broader activities of government that have remained virtually unchanged over many years so that as specific programs expand and contract they will remain useful for analytical purposes. Medicaid, for example, is a well-known program that is included in the larger public welfare function, specifically as a medical vendor payment, along with all other social welfare activities" (p. viii).

[Dollar amounts in thousands]

City	Social service and income maintenance expenditures		
	Public welfare	Hospitals	Health
Albany	55	-	127
Amherst town	8,214	-	-
Babylon town	5,175	-	1,267
Brookhaven town	-	-	1,575
Buffalo	-	-	1,824
Clarkstown town	-	-	1,238
Colonietown	562	-	1,149
Greenburgh town	144	-	173
Hempstead town	1,427	-	755
Huntington town	13	-	1,479
Islip town	305	-	2,633
New York City	6,527,606	3,118,581	576,847
North Hempstead town	152	-	107
Ramapo town	-	-	2,182
Smithtown town	310	-	268

[Continued]

★ 452 ★

Local Government Spending on Health Care in New York: 1990-1991
[Continued]

City	Social service and income maintenance expenditures		
	Public welfare	Hospitals	Health
Tonawanda town	-	-	510
Yonkers	-	-	1,037

Source: U.S. Bureau of the Census. *City Government Finances, 1990-1991.* Series GF/91-4. Washington, DC: U.S. Government Printing Office, 1993, pp. 31-34. "Data in this report pertain to government fiscal years that ended between July 1, 1990, and June 30, 1991.... About three-fourths of all city governments in the nation had a fiscal year ending in either December (42 percent) or June (32 percent). September and April were the next most common months in which city governments ended their fiscal years. Of all townships, three-fifths had fiscal years corresponding directly with the calendar year 1990 (i.e., they ended their fiscal years on December 31, 1990). March, February, and June had the next most common fiscal year ending dates for townships" (p. vi). *Notes:* Detail may not add to total due to rounding. The Public Welfare heading covers the support of and assistance to needy persons contingent upon their need, excluding pensions to former employees and other benefits not contingent upon need. Among the expenditures in this category are: Cash assistance paid directly to needy persons under categorical programs (e.g., Old Age Assistance, Aid to Families With Dependent Children, Aid to the Blind, and Aid to the Disabled) or under any welfare programs; vendor payments made directly to private purveyors for medical care, burial, and other commodities and services provided under welfare programs; and provision and operation by the city of welfare institutions. Hospital data reflects spending for hospital facilities established or operated directly by city and township governments, the provision of health care, and support of other public or private hospitals. The Health category covers outpatient health services other than hospital care, including public health administration; research and education; categorical health programs; treatment and immunization clinics; nursing; environmental health activities (e.g., air and water pollution control); ambulance service provided separately from fire protection services; school health services provided by health agencies; other general public health activities (e.g., mosquito abatement). Health and hospital services provided directly by the city through its own hospitals and health agencies and any payments to other governments for such purposes are classed under those functional headings.

★ 453 ★

Government Spending: Local

Local Government Spending on Health Care in North Carolina: 1990-1991

Local government spending for social service and income maintenance items is provided below. Data reflect city, urban town, and township government expenditures by function, thus grouping health-related activities (public welfare, hospitals, social insurance, and veterans' services) to provide a comprehensive picture of spending. Totals for these categories are not provided since they are meant only as presentational guidelines. According to the source: "Functions cannot be equated specifically with a single federal or state government program. Instead they represent broader activities of government that have remained virtually unchanged over many years so that as specific programs expand and contract they will remain useful for analytical purposes. Medicaid, for example, is a well-known program that is included in the larger public welfare function, specifically as a medical vendor payment, along with all other social welfare activities" (p. viii).

[Dollar amounts in thousands]

City	Social service and income maintenance expenditures		
	Public welfare	Hospitals	Health
Charlotte	268	-	2,702
Greensboro	-	-	373
Raleigh	715	-	199
Winston-Salem	-	-	245

Source: U.S. Bureau of the Census. *City Government Finances, 1990-1991.* Series GF/91-4. Washington, DC: U.S. Government Printing Office, 1993, p. 34-35. "Data in this report pertain to government fiscal years that ended between July 1, 1990, and June 30, 1991.... About three-fourths of all city governments in the nation had a fiscal year ending in either December (42 percent) or June (32 percent). September and April were the next most common months in which city governments ended their fiscal years. Of all townships, three-fifths had fiscal years corresponding directly with the calendar year 1990 (i.e., they ended their fiscal years on December 31, 1990). March, February, and June had the next most common fiscal year ending dates for townships" (p. vi). *Notes:* Detail may not add to total due to rounding. The Public Welfare heading covers the support of and assistance to needy persons contingent upon their need, excluding pensions to former employees and other benefits not contingent upon need. Among the expenditures in this category are: Cash assistance paid directly to needy persons under categorical programs (e.g., Old Age Assistance, Aid to Families With Dependent Children, Aid to the Blind, and Aid to the Disabled) or under any welfare programs; vendor payments made directly to private purveyors for medical care, burial, and other commodities and services provided under welfare programs; and provision and operation by the city of welfare institutions. Hospital data reflects spending for hospital facilities established or operated directly by city and township governments, the provision of health care, and support of other public or private hospitals. The Health category covers outpatient health services other than hospital care, including public health administration; research and education; categorical health programs; treatment and immunization clinics; nursing; environmental health activities (e.g., air and water pollution control); ambulance service provided separately from fire protection services; school health services provided by health agencies; other general public health activities (e.g., mosquito abatement). Health and hospital services provided directly by the city through its own hospitals and health agencies and any payments to other governments for such purposes are classed under those functional headings.

★ 454 ★

Government Spending: Local

Local Government Spending on Health Care in North Dakota: 1990-1991

Local government spending for social service and income maintenance items is provided below. Data reflect city, urban town, and township government expenditures by function, thus grouping health-related activities (public welfare, hospitals, social insurance, and veterans' services) to provide a comprehensive picture of spending. Totals for these categories are not provided since they are meant only as presentational guidelines. According to the source: "Functions cannot be equated specifically with a single federal or state government program. Instead they represent broader activities of government that have remained virtually unchanged over many years so that as specific programs expand and contract they will remain useful for analytical purposes. Medicaid, for example, is a well-known program that is included in the larger public welfare function, specifically as a medical vendor payment, along with all other social welfare activities" (p. viii).

[Dollar amounts in thousands]

| City | Social service and income maintenance expenditures | | |
	Public welfare	Hospitals	Health
Fargo	198	-	1,685

Source: U.S. Bureau of the Census. *City Government Finances, 1990-1991.* Series GF/91-4. Washington, DC: U.S. Government Printing Office, 1993, p. 35. "Data in this report pertain to government fiscal years that ended between July 1, 1990, and June 30, 1991.... About three-fourths of all city governments in the nation had a fiscal year ending in either December (42 percent) or June (32 percent). September and April were the next most common months in which city governments ended their fiscal years. Of all townships, three-fifths had fiscal years corresponding directly with the calendar year 1990 (i.e., they ended their fiscal years on December 31, 1990). March, February, and June had the next most common fiscal year ending dates for townships" (p. vi). *Notes:* Detail may not add to total due to rounding. The Public Welfare heading covers the support of and assistance to needy persons contingent upon their need, excluding pensions to former employees and other benefits not contingent upon need. Among the expenditures in this category are: Cash assistance paid directly to needy persons under categorical programs (e.g., Old Age Assistance, Aid to Families With Dependent Children, Aid to the Blind, and Aid to the Disabled) or under any welfare programs; vendor payments made directly to private purveyors for medical care, burial, and other commodities and services provided under welfare programs; and provision and operation by the city of welfare institutions. Hospital data reflects spending for hospital facilities established or operated directly by city and township governments, the provision of health care, and support of other public or private hospitals. The Health category covers outpatient health services other than hospital care, including public health administration; research and education; categorical health programs; treatment and immunization clinics; nursing; environmental health activities (e.g., air and water pollution control); ambulance service provided separately from fire protection services; school health services provided by health agencies; other general public health activities (e.g., mosquito abatement). Health and hospital services provided directly by the city through its own hospitals and health agencies and any payments to other governments for such purposes are classed under those functional headings.

★ 455 ★

Government Spending: Local

Local Government Spending on Health Care in Ohio: 1990-1991

Local government spending for social service and income maintenance items is provided below. Data reflect city, urban town, and township government expenditures by function, thus grouping health-related activities (public welfare, hospitals, social insurance, and veterans' services) to provide a comprehensive picture of spending. Totals for these categories are not provided since they are meant only as presentational guidelines. According to the source: "Functions cannot be equated specifically with a single federal or state government program. Instead they represent broader activities of government that have remained virtually unchanged over many years so that as specific programs expand and contract they will remain useful for analytical purposes. Medicaid, for example, is a well-known program that is included in the larger public welfare function, specifically as a medical vendor payment, along with all other social welfare activities" (p. viii).

[Dollar amounts in thousands]

| City | Social service and income maintenance expenditures | | |
	Public welfare	Hospitals	Health
Akron	-	-	7,484
Canton	-	-	2,055
Cincinnati	-	-	31,256
Cleveland	15	-	16,389
Columbus	-	-	22,210
Dayton	444	-	-
Parma	-	-	467
Toledo	-	-	5,735
Youngstown	-	-	1,550

Source: U.S. Bureau of the Census. *City Government Finances, 1990-1991.* Series GF/91-4. Washington, DC: U.S. Government Printing Office, 1993, pp. 35-36. "Data in this report pertain to government fiscal years that ended between July 1, 1990, and June 30, 1991.... About three-fourths of all city governments in the nation had a fiscal year ending in either December (42 percent) or June (32 percent). September and April were the next most common months in which city governments ended their fiscal years. Of all townships, three-fifths had fiscal years corresponding directly with the calendar year 1990 (i.e., they ended their fiscal years on December 31, 1990). March, February, and June had the next most common fiscal year ending dates for townships" (p. vi). *Notes:* Detail may not add to total due to rounding. The Public Welfare heading covers the support of and assistance to needy persons contingent upon their need, excluding pensions to former employees and other benefits not contingent upon need. Among the expenditures in this category are: Cash assistance paid directly to needy persons under categorical programs (e.g., Old Age Assistance, Aid to Families With Dependent Children, Aid to the Blind, and Aid to the Disabled) or under any welfare programs; vendor payments made directly to private purveyors for medical care, burial, and other commodities and services provided under welfare programs; and provision and operation by the city of welfare institutions. Hospital data reflects spending for hospital facilities established or operated directly by city and township governments, the provision of health care, and support of other public or private hospitals. The Health category covers outpatient health services other than hospital care, including public health administration; research and education; categorical health programs; treatment and immunization clinics; nursing; environmental health activities (e.g., air and water pollution control); ambulance service provided separately from fire protection services; school health services provided by health agencies; other general public health activities (e.g., mosquito abatement). Health and hospital services provided directly by the city through its own hospitals and health agencies and any payments to other governments for such purposes are classed under those functional headings.

★ 456 ★

Government Spending: Local

Local Government Spending on Health Care in Oklahoma: 1990-1991

Local government spending for social service and income maintenance items is provided below. Data reflect city, urban town, and township government expenditures by function, thus grouping health-related activities (public welfare, hospitals, social insurance, and veterans' services) to provide a comprehensive picture of spending. Totals for these categories are not provided since they are meant only as presentational guidelines. According to the source: "Functions cannot be equated specifically with a single federal or state government program. Instead they represent broader activities of government that have remained virtually unchanged over many years so that as specific programs expand and contract they will remain useful for analytical purposes. Medicaid, for example, is a well-known program that is included in the larger public welfare function, specifically as a medical vendor payment, along with all other social welfare activities" (p. viii).

[Dollar amounts in thousands]

| City | Social service and income maintenance expenditures | | |
	Public welfare	Hospitals	Health
Lawton[1]	30	-	174
Norman	50	46,248	1,660
Oklahoma City	-	-	1,554
Tulsa	-	-	15,870

Source: U.S. Bureau of the Census. *City Government Finances, 1990-1991.* Series GF/91-4. Washington, DC: U.S. Government Printing Office, 1993, p. 37. "Data in this report pertain to government fiscal years that ended between July 1, 1990, and June 30, 1991.... About three-fourths of all city governments in the nation had a fiscal year ending in either December (42 percent) or June (32 percent). September and April were the next most common months in which city governments ended their fiscal years. Of all townships, three-fifths had fiscal years corresponding directly with the calendar year 1990 (i.e., they ended their fiscal years on December 31, 1990). March, February, and June had the next most common fiscal year ending dates for townships" (p. vi). *Notes:* Detail may not add to total due to rounding. The Public Welfare heading covers the support of and assistance to needy persons contingent upon their need, excluding pensions to former employees and other benefits not contingent upon need. Among the expenditures in this category are: Cash assistance paid directly to needy persons under categorical programs (e.g., Old Age Assistance, Aid to Families With Dependent Children, Aid to the Blind, and Aid to the Disabled) or under any welfare programs; vendor payments made directly to private purveyors for medical care, burial, and other commodities and services provided under welfare programs; and provision and operation by the city of welfare institutions. Hospital data reflects spending for hospital facilities established or operated directly by city and township governments, the provision of health care, and support of other public or private hospitals. The Health category covers outpatient health services other than hospital care, including public health administration; research and education; categorical health programs; treatment and immunization clinics; nursing; environmental health activities (e.g., air and water pollution control); ambulance service provided separately from fire protection services; school health services provided by health agencies; other general public health activities (e.g., mosquito abatement). Health and hospital services provided directly by the city through its own hospitals and health agencies and any payments to other governments for such purposes are classed under those functional headings. 1. Data are for 1989-1990.

★ 457 ★

Government Spending: Local

Local Government Spending on Health Care in Oregon: 1990-1991

Local government spending for social service and income maintenance items is provided below. Data reflect city, urban town, and township government expenditures by function, thus grouping health-related activities (public welfare, hospitals, social insurance, and veterans' services) to provide a comprehensive picture of spending. Totals for these categories are not provided since they are meant only as presentational guidelines. According to the source: "Functions cannot be equated specifically with a single federal or state government program. Instead they represent broader activities of government that have remained virtually unchanged over many years so that as specific programs expand and contract they will remain useful for analytical purposes. Medicaid, for example, is a well-known program that is included in the larger public welfare function, specifically as a medical vendor payment, along with all other social welfare activities" (p. viii).

[Dollar amounts in thousands]

City	Social service and income maintenance expenditures		
	Public welfare	Hospitals	Health
Salem	-	-	1,675

Source: U.S. Bureau of the Census. *City Government Finances, 1990-1991.* Series GF/91-4. Washington, DC: U.S. Government Printing Office, 1993, p. 37. "Data in this report pertain to government fiscal years that ended between July 1, 1990, and June 30, 1991.... About three-fourths of all city governments in the nation had a fiscal year ending in either December (42 percent) or June (32 percent). September and April were the next most common months in which city governments ended their fiscal years. Of all townships, three-fifths had fiscal years corresponding directly with the calendar year 1990 (i.e., they ended their fiscal years on December 31, 1990). March, February, and June had the next most common fiscal year ending dates for townships" (p. vi). *Notes:* Detail may not add to total due to rounding. The Public Welfare heading covers the support of and assistance to needy persons contingent upon their need, excluding pensions to former employees and other benefits not contingent upon need. Among the expenditures in this category are: Cash assistance paid directly to needy persons under categorical programs (e.g., Old Age Assistance, Aid to Families With Dependent Children, Aid to the Blind, and Aid to the Disabled) or under any welfare programs; vendor payments made directly to private purveyors for medical care, burial, and other commodities and services provided under welfare programs; and provision and operation by the city of welfare institutions. Hospital data reflects spending for hospital facilities established or operated directly by city and township governments, the provision of health care, and support of other public or private hospitals. The Health category covers outpatient health services other than hospital care, including public health administration; research and education; categorical health programs; treatment and immunization clinics; nursing; environmental health activities (e.g., air and water pollution control); ambulance service provided separately from fire protection services; school health services provided by health agencies; other general public health activities (e.g., mosquito abatement). Health and hospital services provided directly by the city through its own hospitals and health agencies and any payments to other governments for such purposes are classed under those functional headings.

★ 458 ★

Government Spending: Local

Local Government Spending on Health Care in Pennsylvania: 1990-1991

Local government spending for social service and income maintenance items is provided below. Data reflect city, urban town, and township government expenditures by function, thus grouping health-related activities (public welfare, hospitals, social insurance, and veterans' services) to provide a comprehensive picture of spending. Totals for these categories are not provided since they are meant only as presentational guidelines. According to the source: "Functions cannot be equated specifically with a single federal or state government program. Instead they represent broader activities of government that have remained virtually unchanged over many years so that as specific programs expand and contract they will remain useful for analytical purposes. Medicaid, for example, is a well-known program that is included in the larger public welfare function, specifically as a medical vendor payment, along with all other social welfare activities" (p. viii).

[Dollar amounts in thousands]

City	Social service and income maintenance expenditures		
	Public welfare	Hospitals	Health
Allentown	-	-	2,607
Erie	-	-	218
Philadelphia	216,493	15,493	249,888
Pittsburgh	30	-	6,898
Reading	-	-	2
Scranton	-	-	5
Upper Darby township	-	-	263

Source: U.S. Bureau of the Census. *City Government Finances, 1990-1991.* Series GF/91-4. Washington, DC: U.S. Government Printing Office, 1993, p. 38. "Data in this report pertain to government fiscal years that ended between July 1, 1990, and June 30, 1991.... About three-fourths of all city governments in the nation had a fiscal year ending in either December (42 percent) or June (32 percent). September and April were the next most common months in which city governments ended their fiscal years. Of all townships, three-fifths had fiscal years corresponding directly with the calendar year 1990 (i.e., they ended their fiscal years on December 31, 1990). March, February, and June had the next most common fiscal year ending dates for townships" (p. vi). *Notes:* Detail may not add to total due to rounding. The Public Welfare heading covers the support of and assistance to needy persons contingent upon their need, excluding pensions to former employees and other benefits not contingent upon need. Among the expenditures in this category are: Cash assistance paid directly to needy persons under categorical programs (e.g., Old Age Assistance, Aid to Families With Dependent Children, Aid to the Blind, and Aid to the Disabled) or under any welfare programs; vendor payments made directly to private purveyors for medical care, burial, and other commodities and services provided under welfare programs; and provision and operation by the city of welfare institutions. Hospital data reflects spending for hospital facilities established or operated directly by city and township governments, the provision of health care, and support of other public or private hospitals. The Health category covers outpatient health services other than hospital care, including public health administration; research and education; categorical health programs; treatment and immunization clinics; nursing; environmental health activities (e.g., air and water pollution control); ambulance service provided separately from fire protection services; school health services provided by health agencies; other general public health activities (e.g., mosquito abatement). Health and hospital services provided directly by the city through its own hospitals and health agencies and any payments to other governments for such purposes are classed under those functional headings.

★ 459 ★

Government Spending: Local

Local Government Spending on Health Care in Rhode Island: 1990-1991

Local government spending for social service and income maintenance items is provided below. Data reflect city, urban town, and township government expenditures by function, thus grouping health-related activities (public welfare, hospitals, social insurance, and veterans' services) to provide a comprehensive picture of spending. Totals for these categories are not provided since they are meant only as presentational guidelines. According to the source: "Functions cannot be equated specifically with a single federal or state government program. Instead they represent broader activities of government that have remained virtually unchanged over many years so that as specific programs expand and contract they will remain useful for analytical purposes. Medicaid, for example, is a well-known program that is included in the larger public welfare function, specifically as a medical vendor payment, along with all other social welfare activities" (p. viii).

[Dollar amounts in thousands]

| City | Social service and income maintenance expenditures | | |
	Public welfare	Hospitals	Health
Cranston	1,292	-	100
Providence	14,236	-	127
Warwick	1,867	-	794

Source: U.S. Bureau of the Census. *City Government Finances, 1990-1991.* Series GF/91-4. Washington, DC: U.S. Government Printing Office, 1993, p. 65. "Data in this report pertain to government fiscal years that ended between July 1, 1990, and June 30, 1991. About three-fourths of all city governments in the nation had a fiscal year ending in either December (42 percent) or June (32 percent). September and April were the next most common months in which city governments ended their fiscal years. Of all townships, three-fifths had fiscal years corresponding directly with the calendar year 1990 (i.e., they ended their fiscal years on December 31, 1990). March, February, and June had the next most common fiscal year ending dates for townships" (p. vi). *Notes:* Detail may not add to total due to rounding. The Public Welfare heading covers the support of and assistance to needy persons contingent upon their need, excluding pensions to former employees and other benefits not contingent upon need. Among the expenditures in this category are: Cash assistance paid directly to needy persons under categorical programs (e.g., Old Age Assistance, Aid to Families With Dependent Children, Aid to the Blind, and Aid to the Disabled) or under any welfare programs; vendor payments made directly to private purveyors for medical care, burial, and other commodities and services provided under welfare programs; and provision and operation by the city of welfare institutions. Hospital data reflects spending for hospital facilities established or operated directly by city and township governments, the provision of health care, and support of other public or private hospitals. The Health category covers outpatient health services other than hospital care, including public health administration; research and education; categorical health programs; treatment and immunization clinics; nursing; environmental health activities (e.g., air and water pollution control); ambulance service provided separately from fire protection services; school health services provided by health agencies; other general public health activities (e.g., mosquito abatement). Health and hospital services provided directly by the city through its own hospitals and health agencies and any payments to other governments for such purposes are classed under those functional headings.

★ 460 ★
Government Spending: Local

Local Government Spending on Health Care in South Carolina: 1990-1991

Local government spending for social service and income maintenance items is provided below. Data reflect city, urban town, and township government expenditures by function, thus grouping health-related activities (public welfare, hospitals, social insurance, and veterans' services) to provide a comprehensive picture of spending. Totals for these categories are not provided since they are meant only as presentational guidelines. According to the source: "Functions cannot be equated specifically with a single federal or state government program. Instead they represent broader activities of government that have remained virtually unchanged over many years so that as specific programs expand and contract they will remain useful for analytical purposes. Medicaid, for example, is a well-known program that is included in the larger public welfare function, specifically as a medical vendor payment, along with all other social welfare activities" (p. viii).

[Dollar amounts in thousands]

| City | Social service and income maintenance expenditures | | |
	Public welfare	Hospitals	Health
Charleston	142	-	76
Columbia	-	-	424

Source: U.S. Bureau of the Census. *City Government Finances, 1990-1991.* Series GF/91-4. Washington, DC: U.S. Government Printing Office, 1993, p. 39. "Data in this report pertain to government fiscal years that ended between July 1, 1990, and June 30, 1991.... About three-fourths of all city governments in the nation had a fiscal year ending in either December (42 percent) or June (32 percent). September and April were the next most common months in which city governments ended their fiscal years. Of all townships, three-fifths had fiscal years corresponding directly with the calendar year 1990 (i.e., they ended their fiscal years on December 31, 1990). March, February, and June had the next most common fiscal year ending dates for townships" (p. vi). *Notes:* Detail may not add to total due to rounding. The Public Welfare heading covers the support of and assistance to needy persons contingent upon their need, excluding pensions to former employees and other benefits not contingent upon need. Among the expenditures in this category are: Cash assistance paid directly to needy persons under categorical programs (e.g., Old Age Assistance, Aid to Families With Dependent Children, Aid to the Blind, and Aid to the Disabled) or under any welfare programs; vendor payments made directly to private purveyors for medical care, burial, and other commodities and services provided under welfare programs; and provision and operation by the city of welfare institutions. Hospital data reflects spending for hospital facilities established or operated directly by city and township governments, the provision of health care, and support of other public or private hospitals. The Health category covers outpatient health services other than hospital care, including public health administration; research and education; categorical health programs; treatment and immunization clinics; nursing; environmental health activities (e.g., air and water pollution control); ambulance service provided separately from fire protection services; school health services provided by health agencies; other general public health activities (e.g., mosquito abatement). Health and hospital services provided directly by the city through its own hospitals and health agencies and any payments to other governments for such purposes are classed under those functional headings.

★ 461 ★

Government Spending: Local

Local Government Spending on Health Care in South Dakota: 1990-1991

Local government spending for social service and income maintenance items is provided below. Data reflect city, urban town, and township government expenditures by function, thus grouping health-related activities (public welfare, hospitals, social insurance, and veterans' services) to provide a comprehensive picture of spending. Totals for these categories are not provided since they are meant only as presentational guidelines. According to the source: "Functions cannot be equated specifically with a single federal or state government program. Instead they represent broader activities of government that have remained virtually unchanged over many years so that as specific programs expand and contract they will remain useful for analytical purposes. Medicaid, for example, is a well-known program that is included in the larger public welfare function, specifically as a medical vendor payment, along with all other social welfare activities" (p. viii).

[Dollar amounts in thousands]

City	Social service and income maintenance expenditures		
	Public welfare	Hospitals	Health
Sioux Falls	-	-	1,842

Source: U.S. Bureau of the Census. *City Government Finances, 1990-1991.* Series GF/91-4. Washington, DC: U.S. Government Printing Office, 1993, p. 39. "Data in this report pertain to government fiscal years that ended between July 1, 1990, and June 30, 1991.... About three-fourths of all city governments in the nation had a fiscal year ending in either December (42 percent) or June (32 percent). September and April were the next most common months in which city governments ended their fiscal years. Of all townships, three-fifths had fiscal years corresponding directly with the calendar year 1990 (i.e., they ended their fiscal years on December 31, 1990). March, February, and June had the next most common fiscal year ending dates for townships" (p. vi). *Notes:* Detail may not add to total due to rounding. The Public Welfare heading covers the support of and assistance to needy persons contingent upon their need, excluding pensions to former employees and other benefits not contingent upon need. Among the expenditures in this category are: Cash assistance paid directly to needy persons under categorical programs (e.g., Old Age Assistance, Aid to Families With Dependent Children, Aid to the Blind, and Aid to the Disabled) or under any welfare programs; vendor payments made directly to private purveyors for medical care, burial, and other commodities and services provided under welfare programs; and provision and operation by the city of welfare institutions. Hospital data reflects spending for hospital facilities established or operated directly by city and township governments, the provision of health care, and support of other public or private hospitals. The Health category covers outpatient health services other than hospital care, including public health administration; research and education; categorical health programs; treatment and immunization clinics; nursing; environmental health activities (e.g., air and water pollution control); ambulance service provided separately from fire protection services; school health services provided by health agencies; other general public health activities (e.g., mosquito abatement). Health and hospital services provided directly by the city through its own hospitals and health agencies and any payments to other governments for such purposes are classed under those functional headings.

★ 462 ★

Government Spending: Local

Local Government Spending on Health Care in Tennessee: 1990-1991

Local government spending for social service and income maintenance items is provided below. Data reflect city, urban town, and township government expenditures by function, thus grouping health-related activities (public welfare, hospitals, social insurance, and veterans' services) to provide a comprehensive picture of spending. Totals for these categories are not provided since they are meant only as presentational guidelines. According to the source: "Functions cannot be equated specifically with a single federal or state government program. Instead they represent broader activities of government that have remained virtually unchanged over many years so that as specific programs expand and contract they will remain useful for analytical purposes. Medicaid, for example, is a well-known program that is included in the larger public welfare function, specifically as a medical vendor payment, along with all other social welfare activities" (p. viii).

[Dollar amounts in thousands]

| City | Social service and income maintenance expenditures | | |
	Public welfare	Hospitals	Health
Chattanooga	6,580	-	2,320
Clarksville	28	-	87
Knoxville	-	-	4,513
Memphis	-	8,856	6,259
Nashville-Davidson	8,553	49,836	19,031

Source: U.S. Bureau of the Census. *City Government Finances, 1990-1991.* Series GF/91-4. Washington, DC: U.S. Government Printing Office, 1993, pp. 39-40. "Data in this report pertain to government fiscal years that ended between July 1, 1990, and June 30, 1991.... About three-fourths of all city governments in the nation had a fiscal year ending in either December (42 percent) or June (32 percent). September and April were the next most common months in which city governments ended their fiscal years. Of all townships, three-fifths had fiscal years corresponding directly with the calendar year 1990 (i.e., they ended their fiscal years on December 31, 1990). March, February, and June had the next most common fiscal year ending dates for townships" (p. vi). *Notes:* Detail may not add to total due to rounding. The Public Welfare heading covers the support of and assistance to needy persons contingent upon their need, excluding pensions to former employees and other benefits not contingent upon need. Among the expenditures in this category are: Cash assistance paid directly to needy persons under categorical programs (e.g., Old Age Assistance, Aid to Families With Dependent Children, Aid to the Blind, and Aid to the Disabled) or under any welfare programs; vendor payments made directly to private purveyors for medical care, burial, and other commodities and services provided under welfare programs; and provision and operation by the city of welfare institutions. Hospital data reflects spending for hospital facilities established or operated directly by city and township governments, the provision of health care, and support of other public or private hospitals. The Health category covers outpatient health services other than hospital care, including public health administration; research and education; categorical health programs; treatment and immunization clinics; nursing; environmental health activities (e.g., air and water pollution control); ambulance service provided separately from fire protection services; school health services provided by health agencies; other general public health activities (e.g., mosquito abatement). Health and hospital services provided directly by the city through its own hospitals and health agencies and any payments to other governments for such purposes are classed under those functional headings.

★ 463 ★

Government Spending: Local

Local Government Spending on Health Care in Texas: 1990-1991

Local government spending for social service and income maintenance items is provided below. Data reflect city, urban town, and township government expenditures by function, thus grouping health-related activities (public welfare, hospitals, social insurance, and veterans' services) to provide a comprehensive picture of spending. Totals for these categories are not provided since they are meant only as presentational guidelines. According to the source: "Functions cannot be equated specifically with a single federal or state government program. Instead they represent broader activities of government that have remained virtually unchanged over many years so that as specific programs expand and contract they will remain useful for analytical purposes. Medicaid, for example, is a well-known program that is included in the larger public welfare function, specifically as a medical vendor payment, along with all other social welfare activities" (p. viii).

[Dollar amounts in thousands]

City	Social service and income maintenance expenditures		
	Public welfare	Hospitals	Health
Abiliene	-	-	2,698
Amarillo	-	-	2,090
Arlington	860	-	1,253
Austin	1,720	88,405	32,325
Beaumont	405	-	2,772
Brownsville	12	-	1,223
Carrollton	-	-	829
Corpus Christi	-	-	6,651
Dallas	-	-	18,330
El Paso	-	-	12,534
Fort Worth	-	-	9,540
Garland	-	-	1,073
Grand Prairie	-	-	1,154
Houston	-	-	53,113
Irving	-	-	987
Laredo	1,816	-	2,553
Lubbock	-	-	2,696
McAllen	170	-	272
Mesquite	3	-	860
Midland	77	-	1,522
Odessa	468	-	-
Pasadena	-	-	828
Plano	-	-	597
Richardson	-	-	645
San Angelo	1,323	-	2,389
San Antonio	4,608	-	17,493
Tyler	681	-	1,042

[Continued]

★ 463 ★

Local Government Spending on Health Care in Texas:
1990-1991
[Continued]

City	Social service and income maintenance expenditures		
	Public welfare	Hospitals	Health
Waco	981	-	1,735
Wichita Falls	-	-	1,661

Source: U.S. Bureau of the Census. *City Government Finances, 1990-1991.* Series GF/91-4. Washington, DC: U.S. Government Printing Office, 1993, pp. 40-43. "Data in this report pertain to government fiscal years that ended between July 1, 1990, and June 30, 1991.... About three-fourths of all city governments in the nation had a fiscal year ending in either December (42 percent) or June (32 percent). September and April were the next most common months in which city governments ended their fiscal years. Of all townships, three-fifths had fiscal years corresponding directly with the calendar year 1990 (i.e., they ended their fiscal years on December 31, 1990). March, February, and June had the next most common fiscal year ending dates for townships" (p. vi). *Notes:* Detail may not add to total due to rounding. The Public Welfare heading covers the support of and assistance to needy persons contingent upon their need, excluding pensions to former employees and other benefits not contingent upon need. Among the expenditures in this category are: Cash assistance paid directly to needy persons under categorical programs (e.g., Old Age Assistance, Aid to Families With Dependent Children, Aid to the Blind, and Aid to the Disabled) or under any welfare programs; vendor payments made directly to private purveyors for medical care, burial, and other commodities and services provided under welfare programs; and provision and operation by the city of welfare institutions. Hospital data reflects spending for hospital facilities established or operated directly by city and township governments, the provision of health care, and support of other public or private hospitals. The Health category covers outpatient health services other than hospital care, including public health administration; research and education; categorical health programs; treatment and immunization clinics; nursing; environmental health activities (e.g., air and water pollution control); ambulance service provided separately from fire protection services; school health services provided by health agencies; other general public health activities (e.g., mosquito abatement). Health and hospital services provided directly by the city through its own hospitals and health agencies and any payments to other governments for such purposes are classed under those functional headings.

★ 464 ★

Government Spending: Local

Local Government Spending on Health Care in Utah: 1990-1991

Local government spending for social service and income maintenance items is provided below. Data reflect city, urban town, and township government expenditures by function, thus grouping health-related activities (public welfare, hospitals, social insurance, and veterans' services) to provide a comprehensive picture of spending. Totals for these categories are not provided since they are meant only as presentational guidelines. According to the source: "Functions cannot be equated specifically with a single federal or state government program. Instead they represent broader activities of government that have remained virtually unchanged over many years so that as specific programs expand and contract they will remain useful for analytical purposes. Medicaid, for example, is a well-known program that is included in the larger public welfare function, specifically as a medical vendor payment, along with all other social welfare activities" (p. viii).

[Dollar amounts in thousands]

City	Social service and income maintenance expenditures		
	Public welfare	Hospitals	Health
Salt Lake City	-	-	24

Source: U.S. Bureau of the Census. *City Government Finances, 1990-1991.* Series GF/91-4. Washington, DC: U.S. Government Printing Office, 1993, p. 44. "Data in this report pertain to government fiscal years that ended between July 1, 1990, and June 30, 1991.... About three-fourths of all city governments in the nation had a fiscal year ending in either December (42 percent) or June (32 percent). September and April were the next most common months in which city governments ended their fiscal years. Of all townships, three-fifths had fiscal years corresponding directly with the calendar year 1990 (i.e., they ended their fiscal years on December 31, 1990). March, February, and June had the next most common fiscal year ending dates for townships" (p. vi). *Notes:* Detail may not add to total due to rounding. The Public Welfare heading covers the support of and assistance to needy persons contingent upon their need, excluding pensions to former employees and other benefits not contingent upon need. Among the expenditures in this category are: Cash assistance paid directly to needy persons under categorical programs (e.g., Old Age Assistance, Aid to Families With Dependent Children, Aid to the Blind, and Aid to the Disabled) or under any welfare programs; vendor payments made directly to private purveyors for medical care, burial, and other commodities and services provided under welfare programs; and provision and operation by the city of welfare institutions. Hospital data reflects spending for hospital facilities established or operated directly by city and township governments, the provision of health care, and support of other public or private hospitals. The Health category covers outpatient health services other than hospital care, including public health administration; research and education; categorical health programs; treatment and immunization clinics; nursing; environmental health activities (e.g., air and water pollution control); ambulance service provided separately from fire protection services; school health services provided by health agencies; other general public health activities (e.g., mosquito abatement). Health and hospital services provided directly by the city through its own hospitals and health agencies and any payments to other governments for such purposes are classed under those functional headings.

★ 465 ★

Government Spending: Local

Local Government Spending on Health Care in Vermont: 1990-1991

Local government spending for social service and income maintenance items is provided below. Data reflect city, urban town, and township government expenditures by function, thus grouping health-related activities (public welfare, hospitals, social insurance, and veterans' services) to provide a comprehensive picture of spending. Totals for these categories are not provided since they are meant only as presentational guidelines. According to the source: "Functions cannot be equated specifically with a single federal or state government program. Instead they represent broader activities of government that have remained virtually unchanged over many years so that as specific programs expand and contract they will remain useful for analytical purposes. Medicaid, for example, is a well-known program that is included in the larger public welfare function, specifically as a medical vendor payment, along with all other social welfare activities" (p. viii).

[Dollar amounts in thousands]

City	Social service and income maintenance expenditures		
	Public welfare	Hospitals	Health
Burlington	-	-	543

Source: U.S. Bureau of the Census. *City Government Finances, 1990-1991.* Series GF/91-4. Washington, DC: U.S. Government Printing Office, 1993, p. 44. "Data in this report pertain to government fiscal years that ended between July 1, 1990, and June 30, 1991.... About three-fourths of all city governments in the nation had a fiscal year ending in either December (42 percent) or June (32 percent). September and April were the next most common months in which city governments ended their fiscal years. Of all townships, three-fifths had fiscal years corresponding directly with the calendar year 1990 (i.e., they ended their fiscal years on December 31, 1990). March, February, and June had the next most common fiscal year ending dates for townships" (p. vi). *Notes:* Detail may not add to total due to rounding. The Public Welfare heading covers the support of and assistance to needy persons contingent upon their need, excluding pensions to former employees and other benefits not contingent upon need. Among the expenditures in this category are: Cash assistance paid directly to needy persons under categorical programs (e.g., Old Age Assistance, Aid to Families With Dependent Children, Aid to the Blind, and Aid to the Disabled) or under any welfare programs; vendor payments made directly to private purveyors for medical care, burial, and other commodities and services provided under welfare programs; and provision and operation by the city of welfare institutions. Hospital data reflects spending for hospital facilities established or operated directly by city and township governments, the provision of health care, and support of other public or private hospitals. The Health category covers outpatient health services other than hospital care, including public health administration; research and education; categorical health programs; treatment and immunization clinics; nursing; environmental health activities (e.g., air and water pollution control); ambulance service provided separately from fire protection services; school health services provided by health agencies; other general public health activities (e.g., mosquito abatement). Health and hospital services provided directly by the city through its own hospitals and health agencies and any payments to other governments for such purposes are classed under those functional headings.

★ 466 ★
Government Spending: Local

Local Government Spending on Health Care in Virginia: 1990-1991

Local government spending for social service and income maintenance items is provided below. Data reflect city, urban town, and township government expenditures by function, thus grouping health-related activities (public welfare, hospitals, social insurance, and veterans' services) to provide a comprehensive picture of spending. Totals for these categories are not provided since they are meant only as presentational guidelines. According to the source: "Functions cannot be equated specifically with a single federal or state government program. Instead they represent broader activities of government that have remained virtually unchanged over many years so that as specific programs expand and contract they will remain useful for analytical purposes. Medicaid, for example, is a well-known program that is included in the larger public welfare function, specifically as a medical vendor payment, along with all other social welfare activities" (p. viii).

[Dollar amounts in thousands]

City	Social service and income maintenance expenditures		
	Public welfare	Hospitals	Health
Alexandria	18,253	700	13,698
Chesapeake	8,743	-	9,790
Hampton	7,305	-	2,653
Newport News	13,532	-	3,804
Norfolk	30,298	11,394	17,543
Portsmouth	16,581	-	7,912
Richmond	39,915	-	17,183
Roanoke	12,139	-	979
Virginia Beach	14,279	-	17,174

Source: U.C. Bureau of the Census. *City Government Finances, 1990-1991,* Series GF/91-4. Washington, DC: U.S. Government Printing Office, 1993, pp. 44-45. "Data in this report pertain to government fiscal years that ended between July 1, 1990, and June 30, 1991.... About three-fourths of all city governments in the nation had a fiscal year ending in either December (42 percent) or June (32 percent). September and April were the next most common months in which city governments ended their fiscal years. Of all townships, three-fifths had fiscal years corresponding directly with the calendar year 1990 (i.e., they ended their fiscal years on December 31, 1990). March, February, and June had the next most common fiscal year ending dates for townships" (p. vi). *Notes:* Detail may not add to total due to rounding. The Public Welfare heading covers the support of and assistance to needy persons contingent upon their need, excluding pensions to former employees and other benefits not contingent upon need. Among the expenditures in this category are: Cash assistance paid directly to needy persons under categorical programs (e.g., Old Age Assistance, Aid to Families With Dependent Children, Aid to the Blind, and Aid to the Disabled) or under any welfare programs; vendor payments made directly to private purveyors for medical care, burial, and other commodities and services provided under welfare programs; and provision and operation by the city of welfare institutions. Hospital data reflects spending for hospital facilities established or operated directly by city and township governments, the provision of health care, and support of other public or private hospitals. The Health category covers outpatient health services other than hospital care, including public health administration; research and education; categorical health programs; treatment and immunization clinics; nursing; environmental health activities (e.g., air and water pollution control); ambulance service provided separately from fire protection services; school health services provided by health agencies; other general public health activities (e.g., mosquito abatement). Health and hospital services provided directly by the city through its own hospitals and health agencies and any payments to other governments for such purposes are classed under those functional headings.

★ 467 ★

Government Spending: Local

Local Government Spending on Health Care in Washington: 1990-1991

Local government spending for social service and income maintenance items is provided below. Data reflect city, urban town, and township government expenditures by function, thus grouping health-related activities (public welfare, hospitals, social insurance, and veterans' services) to provide a comprehensive picture of spending. Totals for these categories are not provided since they are meant only as presentational guidelines. According to the source: "Functions cannot be equated specifically with a single federal or state government program. Instead they represent broader activities of government that have remained virtually unchanged over many years so that as specific programs expand and contract they will remain useful for analytical purposes. Medicaid, for example, is a well-known program that is included in the larger public welfare function, specifically as a medical vendor payment, along with all other social welfare activities" (p. viii).

[Dollar amounts in thousands]

City	Social service and income maintenance expenditures		
	Public welfare	Hospitals	Health
Bellevue	51	-	1,475
Seattle	-	-	13,751
Spokane	-	-	1,358
Tacoma	1,393	-	2,934

Source: U.S. Bureau of the Census. *City Government Finances, 1990-1991.* Series GF/91-4. Washington, DC: U.S. Government Printing Office, 1993, pp. 45-46. "Data in this report pertain to government fiscal years that ended between July 1, 1990, and June 30, 1991.... About three-fourths of all city governments in the nation had a fiscal year ending in either December (42 percent) or June (32 percent). September and April were the next most common months in which city governments ended their fiscal years. Of all townships, three-fifths had fiscal years corresponding directly with the calendar year 1990 (i.e., they ended their fiscal years on December 31, 1990). March, February, and June had the next most common fiscal year ending dates for townships" (p. vi). *Notes:* Detail may not add to total due to rounding. The Public Welfare heading covers the support of and assistance to needy persons contingent upon their need, excluding pensions to former employees and other benefits not contingent upon need. Among the expenditures in this category are: Cash assistance paid directly to needy persons under categorical programs (e.g., Old Age Assistance, Aid to Families With Dependent Children, Aid to the Blind, and Aid to the Disabled) or under any welfare programs; vendor payments made directly to private purveyors for medical care, burial, and other commodities and services provided under welfare programs; and provision and operation by the city of welfare institutions. Hospital data reflects spending for hospital facilities established or operated directly by city and township governments, the provision of health care, and support of other public or private hospitals. The Health category covers outpatient health services other than hospital care, including public health administration; research and education; categorical health programs; treatment and immunization clinics; nursing; environmental health activities (e.g., air and water pollution control); ambulance service provided separately from fire protection services; school health services provided by health agencies; other general public health activities (e.g., mosquito abatement). Health and hospital services provided directly by the city through its own hospitals and health agencies and any payments to other governments for such purposes are classed under those functional headings.

★ 468 ★

Government Spending: Local

Local Government Spending on Health Care in West Virginia: 1990-1991

Local government spending for social service and income maintenance items is provided below. Data reflect city, urban town, and township government expenditures by function, thus grouping health-related activities (public welfare, hospitals, social insurance, and veterans' services) to provide a comprehensive picture of spending. Totals for these categories are not provided since they are meant only as presentational guidelines. According to the source: "Functions cannot be equated specifically with a single federal or state government program. Instead they represent broader activities of government that have remained virtually unchanged over many years so that as specific programs expand and contract they will remain useful for analytical purposes. Medicaid, for example, is a well-known program that is included in the larger public welfare function, specifically as a medical vendor payment, along with all other social welfare activities" (p. viii).

[Dollar amounts in thousands]

City	Social service and income maintenance expenditures		
	Public welfare	Hospitals	Health
Huntington	-	-	94

Source: U.S. Bureau of the Census. *City Government Finances, 1990-1991.* Series GF/91- 4. Washington, DC: U.S. Government Printing Office, 1993, p. 46. "Data in this report pertain to government fiscal years that ended between July 1, 1990, and June 30, 1991.... About three-fourths of all city governments in the nation had a fiscal year ending in either December (42 percent) or June (32 percent). September and April were the next most common months in which city governments ended their fiscal years. Of all townships, three-fifths had fiscal years corresponding directly with the calendar year 1990 (i.e., they ended their fiscal years on December 31, 1990). March, February, and June had the next most common fiscal year ending dates for townships" (p. vi). *Notes:* Detail may not add to total due to rounding. The Public Welfare heading covers the support of and assistance to needy persons contingent upon their need, excluding pensions to former employees and other benefits not contingent upon need. Among the expenditures in this category are: Cash assistance paid directly to needy persons under categorical programs (e.g., Old Age Assistance, Aid to Families With Dependent Children, Aid to the Blind, and Aid to the Disabled) or under any welfare programs; vendor payments made directly to private purveyors for medical care, burial, and other commodities and services provided under welfare programs; and provision and operation by the city of welfare institutions. Hospital data reflects spending for hospital facilities established or operated directly by city and township governments, the provision of health care, and support of other public or private hospitals. The Health category covers outpatient health services other than hospital care, including public health administration; research and education; categorical health programs; treatment and immunization clinics; nursing; environmental health activities (e.g., air and water pollution control); ambulance service provided separately from fire protection services; school health services provided by health agencies; other general public health activities (e.g., mosquito abatement). Health and hospital services provided directly by the city through its own hospitals and health agencies and any payments to other governments for such purposes are classed under those functional headings.

★ 469 ★

Government Spending: Local

Local Government Spending on Health Care in Wisconsin: 1990-1991

Local government spending for social service and income maintenance items is provided below. Data reflect city, urban town, and township government expenditures by function, thus grouping health-related activities (public welfare, hospitals, social insurance, and veterans' services) to provide a comprehensive picture of spending. Totals for these categories are not provided since they are meant only as presentational guidelines. According to the source: "Functions cannot be equated specifically with a single federal or state government program. Instead they represent broader activities of government that have remained virtually unchanged over many years so that as specific programs expand and contract they will remain useful for analytical purposes. Medicaid, for example, is a well-known program that is included in the larger public welfare function, specifically as a medical vendor payment, along with all other social welfare activities" (p. viii).

[Dollar amounts in thousands]

| City | Social service and income maintenance expenditures | | |
	Public welfare	Hospitals	Health
Green Bay	-	-	1,400
Kenosha	-	-	3,176
Madison	10	-	5,776
Milwaukee	-	-	9,286
Racine	-	-	1,805

Source: U.S. Bureau of the Census. *City Government Finances, 1990-1991.* Series GF/91-4. Washington, DC: U.S. Government Printing Office, 1993, p. 46. "Data in this report pertain to government fiscal years that ended between July 1, 1990, and June 30, 1991.... About three-fourths of all city governments in the nation had a fiscal year ending in either December (42 percent) or June (32 percent). September and April were the next most common months in which city governments ended their fiscal years. Of all townships, three-fifths had fiscal years corresponding directly with the calendar year 1990 (i.e., they ended their fiscal years on December 31, 1990). March, February, and June had the next most common fiscal year ending dates for townships" (p. vi). *Notes:* Detail may not add to total due to rounding. The Public Welfare heading covers the support of and assistance to needy persons contingent upon their need, excluding pensions to former employees and other benefits not contingent upon need. Among the expenditures in this category are: Cash assistance paid directly to needy persons under categorical programs (e.g., Old Age Assistance, Aid to Families With Dependent Children, Aid to the Blind, and Aid to the Disabled) or under any welfare programs; vendor payments made directly to private purveyors for medical care, burial, and other commodities and services provided under welfare programs; and provision and operation by the city of welfare institutions. Hospital data reflects spending for hospital facilities established or operated directly by city and township governments, the provision of health care, and support of other public or private hospitals. The Health category covers outpatient health services other than hospital care, including public health administration; research and education; categorical health programs; treatment and immunization clinics; nursing; environmental health activities (e.g., air and water pollution control); ambulance service provided separately from fire protection services; school health services provided by health agencies; other general public health activities (e.g., mosquito abatement). Health and hospital services provided directly by the city through its own hospitals and health agencies and any payments to other governments for such purposes are classed under those functional headings.

★ 470 ★

Government Spending: Local

Local Government Spending on Health Care in Wyoming: 1990-1991

Local government spending for social service and income maintenance items is provided below. Data reflect city, urban town, and township government expenditures by function, thus grouping health-related activities (public welfare, hospitals, social insurance, and veterans' services) to provide a comprehensive picture of spending. Totals for these categories are not provided since they are meant only as presentational guidelines. According to the source: "Functions cannot be equated specifically with a single federal or state government program. Instead they represent broader activities of government that have remained virtually unchanged over many years so that as specific programs expand and contract they will remain useful for analytical purposes. Medicaid, for example, is a well-known program that is included in the larger public welfare function, specifically as a medical vendor payment, along with all other social welfare activities" (p. viii).

[Dollar amounts in thousands]

| City | Social service and income maintenance expenditures | | |
	Public welfare	Hospitals	Health
Cheyenne	388	-	1,143

Source: U.S. Bureau of the Census. *City Government Finances, 1990-1991.* Series GF/91-4. Washington, DC: U.S. Government Printing Office, 1993, p. 46. "Data in this report pertain to government fiscal years that ended between July 1, 1990, and June 30, 1991.... About three-fourths of all city governments in the nation had a fiscal year ending in either December (42 percent) or June (32 percent). September and April were the next most common months in which city governments ended their fiscal years. Of all townships, three-fifths had fiscal years corresponding directly with the calendar year 1990 (i.e., they ended their fiscal years on December 31, 1990). March, February, and June had the next most common fiscal year ending dates for townships" (p. vi). *Notes:* Detail may not add to total due to rounding. The Public welfare heading covers the support of and assistance to needy persons contingent upon their need, excluding pensions to former employees and other benefits not contingent upon need. Among the expenditures in this category are: Cash assistance paid directly to needy persons under categorical programs (e.g., Old Age Assistance, Aid to Families With Dependent Children, Aid to the Blind, and Aid to the Disabled) or under any welfare programs; vendor payments made directly to private purveyors for medical care, burial, and other commodities and services provided under welfare programs; and provision and operation by the city of welfare institutions. Hospital data reflects spending for hospital facilities established or operated directly by city and township governments, the provision of health care, and support of other public or private hospitals. The Health category covers outpatient health services other than hospital care, including public health administration; research and education; categorical health programs; treatment and immunization clinics; nursing; environmental health activities (e.g., air and water pollution control); ambulance service provided separately from fire protection services; school health services provided by health agencies; other general public health activities (e.g., mosquito abatement). Health and hospital services provided directly by the city through its own hospitals and health agencies and any payments to other governments for such purposes are classed under those functional headings.

★ 471 ★

Government Spending: Local

Municipalities' Health Care Finances, by Population-Size Groups: 1990-1991

This table presents city government expenditures by function, thus grouping health-related activities (public welfare, hospitals, social insurance, and veterans' services) to provide a comprehensive picture of spending. Totals for these categories are not provided since they are meant only as presentational guidelines. According to the source: "Functions cannot be equated specifically with a single federal or state government program. Instead they represent broader activities of government that have remained virtually unchanged over many years so that as specific programs expand and contract they will remain useful for analytical purposes. Medicaid, for example, is a well-known program that is included in the larger public welfare function, specifically as a medical vendor payment, along with all other social welfare activities" (p. viii).

[Dollar amounts in millions. Detail may not add to total due to rounding.]

Item	All municipalities	Municipalities having a 1990 population of:						
		1 million or more	500,000 to 999,999	300,000 to 499,999	200,000 to 299,999	100,000 to 199,999	75,000 to 99,999	Less than 75,000
Number of municipalities, 1990	19,296	8	16	28	24	119	98	19,003
Population, 1990 (in thousands)	153,827	19,953	10,954	11,088	5,975	16,390	8,455	81,012
Revenue	210,498	61,428	23,521	16,459	8,387	20,397	9,517	70,789
Expenditure	211,506	59,982	23,294	16,404	8,788	21,117	9,833	72,088
Social services and income maintenance								
Public welfare	8,941	6,842	1,170	160	143	241	59	326
Hospitals	7,049	3,134	1,039	288	107	242	210	2,029
Health	2,769	1,093	535	275	136	214	79	437
Other	12	-	12	-	-	-	-	-

Source: U.S. Bureau of the Census. *City Government Finances, 1990-1991.* Series GF/91-4. Washington, DC: U.S. Government Printing Office, 1993, p. 3. "Data in this report pertain to government fiscal years that ended between July 1, 1990, and June 30, 1991.... About three-fourths of all city governments in the nation had a fiscal year ending in either December (42 percent) or June (32 percent). September and April were the next most common months in which city governments ended their fiscal years. Three-fifths of all townships had fiscal years corresponding directly with the calendar year 1990 (i.e., they ended their fiscal years on December 31, 1990). March, February, and June had the next most common fiscal year ending dates for townships" (p.vi). *Notes:* Municipalities were distributed according to their 1990 estimated populations. The Public Welfare heading covers the support of and assistance to needy persons contingent upon their need, excluding pensions to former employees and other benefits not contingent upon need. Among the expenditures in this category are: Cash assistance paid directly to needy persons under categorical programs (e.g., Old Age Assistance, Aid to Families With Dependent Children, Aid to the Blind, and Aid to the Disabled) or under any welfare programs; vendor payments made directly to private purveyors for medical care, burial, and other commodities and services provided under welfare programs; and provision and operation by the city of welfare institutions. Hospital data reflects spending for hospital facilities established or operated directly by city and township governments, the provision of health care, and support of other public or private hospitals. The Health category covers outpatient health services other than hospital care, including public health administration; research and education; categorical health programs; treatment and immunization clinics; nursing; environmental health activities (e.g., air and water pollution control); ambulance service provided separately from fire protection services; school health services provided by health agencies; other general public health activities (e.g., mosquito abatement). Health and hospital services provided directly by the city through its own hospitals and health agencies and any payments to other governments for such purposes are classed under those functional headings.

★ 472 ★

Government Spending: Local

Per Capita Amounts of City Government Health Care Finance Items: 1990-1991

This table presents city government expenditures by function, thus grouping health-related activities (public welfare, hospitals, social insurance, and veterans' services) to provide a comprehensive picture of spending. Totals for these categories are not provided since they are meant only as presentational guidelines. According to the source: "Functions cannot be equated specifically with a single federal or state government program. Instead they represent broader activities of government that have remained virtually unchanged over many years so that as specific programs expand and contract they will remain useful for analytical purposes. Medicaid, for example, is a well-known program that is included in the larger public welfare function, specifically as a medical vendor payment, along with all other social welfare activities" (p. viii). Data are provided by population-size groups.

[Detail may not add to total due to rounding.]

Item	All municipalities	Municipalities having a 1990 population of:						
		1 million or more	500,000 to 999,999	300,000 to 499,999	200,000 to 299,999	100,000 to 199,999	75,000 to 99,999	Less than 75,000
Revenue	1,368.40	3,078.59	2,147.25	1,484.44	1,403.80	1,244.43	1,125.59	873.81
Expenditure	1,374.96	3,006.15	2,126.48	1,479.45	1,470.92	1,288.35	1,162.89	889.85
Social services and income maintenance								
Public welfare	58.12	342.91	106.84	14.43	23.97	14.73	6.93	4.01
Hospitals	45.83	157.07	94.83	25.93	17.92	14.76	24.79	25.06
Health	18.00	54.76	48.84	24.82	22.81	13.06	9.38	5.38
Other	.08	-	1.05	-	-	-	-	-

Source: U.S. Bureau of the Census. *City Government Finances, 1990-1991.* Series GF/91-4. Washington, DC: U.S. Government Printing Office, 1993, p. 4. "Data in this report pertain to government fiscal years that ended between July 1, 1990, and June 30, 1991.... About three-fourths of all city governments in the nation had a fiscal year ending in either December (42 percent) or June (32 percent). September and April were the next most common months in which city governments ended their fiscal years. Of all the townships, three-fifths had fiscal years corresponding directly with the calendar year 1990 (i.e., they ended their fiscal years on December 31, 1990). March, February, and June had the next most common fiscal year ending dates for townships" (p. vi). *Notes:* Municipalities were distributed according to their 1990 estimated populations. The Public Welfare heading covers the support of and assistance to needy persons contingent upon their need, excluding pensions to former employees and other benefits not contingent upon need. Among the expenditures in this category are: Cash assistance paid directly to needy persons under categorical programs (e.g., Old Age Assistance, Aid to Families With Dependent Children, Aid to the Blind, and Aid to the Disabled) or under any welfare programs; vendor payments made directly to private purveyors for medical care, burial, and other commodities and services provided under welfare programs; and provision and operation by the city of welfare institutions. Hospital data reflects spending for hospital facilities established or operated directly by city and township governments, the provision of health care, and support of other public or private hospitals. The Health category covers outpatient health services other than hospital care, including public health administration; research and education; categorical health programs; treatment and immunization clinics; nursing; environmental health activities (e.g., air and water pollution control); ambulance service provided separately from fire protection services; school health services provided by health agencies; other general public health activities (e.g., mosquito abatement). Health and hospital services provided directly by the city through its own hospitals and health agencies and any payments to other governments for such purposes are classed under these functional headings.

★ 473 ★

Government Spending: Local

Percent Distribution of City Government Health Care Finance Items: 1990-1991

This table presents city government expenditures by function, thus grouping health-related activities (public welfare, hospitals, social insurance, and veterans' services) to provide a comprehensive picture of spending. Totals for these categories are not provided since they are meant only as presentational guidelines. According to the source: "Functions cannot be equated specifically with a single federal or state government program. Instead they represent broader activities of government that have remained virtually unchanged over many years so that as specific programs expand and contract they will remain useful for analytical purposes. Medicaid, for example, is a well-known program that is included in the larger public welfare function, specifically as a medical vendor payment, along with all other social welfare activities" (p. viii). Data are provided by population-size groups.

[Detail may not add to total due to rounding.]

Item	All municipalities	Municipalities having a 1990 population of:						
		1 million or more	500,000 to 999,999	300,000 to 499,999	200,000 to 299,999	100,000 to 199,999	75,000 to 99,999	Less than 75,000
Revenue	100.0	29.2	11.2	7.8	4.0	9.7	4.5	33.6
Expenditure	100.0	28.4	11.0	7.8	4.2	10.0	4.6	34.1
Social services and income maintenance								
Public welfare	100.0	76.5	13.1	1.8	1.6	2.7	.7	3.6
Hospitals	100.0	44.5	14.7	4.1	1.5	3.4	3.0	28.8
Health	100.0	39.5	19.3	9.9	4.9	7.7	2.9	15.7
Other	100.0	-	100.0	-	-	-	-	-

Source: U.S. Bureau of the Census. *City Government Finances, 1990-1991.* Series GF/91-4. Washington, DC: U.S. Government Printing Office, 1993, p. 5. "Data in this report pertain to government fiscal years that ended between July 1, 1990, and June 30, 1991.... About three-fourths of all city governments in the nation had a fiscal year ending in either December (42 percent) or June (32 percent). September and April were the next most common months in which city governments ended their fiscal years. Of all townships, three-fifths had fiscal years corresponding directly with the calendar year 1990 (i.e., they ended their fiscal years on December 31, 1990). March, February, and June had the next most common fiscal year ending dates for townships" (p. vi). *Notes:* Municipalities were distributed according to their 1988 estimated populations. The Public Welfare heading covers the support of and assistance to needy persons contingent upon their need, excluding pensions to former employees and other benefits not contingent upon need. Among the expenditures in this category are: Cash assistance paid directly to needy persons under categorical programs (e.g., Old Age Assistance, Aid to Families With Dependent Children, Aid to the Blind, and Aid to the Disabled) or under any welfare programs; vendor payments made directly to private purveyors for medical care, burial, and other commodities and services provided under welfare programs; and provision and operation by the city of welfare institutions. Hospital data reflects spending for hospital facilities established or operated directly by city and township governments, the provision of health care, and support of other public or private hospitals. The Health category covers outpatient health services other than hospital care, including public health administration; research and education; categorical health programs; treatment and immunization clinics; nursing; environmental health activities (e.g., air and water pollution control); ambulance service provided separately from fire protection services; school health services provided by health agencies; other general public health activities (e.g., mosquito abatement). Health and hospital services provided directly by the city through its own hospitals and health agencies and any payments to other governments for such purposes are classed under those functional headings.

★ 474 ★

Government Spending: Local

Summary of City Government Health Care Finances: 1990-1991 and Prior Periods

This table presents city government expenditures by function, thus grouping health-related activities (public welfare, hospitals, social insurance, and veterans' services) to provide a comprehensive picture of spending. Totals for these categories are not provided since they are meant only as presentational guidelines. According to the source: "Functions cannot be equated specifically with a single federal or state government program. Instead they represent broader activities of government that have remained virtually unchanged over many years so that as specific programs expand and contract they will remain useful for analytical purposes. Medicaid, for example, is a well-known program that is included in the larger public welfare function, specifically as a medical vendor payment, along with all other social welfare activities" (p. viii).

[Dollar amounts in millions. Detail may not add to total due to rounding.]

Item	1990-1991	1989-1990	1988-1989	1987-1988	Percent change 1989-1990 to 1990-1991	Percent distribution 1990-1991
Revenue	210,498	202,393	184,770	176,664	4.0	(x)
Expenditure	211,506	198,822	182,763	174,674	6.4	100.0
Social services and income maintenance						
Public welfare	8,941	7,890	7,129	6,537	13.3	5.4
Cash assistance payments	2,549	2,212	2,099	2,043	15.2	1.6
Medical vendor payments	386	384	361	344	.5	.2
Other	6,006	5,294	4,669	4,150	13.4	3.7
Hospitals	7,049	6,581	6,097	5,866	7.1	4.3
Own	6,441	6,024	5,576	5,424	6.9	3.9
Capital outlay	387	338	301	338	14.5	.2
Other	608	557	521	443	9.2	.4
Health	2,769	2,560	2,221	2,175	8.2	1.7

Source: U.S. Bureau of the Census. *City Government Finances, 1990-1991.* Series GF/91-4. Washington, DC: U.S. Government Printing Office, 1993, p. 1. *Notes:* The classification of medical vendor payments varies somewhat between public welfare and hospitals according to the situation; private purveyor payments made under welfare programs are classed as public welfare, but any services provided directly by a government through its hospital agency is included under the Hospitals heading. Hospital data reflects spending for hospital facilities established or operated directly by city and township governments, the provision of health care, and support of other public or private hospitals. "Own" hospitals comprise those administered by the government concerned, but exclude payments to other governments and to private agencies for hospital support and services that are classified under "Other" hospitals. The Public Welfare heading covers the support of and assistance to needy persons contingent upon their need, excluding pensions to former employees and other benefits not contingent upon need. Among the expenditures in this category are: Cash assistance paid directly to needy persons under categorical programs (e.g., Old Age Assistance, Aid to Families With Dependent Children, Aid to the Blind, and Aid to the Disabled) or under any welfare programs; vendor payments made directly to private purveyors for medical care, burial, and other commodities and services provided under welfare programs; and provision and operation by the city of welfare institutions. "Other" public welfare includes payments to other governments for welfare purposes, amounts for administration, support of private welfare agencies, and other services such as vendor payments under various public welfare programs (e.g., Medicaid, the federally supported medical care program). The Health category covers outpatient health services other than hospital care, including public health administration; research and education; categorical health programs; treatment and immunization clinics; nursing; environmental health activities (e.g., air and water pollution control); ambulance service provided separately from fire protection services; school health services provided by health agencies; other general public health activities (e.g., mosquito abatement). Health and hospital services provided directly by the city through its own hospitals and health agencies and any payments to other governments for such purposes are classed under those functional headings. These data are estimates subject to sampling variation. In particular, some estimates are based upon a limited sample and may be subject to relatively sizable sampling variations. Minor corrections of less than 1 percent are not reflected in this table.

Government Spending: State

★ 475 ★

State and Local Government Health-Related Expenditures: 1970-1971 and 1980-1990

The table below reflects health-related expenditures of state and local governments.

Social services and income maintenance expenditures[1]	1970-1971	1980-1981	1988-1989	1989-1990
	In millions ($)			
General expenditures[2]	150,674	407,449	762,360	834,786
Public welfare	18,226	54,121	97,879	110,518
Hospitals and health	11,205	36,101	67,757	74,635
Social insurance administration	945	2,276	2,947	3,014
	Percentage distribution			
General expenditures[2]	100.0	100.0	100.0	100.0
Public welfare	12.1	13.3	12.8	13.2
Hospitals and health	7.4	8.9	8.9	8.9
Social insurance administration	0.6	0.6	0.4	0.4

Source: U.S. Department of Education. Office of Educational Research and Improvement. National Center for Education Statistics. *Digest of Education Statistics, 1992*. Washington, DC: U.S. Government Printing Office, 1992, p. 37. Primary source: U.S. Department of Commerce. Bureau of the Census. *Government Finances, 1989-1990*. Series GF/90-5. This table was prepared in February 1992. *Notes:* 1. General expenditures include expenditures through the federal government ($2,106,000 in 1985-1986), which are excluded from general expenditures. 2. Excludes duplicative intergovernmental transactions.

★ 476 ★

Government Spending: State

State and Local Government Health Services and Supply Expenditures and Percent Distribution for Selected Years: 1965-1991

This table profiles the health expenditures of state and local governments. See corresponding charts on business, federal government, and household spending for profiles of other sources of health care spending.

Type of Payer	1965	1967	1970	1975	1980	1985	1987	1988	1989	1990	1991
	Amount in billion dollar[1]s										
Total[1]	38.2	47.9	69.1	124.7	238.9	407.2	476.9	526.2	583.6	652.4	728.6
Public	7.9	12.8	18.9	38.5	76.8	128.2	149.4	163.7	185.4	215.8	254.5
State and local governments	4.5	5.8	8.5	17.2	34.2	59.3	72.4	79.4	88.8	102.1	120.7
Employer contributions to private health insurance	0.3	0.4	0.6	1.9	6.7	16.0	17.9	20.4	23.6	26.3	29.7
Other[2]	4.2	5.5	7.9	15.2	27.5	43.3	54.5	59.1	65.2	75.8	91.0
	Percent distribution										
Total	100.0	100.0	100.0	100.0	100.0	100.0	100.0	100.0	100.0	100.0	100.0
Public	20.7	26.8	27.4	30.8	32.2	31.5	31.3	31.1	31.8	33.1	34.9
State and local governments	11.7	12.2	12.3	13.8	14.3	14.6	15.2	15.1	15.2	15.6	16.6

[Continued]

★ 476 ★

State and Local Government Health Services and Supply Expenditures and Percent Distribution for Selected Years: 1965-1991

[Continued]

Type of Payer	1965	1967	1970	1975	1980	1985	1987	1988	1989	1990	1991
Employer contributions to private health insurance	0.7	0.8	0.9	1.5	2.8	3.9	3.7	3.9	4.0	4.0	4.1
Other[2]	11.0	11.4	11.4	12.2	11.5	10.6	11.4	11.2	11.2	11.6	12.5

Source: U.S. Department of Health and Human Services. Public Health Service. Centers for Disease Control and Prevention. National Center for Health Statistics. *Health, United States, 1992.* Hyattsville, MD: Public Health Service, 1993, pp. 170-171. Primary source: Health Care Financing Administration. Office of National Health Statistics. Office of the Actuary. "Business, Households, and Governments—Health Spending 1991." *Health Care Financing Review* 14, no.3 (winter 1993). *Notes:* Data are compiled by the Health Care Financing Administration. 1. Excludes research and construction. 2. Includes expenditures for state and local programs such as Medicaid and maternal and child health, and employer contributions to Medicare hospital insurance trust fund.

★ 477 ★

Government Spending: State

State Government Health-Related Finances, by State: 1989-1990

[In thousand dollars]

State	Social services and income maintenance						Social insurance administration	Veterans' services
	Public welfare	Cash assistance payments	Vendor payments	Other public welfare	Hospitals	Health		
United States	83,200,542	11,971,052	57,085,414	14,144,076	22,551,710	12,868,305	3,003,319	151,682
Alabama	1,044,636	140,581	734,564	169,491	594,933	286,757	34,179	4,613
Alaska	295,972	68,601	163,208	64,163	29,765	93,286	22,374	641
Arizona	1,077,045	155,892	759,087	162,066	75,311	219,561	20,611	1,647
Arkansas	787,518	80,466	529,588	177,464	191,302	97,166	30,482	2,078
California	6,998,420	-	5,726,277	1,272,143	2,058,956	967,464	270,197	19,206
Colorado	613,382	-	494,816	118,566	149,561	173,853	51,315	-
Connecticut	1,623,515	363,466	991,791	268,258	644,852	285,704	55,567	-
Delaware	227,169	29,022	96,559	101,588	45,975	101,296	7,277	150
District of Columbia	-	-	-	-	-	-	-	-
Florida	3,528,923	576,085	2,447,068	505,770	476,379	1,227,473	29,687	6,812
Georgia	2,125,244	323,342	1,452,166	349,736	481,328	193,876	77,780	5,140
Hawaii	420,921	112,854	210,535	97,532	151,417	159,135	17,238	2,102
Idaho	228,382	24,184	133,740	70,458	27,574	48,177	11,537	804
Illinois	4,277,720	1,084,068	2,285,851	907,801	599,279	742,812	173,730	13,284
Indiana	1,668,021	12,850	1,456,283	198,888	416,771	265,313	63,041	360
Iowa	1,076,865	152,933	559,946	363,986	426,136	67,696	41,115	2
Kansas	731,966	138,733	422,468	170,765	274,454	66,788	16,250	1,502
Kentucky	1,412,989	175,477	1,008,523	228,989	262,801	101,102	41,542	1,385
Louisiana	1,312,702	210,078	898,511	204,113	618,881	228,162	53,593	5,116
Maine	671,572	119,313	440,576	111,683	67,914	89,455	18,822	2,119
Maryland	1,863,573	376,746	1,142,307	344,520	328,665	149,210	24,769	3,335
Massachusetts	4,370,117	787,674	2,686,764	895,679	841,464	792,214	89,735	2,802
Michigan	4,248,373	1,399,600	1,773,959	1,074,814	1,098,202	707,457	147,243	648
Minnesota	1,467,451	908	1,388,071	78,472	503,409	205,076	84,861	3,103
Mississippi	692,444	60,838	492,287	139,319	211,070	106,028	33,267	2,824
Missouri	1,367,460	216,259	880,783	270,418	386,297	279,917	62,742	1,590
Montana	266,914	38,218	174,159	54,537	33,063	58,352	9,052	462
Nebraska	494,843	61,507	286,661	146,675	191,610	32,620	21,859	1,305
Nevada	211,339	26,687	135,003	49,649	44,225	47,654	18,559	1,622
New Hampshire	288,768	36,604	163,724	88,440	45,043	97,341	14,092	195

[Continued]

★ 477 ★

State Government Health-Related Finances, by State: 1989-1990

[Continued]

| State | Social services and income maintenance | | | | | | | |
	Public welfare	Cash assistance payments	Vendor payments	Other public welfare	Hospitals	Health	Social insurance administration	Veterans' services
New Jersey	2,670,913	-	2,194,473	476,440	740,424	375,668	58,744	3,697
New Mexico	435,600	60,342	238,451	136,807	187,300	130,411	46,533	957
New York	8,757,524	-	8,333,748	423,776	3,290,289	1,155,269	318,660	14,303
North Carolina	1,544,441	309,485	1,117,648	117,308	541,417	174,933	47,943	2,510
North Dakota	221,920	18,162	176,007	27,751	61,229	18,081	3,750	402
Ohio	4,160,204	883,150	2,923,385	353,669	964,706	312,024	141,120	588
Oklahoma	1,088,312	175,346	674,448	238,518	293,015	124,769	39,249	1,664
Oregon	933,856	136,040	516,713	281,103	304,383	82,079	31,267	17,341
Pennsylvania	4,265,236	1,054,241	2,181,600	1,029,395	927,808	254,224	137,444	2,662
Rhode Island	516,625	95,320	305,639	115,666	121,364	135,132	22,865	-
South Carolina	1,068,311	108,198	613,995	346,118	405,609	364,353	58,772	634
South Dakota	186,121	25,463	123,428	37,230	34,827	55,043	11,555	569
Tennessee	1,304,195	194,366	888,220	221,609	367,694	275,989	58,257	1,608
Texas	4,188,589	762,244	2,643,921	782,424	1,140,697	373,884	211,931	9,544
Utah	455,189	83,338	270,435	101,416	223,956	71,881	32,293	70
Vermont	264,819	48,233	138,074	78,512	22,549	43,083	8,721	93
Virginia	1,137,453	218,816	848,474	70,163	832,814	421,028	64,614	2,577
Washington	1,935,488	483,563	1,040,377	411,548	362,388	388,763	72,977	1,320
West Virginia	631,538	118,671	397,916	114,951	96,522	87,113	20,809	824
Wisconsin	1,934,461	403,481	1,466,569	64,411	324,761	94,227	61,590	5,472
Wyoming	105,503	19,607	56,618	29,278	31,288	39,406	11,676	-

Source: U.S. Department of Commerce. Economics and Statistics Administration. Bureau of the Census. *Government Finances, 1989-1990: Preliminary Report.* Series GF-90-5P. Washington, DC: U.S. Government Printing Office, September 1991, pp. 1-52. *Note:* Detail may not add to total because of rounding.

Trends and Projections

★ 478 ★

Average Annual Percent Change in Consumer Price Index for Medical Care and Selected Items: 1950-1992

Data are based on reporting by samples of providers and other retail outlets.

[1982-1984 = 100]

Year	All items	Medical care	Food	Apparel and upkeep	Housing	Energy	Personal care
1950-92	4.3	6.2	4.1	2.9	6.2[1]	4.9[2]	4.0
1950-55	2.1	3.8	1.8	1.3	-	-	2.7
1955-60	2.0	4.1	1.5	1.3	-	-	3.0
1960-65	1.3	2.5	1.4	0.9	-	0.4	1.1

[Continued]

★ 478 ★

Average Annual Percent Change in Consumer Price Index for Medical Care and Selected Items: 1950-1992
[Continued]

Year	All items	Medical care	Food	Apparel and upkeep	Housing	Energy	Personal care
1965-70	4.3	6.2	4.0	4.4	-	2.2	3.5
1970-75	6.8	6.9	8.8	4.1	6.9	10.5	5.9
1975-80	8.9	9.5	7.7	4.6	9.9	15.4	7.2
1975-76	5.8	9.5	3.0	3.7	6.1	7.1	6.6
1976-77	6.5	9.6	6.3	4.5	6.7	9.5	6.5
1977-78	7.6	8.4	9.9	3.6	8.7	6.3	6.4
1978-79	11.3	9.2	11.0	4.3	12.3	25.1	7.6
1979-80	13.5	11.0	8.6	7.1	15.7	30.9	8.9
1980-85	5.5	8.7	4.0	2.9	5.8	3.4	5.7
1980-81	10.3	10.7	7.8	4.8	11.5	13.6	8.8
1981-82	6.2	11.6	4.1	2.6	7.2	1.5	7.1
1982-83	3.2	8.8	2.1	2.5	2.7	0.7	5.1
1983-84	4.3	6.2	3.8	1.9	4.1	1.0	4.0
1984-85	3.6	6.3	2.3	2.8	4.0	0.7	3.8
1985-90	4.0	7.5	4.6	3.4	3.6	0.1	3.8
1985-86	1.9	7.5	3.2	0.9	3.0	-13.2	3.3
1986-87	3.6	6.6	4.1	4.4	3.0	0.5	2.9
1987-88	4.1	6.5	4.1	4.3	3.8	0.8	3.7
1988-89	4.8	7.7	5.8	2.8	3.8	5.6	4.7
1989-90	5.4	9.0	5.8	4.6	4.5	8.3	4.3
1990-91	4.2	8.7	2.9	3.7	4.0	0.4	3.5
1991-92	3.0	7.4	1.2	2.5	2.9	0.5	2.5

Source: U.S. Department of Health and Human Services. Public Health Service. Centers for Disease Control and Prevention. National Center for Health Statistics. *Health, United States, 1992.* Hyattsville, MD: Public Health Service, 1993, p. 164. Primary source: U.S. Department of Labor. Bureau of Labor Statistics. Consumer Price Index (various releases). *Notes:* 1. Data are for 1970-1992. 2. Data are for 1960-1992.

★ 479 ★

Trends and Projections

Average Annual Percent Change in Consumer Price Index for Medical Care Components: 1950-1992

Date are based on reporting by samples of providers and other retail outlets.

[1982-1984 = 100, except where noted]

Item and medical care component	1950-1960	1960-1965	1965-1970	1970-1975	1975-1980	1980-1985	1985-1989	1989-1990	1990-1991	1991-1992
CPI, all items	2.1	1.3	4.3	6.8	8.9	5.5	3.6	5.4	4.2	3.0
Less medical care	-	1.2	4.1	6.7	8.8	5.3	3.4	5.2	3.9	2.8
CPI, all services	3.6	2.0	5.6	6.5	10.2	7.1	4.7	5.5	5.1	3.9
All medical care	4.0	2.5	6.2	6.9	9.5	8.7	7.1	9.0	8.7	7.4
Medical care services	4.3	3.1	7.3	7.6	9.9	8.6	7.1	9.3	8.9	7.6
Professional medical services	-	-	-	6.5	8.9	7.8	6.6	6.6	6.1	6.1
Physicians' services	3.4	2.8	6.6	6.9	9.7	8.2	7.3	7.1	6.0	6.3
Dental services	2.5	2.3	5.3	6.3	8.2	7.7	6.4	6.6	7.4	6.8
Eye care[1]	-	-	-	-	-	-	-	4.4	3.9	4.2
Services by other medical professionals[1]	-	-	-	-	-	-	-	5.3	5.3	4.0
Hospital and related services	-	-	-	-	-	10.9	8.4	10.9	10.2	9.1
Hospital rooms	6.6	5.8	13.9	10.2	12.2	11.2	8.2	10.9	9.4	8.8
Other inpatient services[1]	-	-	-	-	-	-	-	10.7	10.7	9.1
Outpatient services[1]	-	-	-	-	-	-	-	11.2	10.6	10.0
Medical care commodities	1.7	-0.8	0.7	2.8	7.2	8.8	7.0	8.4	8.2	6.4
Prescription drugs	2.2	-2.4	-0.2	1.6	7.2	10.6	8.3	10.0	9.9	7.5
Nonprescription drugs and medical supplies[1]	-	-	-	-	-	-	-	5.2	4.7	3.9
Internal and respiratory over-the-counter drugs	-	-	1.6	4.1	7.7	8.4	5.5	5.1	4.5	3.8
Nonprescription medical equipment and supplies	-	-	-	-	-	6.7	4.6	5.3	5.1	4.1

Source: U.S. Department of Health and Human Services. Public Health Service. Centers for Disease Control and Prevention. National Center for Health Statistics. *Health, United States, 1992.* Hyattsville, MD: Public Health Service, 1993, p. 165. Primary source: U.S. Department of Labor. Bureau of Labor Statistics. Consumer Price Index. Various releases. *Notes:* CPI is an acronym for Consumer Price Index. 1. December 1986 = 100.

★ 480 ★

Trends and Projections

Average Annual Rate of Price Inflation of Medical Care Services and Other Items for Selected Years: 1960-1990

[In percentages]

Period	Medical care services	All items	Personal care
1960-65	2.5	1.3	1.1
1965-70	6.2	4.3	3.5
1970-75	6.9	6.8	5.9
1975-80	9.5	8.9	7.2
1980-85	8.7	5.5	5.7
1985-90	7.5	4.0	3.8
1980-81	10.8	10.3	8.9
1981-82	11.6	6.1	7.0
1982-83	8.7	3.2	5.1
1983-84	6.2	4.3	4.0
1984-85	6.2	3.5	3.9
1985-86	7.5	1.9	3.3

[Continued]

★ 480 ★

Average Annual Rate of Price Inflation of Medical Care Services and Other Items for Selected Years: 1960-1990

[Continued]

Period	Medical care services	All items	Personal care
1986-87	6.6	3.7	2.9
1987-88	6.5	4.1	3.8
1988-89	7.6	4.8	4.7
1989-90	9.1	5.4	4.3

Source: U.S. Department of Labor. Pension and Welfare Benefits Administration. *Trends in Health Benefits.* Washington, DC: U.S. Government Printing Office, 1993, p. 81. Primary source: Bureau of Labor Statistics.

★ 481 ★
Trends and Projections

Consumer Price Index for Medical Care and Selected Items: 1950-1992

| 1992 - 190.1 |
| 1991 - 177.0 |
| 1990 - 162.8 |
| 1989 - 149.3 |
| 1988 - 138.6 |
| 1987 - 130.1 |
| 1986 - 122.0 |
| 1985 - 113.5 |
| 1984 - 106.8 |
| 1983 - 100.6 |
| 1982 - 92.5 |
| 1981 - 82.9 |
| 1980 - 74.9 |
| 1979 - 67.5 |
| 1978 - 61.8 |
| 1977 - 57.0 |
| 1976 - 52.0 |
| 1975 - 47.5 |
| 1970 - 34.0 |
| 1965 - 25.2 |
| 1960 - 22.3 |
| 1955 - 18.2 |
| 1950 - 15.1 |

Chart shows data from column 2.

Data are based on reporting by samples of providers and other retail outlets.

[1982-1984 = 100]

Year	All items	Medical care	Food	Apparel and upkeep	Housing	Energy	Personal care
1950	24.1	15.1	25.4	40.3	-	-	26.2
1955	26.8	18.2	27.8	42.9	-	-	29.9
1960	29.6	22.3	30.0	45.7	-	22.4	34.6
1965	31.5	25.2	32.2	47.8	-	22.9	36.6
1970	38.8	34.0	39.2	59.2	36.4	25.5	43.5
1975	53.8	47.5	59.8	72.5	50.7	42.1	57.9
1976	56.9	52.0	61.6	75.2	53.8	45.1	61.7
1977	60.6	57.0	65.5	78.6	57.4	49.4	65.7
1978	65.2	61.8	72.0	81.4	62.4	52.5	69.9

[Continued]

★ 481 ★

Consumer Price Index for Medical Care and Selected Items: 1950-1992

[Continued]

Year	All items	Medical care	Food	Apparel and upkeep	Housing	Energy	Personal care
1979	72.6	67.5	79.9	84.9	70.1	65.7	75.2
1980	82.4	74.9	86.8	90.9	81.1	86.0	81.9
1981	90.9	82.9	93.6	95.3	90.4	97.7	89.1
1982	96.5	92.5	97.4	97.8	96.9	99.2	95.4
1983	99.6	100.6	99.4	100.2	99.5	99.9	100.3
1984	103.9	106.8	103.2	102.1	103.6	100.9	104.3
1985	107.6	113.5	105.6	105.0	107.7	101.6	108.3
1986	109.6	122.0	109.0	105.9	110.9	88.2	111.9
1987	113.6	130.1	113.5	110.6	114.2	88.6	115.1
1988	118.3	138.6	118.2	115.4	118.5	89.3	119.4
1989	124.0	149.3	125.1	118.6	123.0	94.3	125.0
1990	130.7	162.8	132.4	124.1	128.5	102.1	130.4
1991	136.2	177.0	136.3	128.7	133.6	102.5	134.9
1992	140.3	190.1	137.9	131.9	137.5	103.0	138.3

Source: U.S. Department of Health and Human Services. Public Health Service. Centers for Disease Control and Prevention. National Center for Health Statistics. *Health, United States, 1992.* Hyattsville, MD: Public Health Service, 1993, p. 164. Primary source: U.S. Department of Labor. Bureau of Labor Statistics. Consumer Price Index (various releases).

★ 482 ★

Trends and Projections

Consumer Price Index for Medical Care Components: 1950-1992

Date are based on reporting by samples of providers and other retail outlets.

[1982-1984 = 100, except where noted]

Item and medical care component	1950	1960	1965	1970	1975	1980	1985	1989	1990	1991	1992
CPI, all items	24.1	29.6	31.5	38.8	53.8	82.4	107.6	124.0	130.7	136.2	140.3
Less medical care	-	30.2	32.0	39.2	54.3	82.8	107.2	122.4	128.8	133.8	137.5
CPI, all services	16.9	24.1	26.6	35.0	48.0	77.9	109.9	131.9	139.2	146.3	152.0
All medical care	15.1	22.3	25.2	34.0	47.5	74.9	113.5	149.3	162.8	177.0	190.1
Medical care services	12.8	19.5	22.7	32.3	46.6	74.8	113.2	148.9	162.7	177.1	190.5
Professional medical services	-	-	-	37.0	50.8	77.9	113.5	146.4	156.1	165.7	175.8
Physicians' services	15.7	21.9	25.1	34.5	48.1	76.5	113.3	150.1	160.8	170.5	181.2
Dental services	21.0	27.0	30.3	39.2	53.2	78.9	114.2	146.1	155.8	167.4	178.7
Eye care[1]	-	-	-	-	-	-	-	112.4	117.3	121.9	127.0
Services by other medical professionals[1]	-	-	-	-	-	-	-	114.2	120.2	126.6	131.7
Hospital and related services	-	-	-	-	-	69.2	116.1	160.5	178.0	196.1	214.0
Hospital rooms	4.9	9.3	12.3	23.6	38.3	68.0	115.4	158.1	175.4	191.9	208.7
Other inpatient services[1]	-	-	-	-	-	-	-	128.9	142.7	158.0	172.3

[Continued]

★ 482 ★

Consumer Price Index for Medical Care Components: 1950-1992

[Continued]

Item and medical care component	1950	1960	1965	1970	1975	1980	1985	1989	1990	1991	1992
Outpatient services[1]	-	-	-	-	-	-	-	124.7	138.7	153.4	168.7
Medical care commodities	39.7	46.9	45.0	46.5	53.3	75.4	115.2	150.8	163.4	176.8	188.1
Prescription drugs	43.4	54.0	47.8	47.4	51.2	72.5	120.1	165.2	181.7	199.7	214.7
Nonprescription drugs and medical supplies[1]	-	-	-	-	-	-	-	114.6	120.6	126.3	131.2
Internal and respiratory over-the-counter drugs	-	-	39.0	42.3	51.8	74.9	112.2	138.8	145.9	152.4	158.2
Nonprescription medical equipment and supplies	-	-	-	-	-	79.2	109.6	131.1	138.0	145.0	150.9

Source: U.S. Department of Health and Human Services. Public Health Service. Centers for Disease Control and Prevention. National Center for Health Statistics. *Health, United States, 1992.* Hyattsville, MD: Public Health Service, 1993, p. 165. Primary source: U.S. Department of Labor. Bureau of Labor Statistics. Consumer Price Index. Various releases. *Notes:* CPI is an acronym for Consumer Price Index. 1. December 1986=100.

★ 483 ★

Trends and Projections

Factors Affecting the Growth of Personal Health Care Expenditures: 1960-1991

Table below reflects average annual percent change and percent distribution for factors affecting the growth of personal health care expenditures. These data are compiled by the Health Care Financing Administration and include revisions dating from 1960.

Period	Average annual percent change	Percent distribution			
		All factors	Prices	Population	Intensity[1]
1960-91	11.3	100	57	10	33
1960-61	6.1	100	31	27	42
1961-62	7.6	100	32	20	48
1962-63	9.3	100	22	16	62
1963-64	9.9	100	29	14	57
1964-65	8.6	100	37	15	48
1965-66	10.5	100	45	11	44
1966-67	13.6	100	43	8	49
1967-68	13.1	100	45	8	47
1968-69	13.0	100	51	8	41
1969-70	13.7	100	50	8	42
1970-71	9.9	100	65	11	24
1971-72	11.3	100	39	9	52
1972-73	11.7	100	38	7	55
1973-74	14.6	100	63	6	31
1974-75	14.7	100	75	6	19

[Continued]

★ 483 ★

Factors Affecting the Growth of Personal Health Care Expenditures: 1960-1991

[Continued]

Period	Average annual percent change	Percent distribution			
		All factors	Prices	Population	Intensity[1]
1975-76	14.0	100	62	6	32
1976-77	12.3	100	63	7	30
1977-78	12.2	100	66	8	26
1978-79	13.0	100	70	8	22
1979-80	15.9	100	73	6	21
1980-81	16.2	100	70	6	24
1981-82	12.4	100	77	8	15
1982-83	10.0	100	72	10	18
1983-84	8.4	100	75	12	13
1984-85	8.3	100	66	12	22
1985-86	8.4	100	60	12	28
1986-87	9.6	100	61	11	28
1987-88	9.9	100	68	10	22
1988-89	10.0	100	70	10	20
1989-90	11.4	100	58	9	33
1990-91	11.6	100	54	9	37

Source: U.S. Department of Health and Human Services. Public Health Service. Centers for Disease Control and Prevention. National Center for Health Statistics. *Health, United States, 1992.* Hyattsville, MD: Public Health Service, 1993, p. 163. Primary source: Health Care Financing Administration. Office of National Health Statistics. Office of the Actuary. "National Health Expenditures, 1991." *Health Care Financing Review* 14, no. 2 (winter 1992). *Note:* 1. Represents changes in use or kinds of services and supplies.

★ 484 ★

Trends and Projections

Government Health-Related Expenditures: 1970-1971 and 1980-1990

The table below reflects health-related expenditures of federal, state, and local governments.

Social services and income maintenance expenditures[1]	1970-1971	1980-1981	1986-1987	1987-1988	1988-1989	1989-1990
	In millions ($)					
General expenditures[1]	301,096	827,877	1,375,367	1,461,880	1,542,583	1,686,774
Public welfare	20,446	74,643	106,407	115,113	126,132	140,734
Hospitals and health	14,835	47,378	72,604	78,789	85,091	92,487
Social insurance administration	2,031	5,075	6,775	7,166	7,352	7,716
	Percentage distribution					
General expenditures[1]	100.0	100.0	100.0	100.0	100.0	100.0
Public welfare	6.8	9.0	7.7	7.9	8.2	8.3

[Continued]

★ 484 ★

Government Health-Related Expenditures: 1970-1971 and 1980-1990
[Continued]

Social services and income maintenance expenditures[1]	1970-1971	1980-1981	1986-1987	1987-1988	1988-1989	1989-1990
Hospitals and health	4.9	5.7	5.3	5.4	5.5	5.5
Social insurance administration	0.7	0.6	0.5	0.5	0.5	0.5

Source: U.S. Department of Education. Office of Educational Research and Improvement. National Center for Education Statistics. *Digest of Education Statistics, 1992.* Washington, DC: U.S. Government Printing Office, 1992, p. 37. Primary source: U.S. Department of Commerce. Bureau of the Census. *Government Finances, 1989-1990.* Series GF/90-5. This table was prepared in February 1992. *Note:* 1. Excludes duplicative governmental transactions.

★ 485 ★

Trends and Projections

Gross Domestic Product, National Health Expenditures, and Federal, State, and Local Government Expenditures for Selected Years: 1960-1991

Data are compiled by the Health Care Financing Administration and include revisions in health expenditures dating from 1985 and in population from 1960. Data reflect Bureau of Economic Analysis revisions to the Gross Domestic Product (GDP) and federal, state, and local government expenditures and Social Security Administration population revisions as of July 1992.

Year	Gross Domestic Product in billions ($)	National health expenditures			Federal government expenditures			State and local government expenditures		
		Amount in billions ($)	Percent of Gross Domestic Product	Amount per capita ($)	Total in billions ($)	Health in billions ($)	Health as a percent of total	Total in billions ($)	Health in billions ($)	Health as a percent of total
1960	513.4	27.1	5.3	143	93.4	2.9	3.1	48.3	3.7	7.8
1965	702.7	41.6	5.9	204	124.6	4.8	3.9	72.3	5.5	7.6
1966	769.8	45.9	6.0	222	144.9	7.5	5.2	81.1	6.1	7.5
1967	814.3	51.7	6.3	248	165.2	12.2	7.4	90.9	6.9	7.6
1968	889.3	58.5	6.6	278	181.5	14.1	7.8	102.6	7.7	7.5
1969	959.5	65.7	6.9	309	191.0	16.1	8.4	113.3	8.5	7.5
1970	1,010.7	74.4	7.4	346	208.5	17.7	8.5	127.2	9.9	7.8
1971	1,097.2	82.3	7.5	379	224.3	20.4	9.1	142.8	10.8	7.6
1972	1,207.0	92.3	7.6	421	249.3	22.9	9.2	156.3	12.2	7.8
1973	1,349.6	102.5	7.6	464	270.3	25.2	9.3	171.9	14.1	8.2
1974	1,458.6	116.1	8.0	521	305.6	30.5	10.0	193.5	16.1	8.3
1975	1,585.9	132.9	8.4	592	364.2	36.4	10.0	221.0	18.7	8.5
1976	1,768.4	152.2	8.6	672	392.7	42.9	10.9	239.3	19.5	8.1
1977	1,974.1	172.0	8.7	753	426.4	47.6	11.2	256.3	22.5	8.8
1978	2,232.7	193.7	8.7	840	469.3	54.3	11.6	278.2	25.5	9.1
1979	2,488.6	217.2	8.7	933	520.3	61.4	11.8	305.4	28.9	9.5
1980	2,708.0	250.1	9.2	1,064	613.1	72.0	11.7	336.6	33.2	9.9
1981	3,030.6	290.2	9.6	1,222	697.8	84.0	12.0	362.3	37.8	10.4
1982	3,149.6	326.1	10.4	1,359	770.9	93.3	12.1	382.1	41.5	10.9
1983	3,405.0	358.6	10.5	1,480	840.0	103.2	12.3	403.2	44.4	11.0
1984	3,777.2	389.6	10.3	1,592	892.7	112.6	12.6	434.1	47.0	10.8
1985	4,038.7	422.6	10.5	1,711	969.9	123.5	12.7	472.6	51.2	10.8
1986	4,268.6	454.9	10.7	1,824	1,028.2	132.5	12.9	517.0	57.2	11.1
1987	4,539.9	494.2	10.9	1,962	1,065.6	143.6	13.5	554.2	64.4	11.6
1988	4,900.4	546.1	11.1	2,146	1,109.0	156.6	14.1	593.0	70.5	11.9
1989	5,250.8	604.3	11.5	2,352	1,181.6	175.0	14.8	636.7	78.3	12.3

[Continued]

★ 485 ★

Gross Domestic Product, National Health Expenditures, and Federal, State, and Local Government Expenditures for Selected Years: 1960-1991

[Continued]

Year	Gross Domestic Product in billions ($)	National health expenditures			Federal government expenditures			State and local government expenditures		
		Amount in billions ($)	Percent of Gross Domestic Product	Amount per capita ($)	Total in billions ($)	Health in billions ($)	Health as a percent of total	Total in billions ($)	Health in billions ($)	Health as a percent of total
1990	5,522.2	675.0	12.2	2,601	1,273.6	194.5	15.3	699.2	90.5	12.9
1991	5,677.5	751.8	13.2	2,868	1,332.7	222.9	16.7	760.7	107.1	14.1

Source: U.S. Department of Health and Human Services. Public Health Service. Centers for Disease Control and Prevention. National Center for Health Statistics. *Health, United States, 1992.* Hyattsville, MD: Public Health Service, 1993, p. 160. Primary source: Health Care Financing Administration. Office of National Health Statistics. Office of the Actuary. "National Health Expenditures, 1991." *Health Care Financing Review* 14, no. 2 (winter 1992).

★ 486 ★

Trends and Projections

Miscellaneous Personal Health Care Expenditures and Percent Distribution According to Source of Funds for Selected Years: 1960-1991

Data were compiled by the Health Care Financing Administration. Table excludes expenditures for hospital care, nursing home care, and physician services. See separate tables for data on these expenditures.

Personal health care[2]	Total in billions	Out-of-pocket payments	Private health insurance	Other private funds	Government		
					Total[1]	Medicaid	Medicare
		Percent distribution					
1960	8.4	87.8	1.4	2.7	8.0	-	-
1965	11.7	87.4	2.2	2.6	7.8	-	-
1970	18.5	80.6	4.3	2.7	12.4	4.4	0.7
1975	31.0	72.2	8.5	3.0	16.4	6.2	1.7
1980	55.1	62.1	17.5	3.5	16.9	6.0	3.1
1984	85.5	57.4	21.9	4.0	16.7	6.1	4.7
1985	93.4	56.6	21.9	4.3	17.2	6.5	4.8
1986	102.2	56.1	22.2	4.1	17.7	6.9	4.8
1987	112.4	55.3	22.9	3.9	17.9	7.3	4.7
1988	122.9	54.3	23.7	3.9	18.1	7.6	4.7
1989	135.0	53.2	23.6	4.0	19.1	8.4	5.2
1990	151.2	51.5	23.6	4.3	20.7	9.0	5.9
1991	169.7	48.8	23.8	4.5	22.9	10.5	6.8

Source: U.S. Department of Health and Human Services. Public Health Service. Centers for Disease Control and Prevention. National Center for Health Statistics. *Health, United States, 1992.* Hyattsville, MD: Public Health Service, 1993, p. 172. Primary source: Health Care Financing Administration. Office of National Health Statistics. Office of the Actuary. "National Health Expenditures, 1991." *Health Care Financing Review* 14, no. 2 (winter 1992). *Notes:* 1. Includes other government expenditures for these health care services; for example, care funded by the U.S. Department of Veterans Affairs and state and locally financed subsidies to hospitals. 2. Includes expenditures for dental services, other professional services, home health care, drugs and other medical nondurables, vision products and other medical durables, and other personal health care.

★ 487 ★

Trends and Projections

National Health Care Expenditures According to Source of Funds for Selected Years: 1929-1991

Data for this table were compiled by the Health Care Financing Administration. Data include revisions in health expenditures dating from 1985 and in population dating from 1960, and reflect Social Security Administration population revisions as of July 1992.

Year	All health expenditures (in billions of dollars)	Private funds			Public funds		
		Amount (in billions of dollars)	Amount per capita	Percent of total	Amount (in billions of dollars)	Amount per capita	Percent of total
1929	3.6	3.2	25	86.4	0.5	4	13.6
1935	2.9	2.4	18	80.8	0.6	4	19.2
1940	4.0	3.2	23	79.7	0.8	6	20.3
1950	12.7	9.2	58	72.8	3.4	22	27.2
1955	17.7	13.2	75	74.3	4.6	27	25.7
1960	27.1	20.5	108	75.5	6.7	35	24.5
1965	41.6	31.3	154	75.3	10.3	50	24.7
1966	45.9	32.3	157	70.4	13.6	66	29.6
1967	51.7	32.5	156	62.9	19.2	92	37.1
1968	58.5	36.7	174	62.8	21.8	103	37.2
1969	65.7	41.1	193	62.5	24.6	116	37.5
1970	74.4	46.7	217	62.8	27.7	129	37.2
1971	82.3	51.1	235	62.1	31.2	144	37.9
1972	92.3	57.2	261	62.0	35.1	160	38.0
1973	102.5	63.2	286	61.6	39.3	178	38.4
1974	116.1	69.4	312	59.8	46.6	209	40.2
1975	132.9	77.8	346	58.5	55.1	246	41.5
1976	152.2	89.8	396	59.0	62.4	276	41.0
1977	172.0	102.0	446	59.3	70.1	307	40.7
1978	193.7	113.9	494	58.8	79.8	346	41.2
1979	217.2	126.9	545	58.4	90.4	388	41.6
1980	250.1	145.0	617	58.0	105.2	447	42.0
1981	290.2	168.5	709	58.0	121.8	513	42.0
1982	326.1	191.3	797	58.7	134.8	562	41.3
1983	358.6	211.0	871	58.8	147.6	609	41.2
1984	389.6	230.0	940	59.0	159.6	652	41.0
1985	422.6	248.0	1,004	58.7	174.6	707	41.3
1986	454.9	265.2	1,063	58.3	189.6	760	41.7
1987	494.2	286.2	1,136	57.9	208.0	826	42.1
1988	546.1	319.0	1,254	58.4	227.1	893	41.6
1989	604.3	351.0	1,366	58.1	253.3	986	41.9

[Continued]

★ 487 ★

National Health Care Expenditures According to Source of Funds for Selected Years: 1929-1991
[Continued]

Year	All health expenditures (in billions of dollars)	Private funds			Public funds		
		Amount (in billions of dollars)	Amount per capita	Percent of total	Amount (in billions of dollars)	Amount per capita	Percent of total
1990	675.0	390.0	1,502	57.8	285.1	1,098	42.2
1991	751.8	421.8	1,609	56.1	330.0	1,259	43.9

Source: U.S. Department of Health and Human Services. Public Health Service. Centers for Disease Control and Prevention. National Center for Health Statistics. *Health, United States, 1992.* Hyattsville, MD: Public Health Service, 1993, p. 168. Primary source: Health Care Financing Administration. Office of National Health Statistics. Office of the Actuary. "National Health Expenditures: 1991." *Health Care Financing Review* 14, no. 2 (winter 1992).

★ 488 ★

Trends and Projections

National Health Care Expenditures and Percent Distribution According to Type of Expenditure for Selected Years: 1960-1991

Data for this table were compiled by the Health Care Financing Administration. Data include revisions in health expenditures dating from 1985.

Type of expenditures	1960	1965	1970	1975	1980	1985	1987	1988	1989	1990	1991
	Amount in billions ($)										
Total	27.1	41.6	74.4	132.9	250.1	422.6	494.2	546.1	604.3	675.0	751.8
	Percent distribution										
All expenditures	100.0	100.0	100.0	100.0	100.0	100.0	100.0	100.0	100.0	100.0	100.0
Health services and supplies	93.7	91.7	92.8	93.8	95.5	96.4	96.5	90.4	90.0	90.0	90.0
Personal health care	88.1	85.6	87.3	87.7	87.7	87.5	88.9	88.4	87.9	87.6	87.8
Hospital care	34.2	33.7	37.6	39.4	40.9	39.8	39.3	38.8	38.5	38.2	38.4
Physician services	19.5	19.7	18.3	17.5	16.7	17.5	18.8	19.3	19.2	19.1	18.9
Dentist services	7.2	6.7	6.3	6.2	5.7	5.5	5.5	5.4	5.2	5.0	4.9
Nursing home care	3.6	4.1	6.5	7.5	8.0	8.1	8.0	7.8	7.9	7.9	8.0
Other professional services	2.2	2.1	2.0	2.6	3.5	3.9	4.3	4.4	4.5	4.5	4.8
Home health care	0.1	0.1	0.2	0.3	0.5	0.9	0.8	0.8	0.9	1.1	1.3
Drugs and other medical nondurables	15.7	14.2	11.8	9.8	8.6	8.6	8.7	8.5	8.4	8.2	8.1
Vision products and other medical durables	3.0	3.0	2.7	2.3	1.8	1.7	1.8	1.9	1.7	1.7	1.6
Other personal health care	2.6	2.0	1.8	2.0	1.8	1.5	1.6	1.6	1.6	1.7	1.9
Program administration and net cost of health insurance	4.3	4.6	3.7	3.8	4.9	6.0	4.7	4.9	5.6	5.8	5.8
Government public health activities	1.4	1.5	1.9	2.3	2.9	2.9	3.0	3.0	3.1	3.3	3.3
Research and construction	6.3	8.3	7.2	6.2	4.5	3.6	3.5	3.6	3.4	3.4	3.1
Noncommercial research	2.6	3.7	2.6	2.5	2.2	1.8	1.8	1.9	1.8	1.8	1.7
Construction	3.7	4.6	4.5	3.7	2.3	1.8	1.7	1.7	1.6	1.6	1.4

Source: U.S. Department of Health and Human Services. Public Health Service. Centers for Disease Control and Prevention. National Center for Health Statistics. *Health, United States, 1992.* Hyattsville, MD: Public Health Service, 1993, p. 162. Primary source: Health Care Financing Administration. Office of National Health Statistics. Office of the Actuary. "National Health Expenditures, 1991." *Health Care Financing Review* 14, no. 2 (winter 1992).

★ 489 ★

Trends and Projections

National Health Care Expenditures Average Annual Percent Change According to Source of Funds for Selected Years: 1929-1991

Data for this table were compiled by the Health Care Financing Administration. Data include revisions in health expenditures dating from 1985 and in population dating from 1960, and reflect Social Security Administration population revisions as of July 1992.

Year	All health expenditures (in billions of dollars)	Private funds		Public funds	
		Amount (in billions of dollars)	Amount per capita	Amount (in billions of dollars)	Amount per capita
1929-65	7.0	6.6	5.2	8.8	7.3
1965-91	11.8	10.5	9.5	14.3	13.2
1929-35	-3.6	-4.6	-5.1	2.2	1.4
1935-40	6.3	6.0	4.7	7.6	6.8
1940-50	12.2	11.2	9.7	15.5	13.8
1950-55	7.0	7.4	5.3	5.8	4.2
1955-60	8.9	9.2	7.5	7.9	5.3
1960-65	8.9	8.9	7.3	9.1	7.6
1965-70	12.3	8.3	7.2	21.9	20.6
1970-75	12.3	10.7	9.8	14.8	13.8
1975-80	13.5	13.3	12.2	13.8	12.7
1980-85	11.1	11.3	10.2	10.7	9.6
1980-81	16.0	16.2	15.1	15.8	14.6
1981-82	12.4	13.6	12.4	10.7	9.6
1982-83	10.0	10.3	9.2	9.5	8.5
1983-84	8.7	9.0	8.0	8.1	7.1
1984-85	8.5	7.8	6.8	9.4	8.3
1985-90	9.8	9.5	8.4	10.3	9.2
1985-86	7.6	7.0	5.9	8.6	7.6
1986-87	8.6	7.9	6.9	9.7	8.6
1987-88	10.5	11.5	10.4	9.2	8.1
1988-89	10.7	10.0	8.9	11.5	10.4
1989-90	11.7	11.1	10.0	12.5	11.4
1990-91	11.4	8.2	7.1	15.7	14.6

Source: U.S. Department of Health and Human Services. Public Health Service. Centers for Disease Control and Prevention. National Center for Health Statistics. *Health, United States, 1992.* Hyattsville, MD: Public Health Service, 1993, p. 168. Primary source: Health Care Financing Administration. Office of National Health Statistics. Office of the Actuary. "National Health Expenditures, 1991." *Health Care Financing Review* 14, no. 2 (winter 1992).

★ 490 ★

Trends and Projections

National Health Care Expenditures Average Annual Percent Change According to Type of Expenditure for Selected Years: 1960-1991

Data for this table were compiled by the Health Care Financing Administration. Data include revisions in health expenditures dating from 1985.

Type of expenditures	1960-1965	1965-1970	1970-1975	1975-1080	1980-1985	1985-1987	1987-1988	1988-1989	1989-1990	1990-1991
					Average annual percent change					
All expenditures	8.9	12.3	12.3	13.5	11.1	8.1	10.5	10.7	11.7	11.4
Health services and supplies	8.5	12.6	12.5	13.9	11.3	8.2	10.3	10.9	11.8	11.7
Personal health care	8.3	12.8	12.4	13.5	11.0	9.0	9.9	10.0	11.4	11.6
Hospital care	8.6	14.7	13.4	14.3	10.4	7.4	9.2	9.6	11.1	11.8
Physician services	9.2	10.6	11.4	12.5	12.1	12.1	13.1	10.4	11.0	10.2
Dentist services	7.3	10.8	12.1	11.7	10.1	8.0	8.5	7.5	7.7	8.8
Nursing home care	11.6	23.4	15.4	15.0	11.3	7.8	7.8	11.1	12.3	12.4
Other professional services	7.4	11.8	18.3	19.9	13.8	12.8	12.4	13.8	13.5	16.7
Home health care	9.6	19.7	23.2	27.2	23.3	3.6	9.9	24.4	34.4	29.0
Drugs and other medical nondurables	6.8	8.4	8.1	10.7	10.8	9.3	7.2	9.1	10.3	9.0
Vision products and other medical durables	9.0	10.1	8.8	8.2	9.4	12.7	11.8	8.0	12.0	5.4
Other personal health care	3.5	10.7	14.6	11.0	6.9	10.6	12.1	11.8	17.4	21.9
Program administration and net cost of										
health insurance	10.5	7.5	12.8	19.3	15.5	-4.4	16.8	25.7	15.3	12.7
Government public health activities	10.8	17.1	17.0	18.9	11.3	8.9	13.5	14.3	16.0	11.6
Research and construction	15.2	9.0	9.2	6.4	6.4	5.9	14.9	4.2	9.6	2.1
Noncommercial research	17.1	5.1	11.2	10.4	7.4	7.8	14.5	6.2	8.0	6.1
Construction	13.9	11.8	8.0	3.3	5.4	4.2	15.3	1.9	11.5	-2.2

Source: U.S. Department of Health and Human Services. Public Health Service. Centers for Disease Control and Prevention. National Center for Health Statistics. *Health, United States, 1992.* Hyattsville, MD: Public Health Service, 1993, p. 162. Primary source: Health Care Financing Administration. Office of National Health Statistics. Office of the Actuary. "National Health Expenditures, 1991." *Health Care Financing Review* 14, no. 2 (winter 1992).

★ 491 ★

Trends and Projections

National Health Care Spending Projections: 1993, 1995 and 2000

	Calendar year		
	1993	1995	2000
National total in billions ($)	903.3	1,101.9	1,739.8
Percent of GDP	14.4	15.6	18.1
Per capita amount ($)	3,380	4,050	6,148
	Percent of total		
Source of funds			
Private	53.4	52.0	49.4
Public	46.6	48.0	50.6
Federal	32.1	33.2	35.5
State/local	14.5	14.8	15.1

Source: U.S. Department of Health and Human Services. Health Care Financing Administration (HCFA). Bureau of Data Management and Strategy. *1993 HCFA Statistics.* HCFA Pub. No. 03341. Washington, DC: U.S. Department of Health and Human Services, June 1993, p. 26. Primary source: Health Care Financing Administration. Office of the Actuary. Office of National Health Statistics. "National Health Expenditures Projections Through 2030." *Health Care Financing Administration Review* (fall 1992). *Note:* GDP is an acronym for Gross Domestic Product.

★ 492 ★
Trends and Projections

Personal Health Care Expenditures and Percent Distribution According to Source of Funds for Selected Years: 1929-1991

These data, compiled by the Health Care Financing Administration, include revisions in health expenditures dating from 1985 and in population dating from 1960. They reflect Social Security Administration population revisions as of July 1992.

Year	Total in billions[1] ($)	Per capita ($)	Percent distribution						
			All sources	Out-of-pocket payments	Private health insurance	Other private funds	Government		
							Total	Federal	State and local
1929	3.2	26	100.0	88.4[2]	[2]	2.6	9.0	2.7	6.3
1935	2.7	21	100.0	82.4[2]	[2]	2.8	14.7	3.4	11.3
1940	3.5	26	100.0	81.3[2]	[2]	2.6	16.1	4.1	12.0
1950	10.9	70	100.0	65.5	9.1	2.9	22.4	10.4	12.0
1955	15.7	93	100.0	58.1	16.1	2.8	23.0	10.5	12.5
1960	23.9	126	100.0	55.9	21.0	1.7	21.4	8.9	12.5
1965	35.6	175	100.0	53.4	24.3	1.9	20.4	8.3	12.0
1970	64.9	302	100.0	39.5	23.4	2.6	34.6	22.6	12.0
1971	71.3	329	100.0	38.0	23.8	2.6	35.6	23.7	11.9
1972	79.4	362	100.0	37.5	23.6	2.7	36.1	24.0	12.2
1973	88.6	401	100.0	37.1	23.9	2.6	36.4	23.8	12.6
1974	101.6	456	100.0	35.0	24.6	2.5	37.8	25.6	12.2
1975	116.6	519	100.0	33.1	25.6	2.5	38.9	26.6	12.3
1976	132.8	587	100.0	32.0	26.4	3.0	38.6	27.6	11.0
1977	149.2	653	100.0	31.0	27.3	2.9	38.8	27.6	11.2
1978	167.5	726	100.0	30.0	27.9	3.0	39.1	28.0	11.1
1979	189.3	813	100.0	28.6	28.9	3.0	39.5	28.4	11.1
1980	219.4	933	100.0	27.1	29.7	3.5	39.7	28.9	10.8
1981	254.8	1,073	100.0	26.4	30.3	3.5	39.9	29.4	10.5
1982	286.4	1,194	100.0	25.9	30.9	3.6	39.6	29.3	10.3
1983	314.9	1,300	100.0	25.8	30.9	3.5	39.8	29.7	10.1
1984	341.2	1,395	100.0	25.7	31.2	3.4	39.8	29.8	9.9
1985	369.7	1,497	100.0	25.5	30.9	3.5	40.1	30.2	9.9
1986	400.8	1,607	100.0	25.2	31.0	3.5	40.3	30.0	10.3
1987	439.3	1,744	100.0	24.8	31.4	3.4	40.4	29.7	10.7
1988	482.8	1,898	100.0	24.5	32.1	3.5	39.9	29.3	10.5
1989	530.9	2,066	100.0	23.8	32.1	3.6	40.5	29.9	10.6
1990	591.5	2,279	100.0	23.1	32.3	3.6	41.0	29.9	11.0
1991	660.2	2,518	100.0	21.9	31.7	3.6	42.9	30.9	12.0

Source: U.S. Department of Health and Human Services. Public Health Service. Centers for Disease Control and Prevention. National Center for Health Statistics. *Health, United States, 1992.* Hyattsville, MD: Public Health Service, 1993, p. 169. Primary source: Health Care Financing Administration. Office of National Health Statistics. Office of the Actuary. "National Health Expenditures, 1991." *Health Care Financing Review* 14, no. 2 (winter 1992). *Notes:* 1. Includes all expenditures for health services and supplies other than expenses for program administration and net cost of private health insurance and government public health activities. 2. Out-of-pocket payments and private health insurance are combined for these years.

Chapter 7
HEALTH CARE PROGRAMS

A variety of social programs exist to provide health-related assistance to needy individuals. The Social Security Administration reported that "in December 1992, 41.5 million persons—73 percent of them aged 65 or older—were receiving benefits under the largest single program—Old-Age, Survivors, and Disability Insurance (OASDI). As of July 1, 1992, the Medicare program covered 31.6 million persons aged 65 or older and 3.6 million disabled persons under the age 65. Medicaid benefits were paid on behalf of 31.2 million persons in fiscal year 1992, and the Food Stamp program had 25.4 million participants in fiscal year 1992. Federally administered Supplemental Security Income (SSI) payments in December 1992 were made to 5.6 million persons, of whom 2.1 million were aged 65 or older. Finally, Aid to Families With Dependent Children (AFDC) payments were received by 14.0 million children and adults in 4.9 million families in December 1992" (U.S. Department of Health and Human Services. Social Security Administration. "Social Security Programs in the United States, 1993." *Social Security Bulletin* 4, no. 4, 22 December 1993). This chapter contains tables that show the availability and use of selected administrative, financial, and delivery programs promoting the health and well-being of Americans. Tables cover widespread efforts such as Medicaid and more focused programs such as compensation to disabled veterans. Tables on expenditures for specific social welfare programs will be found in this chapter as well. Workers' compensation, however, has been omitted. Tables related to this and other occupational programs are included in the chapter on Health in the Workplace.

Medicaid: Benefits and Beneficiaries

★ 493 ★

Medicaid Outlays: 1992

From the source: "Medicaid is a federal-state matching entitlement program, which provides medical assistance for certain individuals and families with low incomes and resources. It is a jointly funded cooperative venture between the federal and state governments to assist states in the provision of more adequate medical care to eligible needy persons. Medicaid is the largest program providing medical and health-related services to America's poorest people.... In 1992, the Medicaid program provided health care services to over 31 million recipients who were aged, blind, or disabled persons; pregnant women; or certain individuals in families with dependent children."

[In billion dollars]

Outlays	Amount
Total outlays	114.5
Federal funds[1]	65.9
State funds[1]	48.6
Outlays include:	
Vendor payments	91.5
Premium payments	6.0
Payments to disproportionate share hospitals[2]	17.0

Source: U.S. Department of Health and Human Services. Social Security Administration (SSA). "Social Security Programs in the United States, 1993." *Social Security Bulletin* 4, no. 4 (22 December 1993), n.p. *Notes:* 1. Plus administrative costs. 2. Special payments to certain hospitals with large proportions of low-income and Medicaid patients.

★ 494 ★

Medicaid: Benefits and Beneficiaries

Medicaid Outlays, by Types of Patients and Care

Medicaid is commonly thought of as assistance for welfare mothers and children; however, a significant portion of Medicaid spending is devoted to older Americans and disabled members of the population. The table below illustrates Medicaid spending by type of patient and by type of care.

Patient/care	Percent
Types of patients	
Disabled or aged	66
Other	34
Types of care	
Long-term	40
Other	60

Source: "Where Medicaid Dollars Go." *Washington Post National Weekly Edition,* 14-20 February 1994, p. 10. Primary sources: 1) Congressional Research Service. 2) Health Care Financing Administration.

★ 495 ★

Medicaid: Benefits and Beneficiaries

Medicaid Recipients and Payments, by State: 1991

Data are preliminary estimates, provided by state or other area.

Region, division, and state	Medicaid[1]	
	Recipients[2] (1,000)	Payments[3] (million dollars)
All areas	28,280	77,048
United States[4]	27,067	76,898
Northeast	5,721	26,030
New England	1,368	6,141
Maine	151	536
New Hampshire	60	292
Vermont	71	197
Massachusetts	651	2,828
Rhode Island	164	657
Connecticut	272	1,630
Middle Atlantic	4,353	19,889
New York	2,462	13,728
New Jersey	614	2,725
Pennsylvania	1,277	3,436
Midwest	6,026	16,869
East North Central	4,387	12,057
Ohio	1,299	3,653
Indiana	415	1,662
Illinois	1,144	2,731

[Continued]

★ 495 ★

Medicaid Recipients and Payments, by State: 1991
[Continued]

Region, division, and state	Medicaid[1]	
	Recipients[2] (1,000)	Payments[3] (million dollars)
Michigan	1,113	2,540
Wisconsin	416	1,471
West North Central	1,639	4,811
Minnesota	422	1,561
Iowa	261	766
Missouri	503	1,118
North Dakota	53	227
South Dakota	57	196
Nebraska	134	390
Kansas	209	553
South	9,331	22,130
South Atlantic	4,277	11,127
Delaware	51	186
Maryland	363	1,292
District of Columbia	100	446
Virginia	442	1,218
West Virginia	284	542
North Carolina	667	1,788
South Carolina	375	910
Georgia	746	1,799
Florida	1,249	2,944
East South Central	2,096	4,246
Kentucky	525	1,200
Tennessee	697	1,485
Alabama	403	805
Mississippi	470	755
West South Central	2,959	6,758
Arkansas	285	688
Louisiana	641	1,723
Oklahoma	305	814
Texas	1,729	3,532
West	5,989	11,869
Mountain	1,058	2,095
Montana	64	193
Idaho	70	223
Wyoming	37	90
Colorado	223	673
New Mexico	162	342
Arizona	313	84
Utah	129	311
Nevada	59	178
Pacific	4,931	9,774
Washington	506	1,131
Oregon	263	667

[Continued]

★ 495 ★

Medicaid Recipients and Payments, by State: 1991

[Continued]

Region, division, and state	Medicaid[1]	
	Recipients[2] (1,000)	Payments[3] (million dollars)
California	4,019	7,579
Alaska	51	160
Hawaii	91	238
PR	1,201	146
Outlying areas	12[5]	4[5]
Foreign	(X)	(X)

Source: 1993 Statistical Abstract of the United States on CD-ROM [machine-readable datafiles]. CD-ABSTR-93. Washington, DC: U.S. Department of Commerce, Economics and Statistics Administration, Bureau of the Census, Data User Services Division, 1993. Primary source: Health Care Financing Administration, unpublished data. Notes: "X" represents "not applicable." 1. For fiscal year ending September 30. 2. Persons receiving Medicaid at any time during the year. 3. Payments are for calendar year and represent disbursements from federal hospital and medical insurance trust funds. Estimates of distribution by state based on preliminary billing data. 4. Includes data for enrollees with residence unknown. 5. Virgin Islands only.

★ 496 ★

Medicaid: Benefits and Beneficiaries

Medicaid Recipients and Payments, by Type of Beneficiary: 1972-1991

Data show the unduplicated number of recipients, total vendor payments, and average amounts spent on each group by type of eligibility category for fiscal years 1972 through 1991. Fiscal year 1977 began in October 1976 and was the first year of the new federal fiscal cycle. Before 1977, the fiscal year began in July. Beginning in fiscal year 1980, recipients categories do not add to unduplicated total because of the small number of recipients that are in more than 1 category during the year. Data are provided by category of recipient.

Fiscal year	Total	Aged 65 or older	Blindness	Permanent and total disability	Dependent children under age 21	Adults in families with dependent children	Other
				Number (in thousands)			
1972	17,606	3,318	108	1,625	7,841	3,137	1,576
1975	22,007	3,615	109	2,355	9,598	4,529	1,800
1976	22,815	3,612	97	2,572	9,924	4,774	1,836
1977	22,832	3,636	92	2,710	9,651	4,785	1,959
1978	21,965	3,376	82	2,636	9,376	4,643	1,852
1979	21,520	3,364	79	2,674	9,106	4,570	1,727
1980	21,605	3,440	92	2,819	9,333	4,877	1,499
1981	21,980	3,367	86	2,993	9,581	5,187	1,364
1982	21,603	3,240	84	2,806	9,563	5,356	1,434
1983	21,554	3,371	77	2,844	9,535	5,592	1,129
1984	21,607	3,238	79	2,834	9,684	5,600	1,187

[Continued]

★ 496 ★

Medicaid Recipients and Payments, by Type of Beneficiary: 1972-1991
[Continued]

Fiscal year	Total	Aged 65 or older	Blindness	Permanent and total disability	Dependent children under age 21	Adults in families with dependent children	Other
1985	21,814	3,061	80	2,937	9,757	5,518	1,214
1986	22,515	3,140	82	3,100	10,029	5,647	1,362
1987	23,109	3,224	85	3,296	10,168	5,599	1,418
1988	22,907	3,159	86	3,401	10,037	5,503	1,343
1989	23,511	3,132	95	3,496	10,318	5,717	1,175

Amount (in millions)

1972	$6,300	$1,925	$45	$1,354	$1,139	$962	$875
1975	12,242	4,358	93	3,052	2,186	2,062	492
1976	14,091	4,910	96	3,824	2,431	2,288	542
1977	16,239	5,499	116	4,767	2,610	2,606	641
1978	17,992	6,308	116	5,505	2,748	2,673	643
1979	20,472	7,046	108	6,774	2,884	3,021	638
1980	23,311	8,739	124	7,497	3,123	3,231	596
1981	27,204	9,926	154	9,301	3,508	3,763	552
1982	29,399	10,739	172	10,233	3,473	4,093	689
1983	32,391	11,954	183	11,184	3,836	4,487	747
1984	33,891	12,815	219	11,758	3,979	4,420	700
1985	37,508	14,096	249	13,203	4,414	4,746	798
1986	41,005	15,097	277	14,635	5,135	4,880	980
1987	45,050	16,037	309	16,507	5,508	5,592	1,078
1988	48,710	17,135	344	18,250	5,848	5,883	1,198
1989	54,500	18,558	409	20,476	6,892	6,897	1,268
1990	64,859	21,508	434	23,969	9,100	8,590	1,257
1991	77,048	25,453	475	27,798	11,690	10,439	1,193

Average amount

1972	$358	$580	$417	$833	$145	$307	$555
1975	556	1,205	850	1,296	228	455	273
1976	618	1,359	990	1,487	245	479	295
1977	711	1,512	1,258	1,759	270	545	327
1978	819	1,869	1,412	2,088	293	576	347
1979	951	2,094	1,369	2,534	317	661	369
1980	1,079	2,540	1,358	2,659	335	663	398
1981	1,238	2,948	1,784	3,108	366	725	405
1982	1,361	3,315	2,047	3,646	363	764	480
1983	1,503	3,545	2,379	3,932	402	802	662
1984	1,569	3,957	2,766	4,149	411	789	590

[Continued]

★ 496 ★

Medicaid Recipients and Payments, by Type of Beneficiary: 1972-1991
[Continued]

Fiscal year	Total	Aged 65 or older	Blindness	Permanent and total disability	Dependent children under age 21	Adults in families with dependent children	Other
1985	1,719	4,605	3,104	4,496	452	860	658
1986	1,821	4,808	3,401	4,721	512	864	719
1987	1,949	4,975	3,644	5,008	542	999	761
1988	2,126	5,425	4,005	5,366	583	1,069	891
1989	2,318	5,926	4,317	5,858	668	1,206	1,079
1990	2,568	6,717	5,212	6,595	811	1,429	1,138
1991	2,725	7,577	5,572	6,979	871	1,540	1,813

Source: U.S. Department of Health and Human Services. Social Security Administration (SSA). *Annual Statistical Supplement to the "Social Security Bulletin," 1992.* SSA Publication No. 13-11700. Washington, DC: U.S. Department of Health and Human Services, Social Security Administration, Office of Research and Statistics, 1993, p. 309.

★ 497 ★

Medicaid: Benefits and Beneficiaries

Medicaid Recipients and Payments, by Type of Service: 1980-1991

For fiscal year ending in year shown. Includes Puerto Rico and outlying areas. Medical vendor payments are those made directly to suppliers of medical care. Data are provided by basis of eligibility and by type of service.

Basis of eligibility and type of service	Recipients (1,000)					Payments (million dollars)				
	1980	1985	1989	1990	1991	1980	1985	1989	1990	1991
Total[1]	21,605	21,814	23,511	25,255	28,280	23,311	37,508	54,500	64,859	77,048
Age 65 and over	3,440	3,061	3,132	3,202	3,359	8,739	14,096	18,558	21,508	25,453
Blindness	92	80	95	83	85	124	249	409	434	475
Disabled[2]	2,819	2,937	3,496	3,635	3,983	7,497	13,203	20,476	23,969	27,798
AFDC program[3]	14,210	15,275	16,036	17,230	20,194	6,354	9,160	13,788	17,690	22,129
Other and unknown	1,499	1,214	1,175	1,105	658	596	798	1,268	1,257	1,193
Inpatient services in–										
General hospital	3,680	3,434	4,170	4,593	5,072	6,412	9,453	13,378	16,674	19,891
Mental hospital	66	60	90	92	65	775	1,192	1,470	1,714	2,010
Intermediate care facilities:										
Mentally retarded	121	147	148	147	146	1,989	4,731	6,649	7,354	7,680
Nursing facility services[4]	1,398	1,375	1,452	1,461	1,500	7,887	11,587	15,531	17,693	20,709
Physicians	13,765	14,387	15,686	17,078	19,321	1,875	2,346	3,408	4,018	4,952
Dental	4,652	4,672	4,214	4,552	5,209	462	458	498	593	710
Other practitioner	3,234	3,357	3,555	3,873	4,282	198	251	317	372	437
Outpatient hospital	9,705	10,072	11,344	12,370	14,137	1,101	1,789	2,837	3,324	4,283
Clinic	1,531	2,121	2,391	2,804	3,511	320	714	1,249	1,688	2,211
Laboratory[5]	3,212	6,354	7,759	8,959	10,505	121	337	590	721	897
Home health	392	535	609	719	813	332	1,120	2,572	3,404	4,101

[Continued]

★ 497 ★

Medicaid Recipients and Payments, by Type of Service: 1980-1991

[Continued]

Basis of eligibility and type of service	Recipients (1,000)					Payments (million dollars)				
	1980	1985	1989	1990	1991	1980	1985	1989	1990	1991
Prescribed drugs	13,707	13,921	15,916	17,294	19,602	1,318	2,315	3,689	4,420	5,424
Family planning	1,129	1,636	1,564	1,752	2,185	81	195	227	265	359

Source: 1993 Statistical Abstract of the United States on CD-ROM [machine-readable datafiles]. CD-ABSTR-93. Washington, DC: U.S. Department of Commerce, Economics and Statistics Administration, Bureau of the Census, Data User Services Division, 1993. Primary source: Health Care Financing Administration. Health Care Review (quarterly). Notes: 1. Recipient data do not add due to small number of recipients that are reported in more than one category. Includes recipients of, and payments for other care not shown separately. 2. Permanently and totally. 3. Aid to Families With Dependent Children (AFDC). 4. Nursing facility services includes skilled nursing facility services and intermediate care facility services for all other than the mentally retarded 5. Includes radiological services.

★ 498 ★

Medicaid: Benefits and Beneficiaries

Medicaid Recipients, by Selected Characteristics: 1980-1991

Represents number of persons as of March of following year who were enrolled at any time in year shown. Person did not have to receive medical care paid for by Medicaid in order to be counted.

In thousands, except percentages]

Poverty status	1980	1985	1990	1991							
				Total[1]	White	Black	Hispanic[2]	Under 18 years old	18-44 years old	45-64 years old	65 years old and older
Persons covered, total	18,966	19,204	24,160	26,739	16,990	8,282	4,577	13,374	8,055	2,420	2,891
Below poverty level	11,113	12,652	15,175	16,888	9,782	6,241	3,022	9,388	5,011	1,301	1,187
Above poverty level	7,854	6,552	8,985	9,851	7,208	2,041	1,555	3,986	3,044	1,119	1,704
Percent of total population	8.4	8.1	9.7	10.6	8.1	26.5	20.7	20.3	7.6	5.0	9.5
Below poverty level	39.1	39.7	45.2	47.3	41.2	60.9	47.7	65.5	37.7	30.2	31.4
Above poverty level	4.0	3.2	4.2	4.6	3.9	9.7	9.9	7.7	3.3	2.6	6.4

Source: 1993 Statistical Abstract of the United States on CD-ROM [machine-readable datafiles]. CD-ABSTR-93. Washington, DC: U.S. Department of Commerce, Economics and Statistics Administration, Bureau of the Census, Data User Services Division, 1993. Primary source: Bureau of the Census. Current Population Reports. P60-181; also earlier reports and unpublished data. Notes: 1. Includes other races not shown separately. 2. Persons of Hispanic origin may be of any race.

★ 499 ★

Medicaid: Benefits and Beneficiaries

Medicaid Recipients, by Selected Cities: 1992

Data below present Medicaid recipients in Health Care Financing Administration (HCFA) regions.

[In thousands]

Regions	Resident population[1]	Medicaid recipients[2]	Recipients as percent of population
All regions	255,081[3]	31,150	12.2
Boston, Massachusetts	13,200	1,527	11.6
New York, New York	25,908	4,153	16.0
Philadelphia, Pennsylvania	26,384	2,768	10.5
Atlanta, Georgia	46,214	5,940	12.9
Chicago, Illinois	47,233	5,238	11.1
Dallas, Texas	29,135	3,620	12.4
Kansas City, Missouri	12,134	1,211	10.0
Denver, Colorado	7,920	620	7.8
San Francisco, California	33,354[4]	5,065	15.2
Seattle, Washington	9,767	1,008	10.3

Source: U.S. Department of Health and Human Services. Health Care Financing Administration (HCFA). Bureau of Data Management and Strategy. *1993 HCFA Statistics.* HCFA Pub. No. 03341 Washington, DC: U.S. Department of Health and Human Services, June 1993, p. 13. Primary sources: Health Care Financing Administration, Bureau of Data Management and Strategy, Office of Program Statistics, Division of Medicaid Statistics; U.S. Bureau of the Census, Population Division, Population Estimates Branch. *Notes:* Numbers may not add to totals because of rounding. 1. Population estimates shown are based on the July 1, 1992, population. 2. Medicaid recipient data are as of fiscal year 1992. 3. Excludes persons in outlying areas, those with unknown state of residence and those living in foreign countries. 4. Excludes Arizona, which operates a medical assistance program under a Section 1115 demonstration project.

Medicaid: Coverage

★ 500 ★

Medicaid Utilization Measures: 1975-1991

For fiscal years ending in year shown. Includes Virgin Islands. Data are provided by type of facility.

[In thousands]

Measure	1975	1980	1985	1986	1987	1988	1989	1990	1991
General hospitals:									
Total discharges	3,031	3,203	3,616	3,713	3,558	3,905	3,734	4,823	5,281
Recipients discharged	2,336	2,255	2,390	2,564	2,525	2,640	2,701	3,261	3,638
Total days of care	22,941	24,089	29,562	29,517	23,124	24,022	22,754	27,471	28,998

[Continued]

★ 500 ★

Medicaid Utilization Measures: 1975-1991
[Continued]

Measure	1975	1980	1985	1986	1987	1988	1989	1990	1991
Nursing facilities:[1]									
Total recipients	1,212	1,395	1,375	1,399	1,371	1,445	1,438	1,461	1,500
Total days of care	199,715	273,497	277,996	334,016	328,758	344,693	367,228	360,044	387,621
Intermediate care facilities:[2]									
Total recipients	69	121	147	145	140	145	147	146	146
Total days of care	9,060	250,124	47,324	48,418	45,611	46,825	50,276	49,730	50,223

Source: 1993 Statistical Abstract of the United States on CD-ROM [machine-readable datafiles]. CD-ABSTR-93. Washington, DC: U.S. Department of Commerce, Economics and Statistics Administration, Bureau of the Census, Data User Services Division, 1993. Primary source: Health Care Financing Administration, unpublished data. Notes: 1. Includes skilled nursing facilities and intermediate care facilities for all other than the mentally retarded. 2. Mentally retarded.

★ 501 ★

Medicaid: Coverage

Prescription Drug Medicaid Co-Pays

Data below reflect the monthly Medicaid co-pays for prescription drugs in selected states.

State	Co-pay
Connecticut	10.00
Pennsylvania	6.00
Maryland	5.00
New Jersey	5.00
Maine	3.00-5.00
Illinois	25.00
New York	23.00

Source: Glaser, Martha. "Medicaid Prices Closing in on $20 Per Prescription." Drug Topics 136, no. 21, 9 November 1992, p. 96. Primary source: National Pharmaceutical Council.

Medicare: Benefits and Beneficiaries

★ 502 ★

Medicare Beneficiaries, by Age

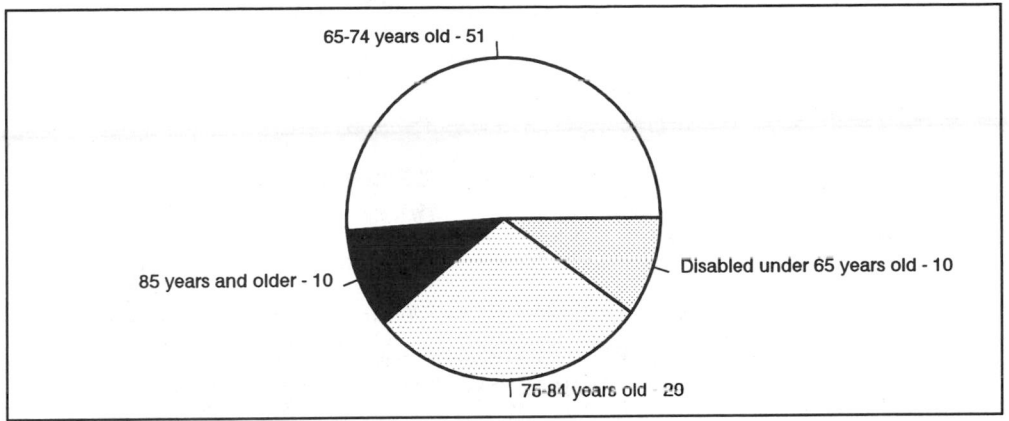

The table below shows the users of Medicare funds. Data are provided by age.

Age	Percent
Disabled under 65 years old	10
65-74 years old	51
75-84 years old	29
85 years and older	10

Source: "Who Uses Medicare." *USA TODAY*, 10 March 1993, final edition, p. 1A. Primary source: Health Care Financing Administration.

★ 503 ★

Medicare: Benefits and Beneficiaries

Medicare Beneficiaries, by Selected Cities: 1992

Data below present the number of persons served by Medicare in Health Care Financing Administration (HCFA) regions.

Regions	Aged persons served (in thousands)	Aged persons served (per 1,000 enrollees)	Disabled persons served (in thousands)	Disabled persons served (per 1,000 enrollees)
All regions	25,178	800	2,465	732
Boston, Massachusetts	1,459	831	123	753
New York, New York	2,943	803	285	682
Philadelphia, Pennsylvania	2,878	844	261	749

[Continued]

★ 503 ★

Medicare Beneficiaries, by Selected Cities: 1992
[Continued]

Regions	Aged persons served (in thousands)	Aged persons served (per 1,000 enrollees)	Disabled persons served (in thousands)	Disabled persons served (per 1,000 enrollees)
Atlanta, Georgia	4,972	830	566	761
Chicago, Illinois	4,820	824	458	734
Dallas, Texas	2,556	824	258	727
Kansas City, Missouri	1,408	827	117	745
Denver, Colorado	661	791	57	682
San Francisco, California	2,643	699	266	717
Seattle, Washington	839	701	74	698

Source: U.S. Department of Health and Human Services. Health Care Financing Administration (HCFA). Bureau of Data Management and Strategy. 1993 HCFA Statistics. HCFA Pub. No. 03341. Washington, DC: U.S. Department of Health and Human Services, June 1993, p. 35. Primary sources: Health Care Financing Administration. Bureau of Data Management and Strategy. Data from the Decision Support System. Notes: Data as of calendar year 1991 for persons served under Hospital Insurance and/or Supplementary Medical Insurance. Based on utilization for fee-for-service and excludes utilization under alternative payment systems such as health maintenance organizations. Numbers may not add to totals because of rounding. 1. Excludes residents of foreign countries.

★ 504 ★

Medicare: Benefits and Beneficiaries

Medicare Beneficiaries, by Type: 1983-1991
[Number of beneficiaries in thousands]

Fiscal year	Medicare aged beneficiaries	Medicare disabled beneficiaries
1983	26,670	2,918
1984	27,112	2,884
1985	27,123	2,944
1986	27,728	2,986
1987	28,239	3,042
1988	28,779	3,115
1989	29,358	3,200
1990[1]	29,951	3,251
1991[1]	30,480	3,297

Source: Medicare and Medicaid's 25th Anniversary—Much Promised, Accomplished, and Left Unfinished: A Report Presented by the Chairman of the Select Committee on Aging. Washington, DC: U.S. Government Printing Office, 1990, n.p. Primary source: Health Care Financing Administration and Congressional Budget Office, 1990. Note: 1. Estimate.

★ 505 ★

Medicare: Benefits and Beneficiaries

Medicare Enrollment and Benefits, by Program: 1992

From the source: "The Social Security Amendments of 1965 established two separate but coordinated health insurance plans for persons aged 65 or older. The compulsory program of Hospital Insurance (HI) is Part A of Medicare and a voluntary program of Supplementary Medical Insurance (SMI) is Part B. Benefits were first available in July 1966, although post-hospital extended care services in skilled-nursing facilities (SNF) were not covered until January 1967. The 1972 Amendments extended Medicare coverage to certain severely disabled persons under age 65 and to certain persons suffering from kidney disease."

Program	Enrollees	Benefit payments
Hospital Insurance (Part A)	35.2 million	$83.9 billion
Supplementary Medical Insurance (Part B)	33.9 million	$49.3 billion

Source: U.S. Department of Health and Human Services. Social Security Administration (SSA). "Social Security Programs in the United States, 1993." *Social Security Bulletin* 4, no. 4 (22 December 1993), n.p.

★ 506 ★

Medicare: Benefits and Beneficiaries

Medicare Enrollment and Benefits, by State: 1991

Data are preliminary estimates, provided by state or other areas.

Region, division, and state	Enrollment[1] (1,000)	Payments[2] (million dollars)
All areas	34,870	118,546
United States[3]	34,153	117,926
Northeast	7,541	28,768
New England	1,918	6,739
Maine	186	520
New Hampshire	141	400
Vermont	76	200
Massachusetts	879	3,418
Rhode Island	161	526
Connecticut	476	1,676
Middle Atlantic	5,623	22,029
New York	2,529	10,345
New Jersey	1,109	3,834
Pennsylvania	1,985	7,850
Midwest	8,548	28,759
East North Central	5,879	20,867
Ohio	1,571	5,959
Indiana	775	2,488

[Continued]

★ 506 ★

Medicare Enrollment and Benefits, by State: 1991
[Continued]

Region, division, and state	Enrollment[1] (1,000)	Payments[2] (million dollars)
Illinois	1,553	5,531
Michigan	1,257	4,808
Wisconsin	723	2,081
West North Central	2,669	7,892
Minnesota	597	1,509
Iowa	461	1,294
Missouri	792	2,698
North Dakota	100	293
South Dakota	111	293
Nebraska	240	635
Kansas	368	1,169
South	11,780	40,235
South Atlantic	6,298	21,160
Delaware	91	315
Maryland	554	2,326
District of Columbia	78	381
Virginia	741	2,341
West Virginia	312	949
North Carolina	917	2,607
South Carolina	454	1,212
Georgia	750	2,588
Florida	2,402	8,443
East South Central	2,213	7,482
Kentucky	543	1,801
Tennessee	706	2,405
Alabama	593	2,124
Mississippi	371	1,154
West South Central	3,269	11,592
Arkansas	397	1,257
Louisiana	541	2,283
Oklahoma	458	1,488
Texas	1,873	6,564
West	6,270	20,146
Mountain	1,697	5,027
Montana	120	345
Idaho	135	344
Wyoming	53	158
Colorado	369	1,041
New Mexico	186	509
Arizona	517	1,717
Utah	166	436
Nevada	151	477
Pacific	4,573	15,119
Washington	630	1,827

[Continued]

★ 506 ★

Medicare Enrollment and Benefits, by State: 1991

[Continued]

Region, division, and state	Enrollment[1] (1,000)	Payments[2] (million dollars)
Oregon	434	1,035
California	3,352	11,871
Alaska	27	93
Hawaii	131	293
PR	437	581
Outlying areas	9	16
Foreign	272	28

Source: 1993 Statistical Abstract of the United States on CD-ROM [machine-readable datafiles]. CD-ABSTR-93. Washington, DC: U.S. Department of Commerce, Economics and Statistics Administration, Bureau of the Census, Data User Services Division, 1993. Primary source: Health Care Financing Administration, unpublished data. Notes: "X" represents "not applicable." 1. Hospital and/or medical insurance enrollment as of July 1. 2. Benefit payments are for calendar year. Payments for "All Areas" represent actual Trust Fund disbursements as shown in the 1990 Trustees Reports, and other actuarial data. Distribution by state is based on interim payment as reflected on claims for services rendered in 1989 and recorded in central office through December 1990. Payments have been adjusted to include estimated Prospective Payment System (PPS) pass-through amounts, but exclude retroactive cost-based adjustments and administrative expenses. Data reflect state of residence of beneficiary. 3. Includes data for enrollees with residence unknown.

★ 507 ★

Medicare. Benefits and Beneficiaries

Medicare Enrollment and Benefits, by Type of Insurance: 1970-1991

Enrollment as of July 1, payments for calendar year. Benefit payments represent trust fund outlays. Includes Puerto Rico, outlying areas, and enrollees in foreign countries. Data are provided for selected years.

Type of insurance	Unit	1970	1975	1980	1985	1986	1987	1988	1989	1990	1991
HOSPITAL AND/OR MEDICAL INSURANCE											
Enrollment, total	1,000	20,491	24,959	28,478	31,083	31,750	32,411	32,980	33,579	34,203	34,870
Benefit payments	Million $	7,099	15,588	35,699	70,527	75,997	80,316	86,487	98,305	108,707	118,778
HOSPITAL INSURANCE											
Enrollment, total	1,000	20,361	24,640	28,067	30,589	31,216	31,853	32,413	33,040	33,719	34,429
Persons 65 and over	1,000	20,361	22,472	25,104	27,683	28,257	28,822	29,312	29,869	30,464	31,043
Disabled persons[1]	1,000	(X)	2,168	2,963	2,907	2,959	3,031	3,101	3,171	3,255	3,385
Benefit payments	Million $	5,124	11,315	25,064	47,580	49,758	49,496	52,517	60,011	66,239	71,549
MEDICAL INSURANCE											
Enrollment, total	1,000	19,584	23,904	27,400	29,989	30,590	31,170	31,617	32,099	32,629	33,237
Persons 65 and over	1,000	19,584	21,945	24,680	27,311	27,863	28,382	28,780	29,216	29,686	30,185

[Continued]

★ 507 ★

Medicare Enrollment and Benefits, by Type of Insurance: 1970-1991
[Continued]

Type of insurance	Unit	1970	1975	1980	1985	1986	1987	1988	1989	1990	1991
Disabled persons[1]	1,000	(X)	1,959	2,719	2,678	2,727	2,788	2,837	2,883	2,943	3,052
Benefit payments	Million $	1,975	4,273	10,635	22,947	26,239	30,820	33,970	38,294	42,468	47,229

Source: 1993 Statistical Abstract of the United States on CD-ROM [machine-readable datafiles]. CD-ABSTR-93. Washington, DC: U.S. Department of Commerce, Economics and Statistics Administration, Bureau of the Census, Data User Services Division, 1993. Primary source: U.S. Health Care Financing Administration. Published in U.S. Social Security Administration's *Annual Statistical Supplement to the "Social Security Bulletin." Notes:* "X" indicates "not applicable." 1. Age under 65; includes persons enrolled because of end-stage renal disease (ESRD) only.

★ 508 ★

Medicare: Benefits and Beneficiaries

Medicare Enrollment and Reimbursements, by Type of Coverage and Service: 1980-1990

Persons served are enrollees who used covered services, incurred expenses greater than the applicable deductible amounts, and for whom Medicare paid benefits. Reimbursements are amounts paid to providers for covered services. Excluded are retroactive adjustments resulting from end of fiscal year cost settlements and certain lump-sum interim payments. Also excluded are beneficiary (or third-party payor) liabilities for applicable deductibles, coinsurance amounts, and charges for noncovered services. Includes data for enrollees living in outlying territories and foreign countries.

Type of coverage and service	Unit	Persons 65 years old and over				Disabled persons[1]			
		1980	1985	1989	1990	1980	1985	1989	1990
Persons served, total[2]	1,000	16,271	20,347	23,868	24,809	1,760	1,944	2,287	2,390
Hospital Insurance[2]	1,000	6,024	6,058	6,155	6,367	728	662	659	680
Inpatient hospital	1,000	5,951	5,714	5,725	5,906	721	636	627	644
Skilled-nursing services	1,000	248	304	613	615	9	10	23	23
Home health services[3]	1,000	675	1,448	1,580	1,818	51	101	105	122
Supplementary Medical Insurance[2]	1,000	16,099	20,186	23,746	24,687	1,723	1,916	2,263	2,365
Physicians' and other medical services	1,000	15,627	19,590	23,283	24,193	1,631	1,820	2,159	2,249
Outpatient services	1,000	6,629	9,889	13,291	14,055	909	1,096	1,415	1,496
Home health services[3]	1,000	302	27	36	38	25	-	-	-
Persons served per 1,000 enrollees, total[2]	Rate	638	722	785	802	594	669	721	734
Hospital Insurance[2]	Rate	240	219	206	209	246	228	208	209
Inpatient hospital	Rate	237	206	192	194	243	219	198	198
Skilled-nursing services	Rate	10	11	21	20	3	4	7	7
Home health services[3]	Rate	27	52	53	60	17	35	33	38
Supplementary Medical Insurance[2]	Rate	652	739	813	832	634	716	785	804
Physicians' and other medical services	Rate	633	717	797	815	600	680	749	764
Outpatient services	Rate	269	362	455	474	334	409	491	508
Home health services[3]	Rate	12	1	1	1	9	-	-	-
Reimbursements, total	Million $	29,134	56,199	82,222	88,778	4,478	7,495	10,363	11,239
Hospital Insurance	Million $	20,353	37,360	50,448	54,244	2,765	4,785	6,253	6,694
Inpatient hospital	Million $	19,583	35,313	45,439	48,952	2,714	4,638	5,936	6,346
Skilled-nursing services	Million $	331	464	2,806	1,886	13	17	143	85
Home health services[3]	Million $	440	1,583	2,202	3,406	38	130	173	264
Supplementary Medical Insurance	Million $	8,781	18,839	31,774	34,533	1,713	2,709	4,111	4,545
Physicians' and other medical services	Million $	7,361	15,309	25,310	27,379	997	1,712	2,623	2,831
Outpatient services	Million $	1,261	3,499	6,407	7,077	701	997	1,489	1,714
Home health services[3]	Million $	159	31	57	78	16	-	-	-

[Continued]

★ 508 ★

Medicare Enrollment and Reimbursements, by Type of Coverage and Service: 1980-1990

[Continued]

Type of coverage and service	Unit	Persons 65 years old and over				Disabled persons[1]			
		1980	1985	1989	1990	1980	1985	1989	1990
Reimbursements, per person served, total	$	1,791	2,762	3,445	3,578	2,544	3,855	4,531	4,703
Hospital Insurance	$	3,379	6,167	8,196	8,520	3,798	7,224	9,482	9,847
Inpatient hospital	$	3,291	6,181	7,937	8,289	3,765	7,295	9,455	9,849
Skilled-nursing services	$	1,336	1,525	4,580	3,068	1,571	1,681	6,107	3,702
Home health services[3]	$	652	1,093	1,394	1,874	733	1,288	1,645	2,156
Supplementary Medical Insurance	$	545	933	1,338	1,399	994	1,414	1,817	1,922
Physicians' and other medical services	$	471	781	1,087	1,132	611	941	1,215	1,259
Outpatient services	$	190	354	482	503	771	909	1,051	1,146
Home health services[3]	$	526	1,122	1,614	2,033	619	-	-	-

Source: 1993 Statistical Abstract of the United States on CD-ROM [machine-readable datafiles]. CD-ABSTR-93. Washington, DC: U.S. Department of Commerce, Economics and Statistics Administration, Bureau of the Census, Data User Services Division, 1993. Primary source: U.S. Health Care Financing Administration. *Medicare Program Statistics* (annual); and unpublished data. *Notes:* "-" represents or rounds to zero. 1. Age under 65; includes persons enrolled because of end-stage renal disease (ESRD) only. 2. Persons are counted once for each type of covered service used, but are not double counted in totals. 3. Beginning 1982, a change in legislation resulted in virtually all home health services being paid under hospital insurance.

Medicare: Coverage

★ 509 ★

Medicare Denial Rates

Carriers processing Medicare's 112 million Part B (Supplementary Medical Insurance) claims denied about 9 percent on grounds of medical necessity. The U.S. General Accounting Office (GAO), however, did not find the denials uniformly distributed. The table below represents the services denied for medical necessity per 1,000 services allowed for selected states or regions within states.

Place	Services denied for medical necessity per 1,000 allowed
Southern California	23.1
Illinois	14.1
Wisconsin	12.0
Northern California	4.4

[Continued]

★ 509 ★

Medicare Denial Rates
[Continued]

Place	Services denied for medical necessity per 1,000 allowed
North Carolina	4.0
South Carolina	1.4

Source: Culhane, Charles. "Medicare Denial Rates Vary Widely; Carriers Inconsistent in Judging Medical Necessity." *American Medical News,* 18 April 1994, p. 3. Primary source: GAO, 1994. *Note:* Based on 5 percent sample of Medicare Part B claims.

★ 510 ★

Medicare: Coverage

Medicare Hospital Insurance Bills Approved and Reimbursed: 1966-1991

The table below shows the number of bills approved for payment and the amount reimbursed through Medicare's Hospital Insurance (HI) program. Data are provided by type of benefit and type of beneficiary for 1966 through 1991.

[Number in thousands]

Year approved	Total[1]		Inpatient hospital[2]		Home health		Skilled nursing facilities[3]	
	Number	Amount reimbursed	Number	Amount reimbursed	Number	Amount reimbursed	Number	Amount reimbursed
All persons								
1966	1,979	824,367	1,866	821,362	34	2,113	...	...
1970	7,512	4,855,161	6,313	4,578,080	571	46,896	627	230,183
1975	10,318	10,414,195	8,687	10,006,206	1,078	145,631	553	262,358
1979	12,831	19,321,096	10,314	18,615,371	1,997	377,732	520	327,992
1980	13,866	23,200,897	11,088	22,367,454	2,266	473,805	512	359,638
1981	14,896	27,701,752	11,508	26,639,308	2,875	666,260	513	396,185
1982	16,737	33,080,071	11,996	31,579,763	4,223	1,068,162	518	432,147
1983	17,312	36,133,754	12,107	34,337,127	4,661	1,337,527	543	459,100
1984	16,483	36,046,031	10,985	34,007,966	4,958	1,577,714	540	460,351
1985	15,615	37,533,351	10,352	35,414,544	4,747	1,656,411	515	462,396
1986	16,000	39,045,165	10,474	36,679,676	4,974	1,829,759	551	535,730
1987	15,406	39,584,874	10,262	37,225,007	4,663	1,807,762	481	552,105
1988	15,391	40,859,263	10,180	38,216,668	4,614	1,891,160	597	751,435
1989	16,325	44,955,779	9,940	40,144,211	4,979	2,224,408	1,406	2,587,160
1990	18,232	49,331,647	10,395	43,779,106	6,431	3,330,256	1,406	2,222,285
1991	20,428	55,258,108	10,658	47,969,767	8,388	5,047,391	1,381	2,240,950

[Continued]

★ 510 ★

Medicare Hospital Insurance Bills Approved and Reimbursed: 1966-1991
[Continued]

Year approved	Total[1]		Inpatient hospital[2]		Home health		Skilled nursing facilities[3]	
	Number	Amount reimbursed	Number	Amount reimbursed	Number	Amount reimbursed	Number	Amount reimbursed
Persons aged 65 or older [4]								
1973	8,080	6,550,708	6,980	6,297,814	624	60,549	476	192,345
1975	9,389	9,429,866	7,844	9,041,321	1,009	135,687	536	252,859
1979	11,385	16,999,417	9,040	16,337,003	1,847	347,921	502	314,493
1980	12,287	20,357,667	9,705	19,580,817	2,097	436,589	485	340,250
1981	13,254	24,378,817	10,098	23,384,330	2,661	613,719	495	380,769
1982	14,962	29,170,229	10,555	27,772,783	3,906	981,067	501	416,380
1983	15,540	31,959,130	10,700	30,284,469	4,315	1,231,532	525	443,129
1984	14,871	32,040,872	9,754	30,139,771	4,595	1,456,125	523	444,976
1985	14,063	33,325,618	9,160	31,348,094	4,404	1,530,937	499	446,587
1986	14,363	34,579,907	9,218	32,373,793	4,612	1,690,046	532	516,068
1987	13,882	35,322,516	9,090	33,119,345	4,327	1,671,678	465	531,493
1988	13,917	36,602,037	9,047	34,124,594	4,294	1,754,560	577	722,883
1989	14,751	40,044,850	8,774	35,522,207	4,630	2,060,815	1,347	2,461,828
1990	16,525	44,015,084	9,191	38,806,251	5,984	3,086,110	1,350	2,122,723
1991	18,548	49,332,113	9,406	42,498,728	7,812	4,682,130	1,331	2,151,255
Disabled persons[5]								
1973	215	173,178	206	170,850	6	692	4	1,637
1975	929	984,329	843	964,885	69	9,944	17	9,499
1979	1,443	2,321,679	1,274	2,278,368	150	29,811	18	13,499
1980	1,545	2,773,750	1,357	2,722,587	168	37,199	18	13,065
1981	1,642	3,322,935	1,410	3,254,978	214	52,541	18	15,416
1982	1,775	3,909,842	1,441	3,806,980	317	87,095	17	15,767
1983	1,772	4,174,624	1,407	4,052,658	346	105,995	18	15,971
1984	1,612	4,005,159	1,232	3,868,195	363	121,589	17	15,375
1985	1,552	4,207,733	1,192	4,066,450	343	125,474	16	15,809
1986	1,637	4,465,258	1,256	4,305,883	362	139,713	19	19,662
1987	1,524	4,262,358	1,172	4,105,662	335	136,084	16	20,612
1988	1,474	4,257,226	1,135	4,092,074	321	136,600	20	28,552
1989	1,574	4,910,929	1,166	4,622,004	349	163,593	59	125,332

[Continued]

★ 510 ★

Medicare Hospital Insurance Bills Approved and Reimbursed: 1966-1991
[Continued]

Year approved	Total[1]		Inpatient hospital[2]		Home health		Skilled nursing facilities[3]	
	Number	Amount reimbursed	Number	Amount reimbursed	Number	Amount reimbursed	Number	Amount reimbursed
1990	1,706	5,316,563	1,203	4,972,855	447	244,146	56	99,562
1991	1,879	5,925,995	1,253	5,471,039	577	365,261	50	89,695

Source: U.S. Department of Health and Human Services. Social Security Administration (SSA). *Annual Statistical Supplement to the "Social Security Bulletin," 1992.* SSA Publication No. 13-11700. Washington, DC: U.S. Department of Health and Human Services, Social Security Administration, Office of Research and Statistics, 1993, p. 299. *Notes:* Three dots (...) means not applicable. 1. Included in total but not shown separately are data on approved bills for outpatient diagnostic services rendered before April 1, 1968. Beginning in April 1968, outpatient diagnostic services, formerly covered under Hospital Insurance are covered under Supplementary Medical Insurance. 2. The Social Security Amendments of 1983 (Public Law 98-21) replace (for most hospitals) the retrospective cost reimbursement system and the cost-per-case limits and rate of increase ceiling created by the Tax Equity and Fiscal Responsibility Act of 1982. Effective with hospital cost-reporting periods beginning on or after October 1, 1983, Medicare payments for inpatient operating costs are to be based on a fixed amount, determined in advance, for each case, according to one of 475 diagnosis- related groups (DRG's) into which a case is classified. The prospective payment is considered payment in full; hospitals are prohibited from charging beneficiaries more than the statutory deductible and coinsurance. Additional payments, determined by nondiagnostic criteria, are made to hospitals by the program for various "pass-through" costs and additional adjustments. These additional payments are not included in the inpatient hospital billing amounts reimbursed shown in this table. 3. Coverage began January 1, 1967. Benefit payments shown for 1985 are incomplete due to billing lags. 4. Beginning October 1, 1978, includes a relatively small number of persons entitled to benefits solely because of end-stage renal disease. 5. Includes a relatively small number of persons under age 65 entitled to benefits solely because of end-stage renal disease.

★ 511 ★

Medicare: Coverage

Short-Stay Hospital Charges Covered by Medicare Through Hospital Insurance: 1975-1991

Data below reflect the average covered charges per day of care paid by Medicare through Hospital Insurance (HI). Data are based on bills approved in each year and recorded in the Health Care Financing Administration before December 27, 1991. Table includes data for services rendered to both aged and disabled persons. Data are provided by state, geographic division, and outside area.

Census division and state[1]	Short-stay hospitals							
	1975	1980	1985	1987[2]	1988[2]	1989[2]	1990[2]	1991[2]
Total[3]	$143	$292	$584	$707	$868	$999	$1,105	$1,279
United States[4]	144	293	586	709	871	1,003	1,110	1,285
New England	159	298	546	638	749	860	988	1,142
Connecticut	167	287	559	683	846	983	1,177	1,367
Maine	133	284	572	587	697	802	924	1,069
Massachusetts	168	316	553	655	741	829	940	1,079
New Hampshire	123	264	533	610	758	904	1,021	1,186
Rhode Island	154	284	486	540	634	750	852	972
Vermont	124	230	487	572	694	814	922	1,069
Middle Atlantic	163	304	536	619	738	896	943	1,075
New Jersey	157	300	464	514	593	637	725	893
New York	176	301	516	564	656	736	836	927
Pennsylvania	145	312	705	777	936	1,446	1,236	1,371

[Continued]

★ 511 ★

Short-Stay Hospital Charges Covered by Medicare Through Hospital Insurance: 1975-1991

[Continued]

Census division and state[1]	Short-stay hospitals							
	1975	1980	1985	1987[2]	1988[2]	1989[2]	1990[2]	1991[2]
East North Central	140	294	604	710	864	978	1,097	1,250
Illinois	148	322	649	757	942	1,071	1,203	1,388
Indiana	116	236	524	633	772	892	997	1,153
Michigan	156	332	650	807	958	1,070	1,193	1,360
Ohio	134	277	545	665	809	911	1,031	1,145
Wisconsin	128	251	543	591	714	822	933	1,080
West North Central	117	248	594	670	817	919	1,052	1,224
Iowa	110	239	490	606	718	800	901	1,049
Kansas	113	244	605	679	827	934	1,093	1,263
Minnesota	124	248	605	684	858	979	1,132	1,297
Missouri	119	257	603	702	864	976	1,108	1,286
Nebraska	116	251	585	654	806	883	1,045	1,251
North Dakota	118	237	571	651	782	854	937	1,081
South Dakota	107	228	566	597	703	811	915	1,106
South Atlantic	135	273	544	693	866	979	1,106	1,290
Delaware	153	274	562	679	827	972	1,191	1,348
District of Columbia	174	373	710	832	1,063	1,215	1,374	1,524
Florida	161	321	689	850	1,058	1,209	1,361	1,585
Georgia	125	258	573	676	838	940	1,081	1,238
Maryland	164	274	495	571	675	735	813	913
North Carolina	101	214	466	555	696	806	932	1,093
South Carolina	106	229	530	606	780	913	1,020	1,191
Virginia	118	247	507	604	781	890	1,023	1,207
West Virginia	108	247	557	660	800	902	1,009	1,155
East South Central	115	243	533	644	806	908	1,021	1,183
Alabama	126	282	604	753	935	1,063	1,179	1,367
Kentucky	107	216	520	600	764	869	967	1,111
Mississippi	98	213	451	549	679	768	866	993
Tennessee	122	250	559	644	807	891	1,013	1,181
West South Central	117	253	603	714	874	999	1,139	1,317
Arkansas	104	231	554	594	710	799	927	1,036
Louisiana	116	265	616	740	905	1,025	1,180	1,343
Oklahoma	128	271	592	681	790	878	997	1,126
Texas	118	250	612	743	925	1,075	1,212	1,429
Mountain	142	305	673	823	1,026	1,192	1,350	1,558
Arizona	155	325	682	879	1,078	1,273	1,443	1,677
Colorado	144	288	623	789	981	1,140	1,308	1,558
Idaho	129	273	611	723	882	1,017	1,140	1,318
Montana	116	262	620	680	832	929	1,037	1,184
Nevada	177	424	994	1,216	1,543	1,753	2,030	2,197

[Continued]

★ 511 ★

Short-Stay Hospital Charges Covered by Medicare Through Hospital Insurance: 1975-1991

[Continued]

Census division and state[1]	Short-stay hospitals							
	1975	1980	1985	1987[2]	1988[2]	1989[2]	1990[2]	1991[2]
New Mexico	133	293	684	782	913	1,055	1,140	1,328
Utah	142	316	620	748	1,001	1,141	1,283	1,437
Wyoming	109	245	614	662	813	942	1,094	1,251
Pacific	196	416	852	1,022	1,280	1,463	1,650	1,974
Alaska	228	379	706	897	1,252	1,330	1,477	1,555
California	206	448	893	1,087	1,377	1,576	1,796	2,151
Hawaii	148	333	713	854	1,031	1,142	1,224	1,539
Oregon	158	329	741	838	981	1,136	1,275	1,491
Washington	163	293	646	744	912	1,021	1,162	1,339
Outlying areas	77	152	283	421	502	745	910	1,211
Puerto Rico	77	151	311	362	436	475	505	555
Virgin Islands	92	161	264	401	385	498	747	901
Other	88	263	273	501	685	1,263	1,478	2,178

Source: U.S. Department of Health and Human Services. Social Security Administration (SSA). *Annual Statistical Supplement to the "Social Security Bulletin," 1992.* SSA Publication No. 13-11700. Washington, DC: U.S. Department of Health and Human Services, Social Security Administration, Office of Research and Statistics, 1993, p. 301.

★ 512 ★

Medicare: Coverage

Skilled Nursing Facility Charges Covered by Medicare Through Hospital Insurance: 1975-1991

Table below reflects the average covered charges per day of care paid by Medicare through Hospital Insurance (HI). Data are based on bills approved in each year and recorded in the Health Care Financing Administration before December 27, 1991. Data are for services rendered to both aged and disabled persons. Data are provided by state.

Census division and state[1]	Skilled nursing facilities							
	1975	1980	1985	1987[2]	1988[2]	1989[2]	1990[2]	1991[2]
Total[3]	$43	$70	$119	$163	$171	$156	$184	$228
New England	50	77	115	141	147	140	164	189
Connecticut	35	51	95	108	125	133	156	183
Maine	52	100	146	216	244	230	282	239
Massachusetts	63	98	139	177	182	145	173	194
New Hampshire	41	86	129	165	181	178	212	246
Rhode Island	43	59	93	102	110	113	128	146
Vermont	38	62	105	119	139	123	145	197
Middle Atlantic	50	73	115	149	145	143	164	189
New Jersey	45	81	124	285	144	135	157	184
New York	61	80	120	136	144	148	165	182

[Continued]

★512★

Skilled Nursing Facility Charges Covered by Medicare Through Hospital Insurance: 1975-1991
[Continued]

Census division and state[1]	Skilled nursing facilities							
	1975	1980	1985	1987[2]	1988[2]	1989[2]	1990[2]	1991[2]
Pennsylvania	40	65	105	135	148	139	165	196
East North Central	40	68	108	145	149	136	159	196
Illinois	37	77	118	209	210	183	206	248
Indiana	35	60	101	124	139	141	172	215
Michigan	45	60	93	108	109	107	126	146
Ohio	41	69	114	146	144	129	148	188
Wisconsin	35	64	111	133	140	130	144	169
West North Central	45	82	148	205	185	159	187	225
Iowa	46	84	175	217	236	233	263	296
Kansas	39	66	151	171	209	221	249	284
Minnesota	46	94	137	213	109	102	119	148
Missouri	47	95	163	263	281	231	255	297
Nebraska	41	71	127	160	180	182	202	222
North Dakota	43	49	88	108	118	105	114	136
South Dakota	33	61	106	161	156	141	159	165
South Atlantic	34	59	97	129	148	136	158	204
Delaware	31	50	76	91	98	104	124	176
District of Columbia	34	64	110	129	152	159	177	246
Florida	34	59	101	138	166	151	182	238
Georgia	34	71	108	129	135	120	138	179
Maryland	37	56	99	116	129	121	134	173
North Carolina	31	52	91	110	120	113	128	151
South Carolina	26	46	74	138	158	129	150	182
Virginia	42	68	103	135	143	142	163	195
West Virginia	36	64	91	120	135	131	157	218
East South Central	37	56	98	122	138	122	147	188
Alabama	33	38	73	106	123	108	134	172
Kentucky	36	58	114	117	131	123	147	182
Mississippi	45	105	124	157	174	136	150	192
Tennessee	41	70	99	125	142	132	155	205
West South Central	45	94	159	228	257	210	260	323
Arkansas	44	84	163	222	238	181	228	258
Louisiana	43	83	231	353	408	330	363	477
Oklahoma	60	145	176	296	328	286	315	353
Texas	43	78	117	167	197	181	229	288
Mountain	38	64	126	158	190	176	214	265
Arizona	41	71	130	172	183	178	225	279
Colorado	42	73	143	182	234	206	246	306
Idaho	27	46	83	120	136	129	146	186

[Continued]

★512★

Skilled Nursing Facility Charges Covered by Medicare Through Hospital Insurance: 1975-1991
[Continued]

Census division and state[1]	Skilled nursing facilities							
	1975	1980	1985	1987[2]	1988[2]	1989[2]	1990[2]	1991[2]
Montana	30	44	87	104	117	104	120	143
Nevada	37	66	132	159	166	164	221	276
New Mexico	57	122	122	202	240	233	260	293
Utah	36	75	128	162	209	216	257	288
Wyoming	36	49	121	136	164	165	199	270
Pacific	45	81	142	194	215	204	253	329
Alaska	68	115	130	270	271	266	272	335
California	46	87	150	202	225	215	269	355
Hawaii	49	83	152	161	184	168	196	260
Oregon	40	63	119	151	166	164	197	240
Washington	34	62	111	144	158	153	186	228
Outlying areas	51	96	92	160	176	161	200	237
Puerto Rico	51	97	101	115	126	164	189	220
Virgin Islands	43	104	82	214	236	161	214	299
Other	52	79	94	151	165	157	195	192

Source: U.S. Department of Health and Human Services. Social Security Administration (SSA). *Annual Statistical Supplement to the "Social Security Bulletin," 1992.* SSA Publication No. 13-11700. Washington, DC: U.S. Department of Health and Human Services, Social Security Administration, Office of Research and Statistics, 1993, p. 302.

Medicare: Providers

★513★

Doctor Participation in Medicare

The table below reflects the percent of total medical doctors (MDs) and osteopaths (DOs), as well as limited-license practitioners, who participate in Medicare. Approximately 60 percent of all doctors participate. Data are provided by selected states representing the high and low percentages of participation.

State	Percent
Alabama	85.1
Nevada	84.9
Rhode Island	80.9
Utah	80.3
Minnesota	44.4
Louisiana	44.0
New Hampshire	43.0

[Continued]

★ 513 ★

Doctor Participation in Medicare
[Continued]

State	Percent
New York	40.7
Idaho	37.1
South Dakota	31.6

Source: "More Doctors Sign Up to Participate in Medicare." *American Medical News,* 23-30 August 1993, p. 5.

★ 514 ★

Medicare: Providers

Health Agencies Participating in Medicare: 1967-1991

The table below indicates the number of health care agencies and organizations that participate in Medicare programs. Data are provided by type of facility.

Year	Hospitals			Skilled nursing facilities	Home health agencies	Independent laboratories
	All hospitals	General[1]	Psychiatric			
Facilities						
1967	6,829	6,501	328	4,405	1,890	2,355
1968	6,831	6,492	339	4,787	2,173	2,645
1969	6,791	6,447	344	4,786	2,311	2,676
1970	6,779	6,444	335	4,494	2,333	2,750
1971	6,741	6,401	340	4,084	2,256	2,808
1972	6,744	6,392	352	3,981	2,212	2,906
1973	6,746	6,388	358	3,981	2,222	2,901
1974	6,707	6,349	358	3,892	2,254	2,991
1975	6,770	6,383	387	3,932	2,290	3,174
1976	6,774	6,368	406	3,992	2,353	3,156
1977	6,755	6,353	402	4,461	2,496	3,249
1978	6,848	6,432	416	4,982	2,715	3,384
1979	6,780	6,372	408	5,055	2,858	3,448
1980	6,736	6,325	411	5,155	3,012	3,374
1981	6,749	6,335	414	5,295	3,169	3,511
1982	6,737	6,321	416	5,510	3,627	3,643
1983	6,687	6,257	430	5,760	4,235	3,708
1984	6,676	6,228	448	6,183	5,237	3,890
1985	6,710	6,209	501	6,725	5,932	4,029
1986	6,731	6,189	542	7,148	5,953	4,298
1987	6,715	6,130	585	7,379	5,769	4,487
1988	6,658	6,044	614	7,683	5,673	4,676
1989	6,547	5,891	656	8,688	5,661	4,828

[Continued]

★514★

Health Agencies Participating in Medicare: 1967-1991
[Continued]

Year	Hospitals			Skilled nursing facilities	Home health agencies	Independent laboratories
	All hospitals	General[1]	Psychiatric			
1990	6,522	5,848	674	9,008	5,730	4,881
1991	6,471	5,759	712	10,061	5,963	4,898

Beds

Year	All hospitals	General[1]	Psychiatric	Skilled nursing facilities	Home health agencies	Independent laboratories
1967	1,141,155	837,211	303,944	308,843	...	...
1968	1,166,173	852,643	313,530	337,937	...	...
1969	1,182,843	863,876	318,967	360,049	...	...
1970	1,190,309	878,509	311,800	325,415	...	...
1971	1,172,353	888,205	284,148	296,090	...	...
1972	1,155,270	906,280	248,990	287,533	...	...
1973	1,147,501	919,832	227,669	290,060	...	...
1974	1,132,435	925,772	206,663	289,416	...	...
1975	1,136,908	939,717	197,191	287,468	...	...
1976	1,169,433	980,805	188,628	332,515	...	...
1977	1,130,519	976,465	154,054	381,715	...	...
1978	1,154,250	1,015,645	138,605	414,188	...	...
1979	1,152,088	1,016,525	135,563	433,715	...	...
1980	1,145,245	1,017,794	127,451	448,007	...	...
1981	1,152,877	1,032,042	120,835	463,715	...	...
1982	1,146,480	1,044,427	102,053	497,056	...	...
1983	1,143,544	1,046,674	96,870	519,551	...	...
1984	1,146,093	1,050,832	95,261	548,201	...	...
1985	1,144,589	1,046,889	97,700	[2]	...	...
1986	1,137,853	1,043,430	94,423	444,326	...	...
1987	1,124,928	1,030,556	94,372	449,867	...	...
1988	1,115,809	1,022,116	93,693	476,447	...	...
1989	1,106,295	1,008,845	97,450	507,475	...	...
1990	1,104,703	1,005,480	99,223	512,107	...	...
1991	1,102,286	1,003,147	99,139	583,116	...	...

Source: U.S. Department of Health and Human Services. Social Security Administration (SSA). *Annual Statistical Supplement to the "Social Security Bulletin," 1992.* SSA Publication No. 13-11700. Washington, DC: U.S. Department of Health and Human Services, Social Security Administration, Office of Research and Statistics, 1993, p. 305. *Notes:* Three dots (...) stands for not applicable. 1. Includes short-stay and other long-stay hospitals. 2. Data not available.

★ 515 ★

Medicare: Providers

Hospitals Participating in Medicare's Hospital Insurance Program: 1991

Table indicates the number of hospitals and the number of hospital beds per 1,000 Medicare enrollees. Facilities included are participants in Medicare's Hospital Insurance (HI) program. Data are provided by state.

Census division and state	All hospitals		Short stay			Long stay	
	Hospitals	Beds	Hospitals	Beds	Beds per 1,000 enrollees[1]	Hospitals	Beds
Total	6,471	1,102,286	5,450	965,357	31.1	1,021	136,929
United States	6,411	1,091,206	5,393	954,962	31.4	1,018	136,244
New England	299	57,272	226	45,215	25.9	73	12,057
Connecticut	52	14,429	35	11,131	25.4	17	3,298
Maine	42	4,593	39	4,390	26.6	3	203
Massachusetts	141	28,099	99	21,186	26.5	42	6,913
New Hampshire	31	3,758	26	3,168	24.7	5	590
Rhode Island	16	4,220	12	3,341	23.0	4	879
Vermont	17	2,173	15	1,999	29.3	2	174
Middle Atlantic	678	177,901	554	142,081	28.1	124	35,820
New Jersey	115	35,242	91	30,332	30.3	24	4,910
New York	289	91,997	244	69,904	31.4	45	22,093
Pennsylvania	274	50,662	219	41,845	23.0	55	8,817
East North Central	947	194,821	814	178,812	34.0	133	16,009
Illinois	232	52,827	206	49,871	35.7	26	2,956
Indiana	153	28,638	116	25,904	37.3	37	2,734
Michigan	194	35,944	175	33,203	29.9	19	2,741
Ohio	219	55,485	188	50,187	36.0	31	5,298
Wisconsin	149	21,927	129	19,647	29.9	20	2,280
West North Central	805	92,710	739	84,383	34.7	66	8,327
Iowa	127	14,220	123	13,530	31.9	4	690
Kansas	146	13,854	131	12,096	35.7	15	1,758
Minnesota	161	19,649	151	17,509	31.9	10	2,140
Missouri	156	28,734	132	26,419	37.3	24	2,315
Nebraska	100	8,289	92	7,432	33.5	8	857
North Dakota	54	4,355	51	3,925	43.0	3	430
South Dakota	61	3,609	59	3,472	33.9	2	137
South Atlantic	996	189,640	807	166,168	29.6	189	23,472
Delaware	11	2,479	7	2,174	26.7	4	305
District of Columbia	14	5,043	10	3,946	59.3	4	1,097
Florida	286	59,350	219	53,925	24.3	67	5,425
Georgia	192	28,808	162	25,265	39.1	30	3,543
Maryland	69	18,201	51	13,621	27.5	18	4,580
North Carolina	149	27,902	129	24,282	30.5	20	3,620
South Carolina	83	13,690	70	11,944	31.0	13	1,746
Virginia	122	23,914	99	21,418	33.1	23	2,496
West Virginia	70	10,253	60	9,593	36.0	10	660

[Continued]

★ 515 ★

Hospitals Participating in Medicare's Hospital Insurance Program: 1991
[Continued]

Census division and state	All hospitals		Short stay			Long stay	
	Hospitals	Beds	Hospitals	Beds	Beds per 1,000 enrollees[1]	Hospitals	Beds
East South Central	519	80,843	461	75,340	39.9	58	5,503
Alabama	128	21,074	115	20,015	39.6	13	1,059
Kentucky	121	18,310	104	16,352	36.0	17	1,958
Mississippi	111	13,146	105	12,683	40.6	6	463
Tennessee	159	28,313	137	26,290	42.7	22	2,023
West South Central	939	122,728	760	107,608	37.2	179	15,120
Arkansas	101	12,995	84	11,222	32.4	17	1,773
Louisiana	178	25,615	141	21,945	48.1	37	3,670
Oklahoma	147	16,845	126	15,120	36.4	21	1,725
Texas	513	67,273	409	59,321	35.4	104	7,952
Mountain	460	50,742	373	41,980	27.6	87	8,762
Arizona	90	12,722	69	10,864	23.3	21	1,858
Colorado	88	14,529	66	10,615	32.4	22	3,914
Idaho	51	3,177	44	2,814	22.7	7	363
Montana	61	3,378	57	3,208	29.9	4	170
Nevada	30	3,754	25	3,307	24.3	5	447
New Mexico	57	5,597	45	4,918	30.5	12	679
Utah	51	5,682	40	4,492	29.9	11	1,190
Wyoming	32	1,903	27	1,762	36.2	5	141
Pacific	768	124,549	659	113,375	28.1	109	11,174
Alaska	25	1,646	22	1,392	60.5	3	254
California	544	96,718	453	88,454	30.2	91	8,264
Hawaii	26	2,745	22	2,344	19.7	4	401
Oregon	71	8,622	66	8,184	20.7	5	438
Washington	102	14,818	96	13,001	22.9	6	1,817
Outlying areas	60	11,080	57	10,395	29.7	3	685
Puerto Rico	56	10,581	53	9,896	28.8	3	685
Virgin Islands	1	160	1	160	24.4	...	...
Other	3	339	3	339	1.5	...	...

Source: U.S. Department of Health and Human Services. Social Security Administration (SSA). *Annual Statistical Supplement to the "Social Security Bulletin,"* 1992. SSA Publication No. 13-11700. Washington, DC: U.S. Department of Health and Human Services, Social Security Administration, Office of Research and Statistics, 1993, p. 306. *Notes:* Three dots (...) means not applicable. 1. Based on number of persons aged 65 or older enrolled in the Hospital Insurance program as of July 1, 1991.

★516★

Medicare: Providers

Medicare Hospital Utilization and Hospital and Physician Charges: 1970-1991

Data reflect date expense was incurred based on bills submitted for payment and recorded in Health Care Financing Administration central records through May 1992. Includes Puerto Rico, Virgin Islands, Guam, other outlying areas, and enrollees in foreign countries.

Item	Unit	Persons 65 years old and older					Disabled persons[1]				
		1970	1980	1985	1990	1991	1975	1980	1985	1990	1991
Hospital inpatient care:											
Admissions[2]	1,000	6,141	9,258	9,751	9,216	9,653	822	1,271	1,319	1,257	1,316
Per 1,000 enrollees[3]	Rate	302	369	352	303	311	379	429	454	386	389
Covered days of care	Millions	79	98	80	82	83	9	13	11	11	12
Per 1,000 enrollees[3]	Rate	3,902	3,885	2,882	2,702	2,674	4,198	4,549	3,739	3,464	3,545
Per admission	Days	12.9	10.5	8.2	8.9	10.0	11.1	10.6	8.2	8.8	9.1
Hospital covered charges	Million $	5,968	28,615	49,236	90,846	105,596	1,371	4,087	6,582	11,910	14,114
Per covered day	$	75	293	617	1,104	1,272	151	303	606	1,057	1,176
Percent of covered charges reimbursed[4]	Percent	78.0	70.0	65.6	47.5	46.0	73.6	68.6	64.4	46.5	44.7
Physician allowed charges	Million $	2,310	9,011	17,743	30,447	32,138	367	1,112	1,823	2,907	3,065
Percent reimbursed	Percent	71.9	78.0	78.8	76.9	76.7	76.1	78.7	78.7	75.7	75.9

Source: *1993 Statistical Abstract of the United States on CD-ROM* [machine-readable datafiles]. CD-ABSTR-93. Washington, DC: U.S. Department of Commerce, Economics and Statistics Administration, Bureau of the Census, Data User Services Division, 1993. Primary source: U.S. Health Care Financing Administration, unpublished data. *Notes:* 1. Disabled persons under age 65 and persons enrolled solely because of end-stage renal disease. 2. Beginning 1990, represents number of discharges and includes pass-through amounts, except for kidney acquisition. 3. Based on Hospital Insurance (HI) enrollment as of July 1. 4. Billing reimbursements exclude: (1) Prospective Payment System (PPS) pass-through amounts for capital, direct medical education, kidney acquisitions, and bad debts by Medicare patients; (2) certain lump-sum interim payments; and (3) retroactive adjustments resulting from end-of-fiscal year cost reports.

★517★

Medicare: Providers

Skilled Nursing and Other Health Care Facilities Participating in Medicare: 1991

Data show the number of skilled nursing facilities, home health agencies, independent laboratories, and end-stage renal disease facilities that participate in Medicare Hospital Insurance (HI) and Supplementary Medical Insurance (SMI) programs. Data are provided by state.

Census division and state	Skilled-nursing facilities			Home health agencies	Independent laboratories	End-stage renal disease facilities
	Number	Beds	Beds per 1,000 enrollees[1]			
Total	10,061	583,116	18.8	5,963	4,898	2,211
United States	10,054	582,790	19.1	5,919	4,622	2,187
New England	728	47,411	27.2	338	341	80
Connecticut	211	21,013	48.0	101	91	20
Maine	34	1,076	6.5	22	19	6

[Continued]

★517★

Skilled Nursing and Other Health Care Facilities Participating in Medicare: 1991
[Continued]

Census division and state	Skilled-nursing facilities			Home health agencies	Inde-pendent labor-atories	End-stage renal disease facilities
	Number	Beds	Beds per 1,000 enrollees[1]			
Massachusetts	354	19,991	25.0	152	162	40
New Hampshire	18	394	3.1	36	20	6
Rhode Island	86	3,775	25.9	14	46	6
Vermont	25	1,162	17.0	13	3	2
Middle Atlantic	1,434	163,220	32.3	510	633	274
New Jersey	219	19,303	19.3	56	100	37
New York	588	99,870	44.8	202	256	116
Pennsylvania	627	44,047	24.2	252	277	121
East North Central	1,827	95,840	18.2	955	557	271
Illinois	420	10,843	7.8	255	161	92
Indiana	289	9,154	13.2	142	69	38
Michigan	329	21,111	19.0	158	126	53
Ohio	579	42,692	30.6	247	148	53
Wisconsin	210	12,040	18.3	153	53	35
West North Central	1,052	57,718	23.7	757	262	152
Iowa	63	1,679	4.0	153	29	16
Kansas	90	1,740	5.1	126	58	18
Minnesota	424	38,151	69.5	194	33	34
Missouri	300	6,688	9.5	187	86	54
Nebraska	58	1,816	8.2	49	24	13
North Dakota	82	6,883	75.4	29	19	10
South Dakota	35	761	7.4	19	13	7
South Atlantic	1,655	79,269	14.1	846	713	515
Delaware	33	2,243	27.6	18	22	7
District of Columbia	11	508	7.6	14	12	21
Florida	523	20,864	9.4	254	278	152
Georgia	215	6,771	10.5	78	104	81
Maryland	168	15,062	30.4	75	110	53
North Carolina	326	14,366	18.1	132	70	65
South Carolina	150	11,469	29.8	55	26	46
Virginia	164	4,521	7.0	161	58	75
West Virginia	65	3,465	13.0	59	33	15
East South Central	630	28,546	15.1	556	340	168
Alabama	211	9,838	19.5	126	98	42
Kentucky	216	9,799	21.6	103	89	28
Mississippi	49	1,388	4.4	79	51	33
Tennessee	154	7,521	12.2	248	102	65

[Continued]

★517★

Skilled Nursing and Other Health Care Facilities Participating in Medicare: 1991

[Continued]

Census division and state	Skilled-nursing facilities			Home health agencies	Independent laboratories	End-stage renal disease facilities
	Number	Beds	Beds per 1,000 enrollees[1]			
West South Central	631	18,485	6.4	1,002	520	298
Arkansas	66	2,136	6.2	176	40	37
Louisiana	75	3,688	8.1	229	89	73
Oklahoma	39	699	1.7	92	53	34
Texas	451	11,962	7.1	505	338	154
Mountain	599	23,382	15.4	412	240	121
Arizona	131	3,078	6.6	63	65	45
Colorado	151	3,700	11.3	118	62	19
Idaho	71	2,143	17.3	32	19	7
Montana	92	3,968	37.0	44	11	7
Nevada	35	3,554	26.1	24	26	6
New Mexico	29	569	3.5	56	25	19
Utah	63	5,497	36.6	41	19	16
Wyoming	27	873	17.9	34	13	2
Pacific	1,498	68,919	17.1	543	1,016	308
Alaska	7	235	10.2	9	7	2
California	1,147	59,788	20.4	395	835	254
Hawaii	31	1,937	16.3	23	30	12
Oregon	110	2,044	5.2	61	51	16
Washington	203	4,915	8.7	55	93	24
Outlying areas	7	326	.9	44	276	24
Puerto Rico	6	290	.8	42	270	21
Virgin Islands	...	...	...	1	...	...
Other	1	36	51.1	1	6	3

Source: U.S. Department of Health and Human Services. Social Security Administration (SSA). *Annual Statistical Supplement to the "Social Security Bulletin," 1992.* SSA Publication No. 13-11700. Washington, DC: U.S. Department of Health and Human Services, Social Security Administration, Office of Research and Statistics, 1993, p. 307. *Notes:* Three dots (...) means not applicable. 1. Based on number of persons aged 65 or older enrolled in the Hospital Insurance program as of July 1, 1991.

Medicare: Spending

★518★

Medicare Administrative Costs: 1991

The table below indicates the administrative costs associated with Medicare Hospital Insurance (HI; Part A) and Supplementary Medical Insurance (SMI; Part B) programs. Data provided for 1991.

Program	Number
Hospital Insurance	$1.0 billion
As a percent of total benefits paid	1.4 percent
Supplementary Medical Insurance	$1.5 billion
As a percent of total benefits paid	3.3 percent

Source: U.S. Department of Health and Human Services. Social Security Administration (SSA). *Annual Statistical Supplement to the "Social Security Bulletin," 1992.* SSA Publication No. 13-11700. Washington, DC: U.S. Department of Health and Human Services, Social Security Administration, Office of Research and Statistics, 1993, p. 3.

★519★

Medicare: Spending

Percent of Federal Budget Spent on Medicare Programs: 1980-1997

	1980	1985	1990	1991	1992	1993	1994	1995	1996	1997
Total Social Security and Medicare	25.5	27.1	28.3	28.8	28.4	29.4	31.2	33.2	34.5	34.4
Medicare	5.8	7.4	8.5	8.6	8.8	9.5	10.4	11.5	12.4	12.7

Source: "Entitlements for the Retired Take Ever More Money." *New York Times*, 30 August 1992, p. 4E. Primary source: Congressional Budget Office. *Note:* Numbers may not add due to rounding.

★ 520 ★

Medicare: Spending

Projected Percent Increase in Spending on Medicare: 1992-1997

Data below indicate the anticipated percent increases in spending for Medicare for each fiscal year.

Year	Increase
1992	12.3
1993	10.9
1994	11.3
1995	11.4
1996	11.4
1997	11.2

Source: "Entitlements for the Retired Take Ever More Money." *New York Times,* 30 August 1992, p. 4E. Primary source: Social Security Administration.

Social Security: Benefits and Beneficiaries

★ 521 ★

Social Security Annual Payments and Average Monthly Benefits: 1970-1991

Based on average monthly benefit as of December.

Year, division, state, and other area	Annual Payments (1,000)				Average monthly benefit (in dollars)		
	Total	Retired workers and dependents[1]	Survivors[2]	Disabled workers and dependents	Retired workers[0]	Disabled workers	Widows and widowers[4]
1970	31,863	21,076	7,721	3,067	118	131	102
1980	120,472	78,025	27,010	15,437	341	371	311
1983	167,033	114,133	35,369	17,530	441	456	396
1984	175,762	121,023	36,839	17,900	461	471	415
1985	186,195	128,536	38,824	18,836	479	484	433
1986	196,692	135,949	40,896	19,847	489	488	444
1987	204,156	141,329	42,315	20,512	513	508	468
1988	217,214	150,526	44,996	21,692	537	530	493
1989	230,850	160,352	47,625	22,873	567	556	522
1990	247,796	172,042	50,951	24,803	603	587	557
1991, total	268,098	185,545	54,891	27,662	629	609	584
United States	264,049	183,287	53,806	26,956	(NA)	(NA)	(NA)
New England	14,955	10,933	2,701	1,321	(NA)	(NA)	(NA)
Maine	1,345	932	265	148	578	556	551
New Hampshire	1,127	830	199	98	632	605	605
Vermont	586	407	117	62	617	594	585

[Continued]

★521★

Social Security Annual Payments and Average Monthly Benefits: 1970-1991
[Continued]

Year, division, state, and other area	Annual Payments (1,000)				Average monthly benefit (in dollars)		
	Total	Retired workers and dependents[1]	Survivors[2]	Disabled workers and dependents	Retired workers[3]	Disabled workers	Widows and widowers[4]
Massachusetts	6,719	4,851	1,246	622	632	595	614
Rhode Island	1,240	920	210	110	629	580	607
Connecticut	3,938	2,993	664	281	691	613	651
Middle Atlantic	45,320	32,453	8,873	3,994	(NA)	(NA)	(NA)
New York	20,451	14,648	3,828	1,975	673	636	627
New Jersey	9,125	6,706	1,677	742	689	634	642
Pennsylvania	15,744	11,099	3,368	1,277	648	630	615
East North Central	48,096	33,051	10,253	4,792	(NA)	(NA)	(NA)
Ohio	12,501	8,340	2,872	1,289	645	635	613
Indiana	6,387	4,397	1,335	655	655	631	618
Illinois	12,591	8,837	2,622	1,132	668	633	630
Michigan	10,793	7,317	2,297	1,179	672	669	628
Wisconsin	5,824	4,160	1,127	537	646	615	614
West North Central	20,052	14,136	4,171	1,745	(NA)	(NA)	(NA)
Minnesota	4,424	3,172	908	344	614	596	584
Iowa	3,522	2,505	734	283	631	604	595
Missouri	6,012	4,117	1,244	651	615	597	577
North Dakota	698	485	159	54	593	576	550
South Dakota	794	551	175	68	582	550	547
Nebraska	1,786	1,274	377	135	621	591	599
Kansas	2,816	2,032	574	210	645	591	607
South Atlantic	47,205	32,707	9,300	5,198	(NA)	(NA)	(NA)
Delaware	756	538	145	73	656	625	614
Maryland	4,204	2,933	894	377	628	626	594
District of Columbia	456	312	99	45	537	546	495
Virginia	5,387	3,607	1,149	631	595	596	542
West Virginia	2,409	1,422	616	371	622	654	554
North Carolina	6,858	4,599	1,361	898	588	573	512
South Carolina	3,415	2,245	678	492	588	583	506
Georgia	5,550	3,519	1,215	816	587	582	519
Florida	18,170	13,532	3,143	1,495	628	620	602
East South Central	16,086	9,973	3,728	2,385	(NA)	(NA)	(NA)
Kentucky	3,963	2,365	951	647	579	605	520
Tennessee	5,189	3,343	1,143	703	588	577	524
Alabama	4,357	2,706	1,046	605	581	582	512
Mississippi	2,577	1,559	588	430	546	560	471
West South Central	24,389	15,815	5,864	2,710	(NA)	(NA)	(NA)
Arkansas	2,791	1,784	604	403	565	576	502
Louisiana	3,989	2,304	1,085	600	584	617	535
Oklahoma	3,410	2,312	761	337	600	592	555
Texas	14,199	9,415	3,414	1,370	610	600	564
Mountain	13,090	9,203	2,485	1,402	(NA)	(NA)	(NA)
Montana	915	617	185	113	611	623	589

[Continued]

★ 521 ★

Social Security Annual Payments and Average Monthly Benefits: 1970-1991

[Continued]

Year, division, state, and other area	Annual Payments (1,000)				Average monthly benefit (in dollars)		
	Total	Retired workers and dependents[1]	Survivors[2]	Disabled workers and dependents	Retired workers[3]	Disabled workers	Widows and widowers[4]
Idaho	1,035	733	202	100	611	612	586
Wyoming	426	299	86	41	628	613	599
Colorado	2,803	1,915	571	317	613	603	587
New Mexico	1,364	907	292	165	592	595	546
Arizona	4,066	2,939	702	425	637	641	607
Utah	1,288	924	248	116	635	595	613
Nevada	1,193	869	199	125	631	643	609
Pacific	34,856	25,016	6,431	3,409	(NA)	(NA)	(NA)
Washington	5,021	3,638	906	477	653	624	619
Oregon	3,437	2,530	610	297	641	618	611
California	25,200	17,948	4,713	2,539	643	611	609
Alaska	227	147	52	28	626	607	556
Hawaii	971	753	150	68	619	602	559
Puerto Rico	2,335	1,203	526	606	402	502	362
Guam	24	12	9	3	450	482	424
American Samoa	13	5	5	3	393	442	324
Virgin Islands	52	33	13	6	531	569	492
Abroad	1,625	1,005	534	85	448	535	448

Source: 1993 Statistical Abstract of the United States on CD-ROM [machine-readable datafiles]. CD-ABSTR-93. Washington, DC: U.S. Department of Commerce, Economics and Statistics Administration, Bureau of the Census, Data User Services Division, 1993. Primary source: U.S. Social Security Administration. *Social Security Bulletin* (quarterly). *Notes:* "NA" represents "not available." "Z" represents less than 500. 1. Includes special benefits. 2. Includes lump-sum payments to survivors of deceased workers. 3. Excludes persons with special benefits. 4. Nondisabled only.

★ 522 ★

Social Security: Benefits and Beneficiaries

Social Security Beneficiaries: 1970-1991

Number of beneficiaries in current-payment status as of December.

Year, division, state, and other area	Beneficiaries (1,000)[1]			
	Total	Retired workers and dependents[2]	Survivors	Disabled workers and dependents
1970	26,229	17,093	6,470	2,665
1980	35,585	23,309	7,598	4,678
1983	36,085	25,021	7,251	3,813
1984	36,479	25,474	7,182	3,822
1985	37,058	25,989	7,162	3,907
1986	37,703	26,541	7,166	3,995
1987	38,190	26,988	7,157	4,045

[Continued]

★ 522 ★

Social Security Beneficiaries: 1970-1991
[Continued]

Year, division, state, and other area	Beneficiaries (1,000)[1]			
	Total	Retired workers and dependents[2]	Survivors	Disabled workers and dependents
1988	38,627	27,390	7,163	4,074
1989	39,151	27,853	7,170	4,129
1990	39,832	28,367	7,197	4,266
1991, total	40,568	28,812	7,246	4,515
United States	39,621	28,241	7,028	4,352
New England	2,182	1,633	335	213
Maine	218	156	36	26
New Hampshire	167	126	25	16
Vermont	90	64	15	10
Massachusetts	989	735	154	100
Rhode Island	184	139	27	18
Connecticut	534	413	78	43
Middle Atlantic	6,375	4,687	1,088	600
New York	2,868	2,094	476	298
New Jersey	1,242	933	200	109
Pennsylvania	2,265	1,660	412	193
East North Central	6,883	4,889	1,256	737
Ohio	1,827	1,271	356	200
Indiana	919	652	164	103
Illinois	1,772	1,279	319	174
Michigan	1,515	1,062	278	174
Wisconsin	850	625	139	86
West North Central	3,054	2,228	537	289
Minnesota	677	505	116	56
Iowa	527	389	92	46
Missouri	922	651	164	107
North Dakota	112	82	21	9
South Dakota	130	93	24	13
Nebraska	272	201	48	23
Kansas	414	307	72	35
South Atlantic	7,343	5,214	1,280	852
Delaware	108	79	18	11
Maryland	625	452	116	57
District of Columbia	78	56	16	7
Virginia	857	593	159	105
West Virginia	373	230	82	61
North Carolina	1,111	758	201	152
South Carolina	558	371	104	84
Georgia	905	583	181	141
Florida	2,728	2,092	403	234
East South Central	2,685	1,706	555	424
Kentucky	658	407	139	113
Tennessee	846	557	165	123

[Continued]

★ 522 ★

Social Security Beneficiaries: 1970-1991
[Continued]

Year, division, state, and other area	Beneficiaries (1,000)[1]			
	Total	Retired workers and dependents[2]	Survivors	Disabled workers and dependents
Alabama	722	460	155	107
Mississippi	459	282	96	81
West South Central	3,924	2,625	824	474
Arkansas	473	311	91	72
Louisiana	663	397	157	108
Oklahoma	539	379	104	56
Texas	2,249	1,538	472	238
Mountain	2,013	1,456	329	229
Montana	142	99	24	19
Idaho	161	118	27	17
Wyoming	64	46	11	7
Colorado	434	308	75	52
New Mexico	227	154	43	30
Arizona	609	453	91	65
Utah	198	144	33	21
Nevada	178	134	25	18
Pacific	5,161	3,805	822	534
Washington	728	543	112	74
Oregon	509	385	76	47
California	3,738	2,735	606	397
Alaska	35	23	7	5
Hawaii	151	119	21	11
Puerto Rico	570	316	115	139
Guam	6	3	2	1
American Samoa	4	2	2	1
Virgin Islands	10	6	3	1
Abroad	361	244	96	21

Source: 1993 Statistical Abstract of the United States on CD-ROM [machine-readable datafiles]. CD-ABSTR-93. Washington, DC: U.S. Department of Commerce, Economics and Statistics Administration, Bureau of the Census, Data User Services Division, 1993. Primary source: U.S. Social Security Administration. *Social Security Bulletin* (quarterly). *Notes:* "NA" represents "not available." "Z" represents less than 500. 1. Data for 1991 based on 10-percent sample. 2. Includes special benefits.

★ 523 ★

Social Security: Benefits and Beneficiaries

Social Security Trends and Projections

The table below reflects past numbers and projections of workers covered by and beneficiaries of Social Security.

Year	Covered workers (in millions)	Beneficiaries (in millions)	Covered workers per OASI[1] beneficiary
1950	48.3	2.9	16.5
1970	93.1	22.6	4.1
1980	112.2	30.4	3.7
1990	133.5	35.3	3.8
2000			
Optimisitic projection	149.2	38.6	3.9
Intermediate projection	145.2	39.1	3.7
Pessimistic projection	141.6	39.6	3.6
2030			
Optimisitic projection	143.2	67.1	2.1
Intermediate projection	140.4	69.6	2.0
Pessimistic projection	135.8	72.6	1.9
2060			
Optimisitic projection	151.7	75.9	2.0
Intermediate projection	146.9	79.3	1.9
Pessimistic projection	142.8	86.5	1.7

Source: "Will Social Security Be There When You Need It?" *LAN* (August 1992), p. 34. Primary sources: U.S. Department of Health and Human Services, Social Security Administration; Employee Benefit Research Institute. *Note:* 1. Old-Age and Survivors Insurance.

Social Security: Programs

★ 524 ★

OASDI Administrative Costs: 1991

Data provide Old-Age, Survivors, and Disability Insurance (OASDI) administrative costs for 1991.

[In dollars, except as noted]

Program	Cost
Old-Age and Survivors Insurance	1.8 billion
As a percent of total benefits paid	.7%
Disability Insurance	794 million
As a percent of total benefits paid	2.9%

Source: U.S. Department of Health and Human Services. Social Security Administration (SSA). *Annual Statistical Supplement to the "Social Security Bulletin," 1992.* SSA Publication No. 13-11700. Washington, DC: U.S. Department of Health and Human Services, Social Security Administration, Office of Research and Statistics, 1993, p. 2.

★ 525 ★

Social Security: Programs

OASDI Benefits: 1970-1991

The table below reflects the types of beneficiaries of Old-Age, Survivors, and Disability Insurance (OASDI). A person eligible to receive more than one type of benefit is generally classified or counted only once as a retired-worker beneficiary.

Type of beneficiary	1970	1980	1985	1990	1991
Benefits in current-payment status (end of year)[1]					
Number of benefits (1,000)	26,229	35,585	37,058	39,832	40,592
Retired workers (1,000)[2]	13,349	19,562	22,432	24,838	25,289
Disabled workers (1,000)[3]	1,493	2,859	2,657	3,011	3,195
Wives and husbands[4] (1,000)[2]	2,952	3,477	3,375	3,367	3,370
Children (1,000)	4,122	4,607	3,319	3,187	3,268
Under age 18	3,315	3,423	2,699	2,497	2,558
Disabled children[5]	271	450	526	600	616
Students[6]	537	733	94	89	95
Of retired workers	546	639	457	422	426
Of deceased workers	2,688	2,610	1,917	1,776	1,791
Of disabled workers	889	1,358	945	989	1,052
Widowed mothers (1,000)[7]	523	562	372	304	301
Widows and widowers[8] (1,000)[2]	3,227	4,411	4,863	5,111	5,158
Parents (1,000)[2]	29	15	10	6	5
Special benefits (1,000)[9]	534	93	32	7	5

[Continued]

★ 525 ★

OASDI Benefits: 1970-1991
[Continued]

Type of beneficiary	1970	1980	1985	1990	1991
Average monthly benefit, current dollars:					
Retired workers[2]	118	341	479	603	629
Retired worker and wife[2]	199	567	814	1,027	1,072
Disabled workers[3]	131	371	484	587	609
Wives and husbands[2][4]	59	164	236	298	311
Children of retired workers	45	140	198	259	273
Children of deceased workers	82	240	330	406	420
Children of disabled workers	39	110	142	164	168
Widowed mothers[7]	87	246	332	409	424
Widows and widowers, nondisabled[2]	102	311	433	557	584
Parents[2]	103	276	378	482	506
Special benefits[9]	45	105	138	167	173
Average monthly benefit, constant (1991) dollars:[10]					
Retired workers[2]	409	545	604	621	629
Retired worker and wife[2]	690	906	1,027	1,058	1,072
Disabled workers[3]	454	593	611	605	609
Wives and husbands[2][4]	204	262	298	307	311
Children of deceased workers	284	383	418	418	420
Widowed mothers[7]	301	393	419	422	424
Widows and widowers, nondisabled[2]	353	497	546	573	584
Number of benefits awarded during year (1,000)					
Total	3,722	4,215	3,796	3,717	3,865
Retired workers[2]	1,338	1,620	1,690	1,665	1,695
Disabled workers[3]	350	389	377	468	536
Wives and husbands[2][4]	436	469	440	379	380
Children	1,091	1,174	714	695	727
Widowed mothers[7]	112	108	72	58	58
Widows and widowers[2][8]	363	452	502	452	469
Parents[2]	2	1	(Z)	(Z)	(Z)
Special benefits[9]	30	1	1	(Z)	(Z)
Benefit payments during year (billion dollars)					
Total amount[11]	31.9	120.5	186.2	247.8	268.1
Monthly benefits[12]	31.6	120.1	186.0	247.6	267.9
Retired workers[2]	18.4	70.4	116.8	156.8	169.1
Disabled workers[3]	2.4	12.8	16.5	22.1	24.7
Wives and husbands[2][4]	2.2	7.0	11.1	14.5	15.5
Children	3.5	10.5	10.7	12.0	12.8
Under age 18	2.7	7.4	8.5	9.0	9.5
Disabled children[5]	0.3	1.0	1.8	2.5	2.8
Students[6]	0.6	2.1	0.4	0.5	0.5

[Continued]

★ 525 ★

OASDI Benefits: 1970-1991
[Continued]

Type of beneficiary	1970	1980	1985	1990	1991
Of retired workers	0.3	1.1	1.1	1.3	1.4
Of deceased workers	2.8	7.4	7.8	8.6	9.0
Of disabled workers	0.5	2.0	1.8	2.2	2.4
Widowed mothers[7]	0.6	1.6	1.5	1.4	1.5
Widows and widowers[2] [8]	4.1	17.6	29.3	40.7	44.1
Parents[2]	(Z)	0.1	0.1	(Z)	(Z)
Special benefits[9]	0.3	0.1	0.1	(Z)	(Z)
Lump sum	0.3	0.4	0.2	0.2	0.2

Source: 1993 Statistical Abstract of the United States on CD-ROM [machine-readable datafiles]. CD-ABSTR-93. Washington, DC: U.S. Department of Commerce, Economics and Statistics Administration, Bureau of the Census, Data User Services Division, 1993. Primary source: U.S. Social Security Administration. *Annual Statistical Supplement to the "Social Security Bulletin";* and unpublished data. *Notes:* Z represents fewer than 500 or less than $50 million. 1. Benefit payment actually being made at a specified time with no deductions or with deductions amounting to less than a month's benefits; i.e., the benefits actually being received. 2. 62 years and over. 3. Disabled workers under age 65. 4. Includes wife beneficiaries with entitled children in their care and entitled divorced wives. 5. 18 years old and over. Disability began before age 18 and, beginning 1973, before age 22. 6. Full-time students aged 18-21 through 1984 and aged 18 and 19 beginning 1985. 7. Includes surviving divorced mothers with entitled children in their care and, beginning 1980, widowed fathers with entitled children in their care. 8. Includes widows aged 60-61, surviving divorced wives aged 60 and over, disabled widows and widowers aged 50 and over; and beginning 1980, widowers aged 60-61. 9. Benefits for persons aged 72 and over not insured under regular or transitional provisions of Social Security Act. 10. Constant dollar figures are based on the consumer price index for December as published by the U.S. Bureau of Labor Statistics. 11. Represents total disbursements of benefit checks by the U.S. Department of the Treasury during the years specified. 12. Distribution by type estimated.

★ 526 ★

Social Security Programs

OASDI Covered Employment

In 1991, there were 132.3 million workers in employment covered by Old-Age, Survivors, and Disability Insurance (OASDI). According to the source, "OASDI benefits increased by a 3.0 percent cost-of-living adjustment effective for December 1992. Amounts fo taxable and creditable earnings increased in 1993 to $57,600 for OASDI and $135,000 for Hospital Insurance (HI). In 1993, the amount of earnings required for a quarter of coverage increased to $590. The retirement test exempt amounts increased to $10,560 for persons aged 65-69 and $7,680 for those under age 65" (p. 2). The table below provides an overview of Old-Age, Survivors, and Disability Insurance (OASDI) as related to earnings.

Earnings	Amounts	
Estimated average earnings, 1991	$21,107	
Earnings required in 1993 for:		
1 quarter of coverage	$590	
Maximum 4 quarters of coverage	$2,360	

[Continued]

★ 526 ★

OASDI Covered Employment
[Continued]

Earnings	Amounts	
Earnings test exempt amounts for 1993:		
Under age 65	$7,680	$640/month
Aged 65-69	$10,560	$880/month

Source: U.S. Department of Health and Human Services. Social Security Administration (SSA). *Annual Statistical Supplement to the "Social Security Bulletin," 1992.* SSA Publication No. 13-11700. Washington, DC: U.S. Department of Health and Human Services, Social Security Administration, Office of Research and Statistics, 1993, p. 2.

★ 527 ★

Social Security: Programs

Social Security Trust Funds: 1970-1991

[In billions of dollars, except percentages]

Type of trust fund	1970	1980	1982	1983	1984	1985	1986	1987	1988	1989	1990	1991
Old-Age and Survivors Insurance												
Net contribution income[1]	30.3	103.5	123.7	138.3	167.0	180.2	194.2	206.0	233.2	252.6	272.4	278.4
Interest received[2]	1.5	1.8	0.8	6.7	2.6	1.9	3.1	4.7	7.6	12.0	16.4	20.8
Benefit payments[3]	28.8	105.1	138.8[4]	149.2	157.8	167.2	176.8	183.6[4]	195.5[4]	208.0	223.0	240.5
Assets, end of year	32.5	22.8	22.1[5]	19.7[5]	27.1[5]	35.8[5]	39.1	62.1	102.9	155.1	214.2	267.8
Reserve ratio (percent)[6]	111	21	16	13	17	21	22	33	52	74	96	111
Disability Insurance												
Net contribution income[1]	4.5	13.3	22.0	18.0	16.1	17.4	18.6	19.7	22.1	24.1	28.7	29.3
Interest received[2]	0.3	0.5	0.5	1.6	1.2	0.9	0.8	0.6	0.6	0.7	0.9	1.1
Benefit payments[3]	3.1	15.5	17.4[4]	17.5	17.9	18.8	19.9	20.5[4]	21.7[4]	22.9	24.8	27.7
Assets, end of year	5.6	3.6	2.7[7]	5.2[7]	4.0[7]	6.3[7]	7.8	6.7	6.9	7.9	11.1	12.9
Reserve ratio (percent)[6]	174	23	15	29	21	33	38	31	31	33	45	47
Hospital Insurance												
Net contribution income[18]	4.9	23.9	34.6	38.2	42.5	47.7	54.7	58.8	62.6	68.5	71.1	78.4
Interest received[2]	0.2	1.1	2.0	2.6	3.0	3.4	3.6	4.5	5.8	7.3	8.5	9.5
Benefit payments	5.1	25.1	35.6	39.3	43.3	47.5	49.8	49.5	52.5	60.0	66.2	71.5
Assets, end of year	3.2	13.7	8.2[9]	12.9[9]	15.7[9]	20.5[9]	40.0	53.7	69.6	85.6	98.9	115.2
Reserve ratio (percent)[6]	61	54	23	32	36	42	79	107	131	141	148	161
Supplementary Medical Insurance												
Net premium income	1.1	3.0	3.7[10]	4.2	5.2	5.6	5.7	7.4	8.8	10.8	11.3	11.9
Transfers from general revenue	1.1	7.5	12.3[10]	14.9	17.1	18.3	17.8	23.6	26.2	30.9	33.0	37.6
Interest received	(Z)	0.4	0.6	0.7	1.0	1.2	1.1	0.9	0.9	1.1	1.6	1.7
Benefit payments	2.0	10.6	15.5	18.1	19.7	22.9	26.2	30.8	34.0	38.4	42.5	47.2

[Continued]

★ 527 ★

Social Security Trust Funds: 1970-1991
[Continued]

Type of trust fund	1970	1980	1982	1983	1984	1985	1986	1987	1988	1989	1990	1991
Assets, end of year	0.2	4.5	6.2	7.1	9.7	10.9	8.3	8.4	9.0	12.2	15.5	17.9
Reserve ratio (percent)[6]	8	40	38	37	47	46	30	26	26	31	35	38

Source: 1993 Statistical Abstract of the United States on CD-ROM [machine-readable datafiles]. CD-ABSTR-93. Washington, DC: U.S. Department of Commerce, Economics and Statistics Administration, Bureau of the Census, Data User Services Division, 1993. Primary source: U.S. Social Security Administration. *Annual Report of Board of Trustees, OASI, DI, HI, and SMI Trust Funds.* Also published in *Social Security Bulletin* (quarterly). *Notes:* "Z" represents less than $500 million. 1. Includes deposits by states and deductions for refund of estimated employee-tax overpayment. Beginning in 1983, includes government contributions on deemed wage credits for military service in 1957 and later. Beginning 1984 includes tax credits on wages paid in 1984 and net earnings from self-employment in 1984-89; and taxation of benefits (Old-Age and Survivors Insurance [OASI] and Disability Insurance [DI], only). 2. Beginning in 1983, includes interest on advance tax transfers and interest on reimbursement for unnegotiated checks. Data for 1983 and 1984 reflect interest on deemed wage credits for military service performed after 1956. Data for 1983-1986 reflect interest on interfund borrowing. 3. Includes payments for vocational rehabilitation services furnished to disabled persons receiving benefits because of their disabilities. Beginning in 1983, amounts reflect deductions for unnegotiated benefit checks. 4. Data adjusted to reflect 12 months of benefit payments. 5. Includes $18 billion borrowed from the Disability Insurance (DI) and Hospital Insurance (HI) Trust Funds. Repayments on Jan. 31, 1985, reduced such amounts to $13.2 billion. 6. Assets at end of year as a percentage of benefit payments and administrative expenses during the year. 7. Excludes $5 billion lent to the Old-Age and Survivors Insurance (OASI) Trust Fund. Repayment on Jan. 31, 1985, reduced the total to $2.5 billion. 8. Beginning in 1980, includes premiums from aged ineligibles enrolled in HI. 9. Excludes $12 billion lent to the OASI Trust Fund. Repayment on January 31, 1985, reduced the total to $10.6 billion. 10. Data adjusted to reflect 12 months of premium and general revenue income.

Social Security: Spending

★ 528 ★

Percent of Federal Budget Spent on Social Security Programs: 1980-1997

	1980	1985	1990	1991	1992	1993	1994	1995	1996	1997
Total Social Security and Medicare	25.5	27.1	28.3	28.8	28.4	29.4	31.2	33.2	34.5	34.4
Social Security	19.8	19.7	19.7	20.2	19.6	19.9	20.8	21.7	22.1	21.7

Source: "Entitlements for the Retired Take Ever More Money." *New York Times*, 30 August 1992, p. 4E. Primary source: Congressional Budget Office. *Note:* Numbers may not add due to rounding.

★ 529 ★

Social Security: Spending

Projected Percent Increase in Spending on Social Security: 1992-1997

Data below indicate the anticipated percent increases in spending for Social Security for each fiscal year.

[In percentages]

Year	Increase
1992	6.7
1993	5.6
1994	5.6
1995	5.7
1996	5.4
1997	5.6

Source: "Entitlements for the Retired Take Ever More Money." *New York Times,* 30 August 1992, p. 4E. Primary source: Social Security Administration.

Social Welfare: Miscellaneous Programs

★ 530 ★

Black Lung Benefit Program Rates: 1994

The Black Lung Benefit Program was instituted in 1969 with the Federal Coal Mine Health and Safety Act. The program offers a monthly benefit payment to miners disabled by black lung (pneumoconiosis) or to their widows and dependents. The table below reflects the monthly benefit rates for the Black Lung Progam, effective January through September 1994.

[In dollars]

Beneficiary	Rate
Miner or widow	427.40
Miner or widow and one dependent	641.10
Miner or widow and two dependents	748.00
Miner or widow and three or more dependents	854.80

Source: U.S. Department of Health and Human Services. Social Security Administration (SSA). "Social Security Programs in the United States, 1993." *Social Security Bulletin* 4, no. 4 (22 December 1993), n.p.

★ 531 ★

Social Welfare: Miscellaneous Programs

Emergency Fund for the Medically Indigent: 1985-1991

The table below presents an overview of the Emergency Fund for the Medically Indigent, Inc. (EFMI) Program. The EFMI is a United Way agency.

Year	Total income ($)	Total patients	Patient cost ($)[1]	Pharmacy patients	Pharmacy cost ($)
1985	2,154.00	114	1,731.00	46	515.68
1986	3,477.28	193	3,008.64	76	1,245.39
1987	4,840.31	253	4,007.17	129	1,944.54
1988	5,571.24	253	4,709.01	151	3,096.36
1989	7,460.04	276	5,812.87	169	3,920.62
1990	7,471.27	379	8,819.61[2]	270	6,877.11
1991	9,309.73	414	10,462.38[2]	290	8,589.38

Source: U.S. Senate Special Committee on Aging. *The Effects of Escalating Drug Costs on the Elderly: Hearing Before the Special Committee on Aging.* 102d Cong., 2nd sess., 22 April 1992. Serial no. 102-21. Washington, DC: U.S. Government Printing Office, 1992, p. 28. Primary source: Emergency Fund for the Medically Indigent, Inc., 141 Lakeshore Circle N.E., Milledgeville, GA 31061. *Notes:* 1. Does not include administrative costs, which are about $150 per year. 2. Deficit covered by money ($2,000) from Governor's Contingency Fund awarded in August 1989.

★ 532 ★

Social Welfare: Miscellaneous Programs

Head Start Programs: 1991

The table below presents data regarding U.S. Department of Health and Human Services allocations for Head Start or for enrollment in Head Start. Data are provided by state or other area for fiscal year 1991.

[In thousands]

State	Head Start allocations (in thousands)	Head Start enrollment[1]
Total	$1,951,775	583,471
Alabama	36,102	12,463
Alaska	3,887	970
Arizona	17,695	5,344
Arkansas	19,778	7,761
California	192,555	49,945
Colorado	17,043	6,124
Connecticut	16,813	5,051
Delaware	3,771	1,199
District of Columbia	9,108	2,560
Florida	58,817	19,034
Georgia	46,208	14,978
Hawaii	6,739	1,846
Idaho	5,834	1,502

[Continued]

★ 532 ★

Head Start Programs: 1991
[Continued]

State	Head Start allocations (in thousands)	Head Start enrollment[1]
Illinois	88,580	27,184
Indiana	27,371	9,543
Iowa	14,563	4,971
Kansas	11,958	4,332
Kentucky	34,165	11,772
Louisiana	42,049	14,558
Maine	8,037	2,928
Maryland	24,435	7,234
Massachusetts	37,634	9,624
Michigan	73,505	24,914
Minnesota	21,155	6,654
Mississippi	66,198	21,511
Missouri	31,661	11,348
Montana	5,366	1,786
Nebraska	8,901	2,820
Nevada	3,566	911
New Hampshire	3,595	945
New Jersey	48,996	11,051
New Mexico	11,960	4,647
New York	137,040	32,492
North Carolina	39,459	13,438
North Dakota	3,501	1,208
Ohio	76,276	27,794
Oklahoma	21,587	8,562
Oregon	15,623	3,634
Pennsylvania	75,220	21,247
Rhode Island	6,152	2,197
South Carolina	24,556	8,544
South Dakota	4,750	1,569
Tennessee	34,272	11,546
Texas	98,971	33,615
Utah	9,295	3,097
Vermont	3,814	1,041
Virginia	28,719	8,345
Washington	24,005	5,923
West Virginia	16,273	5,386
Wisconsin	27,651	9,161
Wyoming	2,777	990
Outlying areas:		
Puerto Rico	83,566	26,875
Pacific territories	5,609	5,176
Virgin Islands	3,814	1,352

[Continued]

★ 532 ★

Head Start Programs: 1991
[Continued]

State	Head Start allocations (in thousands)	Head Start enrollment[1]
Migrant programs[1]	141,140	42,769
Special projects	69,656	-

Source: U.S. Department of Education. Office of Educational Research and Improvement. National Center for Education Statistics. *Digest of Education Statistics, 1992.* Washington, DC: U.S. Government Printing Office, 1992, p. 381. This table was prepared March 1992. Primary source: U.S. Department of Health and Human Services. Office of Development Services. *Notes:* Because of rounding, details may not add to totals. "—" represents "not applicable." 1. The distribution of enrollment by age was: 7 percent were 5 years old and older; 63 percent were 4 years old; 27 percent were 3 years old; and 3 percent were under 3 years old. Handicapped children accounted for 13.1 percent in Head Start programs. The racial/ethnic composition was: 4 percent Native American; 22 percent Hispanic, 38 percent black, 33 percent white, and 3 percent Asian. 2. Includes Native American and migrant programs.

★ 533 ★

Social Welfare: Miscellaneous Programs

Low-Income Home Energy Assistance Program: 1991

During the 1991 fiscal year, states utilized $1.32 billion in Low-Income Home Energy Assistance Program (LIHEAP) funds to assist their residents with heating costs. Approximately 6.1 million households received aid through this program.

Source: U.S. Department of Health and Human Services. Social Security Administration (SSA). *Annual Statistical Supplement to the "Social Security Bulletin," 1992.* SSA Publication No. 13-11700. Washington, DC: U.S. Department of Health and Human Services, Social Security Administration, Office of Research and Statistics, 1993, p. 4.

★ 534 ★

Social Welfare: Miscellaneous Programs

U.S. Food and Drug Administration Inspection Responsibilities

Foods - 46,205

Medical devices - 16,758

Human drugs - 13,899

Animal drugs and feed - 4,772

Conveyances - 4,314

Biologics - 3,816

Radiological health - 3,507

Cosmetics - 1,767

Vitamins - 1,757

Other establishments - 1,488

Color additives - 134

The U.S. Food and Drug Administration (FDA) conducts regular regulatory inspections of certain products, such as drugs amd medical devices. As of February 1992, the FDA's inspection responsibilities encompassed 90,175 establishments. The table below enumerates the enterprises in each area of the FDA's jurisdiction.

Establishments	Number
Animal drugs and feed	4,772
Biologics	3,816
Color additives	134
Conveyances	4,314
Cosmetics	1,767
Foods	46,205
Human drugs	13,899
Medical devices	16,758
Radiological health	3,507
Vitamins	1,757
Other establishments	1,488

Source: "New Unit Fights Crime." *FDA Consumer* (June 1992), p. 18. *Notes:* The sum of all categories is greater than the total because some establishments do business in more than one category. The FDA defines an establishment as a business or other facility under one ownership and at one geographic location or address that processes, manufactures, labels, repacks, stores, distributes, tests, or otherwise manipulates products under the jurisdiction of the FDA. In addition, certain individuals or groups of individuals whose activities fall under the jurisdiction of the FDA are also establishments.

Social Welfare: Nutrition Programs

★ 535 ★

Child Nutrition Program Obligations: 1990-1991

The table below presents data regarding U.S. Department of Agriculture obligations for child nutrition programs. Data are provided by state or other area for fiscal years 1990 and 1991.

[In thousands]

State	Total, fiscal year 1990	Fiscal year 1991								
		Total	Special milk	School lunch[1]	School breakfast	State administrative expenses	Commodities and cash in lieu of commodities[2]	Child and adult care	Summer food service	Nutrition education and training
Alabama	127,348	134,574	40	81,166	14,917	1,390	14,578	17,393	4,973	117
Alaska	13,955	15,364	6	8,976	1,136	311	977	3,897	5	56
Arizona	78,376	87,627	182	53,159	12,403	939	4,205	14,382	2,262	95
Arkansas	68,024	81,293	36	43,908	10,637	817	14,857	9,765	1,206	67
California	640,913	735,286	942	440,400	95,810	6,681	68,088	111,217	11,367	781
Colorado	60,954	66,007	146	34,078	3,526	917	6,959	19,071	1,221	88
Connecticut	43,326	47,403	652	25,505	4,029	582	5,958	8,892	1,704	81
Delaware	13,736	15,107	44	6,232	1,305	308	1,384	4,445	1,333	56
District of Columbia	16,036	17,571	16	10,543	2,293	322	1,969	1,860	512	56
Florida	265,757	300,655	117	181,357	39,437	2,560	29,580	32,409	14,900	295
Georgia	178,800	195,605	47	116,864	25,245	1,859	23,002	22,590	5,815	180
Hawaii	24,623	25,167	8	14,653	2,575	350	3,470	3,682	373	56
Idaho	20,671	22,897	172	15,461	1,214	322	2,608	2,753	311	56
Illinois	214,191	233,472	2,806	143,461	16,752	2,297	26,877	32,484	8,476	319
Indiana	89,596	95,488	356	58,187	5,841	975	14,349	14,261	1,363	156
Iowa	54,141	61,500	250	33,600	3,324	680	12,219	10,451	899	78
Kansas	68,420	64,459	324	30,945	2,064	797	6,701	23,016	545	67
Kentucky	99,820	112,236	274	67,324	18,713	1,068	13,280	9,203	2,270	104
Louisiana	165,161	175,016	78	110,362	22,725	1,817	14,818	19,592	5,485	139
Maine	22,518	24,316	142	12,495	1,680	402	2,161	6,974	405	56
Maryland	73,254	79,204	383	42,426	7,819	892	9,216	16,206	2,143	119
Massachusetts	99,732	117,909	568	47,499	10,394	2,440	26,888	27,719	2,256	145
Michigan	145,538	158,596	1,382	90,945	7,476	1,730	17,471	35,080	4,250	263
Minnesota	101,871	111,601	1,164	45,759	4,682	1,475	12,194	44,526	1,679	121
Mississippi	128,678	134,209	16	79,858	19,173	1,511	11,048	17,691	4,828	83
Missouri	100,148	108,382	591	62,278	10,689	1,134	13,354	17,928	2,270	138
Montana	17,612	19,402	66	10,505	1,046	370	2,077	4,933	349	56
Nebraska	36,388	48,117	245	19,143	1,808	563	12,384	13,517	400	56
Nevada	13,404	15,780	69	9,298	2,128	262	1,788	2,038	142	56
New Hampshire	12,836	12,648	213	7,100	648	273	2,115	2,013	230	56
New Jersey	102,859	118,159	1,039	67,526	6,781	1,476	17,736	18,256	5,152	194
New Mexico	56,148	62,030	19	30,908	5,239	726	5,340	13,866	5,875	56
New York	410,097	449,662	1,610	249,938	49,045	2,864	55,395	55,808	34,537	465
North Carolina	154,372	169,902	138	98,396	25,667	1,604	20,536	19,885	3,505	172
North Dakota	18,237	20,043	71	8,739	680	384	2,243	7,378	492	56
Ohio	186,369	195,296	1,128	113,916	21,121	2,002	24,882	28,389	3,560	299
Oklahoma	78,927	86,035	137	50,344	11,989	946	9,356	12,118	1,057	88
Oregon	44,131	50,017	257	28,896	3,896	633	3,591	11,788	883	74
Pennsylvania	173,400	188,252	792	110,111	13,170	1,845	24,524	26,473	11,033	303
Rhode Island	13,686	14,269	110	8,154	958	275	1,312	2,333	1,072	56
South Carolina	99,085	108,557	26	65,448	15,160	985	10,952	10,251	5,635	99
South Dakota	21,744	23,125	53	12,463	1,966	329	3,753	3,657	847	56
Tennessee	115,115	123,401	35	72,886	19,092	1,217	15,408	12,134	2,498	131
Texas	507,604	558,822	103	334,310	89,071	5,131	50,382	70,190	9,117	519
Utah	44,867	52,847	71	26,599	1,189	585	6,844	16,650	845	64
Vermont	9,151	10,169	186	4,814	507	293	1,170	3,069	73	56
Virginia	101,339	111,147	245	65,355	13,259	767	15,387	13,895	2,082	156

[Continued]

★ 535 ★

Child Nutrition Program Obligations: 1990-1991
[Continued]

State	Total, fiscal year 1990	Fiscal year 1991								
		Total	Special milk	School lunch[1]	School breakfast	State administrative expenses	Commodities and cash in lieu of commodities[2]	Child and adult care	Summer food service	Nutrition education and training
Washington	80,918	93,112	286	48,421	9,097	1,087	8,593	23,965	1,538	127
West Virginia	49,393	55,589	22	30,584	10,743	600	8,152	4,737	694	56
Wisconsin	76,830	82,426	1,907	48,544	3,683	895	11,621	14,339	1,299	138
Wyoming	9,863	11,436	17	5,832	502	290	1,678	2,941	120	56

Source: U.S. Department of Education. Office of Educational Research and Improvement. National Center for Education Statistics. *Digest of Education Statistics, 1992.* Washington, DC: U.S. Government Printing Office, 1992, p. 380. This table was prepared February 1992. Primary source: U.S. Department of Agriculture, Food and Nutrition Service, Budget Division. Unpublished data. *Notes:* Data are based on obligations as reported as of September 30, 1991. Because of rounding, details may not add to totals. 1. Special Meal Assistance program is combined with School Lunch programs. 2. Commodities are based on preliminary food orders for fiscal year 1991.

★ 536 ★

Social Welfare: Nutrition Programs

Child Nutrition Programs: 1992-1994

The table below indicates funding for federal child nutrition programs for 1992, 1993, and 1994. Data for 1993 and 1994 are estimates.

[In thousands of dollars]

Program	1992	1993 (estimated)	1994 (estimated)
School lunch	3,870,098	4,131,424	4,328,214
School breakfast	801,191	891,163	980,352
Child and adult care feeding	1,089,627	1,273,160	1,528,446
Summer feeding	202,927	230,394	254,612
State administrative expenses	68,766	79,932	86,738
Commodity procurement	203,254	221,702	241,033
Coordinated review effort	4,111	4,241	3,843
Nutrition studies and surveys	3,829	3,835	3,939
Nutrition education and training	10,000	10,000	10,270
Food Service Management Institute	1,322	1,661	1,706
Dietary guidelines	-	2,000	2,054
Miscellaneous	-	-	3,700
Total	6,255,125	6,849,512	7,444,907

Source: "DC School Foodservice Not Going to Contract." *Food Management* (July 1993), p. 60. Primary source: Community Nutrition Institute.

★537★
Social Welfare: Nutrition Programs

Federal Food Programs: 1980-1992

For fiscal years ending in years shown. Program data include Puerto Rico, Virgin Islands, Guam, American Samoa, Northern Marianas, and the former Trust Territory when a federal food program was operated in these areas. Participation data are average monthly figures except as noted. Participants are not reported for the special milk program, the nutrition program for the elderly, and the commodity distribution programs. Cost data are direct federal benefits to recipients; they exclude federal administrative payments and applicable state and local contributions. Federal costs for commodities and cash-in-lieu of commodities are shown separately from direct cash benefits for those programs receiving both.

Program	Unit	1980	1985	1990	1991	1992 (preliminary)
Food stamps						
Participants	Million	21.1	19.9	20.1	22.6	25.4
Federal cost	Million $	8,721	10,744	14,187	17,339	20,891
Monthly average coupon value per recipient	$	34.47	44.99	58.93	63.86	68.53
Nutrition assistance program for Puerto Rico:[1]						
Federal cost	Million $	(X)	825	937	963	1,002
National School Lunch Program (NSLP):[2]						
Free lunches served	Million	1,671	1,657	1,662	1,749	1,880
Reduced-price lunches served	Million	308	255	273	293	284
Children participating[3]	Million	26.6	23.6	24.1	24.2	24.5
Federal cost	Million $	2,279	2,578	3,214	3,525	3,840
School Breakfast (SB):						
Children participating[0]	Million	3.6	3.4	4.1	4.4	4.9
Federal cost	Million $	288	379	596	685	783
Special school milk:						
Federal cost	Million $	145	16	19	20	20
Special supplemental food program (WIC):[4]						
Participants	Million	1.9	3.1	4.5	4.9	5.4
Federal cost	Million $	584	1,193	1,637	1,752	1,959
Commodity supplemental food program:[5]						
Participants	Million	0.1	0.2	0.3	0.3	0.3
Federal cost	Million $	19	42	71	76	87
Child and adult care (CC):[6]						
Participants[7]	Million	0.7	1.0	1.5	1.6	1.8
Federal cost	Million $	207	390	720	834	966
Summer Feeding (SF):[8]						
Children participating[9]	Million	1.9	1.5	1.7	1.8	1.9
Federal cost	Million $	104	103	145	160	183
Needy family commodity:						
Participants	Million	0.1	0.1	0.1	0.1	0.1
Federal cost	Million $	24	47	51	49	45
Nutrition program for the elderly:						
Meals served	Million	166	225	246	245	245
Federal cost	Million $	75	134	142	140	152
Federal cost of commodities donated to:[10]						
Child nutrition (NSLP, CC, SF and SB)	Million $	930	840	646	701	755

[Continued]

★ 537 ★

Federal Food Programs: 1980-1992

[Continued]

Program	Unit	1980	1985	1990	1991	1992 (preliminary)
Charitable institutions, summer camps	Million $	71	170	104	93	111
Emergency feeding[11]	Million $	(X)	973	286	252	225

Source: 1993 Statistical Abstract of the United States on CD-ROM [machine-readable datafiles]. CD-ABSTR-93. Washington, DC: U.S. Department of Commerce, Economics and Statistics Administration, Bureau of the Census, Data User Services Division, 1993. Primary source: U.S. Department of Agriculture. Food and Nutrition Service (FNS). *Annual Historical Review of FNS Programs;* and unpublished data. *Notes:* "X" represents "not applicable." 1. Puerto Rico was included in the food stamp program until June 30, 1982. 2. See related table on National School Lunch Program (NSLP). 3. Nine month (September through May) average daily meals (lunches or breakfasts) served divided by the ratio of average daily attendance to enrollment. 4. Special Supplemental Food Program (WIC) serves women, infants, and children. 5. Program provides commodities to women, infants, children, and the elderly. 6. Program provides year-round subsidies to feed preschool children in child care centers and family day care homes. Certain care centers serving disabled or elderly adults also receive meal subsidies. 7. Quarterly average daily attendance at participating institutions. 8. Program provides free meals to children in poor areas during summer months. 9. Peak month (July) average daily attendance at participating institutions. 10. Includes the federal cost of commodity entitlements, cash-in-lieu of commodities, and bonus foods. 11. Provides free commodities to needy persons for home consumption through food banks, hunger centers, soup kitchens, and similar nonprofit agencies. Includes the Emergency Food Assistance Program and the commodity purchases for soup kitchens/food banks program.

★ 538 ★

Social Welfare: Nutrition Programs

Federal Food Stamp Benefits: 1992

The federal food stamp program began in 1964. In 1992, its monthly enrollment was approximately 25 million people, or 10.4 percent of the population—the highest number since its inception. The table below indicates the average and maximum family benefits for 1992.

[In dollars]

Benefit	Amount
Average family benefit	173
Maximum benefit	370

Source: De Parle, Jason. "Food Stamp Users up Sharply in Sign of Weak Recovery." *New York Times,* 2 March 1993, pp. A1, A18.

★ 539 ★

Social Welfare: Nutrition Programs

Federal Food Stamp Program, by State: 1990-1992

Cost data for years ending September 30. Data on food stamp households and persons are average monthly number participating in year ending September 30. Food Stamp costs are for benefits only and exclude administrative expenditures. Data are provided by state or area. Figures for 1992 are preliminary.

Region, division, and state	Households participating (1,000)		Persons (1,000)			Cost (million dollars)		
	1991	1992	1990	1991	1992	1990	1991	1992
Total[1]	8,880	10,058	20,067	22,625	25,404	14,187	17,339	20,891
United States	8,872	10,048	20,036	22,599	25,370	14,153	17,306	20,842
Northeast	1,777	1,964	3,589	4,066	4,480	2,462	3,023	3,641
New England	368	413	707	857	963	426	575	706
Maine	51	58	94	116	133	63	85	109
New Hampshire	20	25	31	47	58	20	34	45
Vermont	21	23	38	48	54	22	30	37
Massachusetts	172	183	347	397	429	207	269	315
Rhode Island	34	38	64	78	87	42	57	69
Connecticut	70	86	133	171	202	72	100	131
Middle Atlantic	1,409	1,551	2,882	3,209	3,517	2,036	2,448	2,935
New York	777	855	1,548	1,716	1,885	1,086	1,290	1,586
New Jersey	176	201	382	441	495	289	366	433
Pennsylvania	456	495	952	1,052	1,137	661	792	916
Midwest	2,113	2,271	4,806	5,218	5,616	3,566	4,206	4,738
East North Central	1,598	1,705	3,616	3,914	4,183	2,765	3,254	3,626
Ohio	499	529	1,089	1,171	1,251	861	984	1,102
Indiana	131	160	311	375	448	226	294	373
Illinois	460	488	1,013	1,096	1,156	835	961	1,069
Michigan	408	405	917	978	994	663	808	846
Wisconsin	100	123	286	294	334	180	207	236
West North Central	515	566	1,190	1,304	1,433	801	952	1,112
Minnesota	120	128	263	286	309	165	202	234
Iowa	72	76	170	180	192	109	123	143
Missouri	190	214	431	490	549	312	380	447
North Dakota	16	18	39	41	46	25	28	35
South Dakota	18	19	50	52	55	35	39	42
Nebraska	39	43	95	99	107	59	67	78
Kansas	60	68	142	156	175	96	113	133
South	3,447	4,024	8,040	9,218	10,575	5,928	7,261	8,892
South Atlantic	1,416	1,737	2,993	3,631	4,402	2,223	2,873	3,776
Delaware	15	19	33	41	51	25	32	42
Maryland	130	147	255	304	343	203	259	312
District of Columbia	32	38	62	72	82	43	54	70
Virginia	171	206	346	414	495	247	321	406
West Virginia	105	117	262	281	310	192	220	255
North Carolina	201	236	419	517	597	282	378	461
South Carolina	116	133	299	329	369	240	239	297
Georgia	244	288	536	648	751	382	505	627
Florida	402	553[2]	781	1,025	1,404[2]	609	865	1,306[2]
East South Central	795	881	1,938	2,128	2,317	1,386	1,629	1,864
Kentucky	183	197	458	496	529	334	387	430
Tennessee	239	280	527	608	702	372	459	562

[Continued]

★ 539 ★

Federal Food Stamp Program, by State: 1990-1992
[Continued]

Region, division, and state	Households participating (1,000)		Persons (1,000)			Cost (million dollars)		
	1991	1992	1990	1991	1992	1990	1991	1992
Alabama	186	208	454	504	550	328	394	451
Mississippi	187	196	499	520	536	352	389	421
West South Central	1,236	1,406	3,109	3,459	3,856	2,319	2,759	3,252
Arkansas	94	102	235	258	277	155	183	207
Louisiana	261	278[2]	727	742	779[2]	549	598	666[2]
Oklahoma	117	135	267	298	346	186	224	276
Texas	764	891	1,880	2,161	2,454	1,429	1,754	2,103
West	1,535	1,789	3,601	4,097	4,699	2,197	2,816	3,571
Mountain	422	488	988	1,147	1,312	726	900	1,079
Montana	23	25	57	61	66	41	47	52
Idaho	23	26	59	65	72	40	47	53
Wyoming	11	12	28	31	33	21	23	26
Colorado	95	102	221	241	260	156	187	219
New Mexico	64	77	157	188	221	117	147	182
Arizona	138	166	317	388	457	239	310	377
Utah	40	44	99	110	123	71	83	96
Nevada	28	36	50	63	80	41	56	74
Pacific	1,113	1,301	2,613	2,950	3,387	1,471	1,916	2,492
Washington	158	178	340	385	432	229	278	344
Oregon	103	114	216	240	265	168	197	226
California	807	958	1,955	2,212	2,558	968	1,307	1,759
Alaska	10	12	25	30	38	25	34	41
Hawaii	35	39[2]	77	83	94[2]	81	100	122[2]

Source: 1993 Statistical Abstract of the United States on CD-ROM [machine-readable datafiles]. CD-ABSTR-93. Washington, DC: U.S. Department of Commerce, Economics and Statistics Administration, Bureau of the Census, Data User Services Division, 1993. Primary source: U.S. Department of Agriculture. Food and Nutrition Service (FNS). Annual Historical Review of FNS Programs; and unpublished data. Notes: "NA" represents "not available." 1. Includes Puerto Rico (when applicable), other outlying areas and U.S. Department of Defense overseas. 2. Includes hurricane disaster relief.

★ 540 ★

Social Welfare: Nutrition Programs

National School Lunch Program: 1990-1992

Cost data for years ending September 30. Data on pupils participating in National School Lunch Program (NSLP) are for month in which the highest number of children participated nationwide. Data for National School Lunch Program cover public and private elementary and secondary schools and residential child care institutions. National School Lunch Program costs include federal cash reimbursements at rates set by law for each meal served; they do not include the value of U.S. Department of Agriculture donated commodities utilized in this program. Data are provided by state or area. Figures for 1992 are preliminary.

Region, division, and state	NATIONAL SCHOOL LUNCH PROGRAM					
	Persons (1,000)			Cost (million dollars)		
	1990	1991	1992 preliminary	1990	1991	1992 preliminary
Total[1]	24,589	24,656	25,095	3,214	3,525	3,840
United States	24,019	24,080	24,528	3,008	3,404	3,721
Northeast	4,033	3,955	4,023	489	531	589
New England	991	942	954	95	105	119
Maine	108	105	106	11	12	14
New Hampshire	91	85	90	6	7	8
Vermont	47	47	48	4	4	5
Massachusetts	454	430	429	44	48	53
Rhode Island	60	56	61	7	8	10
Connecticut	231	219	220	23	26	29
Middle Atlantic	3,042	3,013	3,069	393	426	470
New York	1,546	1,548	1,577	232	249	270
New Jersey	507	504	513	60	67	77
Pennsylvania	990	961	979	102	110	123
Midwest	5,806	5,810	5,911	619	673	724
East North Central	3,687	3,700	3,743	421	459	495
Ohio	919	956	953	109	116	126
Indiana	635	610	610	54	59	64
Illinois	932	937	955	131	144	155
Michigan	733	723	745	82	91	97
Wisconsin	468	474	480	45	49	53
West North Central	2,119	2,110	2,168	197	214	229
Minnesota	489	493	505	42	46	48
Iowa	392	376	396	31	34	36
Missouri	547	547	557	58	63	68
North Dakota	94	93	94	8	9	9
South Dakota	102	104	106	12	12	13
Nebraska	191	193	197	18	19	21
Kansas	302	304	313	29	31	34
South	9,890	9,941	10,079	1,334	1,457	1,600
South Atlantic	4,454	4,451	4,515	558	618	683
Delaware	59	59	59	6	6	7
Maryland	347	337	352	40	43	48
District of Columbia	47	47	47	10	10	11
Virginia	586	576	589	60	65	72
West Virginia	198	217	184	29	31	31
North Carolina	749	740	750	91	99	107
South Carolina	451	453	458	60	65	72

[Continued]

★ 540 ★

National School Lunch Program: 1990-1992
[Continued]

| Region, division, and state | NATIONAL SCHOOL LUNCH PROGRAM | | | | | |
| | Persons (1,000) | | | Cost (million dollars) | | |
	1990	1991	1992 preliminary	1990	1991	1992 preliminary
Georgia	908	910	927	106	117	131
Florida	1,110	1,112	1,149	158	182	204
East South Central	2,085	2,100	2,102	281	301	324
Kentucky	498	515	523	61	67	73
Tennessee	590	592	592	68	73	80
Alabama	570	568	567	77	81	87
Mississippi	428	425	420	76	80	84
West South Central	3,351	3,390	3,462	495	538	593
Arkansas	292	294	310	41	44	46
Louisiana	694	695	691	104	110	116
Oklahoma	362	363	370	46	50	55
Texas	2,003	2,038	2,091	304	334	376
West	4,289	4,383	4,515	657	743	808
Mountain	1,362	1,382	1,415	170	188	210
Montana	84	86	88	10	10	11
Idaho	131	134	135	14	15	17
Wyoming	57	59	59	5	6	6
Colorado	282	282	290	31	35	37
New Mexico	179	179	183	30	33	36
Arizona	331	336	356	47	53	61
Utah	233	229	221	24	27	30
Nevada	67	77	83	8	9	12
Pacific	2,927	3,001	3,100	487	555	598
Washington	361	377	395	43	49	55
Oregon	234	237	246	26	30	33
California	2,147	2,201	2,268	396	452	484
Alaska	39	40	43	8	9	10
Hawaii	145	146	148	14	15	16

Source: 1993 Statistical Abstract of the United States on CD-ROM [machine-readable datafiles]. CD-ABSTR-93. Washington, DC: U.S. Department of Commerce, Economics and Statistics Administration, Bureau of the Census, Data User Services Division, 1993. Primary source: U.S. Department of Agriculture, Food Nutrition Service (FNS). Annual Historical Review of FNS Programs and unpublished data. Notes: "NA" represents "not available." 1. Includes Puerto Rico (for NSLP), other outlying areas and Department of Defense overseas.

★ 541 ★
Social Welfare: Nutrition Programs

School Breakfast Program: 1982-1992

Figures indicate the numbers of schools and children participating in school breakfast programs.

Year	Number of schools[1] (in thousands)	Daily participation (million children)			
		Free	Reduced price	Full price	Total
1982	34.3	2.80	0.16	0.36	3.32
1983	33.5	2.87	0.15	0.34	3.36
1984	33.8	2.91	0.15	0.37	3.43
1985	34.8	2.88	0.16	0.40	3.44
1986	35.2	2.93	0.16	0.41	5.50
1987	37.2	3.01	0.17	0.43	3.61
1988	38.8	3.03	0.18	0.47	3.68
1989	40.0	3.10	0.20	0.51	3.81
1990	42.8	3.30	0.22	0.55	4.07
1991	46.1	3.61	0.25	0.58	4.44
1992	50.2	4.05	0.26	0.60	4.92

Source: "School Breakfast Program Serves Almost 5 Million Children in 50,000 Schools." *FoodReview* 16, no. 3 (September-December 1993), p. 42. *Note:* 1. Includes schools and residential childcare institutions.

Social Welfare: Public Aid

★ 542 ★

Aid to Families With Dependent Children and Supplemental Security Income Recipients and Payments: 1980-1991

Recipients as of December. Data for Supplemental Security Income (SSI) cover federal SSI payments and/or federally administered state supplementation, except as noted. Aid to Families With Dependent Children is commonly represented as AFDC.

Division and state or other area	AFDC								SSI			
	Recipients (1,000)[1]			Payments for year (million dollars)			Monthly payments per family		Recipients (1,000)		Payments for year (million dollars)	
	1980	1990	1991	1980	1990	1991	1990	1991	1990	1991	1990	1991
Total	11,101	12,159	13,489	12,475	19,078	20,931	$392	$390	4,817[2]	5,118[2]	16,133	17,996
U.S	10,923	11,958	13,285	12,409	18,995	20,843	396	394	4,817	5,118	16,133	17,996
New England	647	577	653	910	1,250	1,383	535	522	209	222	652	739
Maine	58	62	69	60	104	116	422	416	24	24	56	62
New Hampshire	24	21	28	27	35	49	431	443	7[4]	7[4]	19[4]	22[4]
Vermont	24	25	29	32	51	59	527	524	10	11	31	35
Massachusetts	348	282	311	510	647	682	556	532	119	127	397	450
Rhode Island	54	52	59	72	104	122	499	510	17	18	53	59
Connecticut	140	135	157	209	309	355	571	565	32[4]	34[4]	96[4]	112[4]

[Continued]

★ 542 ★

Aid to Families With Dependent Children and Supplemental Security Income Recipients and Payments: 1980-1991
[Continued]

Division and state or other area	AFDC								SSI			
	Recipients (1,000)[1]			Payments for year (million dollars)			Monthly payments per family		Recipients (1,000)		Payments for year (million dollars)	
	1980	1990	1991	1980	1990	1991	1990	1991	1990	1991	1990	1991
Middle Atlantic	2,216	1,9	2,062	2,954	3,623	3,873	472	466	711	758	2,533	2,866
New York	1,110	1,0	1,108	1,623	2,337	2,496	556	550	415	445	1,557	1,762
New Jersey	469	323	364	560	459	496	352	342	105	112	340	387
Pennsylvania	637	549	590	771	827	881	382	380	191	202	635	717
East North Central	2,419	2,3	2,560	2,838	3,611	3,701	379	367	622	669	2,021	2,320
Ohio	572	657	746	561	896	955	328	325	156	169	483	564
Indiana	170	164	195	139	174	202	263	267	60[4]	66[4]	174[4]	204[4]
Illinois	691	656	698	722	868	929	342	346	177[4]	192[4]	593[4]	688[4]
Michigan	753	684	680	1,063	1,232	1,163	464	424	143	151	483	538
Wisconsin	232	236	241	353	441	452	464	466	86	91	288	326
West North Central	614	647	705	697	955	1,030	366	372	216	230	584	669
Minnesota	146	177	183	207	355	379	512	524	40[4]	44[4]	110[4]	129[4]
Iowa	111	96	103	144	154	162	371	380	33	34	86	96
Missouri	216	218	249	182	237	265	274	280	85[4]	90[4]	237[4]	269[4]
North Dakota	13	16	18	16	24	26	359	360	7[4]	8[4]	18[4]	20[4]
South Dakota	19	19	20	19	22	24	272	286	10	11	26	30
Nebraska	38	44	48	42	60	63	336	332	16[4]	17[4]	42[4]	48[4]
Kansas	72	77	84	87	103	111	332	341	25	26	65	76
South Atlantic	1,463	1,6	1,985	1,125	1,844	2,170	272	273	847	898	2,370	2,662
Delaware	34	22	26	32	30	34	292	291	8	8	22	25
Maryland	220	198	220	214	304	337	370	372	60	63	185	209
District of Columbia	82	54	61	92	87	100	380	386	16	17	544	59
Virginia	176	158	185	160	181	208	265	270	95[4]	101[4]	257[4]	290[4]
West Virginia	80	109	119	60	112	116	249	252	47[5]	50[5]	146[5]	165[5]
North Carolina	202	255	308	154	257	312	237	238	149[4]	157[4]	403[4]	444[4]
South Carolina	156	118	137	72	97	111	203	203	90[4]	93[4]	234[4]	257[4]
Georgia	234	320	383	138	333	392	265	267	159	166	415	462
Florida	279	420	546	203	443	560	263	267	222	241	653	751
East South Central	704	742	816	366	510	569	168	171	501	524	1,371	1,539
Kentucky	175	204	230	136	185	208	224	217	115[4]	122[4]	337[4]	382[4]
Tennessee	174	230	266	85	176	200	186	187	140	147	384	433
Alabama	178	132	142	84	63	73	115	125	133[4]	137[4]	351[4]	387[4]
Mississippi	176	176	178	61	86	88	120	122	114	118	300	337
West South Central	716	1,1	1,238	401	811	895	180	183	564	596	1,478	1,678
Arkansas	85	73	76	51	57	60	190	191	76	79	187	211
Louisiana	219	279	276	124	188	189	167	170	133	140	378	428
Oklahoma	92	129	133	92	135	157	279	301	60[4]	62[4]	158[4]	174[4]
Texas	320	673	753	134	431	489	165	166	295[5]	315[5]	755[5]	865[5]
Mountain	302	454	544	274	523	643	297	314	162	178	476	559
Montana	20	29	32	19	40	43	344	347	10	11	29	33
Idaho	20	17	19	24	20	23	266	276	10[4]	11[4]	29[4]	35[4]
Wyoming	7	16	19	9	20	26	313	351	3[4]	4[4]	9[4]	11[4]
Colorado	81	109	127	81	138	154	320	322	38[4]	42[4]	110[4]	131[4]
New Mexico	56	67	86	42	66	92	273	304	32[4]	34[4]	90[4]	102[4]
Arizona	60	144	178	40	146	197	268	299	45[4]	50[4]	139[4]	162[4]
Utah	44	47	51	48	65	73	347	359	13	14	38	46
Nevada	14	25	32	11	28	35	278	287	11	13	33	39
Pacific	1,843	2,4	2,723	2,844	5,866	6,577	606	609	984	1,041	4,646	4,962
Washington	173	237	269	251	447	533	452	492	62	67	208	242
Oregon	94	99	117	147	150	187	374	401	32[4]	34[4]	95[4]	110[4]
California	1,498	2,023	2,258	2,328	5,107	5,664	637	632	873	920	4,278	4,537
Alaska	16	24	30	27	62	81	651	691	5[4]	5[4]	14[4]	16[4]
Hawaii	61	44	49	91	100	112	581	613	14	14	51	56

[Continued]

★ 542 ★

Aid to Families With Dependent Children and Supplemental Security Income Recipients and Payments: 1980-1991

[Continued]

Division and state or other area	AFDC								SSI			
	Recipients (1,000)[1]			Payments for year (million dollars)			Monthly payments per family		Recipients (1,000)		Payments for year (million dollars)	
	1980	1990	1991	1980	1990	1991	1990	1991	1990	1991	1990	1991
Puerto Rico	170	193	195	60	74	77	103	105	(X)	(X)	(X)	(X)
Guam	5	4	5	3	6	7	418	505	(X)	(X)	(X)	(X)
Virgin Islands	3	3	4	2	3	3	279	285	(X)	(X)	(X)	(X)
N. Mariana	(X)	(X)	(X)	(X)	(X)	(X)	(X)	(X)	1[5]	1[5]	2[5]	2[5]

Source: 1993 Statistical Abstract of the United States on CD-ROM [machine-readable datafiles]. CD-ABSTR-93. Washington, DC: U.S. Department of Commerce, Economics and Statistics Administration, Bureau of the Census, Data User Services Division, 1993. Primary source: U.S. Social Security Administration. *Social Security Bulletin* (quarterly) and *Annual Statistical Supplement to the "Social Security Bulletin"*; U.S. Administration for Children and Families. *Quarterly Public Assistance Statistics* (annual). *Notes:* "NA" represents "not available." "X" represents "not applicable." 1. Includes the children and one or both parents, or one caretaker relative other than a parent, in families where the needs of such adults were considered in determining the amount of assistance. 2. Includes small number of recipients whose residence was "unknown." 3. 1980 figures include payments to Indochina refugees (total, $24 million) which were not available by state. 4. Data for persons with federal SSI payments only; state has state-administered supplementation. 5. Data for persons with federal SSI payments only; state supplementary payments not made.

★ 543 ★

Social Welfare: Public Aid

Cash and Noncash Social Welfare Benefits for Persons With Limited Income: 1985-1990

Figures indicate expenditures for years ending September 30, except as noted. Programs covered provide cash, goods, or services to persons who make no payment and render no service in return. In case of job and training programs and some educational benefits, recipients must work or study for wages, training allowances, stipends, grants, or loans. Most of the programs base eligibility on individual, household, or family income, but some use group or area income tests; and a few offer help on the basis of presumed need.

[In millions of dollars]

Program	Total expenditures[1]									
	1985	1987	1988	1989	1990	1985	1987	1988	1989	1990
Total	143,606	158,953	172,508	186,449	210,630	105,064	114,789	125,047	134,715	152,166
Medical care[2]	49,752	60,505	66,644	73,554	86,197	27,880	35,098	38,608	42,393	50,211
Medicaid[3]	41,258	49,329	54,304	60,896	72,228	22,844	27,960	30,567	34,384	41,195
Veterans[4][5]	3,053	5,035	5,855	5,678	6,458	3,053	5,035	5,855	5,678	6,458
General assistance[5]	3,125	3,722	3,966	4,300	4,600	0	0	0	0	0
Indian Health Services	862	929	1,006	1,082	1,250	862	929	1,006	1,082	1,250
Maternal and child health services	783	812	860	903	907	478	496	527	554	554
Community health centers	383	420	396	435	478	383	420	396	435	478
Cash aid[2]	37,636	42,279	45,707	49,652	55,136	24,486	27,459	30,314	33,163	37,044
Aid to Families With Dependent Children[3][6]	16,736	18,454	19,016	19,662	21,196	8,909	9,996	10,319	10,647	11,505
Supplemental Security Income[3]	11,857	13,744	14,684	15,757	17,232	9,603[7]	10,893[7]	11,648[7]	12,417[7]	13,606[7]
Earned income tax credit (refunded portion)	1,162	1,488	2,930	4,257	5,902	1,162	1,488	2,930	4,257	5,902
Pensions for needy veterans[8]	3,842	3,790	3,935	4,024	3,954	3,842	3,790	3,935	4,024	3,954
General assistance	2,499	2,642	2,624	2,819	3,184	0	0	0	0	0
Food benefits[2]	20,391	21,060	21,355	21,997	25,257	19,362	19,893	20,216	20,835	24,011
Food stamps[3][9]	13,470	13,535	14,369	14,916	17,702	12,599	12,539	13,289	13,815	16,517
School lunch program[10][11]	2,665	3,281	2,937	3,082	3,250	2,665	3,281	2,937	3,082	3,250
Women, infants and children[12]	1,500	1,664	1,800	1,924	2,119	1,500	1,664	1,800	1,924	2,119
Nutrition program for elderly[13]	614	649	561	582	578	456	478	502	521	517
Housing benefits[2]	14,113	13,211	14,701	15,925	17,544	14,113	13,211	14,701	15,925	17,544
Lower-income housing assistance (Sec.8)	6,818	8,125	9,133	9,918	10,577	6,818	8,125	9,133	9,918	10,577
Low-rent public housing	3,408	2,161	2,526	3,043	3,918	3,408	2,161	2,526	3,043	3,918
Rural housing loans[14]	1,790	1,144	1,271	1,267	1,311	1,790	1,144	1,271	1,267	1,311

[Continued]

★ 543 ★

Cash and Noncash Social Welfare Benefits for Persons With Limited Income: 1985-1990
[Continued]

Program	Total expenditures[1]									
	1985	1987	1988	1989	1990	1985	1987	1988	1989	1990
Interest reduction payments	619	638	628	611	630	619	638	628	611	630
Rural rental housing loans[14]	903	555	555	555	572	903	555	555	555	572
Education aid[2]	9,970	10,279	11,691	13,029	14,375	9,516	9,768	11,147	12,484	13,746
Stafford loans[15]	3,888	3,179	3,775	5,012	5,648	3,888	3,179	3,775	5,012	5,648
Pell grants[16]	2,800	3,580	4,187	4,260	4,484	2,800	3,580	4,187	4,260	4,484
Head Start	1,309	1,413	1,508	1,544	1,940	1,047	1,130	1,206	1,235	1,552
College Work-Study Program[16]	555	593	593	588	610	555	593	593	588	610
Supplemental Educational Opportunity Grants[16]	375	395	413	408	438	375	395	413	408	438
Services[2]	5,476	5,587	5,659	5,671	5,801	3,551	3,607	3,559	3,571	3,661
Social services (Title 20)[17]	4,650	4,680	4,800	4,800	4,902	2,725	2,700	2,700	2,700	2,762
Community services block grant	372	409	382	381	389	372	409	382	381	389
Jobs and training[2]	3,976	3,853	3,820	3,912	4,215	3,895	3,782	3,748	3,815	3,966
Training for disadvantaged adults and youth [18] [19]	1,886	1,840	1,810	1,788	1,745	1,886	1,840	1,810	1,788	1,745
Job Corps [18] [19]	617	656	716	742	803	617	656	716	742	803
Summer youth employment program [18] [19]	725	750	718	709	700	725	750	718	709	700
Work incentive program	297	140	103	186	452	267	126	93	148	265
Senior community service employment program[19]	362	373	368	382	408	326	336	331	344	367
Energy assistance[2]	2,292	2,179	2,001	1,809	1,802	2,261	1,971	1,824	1,629	1,680
Low-income energy assistance [3] [20]	2,095	2,013	1,840	1,648	1,641	2,070	1,810	1,663	1,468	1,519
Other[21]	(X)	(X)	930	900	303	(X)	(X)	930	900	303

Source: 1993 Statistical Abstract of the United States on CD-ROM [machine-readable datafiles]. CD-ABSTR-93. Washington, DC: U.S. Department of Commerce, Economics and Statistics Administration, Bureau of the Census, Data User Services Division, 1993. Primary source: Library of Congress. Congressional Research Service. Cash and Noncash Benefits for Persons With Limited Income: Eligibility Rules, Recipient and Expenditure Data, Fiscal Year 1988-1990. Report No. 91-741 EPW. 30 September 1991; and earlier reports. Notes: "X" represents "not applicable." 1. Includes state and local government expenditures not shown separately. 2. Includes other programs not shown separately. 3. Includes administrative expenses. 4. Medical care for veterans with a non-service-connected disability. 5. Estimated. 6. Aid to Families with Dependent Children program. Excludes data for foster care program and child support operations (cost and collections). 7. Excludes federal sums spent for Supplementary Social Insurance (SSI; state supplements) to Indochinese refugees. 8. Includes dependents and survivors. 9. Includes Puerto Rico's nutritional assistance program. 10. Free and reduced-price segments. 11. Includes estimate of commodity assistance. 12. Special supplemental food program for women, infants and children (WIC). 13. No income test required but preference given to those with greatest need. 14. Amount of loans obligated. 15. Formerly Guaranteed Student Loans. 16. Appropriation available for school year ending the fiscal year named. 17. Non-federal expenditure data are rough estimates. 18. Programs represent specific titles under the Job Training and Partnership Act (JTPA). 19. Federal funds are appropriations. 20. Federal funds include amounts transferred to other programs serving the needy. State spending includes funds received as "oil overcharge" settlements. 21. Represents State Legalization Impact Assistance Grants, offered between 1988 and 1992, to offset state and local costs of welfare, health care, and education provided to legalized aliens.

★ 544 ★

Social Welfare: Public Aid

Households Receiving Means-Tested Noncash Social Welfare Benefits: 1980-1991

Households as of March of following year. Covers civilian noninstitutional population, including persons in the Armed Forces living off post or with their families on post. A means-tested benefit program requires that the household's income and/or assets fall below specified guidelines in order to qualify for benefits. The means-tested noncash benefits covered are food stamps, free or reduced-price school lunches, public or subsidized housing, and Medicaid. There are general trends toward under-estimation of noncash beneficiaries. Households are classified according to poverty status of family or nonfamily householder.

[In thousands, except percentages]

Type of benefit received	1980	1985	1990	1991			
				Total	Below poverty level		Above poverty level
					Number	Percent distribution	
Total households	82,368	88,458	94,312	95,669	12,949	100	82,720
Receiving at least one noncash benefit	14,266	14,466	16,098	17,387	8,262	64	9,125
Not receiving cash public assistance	7,860	7,860	8,819	9,539	3,362	26	6,177
Receiving cash public assistance[1]	6,407	6,607	7,279	7,849	4,900	38	2,949
Total households receiving–							
Food stamps	6,769	6,779	7,163	7,839	5,489	42	2,350
School lunch	5,532	5,752	6,252	6,922	3,677	28	3,245
Public housing	2,777	3,799	4,339	4,511	2,765	21	1,746
Medicaid	8,287	8,178	10,321	11,458	6,220	48	5,238

Source: 1993 Statistical Abstract of the United States on CD-ROM [machine-readable datafiles]. CD-ABSTR-93. Washington, DC: U.S. Department of Commerce, Economics and Statistics Administration, Bureau of the Census, Data User Services Division, 1993. Primary source: U.S. Bureau of the Census. *Current Population Reports.* Series P60-155; earlier reports; and unpublished data. *Notes:* 1. Households receiving money from Aid to Families With Dependent Children (AFDC) program, Supplemental Security Income (SSI) program or other public assistance programs.

★ 545 ★

Social Welfare: Public Aid

Persons With Limited Incomes Receiving Cash and Noncash Social Welfare Benefits: 1985-1990

The table below reflects the average number of monthly participants in social welfare programs. Data are for years ending September 30, except as noted. Programs covered provide cash, goods, or services to persons who make no payment and render no service in return. In case of job and training programs and some educational benefits, recipients must work or study for wages, training allowances, stipends, grants, or loans. Most of the programs base eligibility on individual, household, or family income, but some use group or area income tests; and a few offer help on the basis of presumed need.

[In thousands]

Program	1985	1986	1987	1988	1989	1990
Medical care						
Medicaid[1]	21,814	22,518	23,183	22,907	23,511	25,255
Veterans [2][3]	504	465	570	585	569	585
Indian Health Services[4]	931	990	1,000	1,000	1,100	1,100
Community health centers[4]	5,200	5,350	5,500	5,250	5,350	5,350

[Continued]

★ 545 ★

Persons With Limited Incomes Receiving Cash and Noncash Social Welfare Benefits: 1985-1990
[Continued]

Program	1985	1986	1987	1988	1989	1990
Cash aid						
Aid to Families With Dependent Children[5]	10,813	10,995	11,065	10,920	10,935	11,439
Supplemental Security Income	4,305	4,450	4,569	4,469	4,753	4,913
Earned income tax credit[6]	17,313	19,197	22,311	26,214	33,444	33,693
Pensions for needy veterans [7][8]	1,489	1,397	1,267	1,201	1,139	1,080
General assistance[6]	1,323	1,334	1,193	1,115	1,091	1,205
Food benefits						
Food stamps[9]	21,400	20,900	20,600	20,100	20,200	21,500
School lunch program[10][11]	11,500	11,600	11,600	11,600	11,700	11,600
Women, infants and children[12]	3,138	3,312	3,430	3,600	4,100	4,500
Nutrition program for elderly[4][13]	3,630	3,584	3,496	3,494	3,538	3,548
Housing benefits						
Lower-income housing assistance (Sec. 8)[14]	2,010	2,143	2,240	2,338	2,420	2,500
Low-rent public housing[14]	1,355	1,380	1,390	1,398	1,404	1,405
Rural housing loans[15]	41	26	24	26	25	25
Interest reduction payments[15]	528	529	528	528	528	531
Rural rental housing loans[15]	26	21	17	17	16	16
Education aid						
Stafford loans[16][17]	3,477	3,242	3,300	3,619	3,682	3,624
Pell grants[16]	2,797	2,881	2,660	2,882	3,198	3,434
Head Start	448	448	447	448	451	541
College Work-Study Program[16]	737	728	738	686	785	835
Supplemental Educational Opportunity Grants[16]	720	686	689	635	660	633
Jobs and training						
Training for disadvantaged adults and youth[18][19]	350	337	393	384	397	416
Job Corps[18]	41	41	41	41	41	40
Summer youth employment program[18][20]	785	634	723	706	605	625
Work incentive program[21]	1,013	870	914	(NA)	1,700	444
Senior community service employment program[22]	64	61	66	65	66	65
Energy aid						
Low-income energy assistance[23]	6,800	6,700	6,800	6,200	5,900	5,800

Source: 1993 Statistical Abstract of the United States on CD-ROM [machine-readable datafiles]. CD-ABSTR-93. Washington, DC: U.S. Department of Commerce, Economics and Statistics Administration, Bureau of the Census, Data User Services Division, 1993. Primary source: Library of Congress. Congressional Research Service. *Cash and Noncash Benefits for Persons With Limited Income: Eligibility Rules, Recipient and Expenditure Data, Fiscal Year 1988-1990.* Report No. 91-741 EPW. September 1991; and earlier reports. *Notes:* 1. Unduplicated annual number. 2. Medical care for veterans with a non-service-connected disability. 3. For 1985, estimated number of patients discharged from hospital during year. For other years, estimated number of inpatients. 4. Annual numbers. 5. Aid to Families with Dependent Children program. Excludes data for foster care program and child support operations (cost and collections). 6. Estimated. 7. Includes dependents and survivors. 8. Estimate as of September. 9. Includes Puerto Rico's nutritional assistance program. 10. Free and reduced-price segments. 11. Estimated daily average. 12. Special supplemental food program for women, infants, and children (WIC). 13. No income test required but preference given to those with greatest need. 14. Units eligible for payment at end of year. 15. Represents total families or dwelling units during year. 16. Total numbers for the school year ending in year shown. 17. Formerly Guaranteed Student Loans. 18. Programs represent specific titles under the Job Training and Partnership Act (JTPA). 19. Average monthly enrollment for program year. 20. Total participants (June-August). 21. New registrants only. 22. Annual number of jobs authorized. 23. Number of households that received heating and winter crisis aid.

★ 546 ★

Social Welfare: Public Aid

Public Aid Payments: 1970-1990

Supplemental Security Income (SSI) data cover federally and state-administered payments.

[In million dollars]

Program	1970	1975	1980	1985	1986	1987	1988	1989	1990	1991
Payments, total[1]	8,443	16,313	21,994	26,431	28,311	29,556	30,910	32,762	36,047	39,788
Supplemental Security Income[2]	(X)	5,878	7,941	11,060	12,081	12,951	13,786	14,980	16,599	18,524
Aged	(X)	2,605	2,734	3,035	3,096	3,194	3,299	3,476	3,736	3,890
Blind	(X)	131	190	264	277	291	302	316	334	347
Disabled	(X)	3,142	5,014	7,755	8,700	9,458	10,177	11,180	12,521	14,268
Public assistance[1]	8,443	10,434	14,048	15,371	16,230	16,605	17,124	17,782	19,448	21,264
Old-age assistance	1,862	5	9	8	8	7	7	7	7	11
Blind	98	(Z)	(Z)	(Z)	(Z)	(Z)	(Z)	(Z)	(Z)	(Z)
Permanently, totally disabled	1,000	3	9	10	11	11	11	12	12	19
Families with dependent children	4,853	9,211	12,475	15,196	16,033	16,373	16,827	17,466	19,078	20,931
Emergency assistance	11	78	113	157	178	214	279	297	349	303
General assistance	618	1,138	1,442	(NA)	(NA)	(NA)	(NA)	(NA)	(NA)	(NA)

Source: 1993 Statistical Abstract of the United States on CD-ROM [machine-readable datafiles]. CD-ABSTR-93. Washington, DC: U.S. Department of Commerce, Economics and Statistics Administration, Bureau of the Census, Data User Services Division, 1993. Primary source: U.S. Social Security Administration. *Social Security Bulletin* (quarterly) and *Annual Statistical Supplement to the "Social Security Bulletin"*; and U.S. Administration for Children and Families. *Quarterly Public Assistance Statistics* (annual). *Notes:* "NA" represents "not available." "X" represents "not applicable." "Z" represents less than $500,000. 1. Beginning 1981, excludes general assistance payments. 2. Includes data not available by reason for eligibility.

★ 547 ★

Social Welfare: Public Aid

Public Aid Recipients and Average Monthly Cash Payments Under Supplemental Security Income and Public Assistance: 1975-1991

As of December, except as noted. Public assistance data for all years include Puerto Rico, Guam, and Virgin Islands; Supplemental Social Insurance (SSI) data are for federally administered payments only. Excludes payments made directly to suppliers of medical care.

Program	Recipients (1,000)					Average monthly payments (dollars)				
	1975	1980	1985	1990	1991	1975	1980	1985	1990	1991
SSI, total	4,314	4,142	4,138	4,817	5,118	114	168	226	299	321
Aged	2,307	1,808	1,504	1,454	1,465	91	128	164	213	221
Blind	74	78	82	84	85	147	213	274	342	351
Disabled	1,933	2,256	2,551	3,279	3,569	141	198	261	337	361
Old-age assistance[1]	18	19	18	17	17	21	39	36	45	55
Aid to the blind[1]	(Z)	(Z)	(Z)	(Z)	(Z)	15	36	39	42	56
Aid to permanently, totally disabled[1]	17	21	23	26	27	15	35	38	40	58
AFDC Families[2]	3,568	3,843	3,721	4,218	4,708	229	288	341	392	390
Recipients[3]	11,404	11,101	10,924	12,159	13,489	72	100	118	136	135

[Continued]

★ 547 ★

Public Aid Recipients and Average Monthly Cash Payments Under Supplemental Security Income and Public Assistance: 1975-1991

[Continued]

Program	Recipients (1,000)					Average monthly payments (dollars)				
	1975	1980	1985	1990	1991	1975	1980	1985	1990	1991
Children	8,106	7,599	7,247	8,232	9,126	(NA)	(NA)	(NA)	(NA)	(NA)
General assistance cases	692	796	1,051	1,004	1,106	144	161	(NA)	(NA)	(NA)

Source: 1993 Statistical Abstract of the United States on CD-ROM [machine-readable datafiles]. CD-ABSTR-93. Washington, DC: U.S. Department of Commerce, Economics and Statistics Administration, Bureau of the Census, Data User Services Division, 1993. Primary source: U.S. Social Security Administration. Social Security Bulletin (quarterly) and Annual Statistical Supplement to the "Social Security Bulletin"; and U.S. Administration for Children and Families. Quarterly Public Assistance Statistics (annual). Notes: "NA" represents "not available." "Z" represents fewer than 500. 1. Average monthly recipients and payments for the year. 2. Aid to Families with Dependent Children (AFDC) program. 3. Includes the children and one or both parents, or one caretaker relative other than a parent, in families where the needs of such adults were considered in determining the amount of assistance.

★ 548 ★

Social Welfare: Public Aid

Public Aid Recipients as Percent of Population: 1990 and 1991

Total recipients of Aid to Families With Dependent Children (AFDC) and of federal Supplemental Security Income (SSI) as percent of resident population as of June. Based on estimated resident population as of April 1 for 1990 and as of July 1 for 1991.

Division and state	Public aid recipients as percent of population		SSI recipients		AFDC recipients	
	1990	1991	1990	1991	1990	1991
United States	6.5	7.0	4,702,963	4,959,179	11,411,433	12,640,738
New England	5.6	6.3	205,268	215,819	534,413	617,319
Maine	6.6	7.3	23,397	24,014	57,582	66,199
New Hampshire	2.2	2.9	6,730	7,267	17,498	25,062
Vermont	5.7	6.6	9,837	10,431	22,299	27,154
Massachusetts	6.4	7.0	117,025	123,054	265,298	295,470
Rhode Island	6.4	7.3	17,138	17,778	47,293	55,661
Connecticut	4.7	5.5	31,141	33,275	124,443	147,773
Middle Atlantic	6.7	7.2	688,245	734,663	1,825,582	1,985,392
New York	7.7	8.3	400,067	429,927	991,226	1,068,762
New Jersey	5.3	5.8	102,485	108,564	309,546	344,069
Pennsylvania	6.0	6.4	185,693	196,172	524,810	572,561
East North Central	7.0	7.4	605,340	643,982	2,333,958	2,474,980
Ohio	7.3	7.8	151,564	162,229	636,264	691,625
Indiana	3.9	4.3	58,752	62,852	155,714	180,676
Illinois	7.1	7.5	171,303	184,566	641,655	677,624
Michigan	8.6	8.8	139,432	146,181	662,267	682,828
Wisconsin	6.6	6.7	84,289	88,154	238,058	242,227
West North Central	4.8	5.0	212,271	223,557	639,681	674,765
Minnesota	4.9	5.0	39,432	42,144	174,878	181,046
Iowa	4.7	4.7	32,256	33,903	98,251	97,532
Missouri	5.8	6.2	83,711	87,490	212,247	233,841
North Dakota	3.6	3.8	7,514	7,745	15,380	16,620
South Dakota	4.2	4.4	9,972	10,625	19,125	20,084

[Continued]

★548★

Public Aid Recipients as Percent of Population: 1990 and 1991
[Continued]

Division and state	Public aid recipients as percent of population		SSI recipients		ADFC recipients	
	1990	1991	1990	1991	1990	1991
Nebraska	3.7	3.9	15,412	16,304	43,075	45,593
Kansas	4.1	4.2	23,974	25,346	76,725	80,049
South Atlantic	5.4	6.1	832,783	872,692	1,533,809	1,822,300
Delaware	4.4	4.7	7,925	8,253	21,318	23,892
Maryland	5.1	5.6	58,685	61,790	185,548	209,098
District of Columbia	10.9	12.3	16,118	16,382	49,875	56,777
Virginia	3.9	4.3	93,899	98,376	147,213	173,587
West Virginia	8.8	8.9	46,389	48,485	112,301	112,192
North Carolina	5.7	6.5	145,996	153,309	228,673	284,985
South Carolina	5.8	6.3	89,565	91,604	111,887	130,972
Georgia	7.1	7.9	157,857	162,552	299,438	357,593
Florida	4.6	5.3	216,349	231,941	377,556	473,204
East South Central	7.9	8.5	495,156	512,749	703,163	785,028
Kentucky	7.9	9.1	112,779	118,517	178,770	220,678
Tennessee	7.2	7.9	137,729	143,089	214,394	247,871
Alabama	6.5	6.6	131,620	134,753	129,662	136,879
Mississippi	11.4	11.4	113,028	116,390	180,337	179,600
West South Central	6.2	6.5	554,635	578,459	1,095,406	1,178,906
Arkansas	6.3	6.4	75,141	77,774	72,419	75,063
Louisiana	9.8	9.7	131,435	134,954	281,549	277,007
Oklahoma	5.6	5.8	59,726	61,339	117,593	123,396
Texas	5.4	5.8	288,333	304,392	623,845	703,440
Mountain	4.2	4.7	156,086	170,287	417,646	487,105
Montana	4.9	5.7	9,672	10,484	29,249	35,930
Idaho	2.7	2.8	10,127	10,980	16,978	18,155
Wyoming	3.8	4.7	3,320	3,704	13,879	17,782
Colorado	4.3	4.4	36,802	39,486	103,821	109,696
New Mexico	5.8	7.0	30,401	32,789	57,478	76,072
Arizona	4.7	5.4	42,863	47,534	127,739	153,488
Utah	3.3	3.5	11,930	13,345	44,866	49,254
Nevada	2.9	3.0	10,971	11,965	23,636	26,728
Pacific	8.4	9.1	952,900	1,006,901	2,327,775	2,614,943
Washington	6.0	6.4	59,580	64,686	230,022	256,576
Oregon	4.3	4.9	30,724	33,089	90,587	109,568
California	9.4	10.1	844,526	890,141	1,942,311	2,174,391
Alaska	4.6	5.8	4,505	4,848	20,971	28,130
Hawaii	5.2	5.3	13,565	14,137	43,884	46,278

Source: 1993 Statistical Abstract of the United States on CD-ROM [machine-readable datafiles]. CD-ABSTR-93. Washington, DC: U.S. Department of Commerce, Economics and Statistics Administration, Bureau of the Census, Data User Services Division, 1993. Primary source: Compiled by U.S. Bureau of the Census. Data from U.S. Social Security Administration. *Social Security Bulletin* (quarterly); and U.S. Administration for Children and Families. *Quarterly Public Assistance Statistics* (annual).

★ 549 ★

Social Welfare: Public Aid

Supplemental Security Income

From the source: "Effective January 1, 1993, [there was a] 3.0 percent cost-of-living adjustment to federal benefit rates; new rates are $434 monthly for an individual living in his or her own household and $652 for a couple" (p. 3). Data below reflect the benefits and their recipients for Supplemental Security Income (SSI) in 1991.

	Amounts
Total:	
Benefits paid in 1991	$18.5 billion
Number of recipients[1]	5.2 million
Average benefit[1]	$324.44
Federally administered payments:	
Benefits paid in 1991	$18.0 billion
Number of recipients[1]	5.1 million
Average benefit[1]	$320.53
Federal SSI payments:	
Benefits paid in 1991	$14.8 billion
Number of recipients[1]	4.7 million
Average benefit[1]	$286.03
Federally administered state supplementation:	
Benefits paid in 1991	$3.2 billion
Number of recipients[1]	2.2 million[2]
Average benefit[1]	$130.55
State-administered supplementation:	
Benefits paid in 1991	$0.5 billion
Number of recipients[1]	0.3 million[3]
Average benefit[1]	$150.46

Source: U.S. Department of Health and Human Services. Social Security Administration (SSA). *Annual Statistical Supplement to the "Social Security Bulletin," 1992.* SSA Publication No. 13-11700. Washington, DC: U.S. Department of Health and Human Services, Social Security Administration, Office of Research and Statistics, 1993, p. 3. *Notes:* 1. December 1991. 2. Includes 1.8 million persons receiving federal SSI and state supplementation and 0.4 million persons receiving state supplementation only. 3. Includes 227,000 persons receiving federal SSI and state-administered supplementation and 81,000 persons receiving state supplementation only.

★ 550 ★

Social Welfare: Public Aid

Supplementary Social Insurance Payments, by State: 1990

Figures below represent the amount of federally administered Supplementary Social Insurance (SSI) payments made during 1990, as well as the total number of recipients for that year.

[Dollar amounts in thousands]

State	Total number of persons receiving SSI	Amount of payments			
		Total	Aged	Blind	Disabled
Total	4,817,127[1]	16,132,959	3,559,388	328,949	12,244,622
Alabama	132,824[2]	351,078	83,947	5,026	262,105
Alaska	4,634[2]	13,751	2,298	301	11,152
Arizona	44,780[2]	138,854	23,439	2,377	113,038
Arkansas	75,884	187,290	42,100	3,746	141,444
California	872,772	4,277,847	1,304,385	123,453	2,850,009
Colorado	37,542[2]	109,663	17,095	1,440	91,128
Connecticut	32,042[2]	95,960	14,353	1,551	80,056
Delaware	8,080	22,458	2,951	402	19,105
District of Columbia	16,216	54,424	6,842	759	46,823
Florida	221,754	652,759	199,130	10,402	443,227
Georgia	159,518	415,238	83,685	8,185	323,368
Hawaii	13,776	51,335	17,329	689	33,317
Idaho	10,332[2]	28,959	2,761	478	25,720
Illinois	176,690[2]	593,134	71,064	8,157	513,913
Indiana	60,148[2]	173,927	16,588	3,695	153,644
Iowa	32,724	85,754	11,021	3,122	71,611
Kansas	24,520	65,370	8,112	1,185	56,073
Kentucky	114,700[2]	336,904	50,833	6,539	279,532
Louisiana	133,012	378,012	73,506	7,180	297,326
Maine	23,686	56,469	8,190	811	47,468
Maryland	59,774	185,399	29,125	2,687	153,587
Massachusetts	119,320	396,623	113,059	17,173	266,391
Michigan	143,130	483,254	54,596	8,020	420,638
Minnesota	40,396[2]	110,411	17,191	1,985	91,235
Mississippi	113,854	299,674	70,290	5,017	224,367
Missouri	84,978[2]	236,562	35,572	3,582	197,408
Montana	9,958	28,537	2,578	397	25,562
Nebraska	15,560[2]	41,956	4,708	743	36,505
Nevada	11,334	32,599	9,392	1,764	21,443
New Hampshire	6,870[2]	18,896	2,122	240	16,534
New Jersey	105,312	340,387	75,826	4,040	260,521
New Mexico	31,550[2]	89,874	16,959	1,954	70,961
New York	415,270	1,557,042	341,544	15,232	1,200,266
North Carolina	148,666[2]	403,319	81,209	8,095	314,015
North Dakota	7,494[3]	18,400	3,451	257	14,692
Northern Mariana Islands[3]	538	1,959	835	63	1,061
Ohio	155,736	482,533	40,736	8,067	433,730
Oklahoma	60,430[2]	157,778	32,872	3,127	121,779
Oregon	31,522[2]	95,287	11,229	1,724	82,334

[Continued]

★ 550 ★

Supplementary Social Insurance Payments, by State: 1990

[Continued]

State	Total number of persons receiving SSI	Amount of payments			
		Total	Aged	Blind	Disabled
Pennsylvania	190,470	635,306	86,496	10,156	538,654
Rhode Island	17,420	52,718	10,028	702	41,988
South Carolina	90,334[2]	233,739	47,471	5,714	180,554
South Dakota	10,088	25,880	4,110	472	21,298
Tennessee	139,836	383,634	66,669	6,302	310,663
Texas	294,740[3]	754,954	216,527	16,243	522,184
Utah	12,616[2]	37,870	3,933	944	32,993
Vermont	10,068	30,869	4,591	429	25,849
Virginia	95,490[2]	257,110	51,532	4,739	200,839
Washington	61,538	208,065	26,326	2,807	178,932
West Virginia	47,214[3]	145,802	15,532	2,235	128,035
Wisconsin	85,766	287,982	42,248	4,371	241,363
Wyoming	3,458[2]	9,354	1,002	170	8,182

Source: U.S. Department of Health and Human Services. Social Security Administration (SSA). Office of Research and Statistics. *SSI Recipients by State and County.* Washington, DC: U.S. Department of Health and Human Services, Social Security Administration, Office of Research and Statistics, December 1990, pp. 1, 2. *Notes:* 1. Includes persons with federal SSI payments and/or federally administered state supplementation, unless otherwise indicated. 2. Data for federal SSI payments only; state has state-administered supplementation. 3. Data for federal SSI payments only; state supplementary payment not made.

Social Welfare: Spending

★ 551 ★

Federal Social Welfare Expenditures: 1980-1990

Data are provided by source of funds and by public program.

[In millions of dollars]

Program	1980	1985	1987	1988	1989	1990
Total	303,167	450,788	497,906	527,002	565,170	613,822
Social insurance	191,162	310,175	342,933	360,264	387,280	419,338
Old-age, survivors, disability, health	152,110	257,535	286,340	300,048	324,109	352,362
Health Insurance (Medicare)	34,992	71,384	81,631	83,610	94,552	106,806
Public employee retirement[1]	26,983	40,504	44,092	47,606	50,248	53,514
Railroad employee retirement	4,769	6,276	6,549	6,676	6,971	7,230
Unemployment insurance and employment services[2]	4,408	2,604	2,947	2,965	2,893	3,094
Other railroad employee insurance[3]	224	189	189	100	99	105
State temporary disability insurance[4]	(X)	(X)	(X)	(X)	(X)	(X)
Workers' compensation[5]	2,668	3,067	2,816	2,869	2,960	3,033

[Continued]

★ 551 ★

Federal Social Welfare Expenditures: 1980-1990
[Continued]

Program	1980	1985	1987	1988	1989	1990
Hospital and medical benefits	130	280	348	367	410	433
Public aid	49,394	63,475	70,916	75,934	81,762	92,650
Public assistance[6]	23,542	33,523	39,907	43,431	47,828	54,537
Medical assistance payments[7]	14,550	22,677	27,613	30,771	34,858	40,690
Social services	1,757	2,057	2,023	2,025	2,003	2,065
Supplemental Security Income	6,440	9,605	10,800	11,674	12,469	13,625
Food stamps	9,083	12,513	12,362	13,071	13,589	16,254
Other[8]	10,329	7,834	7,847	7,758	7,876	8,234
Health and medical programs	12,040	18,029	20,806	22,875	24,154	27,515
Hospital and medical care	6,636	9,877	11,861	12,737	12,894	14,733
Civilian programs	2,438	2,455	2,736	3,067	2,736	3,447
Defense Department[9]	4,198	7,422	9,125	9,670	10,158	11,286
Maternal and child health programs	351	422	441	468	494	492
Medical research	4,428	5,992	6,667	7,839	8,548	9,528
Medical facilities construction	210	339	264	0	186	499
Other	1,215	1,399	1,573	1,831	2,032	2,263
Veterans programs	21,255	26,705	27,641	28,845	29,638	30,428
Pensions and compensation	11,306	14,333	14,522	14,914	15,279	15,793
Health and medical programs	6,204	9,493	10,503	11,331	11,663	12,004
Hospital and medical care	5,750	8,809	9,522	10,152	10,782	11,321
Hospital construction	323	458	772	964	646	445
Medical and prosthetic research	131	227	210	215	235	238
Education	2,401	1,171	742	653	647	523
Life insurance[10]	665	796	938	963	1,002	1,038
Welfare and other	679	912	936	984	1,047	1,070
Education[11]	13,452	13,796	16,062	16,966	18,660	18,374
Elementary and secondary[12]	7,430	7,278	8,247	8,826	9,684	9,944
Construction[13]	41	23	21	46	18	23
Higher	4,468	5,102	6,191	6,492	7,404	6,747
Construction	42	32	2	1	22	0
Vocational and adult[13]	1,207	1,087	1,247	1,288	1,209	1,293
Housing	6,278	11,059	11,044	14,006	15,184	16,612
Other social welfare	8,786	7,549	8,504	8,112	8,492	8,905
Vocational rehabilitation	1,006	1,187	1,386	1,489	1,560	1,661
Medical services and research	237	275	319	343	390	415
Institutional care[14]	74	121	130	138	141	143
Child nutrition[15]	4,209	4,349	5,050	4,956	5,197	5,470
Child welfare[16]	57	200	222	239	247	253

[Continued]

★551★

Federal Social Welfare Expenditures: 1980-1990

[Continued]

Program	1980	1985	1987	1988	1989	1990
Special CSA and ACTION programs[17]	2,303	504	520	153	163	169
Welfare, not elsewhere classified[18]	1,137	1,188	1,196	1,137	1,184	1,209

Source: 1993 Statistical Abstract of the United States on CD-ROM [machine-readable datafiles]. CD-ABSTR-93. Washington, DC: U.S. Department of Commerce, Economics and Statistics Administration, Bureau of the Census, Data User Services Division, 1993. Primary source: U.S. Social Security Administration. Social Security Bulletin (winter 1992); and unpublished data. Notes: "X" represents "not applicable." 1. Excludes refunds to those leaving service. Federal data include military retirement. 2. Includes compensation for federal employees and ex-servicemen, trade adjustment and cash training allowance, and payments under extended, emergency, disaster, and special unemployment insurance programs. 3. Unemployment and temporary disability insurance. 4. Cash and medical benefits in five areas. Includes private plans where applicable. 5. Benefits paid by private insurance carriers, state funds, and self-insurers. Federal includes black lung benefit programs. 6. Includes payments under state general assistance programs and work incentive activities, not shown separately. 7. Medicaid payments and state and local general assistance medical payments. 8. Refugee assistance, surplus food for the needy, and work-experience training programs under the Comprehensive Employment and Training Act. Beginning 1985, includes low-income energy assistanprogram. 9. Includes medical care for military dependent families. 10. Excludes servicemen's group life insurance. 11. Federal expenditures include administrative costs (Department of Education) and research, not shown separately. 12. Beginning 1987, all state and local vocational education costs included with elementary-secondary. 13. Construction costs of vocational and adult education programs included under elementary-secondary expenditures. 14. Federal expenditures represent primarily surplus foods for nonprofit institutions. 15. Surplus food for schools and programs under National School Lunch and Child Nutrition Acts. 16. Represents primarily child welfare services under Title V of the Social Security Act. 17. Includes domestic volunteer programs under ACTION and community action and migrant workers programs under Community Services Administration (CSA). Beginning 1988, represents ACTION funds only. 18. Federal expenditures include administrative expenses of the Secretary of Health and Human Services; Indian welfare and guidance; and aging and juvenile delinquency activities. State and local include antipoverty and manpower programs, child care and adoption services, legal assistancand other unspecified welfare services.

★552★

Social Welfare: Spending

Private Expenditures for Social Welfare: 1980-1990

Data are provided by type of expenditure.

[In millions of dollars, except percentages]

Type	1980	1982	1983	1984	1985	1986	1987	1988	1989	1990
Total expenditures	246,000	323,690	362,240	398,403	447,120	495,860	525,919	573,768	623,617	680,868
Percent of gross domestic product	9.1	10.3	10.6	10.5	11.1	11.6	11.6	11.7	11.9	12.3
Health	145,000	191,300	211,000	230,000	247,900	264,600	285,700	318,900	350,200	383,600
Income maintenance	51,169	70,096	82,423	93,235	116,207	140,748	140,354	145,790	152,144	163,559
Private pension plan payments [1][2]	37,560	54,325	66,683	76,683	98,450	122,209	120,442	124,546	129,662	140,142
Short-term sickness and disability[2]	6,280	6,884	6,993	7,497	8,026	8,030	8,896	9,636	9,869	10,372
Long-term disability[2]	1,282	1,688	1,817	1,874	1,937	2,263	2,293	2,295	2,892	3,054
Life insurance and death[3]	5,075	6,269	6,519	6,899	7,489	7,797	8,166	8,418	9,063	9,221
Supplemental unemployment[2]	972	930	411	282	305	449	557	895	658	770
Education	27,055	34,227	37,448	40,469	44,099	47,426	52,436	55,860	61,351	66,872
Welfare and other services	22,776	28,067	31,369	34,699	38,914	43,086	47,429	53,218	59,922	66,837

Source: 1993 Statistical Abstract of the United States on CD-ROM [machine-readable datafiles]. CD-ABSTR-93. Washington, DC: U.S. Department of Commerce, Economics and Statistics Administration, Bureau of the Census, Data User Services Division, 1993. Primary source: U.S. Social Security Administration. Annual Statistical Supplement to the "Social Security Bulletin" (annual). Notes: 1. Covers benefits paid for solely by employers and all benefits of employment-related pension plans to which employee contributions are made. Excludes individual savings plans such as Individual Retirement Accounts (IRAs) and Keogh plans. Pension plan benefits include monthly benefits and lump-sum distributions to retired and disabled employees and their dependents and to survivors of deceased employees. Also includes preretirement lump-sum distributions. 2. Covers wage and salary workers in private industry. 3. Covers all wage and salary workers.

★ 553 ★
Social Welfare: Spending

Social Welfare Expenditures Under Public Programs as Percent of Gross Domestic Product and Total Federal Government Outlays: 1960-1990

For fiscal years ending in years shown. Represents outlays from trust funds (mostly social insurance funds built up by earmarked contributions from insured persons, their employers, or both) and budgetary outlays from general revenues. Includes administrative expenditures, capital outlay, and some expenditures and payments outside the United States.

Year	Total expenditures				Federal government			
	Total (billion dollars)	Percent change[1]	Percent of		Total (billion dollars)	Percent change[1]	Percent of	
			Total GDP[2]	Total government outlays			Total GDP[2]	Total federal outlays
1960	52	10.8	10.3	38.4	25	1.9	4.9	28.1
1970	146	14.6	14.8	46.5	77	13.2	7.8	40.0
1975	289	21.2	19.1	56.6	167	21.9	11.0	53.7
1980	493	14.7	18.6	57.2	303	15.2	11.4	54.4
1985	732	8.0	18.4	52.2	451	7.1	11.3	48.7
1990	702	6.8	18.5	53.3	473	4.9	11.2	48.6
1987	834	6.7	18.7	55.3	498	5.3	11.1	50.2
1988	887	6.4	18.4	54.9	527	5.8	10.9	49.5
1989	957	7.9	18.5	55.2	565	7.2	10.9	49.5
1990	1,045	9.2	19.1	56.6	614	8.7	11.2	51.1

Source: 1993 Statistical Abstract of the United States on CD-ROM [machine-readable datafiles]. CD-ABSTR-93. Washington, DC: U.S. Department of Commerce, Economics and Statistics Administration, Bureau of the Census, Data User Services Division, 1993. Primary source: U.S. Social Security Administration. *Social Security Bulletin* (winter 1992); and unpublished data. *Notes:* 1. Percent change from immediate prior year. 2. Gross domestic product (GDP).

★ 554 ★

Social Welfare: Spending

Social Welfare Expenditures Under Public Programs as Percent of Gross Domestic Product and Total State and Local Government Outlays: 1960-1990

For fiscal years ending in years shown. Represents outlays from trust funds (mostly social insurance funds built up by earmarked contributions from insured persons, their employers, or both) and budgetary outlays from general revenues. Includes administrative expenditures, capital outlay, and some expenditures and payments outside the United States.

Year	Total expenditures				State and local government expenditures			
	Total (billion dollars)	Percent change[1]	Percent of		Total (billion dollars)	Percent change[1]	Percent of	
			Total GDP[2]	Total government outlays			Total GDP[2]	Total state and local government outlays
1960	52	10.8	10.3	38.4	27	19.3	5.4	60.1
1970	146	14.6	14.8	46.5	68	16.3	6.9	57.9
1975	289	21.2	19.1	56.6	122	19.6	8.1	61.6
1980	493	14.7	18.6	57.2	190	13.8	7.2	62.9
1985	732	8.0	18.4	52.2	281	9.3	7.1	59.9
1986	782	6.8	18.5	53.3	309	9.8	7.3	64.2
1987	834	6.7	18.7	55.3	336	8.8	7.6	66.6
1988	887	6.4	18.4	54.9	360	7.2	7.5	67.0
1989	957	7.9	18.5	55.2	392	8.8	7.6	68.0
1990	1,045	9.2	19.1	56.6	432	10.0	7.9	68.2

Source: 1993 Statistical Abstract of the United States on CD-ROM [machine-readable datafiles]. CD-ABSTR-93. Washington, DC: U.S. Department of Commerce, Economics and Statistics Administration, Bureau of the Census, Data User Services Division, 1993. Primary source: U.S. Social Security Administration. *Social Security Bulletin* (winter 1992); and unpublished data. *Notes:* 1. Percent change from immediate prior year. 2. Gross domestic product (GDP).

★ 555 ★

Social Welfare: Spending

Social Welfare Expenditures Under Public Programs, by Type of Program: 1960-1990

For fiscal years ending in years shown. Represents outlays from trust funds (mostly social insurance funds built up by earmarked contributions from insured persons, their employers, or both) and budgetary outlays from general revenues. Includes administrative expenditures, capital outlay, and some expenditures and payments outside the United States.

[In billions of dollars, except as noted]

Year	Total	Social insurance	Public aid	Health and medical programs[2]	Veterans programs	Education	Housing	Other social welfare	All health and medical care[3]
Total:									
1960	52	19	4	4	5	18	(Z)	1	6
1970	146	55	16	10	9	51	1	4	25
1975	289	123	41	17	17	81	3	7	51
1980	493	230	73	27	21	121	7	14	100
1985	732	370	98	39	27	172	13	14	171
1986	782	391	104	44	27	189	12	14	186
1987	834	413	112	48	28	205	13	15	203
1988	887	434	120	53	29	219	17	15	218
1989	957	468	129	57	30	239	18	17	241
1990	1,045	511	147	62	31	258	19	18	272
Federal:									
1960	25	14	2	2	5	1	(Z)	(Z)	3
1970	77	45	10	5	9	6	1	2	16
1975	167	100	27	8	17	9	3	4	33
1980	303	191	49	13	21	13	6	9	69
1985	451	310	63	18	27	14	11	8	122
1986	473	326	67	19	27	15	10	8	131
1987	498	343	71	21	28	16	11	9	141
1988	527	360	76	23	29	17	14	8	149
1989	565	387	82	24	30	19	15	8	166
1990	614	419	93	28	30	18	17	9	188
State and local:									
1960	27	5	2	3	(Z)	17	(Z)	1	3
1970	68	9	7	5	(Z)	45	(Z)	2	9
1975	122	23	14	9	(Z)	72	1	3	18
1980	190	39	23	14	(Z)	108	1	5	31
1985	281	59	35	21	(Z)	158	2	6	49
1986	309	65	37	25	(Z)	174	2	6	55
1987	336	70	41	27	(Z)	188	2	7	62
1988	360	74	44	30	(Z)	202	3	7	68
1989	392	81	47	33	(Z)	220	3	8	75
1990	432	91	53	35	(Z)	240	3	9	84
Percent of total expenditures by type:									
1960	100	37	8	9	11	34	(Z)	2	12
1970	100	38	11	7	6	35	1	3	17

[Continued]

★ 555 ★

Social Welfare Expenditures Under Public Programs, by Type of Program: 1960-1990
[Continued]

Year	Total	Social insurance	Public aid	Health and medical programs[2]	Veterans programs	Education	Housing	Other social welfare	All health and medical care[3]
1980	100	47	15	6	4	25	1	3	20
1985	100	51	13	5	4	24	2	2	24
1986	100	50	13	6	4	24	2	2	24
1987	100	50	13	6	3	25	2	2	25
1988	100	49	13	6	3	25	2	2	25
1989	100	49	13	6	3	25	2	2	25
1990	100	49	14	6	3	25	2	2	26
Percent (federal):									
1960	48	74	52	39	98	5	81	37	46
1970	53	83	59	48	99	12	83	55	65
1980	62	83	68	47	99	11	91	65	69
1985	62	84	64	46	99	8	88	56	71
1986	60	83	64	44	99	8	84	55	70
1987	60	83	62	43	99	8	84	56	69
1988	59	83	63	43	99	8	85	52	68
1989	59	83	63	43	99	8	84	51	69
1990	59	82	64	44	98	7	85	50	69
Per capita (current dollars):[3]									
1960	285	105	22	24	30	96	1	6	35
1970	698	262	79	46	43	244	3	20	120
1980	2,126	990	314	118	92	523	30	59	434
1985	3,008	1,516	405	161	111	708	52	56	705
1986	3,183	1,588	425	179	111	772	49	58	758
1987	3,363	1,662	453	194	112	826	53	62	822
1988	3,538	1,724	479	213	116	878	66	62	871
1989	3,789	1,849	510	226	117	947	72	66	957
1990	4,116	2,008	575	246	120	1,020	77	71	1,072
Per capita (constant 1990 dollars): [34]									
1960	1,182	435	91	100	124	398	4	25	145
1970	2,219	833	251	146	137	776	10	64	382
1980	3,348	1,559	495	186	145	824	47	93	684
1985	3,676	1,853	495	197	136	865	64	68	862
1986	3,796	1,895	507	214	132	921	58	69	904
1987	3,835	1,895	517	221	128	942	60	71	937
1988	3,886	1,893	526	234	127	964	72	68	957

[Continued]

★ 555 ★

Social Welfare Expenditures Under Public Programs, by Type of Program: 1960-1990
[Continued]

Year	Total	Social insurance	Public aid	Health and medical programs[2]	Veterans programs	Education	Housing	Other social welfare	All health and medical care[3]
1989	3,979	1,942	536	237	123	994	76	69	1,005
1990	4,116	2,008	575	246	120	1,020	77	71	1,072

Source: 1993 Statistical Abstract of the United States on CD-ROM [machine-readable datafiles]. CD-ABSTR-93. Washington, DC: U.S. Department of Commerce, Economics and Statistics Administration, Bureau of the Census, Data User Services Division, 1993. Primary source: U.S. Social Security Administration. Social Security Bulletin (winter 1992); and unpublished data. Notes: Z represents less than $500 million or 0.5 percent. 1. Excludes program parts of social insurance, public aid, veterans, and other social welfare. 2. Combines "health and medical programs" with medical services included in social insurance, public aid, veterans, vocational rehabilitation, and antipoverty programs. 3. Excludes payments within foreign countries for education, veterans, Old-Age, Survivors, and Disability Health Insurance (OASDHI), and civil service retirement. 4. Constant dollar figures are based on implicit price deflators for personal consumption expenditures published by U.S. Bureau of Economic Analysis in Survey of Current Business (July 1992).

★ 556 ★
Social Welfare: Spending

State and Local Social Welfare Expenditures: 1980-1990

Data are provided by sources of funds and by public program.

[In millions of dollars]

Program	1980	1985	1987	1988	1989	1990
Total	189,547	281,460	336,227	360,479	392,343	431,552
Social insurance	38,592	59,421	69,941	73,783	80,764	91,279
Old-age, survivors, disability, health	(X)	(X)	(X)	(X)	(X)	(X)
Health Insurance (Medicare)	(X)	(X)	(X)	(X)	(X)	(X)
Public employee retirement[1]	12,507	22,540	28,000	30,442	33,548	36,851
Railroad employee retirement	(X)	(X)	(X)	(X)	(X)	(X)
Unemployment insurance and employment services[2]	13,919	15,740	15,099	13,152	13,488	16,878
Other railroad employee insurance[3]	(X)	(X)	(X)	(X)	(X)	(X)
State temporary disability insurance[4]	1,377	1,944	2,545	2,754	2,886	3,224
Workers' compensation[5]	10,789	19,197	24,237	27,435	30,844	34,326
Hospital and medical benefits	3,596	6,800	9,271	10,743	12,415	13,897
Public aid	23,309	34,882	41,179	43,734	46,921	52,992
Public assistance[6]	21,522	32,647	38,341	40,721	43,567	49,387
Medical assistance payments[7]	13,020	21,182	25,509	27,269	29,725	34,677
Social services	586	686	674	675	668	688
Supplemental Security Income	1,787	2,235	2,838	3,013	3,354	3,605
Food stamps	(X)	(X)	(X)	(X)	(X)	(X)
Other[8]	(X)	(X)	(X)	(X)	(X)	(X)
Health and medical programs	14,423	21,024	27,309	30,221	33,021	34,913
Hospital and medical care	5,667	6,688	10,118	11,190	11,930	12,778
Civilian programs	5,667	6,688	10,118	11,190	11,930	12,778
Defense Department[9]	(X)	(X)	(X)	(X)	(X)	(X)
Maternal and child health programs	519	800	1,198	1,198	1,295	1,392

[Continued]

★ 556 ★

State and Local Social Welfare Expenditures: 1980-1990
[Continued]

Program	1980	1985	1987	1988	1989	1990
Medical research	496	899	1,180	1,293	1,360	1,475
Medical facilities construction	1,450	1,336	1,227	1,444	1,462	1,427
Other	6,291	11,301	13,586	15,096	16,974	17,841
Veterans programs	212	338	410	409	466	488
Pensions and compensation	(X)	(X)	(X)	(X)	(X)	(X)
Health and medical programs	(X)	(X)	(X)	(X)	(X)	(X)
Hospital and medical care	(X)	(X)	(X)	(X)	(X)	(X)
Hospital construction	(X)	(X)	(X)	(X)	(X)	(X)
Medical and prosthetic research	(X)	(X)	(X)	(X)	(X)	(X)
Education	(X)	(X)	(X)	(X)	(X)	(X)
Life insurance[10]	(X)	(X)	(X)	(X)	(X)	(X)
Welfare and other	212	338	410	409	466	488
Education[11]	107,597	158,251	188,486	202,415	220,111	240,011
Elementary and secondary[12]	79,720	113,419	146,655	159,009	173,487	189,333
Construction[13]	6,483	8,335	11,304	11,743	14,566	10,613
Higher	21,708	36,028	41,831	43,406	46,624	50,678
Construction	1,486	2,314	3,084	3,198	3,290	3,953
Vocational and adult[13]	6,169	8,804	([12])	([12])	([12])	([12])
Housing	601	1,540	2,129	2,550	2,943	2,856
Other social welfare	4,813	6,004	6,773	7,367	8,117	9,013
Vocational rehabilitation	245	350	387	416	439	466
Medical services and research	56	85	94	101	110	116
Institutional care[14]	408	259	384	393	446	486
Child nutrition[15]	643	960	1,180	1,294	1,448	1,696
Child welfare[16]	743	(NA)	(NA)	(NA)	(NA)	(NA)
Special CSA and ACTION programs[17]	(X)	(X)	(X)	(X)	(X)	(X)
Welfare, not elsewhere classified[18]	2,774	4,435	4,822	5,264	5,784	6,365

Source: 1993 Statistical Abstract of the United States on CD-ROM [machine-readable datafiles]. CD-ABSTR-93. Washington, DC: U.S. Department of Commerce, Economics and Statistics Administration, Bureau of the Census, Data User Services Division, 1993. Primary source: U.S. Social Security Administration. Social Security Bulletin (winter 1992); and unpublished data. Notes: "NA" represents "not available." "X" represents "not applicable." 1. Excludes refunds to those leaving service. Federal data include military retirement. 2. Includes compensation for federal employees and ex-servicemen, trade adjustment and cash training allowance, and payments under extended, emergency, disaster, and special unemployment insurance programs. 3. Unemployment and temporary disability insurance. 4. Cash and medical benefits in five areas. Includes private plans where applicable. 5. Benefits paid by private insurance carriers, state funds, and self-insurers. Federal includes black lung benefit programs. 6. Includes payments under state general assistance programs and work incentive activities, not shown separately. 7. Medicaid payments and state and local general assistance medical payments. 8. Refugee assistance, surplus food for the needy, and work-experience training programs under the Comprehensive Employment and Training Act. Beginning 1985, includes low-income energy assistanprogram. 9. Includes medical care for military dependent families. 10. Excludes servicemen's group life insurance. 11. Federal expenditures include administrative costs (Department of Education) and research, not shown separately. 12. Beginning 1987, all state and local vocational education costs included with elementary-secondary. 13. Construction costs of vocational and adult education programs included under elementary-secondary expenditures. 14. Federal expenditures represent primarily surplus foods for nonprofit institutions. 15. Surplus food for schools and programs under National School Lunch and Child Nutrition Acts. 16. Represents primarily child welfare services under Title V of the Social Security Act. 17. Includes domestic volunteer programs under ACTION and community action and migrant workers programs under Community Services Administration (CSA). Beginning 1988, represents ACTION funds only. 18. Federal expenditures include administrative expenses of the Secretary of Health and Human Services; Indian welfare and guidance; and aging and juvenile delinquency activities. State and local include antipoverty and manpower programs, child care and adoption services, legal assistancand other unspecified welfare services.

Veterans

★ 557 ★

Veterans Administration Health Care Summary: 1980-1990

For years ending September 30.

Item	Unit	1980	1985	1988	1989	1990
Facilities operating:						
Hospitals	Number	172	172	172	172	172
Domiciliaries	Number	16	16	29	28	32
Outpatient clinics	Number	226	226	233		
Nursing home units	Number	92	115	119	122	126
Employment[1]	1,000	194	203	202	200	202
Obligations[2]	Million $	6,215	9,258	10,540	11,289	11,840
Medical care	Million $	5,972	8,936	10,230	10,949	11,500
Research in health care	Million $	138	227	215	235	238
Prescriptions dispensed	Million	36.7	48.1	58	60	60
Laboratory[3]	Million	215	173	188	183	188
Radiology examinations	Million	5.7	5.4	5.6	6	6
Inpatients treated[4]	1,000	1,359	1,435	1,224	1,152	1,113
VA facilities	1,000	1,275	1,339	1,130	1,072	1,039
Other facilities	1,000	84	96	94	80	74
Average daily inpatients[5]	1,000	105	100	96	90	87
VA facilities	1,000	84	75	70	67	65
Other facilities	1,000	21	25	26	23	22
Outpatient medical visits	Million	18.0	19.6	23.2	23	23
VA staff	Million	15.8	17.8	21.5	21	21
Fee-basis	Million	2.2	1.8	1.8	2	1

Source: 1993 Statistical Abstract of the United States on CD-ROM [machine-readable datafiles]. CD-ABSTR-93. Washington, DC: U.S. Department of Commerce, Economics and Statistics Administration, Bureau of the Census, Data User Services Division, 1993. Primary source: 1) U.S. Department of Veterans Affairs. Annual Report of the Secretary of Veterans Affairs. 2) U.S. Department of Veterans Affairs. Directory of VA Facilities (biennial). 3) Unpublished data. Notes: 1. Net full-time equivalent. 2. 1980, cost-basis; thereafter, obligation-basis. Includes other obligations not shown separately. 3. Total unweighted laboratory workload. 4. Based on the number of discharges and deaths during the fiscal year, plus the number on the rolls bed occupants and patients on authorized leave of absence) at the end of the fiscal year. Excludes interhospital transfers. 5. Patients receiving hospital care, or nursing bed care.

★ 558 ★

Veterans

Veterans Compensation and Pension Benefits: 1980-1992

As of September 30. "Living" refers to veterans receiving compensation for disability incurred or aggravated while on active duty and to war veterans receiving pension and benefits for nonservice connected disabilities. "Deceased" refers to veterans no longer living whose dependents were receiving pensions and compensation benefits. Data present the number on rolls and the average payment by period of service and status.

Period of service and Veteran status	Veterans on rolls (1,000)					Average payment (annual basis; dollars)[1]				
	1980	1985	1990	1991	1992	1980	1985	1990	1991	1992
Total	4,646	4,006	3,584	3,509	3,428	2,370	3,505	4,335	4,552	4,712
Living veterans	3,195	2,931	2,746	2,709	2,674	2,600	3,666	4,320	4,491	4,611
Service connected	2,273	2,240	2,184	2,179	2,181	2,669	3,692	4,250	4,406	4,593
Nonservice connected	922	690	562	530	493	2,428	3,581	4,591	4,837	4,689
Deceased veterans	1,451	1,075	838	800	754	1,863	3,066	4,382	4,761	5,071
Service connected	358	336	320	318	314	3,801	5,836	7,349	7,815	8,244
Nonservice connected	1,093	739	518	482	440	1,228	1,809	2,548	2,748	2,810
Prior to World War I	14	7	4	4	3	1,432	1,855	2,616	2,921	3,073
Living	(Z)	(Z)	(Z)	(Z)	(Z)	2,634	4,436	10,502	10,441	8,176
World War I	692	381	198	172	146	1,683	2,461	3,435	3,674	3,754
Living	198	68	18	13	9	2,669	4,439	6,922	7,239	6,476
World War II	2,520	2,097	1,723	1,638	1,543	2,307	3,317	4,052	4,238	4,334
Living	1,849	1,575	1,294	1,226	1,153	2,462	3,460	4,123	4,278	4,333
Korean Conflict[2]	446	399	390	388	387	2,691	4,114	5,105	5,330	5,462
Living	317	309	305	304	300	2,977	4,260	5,103	5,288	5,390
Peace-time	312	404	495	518	550	3,080	3,973	4,132	4,216	4,292
Living	262	352	444	468	500	2,828	3,589	3,709	3,789	3,866
Vietnam era[3]	662	716	774	789	804	2,795	4,021	4,945	5,242	5,551
Living	569	626	685	698	711	2,709	3,849	4,671	4,936	5,234
Persian Gulf War	(X)	(X)	(X)	(X)	(Z)	(X)	(X)	(X)	(X)	1,673
Living	(X)	(X)	(X)	(X)	(Z)	(X)	(X)	(X)	(X)	1,386

Source: 1993 Statistical Abstract of the United States on CD-ROM [machine-readable datafiles]. CD-ABSTR-93. Washington, DC: U.S. Department of Commerce, Economics and Statistics Administration, Bureau of the Census, Data User Services Division, 1993. Primary source: U.S. Department of Veterans Affairs. *Annual Report of the Secretary of Veterans Affairs;* and unpublished data. *Notes:* "X" represents "not applicable." "Z" represents fewer than 500. 1. Averages calculated by multiplying average monthly payment by 12. 2. Service during period June 27, 1950, to January 31, 1955.

★ 559 ★

Veterans

Veterans Compensation, by Date of Service: 1970-1992

As of end of fiscal year. Represents veterans receiving compensation for service-connected disabilities. "Totally disabled" refers to veterans with any disability, mental or physical, that are deemed to be total and permanent, that prevent the individual from maintaining a livelihood, and that are rated for disability at 100 percent.

[In thousands, except as indicated]

Military service	1970	1975	1980	1985	1986	1987	1988	1989	1990	1991	1992
Disabled, all periods[1]	2,092	2,220	2,274	2,240	2,225	2,212	2,199	2,192	2,184	2,179	2,181
Peace-time	185	194	262	352	367	382	398	421	444	468	500
World War I	85	55	30	12	10	8	6	5	3	3	2
World War II	1,416	1,309	1,193	1,049	1,015	982	947	912	876	841	805
Korea	239	240	236	223	220	218	215	212	209	205	202
Vietnam	167	423	553	604	613	623	633	643	652	662	671
Totally disabled, all periods[1]	124	123	121	136	133	132	131	131	131	131	132
Peace-time	16	16	20	26	26	26	26	26	27	27	28
World War I	11	6	3	1	1	1	1	(Z)	(Z)	(Z)	(Z)
World War II	63	58	51	54	51	49	47	45	43	41	39
Korea	16	16	16	17	16	16	16	16	16	16	15
Vietnam	18	26	31	38	39	40	41	43	44	46	49
Compensation (million dollars)	2,393	3,797	6,104	8,270	8,379	8,424	8,722	8,937	9,284	9,612	10,018

Source: *1993 Statistical Abstract of the United States on CD ROM* [machine readable datafiles]. CD-AB81H-93. Washington, DC: U.S. Department of Commerce, Economics and Statistics Administration, Bureau of the Census, Data User Services Division, 1993. Primary source: U.S. Department of Veterans Affairs. *Annual Report of the Secretary of Veterans Affairs,* and unpublished data. *Notes:* "Z" equals less than 500. 1. Includes Spanish-American War and Mexican Border Service, not shown separately.

Chapter 8
HEALTH CARE INDUSTRIES

The 111 tables in this chapter profile health-related industries in the manufacturing, service, insurance, retail, and wholesale sectors. Data provided include the number of establishments and employees in each industry; industry expenses, receipts, and revenue; sales ratios and gross margins; and market shares and trends. When available, information on the top performers in each industry is presented. Please see the chapter on Medical Professions for employment information related to specific occupations.

Health Care Services

★ 560 ★

Health and Allied Services, Establishments and Employees

Data provided for establishments that offer health-related and allied services, notably blood banks, blood donor stations, childbirth preparation classes, health screening services, hearing test services, insurance physical exam services, medical photography and art services, osteoporosis centers, oxygen tent services, plasmapheresis centers, and sperm banks.

State	Establishments	Rank	Employees	Rank
Alabama	5105	27	57267	23
Alaska	779	49	4772	50
Arizona	6459	21	43849	27
Arkansas	3302	32	32916	32
California	58109	1	463209	1
Colorado	6424	22	47664	25
Connecticut	6063	23	57593	22
Delaware	1094	46	9467	44
D.C.	1431	45	8981	46
Florida	24048	4	227924	4
Georgia	9412	11	92714	11
Hawaii	1981	39	12755	42
Idaho	1619	43	12728	43

[Continued]

★ 560 ★

Health and Allied Services, Establishments and Employees
[Continued]

State	Establishments	Rank	Employees	Rank
Illinois	17576	7	149733	7
Indiana	8156	15	85301	12
Iowa	4130	30	40381	30
Kansas	3669	31	40392	29
Kentucky	4964	28	52092	24
Louisiana	6588	20	68275	19
Maine	1998	38	17352	39
Maryland	8215	14	65359	21
Massachusetts	10265	10	107643	9
Michigan	15382	8	132393	8
Minnesota	5452	25	68168	20
Mississippi	2949	33	27712	33
Missouri	8045	16	78719	13
Montana	1441	44	9314	45
Nebraska	2202	37	21717	35
Nevada	1883	40	18031	38
New Hampshire	1655	42	15137	41
New Jersey	14688	9	105322	10
New Mexico	2320	36	18913	37
New York	30682	2	231299	3
North Carolina	7784	17	74010	17
North Dakota	707	51	8856	47
Ohio	17607	6	164224	5
Oklahoma	5282	26	45901	26
Oregon	5573	24	43257	28
Pennsylvania	19874	5	152000	6
Rhode Island	1832	41	16090	40
South Carolina	4181	29	36518	31
South Dakota	912	47	8007	48
Tennessee	7399	18	75344	16
Texas	26497	3	263574	2
Utah	2942	34	21156	36
Vermont	877	48	6207	49
Virginia	8367	13	78403	14
Washington	8662	12	71413	18
West Virginia	2607	35	21892	34
Wisconsin	6830	19	76038	15
Wyoming	734	50	4420	51
U.S. Total	406753	-	3592482	-

Source: Census of Service Industries on CD-ROM, 1987. Geographic Area Series [machine-readable datafiles]. Prepared by U.S. Bureau of the Census. Washington, DC: The Bureau, 1990. *Note:* Data shown only for businesses subject to federal income taxes.

★ 561 ★

Health Care Services

Health and Allied Services, Expenses: 1990-1991

Figures represent estimated annual expenses and year-to-year percent change in annual expenses for tax-exempt firms.

[In millions of dollars]

Year	Expenses	Percent change
1991	5,175	13.3
1990	4,568	

Source: "1991 Service Annual Survey: Health Services." In CENDATA [online service]. Washington, DC: U.S. Bureau of the Census [issued 26 July 1993]. No. 10.10.4 and No. 10.10.4.7.

★ 562 ★

Health Care Services

Health and Allied Services, Receipts: 1987-1991

Figures represent estimated annual receipts for taxable firms.

[In millions of dollars]

Year	Receipts
1991	12,562
1990	10,618
1989	(NA)
1988	(NA)
1987	(NA)

Source: "1991 Service Annual Survey: Health Services." In CENDATA [online service]. Washington, DC: U.S. Bureau of the Census [issued 26 July 1993]. No. 10.10.4 and No. 10.10.4.7. *Note:* "NA" indicates "not available."

★ 563 ★

Health Care Services

Health and Allied Services, Revenue: 1987-1991

Figures represent estimated annual revenue for tax-exempt firms.

[In millions of dollars]

Year	Revenue
1991	5,010
1990	4,480
1989	(NA)
1988	(NA)
1987	(NA)

Source: "1991 Service Annual Survey: Health Services." In CENDATA [online service]. Washington, DC: U.S. Bureau of the Census [issued 26 July 1993]. No. 10.10.4 and No. 10.10.4.7. *Note:* "NA" indicates "not available."

★ 564 ★

Health Care Services

Health-Related Personal Services, Establishments and Employees

Table below reflects data for establishments providing specialized services to individuals; for example, diet and weight reduction workshops.

State	Establishments	Rank	Employees	Rank
Alabama	32	29	82	30
Arizona	29	31	96	29
Arkansas	33	28	100	28
California	378	1	1874	1
Colorado	64	19	249	19
Connecticut	52	21	179	23
Florida	121	7	383	12
Georgia	55	20	129	26
Illinois	179	4	772	2
Indiana	125	6	456	9
Iowa	37	27	135	25
Kansas	40	25	207	21
Kentucky	75	17	260	18
Louisiana	7	34	18	34
Maryland	46	23	194	22
Massachusetts	98	12	337	13
Michigan	197	3	758	3
Minnesota	113	9	534	8
Mississippi	17	33	0[1]	-
Missouri	92	13	307	14
Nebraska	19	32	46	33
New Jersey	74	18	233	20
New York	128	5	606	5

[Continued]

★ 564 ★

Health-Related Personal Services, Establishments and Employees
[Continued]

State	Establishments	Rank	Employees	Rank
North Carolina	112	10	297	15
Ohio	204	2	697	4
Oklahoma	43	24	81	31
Oregon	47	22	152	24
Pennsylvania	125	6	535	7
South Carolina	38	26	80	32
Tennessee	89	15	281	16
Texas	117	8	564	6
Utah	30	30	122	27
Virginia	90	14	390	11
Washington	106	11	391	10
Wisconsin	82	16	280	17
U.S. Total	3317	-	12595	-

Source: *Census of Service Industries on CD-ROM, 1987.* Geographic Area Series [machine-readable datafiles]. Prepared by U.S. Bureau of the Census. Washington, DC: The Bureau, 1990. *Notes:* Data shown only for businesses subject to federal income taxes. 1. Data are withheld to avoid disclosure of individual companies.

★ 565 ★

Health Care Services

Home Health Care Services, Establishments and Employees

State	Establishments	Rank	Employees	Rank
Alabama	69	22	1979	24
Alaska	3	45	0[1]	-
Arizona	55	25	2003	23
Arkansas	33	30	600	33
California	513	1	13784	4
Colorado	82	20	2435	18
Connecticut	77	21	2983	17
Delaware	14	40	366	40
D.C.	9	42	414	39
Florida	465	2	14690	3
Georgia	140	11	3367	15
Hawaii	3	45	0[1]	-
Idaho	19	37	208	44
Illinois	200	7	7731	6
Indiana	105	16	2310	20
Iowa	37	28	789	30
Kansas	31	31	812	29
Kentucky	64	23	1656	26
Louisiana	130	13	2340	19
Maine	17	38	540	36

[Continued]

★ 565 ★

Home Health Care Services, Establishments and Employees
[Continued]

State	Establishments	Rank	Employees	Rank
Maryland	84	19	1855	25
Massachusetts	138	12	7528	7
Michigan	195	8	6567	9
Minnesota	49	26	2296	21
Mississippi	36	29	476	37
Missouri	107	15	4149	14
Montana	7	43	81	47
Nebraska	21	36	656	32
Nevada	24	34	759	31
New Hampshire	16	39	241	43
New Jersey	178	9	7438	8
New Mexico	22	35	561	34
New York	426	3	29645	1
North Carolina	91	18	2079	22
North Dakota	11	41	255	42
Ohio	174	10	5996	10
Oklahoma	63	24	1576	27
Oregon	42	27	919	28
Pennsylvania	281	5	8894	5
Rhode Island	25	33	544	35
South Carolina	36	29	0[1]	-
South Dakota	5	44	107	46
Tennessee	222	6	5375	11
Texas	399	4	23478	2
Utah	16	39	334	41
Vermont	7	43	0[1]	-
Virginia	117	14	4456	12
Washington	91	18	3199	16
West Virginia	27	32	458	38
Wisconsin	97	17	4313	13
Wyoming	7	43	128	45
U.S. Total	5080	-	184793	-

Source: Census of Service Industries on CD-ROM, 1987. Geographic Area Series [machine-readable datafiles]. Prepared by U.S. Bureau of the Census. Washington, DC: The Bureau, 1990. Notes: Data shown only for businesses subject to federal income taxes. 1. Data are withheld to avoid disclosure of individual companies.

★ 566 ★

Health Care Services

Home Health Care Services, Expenses: 1990-1991

Figures represent estimated annual expenses and year-to-year percent change in annual expenses for tax-exempt firms.

[In millions of dollars]

Year	Expenses	Percent change
1991	3,649	19.4
1990	3,057	

Source: "1991 Service Annual Survey: Health Services." In CENDATA [online service]. Washington, DC: U.S. Bureau of the Census [issued 26 July 1993]. No. 10.10.4 and No. 10.10.4.7.

★ 567 ★

Health Care Services

Home Health Care Services, Receipts: 1987-1991

Figures represent estimated annual receipts for taxable firms.

[In millions of dollars]

Year	Receipts
1991	7,381
1990	6,196
1989	(NA)
1988	(NA)
1987	(NA)

Source: "1991 Service Annual Survey: Health Services." In CENDATA [online service]. Washington, DC: U.S. Bureau of the Census [issued 26 July 1993]. No. 10.10.4 and No. 10.10.4.7. *Note:* "NA" indicates "not available."

★ 568 ★

Health Care Services

Home Health Care Services, Revenue: 1987-1991

Figures represent estimated annual revenue for tax-exempt firms.

[In millions of dollars]

Year	Revenue
1991	3,859
1990	3,233
1989	(NA)
1988	(NA)
1987	(NA)

Source: "1991 Service Annual Survey: Health Services." In CENDATA [online service]. Washington, DC: U.S. Bureau of the Census [issued 26 July 1993]. No. 10.10.4 and No. 10.10.4.7. *Note:* "NA" indicates "not available."

★ 569 ★

Health Care Services

Home Health Care Services, Top Providers: 1993

Based on 1993 total revenues.

[In billion dollars]

Type of service	Revenue
Home nursing and aides 　Olsten (Westbury, New York) 　Interim Healthcare (Fort Lauderdale, Florida) 　Visiting Nurse Services of New York (New York, New York)	21
Durable medical equipment 　Homedco Group (Fountain Valley, California) 　Abbey Healthcare Group (Costa Mesa, California) 　Lincare (Clearwater, Florida)	6
Home infusion therapy 　Caremark International (Northbrook, Illinois) 　T2 Medical (Alpharetta, Georgia) 　Medical Care America (Dallas, Texas)	4

Source: "Who's Big in Home Care." *Business Week,* 14 March 1994, p. 72. Primary sources: National Association for Home Care; U.S. Department of Commerce; *Home Health Line.*

★ 570 ★

Health Care Services

Kidney Dialysis Centers, Establishments and Employees

State	Establishments	Rank	Employees	Rank
Alabama	26	8	281	14
Alaska	0	-	0	-
Arizona	10	14	160	16
Arkansas	7	17	71	22
California	126	1	2262	1
Colorado	6	18	127	18
Connecticut	2	22	0^1	-
Delaware	1	23	0^1	-
D.C.	8	16	0^1	-
Florida	69	3	1085	3
Georgia	41	5	698	6
Hawaii	0	-	0	-
Idaho	0	-	0	-
Illinois	25	9	428	9
Indiana	6	18	0^1	-
Iowa	1	23	0^1	-
Kansas	4	20	61	23
Kentucky	3	21	0^1	-
Louisiana	39	6	629	7
Maine	3	21	0^1	-
Maryland	20	12	354	13
Massachusetts	9	15	387	11
Michigan	7	17	0^1	-
Minnesota	0	-	0	-
Mississippi	5	19	84	21
Missouri	7	17	85	20
Montana	0	-	0	-
Nebraska	0	-	0	-
Nevada	2	22	0^1	-
New Hampshire	2	22	0^1	-
New Jersey	9	15	0^1	-
New Mexico	5	19	85	20
New York	20	12	761	5
North Carolina	21	11	425	10
North Dakota	0	-	0	-
Ohio	9	15	152	17
Oklahoma	4	20	46	24
Oregon	3	21	0^1	-
Pennsylvania	48	4	981	4
Rhode Island	2	22	0^1	-
South Carolina	23	10	357	12
South Dakota	0	-	0	-
Tennessee	16	13	184	15
Texas	80	2	1451	2
Utah	3	21	0^1	-
Vermont	0	-	0	-

[Continued]

★ 570 ★

Kidney Dialysis Centers, Establishments and Employees
[Continued]

State	Establishments	Rank	Employees	Rank
Virginia	28	7	455	8
Washington	1	23	0^1	-
West Virginia	6	18	110	19
Wisconsin	4	20	0^1	-
Wyoming	0	-	0	-
U.S. Total	711	-	13102	-

Source: Census of Service Industries on CD-ROM, 1987. Geographic Area Series [machine-readable datafiles]. Prepared by U.S. Bureau of the Census. Washington, DC: The Bureau, 1990. Notes: Data shown only for businesses subject to federal income taxes. 1. Data are withheld to avoid disclosure of individual companies.

★ 571 ★

Health Care Services

Kidney Dialysis Centers, Expenses: 1990-1991

Figures represent estimated annual expenses and year-to-year percent change in annual expenses for tax-exempt firms.

[In millions of dollars]

Year	Expenses	Percent change
1991	398	16.4
1990	342	

Source: "1991 Service Annual Survey: Health Services." In CENDATA [online service]. Washington, DC: U.S. Bureau of the Census [issued 26 July 1993]. No. 10.10.4 and No. 10.10.4.7.

★ 572 ★

Health Care Services

Kidney Dialysis Centers, Receipts: 1987-1991

Figures represent estimated annual receipts for taxable firms.

[In millions of dollars]

Year	Receipts
1991	1,505
1990	1,272
1989	(NA)
1988	(NA)
1987	(NA)

Source: "1991 Service Annual Survey: Health Services." In CENDATA [online service]. Washington, DC: U.S. Bureau of the Census [Issued 26 July 1993]. No. 10.10.4 and No. 10.10.4.7. *Note:* "NA" indicates "not available."

★ 573 ★

Health Care Services

Kidney Dialysis Centers, Revenue: 1987-1991

Figures represent estimated annual revenue for tax-exempt firms.

[In millions of dollars]

Year	Revenue
1991	319
1990	273
1989	(NA)
1988	(NA)
1987	(NA)

Source: "1991 Service Annual Survey: Health Services." In CENDATA [online service]. Washington, DC: U.S. Bureau of the Census [Issued 26 July 1993]. No. 10.10.4 and No. 10.10.4.7. *Note:* "NA" indicates "not available."

★ 574 ★

Health Care Services

Medical Equipment Rental and Leasing, Establishments and Employees

State	Establishments	Rank	Employees	Rank
Alabama	46	17	247	18
Alaska	0	-	0	-
Arizona	38	18	260	15
Arkansas	54	14	253	17
California	214	1	2258	1
Colorado	26	24	178	27
Connecticut	21	27	90	35
Delaware	3	35	0^1	-
D.C.	1	37	0^1	-
Florida	172	2	1090	5
Georgia	62	12	479	12
Hawaii	3	35	7	45
Idaho	2	36	0^1	-
Illinois	97	6	1474	3
Indiana	68	11	759	8
Iowa	37	19	224	22
Kansas	24	25	183	25
Kentucky	54	14	232	21
Louisiana	31	21	180	26
Maine	19	28	106	33
Maryland	29	23	258	16
Massachusetts	51	16	260	15
Michigan	79	7	894	6
Minnesota	30	22	290	14
Mississippi	24	25	99	34
Missouri	60	13	436	13
Montana	14	30	37	40
Nebraska	22	26	155	29
Nevada	13	31	75	38
New Hampshire	15	29	76	37
New Jersey	75	9	688	10
New Mexico	19	28	135	31
New York	127	5	816	7
North Carolina	46	17	246	19
North Dakota	7	33	21	43
Ohio	72	10	727	9
Oklahoma	53	15	207	23
Oregon	13	31	143	30
Pennsylvania	145	4	1452	4
Rhode Island	5	34	14	44
South Carolina	24	25	110	32
South Dakota	7	33	78	36
Tennessee	77	8	597	11
Texas	155	3	1482	2
Utah	13	31	42	39
Vermont	7	33	36	41

[Continued]

★ 574 ★

Medical Equipment Rental and Leasing, Establishments and Employees
[Continued]

State	Establishments	Rank	Employees	Rank
Virginia	53	15	253	17
Washington	29	23	165	28
West Virginia	37	19	245	20
Wisconsin	34	20	206	24
Wyoming	10	32	32	42
U.S. Total	2317	-	18377	-

Source: Census of Service Industries on CD-ROM, 1987. Geographic Area Series [machine-readable datafiles]. Prepared by U.S. Bureau of the Census. Washington, DC: The Bureau, 1990. *Notes:* Data shown only for businesses subject to federal income taxes. 1. Data are withheld to avoid disclosure of individual companies.

★ 575 ★
Health Care Services

Medical Equipment Rental and Leasing, Receipts: 1987-1991

Figures represent estimated annual receipts for taxable firms.

[In millions of dollars]

Year	Receipts
1991	2,424
1990	2,270
1989	NA
1988	NA
1987	NA

Source: "1991 Service Annual Survey: Business and Selected Professional Services." In CENDATA [online service]. Washington, DC: U.S. Bureau of the Census [issued 26 July 1993]. No. 10.10.4 and No. 10.10.4.4. *Note:* "NA" indicates "not available."

★ 576 ★

Health Care Services

Specialty Outpatient Facilities, Expenses: 1990-1991

Figures represent estimated annual expenses and year-to-year percent change in annual expenses for tax-exempt firms.

[In millions of dollars]

Year	Expenses	Percent change
1991	3,330	11.6
1990	2,983	

Source: "1991 Service Annual Survey: Health Services." In CENDATA [online service]. Washington, DC: U.S. Bureau of the Census [issued 26 July 1993]. No. 10.10.4 and No. 10.10.4.7.

★ 577 ★

Health Care Services

Specialty Outpatient Facilities, Receipts: 1987-1991

Figures represent estimated annual receipts for taxable firms.

[In millions of dollars]

Year	Receipts
1991	6,426
1990	5,258
1989	(NA)
1988	(NA)
1987	(NA)

Source: "1991 Service Annual Survey: Health Services." In CENDATA [online service]. Washington, DC: U.S. Bureau of the Census [issued 20 July 1993]. No. 10.10.4 and No. 10.10.4.7. *Note:* "NA" indicates "not available."

★ 578 ★

Health Care Services

Specialty Outpatient Facilities, Revenue: 1987-1991

Figures represent estimated annual revenue for tax-exempt firms.

[In millions of dollars]

Year	Revenue
1991	3,289
1990	3,018
1989	(NA)
1988	(NA)
1987	(NA)

Source: "1991 Service Annual Survey: Health Services." In CENDATA [online service]. Washington, DC: U.S. Bureau of the Census [issued 26 July 1993]. No. 10.10.4 and No. 10.10.4.7. *Note:* "NA" indicates "not available."

Hospitals

★ 579 ★

For-Profit Hospitals, by Size

Table ranks for-profit hospitals by number of beds.

Hospital companies	Beds
Columbia-HCA (Nashville, Tennessee; Louisville, Kentucky)	42,000
Quorum Health Group (Brentwood, Tennessee)	25,564
Health Trust Inc. (Nashville, Tennessee)	9,700
Charter Medical Corp. (Macon, Georgia)	7,186
American Medical International (Dallas, Texas)	7,030
National Medical Enterprises (Santa Monica, California)	5,614
Community Psychiatric Centers (Santa Monica, California)	4,113

Source: Day, Kathleen. "Thinning the Health Care Herd." *Washington Post,* 5 October 1993, p. C1. Primary source: HCIA.

★ 580 ★

Hospitals

General Medical and Surgical Hospitals, Establishments and Employees

State	Establishments	Rank	Employees	Rank
Alabama	43	6	0[1]	-
Alaska	2	20	0[1]	-
Arizona	10	13	3386	16
Arkansas	17	9	3052	17
California	144	2	53596	1
Colorado	8	15	0[1]	-
Connecticut	0	-	0	-
Delaware	0	-	0	-
D.C.	0	-	0	-
Florida	98	3	44776	3
Georgia	39	7	10057	7
Hawaii	1	21	0[1]	-
Idaho	3	19	0[1]	-
Illinois	14	12	5344	9
Indiana	6	17	2181	20
Iowa	3	19	0[1]	-
Kansas	7	16	0[1]	-
Kentucky	27	8	0[1]	-
Louisiana	49	5	11741	5
Maine	0	-	0	-
Maryland	3	19	0[1]	-
Massachusetts	3	19	994	23
Michigan	2	20	0[1]	-
Minnesota	5	18	0[1]	-
Mississippi	14	12	2486	19
Missouri	14	12	4870	10
Montana	3	19	0[1]	-
Nebraska	2	20	0[1]	-
Nevada	8	15	4022	13
New Hampshire	2	20	0[1]	-
New Jersey	1	21	0[1]	-
New Mexico	7	16	3737	14
New York	16	10	10405	6
North Carolina	15	11	4207	12
North Dakota	1	21	0[1]	-
Ohio	2	20	0[1]	-
Oklahoma	15	11	3620	15
Oregon	8	15	1979	21
Pennsylvania	5	18	1044	22
Rhode Island	0	-	0	-
South Carolina	16	10	4779	11
South Dakota	0	-	0	-
Tennessee	58	4	13283	4
Texas	164	1	46497	2
Utah	7	16	0[1]	-
Vermont	0	-	0	-

[Continued]

★ 580 ★

General Medical and Surgical Hospitals, Establishments and Employees
[Continued]

State	Establishments	Rank	Employees	Rank
Virginia	16	10	9092	8
Washington	9	14	2907	18
West Virginia	14	12	0[1]	-
Wisconsin	2	20	0[1]	-
Wyoming	2	20	0[1]	-
U.S. Total	885	-	294133	-

Source: Census of Service Industries on CD-ROM, 1987. Geographic Area Series [machine-readable datafiles]. Prepared by U.S. Bureau of the Census. Washington, DC: The Bureau, 1990. Notes: Data shown only for businesses subject to federal income taxes. 1. Data are withheld to avoid disclosure of individual companies.

★ 581 ★

Hospitals

General Medical and Surgical Hospitals, Expenses: 1990-1991

Figures represent estimated annual expenses and year-to-year percent change in annual expenses for tax-exempt firms.

[In millions of dollars]

Year	Expenses	Percent change
1991	217,961	9.9
1990	198,238	

Source: "1991 Service Annual Survey: Health Services." In CENDATA [online service]. Washington, DC: U.S. Bureau of the Census [issued 26 July 1993]. No. 10.10.4 and No. 10.10.4.7.

★ 582 ★

Hospitals

General Medical and Surgical Hospitals, Receipts: 1987-1991

Figures represent estimated annual receipts for taxable firms.

[In millions of dollars]

Year	Receipts
1991	24,518
1990	22,579
1989	(NA)
1988	(NA)
1987	(NA)

Source: "1991 Service Annual Survey: Health Services." In CENDATA [online service]. Washington, DC: U.S. Bureau of the Census [issued 26 July 1993]. No. 10.10.4 and No. 10.10.4.7. *Note:* "NA" indicates "not available."

★ 583 ★

Hospitals

General Medical and Surgical Hospitals, Revenue: 1987-1991

Figures represent estimated annual revenue for tax-exempt firms.

[In millions of dollars]

Year	Revenue
1991	250,588
1990	225,344
1989	(NA)
1988	(NA)
1987	(NA)

Source: "1991 Service Annual Survey: Health Services." In CENDATA [online service]. Washington, DC: U.S. Bureau of the Census [issued 26 July 1993]. No. 10.10.4 and No. 10.10.4.7. *Note:* "NA" indicates "not available."

★ 584 ★

Hospitals

Hospitals, Establishments and Employees

Hospitals provide diagostic services, treatment, surgical services, and continuous nursing care. See separate tables for data on medical and surgical hospitals, psychiatric hospitals, and specialty hospitals.

State	Establishments	Rank	Employees	Rank
Alabama	48	7	10604	10
Alaska	4	28	0[1]	-
Arizona	21	16	4039	23
Arkansas	23	14	3544	24
California	214	2	61927	1
Colorado	14	21	4226	22
Connecticut	2	30	0[1]	-
Delaware	3	29	0[1]	-
D.C.	1	31	0[1]	-
Florida	142	3	50056	3
Georgia	60	6	12833	7
Hawaii	2	30	0[1]	-
Idaho	9	25	1612	34
Illinois	24	13	7274	11
Indiana	12	23	3081	27
Iowa	3	29	0[1]	-
Kansas	13	22	4646	16
Kentucky	36	8	11020	9
Louisiana	72	4	15172	4
Maine	1	31	0[1]	-
Maryland	9	25	3190	26
Massachusetts	19	17	5030	15
Michigan	12	23	4638	17
Minnesota	6	26	1305	35
Mississippi	19	17	3005	28
Missouri	23	14	6148	13
Montana	5	27	425	38
Nebraska	4	28	0[1]	-
Nevada	14	21	4599	18
New Hampshire	11	24	2097	33
New Jersey	4	28	2218	32
New Mexico	15	20	4356	20
New York	32	10	14567	6
North Carolina	29	11	6235	12
North Dakota	1	31	0[1]	-
Ohio	9	25	1043	36
Oklahoma	22	15	4532	19
Oregon	15	20	2472	31
Pennsylvania	25	12	4295	21
Rhode Island	0	-	0	-
South Carolina	21	16	5472	14
South Dakota	0	-	0	-
Tennessee	66	5	15159	5
Texas	237	1	56707	2
Utah	16	19	2638	30

[Continued]

★ 584 ★

Hospitals, Establishments and Employees
[Continued]

State	Establishments	Rank	Employees	Rank
Vermont	0	-	0	-
Virginia	33	9	12340	8
Washington	17	18	3440	25
West Virginia	17	18	2869	29
Wisconsin	6	26	796	37
Wyoming	4	28	422	39
U.S. Total	1395	-	366495	-

Source: *Census of Service Industries on CD-ROM, 1987.* Geographic Area Series [machine-readable datafiles]. Prepared by U.S. Bureau of the Census. Washington, DC: The Bureau, 1990. *Notes:* Data shown only for businesses subject to federal income taxes. 1. Data are withheld to avoid disclosure of individual companies.

★ 585 ★
Hospitals

Hospitals, Expenses: 1990-1991

Figures represent estimated annual expenses and year-to-year percent change in annual expenses for tax-exempt firms.

[In millions of dollars]

Year	Expenses	Percent change
1991	238,636	9.8
1990	217,389	

Source: "1991 Service Annual Survey: Health Services." In CENDATA [online service]. Washington, DC: U.S. Bureau of the Census [issued 26 July 1993]. No. 10.10.4 and No. 10.10.4.7.

★ 586 ★

Hospitals

Hospitals, Receipts: 1987-1991

Figures represent estimated annual receipts for taxable firms.

[In millions of dollars]

Year	Receipts
1991	31,523
1990	29,059
1989	25,023
1988	22,777
1987	19,720

Source: "1991 Service Annual Survey: Health Services." In CENDATA [online service]. Washington, DC: U.S. Bureau of the Census [issued 26 July 1993]. No. 10.10.4 and No. 10.10.4.7.

★ 587 ★

Hospitals

Hospitals, Revenue: 1987-1991

Figures represent estimated annual revenue for tax-exempt firms.

[In millions of dollars]

Year	Revenue
1991	274,447
1990	247,214
1989	(NA)
1988	(NA)
1987	(NA)

Source: "1991 Service Annual Survey: Health Services." In CENDATA [online service]. Washington, DC: U.S. Bureau of the Census [issued 26 July 1993]. No. 10.10.4 and No. 10.10.4.7. *Note:* "NA" indicates "not available."

★ 588 ★

Hospitals

Psychiatric Hospitals, Establishments and Employees

These establishments provide diagnostic services and treatment of mental illnesses. Mental hospitals are included in this data.

State	Establishments	Rank	Employees	Rank
Alabama	5	13	0^1	-
Alaska	2	16	0^1	-
Arizona	7	11	580	13
Arkansas	5	13	0^1	-
California	47	2	6257	2
Colorado	6	12	0^1	-
Connecticut	2	16	0^1	-
Delaware	2	16	0^1	-
D.C.	1	17	0^1	-
Florida	29	3	3587	3
Georgia	14	5	1929	6
Hawaii	1	17	0^1	-
Idaho	6	12	0^1	-
Illinois	8	10	0^1	-
Indiana	5	13	0^1	-
Iowa	0	-	0	-
Kansas	5	13	0^1	-
Kentucky	8	10	0^1	-
Louisiana	21	4	0^1	-
Maine	1	17	0^1	-
Maryland	4	14	0^1	-
Massachusetts	8	10	1858	8
Michigan	0	12	0^1	-
Minnesota	1	17	0^1	-
Mississippi	4	14	0^1	-
Missouri	9	9	1278	11
Montana	2	16	0^1	-
Nebraska	2	16	0^1	-
Nevada	5	13	0^1	-
New Hampshire	4	14	647	12
New Jersey	2	16	0^1	-
New Mexico	7	11	0^1	-
New York	12	7	3272	4
North Carolina	11	8	1784	9
North Dakota	0	-	0	-
Ohio	4	14	517	14
Oklahoma	6	12	0^1	-
Oregon	5	13	0^1	-
Pennsylvania	9	9	1654	10
Rhode Island	0	-	0	-
South Carolina	4	14	0^1	-
South Dakota	0	-	0	-
Tennessee	8	10	1876	7
Texas	58	1	7899	1
Utah	7	11	0^1	-

[Continued]

★ 588 ★

Psychiatric Hospitals, Establishments and Employees
[Continued]

State	Establishments	Rank	Employees	Rank
Vermont	0	-	0	-
Virginia	13	6	2585	5
Washington	3	15	273	15
West Virginia	1	17	0[1]	-
Wisconsin	1	17	0[1]	-
Wyoming	2	16	0[1]	-
U.S. Total	373	-	54358	-

Source: Census of Service Industries on CD-ROM, 1987. Geographic Area Series [machine-readable datafiles]. Prepared by U.S. Bureau of the Census. Washington, DC: The Bureau, 1990. *Notes:* Data shown only for businesses subject to federal income taxes. 1. Data are withheld to avoid disclosure of individual companies.

★ 589 ★
Hospitals

Psychiatric Hospitals, Expenses: 1990-1991

Figures represent estimated annual expenses and year-to-year percent change in annual expenses for tax-exempt firms.

[In millions of dollars]

Year	Expenses	Percent change
1991	8,138	2.9
1990	7,908	

Source: "1991 Service Annual Survey: Health Services." In CENDATA [online service]. Washington, DC: U.S. Bureau of the Census [issued 26 July 1993]. No. 10.10.4 and No. 10.10.4.7.

★ 590 ★
Hospitals

Psychiatric Hospitals, Receipts: 1987-1991

Figures represent estimated annual receipts for taxable firms.

[In millions of dollars]

Year	Receipts
1991	5,436
1990	5,095
1989	(NA)
1988	(NA)
1987	(NA)

Source: "1991 Service Annual Survey: Health Services." In CENDATA [online service]. Washington, DC: U.S. Bureau of the Census [issued 26 July 1993]. No. 10.10.4 and No. 10.10.4.7. *Note:* "NA" indicates "not available."

★ 591 ★
Hospitals

Psychiatric Hospitals, Revenue: 1987-1991

Figures represent estimated annual revenue for tax-exempt firms.

[In millions of dollars]

Year	Revenue
1991	9,932
1990	9,544
1989	(NA)
1988	(NA)
1987	(NA)

Source: "1991 Service Annual Survey: Health Services." In CENDATA [online service]. Washington, DC: U.S. Bureau of the Census [issued 26 July 1993]. No. 10.10.4 and No. 10.10.4.7. *Note:* "NA" indicates "not available."

★ 592 ★

Hospitals

Specialty Hospitals, Except Psychiatric, Establishments and Employees

Specialty hospitals include those establishments that provide diagnsotic services and treatment for various diseases and conditions, excluding mental illnesses; for example: alcoholism rehabilitation hospitals; cancer hospitals; children's hospitals; chronic disease hospitals; drug rehabilitation hospitals; eye, ear, nose, and throat hospitals; maternity hospitals; orthopedic hospitals; and tuberculosis and respiratory illness hospitals. See tables for psychiatric hospitals and skilled nursing care facilities for establishments treating mental disorders.

State	Establishments	Rank	Employees	Rank
Alabama	0	-	0	-
Alaska	0	-	0	-
Arizona	4	7	73	12
Arkansas	1	10	0[1]	-
California	23	1	2074	3
Colorado	0	-	0	-
Connecticut	0	-	0	-
Delaware	1	10	0[1]	-
D.C.	0	-	0	-
Florida	15	2	1693	4
Georgia	7	5	847	7
Hawaii	0	-	0	-
Idaho	0	-	0	-
Illinois	2	9	0[1]	-
Indiana	1	10	0[1]	-
Iowa	0	-	0	-
Kansas	1	10	0[1]	-
Kentucky	1	10	0[1]	-
Louisiana	2	9	0[1]	-
Maine	0	-	0	-
Maryland	2	9	0[1]	-
Massachusetts	8	4	2178	2
Michigan	4	7	0[1]	-
Minnesota	0	-	0	-
Mississippi	1	10	0[1]	-
Missouri	0	-	0	-
Montana	0	-	0	-
Nebraska	0	-	0	-
Nevada	1	10	0[1]	-
New Hampshire	5	6	0[1]	-
New Jersey	1	10	0[1]	-
New Mexico	1	10	0[1]	-
New York	4	7	890	6
North Carolina	3	8	244	10
North Dakota	0	-	0	-
Ohio	3	8	0[1]	-
Oklahoma	1	10	0[1]	-
Oregon	2	9	0[1]	-
Pennsylvania	11	3	1597	5

[Continued]

★ 592 ★

Specialty Hospitals, Except Psychiatric, Establishments and Employees
[Continued]

State	Establishments	Rank	Employees	Rank
Rhode Island	0	-	0	-
South Carolina	1	10	0^1	-
South Dakota	0	-	0	-
Tennessee	0	-	0	-
Texas	15	2	2311	1
Utah	2	9	0^1	-
Vermont	0	-	0	-
Virginia	4	7	663	8
Washington	5	6	260	9
West Virginia	2	9	0^1	-
Wisconsin	3	8	100	11
Wyoming	0	-	0	-
U.S. Total	137	-	18004	-

Source: Census of Service Industries on CD-ROM, 1987. Geographic Area Series [machine-readable datafiles]. Prepared by U.S. Bureau of the Census. Washington, DC: The Bureau, 1990. *Notes:* Data shown only for businesses subject to federal income taxes. 1. Data are withheld to avoid disclosure of individual companies.

★ 593 ★

Hospitals

Specialty Hospitals, Except Psychiatric, Expenses: 1990-1991

Figures represent estimated annual expenses and year-to-year percent change in annual expenses for tax-exempt firms.

[In millions of dollars]

Year	Expenses	Percent change
1991	12,537	11.5
1990	11,243	

Source: "1991 Service Annual Survey: Health Services." In CENDATA [online service]. Washington, DC: U.S. Bureau of the Census [issued 26 July 1993]. No. 10.10.4 and No. 10.10.4.7.

★ 594 ★

Hospitals

Specialty Hospitals, Except Psychiatric, Receipts: 1987-1991

Figures represent estimated annual receipts for taxable firms.

[In millions of dollars]

Year	Receipts
1991	1,569
1990	1,385
1989	(NA)
1988	(NA)
1987	(NA)

Source: "1991 Service Annual Survey: Health Services." In CENDATA [online service]. Washington, DC: U.S. Bureau of the Census [issued 26 July 1993]. No. 10.10.4 and No. 10.10.4.7. *Note:* "NA" indicates "not available."

★ 595 ★

Hospitals

Specialty Hospitals, Except Psychiatric, Revenue: 1987-1991

Figures represent estimated annual revenue for tax-exempt firms.

[In millions of dollars]

Year	Revenue
1991	13,927
1990	12,326
1989	(NA)
1988	(NA)
1987	(NA)

Source: "1991 Service Annual Survey: Health Services." In CENDATA [online service]. Washington, DC: U.S. Bureau of the Census [issued 26 July 1993]. No. 10.10.4 and No. 10.10.4.7. *Note:* "NA" indicates "not available."

Insurance Carriers

★ 596 ★

Leading Claims Administrators

Table shows the top ten claims administrators. Data are provided by claims paid.

	Claims paid for self-insurers (in million dollars)	Number of self-Insured administration clients	Types of claims for self-insurers					Staff serving self-insurers	1993 gross revenues (in millions)	
			Health[1]	Non-health benefits[2]	Workers' compensation	General liability	All other		Total	From claims administration
First Health Strategies Inc.	3,040.0	1,205	96.3	3.7	0.0	0.0	0.0	2,800	166.0	135.0
CoreSource Inc.	2,112.0	2,322	74.0	1.0	20.0	2.0	3.0	N/A	N/A	N/A
EBP HealthPlans Inc.	2,100.0	2,650	96.0	3.0	1.0	0.0	0.0	1,050	253.0	82.0
Crawford & Co.	2,072.8	1,550	0.0	0.0	58.4	21.0	20.6	N/A	584.9	225.7
Harrington Services Corp.	1,635.0	482	85.0	12.0	3.0	0.0	0.0	1,200	65.0	53.5
Travelers Plan Administrators Inc.	1,562.1	687	85.0	15.0	0.0	0.0	0.0	803	62.0	60.8
Preferred Works Inc.[3]	1,364.9	1,427	10.0	7.0	51.0	0.0	32.0	485	44.8	N/A
Sedgwick James Inc. Claims Management Services	1,323.0	3,467	0.0	0.0	94.0	4.0	2.0	812	N/A	N/A
Gallagher Bassett Services Inc.	1,270.9	1,726	27.0	0.0	44.0	15.0	14.0	N/A	104.4	94.4
Alexsis Inc.	1,200.0	1,068	0.0	0.0	70.0	20.0	10.0	1,321	95.0	85.6

Source: Marley, Sara. "Self-Insurance: P/C Self-Insurance Growth Slows, But Efforts to Control Costs Grow." *Business Insurance,* 7 February 1994, p. 3. Primary source: *Business Insurance* survey. *Notes:* "N/A" stands for "not available." 1. Includes medical, dental, vision, and prescription drug plans. 2. Includes pensions, flexible compensation, disability, and life. 3. Formerly Adjustco Inc.

★ 597 ★

Insurance Carriers

Leading Group Accident and Health Insurers: 1991

Commercial group accident and health insurers are ranked by net premiums earned in 1991.

Company	Premiums ($ bil.)	Group share (%)
Prudential	6.1	27.5
Principal Mutual	2.4	10.8
Aetna	2.3	10.4
Guardian	2.0	9.0
Travelers	1.9	8.6
Metropolitan	1.9	8.6
Connecticut General	1.9	8.6
Continental	1.7	7.7
Employers Health	1.1	5.0
Mutual of Omaha	0.9	4.1

Source: Boston Globe, 30 May 1993, p. 65. Primary source: National Underwriters Co. *1992 Profiles/Health Insurers.*

★ 598 ★

Insurance Carriers

Leading HMOs: 1993

Table below ranks the top 10 general service Health Maintenance Organizations (HMOs) by number of employees and dependents in employer groups as of June 30, 1993.

	Employees and dependents in employer groups	Participating employer/payer groups
Kaiser Foundation Health Plan Inc. (Oakland, California)	5.8 million	52,953
Prudential Health Care Plan Inc. (Roseland, New Jersey)	3.3 million	12,695
CIGNA HealthCare Inc. (Hartford, Connecticut)	2.7 million	N/A
United HealthCare Corp. (Minneapolis, Minnesota)	1.9 million	10,000
U.S. Healthcare Inc. (Blue Bell, Pennsylvania)	1.5 million	N/A
Aetna Health Plans (Middletown, Connecticut)	1.3 million	N/A
Health Insurance Plan of Greater New York (New York, New York)	1.0 million	10,000
Humana Health Care Plans (Louisville, Kentucky)	964,500	N/A
Health Net (Woodland Hills, California)	916,006	2,146
PacifiCare Health Systems (Cypress, California)	818,795	3,290

Source: Wojcik, Joanne. "Managed Care Evolving Despite Clinton Proposal to Reform System." *Business Insurance,* 21 December 1993, p. 1. Primary source: *Busines Insurance* survey. *Notes:* 1. Figures include Point-of-Service plans. 2. Figures may include individuals services through HMOs managed by the ranked organization. 3. Blue Cross/Blue Shield Association is not ranked because network members are independently owned and operated.

★ 599 ★

Insurance Carriers

Leading PPOs: 1993

Table below ranks the top 10 general service Preferred Provider Organizations (PPOs) by number of employees and dependents in employer groups as of June 30, 1993.

	Employees and dependents in employer groups	Participating employer/payer groups
USA Health Network (Phoenix, Arizona)	10,839,529	483
AFFORDABLE Medical Networks (Downers Grove, Illinois)	8,300,000	2,590
Admar Corp. (Santa Ana, California)	7,119,527	134
MultiPlan Inc. (New York, New York)	6,000,000	30,000
Preferred Health Network (Long Beach, California)	5,133,000	32,140
Beech Street of California Inc. (Irvine, California)	4,377,108	480
CAPP CARE Inc. (Newport Beach, California)	3,000,000	150
Anthem Health Systems (Indianapolis, Indiana)	2,942,108	5,593
Private Healthcare Systems Inc. (Waltham, Massachusetts)	2,758,221	42,855
Aetna Health Plans (Middletown, Connecticut)	2,314,748	11,067

Source: Wojcik, Joanne. "Managed Care Evolving Despite Clinton Proposal to Reform System." *Business Insurance,* 21 December 1993, p. 1. Primary source: *Busines Insurance* survey. *Notes:* Blue Cross/Blue Shield Association is not ranked because network members are independently owned and operated.

★ 600 ★

Insurance Carriers

Market Shares of Health Plans: 1991

Plan	Percent
Indemnity/UR	43
PPO	24
Traditional HMO	23
Indemnity	10
POS	1

Source: "At a Glance: Snapshots of the Workplace Health Industry." *Workplace Health* (January 1993), p. 15. Primary source: KPMG survey of employers, 1991; InterStudy Edge, 1992; *HMO Magazine. Notes:* "UR" indicates "utilization review"; "PPO" stands for "Preferred Provider Organziation"; "HMO" represents "Health Maintenance Organization"; "POS" indicates "Point-of-Service Plan."

★ 601 ★

Insurance Carriers

Market Shares of Medical Malpractice Insurers: 1967-1991

[In percentages]

Company	1991	1990	1989	1986	1967
National agency companies	25.5	25.5	25.0	26.9	32.0
Regional agency companies	23.8	23.7	24.1	23.2	21.3
Total agency companies	49.3	49.3	49.1	50.1	53.3
Direct writers	50.7	50.7	50.9	49.9	46.7

Source. Ferraiolo, Diane. "General Liability, Medical Malpractice, Surety and Fidelity, 1991." *Best's Review: Property/Casualty Insurance Edition* 93, no. 8 (December 1992), p. 27.

★ 602 ★

Insurance Carriers

Medicare Carrier Ratings: 1992

The table below presents the top- and bottom-rated Medicare Part B carriers. Carriers must achieve 90 out of 100 points for a passing rating from the Health Care Financing Administration.

Carrier	Rating
Top-rated	
Wholehealth Insurance Network (New York)	100
Blue Cross & Blue Shield of Minnesota	99
Travelers Insurance Co. (Connecticut)	99

[Continued]

★ 602 ★

Medicare Carrier Ratings: 1992
[Continued]

Carrier	Rating
Travelers Insurance Co. (Minnesota)	99
Lowest-rated	
Seguros de Servicio de Salud de Puerto Rico	79
Empire Blue Cross & Blue Shield (New York)	76
King County Medical Blue Shield (Washington)	75
Blue Cross & Blue Shield of Maryland	65

Source: Johnsson, Julie, and Mike Mitka. "Medicare Efficiency Ratings Are Down in 1992." *American Medical News,* 19 April 1993, p. 1. Primary source: Health Care Financing Administration.

★ 603 ★
Insurance Carriers

Net Written Premiums of Accident and Health Insurers: 1987-1992

[In billions of dollars]

Item	1987	1988	1989	1990	1991	1992
Total, all lines of insurance	193.2	202.0	208.4	217.8	223.0	227.5
Commercial lines[1]	112.3	115.4	117.2	120.8	120.9	118.6
Workers' compensation	23.4	26.1	28.5	31.0	31.3	29.7
Accident and health	3.8	4.7	4.6	5.0	5.1	5.4

Source: U.S. Department of Commerce. *U.S. Industrial Outlook, 1994: Forecasts for Selected Manufacturing and Service Industries.* Lanham, MD: Bernan Press, 1994, p. 48-4. Primary source: A. M. Best Co. *Best's Aggregates and Averages.* Property-Casualty editions. *Notes:* Detail may not add to total due to rounding 1. May include some personal insurance, such as accident or health, but data cannot be broken out readily.

★ 604 ★
Insurance Carriers

Premium Receipts From Health Insurance: 1970-1992

```
┌──────────────────────────────────────────────────────┐
│  ┌─────────────┐                                       │
│  │ 1992 - 65.5 │                                       │
│  ├─────────────┤                                       │
│  │ 1991 - 60.9 │                                       │
│  ├─────────────┤                                       │
│  │ 1990 - 58.3 │                                       │
│  ├─────────────┤                                       │
│  │ 1989 - 56.1 │                                       │
│  ├─────────────┤                                       │
│  │ 1988 - 52.3 │                                       │
│  ├─────────────┤                                       │
│  │ 1980 - 29.4 │                                       │
│  ├──────┐                                              │
│  │      │  1970 - 11.4                                 │
│  └──────┘                                              │
│            Chart shows data from column 2.             │
└──────────────────────────────────────────────────────┘
```

The table below reflects life insurance company income from health insurance premiums for selected years between 1970 and 1992.

[In billions of dollars]

Year	Total income	Income from health insurance premiums
1970	49.1	11.4
1980	130.9	29.4
1988	338.1	52.3
1989	367.3	56.1
1990	402.2	58.3
1991	411.0	60.9
1992	426.0	65.5

Source: U.S. Department of Commerce. *U.S. Industrial Outlook, 1994: Forecasts for Selected Manufacturing and Service Industries.* Lanham, MD: Bernan Press, 1994, p. 48-2. Primary source: American Council of Life Insurance. *Notes:* Detail may not add to total due to rounding .

Laboratories and Research Firms

★ 605 ★

Commercial Medical and Biological Research Firms, Establishments and Employees

State	Establishments	Rank	Employees	Rank
Alabama	6	25	120	23
Arizona	19	17	95	24
Arkansas	3	28	0[1]	-
California	234	1	5376	1
Colorado	35	11	309	15
Connecticut	20	16	229	16
Florida	48	8	417	14
Georgia	13	20	132	21
Illinois	51	7	567	12
Indiana	11	21	194	18
Iowa	2	29	0[1]	-
Kansas	8	24	0[1]	-
Kentucky	5	26	3	29
Louisiana	10	22	151	20
Maryland	69	4	1835	4
Massachusetts	73	3	2642	2
Michigan	48	8	705	10
Minnesota	23	14	457	13
Mississippi	3	28	5	28
Missouri	9	23	194	18
Nebraska	4	27	19	27
New Jersey	64	6	1012	9
New York	89	2	1899	3
North Carolina	24	13	196	17
Ohio	42	9	702	11
Oklahoma	0	-	0	-
Oregon	14	19	66	25
Pennsylvania	42	9	1583	5
South Carolina	8	24	27	26
Tennessee	10	22	192	19
Texas	67	5	1302	7
Utah	16	18	123	22
Virginia	39	10	1415	6
Washington	27	12	0[1]	-
Wisconsin	22	15	1127	8
U.S. Total	1220	-	25609	-

Source: Census of Service Industries on CD-ROM, 1987. Geographic Area Series [machine-readable datafiles]. Prepared by U.S. Bureau of the Census. Washington, DC: The Bureau, 1990. Notes: Data shown only for businesses subject to federal income taxes. 1. Data are withheld to avoid disclosure of individual companies.

★ 606 ★

Laboratories and Research Firms

Dental Laboratories, Establishments and Employees

The table below includes data for establishments engaged in the making of dentures, artificial teeth, and orthodontic appliances. Providers of dental x-ray lab services are excluded.

State	Establishments	Rank	Employees	Rank
Alabama	138	20	746	20
Alaska	13	44	0[1]	-
Arizona	154	16	597	24
Arkansas	48	33	291	33
California	1277	1	5404	1
Colorado	136	22	562	25
Connecticut	111	25	601	23
Delaware	14	43	0[1]	-
D.C.	9	45	37	48
Florida	507	3	2122	3
Georgia	226	12	1424	9
Hawaii	41	35	200	36
Idaho	36	38	142	43
Illinois	346	5	1953	4
Indiana	163	14	1112	13
Iowa	68	30	424	28
Kansas	64	31	671	22
Kentucky	68	30	310	30
Louisiana	101	26	448	27
Maine	28	41	132	44
Maryland	139	19	771	18
Massachusetts	165	13	839	17
Michigan	300	7	1564	8
Minnesota	137	21	1130	11
Mississippi	50	32	209	35
Missouri	144	18	946	14
Montana	31	40	60	46
Nebraska	42	34	275	34
Nevada	39	36	181	39
New Hampshire	37	37	185	37
New Jersey	269	9	1380	10
New Mexico	48	33	178	40
New York	608	2	4106	2
North Carolina	247	10	885	15
North Dakota	14	43	150	41
Ohio	303	6	1575	7
Oklahoma	74	28	304	31
Oregon	150	17	560	26
Pennsylvania	272	8	1598	6
Rhode Island	41	35	145	42
South Carolina	71	29	301	32
South Dakota	19	42	74	45
Tennessee	155	15	769	19
Texas	438	4	1917	5
Utah	78	27	314	29

[Continued]

★ 606 ★

Dental Laboratories, Establishments and Employees
[Continued]

State	Establishments	Rank	Employees	Rank
Vermont	13	44	41	47
Virginia	127	24	684	21
Washington	229	11	881	16
West Virginia	34	39	182	38
Wisconsin	135	23	1123	12
Wyoming	13	44	26	49
U.S. Total	7970	-	40708	-

Source: Census of Service Industries on CD-ROM, 1987. Geographic Area Series [machine-readable datafiles]. Prepared by U.S. Bureau of the Census. Washington, DC: The Bureau, 1990. *Notes:* Data shown only for businesses subject to federal income taxes. 1. Data are withheld to avoid disclosure of individual companies.

★ 607 ★

Laboratories and Research Firms

Dental Laboratories, Receipts: 1987-1991

Figures represent estimated annual receipts for taxable firms.

[In millions of dollars]

Year	Receipts
1991	1,678
1990	1,663
1989	1,559
1988	1,499
1987	1,596

Source: "1991 Service Annual Survey: Health Services." In CENDATA [online service]. Washington, DC: U.S. Bureau of the Census [issued 26 July 1993]. No. 10.10.4 and No. 10.10.4.7.

★ 608 ★

Laboratories and Research Firms

Laboratory Applications Market: 1980-1993

Data indicate the size of the laboratory applications market for selected years.

[In million dollars]

Year	Size
1980	66.0
1985	225.0
1987	350.0
1989	500.00
1990	600.0
1991	690.0
1993	725.0

Source: "Expected Future Size of the Laboratory Applications Market." *Computers in Healthcare* (September 1993), p. 47.

★ 609 ★

Laboratories and Research Firms

Medical and Dental Laboratories, Establishments and Employees

State	Establishments	Rank	Employees	Rank
Alabama	211	23	2189	19
Alaska	21	45	0[1]	-
Arizona	291	15	1774	22
Arkansas	87	34	559	38
California	2315	1	20166	1
Colorado	241	19	1458	27
Connecticut	270	17	2094	20
Delaware	61	39	474	40
D.C.	27	43	104	47
Florida	971	3	7345	3
Georgia	365	12	3581	11
Hawaii	65	37	807	34
Idaho	64	38	423	42
Illinois	626	5	5773	8
Indiana	330	14	2873	15
Iowa	116	30	1150	29
Kansas	121	28	1556	26
Kentucky	145	27	1259	28
Louisiana	230	20	1633	25
Maine	47	41	348	43
Maryland	291	15	3250	12
Massachusetts	380	10	3893	10

[Continued]

★ 609 ★

Medical and Dental Laboratories, Establishments and Employees
[Continued]

State	Establishments	Rank	Employees	Rank
Michigan	537	8	6020	7
Minnesota	186	25	1692	24
Mississippi	91	33	836	33
Missouri	272	16	2644	16
Montana	49	40	168	46
Nebraska	83	35	1024	32
Nevada	66	36	668	37
New Hampshire	66	36	507	39
New Jersey	518	9	6221	6
New Mexico	114	31	698	36
New York	1073	2	10640	2
North Carolina	362	13	2346	18
North Dakota	23	44	231	45
Ohio	599	7	4440	9
Oklahoma	168	26	1092	30
Oregon	223	21	1710	23
Pennsylvania	614	6	6914	5
Rhode Island	114	31	708	35
South Carolina	112	32	0[1]	-
South Dakota	33	42	323	44
Tennessee	256	18	3013	14
Texas	969	4	7317	4
Utah	119	29	1065	31
Vermont	21	45	102	48
Virginia	216	22	2432	17
Washington	374	11	3221	13
West Virginia	83	35	450	41
Wisconsin	204	24	1857	21
Wyoming	21	45	62	49
U.S. Total	14841	-	131822	-

Source: Census of Service Industries on CD-ROM, 1987. Geographic Area Series [machine-readable datafiles]. Prepared by U.S. Bureau of the Census. Washington, DC: The Bureau, 1990. *Notes:* Data shown only for businesses subject to federal income taxes. 1. Data are withheld to avoid disclosure of individual companies.

★ 610 ★

Laboratories and Research Firms

Medical and Dental Laboratories, Receipts: 1987-1991

Figures represent estimated annual receipts for taxable firms.

[In millions of dollars]

Year	Receipts
1991	10,527
1990	9,872
1989	8,933
1988	8,119
1987	7,114

Source: "1991 Service Annual Survey: Health Services." In CENDATA [online service]. Washington, DC: U.S. Bureau of the Census [issued 26 July 1993]. No. 10.10.4 and No. 10.10.4.7.

★ 611 ★

Laboratories and Research Firms

Medical Laboratories, Establishments and Employees

Data cover establishments that provide professional analytic and/or diagnostic services to medical professionals. Representative establishments include bacteriological laboratories; biological laboratories; blood analysis laboratories; dental x-ray laboratories; clinical medical laboratories; pathological laboratories; medical testing laboratories; and urinalysis laboratories.

State	Establishments	Rank	Employees	Rank
Alabama	73	25	1443	20
Alaska	8	42	53	47
Arizona	137	16	1177	22
Arkansas	39	33	268	40
California	1038	1	14762	1
Colorado	105	20	896	25
Connecticut	159	12	1493	18
Delaware	47	31	0[1]	-
D.C.	18	39	67	45
Florida	464	4	5223	5
Georgia	139	15	2157	14
Hawaii	24	37	607	33
Idaho	28	35	281	39
Illinois	280	7	3820	8
Indiana	167	11	1761	15
Iowa	48	30	726	31
Kansas	57	28	885	26
Kentucky	77	24	949	24

[Continued]

★ 611 ★

Medical Laboratories, Establishments and Employees
[Continued]

State	Establishments	Rank	Employees	Rank
Louisiana	129	17	1185	21
Maine	19	38	216	42
Maryland	152	13	2479	11
Massachusetts	215	10	3054	9
Michigan	237	9	4456	7
Minnesota	49	29	562	35
Mississippi	41	32	627	32
Missouri	128	18	1698	17
Montana	18	39	108	43
Nebraska	41	32	749	29
Nevada	27	36	487	37
New Hampshire	29	34	322	38
New Jersey	249	8	4841	6
New Mexico	66	27	520	36
New York	465	3	6534	2
North Carolina	115	19	1461	19
North Dakota	9	41	81	44
Ohio	296	6	2865	10
Oklahoma	94	22	788	27
Oregon	73	25	1150	23
Pennsylvania	342	5	5316	4
Rhode Island	73	25	563	34
South Carolina	41	32	0[1]	-
South Dakota	14	40	249	41
Tennessee	101	21	2244	13
Texas	531	2	5400	3
Utah	41	32	751	28
Vermont	8	42	61	46
Virginia	89	23	1748	16
Washington	145	14	2340	12
West Virginia	49	29	268	40
Wisconsin	69	26	734	30
Wyoming	8	42	36	48
U.S. Total	6871	-	91114	-

Source: Census of Service Industries on CD-ROM, 1987. Geographic Area Series [machine-readable datafiles]. Prepared by U.S. Bureau of the Census. Washington, DC: The Bureau, 1990. *Notes:* Data shown only for businesses subject to federal income taxes. 1. Data are withheld to avoid disclosure of individual companies.

★ 612 ★

Laboratories and Research Firms

Medical Laboratories, Receipts: 1987-1991

Figures represent estimated annual receipts for taxable firms.

[In millions of dollars]

Year	Receipts
1991	8,849
1990	8,209
1989	7,374
1988	6,620
1987	5,518

Source: "1991 Service Annual Survey: Health Services." In CENDATA [online service]. Washington, DC: U.S. Bureau of the Census [issued 26 July 1993]. No. 10.10.4 and No. 10.10.4.7.

Medical and Dental Instrument Manufacturers

★ 613 ★

Dental Equipment and Supply Manufacturers, Establishments and Employees

[Employees in thousands]

State	Establishments	Rank	Employees	Rank
California	108	1	2.5	1
Colorado	10	11	0.4	6
Connecticut	10	11	0.6	5
Delaware	1	14	0.4[1]	6
Florida	20	5	0.4[1]	6
Georgia	15	7	0.2[1]	7
Illinois	37	3	1.7[1]	2
Kentucky	3	13	0.2[1]	7
Michigan	12	9	0.4[1]	6
Missouri	14	8	0.4[1]	6
New Jersey	27	4	0.7[1]	4
New York	47	2	1.7[1]	2
North Carolina	10	11	0.7[1]	4
Ohio	11	10	0.4[1]	6
Oregon	20	5	0.7[1]	4
Pennsylvania	27	4	1.3	3
Texas	17	6	0.2[1]	7

[Continued]

★ 613 ★

Dental Equipment and Supply Manufacturers, Establishments and Employees
[Continued]

State	Establishments	Rank	Employees	Rank
Washington	11	10	0.2[1]	7
Wisconsin	8	12	0.4[1]	6

Source: Census of Manufactures on CD-ROM, 1987. Geographic Area Series [machine-readable datafiles]. Prepared by U.S. Bureau of the Census. Washington, DC: The Bureau, 1991. *Note:* 1. Figure shown is the midpoint of a range.

★ 614 ★

Medical and Dental Instrument Manufacturers

Electromedical Equipment Manufacturers, Establishments and Employees
[Employees in thousands]

State	Establishments	Rank	Employees	Rank
California	39	1	6.2	1
Colorado	6	8	2.1	3
Connecticut	9	6	1.3	6
Florida	10	5	0.7[1]	9
Illinois	13	3	0.4[1]	10
Indiana	3	10	0.2[1]	11
Kansas	3	10	0.2[1]	11
Massachusetts	15	2	2.5[2]	2
Minnesota	10	5	1.7[1]	5
Missouri	6	8	0.8	8
New Jersey	8	7	0.7[1]	9
New York	15	2	1.7[1]	5
North Carolina	4	9	0.4[1]	10
Ohio	8	7	0.7[1]	9
Oklahoma	3	10	0.4[1]	10
Oregon	6	8	0.8	8
Pennsylvania	11	4	0.7[1]	9
South Carolina	1	11	0.4[1]	10
Texas	13	3	1.2	7
Utah	3	10	0.2[1]	11
Virginia	3	10	0.2[1]	11
Washington	8	7	2.5[2]	2
Wisconsin	10	5	1.8	4

Source: Census of Manufactures on CD-ROM, 1987. Geographic Area Series [machine-readable datafiles]. Prepared by U.S. Bureau of the Census. Washington, DC: The Bureau, 1991. *Notes:* 1. Figure shown is the midpoint of a range. 2. Figure shown indicates 2,500 or more.

★615★

Medical and Dental Instrument Manufacturers

Medical Instrument and Supply Manufacturers, Establishments and Employees

[Employees in thousands]

State	Establishments	Rank	Employees	Rank
Alabama	27	26	1.0	22
Arizona	34	25	1.3	21
Arkansas	10	33	1.7[1]	20
California	612	1	34.0	1
Colorado	79	13	2.5[2]	17
Connecticut	95	11	7.8	6
Delaware	7	35	1.7[1]	20
Florida	168	6	6.2	9
Georgia	65	17	3.5	16
Idaho	13	31	0.2	26
Illinois	184	3	7.2	8
Indiana	78	14	4.8	11
Iowa	21	28	0.2[1]	26
Kansas	19	29	0.7[1]	24
Kentucky	17	30	1.7[1]	20
Maryland	43	21	0.9	23
Massachusetts	160	8	12.3	2
Michigan	90	12	3.8	15
Minnesota	118	10	7.9	5
Mississippi	12	32	0.5	25
Missouri	68	16	4.5	12
Montana	9	34	0.2	26
Nebraska	13	31	1.7[1]	20
New Hampshire	26	27	0.7[1]	24
New Jersey	163	7	11.6	3
New Mexico	9	34	0.7[1]	24
New York	276	2	2.5[2]	17
North Carolina	76	15	5.6	10
Ohio	150	9	2.5[2]	17
Oklahoma	35	24	0.9	23
Oregon	63	18	1.9	19
Pennsylvania	169	5	11.5	4
Rhode Island	21	28	2.3	18
South Carolina	26	27	4.1	14
South Dakota	2	37	0.7[1]	24
Tennessee	49	20	4.3	13
Texas	171	4	2.5[2]	17
Utah	41	22	4.5	12
Virginia	39	23	1.7[1]	20
Washington	58	19	3.8	15
West Virginia	6	36	0.2[1]	26
Wisconsin	76	15	7.4	7

Source: Census of Manufactures on CD-ROM, 1987. Geographic Area Series [machine-readable datafiles]. Prepared by U.S. Bureau of the Census. Washington, DC: The Bureau, 1991. *Notes:* 1. Figure shown is the midpoint of a range. 2. Figure shown indicates 2,500 or more.

★ 616 ★

Medical and Dental Instrument Manufacturers

Medical Instrument and Supply Manufacturing, by State: 1991

The table below shows manufacturing statistics for each state for the medical instruments and supplies industry. Includes operating manufacturing establishments and auxiliaries. Covers industry groups with 950 or more employees. Data are for 1991.

Area	All employees		Production workers			Value-added by manufacture (million dollars)	Cost of materials[1] (million dollars)	Value of shipments[1] (million dollars)	New capital expenditures (million dollars)	End-of-year inventories (million dollars)
	Number (1,000)	Payroll (million dollars)	Number (1,000)	Hours (millions)	Wages (million dollars)					
United States	240.9	7,217.7	143.4	280.3	3,007.3	21,873.2	11,900.8	33,595.5	1,239.8	5,964.6
Alabama	1.8	28.8	1.3	2.9	20.2	118.4	67.6	184.3	(D)	26.3
Arizona	1.8	49.9	.9	1.9	16.3	177.2	101.0	276.1	21.4	35.4
Arkansas	(D)	(D)	(D)	(D)	(D)	(D)	(D)	(D)	(D)	(D)
California	45.1	1,543.9	23.2	44.5	507.8	4,138.8	2,138.5	6,345.8	249.2	1,094.2
Colorado	(D)	(D)	(D)	(D)	(D)	(D)	(D)	(D)	(D)	(D)
Connecticut	9.5	362.6	6.3	12.0	181.9	1,281.5	495.4	1,707.4	138.6	289.6
Delaware	(D)	(D)	(D)	(D)	(D)	(D)	(D)	(D)	(D)	(D)
Florida	7.7	216.8	4.5	9.4	81.2	550.5	251.8	808.2	25.4	145.8
Georgia	4.0	103.9	2.6	4.7	50.0	332.4	211.4	533.2	9.1	80.2
Illinois	9.1	246.3	5.8	11.3	107.6	649.4	487.5	1,134.4	23.2	202.9
Indiana	7.8	248.9	5.2	11.2	144.4	1,108.7	290.0	1,367.8	58.3	218.3
Kansas	(D)	(D)	(D)	(D)	(D)	(D)	(D)	(D)	(D)	(D)
Kentucky	(D)	(D)	(D)	(D)	(D)	(D)	(D)	(D)	(D)	(D)
Maryland	1.2	34.9	.7	1.3	15.8	71.0	85.6	156.2	(D)	34.3
Massachusetts	15.0	499.9	7.9	15.9	181.1	1,245.3	691.5	1,921.2	47.3	385.9
Michigan	3.6	111.8	2.0	3.7	38.3	331.5	198.3	519.6	12.6	100.6
Minnesota	11.2	354.6	6.2	11.6	133.6	1,152.7	378.5	1,484.4	(D)	252.6
Missouri	6.6	166.0	3.9	8.8	71.6	377.2	262.9	626.6	14.6	119.9
Nebraska	(D)	(D)	(D)	(D)	(D)	(D)	(D)	(D)	(D)	(D)
Nevada	(D)	(D)	(D)	(D)	(D)	(D)	(D)	(D)	(D)	(D)
New Jersey	11.1	402.6	5.5	10.9	145.6	1,041.8	428.0	1,422.7	84.2	366.5
New York	(D)	(D)	(D)	(D)	(D)	(D)	(D)	(D)	(D)	(D)
North Carolina	6.7	159.6	5.0	9.9	91.9	450.3	316.2	770.4	25.5	153.4
Ohio	(D)	(D)	(D)	(D)	(D)	(D)	(D)	(D)	(D)	(D)
Oregon	2.4	85.2	1.2	2.2	31.3	208.0	170.5	378.1	(D)	46.7
Pennsylvania	11.2	331.3	6.9	13.1	150.9	904.7	500.1	1,413.2	67.8	274.6
Rhode Island	2.6	62.3	1.8	3.3	32.8	131.1	122.9	239.9	4.4	53.4
South Carolina	2.4	60.2	1.8	3.6	36.4	144.0	149.1	296.0	7.7	41.1
Tennessee	5.2	143.7	3.4	6.2	61.9	623.2	243.6	872.5	26.3	169.2
Texas	(D)	(D)	(D)	(D)	(D)	(D)	(D)	(D)	(D)	(D)
Utah	4.5	115.5	3.0	6.8	62.8	352.0	223.6	572.7	22.6	121.3
Virginia	(D)	(D)	(D)	(D)	(D)	(D)	(D)	(D)	(D)	(D)
Washington	4.8	176.3	1.6	3.3	35.1	497.1	155.9	648.3	21.4	149.5
Wisconsin	7.7	256.8	4.4	9.1	114.3	1,322.1	966.3	2,290.3	41.7	345.6

Source: U.S. Bureau of the Census. *Annual Survey of Manufactures, 1991. Geographic Area Statistics.* M91(AS)- 3. Washington, DC: U.S. Government Printing Office, February 1993, pp. 3/12-3/129. *Notes:* "D" indicates data withheld to avoid disclosing information for individual companies. 1. Aggregate of cost of materials and value of shipments includes extensive duplication since products of some industries are used as materials by others. 2. See original material for description of standard error of estimate. Percentage standard errors shown are approximate relative standard errors of estimates of level. 3. Manufacturing concerns reported separately for auxiliary units that serve the manufacturing establishments of a company (e.g., administrative offices, storage warehouses, power plants, research laboratories, garages, repair shops, etc.) rather than the general public if these units were at different locations from establishment served or if they serviced more than one manufacturing establishment. Employment and payroll data shown represent total for all such units that primarily serve manufacturing plants.

★ 617 ★

Medical and Dental Instrument Manufacturers

Ophthalmic Goods Manufacturers, Establishments and Employees

[Employees in thousands]

State	Establishments	Rank	Employees	Rank
Arizona	10	11	0.7[1]	5
California	74	1	1.7[1]	4
Florida	33	4	3.1	1
Georgia	9	12	1.7[1]	4
Illinois	30	5	1.7[1]	4
Maryland	8	13	0.7[1]	5
Massachusetts	27	6	2.6	2
Michigan	15	10	0.2[1]	8
Minnesota	9	12	1.7[1]	4
Missouri	7	14	0.4	7
New Hampshire	5	16	0.4[1]	7
New Jersey	21	8	0.7[1]	5
New York	56	2	2.5[2]	3
Ohio	19	9	0.4	7
Pennsylvania	26	7	0.5	6
Rhode Island	2	17	0.7[1]	5
South Carolina	1	18	0.4[1]	7
Tennessee	6	15	0.2	8
Texas	34	3	0.4[1]	7
Virginia	10	11	0.7[1]	5

Source: Census of Manufactures on CD-ROM, 1987. Geographic Area Series [machine-readable datafiles]. Prepared by U.S. Bureau of the Census. Washington, DC. The Bureau, 1991. Notes: 1. Figure shown is the midpoint of a range. 2. Figure shown indicates 2,500 or more.

★ 618 ★

Medical and Dental Instrument Manufacturers

Optical Goods Manufacturing, by State: 1991

The table below shows manufacturing statistics for each state for the optical goods industry. Includes operating manufacturing establishments and auxiliaries. Covers industry groups with 950 or more employees. Data are for 1991.

Area	All employees		Production workers			Value-added by manufacture (million dollars)	Cost of materials[1] (million dollars)	Value of shipments[1] (million dollars)	New capital expenditures (million dollars)	End-of-year inventories (million dollars)
	Number (1,000)	Payroll (million dollars)	Number (1,000)	Hours (millions)	Wages (million dollars)					
United States	26.2	626.9	17.2	34.8	335.6	1,645.2	666.4	2,313.0	120.0	455.4
California	(D)	(D)	(D)	(D)	(D)	(D)	(D)	(D)	(D)	(D)
Florida	3.9	106.6	2.9	6.2	65.8	284.8	100.0	388.5	35.0	68.3
Georgia	(D)	(D)	(D)	(D)	(D)	(D)	(D)	(D)	(D)	(D)
Illinois	(D)	(D)	(D)	(D)	(D)	(D)	(D)	(D)	(D)	(D)
Maryland	(D)	(D)	(D)	(D)	(D)	(D)	(D)	(D)	(D)	(D)
Massachusetts	1.1	26.0	.6	1.3	8.4	116.8	32.6	155.0	(D)	24.6
Minnesota	(D)	(D)	(D)	(D)	(D)	(D)	(D)	(D)	(D)	(D)

[Continued]

★ 618 ★

Optical Goods Manufacturing, by State: 1991
[Continued]

Area	All employees		Production workers			Value-added by manufacture (million dollars)	Cost of materials[1] (million dollars)	Value of shipments[1] (million dollars)	New capital expenditures (million dollars)	End-of-year inventories (million dollars)
	Number (1,000)	Payroll (million dollars)	Number (1,000)	Hours (millions)	Wages (million dollars)					
New Jersey	(D)	(D)	(D)	(D)	(D)	(D)	(D)	(D)	(D)	(D)
New York	(D)	(D)	(D)	(D)	(D)	(D)	(D)	(D)	(D)	(D)
Texas	(D)	(D)	(D)	(D)	(D)	(D)	(D)	(D)	(D)	(D)
Virginia	(D)	(D)	(D)	(D)	(D)	(D)	(D)	(D)	(D)	(D)

Source: U.S. Bureau of the Census. *Annual Survey of Manufactures, 1991. Geographic Area Statistics.* M91(AS)- 3. Washington, DC: U.S. Government Printing Office, February 1993, pp. 3/12-3/129. *Notes:* "D" indicates data withheld to avoid disclosing data for individual companies. 1. Aggregate of cost of materials and value of shipments includes extensive duplication since products of some industries are used as materials by others. 2. See original material for description of standard error of estimate. Percentage standard errors shown are approximate relative standard errors of estimates of level. 3. Manufacturing concerns reported separately for auxiliary units that serve the manufacturing establishments of a company (e.g., administrative offices, storage warehouses, power plants, research laboratories, garages, repair shops, etc.) rather than the general public if these units were at different locations from establishment served or if they serviced more than one manufacturing establishment. Employment and payroll data shown represent total for all such units that primarily serve manufacturing plants.

★ 619 ★

Medical and Dental Instrument Manufacturers

Optical Instrument and Lens Manufacturers, Establishments and Employees

[Employees in thousands]

State	Establishments	Rank	Employees	Rank
California	78	1	6.4	1
Colorado	3	10	0.4[1]	8
Connecticut	8	7	1.9	3
Florida	9	6	0.5	7
Illinois	8	7	0.4[1]	8
Maryland	3	10	0.4[1]	8
Massachusetts	29	3	2.5[2]	2
Mississippi	3	10	0.2[1]	10
Missouri	3	10	0.2[1]	10
New Hampshire	7	8	1.7[1]	4
New Jersey	11	5	0.3	9
New York	30	2	1.3	5
Ohio	3	10	0.7[1]	6
Oregon	5	9	0.7[1]	6
Pennsylvania	14	4	0.5	7
Texas	2	11	0.7[1]	6

Source: Census of Manufactures on CD-ROM, 1987. Geographic Area Series [machine-readable datafiles]. Prepared by U.S. Bureau of the Census. Washington, DC: The Bureau, 1991. *Notes:* 1. Figure shown is the midpoint of a range. 2. Figure shown indicates 2,500 or more.

★ 620 ★

Medical and Dental Instrument Manufacturers

Surgical and Medical Instrument Manufacturers, Establishments and Employees

[Employees in thousands]

State	Establishments	Rank	Employees	Rank
Alabama	5	25	0.4[1]	14
Arizona	10	21	0.2[1]	15
Arkansas	2	27	1.7[1]	10
California	235	1	13.3	1
Colorado	34	10	1.7[1]	10
Connecticut	44	8	3.3	4
Florida	49	6	3.1	5
Georgia	19	15	1.2	12
Illinois	54	5	1.7[1]	10
Indiana	32	11	2.2	9
Maryland	19	15	0.4	14
Massachusetts	79	3	6.2	3
Michigan	22	14	1.7[1]	10
Minnesota	46	7	1.7[1]	10
Missouri	24	12	2.5	8
Nebraska	7	23	1.7[1]	10
New Hampshire	11	20	0.7[1]	13
New Jersey	59	4	2.5	8
New York	90	2	7.1	2
North Carolina	15	18	1.7	10
Ohio	40	9	1.3	11
Oklahoma	9	22	0.2[1]	15
Oregon	16	17	0.2	15
Pennsylvania	46	7	3.1	5
Rhode Island	4	26	0.7[1]	13
South Carolina	6	24	1.7[1]	10
Tennessee	13	19	0.7[1]	13
Texas	54	5	2.9	7
Utah	13	19	3.0	6
Virginia	10	21	0.4[1]	14
Washington	23	13	0.4[1]	14
Wisconsin	18	16	1.7[1]	10

Source: Census of Manufactures on CD-ROM, 1987. Geographic Area Series [machine-readable datafiles]. Prepared by U.S. Bureau of the Census. Washington, DC: The Bureau, 1991. *Note:* 1. Figure shown is the midpoint of a range.

★ 621 ★

Medical and Dental Instrument Manufacturers

Surgical Appliance and Supply Manufacturers, Establishments and Employees

[Employees in thousands]

State	Establishments	Rank	Employees	Rank
Alabama	19	18	0.7[1]	15
Arizona	16	21	1.0	14
California	217	1	9.8	1
Colorado	28	14	0.3	18
Connecticut	27	15	1.9	11
Delaware	4	30	0.7[1]	15
Florida	86	4	1.7[1]	13
Georgia	29	13	1.9	11
Illinois	68	6	2.8	7
Indiana	29	13	1.7[1]	13
Kansas	9	27	0.7[1]	15
Kentucky	12	25	1.7[1]	13
Maryland	18	19	0.3	18
Massachusetts	50	10	1.7[1]	13
Michigan	52	9	1.8	12
Minnesota	57	8	4.3	6
Mississippi	10	26	0.7[1]	15
Missouri	24	17	0.7[1]	15
New Hampshire	13	24	0.4[1]	17
New Jersey	66	7	7.8	2
New Mexico	5	29	0.7[1]	15
New York	117	2	2.5[2]	9
North Carolina	44	11	2.7	8
Ohio	89	3	5.4	4
Oklahoma	16	21	0.3	18
Oregon	19	18	0.2[1]	19
Pennsylvania	83	5	5.8	3
Rhode Island	15	22	1.7[1]	13
South Carolina	16	21	2.5	9
South Dakota	1	31	0.7[1]	15
Tennessee	26	16	2.5[2]	9
Texas	86	4	4.7	5
Utah	14	23	0.2	19
Virginia	17	20	0.5	16
Washington	16	21	0.2	19
West Virginia	6	28	0.2[1]	19
Wisconsin	34	12	2.1	10

Source: Census of Manufactures on CD-ROM, 1987. Geographic Area Series [machine-readable datafiles]. Prepared by U.S. Bureau of the Census. Washington, DC: The Bureau, 1991. *Notes:* 1. Figure shown is the midpoint of a range. 2. Figure shown indicates 2,500 or more.

★ 622 ★

Medical and Dental Instrument Manufacturers

X-Ray Apparatus and Tube Manufacturers, Establishments and Employees

[Employees in thousands]

State	Establishments	Rank	Employees	Rank
California	13	1	0.7[1]	3
Colorado	1	8	0.4[1]	4
Connecticut	5	5	0.7	3
Delaware	1	8	0.4[1]	4
Illinois	12	2	0.7[1]	3
Massachusetts	5	5	0.7[1]	3
New York	7	3	1.1	2
North Carolina	3	6	0.2[1]	5
Ohio	2	7	0.7[1]	3
Pennsylvania	2	7	0.4[1]	4
Utah	2	7	0.7[1]	3
Wisconsin	6	4	1.7[1]	1

Source: Census of Manufactures on CD-ROM, 1987. Geographic Area Series [machine-readable datafiles]. Prepared by U.S. Bureau of the Census. Washington, DC: The Bureau, 1991. *Note:* 1. Figure shown is the midpoint of a range.

Medical Technology

★ 623 ★

Biopharmaceutical Firms, Net Income: 1993

The table below shows the biopharmaceutical firms with the greatest earnings and largest losses for 1993. Data are based on a survey of 106 firms.

[In million dollars]

Firm	Net income
Top 10	
Amgen	374.575
Genentech	58.902
Alza	42.869
Biogen	32.417
Elan	32.332
Life Technologies	16.560
Collagen	9.732
Lunar	5.182
Techne	4.382
Hycor Biomedical	2.275

[Continued]

★ 623 ★

Biopharmaceutical Firms, Net Income: 1993

[Continued]

Firm	Net income
Bottom 10	
Immunex	-425.852
Synergen	-84.196
Gensia	-63.304
Alkermes	-40.147
Regeneron Pharmaceutical	-39.884
Applied Immune Sciences	-39.023
Scios Nova	-36.579
TSI	-32.023
Xoma	-31.307
Cytogen	-29.229

Source: Spalding, B. J. "106 U.S. Biopharmaceutical Firms Lose $1.1 Billion." *Bio/Technology* 12 (April 1994), p. 333.

★ 624 ★

Medical Technology

Biopharmaceutical Firms, Revenue: 1993

The table below shows the biopharmaceutical firms with the most revenues in 1993. Data are based on a survey of 106 firms.

[In million dollars]

Firm	Revenue
Amgen	1,373.842
Genentech	608.189
Alza	234.182
Life Technologies	205.616
Biogen	136.418
Elan	135.752
Immunex	124.185
Genetics Institute	107.791
TSI	58.300
Collagen	49.743

Source: Spalding, B. J. "106 U.S. Biopharmaceutical Firms Lose $1.1 Billion." *Bio/Technology* 12 (April 1994), p. 333.

★ 625 ★

Medical Technology

Biotechnology Companies

The table below presents the location of biotechnology companies throughout the United States.

Location	Number
San Francisco Bay Area	196
New England	175
Mid-Atlantic Area[1]	115
San Diego, California	103
New York	86
Los Angeles/Orange County, California	71
Texas	54
Seattle, Washington	52
Philadelphia/southern New Jersey	52
Northern New Jersey	49
North Carolina	47
Wisconsin	36
Illinois	27
Ohio	27
Michigan	23
Iowa	23
Florida	21
Minnesota	21
Georgia	20
Colorado	20
Oregon	12
Other	64

Source: Waldholz, Michael. "An Industry in Adolescence; Think of Biotechnology as a Teenager: Lots of Promise, Lots of Headaches." *Wall Street Journal,* 20 May 1994, p. R4. Primary source: Ernst & Young. *Note:* 1. Delaware, District of Columbia, Maryland, and Virginia.

★ 626 ★

Medical Technology

Biotechnology Industry: 1989-1993

The table below offers data on key industry areas, including sales, revenue, establishments, and employees. Data are provided for 1989 through 1993.

[Dollar figures in billions]

Industrial indicator	1989	1990	1991	1992	1993
Product sales ($)	2.7	2.9	4.4	6.0	7.0
Total revenue ($)	3.6	4.7	6.3	8.3	10.0
Research and development spending ($)	2.5	2.8	3.4	5.0	5.7
Net loss ($)	(2.1)	(2.2)	(2.6)	(3.4)	(3.6)
Market capitalization ($)	26	35	49	48	45

[Continued]

★ 626 ★

Biotechnology Industry: 1989-1993
[Continued]

Industrial indicator	1989	1990	1991	1992	1993
Companies	1,095	1,100	1,107	1,231	1,272
Employees	59,000	66,000	70,000	79,000	97,000

Source: Waldholz, Michael. "An Industry in Adolescence; Think of Biotechnology as a Teenager: Lots of Promise, Lots of Headaches." *Wall Street Journal,* 20 May 1994, p. R4. Primary source: Ernst & Young.

★ 627 ★

Medical Technology

High Technology Establishments, Employment, and Average Pay: 1991

For workers on private industry payrolls and excludes the self-employed. Based on surveys of the Occupational Employment Statistics Program and subject to sampling error.

Industry	Establishments (1,000)	Employment		Average annual pay
		Total (1,000)	Percent distribution	
All high technology industries[1]	336.5	9,789	100.0	$38,147
Drugs	1.8	268	2.7	43,925
Medical instruments and supplies	4.2	271	2.8	32,075

Source: 1993 Statistical Abstract of the United States on CD-ROM [machine-readable datafiles]. CD-ABSTR-93. Washington, DC: U.S. Department of Commerce, Economics and Statistics Administration, Bureau of the Census, Data User Services Division, 1993. Primary source: U.S. Bureau of Labor Statistics. *Employment and Wages, Annual Averages 1991.* BLS Bulletin 2419. *Notes:* "X" represents "not applicable." 1. Those industries whose proportion of R&D employment is at least equal to the average proportion of all industries surveyed.

★ 628 ★

Medical Technology

U.S. Firms as Suppliers of Medical Technology

```
┌─────────────────────────────────────────────────────────┐
│ ┌───────────────────────────────────────────────────────┐│
│ │ Linear accelerators - 75                              ││
│ └───────────────────────────────────────────────────────┘│
│ ┌───────────────────────────────┐                        │
│ │ Medical devices - 50          │                        │
│ └───────────────────────────────┘                        │
└─────────────────────────────────────────────────────────┘
```

Table indicates the amount of medical technology supplied to the world by U. S. firms.

Technology	Percent
Medical devices	50
Linear accelerators	75

Source: U.S. House Subcommittee on Technology, Environment, and Aviation. *Health Care Reform and Its Possible Effects on Innovative Therapies.* Statement presented by Derrel B. De Passe, Vice President, Worldwide Government Relations Varian Associates, Inc. Washington, DC: Federal Document Clearinghouse Congressional Testimony, 2 February 1994.

Nursing and Personal Care Facilities

★ 629 ★

Intermediate Care Facilities, Establishments and Employees

These establishments provide inpatient nursing and rehabilitative services, although not on a continuous basis. Such facilities are staffed 24-hours a day, with a full-time licensed nurse on duty during each shift. Weekly consultation with a registered nurse on care is required. Intermediate care nursing homes are one such facility.

State	Establishments	Rank	Employees	Rank
Alabama	26	25	910	32
Alaska	0	-	0	-
Arizona	14	34	273	40
Arkansas	24	26	998	29
California	124	4	3167	13
Colorado	14	34	615	36
Connecticut	35	22	2397	20
Delaware	2	39	0[1]	-
D.C.	5	38	0[1]	-
Florida	58	14	2925	15
Georgia	36	21	2524	18
Hawaii	8	36	0[1]	-
Idaho	14	34	174	42
Illinois	106	7	5895	5

[Continued]

★ 629 ★

Intermediate Care Facilities, Establishments and Employees
[Continued]

State	Establishments	Rank	Employees	Rank
Indiana	108	5	6158	4
Iowa	91	8	5399	6
Kansas	71	11	3795	10
Kentucky	61	12	3914	9
Louisiana	59	13	4019	8
Maine	37	20	2303	22
Maryland	29	24	2436	19
Massachusetts	107	6	4427	7
Michigan	71	11	2924	16
Minnesota	79	10	2962	14
Mississippi	20	30	990	30
Missouri	80	9	3285	12
Montana	5	38	0[1]	-
Nebraska	19	31	818	34
Nevada	1	40	0[1]	-
New Hampshire	16	32	0[1]	-
New Jersey	23	27	846	33
New Mexico	9	35	679	35
New York	21	29	1139	27
North Carolina	49	17	2132	24
North Dakota	7	37	186	41
Ohio	265	1	15312	1
Oklahoma	137	3	6878	3
Oregon	53	15	2162	23
Pennsylvania	52	16	2319	21
Rhode Island	15	33	305	39
South Carolina	14	34	457	38
South Dakota	8	36	0[1]	-
Tennessee	44	18	2660	17
Texas	215	2	10540	2
Utah	31	23	1361	26
Vermont	8	36	490	37
Virginia	43	19	3307	11
Washington	36	21	1123	28
West Virginia	22	28	978	31
Wisconsin	35	22	1634	25
Wyoming	0	-	0	-
U.S. Total	2407	-	119829	-

Source: Census of Service Industries on CD-ROM, 1987. Geographic Area Series [machine-readable datafiles]. Prepared by U.S. Bureau of the Census. Washington, DC: The Bureau, 1990. Notes: Data shown only for businesses subject to federal income taxes. 1. Data are withheld to avoid disclosure of individual companies.

★ 630 ★

Nursing and Personal Care Facilities

Intermediate Care Facilities, Expenses: 1990-1991

Figures represent estimated annual expenses and year-to-year percent change in annual expenses for tax-exempt firms.

[In millions of dollars]

Year	Expenses	Percent change
1991	1,604	12.0
1990	1,432	

Source: "1991 Service Annual Survey: Health Services." In CENDATA [online service]. Washington, DC: U.S. Bureau of the Census [issued 26 July 1993]. No. 10.10.4 and No. 10.10.4.7.

★ 631 ★

Nursing and Personal Care Facilities

Intermediate Care Facilities, Receipts: 1987-1991

Figures represent estimated annual receipts for taxable firms.

[In millions of dollars]

Year	Receipts
1991	3,338
1990	2,998
1989	(NA)
1988	(NA)
1987	(NA)

Source: "1991 Service Annual Survey: Health Services." In CENDATA [online service]. Washington, DC: U.S. Bureau of the Census [issued 26 July 1993]. No. 10.10.4 and No. 10.10.4.7. *Note:* "NA" indicates "not available."

★ 632 ★

Nursing and Personal Care Facilities

Intermediate Care Facilities, Revenue: 1987-1991

Figures represent estimated annual revenue for tax-exempt firms.

[In millions of dollars]

Year	Revenue
1991	1,572
1990	1,385
1989	(NA)
1988	(NA)
1987	(NA)

Source: "1991 Service Annual Survey: Health Services." In CENDATA [online service]. Washington, DC: U.S. Bureau of the Census [issued 26 July 1993]. No. 10.10.4 and No. 10.10.4.7. *Note:* "NA" indicates "not available."

★ 633 ★

Nursing and Personal Care Facilities

Leading Long-term Care Facilities: 1993

The table below lists the top 10 assisted-living facilities.

Facility (location)	Beds	Facilities	States[1]	Occupancy rate (%)	Total revenues ($)	Total operating expenses ($)
Beverly Enterprises, Inc. (Fort Smith, Arkansas)	89,298	838	35	88.4	2.6 billion	2.6 billion
Hillhaven Corp. (Tacoma, Washington)	37,402	301	31	93.6	1.2 billion	1.1 billion
Manor HealthCare Corp. (Silver Spring, Maryland)	22,578	162	28	88	830 million	627 million
Living Centers of America Inc. (Houston, Texas)	21,993	242	10	82.6	386 million	NA
Life Care Centers of America, Inc. (Cleveland, Tennessee)	18,562	136	27	92	498 million	NA
Evangelical Lutheran Good Samaritan Society (Sioux Falls, South Dakota)	18,386	240	26	94.5	404 million	390 million
Health Care and Retirement Corp. (Toledo, Ohio)	16,030	125	16	92	545 million	NA
United Health, Inc. (Milwaukee, Wisconsin)	15,886	144	14	92	535 million	NA
Genesis Health Ventures, Inc. (Kennett Square, Pennsylvania)	14,321	94	11	90	NA[2]	NA[2]
ServiceMaster Diversified Health Services/VHA Long Term Care (Memphis, Tennessee)	14,235	95	26	94	NA	NA

Source: Monroe, Stephen M. "'Provider' Surveys Top Chains." *Provider* (January 1994), pp. 37-40. Primary source: American Health Care Association (AHCA). *Notes:* 1. States in which facilities operate. 2. Data does not reflect merger with Meridian Healthcare Inc. Compiled with company-supplied data.

★ 634 ★

Nursing and Personal Care Facilities

Nursing and Personal Care Facilities, Establishments and Employees

Table below reflects establishment and employment data for facilities providing inpatient nursing and health-related personal care. See related tables for data on skilled nursing care and intermediate care facilities.

State	Establishments	Rank	Employees	Rank
Alabama	225	25	14847	26
Alaska	0	-	0	-
Arizona	119	33	7728	33
Arkansas	204	27	12273	29
California	1257	1	86405	1
Colorado	151	30	11209	30
Connecticut	230	23	23672	16
Delaware	27	43	2075	45
D.C.	14	47	1237	47
Florida	543	7	38259	8
Georgia	363	13	25547	12
Hawaii	17	46	0[1]	-
Idaho	66	37	2962	40
Illinois	588	5	45740	5
Indiana	485	8	37398	9
Iowa	306	15	18111	20
Kansas	257	21	13989	27
Kentucky	226	24	14986	25
Louisiana	275	18	18193	19
Maine	127	32	8331	32
Maryland	182	29	17966	21
Massachusetts	592	4	42140	6
Michigan	418	10	32985	10
Minnesota	295	16	24601	14
Mississippi	132	31	8971	31
Missouri	462	9	29021	11
Montana	40	42	2455	44
Nebraska	104	34	6627	35
Nevada	26	44	2597	42
New Hampshire	62	38	4055	38
New Jersey	259	20	24708	13
New Mexico	51	39	3194	39
New York	367	11	49450	4
North Carolina	313	14	20886	17
North Dakota	23	45	1695	46
Ohio	906	3	65693	2
Oklahoma	365	12	17378	22
Oregon	213	26	12883	28
Pennsylvania	576	6	39661	7
Rhode Island	94	36	7169	34
South Carolina	119	33	0[1]	-
South Dakota	47	40	2822	41
Tennessee	238	22	16584	23
Texas	1044	2	61815	3

[Continued]

★ 634 ★

Nursing and Personal Care Facilities, Establishments and Employees
[Continued]

State	Establishments	Rank	Employees	Rank
Utah	104	34	4514	37
Vermont	41	41	2477	43
Virginia	185	28	15398	24
Washington	290	17	20594	18
West Virginia	103	35	5954	36
Wisconsin	272	19	23811	15
Wyoming	12	48	782	48
U.S. Total	13415	-	961598	-

Source: *Census of Service Industries on CD-ROM, 1987.* Geographic Area Series [machine-readable datafiles]. Prepared by U.S. Bureau of the Census. Washington, DC: The Bureau, 1990. *Notes:* Data shown only for businesses subject to federal income taxes. 1. Data are withheld to avoid disclosure of individual companies.

★ 635 ★

Nursing and Personal Care Facilities

Nursing and Personal Care Facilities, Expenses: 1990-1991

Figures represent estimated annual expenses and year-to-year percent change in annual expenses for tax-exempt firms.

[In millions of dollars]

Year	Expenses	Percent change
1991	10,287	11.9
1990	9,193	

Source: "1991 Service Annual Survey: Health Services." In CENDATA [online service]. Washington, DC: U.S. Bureau of the Census [issued 26 July 1993]. No. 10.10.4 and No. 10.10.4.7.

★ 636 ★

Nursing and Personal Care Facilities

Nursing and Personal Care Facilities, Receipts: 1987-1991

Figures represent estimated annual receipts for taxable firms.

[In millions of dollars]

Year	Receipts
1991	28,848
1990	26,446
1989	23,349
1988	21,361
1987	20,063

Source: "1991 Service Annual Survey: Health Services." In CENDATA [online service]. Washington, DC: U.S. Bureau of the Census [issued 26 July 1993]. No. 10.10.4 and No. 10.10.4.7.

★ 637 ★

Nursing and Personal Care Facilities

Nursing and Personal Care Facilities, Revenue: 1987-1991

Figures represent estimated annual revenue for tax-exempt firms.

[In millions of dollars]

Year	Revenue
1991	10,471
1990	9,303
1989	8,844
1988	8,633
1987	8,201

Source: "1991 Service Annual Survey: Health Services." In CENDATA [online service]. Washington, DC: U.S. Bureau of the Census [issued 26 July 1993]. No. 10.10.4 and No. 10.10.4.7.

★ 638 ★

Nursing and Personal Care Facilities

Residential Care Facilities, Establishments and Employees

These facilities provide residential social and personal care for special groups of people, such as children, older Americans, or the mentally ill. Establishments include alcohol rehabilitation centers; children's homes; drug rehabilitation centers; group foster homes; halfway homes; homes for the aged; homes for the deaf or blind; orphanages; rest homes; homes for the mentally ill or emotionally disturbed; self-help group homes; homes for the physically challenged; and residential rehabilitation centers.

State	Establishments	Rank	Employees	Rank
Alabama	60	26	619	30
Arizona	109	18	1412	19
Arkansas	38	30	437	32
California	1984	1	19162	1
Colorado	106	19	983	25
Connecticut	88	21	1018	24
Florida	536	3	5320	5
Georgia	88	21	614	31
Illinois	109	18	2307	15
Indiana	68	22	1036	23
Iowa	64	24	1053	21
Kansas	35	31	331	33
Kentucky	54	27	1045	22
Louisiana	63	25	1132	20
Maryland	66	23	846	28
Massachusetts	201	12	3041	9
Michigan	648	2	4811	6
Minnesota	251	9	3861	7
Mississippi	27	33	263	35
Missouri	279	8	2615	11
Nebraska	28	32	279	34
New Jersey	123	16	1576	17
New York	426	5	7753	2
North Carolina	406	6	5433	4
Ohio	244	10	2571	12
Oklahoma	43	29	668	29
Oregon	360	7	2387	13
Pennsylvania	453	4	5789	3
South Carolina	105	20	968	26
Tennessee	114	17	963	27
Texas	178	15	3700	8
Utah	46	28	2367	14
Virginia	231	11	2850	10
Washington	181	14	2124	16
Wisconsin	188	13	1472	18
U.S. Total	8516	-	98407	-

Source: Census of Service Industries on CD-ROM, 1987. Geographic Area Series [machine-readable datafiles]. Prepared by U.S. Bureau of the Census. Washington, DC: The Bureau, 1990. *Note:* Data shown only for businesses subject to federal income taxes.

★ 639 ★

Nursing and Personal Care Facilities

Skilled Nursing Care Facilities, Establishments and Employees

These establishments provide inpatient nursing and rehabilitative services on a continuous basis. Care is directed by a physician. Facilities are staffed continuously with a licensed nurse and at least one full-time registered nurse during each day shift. Establishments include convalescent homes, extended care facilities, nursing homes, and mental retardation hospitals.

State	Establishments	Rank	Employees	Rank
Alabama	180	21	13483	20
Alaska	0	-	0	-
Arizona	83	33	7177	32
Arkansas	161	25	10391	25
California	1008	1	79933	1
Colorado	125	29	10251	27
Connecticut	182	20	20885	16
Delaware	22	46	1978	42
D.C.	6	50	835	47
Florida	406	5	33883	8
Georgia	299	11	22645	12
Hawaii	8	49	1092	46
Idaho	43	39	2577	39
Illinois	429	4	37594	5
Indiana	351	8	30336	9
Iowa	188	19	11827	23
Kansas	168	23	9730	28
Kentucky	129	28	10256	26
Louisiana	163	24	12293	22
Maine	77	35	5378	35
Maryland	137	26	14920	19
Massachusetts	385	6	34631	6
Michigan	293	12	28524	10
Minnesota	196	17	21378	14
Mississippi	100	31	7650	31
Missouri	334	9	24390	11
Montana	32	42	2382	41
Nebraska	79	34	5620	34
Nevada	24	44	0[1]	-
New Hampshire	39	40	3329	37
New Jersey	202	15	21779	13
New Mexico	28	43	1836	44
New York	302	10	46763	4
North Carolina	190	18	17243	18
North Dakota	16	47	1509	45
Ohio	556	3	47366	3
Oklahoma	199	16	9569	30
Oregon	131	27	9602	29
Pennsylvania	379	7	34437	7
Rhode Island	65	37	6533	33
South Carolina	95	32	0[1]	-
South Dakota	36	41	2405	40

[Continued]

★ 639 ★

Skilled Nursing Care Facilities, Establishments and Employees
[Continued]

State	Establishments	Rank	Employees	Rank
Tennessee	170	22	13314	21
Texas	755	2	48459	2
Utah	63	38	3050	38
Vermont	23	45	1926	43
Virginia	110	30	11606	24
Washington	224	13	18763	17
West Virginia	67	36	4692	36
Wisconsin	212	14	21261	15
Wyoming	12	48	782	48
U.S. Total	9482	-	798425	-

Source: Census of Service Industries on CD-ROM, 1987. Geographic Area Series [machine-readable datafiles]. Prepared by U.S. Bureau of the Census. Washington, DC: The Bureau, 1990. Notes: Data shown only for businesses subject to federal income taxes. 1. Data are withheld to avoid disclosure of individual companies.

★ 640 ★

Nursing and Personal Care Facilities

Skilled Nursing Care Facilities, Expenses: 1990-1991

Figures represent estimated annual expenses and year-to-year percent change in annual expenses for tax-exempt firms.

[In millions of dollars]

Year	Expenses	Percent change
1991	8,024	11.4
1990	7,202	

Source: "1991 Service Annual Survey: Health Services." In CENDATA [online service]. Washington, DC: U.S. Bureau of the Census [issued 26 July 1993]. No. 10.10.4 and No. 10.10.4.7.

★ 641 ★

Nursing and Personal Care Facilities

Skilled Nursing Care Facilities, Receipts: 1987-1991

Figures represent estimated annual receipts for taxable firms.

[In millions of dollars]

Year	Receipts
1991	23,623
1990	21,790
1989	(NA)
1988	(NA)
1987	(NA)

Source: "1991 Service Annual Survey: Health Services." In CENDATA [online service]. Washington, DC: U.S. Bureau of the Census [issued 26 July 1993]. No. 10.10.4 and No. 10.10.4.7. *Note:* "NA" indicates "not available."

★ 642 ★

Nursing and Personal Care Facilities

Skilled Nursing Care Facilities, Revenue: 1987-1991

Figures represent estimated annual revenue for tax-exempt firms.

[In millions of dollars]

Year	Revenue
1991	8,243
1990	7,378
1989	(NA)
1988	(NA)
1987	(NA)

Source: "1991 Service Annual Survey: Health Services." In CENDATA [online service]. Washington, DC: U.S. Bureau of the Census [issued 26 July 1993]. No. 10.10.4 and No. 10.10.4.7. *Note:* "NA" indicates "not available."

Offices and Clinics of Practitioners

★ 643 ★

Clinics of Dentists, Establishments and Employees

Data provided for clinics not owned and operated by associated dentists.

State	Establishments	Rank	Employees	Rank
Alabama	5	17	54	20
Alaska	3	19	0[1]	-
Arizona	9	13	124	12
Arkansas	4	18	26	28
California	82	1	931	1
Colorado	10	12	53	21
Connecticut	1	21	0[1]	-
Delaware	0	-	0	-
D.C.	0	-	0	-
Florida	19	7	171	9
Georgia	10	12	98	15
Hawaii	6	16	8	32
Idaho	3	19	11	31
Illinois	31	4	232	6
Indiana	6	16	59	18
Iowa	4	18	32	25
Kansas	8	14	45	22
Kentucky	2	20	0[1]	-
Louisiana	11	11	83	17
Maine	0	-	0	-
Maryland	8	14	144	10
Massachusetts	18	8	244	5
Michigan	33	3	318	3
Minnesota	13	10	108	13
Mississippi	0	-	0	-
Missouri	5	17	42	23
Montana	3	19	13	30
Nebraska	2	20	0[1]	-
Nevada	2	20	0[1]	-
New Hampshire	1	21	0[1]	-
New Jersey	7	15	87	16
New Mexico	2	20	0[1]	-
New York	23	6	339	2
North Carolina	1	21	0[1]	-
North Dakota	2	20	0[1]	-
Ohio	10	12	53	21
Oklahoma	5	17	28	27
Oregon	23	6	224	7
Pennsylvania	13	10	126	11
Rhode Island	0	-	0	-
South Carolina	0	-	0	-
South Dakota	1	21	0[1]	-
Tennessee	5	17	38	24

[Continued]

★ 643 ★

Clinics of Dentists, Establishments and Employees
[Continued]

State	Establishments	Rank	Employees	Rank
Texas	27	5	173	8
Utah	5	17	29	26
Vermont	2	20	0[1]	-
Virginia	7	15	57	19
Washington	34	2	306	4
West Virginia	2	20	0[1]	-
Wisconsin	15	9	103	14
Wyoming	3	19	16	29
U.S. Total	486	-	4625	-

Source: Census of Service Industries on CD-ROM, 1987. Geographic Area Series [machine-readable datafiles]. Prepared by U.S. Bureau of the Census. Washington, DC: The Bureau, 1990. *Notes:* Data shown only for businesses subject to federal income taxes. 1. Data are withheld to avoid disclosure of individual companies.

★ 644 ★

Offices and Clinics of Practitioners

Clinics of Doctors of Medicine, Establishments and Employees

Data provided for clinics not owned and operated by associated physicians.

State	Establishments	Rank	Employees	Rank
Alabama	71	19	899	25
Alaska	14	37	63	45
Arizona	111	8	3795	4
Arkansas	40	26	1102	10
California	693	1	37290	1
Colorado	81	15	973	21
Connecticut	44	27	779	30
Delaware	12	38	405	39
D.C.	12	38	623	33
Florida	363	2	8943	2
Georgia	94	11	809	28
Hawaii	41	29	605	34
Idaho	16	35	151	41
Illinois	227	4	3235	5
Indiana	70	20	1639	11
Iowa	34	31	371	40
Kansas	33	32	604	35
Kentucky	42	28	788	29
Louisiana	82	14	1170	17
Maine	12	38	143	42
Maryland	68	21	1270	16
Massachusetts	86	12	1672	10
Michigan	155	5	2631	7
Minnesota	49	25	967	22

[Continued]

★ 644 ★

Clinics of Doctors of Medicine, Establishments and Employees
[Continued]

State	Establishments	Rank	Employees	Rank
Mississippi	48	26	788	29
Missouri	105	9	1502	12
Montana	12	38	91	44
Nebraska	15	36	456	38
Nevada	25	33	713	31
New Hampshire	24	34	0[1]	-
New Jersey	80	16	1071	19
New Mexico	24	34	580	36
New York	113	7	2426	8
North Carolina	83	13	1413	14
North Dakota	11	39	92	43
Ohio	151	6	2996	6
Oklahoma	64	22	559	37
Oregon	52	24	966	23
Pennsylvania	155	5	2285	9
Rhode Island	14	37	143	42
South Carolina	61	23	820	27
South Dakota	5	42	0[1]	-
Tennessee	77	17	932	24
Texas	309	3	5183	3
Utah	38	30	1002	20
Vermont	6	41	38	47
Virginia	80	16	881	26
Washington	99	10	1456	13
West Virginia	33	32	639	32
Wisconsin	74	18	1387	15
Wyoming	7	40	46	46
U.S. Total	4224	-	100469	-

Source: Census of Service Industries on CD-ROM, 1987. Geographic Area Series [machine-readable datafiles]. Prepared by U.S. Bureau of the Census. Washington, DC: The Bureau, 1990. *Notes:* Data shown only for businesses subject to federal income taxes. 1. Data are withheld to avoid disclosure of individual companies.

★ 645 ★

Offices and Clinics of Practitioners

Offices and Clinics of Chiropractors, Establishments and Employees

State	Establishments	Rank	Employees	Rank
Alabama	227	26	531	27
Alaska	59	46	202	43
Arizona	471	14	1303	14
Arkansas	178	31	514	28
California	3403	1	9868	1

[Continued]

★ 645 ★

Offices and Clinics of Chiropractors, Establishments and Employees
[Continued]

State	Establishments	Rank	Employees	Rank
Colorado	451	16	1224	17
Connecticut	219	27	0[1]	-
Delaware	36	50	176	45
D.C.	10	51	0[1]	-
Florida	1312	2	3934	2
Georgia	555	12	1516	12
Hawaii	89	40	215	42
Idaho	96	38	309	35
Illinois	798	6	2352	6
Indiana	323	21	961	20
Iowa	350	19	879	22
Kansas	249	25	689	24
Kentucky	182	30	459	30
Louisiana	277	22	902	21
Maine	85	41	300	36
Maryland	146	32	455	31
Massachusetts	384	18	1205	18
Michigan	795	7	2404	4
Minnesota	618	11	1971	10
Mississippi	105	37	256	39
Missouri	519	13	1228	16
Montana	94	39	245	40
Nebraska	120	35	316	34
Nevada	115	36	342	33
New Hampshire	81	44	233	41
New Jersey	777	8	2336	7
New Mexico	137	33	368	32
New York	1203	3	3319	3
North Carolina	341	20	1013	19
North Dakota	62	45	154	46
Ohio	634	9	2273	9
Oklahoma	261	23	742	23
Oregon	398	17	1238	15
Pennsylvania	849	5	2332	8
Rhode Island	45	47	117	47
South Carolina	209	29	498	29
South Dakota	83	43	191	44
Tennessee	253	24	674	25
Texas	855	4	2402	5
Utah	131	34	297	37
Vermont	44	48	105	48
Virginia	215	28	672	26
Washington	631	10	1722	11
West Virginia	84	42	263	38
Wisconsin	465	15	1507	13

[Continued]

★ 645 ★

Offices and Clinics of Chiropractors, Establishments and Employees
[Continued]

State	Establishments	Rank	Employees	Rank
Wyoming	41	49	93	49
U.S. Total	20065	-	58041	-

Source: Census of Service Industries on CD-ROM, 1987. Geographic Area Series [machine-readable datafiles]. Prepared by U.S. Bureau of the Census. Washington, DC: The Bureau, 1990. *Notes:* Data shown only for businesses subject to federal income taxes. 1. Data are withheld to avoid disclosure of individual companies.

★ 646 ★

Offices and Clinics of Practitioners

Offices and Clinics of Chiropractors, Receipts: 1987-1991

Figures represent estimated annual receipts for taxable firms.

[In millions of dollars]

Year	Receipts
1991	4,986
1990	4,828
1989	4,420
1988	3,984
1987	3,275

Source: "1991 Service Annual Survey: Health Services." In CENDATA [online service]. Washington, DC: U.S. Bureau of the Census [issued 26 July 1993]. No. 10.10.4 and No. 10.10.4.7.

★ 647 ★

Offices and Clinics of Practitioners

Offices and Clinics of Dentists, Establishments and Employees

Table reflects number of establishments and employees for offices and clinics owned and operated by associated dentists.

State	Establishments	Rank	Employees	Rank
Alabama	1308	27	6002	26
Alaska	231	49	1164	48
Arizona	1394	26	6344	25
Arkansas	796	33	3241	33
California	13835	1	69240	1
Colorado	1825	21	7689	22

[Continued]

★ 647 ★

Offices and Clinics of Dentists, Establishments and Employees
[Continued]

State	Establishments	Rank	Employees	Rank
Connecticut	1668	22	8431	20
Delaware	210	51	1390	45
D.C.	350	45	1348	46
Florida	4674	6	23570	5
Georgia	2168	14	11011	14
Hawaii	580	36	2846	36
Idaho	446	40	2184	41
Illinois	4771	5	21802	7
Indiana	2096	15	9870	18
Iowa	1171	29	5063	29
Kansas	999	31	4661	31
Kentucky	1396	25	5118	28
Louisiana	1515	24	6360	24
Maine	434	42	1992	43
Maryland	2008	17	9881	17
Massachusetts	2898	10	14728	10
Michigan	4268	8	23823	4
Minnesota	1992	19	10924	15
Mississippi	772	34	3055	34
Missouri	1995	18	8853	19
Montana	426	43	1715	44
Nebraska	716	35	3038	35
Nevada	436	41	2363	40
New Hampshire	481	39	2430	39
New Jersey	3824	9	18364	9
New Mexico	539	38	2475	37
New York	8491	2	36047	2
North Carolina	2034	16	10095	16
North Dakota	259	47	1102	50
Ohio	4447	7	21737	8
Oklahoma	1224	28	4930	30
Oregon	1604	23	7491	23
Pennsylvania	5023	4	22851	6
Rhode Island	395	44	2138	42
South Carolina	1091	30	5190	27
South Dakota	273	46	1145	49
Tennessee	1949	20	8067	21
Texas	5972	3	24839	3
Utah	929	32	3704	32
Vermont	237	48	1199	47
Virginia	2324	12	11150	13
Washington	2633	11	13696	11
West Virginia	575	37	2443	38
Wisconsin	2252	13	11851	12

[Continued]

★ 647 ★

Offices and Clinics of Dentists, Establishments and Employees
[Continued]

State	Establishments	Rank	Employees	Rank
Wyoming	217	50	886	51
U.S. Total	104151	-	491536	-

Source: Census of Service Industries on CD-ROM, 1987. Geographic Area Series [machine-readable datafiles]. Prepared by U.S. Bureau of the Census. Washington, DC: The Bureau, 1990. *Note:* Data shown only for businesses subject to federal income taxes.

★ 648 ★

Offices and Clinics of Practitioners

Offices and Clinics of Dentists, Receipts: 1987-1991

Figures represent estimated annual receipts for taxable firms.

[In millions of dollars]

Year	Receipts
1991	29,731
1990	28,475
1989	26,932
1988	25,550
1987	24,017

Source: "1991 Service Annual Survey: Health Services." In CENDATA [online service]. Washington, DC: U.S. Bureau of the Census [issued 26 July 1993]. No. 10.10.4 and No. 10.10.4.7.

★ 649 ★

Offices and Clinics of Practitioners

Offices and Clinics of Doctors of Medicine, Establishments and Employees

The table below indicates number of establishments and employees for offices and clinics owned and operated by associated physicians.

State	Establishments	Rank	Employees	Rank
Alabama	2527	24	18117	22
Alaska	366	48	2090	47
Arizona	3130	20	16256	23
Arkansas	1591	29	10439	32
California	29641	1	166282	1
Colorado	2739	22	15379	26
Connecticut	2952	21	16040	24
Delaware	576	46	3275	45

[Continued]

★ 649 ★

Offices and Clinics of Doctors of Medicine, Establishments and Employees
[Continued]

State	Establishments	Rank	Employees	Rank
D.C.	867	42	4239	43
Florida	12533	4	72458	3
Georgia	4687	10	28520	10
Hawaii	1029	37	5152	39
Idaho	712	44	4230	44
Illinois	8651	6	48486	7
Indiana	3812	14	23544	16
Iowa	1459	33	11006	31
Kansas	1463	32	11641	30
Kentucky	2441	25	15568	25
Louisiana	3389	18	19788	21
Maine	949	39	4361	42
Maryland	4602	12	24232	15
Massachusetts	4659	11	26805	13
Michigan	6300	9	39171	8
Minnesota	1573	30	20632	19
Mississippi	1472	31	9027	33
Missouri	3371	19	20121	20
Montana	617	45	3275	45
Nebraska	909	41	6744	36
Nevada	962	38	5505	38
New Hampshire	730	43	4805	41
New Jersey	7257	8	34696	9
New Mexico	1092	36	5824	37
New York	16050	2	72464	2
North Carolina	3656	15	26619	14
North Dakota	235	51	4866	40
Ohio	8114	7	49949	6
Oklahoma	2274	27	12167	29
Oregon	2347	26	13476	27
Pennsylvania	9276	5	50610	5
Rhode Island	931	40	4239	43
South Carolina	2138	28	13015	28
South Dakota	349	49	2779	46
Tennessee	3555	16	21739	17
Texas	13646	3	68040	4
Utah	1350	35	7367	35
Vermont	425	47	1928	48
Virginia	4287	13	27006	12
Washington	3487	17	20731	18
West Virginia	1374	34	7992	34
Wisconsin	2615	23	27210	11

[Continued]

★ 649 ★

Offices and Clinics of Doctors of Medicine, Establishments and Employees
[Continued]

State	Establishments	Rank	Employees	Rank
Wyoming	335	50	1698	49
U.S. Total	195502	-	1131603	-

Source: Census of Service Industries on CD-ROM, 1987. Geographic Area Series [machine-readable datafiles]. Prepared by U.S. Bureau of the Census. Washington, DC: The Bureau, 1990. *Note:* Data shown only for businesses subject to federal income taxes.

★ 650 ★

Offices and Clinics of Practitioners

Offices and Clinics of Doctors of Medicine, Receipts: 1987-1991

Figures represent estimated annual receipts for taxable firms.

[In millions of dollars]

Year	Receipts
1991	122,470
1990	115,067
1989	106,300
1988	100,314
1987	90,462

Source: "1991 Service Annual Survey: Health Services." In CENDATA [online service]. Washington, DC: U.S. Bureau of the Census [issued 26 July 1993]. No. 10.10.4 and No. 10.10.4.7.

★ 651 ★

Offices and Clinics of Practitioners

Offices and Clinics of Doctors of Osteopathy, Establishments and Employees

State	Establishments	Rank	Employees	Rank
Alabama	13	32	53	30
Alaska	5	37	15	40
Arizona	262	9	1158	9
Arkansas	16	31	62	27
California	250	10	968	10
Colorado	169	12	694	12
Connecticut	6	36	29	36
Delaware	26	26	0[1]	-

[Continued]

★ 651 ★

Offices and Clinics of Doctors of Osteopathy, Establishments and Employees
[Continued]

State	Establishments	Rank	Employees	Rank
D.C.	1	40	0[1]	-
Florida	610	4	2744	4
Georgia	79	20	352	19
Hawaii	9	34	21	39
Idaho	13	32	58	29
Illinois	122	16	589	13
Indiana	130	14	549	15
Iowa	186	11	0[1]	-
Kansas	92	18	413	18
Kentucky	22	28	97	24
Louisiana	6	36	10	41
Maine	88	19	0[1]	-
Maryland	9	34	28	37
Massachusetts	21	29	39	32
Michigan	1127	1	6989	1
Minnesota	19	30	67	26
Mississippi	8	35	33	33
Missouri	468	6	1973	6
Montana	10	33	31	35
Nebraska	1	40	0[1]	-
Nevada	23	27	59	28
New Hampshire	4	38	15	40
New Jersey	357	7	1948	7
New Mexico	52	23	239	21
New York	144	13	747	11
North Carolina	10	33	31	35
North Dakota	1	40	0[1]	-
Ohio	701	3	3789	3
Oklahoma	309	8	1262	8
Oregon	100	17	426	17
Pennsylvania	870	2	4537	2
Rhode Island	37	25	134	23
South Carolina	2	39	0[1]	-
South Dakota	10	33	92	25
Tennessee	40	24	175	22
Texas	571	5	2438	5
Utah	8	35	40	31
Vermont	9	34	32	34
Virginia	22	28	97	24
Washington	126	15	562	14
West Virginia	66	22	248	20
Wisconsin	76	21	448	16

[Continued]

★ 651 ★

Offices and Clinics of Doctors of Osteopathy, Establishments and Employees

[Continued]

State	Establishments	Rank	Employees	Rank
Wyoming	8	35	26	38
U.S. Total	7314	-	35572	-

Source: Census of Service Industries on CD-ROM, 1987. Geographic Area Series [machine-readable datafiles]. Prepared by U.S. Bureau of the Census. Washington, DC: The Bureau, 1990. *Notes:* Data shown only for businesses subject to federal income taxes. 1. Data are withheld to avoid disclosure of individual companies.

★ 652 ★

Offices and Clinics of Practitioners

Offices and Clinics of Doctors of Osteopathy, Receipts: 1987-1991

Figures represent estimated annual receipts for taxable firms.

[In millions of dollars]

Year	Receipts
1991	2,599
1990	2,513
1989	2,321
1988	2,335
1987	2,119

Source: "1991 Service Annual Survey: Health Services." In CENDATA [online service]. Washington, DC: U.S. Bureau of the Census [issued 26 July 1993]. No. 10.10.4 and No. 10.10.4.7.

★ 653 ★

Offices and Clinics of Practitioners

Offices and Clinics of Optometrists, Establishments and Employees

State	Establishments	Rank	Employees	Rank
Alabama	182	28	561	32
Alaska	37	46	142	46
Arizona	185	27	614	30
Arkansas	185	27	666	28
California	2242	1	8445	1
Colorado	248	20	820	25
Connecticut	206	26	808	26
Delaware	45	44	129	47

[Continued]

★ 653 ★

Offices and Clinics of Optometrists, Establishments and Employees
[Continued]

State	Establishments	Rank	Employees	Rank
D.C.	27	47	0[1]	-
Florida	746	6	2379	8
Georgia	337	16	1205	15
Hawaii	76	37	229	44
Idaho	94	35	293	39
Illinois	632	7	2783	5
Indiana	462	10	1536	10
Iowa	273	19	995	20
Kansas	214	25	887	21
Kentucky	231	23	686	27
Louisiana	206	26	625	29
Maine	117	32	356	35
Maryland	226	24	1050	18
Massachusetts	373	12	1284	14
Michigan	598	8	2725	7
Minnesota	246	21	881	22
Mississippi	138	31	364	34
Missouri	305	17	1111	17
Montana	94	35	010	30
Nebraska	113	33	466	33
Nevada	79	36	343	37
New Hampshire	69	41	238	41
New Jersey	484	9	1740	9
New Mexico	107	34	353	36
New York	751	5	2730	6
North Carolina	425	11	1338	13
North Dakota	60	42	238	41
Ohio	821	4	3129	3
Oklahoma	285	18	876	23
Oregon	232	22	830	24
Pennsylvania	828	3	2912	4
Rhode Island	71	40	235	42
South Carolina	181	29	0[1]	-
South Dakota	73	39	234	43
Tennessee	339	15	998	19
Texas	922	2	3512	2
Utah	75	38	244	40
Vermont	39	45	102	48
Virginia	373	12	1458	11
Washington	347	14	1114	16
West Virginia	164	30	588	31
Wisconsin	353	13	1392	12

[Continued]

★ 653 ★

Offices and Clinics of Optometrists, Establishments and Employees

[Continued]

State	Establishments	Rank	Employees	Rank
Wyoming	56	43	212	45
U.S. Total	15972	-	57900	-

Source: Census of Service Industries on CD-ROM, 1987. Geographic Area Series [machine-readable datafiles]. Prepared by U.S. Bureau of the Census. Washington, DC: The Bureau, 1990. Notes: Data shown only for businesses subject to federal income taxes. 1. Data are withheld to avoid disclosure of individual companies.

★ 654 ★

Offices and Clinics of Practitioners

Offices and Clinics of Optometrists, Receipts: 1987-1991

Figures represent estimated annual receipts for taxable firms.

[In millions of dollars]

Year	Receipts
1991	4,430
1990	4,275
1989	3,864
1988	3,760
1987	3,450

Source: "1991 Service Annual Survey: Health Services." In CENDATA [online service]. Washington, DC: U.S. Bureau of the Census [issued 26 July 1993]. No. 10.10.4 and No. 10.10.4.7.

★ 655 ★

Offices and Clinics of Practitioners

Offices and Clinics of Other Health Practitioners, Establishments and Employees

Table below reflects establishment and employment data for health practitioners such as acupuncturists, audiologists, Christian Science practitioners, dental hygienists, dieticians, hypnotists, inhalation therapists, midwives, naturopaths, registered and practical nurses, nutritionists, occupational therapists, paramedics, physical therapists, physicans' assistants, psychiatric social workers, clinical psychologists, psychotherapists, speech clinicians, and speech pathologists.

State	Establishments	Rank	Employees	Rank
Alabama	547	29	1879	28
Alaska	130	48	420	45
Arizona	1036	19	3113	21
Arkansas	470	32	1530	30
California	8810	1	29957	1
Colorado	1073	17	3179	20
Connecticut	762	25	0[1]	-
Delaware	149	46	551	42
D.C.	121	50	0[1]	-
Florida	3243	3	11090	3
Georgia	1259	12	4239	12
Hawaii	242	42	654	40
Idaho	247	41	769	38
Illinois	2202	7	8112	8
Indiana	1039	18	3783	15
Iowa	781	24	2516	25
Kansas	616	28	2044	27
Kentucky	538	30	1624	29
Louisiana	718	27	2545	23
Maine	295	38	910	36
Maryland	848	23	3339	19
Massachusetts	1322	11	4410	11
Michigan	2184	8	8536	7
Minnesota	1132	15	4212	13
Mississippi	339	35	1435	31
Missouri	1135	14	3661	18
Montana	258	40	792	37
Nebraska	320	36	0[1]	-
Nevada	288	39	1042	34
New Hampshire	240	43	698	39
New Jersey	2024	9	6670	9
New Mexico	389	33	1268	32
New York	3634	2	11511	2
North Carolina	1098	16	3736	17
North Dakota	141	47	496	43
Ohio	2355	6	8944	6
Oklahoma	740	26	2165	26
Oregon	929	21	2967	22
Pennsylvania	2723	5	9421	5
Rhode Island	196	44	634	41

[Continued]

★ 655 ★

Offices and Clinics of Other Health Practitioners, Establishments and Employees
[Continued]

State	Establishments	Rank	Employees	Rank
South Carolina	531	31	0[1]	-
South Dakota	178	45	486	44
Tennessee	853	22	2534	24
Texas	2931	4	9664	4
Utah	344	34	1013	35
Vermont	120	51	290	47
Virginia	989	20	3747	16
Washington	1466	10	4545	10
West Virginia	311	37	1050	33
Wisconsin	1136	13	4103	14
Wyoming	123	49	391	46
U.S. Total	55555	-	188835	-

Source: Census of Service Industries on CD-ROM, 1987. Geographic Area Series [machine-readable datafiles]. Prepared by U.S. Bureau of the Census. Washington, DC: The Bureau, 1990. *Notes:* Data shown only for businesses subject to federal income taxes. 1. Data are withheld to avoid disclosure of individual companies.

★ 656 ★

Offices and Clinics of Practitioners

Offices and Clinics of Other Health Practitioners, Receipts: 1987-1991

Figures represent estimated annual receipts for taxable firms.

[In millions of dollars]

Year	Receipts
1991	15,628
1990	14,802
1989	12,795
1988	12,167
1987	10,340

Source: "1991 Service Annual Survey: Health Services." In CENDATA [online service]. Washington, DC: U.S. Bureau of the Census [issued 26 July 1993]. No. 10.10.4 and No. 10.10.4.7.

★ 657 ★
Offices and Clinics of Practitioners

Offices and Clinics of Podiatrists, Establishments and Employees

State	Establishments	Rank	Employees	Rank
Alabama	44	30	177	27
Alaska	7	45	13	47
Arizona	115	17	335	18
Arkansas	29	35	79	37
California	1032	1	2927	1
Colorado	98	21	219	22
Connecticut	136	14	460	12
Delaware	23	37	91	35
D.C.	36	33	102	34
Florida	439	4	1401	4
Georgia	108	19	354	17
Hawaii	12	42	25	44
Idaho	17	40	51	40
Illinois	377	9	1064	8
Indiana	120	16	401	15
Iowa	66	25	199	25
Kansas	52	28	154	30
Kentucky	40	31	127	32
Louisiana	61	26	170	20
Maine	36	33	87	36
Maryland	176	11	668	10
Massachusetts	206	10	474	11
Michigan	396	6	1539	3
Minnesota	75	22	208	24
Mississippi	19	39	47	41
Missouri	102	20	300	20
Montana	14	41	42	42
Nebraska	37	32	0[1]	-
Nevada	22	38	58	39
New Hampshire	24	36	47	41
New Jersey	386	7	1081	7
New Mexico	40	31	116	33
New York	866	2	2468	2
North Carolina	114	18	322	19
North Dakota	5	46	14	46
Ohio	429	5	1279	6
Oklahoma	72	23	188	26
Oregon	75	22	175	29
Pennsylvania	518	3	1374	5
Rhode Island	51	29	217	23
South Carolina	33	34	0[1]	-
South Dakota	11	43	28	43
Tennessee	68	24	226	21
Texas	378	8	965	9
Utah	56	27	153	31
Vermont	8	44	14	46

[Continued]

★ 657 ★

Offices and Clinics of Podiatrists, Establishments and Employees
[Continued]

State	Establishments	Rank	Employees	Rank
Virginia	142	13	440	13
Washington	145	12	371	16
West Virginia	23	37	64	38
Wisconsin	127	15	405	14
Wyoming	8	44	17	45
U.S. Total	7474	-	21969	-

Source: Census of Service Industries on CD-ROM, 1987. Geographic Area Series [machine-readable datafiles]. Prepared by U.S. Bureau of the Census. Washington, DC: The Bureau, 1990. *Notes:* Data shown only for businesses subject to federal income taxes. 1. Data are withheld to avoid disclosure of individual companies.

★ 658 ★

Offices and Clinics of Practitioners

Offices and Clinics of Podiatrists, Receipts: 1987-1991

Figures represent estimated annual receipts for taxable firms.

[In millions of dollars]

Year	Receipts
1991	1,826
1990	1,689
1989	(NA)
1988	(NA)
1987	(NA)

Source: "1991 Service Annual Survey: Health Services." In CENDATA [online service]. Washington, DC: U.S. Bureau of the Census [issued 26 July 1993]. No. 10.10.4 and No. 10.10.4.7. *Note:* "NA" indicates "not available."

Pharmaceutical Manufacturers

★ 659 ★

Diagnostic Substances Manufacturers, Establishments and Employees

[Employees in thousands]

State	Establishments	Rank	Employees	Rank
California	42	1	2.5	1
Florida	7	6	0.7[1]	4
Georgia	4	8	0.2[1]	6
Indiana	4	8	0.4[1]	5
Iowa	2	10	0.2[1]	6
Kansas	2	10	0.7[1]	4
Maryland	9	5	1.7	2
Massachusetts	9	5	0.7[1]	4
Michigan	3	9	0.4[1]	5
Missouri	4	8	0.2[1]	6
New Jersey	11	3	1.7[1]	2
New York	12	2	1.3	3
Pennsylvania	5	7	0.4[1]	5
Texas	10	4	0.4	5
Virginia	4	8	0.4[1]	5

Source: Census of Manufactures on CD-ROM, 1987. Geographic Area Series [machine-readable datafiles]. Prepared by U.S. Bureau of the Census. Washington, DC: The Bureau, 1991. *Note:* 1. Figure shown is the midpoint of a range.

★ 660 ★

Pharmaceutical Manufacturers

Drug Manufacturers, Establishments and Employees

[Employees in thousands]

State	Establishments	Rank	Employees	Rank
Arizona	14	20	0.7[1]	23
Arkansas	3	27	0.2[1]	26
California	206	1	19.6	2
Colorado	16	18	1.0	21
Connecticut	19	16	2.7	14
Delaware	5	25	0.7[1]	23
Florida	55	6	1.9	16
Georgia	31	12	1.2	20
Illinois	50	7	13.0	6
Indiana	30	13	15.8	3

[Continued]

★ 660 ★

Drug Manufacturers, Establishments and Employees
[Continued]

State	Establishments	Rank	Employees	Rank
Iowa	25	14	1.5	18
Kansas	15	19	1.7	17
Kentucky	9	24	0.2[1]	26
Louisiana	13	21	0.7[1]	23
Maine	12	22	0.3	25
Maryland	33	11	2.8	13
Massachusetts	48	8	3.0	12
Michigan	31	12	6.1	8
Minnesota	25	14	1.0	21
Mississippi	3	27	1.7[1]	17
Missouri	40	9	5.0	9
Nebraska	15	19	1.3	19
New Jersey	140	2	28.4	1
New York	133	3	15.6	5
North Carolina	36	10	8.6	7
North Dakota	1	28	0.4[1]	24
Ohio	36	10	4.2	10
Oklahoma	11	23	0.4[1]	24
Oregon	20	15	0.4	24
Pennsylvania	65	5	15.7	4
South Carolina	18	17	1.5	18
Tennessee	15	19	3.9	11
Texas	68	4	5.0	9
Utah	11	23	0.3	25
Virginia	13	21	2.5[2]	15
Washington	14	20	0.4	24
West Virginia	4	26	0.4[1]	24
Wisconsin	20	15	0.8	22

Source: Census of Manufactures on CD-ROM, 1987. Geographic Area Series [machine-readable datafiles]. Prepared by U.S. Bureau of the Census. Washington, DC: The Bureau, 1991. *Notes:* 1. Figure shown is the midpoint of a range. 2. Figure shown indicates 2,500 or more.

★ 661 ★

Pharmaceutical Manufacturers

Drug Manufacturing, by State: 1991

The table below shows manufacturing statistics for each state for the drug industry. Includes operating manufacturing establishments and auxiliaries. Covers industry groups with 950 or more employees. Data are for 1991.

Area	All employees		Production workers			Value-added by manufacture (million dollars)	Cost of materials[1] (million dollars)	Value of shipments[1] (million dollars)	New capital expenditures (million dollars)	End-of-year inventories (million dollars)
	Number (1,000)	Payroll (million dollars)	Number (1,000)	Hours (millions)	Wages (million dollars)					
United States	184.1	7,197.5	82.6	162.7	2,500.9	43,244.6	18,198.0	60,835.5	2,669.2	7,483.8
California	16.3	612.3	6.9	12.4	179.1	2,447.8	1,816.6	4,206.4	156.0	619.1
Colorado	1.3	41.9	.7	1.5	17.4	127.7	125.7	234.5	12.9	62.5
Connecticut	4.5	238.8	.7	1.3	17.7	799.1	322.2	1,110.7	(D)	130.9
Florida	2.5	70.6	1.4	2.9	27.9	441.0	136.0	574.1	12.7	72.4
Georgia	1.7	64.1	.8	1.5	24.0	185.8	309.6	490.1	35.1	66.6
Illinois	16.6	750.5	3.9	8.0	211.0	1,814.3	677.0	2,426.9	(D)	374.7
Indiana	19.5	961.7	6.6	12.6	260.3	4,917.0	1,653.6	6,554.5	565.4	655.6
Iowa	1.9	48.5	.8	1.2	14.4	267.9	140.9	405.6	(D)	95.5
Kansas	1.8	53.2	.8	1.5	16.9	215.0	116.1	325.4	(D)	68.2
Maryland	3.5	114.6	2.1	4.3	55.0	347.2	235.5	576.6	34.7	112.8
Massachusetts	2.5	90.2	1.1	2.4	26.5	374.3	110.7	468.4	21.9	72.3
Michigan	6.4	229.5	5.2	11.5	176.6	1,903.7	639.6	2,503.1	(D)	418.7
Minnesota	1.1	26.7	.6	1.2	10.9	130.8	80.3	211.1	(D)	21.5
Mississippi	(D)	(D)	(D)	(D)	(D)	(D)	(D)	(D)	(D)	(D)
Missouri	3.8	126.7	1.9	3.7	54.9	1,449.0	421.0	1,836.7	84.8	288.6
Nebraska	1.7	40.1	.9	1.9	16.3	271.4	107.7	375.5	18.1	76.5
New Jersey	28.5	1,202.7	11.8	21.8	399.5	8,145.7	3,310.1	11,249.9	416.1	1,435.7
New York	13.6	478.7	7.3	15.9	221.1	3,458.6	1,108.7	4,492.4	191.2	648.5
North Carolina	11.0	362.9	7.2	13.0	175.6	5,000.2	1,514.1	6,491.4	229.1	761.6
Ohio	1.7	56.7	.8	1.7	24.4	983.3	141.3	1,129.9	(D)	60.4
Pennsylvania	20.7	926.0	7.7	16.1	262.8	5,618.1	2,655.8	8,217.2	215.7	672.2
South Carolina	1.8	45.2	1.3	2.6	30.1	512.3	184.0	697.0	16.5	79.8
Tennessee	3.7	100.0	2.2	3.9	40.8	944.4	341.8	1,296.0	(D)	112.1
Texas	5.6	184.9	3.0	5.9	86.1	638.1	179.3	825.3	(D)	78.5
Utah	1.3	31.3	.8	1.5	16.2	136.4	36.7	169.8	5.6	31.9
Virginia	(D)	(D)	(D)	(D)	(D)	(D)	(D)	(D)	(D)	(D)

Source: U.S. Bureau of the Census. *Annual Survey of Manufactures, 1991. Geographic Area Statistics.* M91(AS)- 3. Washington, DC: U.S. Government Printing Office, February 1993, pp. 3/12-3/129. *Notes:* "D" indicates data withheld to avoid disclosing information on individual companies. 1. Aggregate of cost of materials and value of shipments includes extensive duplication since products of some industries are used as materials by others. 2. See original material for description of standard error of estimate. Percentage standard errors shown are approximate relative standard errors of estimates of level. 3. Manufacturing concerns reported separately for auxiliary units that serve the manufacturing establishments of a company (e.g., administrative offices, storage warehouses, power plants, research laboratories, garages, repair shops, etc.) rather than the general public if these units were at different locations from establishment served or if they serviced more than one manufacturing establishment. Employment and payroll data shown represent total for all such units that primarily serve manufacturing plants.

★ 662 ★

Pharmaceutical Manufacturers

Medicinals and Botanicals Manufacturers, Establishments and Employees

[Employees in thousands]

State	Establishments	Rank	Employees	Rank
California	43	1	1.7[1]	2
Colorado	2	8	0.2[1]	6
Georgia	6	5	0.7[1]	3
Indiana	1	9	0.7[1]	3
Maine	2	8	0.2[1]	6
Michigan	4	6	0.3	5
Missouri	6	5	1.7[1]	2
New Jersey	38	2	4.1	1
New York	20	3	0.7[1]	3
North Carolina	8	4	0.4[1]	4
Pennsylvania	6	5	0.7[1]	3
Virginia	3	7	0.7[1]	3

Source: Census of Manufactures on CD-ROM, 1987. Geographic Area Series [machine-readable datafiles]. Prepared by U.S. Bureau of the Census. Washington, DC: The Bureau, 1991. *Note:* 1. Figure shown is the midpoint of a range.

★ 663 ★

Pharmaceutical Manufacturers

Pharmaceutical Preparation Manufacturers, Establishments and Employees

[Employees in thousands]

State	Establishments	Rank	Employees	Rank
Arizona	9	15	0.7[1]	8
California	94	1	2.5[2]	5
Colorado	10	14	0.7[1]	8
Connecticut	15	11	2.5[2]	5
Delaware	2	20	0.4[1]	9
Florida	26	5	0.7	8
Georgia	18	10	0.3	10
Illinois	33	4	2.5[2]	5
Indiana	20	9	2.5[2]	5
Iowa	11	13	0.4[1]	9
Kansas	6	17	0.7[1]	8
Louisiana	6	17	0.7[1]	8
Maryland	13	12	0.7	8
Massachusetts	23	6	1.7[1]	6
Michigan	18	10	2.5[2]	5
Minnesota	11	13	0.4[1]	9
Mississippi	3	19	1.7[1]	6
Missouri	23	6	3.0	4

[Continued]

★ 663 ★

Pharmaceutical Preparation Manufacturers, Establishments and Employees

[Continued]

State	Establishments	Rank	Employees	Rank
Nebraska	3	19	0.4[1]	9
New Jersey	89	2	22.5	1
New York	94	1	2.5[2]	5
North Carolina	22	7	2.5[2]	5
North Dakota	1	21	0.4[1]	9
Ohio	21	8	2.5[2]	5
Oklahoma	5	18	0.4[1]	9
Oregon	10	14	0.2	11
Pennsylvania	38	3	14.1	2
South Carolina	10	14	1.3	7
Tennessee	7	16	2.5[2]	5
Texas	33	4	4.3	3
Utah	6	17	0.2[1]	11
Virginia	5	18	2.5[2]	5
West Virginia	2	20	0.4[1]	9
Wisconsin	9	15	0.4	9

Source: Census of Manufactures on CD-ROM, 1987. Geographic Area Series [machine-readable datafiles]. Prepared by U.S. Bureau of the Census. Washington, DC: The Bureau, 1991. Notes: 1. Figure shown is the midpoint of a range. 2. Figure shown indicates 2,500 or more.

★ 664 ★

Pharmaceutical Manufacturers

Top Pharmaceutical Companies: 1992

Top 15 pharmaceutical companies are ranked by 1992 pharmaceuticals sales shown in millions of dollars. Shares of the group are shown in percent.

Company	Sales ($ mil.)	% of group
Glaxo	7,247.0	10.3
Merck & Co.	7,225.1	10.2
Bristol-Meyers Squibb	5,908.0	8.4
Hoechst	5,429.3	7.7
Ciba-Geigy	4,611.6	6.5
Sandoz	4,440.7	6.3
SmithKline Beecham	4,370.1	6.2
Bayer	4,309.1	6.1
Roche	4,119.9	5.8
Eli Lilly	4,031.0	5.7
American Home Products	4,018.0	5.7
Rhone-Poulenc Rorer	3,824.3	5.4
Johnson & Johnson	3,795.0	5.4

[Continued]

★ 664 ★

Top Pharmaceutical Companies: 1992

[Continued]

Company	Sales ($ mil.)	% of group
Pfizer	3,770.7	5.3
Abbot	3,512.0	5.0

Source: *Manufacturing Chemist* (December 1992), p. 8.

Retail and Wholesale Trades

★ 665 ★

Annual Retail Sales of Drug and Proprietary Stores: 1992

[In millions of dollars]

Month	1992 sales	
	Not adjusted[1]	Adjusted[1]
January	6,293	6,448
February	6,220	6,466
March	6,365	6,495
April	6,511	6,504
May	6,420	6,465
June	6,273	6,427
July	6,266	6,433
August	6,276	6,457
September	6,056	6,395
October	6,405	6,437
November	6,134	6,311
December	8,066	6,282
Total	77,285	

Source: "Combined Annual and Revised Monthly Retail Trade, January 1983 Through December 1992." In CENDATA [online service]. Washington, DC: U.S. Bureau of the Census [issued 16 April 1993]. No. 10.6.1, No. 10.6.2.1., and No. 10.6.2.2. *Note:* 1. For seasonal, holiday, and trading day differences.

★ 666 ★

Retail and Wholesale Trades

Drug and Proprietary Retailers, Establishment and Employees

State	Establishments	Rank	Employees	Rank
Alabama	1162	16	8822	24
Alaska	55	51	877	50
Arizona	541	31	7799	26
Arkansas	625	29	4009	34
California	4462	1	59311	1
Colorado	470	32	4788	32
Connecticut	727	27	9636	22
Delaware	130	48	1725	45
D.C.	146	46	1728	44
Florida	2690	5	33861	3
Georgia	1660	10	16010	13
Hawaii	112	49	2688	39
Idaho	186	43	1889	43
Illinois	2524	6	32977	4
Indiana	1233	14	20068	10
Iowa	718	28	6692	27
Kansas	551	30	4842	30
Kentucky	1016	19	9177	23
Louisiana	1106	17	10539	20
Maine	261	36	2816	37
Maryland	833	24	11672	15
Massachusetts	1371	12	18643	11
Michigan	1921	8	22953	8
Minnesota	853	23	10633	19
Mississippi	754	26	5414	29
Missouri	1024	18	9913	21
Montana	178	44	1458	48
Nebraska	416	35	3588	35
Nevada	142	47	2132	41
New Hampshire	238	37	2750	38
New Jersey	1642	11	20259	9
New Mexico	226	39	2511	40
New York	4368	2	43078	2
North Carolina	1739	9	17747	12
North Dakota	188	41	1345	49
Ohio	2133	7	24041	7
Oklahoma	773	25	5423	28
Oregon	439	34	4793	31
Pennsylvania	2817	4	28278	6
Rhode Island	229	38	3410	36
South Carolina	890	21	8137	25
South Dakota	187	42	1602	46
Tennessee	1228	15	11176	16
Texas	3208	3	29817	5
Utah	214	40	1919	42
Vermont	149	45	1493	47

[Continued]

★ 666 ★

Drug and Proprietary Retailers, Establishment and Employees
[Continued]

State	Establishments	Rank	Employees	Rank
Virginia	1269	13	12712	14
Washington	869	22	10667	18
West Virginia	450	33	4232	33
Wisconsin	970	20	10859	17
Wyoming	88	50	783	51
U.S. Total	52181	-	573692	-

Source: Census of Retail Trade on CD-ROM, 1987. Geographic Area Series [machine-readable datafiles]. Prepared by U.S. Bureau of the Census. Washington, DC: The Bureau, 1990.

★ 667 ★

Retail and Wholesale Trades

Drugs, Drug Proprietaries, and Druggists' Sundries Wholesalers, Establishments and Employees

State	Establishments	Rank	Employees	Rank
Alabama	59	20	1078	25
Alaska	3	38	0[1]	-
Arizona	51	22	810	28
Arkansas	44	25	1736	19
California	723	1	13405	3
Colorado	79	14	1204	22
Connecticut	76	16	4014	11
Delaware	10	33	1967	16
D.C.	4	37	0[1]	-
Florida	352	4	4882	9
Georgia	143	8	4712	10
Hawaii	40	27	462	34
Idaho	12	32	248	39
Illinois	267	6	20741	1
Indiana	72	18	2391	13
Iowa	43	26	480	33
Kansas	36	28	437	35
Kentucky	44	25	0[1]	-
Louisiana	73	17	1177	23
Maine	6	35	0[1]	-
Maryland	60	19	1379	21
Massachusetts	92	13	3151	12
Michigan	104	11	2276	14
Minnesota	76	16	1822	18
Mississippi	23	30	398	37
Missouri	95	12	1853	17
Montana	9	34	108	42
Nebraska	31	29	528	31

[Continued]

★ 667 ★

Drugs, Drug Proprietaries, and Druggists' Sundries Wholesalers, Establishments and Employees
[Continued]

State	Establishments	Rank	Employees	Rank
Nevada	31	29	279	38
New Hampshire	6	35	0[1]	-
New Jersey	342	5	12780	4
New Mexico	23	30	226	40
New York	577	2	15474	2
North Carolina	79	14	2016	15
North Dakota	4	37	0[1]	-
Ohio	139	9	5945	5
Oklahoma	53	21	1005	26
Oregon	48	23	518	32
Pennsylvania	150	7	5157	8
Rhode Island	12	32	0[1]	-
South Carolina	40	27	596	29
South Dakota	5	36	188	41
Tennessee	111	10	5245	7
Texas	421	3	5613	6
Utah	40	27	552	30
Vermont	6	35	0[1]	-
Virginia	48	23	1529	20
Washington	78	15	1103	24
West Virginia	20	31	403	36
Wisconsin	46	24	864	27
Wyoming	6	35	75	43
U.S. Total	4912	-	133102	-

Source: Census of Wholesale Trade on CD-ROM, 1987. Geographic Area Series [machine-readable datafiles] Prepared by U.S. Bureau of the Census. Washington, DC: The Bureau, 1990. Note: 1. Data are withheld to avoid disclosure of individual companies.

★ 668 ★

Retail and Wholesale Trades

Estimated Purchases, Gross Margins, and Gross Margin/ Sales Ratios of Drugs, Drug Proprietaries, and Druggists' Sundries Wholesalers: 1987-1992

Figures present the estimated annual purchases, gross margins, and gross margin/ sales ratios of merchant wholesalers.

[Purchases and gross margin in millions of dollars]

	1987	1988	1989	1990	1991	1992
Purchases	29,606	34,871	39,616	45,419	52,802	59,917
Gross margin	5,155	5,749	5,819	6,137	7,243	7,253
Gross margin/sales ration	15.17	14.34	12.95	12.01	12.31	10.99

Source: "Combined Annual and Revised Monthly Wholesale Trade, January 1987 Through December 1993." In CENDATA [online service]. Washington, DC: U.S. Bureau of the Census [issued 1 April 1994]. No. 10.7.1 and No. 10.7.23.

★ 669 ★

Retail and Wholesale Trades

Medical, Dental, and Hospital Equipment and Supplies Wholesalers, Establishments and Employees

State	Establishments	Rank	Employees	Rank
Alabama	98	25	1183	22
Alaska	9	46	38	48
Arizona	126	21	1130[2]	24
Arkansas	54	32	386	35
California	1007	1	12003	1
Colorado	156	14	1875	16
Connecticut	128	20	1962	15
Delaware	14	44	105	46
D.C.	7	47	32	49
Florida	550	3	5529	6
Georgia	217	10	3541	10
Hawaii	34	38	271	38
Idaho	18	42	111	45
Illinois	392	5	5981	4
Indiana	120	23	1135	23
Iowa	73	30	632	31
Kansas	86	27	1015	25
Kentucky	83	29	915	28
Louisiana	122	22	0[1]	-
Maine	26	40	223	40
Maryland	132	19	2010	14
Massachusetts	216	11	3378	11

[Continued]

★ 669 ★

Medical, Dental, and Hospital Equipment and Supplies Wholesalers, Establishments and Employees
[Continued]

State	Establishments	Rank	Employees	Rank
Michigan	241	9	3627	9
Minnesota	136	18	2512	12
Mississippi	50	34	534	33
Missouri	186	12	2056	13
Montana	17	43	116	43
Nebraska	46	35	672	30
Nevada	27	39	143	41
New Hampshire	35	37	292	37
New Jersey	351	7	6525	3
New Mexico	34	38	376	36
New York	614	2	7924	2
North Carolina	148	15	1759	18
North Dakota	9	46	114	44
Ohio	334	8	3911	8
Oklahoma	92	26	708	29
Oregon	85	28	940	26
Pennsylvania	382	6	5415	7
Rhode Island	20	41	254	39
South Carolina	55	31	631	32
South Dakota	10	45	117	42
Tennessee	164	13	1852	17
Texas	536	4	5630	5
Utah	53	33	934	27
Vermont	9	46	43	47
Virginia	143	17	1553	20
Washington	147	16	1601	19
West Virginia	40	36	392	34
Wisconsin	113	24	1489	21
Wyoming	2	48	0[1]	-
U.S. Total	7747	-	96848	-

Source: Census of Wholesale Trade on CD-ROM, 1987. Geographic Area Series [machine-readable datafiles]. Prepared by U.S. Bureau of the Census. Washington, DC: The Bureau, 1990. Notes: 1. Data are withheld to avoid disclosure of individual companies. 2. Less than half the units shown.

★ 670 ★

Retail and Wholesale Trades

Ophthalmic Goods Wholesalers, Establishments and Employees

State	Establishments	Rank	Employees	Rank
Alabama	17	23	225	28
Alaska	2	32	0[1]	-
Arizona	24	19	296[2]	26
Arkansas	14	25	150	33
California	249	1	4190	1
Colorado	45	12	353	22
Connecticut	24	19	394	20
Delaware	2	32	0[1]	-
D.C.	0	-	0	-
Florida	143	3	2797	4
Georgia	49	11	523	16
Hawaii	8	29	129	34
Idaho	1	33	0[1]	-
Illinois	82	6	848	10
Indiana	38	14	730	11
Iowa	15	24	184	29
Kansas	14	25	0[1]	-
Kentucky	14	25	250	27
Louisiana	20	22	0[1]	-
Maine	9	28	0[1]	-
Maryland	26	18	366	21
Massachusetts	54	10	653	13
Michigan	73	8	888	9
Minnesota	41	13	944	8
Mississippi	8	29	0[1]	-
Missouri	41	13	351	24
Montana	8	29	0[1]	-
Nebraska	22	21	477	19
Nevada	8	29	0[1]	-
New Hampshire	2	32	0[1]	-
New Jersey	81	7	2878	3
New Mexico	12	26	0[1]	-
New York	217	2	2929	2
North Carolina	34	15	611	14
North Dakota	8	29	0[1]	-
Ohio	63	9	1087	7
Oklahoma	24	19	352	23
Oregon	23	20	582	15
Pennsylvania	95	5	1209	6
Rhode Island	5	30	175	30
South Carolina	14	25	165	31
South Dakota	8	29	0[1]	-
Tennessee	34	15	676	12
Texas	110	4	1760	5
Utah	14	25	163	32
Vermont	4	31	42	35

[Continued]

★ 670 ★

Ophthalmic Goods Wholesalers, Establishments and Employees
[Continued]

State	Establishments	Rank	Employees	Rank
Virginia	29	17	506	17
Washington	33	16	302	25
West Virginia	10	27	0[1]	-
Wisconsin	26	18	478	18
Wyoming	2	32	0[1]	-
U.S. Total	1899	-	30134	-

Source: Census of Wholesale Trade on CD-ROM, 1987. Geographic Area Series [machine-readable datafiles]. Prepared by U.S. Bureau of the Census. Washington, DC: The Bureau, 1990. Notes: 1. Data are withheld to avoid disclosure of individual companies. 2. Less than half the units shown.

Chapter 9
MEDICAL PROFESSIONS

The U.S. Department of Labor forecasts rapid growth in medical-related professions: "Health services will continue to be one of the fastest growing industries in the economy with employment increasing from 9.6 to 13.8 million. Improvements in medical technology, and a growing and aging population, will increase the demand for health services. Employment in home health care services—the second fastest growing industry in the economy—nursing homes, and offices and clinics of physicians and other health practitioners is projected to increase rapidly" (U.S. Department of Labor. *Occupational Outlook Handbook.* 1994-1995 ed. Lincolnwood, IL: VGM Career Horizons, 1994, p. 13). Tables in this chapter illustrate trends in health-related employment. Coverage includes health services managers; health diagnosing practitioners such as chiropractors, physicians, and veterinarians; health assessment and treating occupations, notably dietitians and nurses; health technologists and technicians; and health service occupations. In addition to employment and salary information, tables present data on academic degrees, medical students, medical schools, and other aspects of health education. The chapter also offers data on professional associations. Additional industry-specific employment information is featured in some tables in the chapter on Health Care Industries.

Associations

★ 671 ★

Medical Association Dues

The table below compares the annual membership dues of major medical associations.

[In dollars]

Association	Annual dues
American Academy of Ophthalmology	625
American Academy of Dermatology	450
American Medical Association	420
American Urological Association	350

[Continued]

★ 671 ★

Medical Association Dues
[Continued]

Association	Annual dues
American Dental Association	330
American Veterinary Medical Association	175[1]

Source: "Annual Dues Comparison: Major Medical Associations." DVM Newsmagazine (May 1994), p. 56. Note: 1. Dues as of source's publication; proposed dues is $225/year.

★ 672 ★

Associations

Members of the American Medical Association: 1992

Table below profiles members of the American Medical Association (AMA) by selected characteristics.

[In percentages]

Characteristic	Percent
Sex	
Male	84
Female	16
Age	
Older than 40	62
Younger than 40	38
Training	
U.S. medical graduates	82
International medical graduates	18

Source: Oberman, Linda. "AMA Has Record Membership; Looks to Market Share Gains." American Medical News, 22 February 1993, p. 35. Primary source: AMA Division of Membership. Note: Data are preliminary. Percentages have been rounded.

★ 673 ★
Associations

Physician Participation in the American Medical Association

The American Medical Association (AMA) represents approximately 40 percent of all U.S. physicians. The table below shows the number of physicians who are members of the AMA.

	Number
Physicians in the United States	718,000
Physicians who are members of the AMA	300,000[1]

Source: Wagner, Lynn. "AMA Backs Away From Hard Line on Reform." *Modern Healthcare,* 8 March 1993, p. 3. *Note:* 1. An approximation.

Education: Degrees

★ 674 ★

Allied Health Degrees: 1989-1990

The table presents data on the number of completions of educational programs by type of program and field of study for the 1989-1990 academic year. See also separate tables for specific areas of allied health; for example, diagnostic and treatment services, ophthalmic services, or rehabilitation services.

Instructional program	Awards, curriculums under 1 year	1- to 4-year awards	Associate degrees	Bachelor's degrees (4 or 5 years)	Master's degrees	Doctoral degrees	First-professional degrees
Allied health	61,762	55,451	24,153	12,801	3,698	107	-
Miscellaneous allied health services	15,418	12,845	4,064	783	130	8	-
Central supply technology	166	-	-	-	-	-	-
Medical assisting	12,213	7,969	1,690	-	20	-	-
Medical illustrating	248	-	-	17	51	-	-
Medical office management	1,163	588	153	-	-	-	-
Medical records technology	443	554	1,116	18	-	-	-
Pharmacy assisting	198	993	59	-	-	-	-
Physician assisting	65	226	130	638	31	-	-
Veterinarian assisting	88	1,668	746	14	-	-	-
Health unit coordinating	453	-	4	-	-	-	-
Chiropractic assisting	-	-	31	-	-	-	-
Other	381	336	135	96	28	8	-
Allied health, other	1,446	1,045	641	777	334	12	-

Source: U.S. Department of Labor. Bureau of Labor Statistics. *Occupational Projections and Training Data: A Statistical and Research Supplement to the 1992-1993 "Occupational Outlook Handbook."* 1992 edition. Bulletin 2401. Washington, DC: U.S. Government Printing Office, May 1992, pp. 60-62. Primary source: U.S. Department of Education. National Center for Education. Integrated Postsecondary Education Data System (IPEDS). Completions 1989-1990 Survey. *Note:* "-" indicates data not available.

★ 675 ★

Education: Degrees

Audiology and Speech Pathology Degrees: 1989-1990

The table presents data on the number of completions of educational programs by type of program and field of study for the 1989-1990 academic year.

Instructional program	Awards, curriculums under 1 year	1- to 4-year awards	Associate degrees	Bachelor's degrees (4 or 5 years)	Master's degrees	Doctoral degrees	First-professional degrees
Audiology and speech pathology	-	-	22	2,839	2,920	92	-
Audiology	-	-	19	53	92	1	-
Speech-language pathology/audiology	-	-	3	2,376	2,341	85	-
Speech pathology	-	-	-	298	377	-	-
Other	-	-	-	112	110	6	-

Source: U.S. Department of Labor. Bureau of Labor Statistics. *Occupational Projections and Training Data: A Statistical and Research Supplement to the 1992-1993 "Occupational Outlook Handbook."* 1992 edition. Bulletin 2401. Washington, DC: U.S. Government Printing Office, May 1992, p. 62. Primary source: U.S. Department of Education. National Center for Education. Integrated Postsecondary Education Data System (IPEDS). Completions 1989-1990 Survey. *Note:* "-" indicates data not available.

★ 676 ★

Education: Degrees

Basic Clinical Health Sciences Degrees: 1989-1990

The table presents data on the number of completions of educational programs by type of program and field of study for the 1989-1990 academic year.

Instructional program	Awards, curriculums under 1 year	1- to 4-year awards	Associate degrees	Bachelor's degrees (4 or 5 years)	Master's degrees	Doctoral degrees	First-professional degrees
Basic clinical health sciences	199	-	6	312	117	102	-
Clinical anatomy	-	-	-	-	2	4	-
Clinical biochemistry	-	-	-	16	9	24	-
Clinical microbiology	-	-	-	181	21	20	-
Clinical pathology	-	-	-	-	32	-	-
Clinical physiology	199	-	-	-	6	22	-
Other	-	-	6	115	47	32	-

Source: U.S. Department of Labor. Bureau of Labor Statistics. *Occupational Projections and Training Data: A Statistical and Research Supplement to the 1992-1993 "Occupational Outlook Handbook."* 1992 edition. Bulletin 2401. Washington, DC: U.S. Government Printing Office, May 1992, p. 62. Primary source: U.S. Department of Education. National Center for Education. Integrated Postsecondary Education Data System (IPEDS). Completions 1989-1990 Survey. *Note:* "-" indicates data not available.

★ 677 ★

Education: Degrees

Dentistry and Dental Services Degrees: 1989-1990

The table presents data on the number of completions of educational programs by type of program and field of study for the 1989-1990 academic year.

Instructional program	Awards, curriculums under 1 year	1- to 4-year awards	Associate degrees	Bachelor's degrees (4 or 5 years)	Master's degrees	Doctoral degrees	First-professional degrees
Dentistry	91	-	3	87	449	17	4,159
Dental public health	-	-	-	4	4	-	-
Dentistry, general	-	-	1	83	140	3	4,159
Endodontics	-	-	-	-	16	1	-
Oral/maxial facial surgery	-	-	-	-	4	1	-
Oral pathology	-	-	-	-	1	4	-
Orthodontics	-	-	-	-	92	-	-
Pedodontics	-	-	-	-	9	-	-
Periodontics	-	-	-	-	27	-	-
Prosthodontics	-	-	-	-	23	1	-
Other	91	-	2	-	133	7	-
Dental services	4,620	4,202	3,768	704	31	-	-
Dental assisting	2,656	3,745	359	-	-	-	-
Dental hygiene	14	214	3,140	703	17	-	-
Dental laboratory technology	115	204	267	1	5	-	-
Other	1,835	-	2	-	9	-	-

Source: U.S. Department of Labor. Bureau of Labor Statistics. *Occupational Projections and Training Data: A Statistical and Research Supplement to the 1992-1993 "Occupational Outlook Handbook."* 1992 edition. Bulletin 2401. Washington, DC: U.S. Government Printing Office, May 1992, pp. 60-62. Primary source: U.S. Department of Education. National Center for Education. Integrated Postsecondary Education Data System (IPEDS). Completions 1989-1990 Survey. *Note:* "-" indicates data not available.

★ 678 ★

Education: Degrees

Diagnostic and Treatment Services Degrees: 1989-1990

The table presents data on the number of completions of educational programs by type of program and field of study for the 1989-1990 academic year.

Instructional program	Awards, curriculums under 1 year	1- to 4-year awards	Associate degrees	Bachelor's degrees (4 or 5 years)	Master's degrees	Doctoral degrees	First-professional degrees
Diagnostic and treatment services	12,384	7,648	5,840	753	28	-	-
Cardiovascular technology	621	-	87	102	2	-	-
Dialysis technology	-	-	2	-	-	-	-
Electrocardiograph technology	83	-	13	-	-	-	-
Electroencephalograph technology	8	-	28	-	-	-	-
Emergency medical technician – ambulance	8,224	769	22	25	4	-	-
Emergency medical technician – paramedic	1,812	972	321	6	-	-	-
Medical radiation dosimetry	-	31	27	16	-	-	-
Nuclear medical technology	3	99	178	124	-	-	-
Radiograph medical technology	81	1,884	3,492	374	13	-	-
Respiratory therapy technology	46	1,145	1,194	18	-	-	-
Surgical technology	442	1,854	210	-	-	-	-

[Continued]

★ 678 ★

Diagnostic and Treatment Services Degrees: 1989-1990

[Continued]

Instructional program	Awards, curriculums under 1 year	1- to 4-year awards	Associate degrees	Bachelor's degrees (4 or 5 years)	Master's degrees	Doctoral degrees	First-professional degrees
Diagnostic medical sonography	60	776	154	17	-	-	-
Other	1,004	37	112	71	9	-	-

Source: U.S. Department of Labor. Bureau of Labor Statistics. *Occupational Projections and Training Data: A Statistical and Research Supplement to the 1992-1993 "Occupational Outlook Handbook."* 1992 edition. Bulletin 2401. Washington, DC: U.S. Government Printing Office, May 1992, p. 61. Primary source: U.S. Department of Education. National Center for Education. Integrated Postsecondary Education Data System (IPEDS). Completions 1989-1990 Survey. *Note:* "-" indicates data not available.

★ 679 ★

Education: Degrees

Health Sciences Degrees: 1989-1990

The table presents data on the number of completions of educational programs by type of program and field of study for the 1989-1990 academic year. See also separate tables for specific areas of health science; for example, audiology and speech pathology, medicine, or health services administron.

Instructional program	Awards, curriculums under 1 year	1- to 4-year awards	Associate degrees	Bachelor's degrees (4 or 5 years)	Master's degrees	Doctoral degrees	First-professional degrees
Health sciences	3,299	14,089	41,732	47,234	17,086	1,522	28,821
Chiropractic	-	30	7	-	-	-	2,581
Optometry	-	-	18	252	17	-	1,101
Osteopathic medicine	-	-	-	2	8	-	1,561
Pharmacy	16		7	6,100	287	167	1,191
Podiatry	-	-	-	5	56	-	675
Pre-dentistry	-	-	24	47	-	-	-
Pre-medicine		2	154	004	-	-	-
Pre-veterinary	-	-	106	2	-	-	-
Veterinary medicine	-	-	15	246	104	86	2,160
Other	79	266	99	2,610	1,141	321	-

Source: U.S. Department of Labor. Bureau of Labor Statistics. *Occupational Projections and Training Data: A Statistical and Research Supplement to the 1992-1993 "Occupational Outlook Handbook."* 1992 edition. Bulletin 2401. Washington, DC: U.S. Government Printing Office, May 1992, pp. 62-63. Primary source: U.S. Department of Education. National Center for Education. Integrated Postsecondary Education Data System (IPEDS). Completions 1989-1990 Survey. *Note:* "-" indicates data not available.

★ 680 ★

Education: Degrees

Health Services Administration Degrees: 1989-1990

The table presents data on the number of completions of educational programs by type of program and field of study for the 1989-1990 academic year.

Instructional program	Awards, curriculums under 1 year	1- to 4-year awards	Associate degrees	Bachelor's degrees (4 or 5 years)	Master's degrees	Doctoral degrees	First-professional degrees
Health services administration	361	449	75	3,220	3,000	29	-
Health services administration	150	142	69	2,396	2,475	18	-
Health care planning	145	-	-	14	211	2	-
Medical records administration	51	256	4	621	10	-	-
Other	15	-	2	189	304	9	-

Source: U.S. Department of Labor. Bureau of Labor Statistics. *Occupational Projections and Training Data: A Statistical and Research Supplement to the 1992-1993 "Occupational Outlook Handbook."* 1992 edition. Bulletin 2401. Washington, DC: U.S. Government Printing Office, May 1992, p. 62. Primary source: U.S. Department of Education. National Center for Education. Integrated Postsecondary Education Data System (IPEDS). Completions 1989-1990 Survey. *Note:* "-" indicates data not available.

★ 681 ★

Education: Degrees

Medical Laboratory and Medical Laboratory Technology Degrees: 1989-1990

The table presents data on the number of completions of educational programs by type of program and field of study for the 1989-1990 academic year.

Instructional program	Awards, curriculums under 1 year	1- to 4-year awards	Associate degrees	Bachelor's degrees (4 or 5 years)	Master's degrees	Doctoral degrees	First-professional degrees
Medical laboratory	-	-	8	612	49	1	-
Medical laboratory technologies	758	852	1,912	1,890	39	-	-
Blood bank technology	40	-	2	4	4	-	-
Chemistry technology	-	8	1	9	-	-	-
Clinical animal technology	-	-	6	6	-	-	-
Clinical laboratory aide	267	-	-	-	-	-	-
Clinical laboratory assisting	24	-	14	-	-	-	-
Cytotechnology	2	10	4	75	-	-	-
Hematology	19	-	-	-	-	-	-
Histologic technology	107	-	34	-	-	-	-
Medical laboratory technology	85	334	1,770	127	-	-	-
Medical technology	73	84	30	1,625	30	-	-
Microbiology technology	-	-	1	9	3	-	-
Other	141	168	50	35	2	-	-

Source: U.S. Department of Labor. Bureau of Labor Statistics. *Occupational Projections and Training Data: A Statistical and Research Supplement to the 1992-1993 "Occupational Outlook Handbook."* 1992 edition. Bulletin 2401. Washington, DC: U.S. Government Printing Office, May 1992, pp. 61-62. Primary source: U.S. Department of Education. National Center for Education. Integrated Postsecondary Education Data System (IPEDS). Completions 1989-1990 Survey. *Note:* "-" indicates data not available.

★ 682 ★

Education: Degrees

Medicine Degrees: 1989-1990

The table presents data on the number of completions of educational programs by type of program and field of study for the 1989-1990 academic year.

Instructional program	Awards, curriculums under 1 year	1- to 4-year awards	Associate degrees	Bachelor's degrees (4 or 5 years)	Master's degrees	Doctoral degrees	First-professional degrees
Medicine	706	2,252	248	249	200	178	15,393
Anesthesiology	-	33	-	5	11	-	-
Emergency medicine	3	-	-	-	-	-	-
Family practice	-	-	7	-	1	6	-
Geriatrics	-	-	5	10	17	-	-
Immunology	-	-	-	-	4	20	-
Internal medicine	-	-	-	-	-	16	-
Medicine	-	-	29	94	34	48	15,393
Nuclear medicine	3	-	-	1	-	-	-
Obstetrics and gynecology	110	-	-	-	-	2	-
Orthopedics	-	-	-	-	2	-	-
Otorhinolaryngology/otolaryngology	-	-	-	-	4	2	-
Pathology	-	-	-	-	9	19	-
Pediatrics	-	-	-	-	-	3	-
Preventive medicine	-	-	-	-	27	4	-
Psychiatry	55	-	-	-	-	-	-
Neurology	-	-	-	1	-	1	-
Radiology	19	219	171	5	2	2	-
Surgery	-	810	-	-	7	6	-
Sports medicine	4	-	9	133	50	-	-
Other	512	-	27	-	32	49	-

Source: U.S. Department of Labor. Bureau of Labor Statistics. *Occupational Projections and Training Data: A Statistical and Research Supplement to the 1992-1993 "Occupational Outlook Handbook."* 1992 edition. Bulletin 2401. Washington, DC. U.S. Government Printing Office, May 1992, p. 62. Primary source: U.S. Department of Education. National Center for Education. Integrated Postsecondary Education Data System (IPEDS). Completions 1989-1990 Survey. *Note:* "-" indicates data not available.

★ 683 ★

Education: Degrees

Mental Health and Human Services Degrees: 1989-1990

The table presents data on the number of completions of educational programs by type of program and field of study for the 1989-1990 academic year.

Instructional program	Awards, curriculums under 1 year	1- to 4-year awards	Associate degrees	Bachelor's degrees (4 or 5 years)	Master's degrees	Doctoral degrees	First-professional degrees
Mental health and human services	2,542	1,376	2,502	973	1,289	73	-
Alcohol/drug abuse specialty	354	471	478	75	35	-	-
Community health work	47	-	59	153	306	10	-
Home health aide	740	103	1	-	-	-	-
Mental health/human services assisting	29	134	406	14	-	-	-
Mental health/human services technology	116	280	904	105	48	-	-
Rehabilitation counseling	-	-	7	174	582	14	-
Therapeutic child care work	-	-	34	-	6	-	-

[Continued]

★ 683 ★

Mental Health and Human Services Degrees: 1989-1990
[Continued]

Instructional program	Awards, curriculums under 1 year	1- to 4-year awards	Associate degrees	Bachelor's degrees (4 or 5 years)	Master's degrees	Doctoral degrees	First-professional degrees
Sign language interpreting	21	105	175	16	-	-	-
Other	1,235	246	438	436	312	49	-

Source: U.S. Department of Labor. Bureau of Labor Statistics. *Occupational Projections and Training Data: A Statistical and Research Supplement to the 1992-1993 "Occupational Outlook Handbook."* 1992 edition. Bulletin 2401. Washington, DC: U.S. Government Printing Office, May 1992, p. 61. Primary source: U.S. Department of Education. National Center for Education. Integrated Postsecondary Education Data System (IPEDS). Completions 1989-1990 Survey. *Note:* "-" indicates data not available.

★ 684 ★

Education: Degrees

Nursing and Nursing Specialty Degrees: 1989-1990

The table presents data on the number of completions of educational programs by type of program and field of study for the 1989-1990 academic year.

Instructional program	Awards, curriculums under 1 year	1- to 4-year awards	Associate degrees	Bachelor's degrees (4 or 5 years)	Master's degrees	Doctoral degrees	First-professional degrees
Nursing	1,847	11,024	40,911	29,668	6,797	333	-
Maternal/child care nursing	-	-	-	-	237	3	-
Medical surgical nursing	59	-	30	-	211	-	-
Nurse anesthetists	-	46	-	51	143	-	-
Nursing administration	13	-	39	85	202	1	-
Nursing, general	1,167	9,891	40,099	29,152	4,997	282	
Psychiatric/mental health nursing	160	103	22	5	119	-	-
Public health nursing	-	-	-	15	496	39	-
Other	448	984	721	360	392	8	-
Nursing-related specialty	23,989	25,593	1,040	188	59	-	-
Geriatric aide	1,653	-	50	8	-	-	-
Nursing assisting	18,756	2,228	-	-	-	-	-
Practical nursing	2,463	22,729	617	169	6	-	-
Health unit management	4	-	15	-	-	-	-
Other	1,113	579	358	11	53	-	-

Source: U.S. Department of Labor. Bureau of Labor Statistics. *Occupational Projections and Training Data: A Statistical and Research Supplement to the 1992-1993 "Occupational Outlook Handbook."* 1992 edition. Bulletin 2401. Washington, DC: U.S. Government Printing Office, May 1992, pp. 61-62. Primary source: U.S. Department of Education. National Center for Education. Integrated Postsecondary Education Data System (IPEDS). Completions 1989-1990 Survey. *Note:* "-" indicates data not available.

★ 685 ★

Education: Degrees

Ophthalmic Services Degrees: 1989-1990

The table presents data on the number of completions of educational programs by type of program and field of study for the 1989-1990 academic year.

Instructional program	Awards, curriculums under 1 year	1- to 4-year awards	Associate degrees	Bachelor's degrees (4 or 5 years)	Master's degrees	Doctoral degrees	First-professional degrees
Ophthalmic services	197	177	461	-	-	-	-
Ophthalmic dispensing	62	102	182	-	-	-	-
Optometric technology	1	43	175	-	-	-	-
Other	134	32	104	-	-	-	-

Source: U.S. Department of Labor. Bureau of Labor Statistics. *Occupational Projections and Training Data: A Statistical and Research Supplement to the 1992-1993 "Occupational Outlook Handbook."* 1992 edition. Bulletin 2401. Washington, DC: U.S. Government Printing Office, May 1992, p. 61. Primary source: U.S. Department of Education. National Center for Education. Integrated Postsecondary Education Data System (IPEDS). Completions 1989-1990 Survey. *Note:* "-" indicates data not available.

★ 686 ★

Education: Degrees

Public Health Degrees: 1989-1990

The table presents data on the number of completions of educational programs by type of program and field of study for the 1989-1990 academic year.

Instructional program	Awards, curriculums under 1 year	1- to 4-year awards	Associate degrees	Bachelor's degrees (4 or 5 years)	Master's degrees	Doctoral degrees	First-professional degrees
Public health	-	-	-	350	1,939	196	-
Epidemiology	-	-	-	-	258	54	-
Public health education	-	-	-	19	35	-	-
Public health laboratory science	-	-	-	179	1,236	115	-
Public health practice and management	-	-	-	20	87	17	-
Other	-	-	-	132	323	10	-

Source: U.S. Department of Labor. Bureau of Labor Statistics. *Occupational Projections and Training Data: A Statistical and Research Supplement to the 1992-1993 "Occupational Outlook Handbook."* 1992 edition. Bulletin 2401. Washington, DC: U.S. Government Printing Office, May 1992, pp. 62-63. Primary source: U.S. Department of Education. National Center for Education. Integrated Postsecondary Education Data System (IPEDS). Completions 1989-1990 Survey. *Note:* "-" indicates data not available.

★ 687 ★

Education: Degrees

Rehabilitation Services Degrees: 1989-1990

The table presents data on the number of completions of educational programs by type of program and field of study for the 1989-1990 academic year.

Instructional program	Awards, curriculums under 1 year	1- to 4-year awards	Associate degrees	Bachelor's degrees (4 or 5 years)	Master's degrees	Doctoral degrees	First-professional degrees
Rehabilitation services	408	1,713	3,925	6,733	1,788	14	-
Art therapy	-	-	-	39	124	-	-
Dance therapy	-	-	-	2	44	-	-
Exercise physiology	-	-	24	198	119	-	-
Music therapy	-	-	-	179	20	-	-
Occupational therapy	-	77	132	2,009	379	-	-
Occupational therapy assisting	-	55	800	-	-	-	-
Orthotics/prosthetics	-	-	18	23	-	-	-
Orthopedic assisting	-	-	3	7	-	-	-
Physical therapy	-	110	269	3,532	919	2	-
Physical therapy aide	12	-	27	-	-	-	-
Physical therapy assisting	-	59	1,552	-	-	-	-
Recreational therapy	2	-	51	159	18	-	-
Recreational therapy assisting	-	-	41	4	-	-	-
Respiratory therapy	168	632	957	204	-	-	-
Respiratory therapy assisting	-	148	18	-	-	-	-
Speech/hearing therapy aide	-	-	9	90	47	1	-
Recreational therapy aide	-	-	6	-	-	-	-
Other	226	171	18	287	118	11	-

Source: U.S. Department of Labor. Bureau of Labor Statistics. *Occupational Projections and Training Data: A Statistical and Research Supplement to the 1992-1993 "Occupational Outlook Handbook."* 1992 edition. Bulletin 2401. Washington, DC: U.S. Government Printing Office, May 1992, pp. 61-62. Primary source: U.S. Department of Education. National Center for Education. Integrated Postsecondary Education Data System (IPEDS). Completions 1989-1990 Survey. *Note:* "-" indicates data not available.

Education: Dental Schools

★ 688 ★

Dental School Enrollment: 1978-1991

Data below reflect first-year enrollments.

Year	Enrollments
1978-1979	6,301
1979-1980	6,132
1980-1981	6,030
1981-1982	5,855
1982-1983	5,498
1983-1984	5,274
1984-1985	5,047

[Continued]

★ 688 ★

Dental School Enrollment: 1978-1991
[Continued]

Year	Enrollments
1985-1986	4,843
1986-1987	4,554
1987-1988	4,370
1988-1989	4,196
1989-1990	3,979
1990-1991	4,001

Source: U.S. Deparment of Labor. *Occupational Outlook Handbook.* 1992-1993 edition. Lincolnwood, IL: VGM Career Horizons, p. 143. Primary source: American Dental Association.

Education: Financial Assistance

★ 689 ★

Financial Assistance Programs for Medical Students: 1991-1992

Data reflect the 1991-1992 academic year for 124 medical schools.

Source of assistance	Total amount (million dollars)	Number of programs	Average amount (dollars)
Scholarships			
Administered by schools			
Exceptional financial need	4.0	854	5,782
Medical Scientist Training Program	18.3	783	23,372
School funds	93	24,285	3,828
Financial Aid for Disadvantaged Health Professions Students (FADHPS)	4.1	1,590	2,610
Other scholarships	29.7	9,259	3,203
Not administered by schools			
Armed Forces Health Professions	55.7	2,880	19,336
National Health Services Corps	4.6	238	19,148
Other[1]	2.2	203	10,631
State funded	7.3	875	8,331
Loans			
Administered by schools			
Health Professions Student Loans	35.5	8,641	4,109
Stafford Student Loans	16.2	2,277	7,106
Perkins Loans	32.4	12,660	2,562
Loans from school funds	41.2	11,328	3,638
Not administered by schools			
Stafford Student Loans	319.4	43,489	7,344
Health Education Assistance Loans	113.4	10,632	10,669
Supplemental Loans for Students	86	23,503	3,659

[Continued]

★ 689 ★

Financial Assistance Programs for Medical Students: 1991-1992

[Continued]

Source of assistance	Total amount (million dollars)	Number of programs	Average amount (dollars)
MEDLOANS/ALP	55.2	6,138	8,991
Other loans	15	4,251	3,529
College work-study programs	3.1	1,903	1,610

Source: Krakower, Jack, Janice L. Ganem, and Robert L. Beran. "Medical School Financing, 1991-1992: Comparing Seven Different Types of Schools." *Academic Medicine* 69, no. 1 (January 1994), p. 81. Primary source: Association of American Medical Colleges Institutional Profile System. *Notes:* Totals may not equal the sum of the parts due to rounding. 1. With service commitment.

★ 690 ★

Education: Financial Assistance

Health Education Assistance Loan Defaults: 1987-1992

The table shows the default rate on federal Health Education Assistance Loans (HEAL) for 1987 through 1992. Data are provided by occupation or specialty.

[In percentages]

Occupation or area of specialty	Percent defaulting on student loans
Public health	14.5
Health administration	12.0
Chiropractors	10.3
Pharmacists	9.3
Podiatrists	6.3
Veterinarians	6.1
Clinical psychologists	6.0
Dentists	4.9
Medical doctors	3.0
Optometrists	2.8
Osteopaths	2.4

Source: Page, Leigh. "U.S. Hounds Student Loan Defaulters." *American Medical News,* 20 September 1990, p. 3. Primary source: Health Resources and Services Administration.

Education: Medical Schools/Enrollment

★ 691 ★

Characteristics of Medical School Students: 1991-1993

Student information	1991-1992	1992-1993
Race/ethnicity[1]		
Whites (non-Hispanic)		
Men	7,312	6,993
Women	4,424	4,598
Blacks (non-Hispanic)		
Men	562	561
Women	728	837
Asian/Pacific Islanders		
Men	1,613	1,563
Women	1,089	1,056
Women		
Number of applicants	13,700 (41.4%)	15,619 (41.8%)
Number entering class	6,777 (39.8%)	7,100 (41.8%)
Number enrolled	24,911 (38.0%)	25,933 (39.3%)
Number of graduates[2]	5,483 (35.7%)	5,940 (38.2%)

Source: Jonas, Harry S., Sylvia I. Etzel, and Barbara Barzansky. "Educational Programs in U.S. Medical Schools." *Journal of the American Medical Association (JAMA)* 270, no. 9, 1 September 1993, p. 1065. Primary source for data on women applicants to medical schools: Association of American Medical Colleges. Section for Student Services. *Medical School Admission Requirements.* Washington, DC: Association of American Medical Colleges, Section for Student Services, 1993. *Notes:* 1. Of first-year students; includes repeaters. 2. 1992-1993 figures are estimates (April 1993).

★ 692 ★

Education: Medical Schools/Enrollment

Grade Point Averages of Pre-med Students Entering Medical School: 1988-1992

[In percentages; 4-point scale]

Entering year	Pre-med grade point average			
	A (3.50-4.0)	B (2.60-3.49)	C (1<2.6)	Unknown
1988	44.6	49.0	2.1	4.3
1989	43.7	52.7	2.3	1.3
1990	45.0	52.4	2.2	0.4
1991	46.2	50.5	2.1	1.2
1992	48.3	46.4	1.7	3.6

Source: Jonas, Harry S., Sylvia I. Etzel, and Barbara Barzansky. "Educational Programs in U.S. Medical Schools." *Journal of the American Medical Association (JAMA)* 270, no. 9, 1 September 1993, p. 1063.

★ 693 ★

Education: Medical Schools/Enrollment

International Medical Graduates: 1992

India - 19.5
Pakistan - 11.9
Philippines - 8.8
Former Soviet Union - 3.1
Egypt - 2.6
Dominican Republic - 2.5
Syria - 2.5
United Kingdom - 2.4
Germany - 2.3
Mexico - 1.8

Table lists the 10 top countries from which international medical graduates (IMGs) come. Data reflect graduates by country of medical education, as measured by certificates issued by the Educational Commission for Foreign Medical Graduates.

Country	Percent
India	19.5
Pakistan	11.9
Philippines	8.8
Former Soviet Union	3.1
Egypt	2.6
Dominican Republic	2.5

[Continued]

★ 693 ★

International Medical Graduates: 1992
[Continued]

Country	Percent
Syria	2.5
United Kingdom	2.4
Germany	2.3
Mexico	1.8

Source: "Where IMGs Come From." *American Medical News,* 21 February 1994, p. 8. Primary source: U.S. Medical Licensure Statistics (1993).

★ 694 ★

Education: Medical Schools/Enrollment

Medical Education of Active Physicians, by Location: 1986-2020

Table provides projections as to the countries of medical education of the supply of active medical and osteopathic physicians.

Category	Estimated 1986[1]	Projected			
		1990	2000	2010	2020
	Number of active physicians[4]				
All active physicians	544,830	601,060	721,600	810,160	848,620
MDs	522,020	573,310	682,120	759,630	789,560
U.S. trained	398,880	439,890	527,960	599,620	635,440
Canadian trained	7,200	7,540	7,540	7,530	7,510
Foreign trained[2]	115,940	125,870	146,610	152,480	146,610
DOs	22,810	27,760	30,480	50,530	59,060
Total U.S. trained[3]	421,690	467,640	567,440	650,150	694,500

Source: U.S. Department of Health and Human Services. Public Health Service. Health Resources and Services Administration. *On the Status of Health Personnel in the United States: Seventh Report to the President and Congress.* Rockville, MD: U.S. Department of Health and Human Services, Public Health Service, Health Resources and Services Administration, March 1990, p. VI-45. *Notes:* Population base from U.S. Bureau of the Census's *Current Population Reports,* Series P-25, no. 1035 (February 1989) and no. 1018 (January 1989). 1. Medical doctors (MDs) professionally active in 1986 estimated from American Medical Association (AMA) data and include approximately 90 percent of the physicians who are not classified according to activity status by the AMA and whose addresses are unknown. 2. Includes U.S. citizen foreign medical graduates (FMGs). 3. Includes U.S. trained MDs and doctors of osteopathy (DOs). 4. Figures may not add to totals due to independent rounding.

★ 695 ★

Education: Medical Schools/Enrollment

Medical School Enrollment and Graduates: 1991-1998

Student information	1991-1992	1992-1993	1993-1994	1994-1995	1995-1996	1996-1997	1997-1998
Enrollment							
Number of schools	126	126	-	-	-	-	-
First year	17,027[1]	17,001[1]	16,103	16,136	16,117	16,135	16,138
Intermediate years	33,126[2]	33,414[2]	-	-	-	-	-
Graduates	15,386	15,554[3]	15,958	16,146	16,220	15,885	15,907

Source: Jonas, Harry S., Sylvia I. Etzel, and Barbara Barzansky. "Educational Programs in U.S. Medical Schools." *Journal of the American Medical Association (JAMA)* 270, no. 9, 1 September 1993, p. 1064. Primary source for data on women applicants to medical schools: Association of American Medical Colleges. Section for Student Services. *Medical School Admission Requirements.* Washington, DC: Association of American Medical Colleges, Section for Student Services, 1993. *Notes:* 1. Includes students repeating the year. 2. Includes final year students who did not graduate. 3. 1992-1993 figures are estimates (April 1993).

★ 696 ★

Education: Medical Schools/Enrollment

Medical School Students: 1991-1992

Data are provided by medical school groups.

	All schools (n=126)	Public schools (n=74)	Private schools (n=52)	Community based (n=17)	Research - public (n=7)	Research - private (n=13)	Generalist producers (n=20)	Private, freestanding (n=14)
Medical students	507	506	510	235	660	545	376	568
Graduate students	124	118	129	41	292	258	78	99
Housestaff/clinical fellows	521	489	583	183	811	933	325	372

Source: Krakower, Jack, Janice L. Ganem, and Robert L. Beran. "Medical School Financing, 1991-1992: Comparing Seven Different Types of Schools." *Academic Medicine* 69, no. 1 (January 1994), p. 77. Prepared by the Association of American Medical Colleges, Section for Operational Studies, using data from the Liaison Committee on Medical Education (LCME) Annual Financial Questionnaire, Part 1-A.

Education: Medical Schools/Faculty

★ 697 ★

Environmental Health Professors: 1987 and 1992

The table below presents the estimates of supply, demand, and need for environmental health professors.

Year	Supply	Demand	Need
1987	2,065	2,065	2,275
1992	2,170[1]	2,170[1]	2,629[2]

Source: Anderson, A. C., E. Levine, and B. Stern. "An Estimate of the Need for Environmental Health Academicians in the Workforce." *Public Health Reports* 1990, no. 105 (July/August 1990), pp. 410-414. *Notes:* 1. Based on a 5 percent increase from 1987 to 1992. 2. Based on a conservative estimate of only 25 percent of the total need for new specialists being met by 1992.

★ 698 ★

Education: Medical Schools/Faculty

Geriatrics Faculty: 1991

This table shows the capacity to train physicians as geriatrics faculty and the effect of a decrease in available training faculty due to retirement or entrance into clinical practice. From the source: "Projected net loss in the numbers of geriatrics physician faculty will continue each year in each specialty to the year 2000, ranging from 2 in neurology to 30 in family practice." Data refer to physicians only.

	Specialty				
	Internal medicine	Family practice	Neurology	Psychiatry	Physical medicine
Number of graduating geriatrics fellows (estimated)	66	16	19	40	2
Number of junior faculty entering as faculty[1]	35	8	10	18	1
Number of mid-career entering as faculty	14	7	2	2	1
Total new geriatrics faculty/year	49	15	12	20	2
Number of junior faculty leaving academics[2]	65	38	14	24	6
Number of faculty retiring[3]	10	8	5	8	1
Total geriatrics faculty leaving/year	75	46	29	32	7
Net gain/loss of geriatrics faculty per year	-26	-31	-7	-12	-5

Source: U.S. House of Representatives. *Shortage of Health Care Professions Caring for the Elderly: Recommendations for Change.* 102d Cong., 2nd sess., December 1992. Comm. Pub. No. 102-915. Washington, DC: U.S. Government Printing Office, 1993, p. 11. *Notes:* 1. Based on approximately 50 percent of physicians completing fellowships in geriatrics entering academics. 2. Based on the percent of geriatrics faculty that leave academics before reaching senior faculty status (amortized over 8 years); i.e., 10 percent/year. 3. Based on a 25-year career in academics; i.e., 4 percent retire each year.

★ 699 ★

Education: Medical Schools/Faculty

Medical School Faculty, by Degrees Held: 1992

Data show distribution of U.S. medical school faculty by degree and department for 1992.

Department	Degrees				Department total
	MD[1]	PhD/OHD[2]	MD-PhD MD-OHD	Other	
Family medicine	1,280	281	31	146	1,738
Internal medicine	12,574	1,564	1,003	621	15,762
Neurology	1,330	343	202	121	1,996
Orthopedic surgery	721	126	33	73	953
Physical medicine	417	124	16	119	676

Source: DeLisa, Joel A. "Academic Physiatry: Trends, Opportunities and Challenges." *American Journal of Physical Medicine and Rehabilitation* 72, no. 3 (June 1993), p. 115. *Notes:* Per the source: "This chart was modified from the Association of American Medical Colleges data book (January 1993), *Statistical Information Related to Medical Education,* table C2. This database contains records of approximately 85 percent of all active, full-time U.S. medical school faculty. The 15 percent undercount should be taken into consideration when using the data." 1. Medical doctors (MD). 2. Doctors of philosophy (PhD) or other health doctorates (OHD).

★ 700 ★

Education: Medical Schools/Faculty

Medical School Faculty, by Positions: 1992-1993

Table shows full-time medical school faculty positions by discipline and academic rank for U.S. medical schools. Number and percent of vacant positions are included as well.

	Filled, full-time budgeted positions					Vacant positions	
	Professor	Associate professor	Assistant professor	Instructor and other	Total	Number	Percent
Anatomy	839	728	553	171	2,291	79	3.3
Anesthesiology	529	758	2,079	734	4,100	209	4.8
Biochemistry	879	418	486	151	1,934	78	3.9
Dermatology	182	152	230	55	619	33	5.1
Family medicine	270	514	1,134	269	2,187	135	5.8
Medicine	4,128	4,035	7,300	2,712	18,175	792	4.2
Microbiology	730	484	499	173	1,886	58	3.0
Neurology	577	592	951	305	2,425	120	4.7
Obstetrics and gynecology	711	687	1,373	632	3,403	222	6.1
Ophthalmology	383	322	524	228	1,457	64	4.2
Orthopedics	293	253	533	180	1,259	95	7.0
Otolaryngology	238	189	361	115	903	37	3.9
Pathology	1,355	1,146	1,444	356	4,301	223	4.9
Pediatrics	1,660	1,975	3,569	1,054	8,258	465	5.3
Pharmacology	728	409	435	169	1,741	59	3.3
Physical medicine	101	134	426	162	823	43	5.0
Physiology	824	510	409	120	1,863	54	2.8
Psychiatry	1,292	1,388	2,883	1,324	6,887	304	4.2

[Continued]

★ 700 ★

Medical School Faculty, by Positions: 1992-1993
[Continued]

	Filled, full-time budgeted positions					Vacant positions	
	Professor	Associate professor	Assistant professor	Instructor and other	Total	Number	Percent
Public health and preventive medicine	281	280	398	135	1,094	26	2.4
Radiology	1,234	1,206	2,167	666	5,273	255	4.6
Surgery	1,748	1,481	2,623	778	6,630	413	5.9
Urology	172	107	144	33	456	11	2.3
Other/basic science	492	361	497	213	1,563	36	2.2
Other/clinical science	321	373	974	296	1,964	96	3.1

Source: Jonas, Harry S., Sylvia I. Etzel, and Barbara Barzansky. "Educational Programs in U.S. Medical Schools." *Journal of the American Medical Association (JAMA)* 270, no. 9, 1 September 1993, p. 1062.

★ 701 ★

Education: Medical Schools/Faculty

Medical School Faculty, by Type of School: 1991-1992

Data reflect median numbers of faculty for 1991-1992. Data are provided by medical school groups.

	All schools (n=126)	Public schools (n=74)	Private schools (n=52)	Community based (n=17)	Research - public (n=7)	Research - private (n=13)	Generalist producers (n=20)	Private, freestanding (n=14)
Faculty	550	518	667	167	1,138	1,207	340	452
Basic science	79	80	79	49	103	129	51	65
Clinical science	465	437	568	142	960	1,050	254	383

Source: Krakower, Jack, Janice L. Ganem, and Robert L. Beran. "Medical School Financing, 1991-1992: Comparing Seven Different Types of Schools." *Academic Medicine* 69, no. 1 (January 1994), p. 77. Prepared by the Association of American Medical Colleges, Section for Operational Studies, using data from the Liaison Committee on Medical Education (LCME) Annual Financial Questionnaire, Part I-A.

Education: Medical Schools/Finances

★ 702 ★

Medical School Expenditures: 1991-1992

The table below presents the expenditures of U.S. medical schools, by function, for the 1991-1992 academic year.

Expenditures	Amount (in million dollars)	Percent
Total	22,445	100.0
Instruction	6,293	28.0
Research	5,141	22.9
Science	5,048	22.5
Program support	2,429	10.8
Other functions	1,328	5.9
House staff	1,144	5.1
Operation and maintenance of plant	805	3.6
Scholarships and fellowships	257	1.1

Source: Krakower, Jack, and others. "U.S. Medical School Finances." *Journal of the American Medical Association (JAMA)* 270, no. 9, 1 September 1993, p. 1088. Table prepared by the Association of American Medical Colleges (AAMC) from Liaison Committee on Medical Education (LCME) questionnaires. *Note:* Transfers are not included.

★ 703 ★

Education: Medical Schools/Finances

Medical School Revenues: 1991-1992

Data are provided by revenue sources.

Source	Number of schools[1]	Amount (in million dollars)[2]	Percent
Total revenue	126	23,147	100.0
Federal appropriations	2	105	0.5
State and local governments	109	2,662	11.5
State	108	2,645	11.4
Local	3	18	0.1
Practice plans	113	7,505	32.4
Recovery of indirect costs	125	1,517	6.6
Federal	125	1,309	5.7

[Continued]

★ 703 ★

Medical School Revenues: 1991-1992
[Continued]

Source	Number of schools[1]	Amount (in million dollars)[2]	Percent
State	91	21	0.1
Local	36	11	0.0
Nongovernment	117	175	0.8
Tuition and fees	125	955	4.1
Endowment income	107	401	1.7
Gifts	91	509	2.2
Parent university funds	31	208	0.9
Reimbursements from hospitals	73	2,640	11.4
Other revenues	114	957	4.1
Grants and contracts	126	5,689	24.6
Federal	126	3,748	16.2
State	109	370	1.6
Local	52	216	0.9
Private	122	1,357	5.9

Source: Krakower, Jack, Janice L. Ganem, and Robert L. Beran. "Medical School Financing, 1991-1992: Comparing Seven Different Types of Schools." *Academic Medicine* 69, no. 1 (January 1994), p. 76. Prepared by the Association of American Medical Colleges, Section for Operational Studies, using data from the Liaison Committee on Medical Education (LCME) Annual Financial Questionnaire, Part 1-A. *Notes:* 1. Number of schools reporting nonzero value. 2. Total may not sum due to rounding.

Education: Nursing Schools

★ 704 ★

Nursing Enrollment: 1982-1992

Year	Number
1982	242,035
1984	237,232
1986	193,712
1988	184,924
1990	221,170
1992	257,983

Source: "Nursing Enrollments Hit All-Time High." *AJN* (January 1994), p. 83.

Employment

★ 705 ★

Clinical Laboratory Technologists and Technicians

The table below presents the number of civilians 16 years old or older who reported working as clinical laboratory technologists and technicians during the 1990 Census. Data are provided by total number employed in each Metropolitan Statistical Area (MSA) or Consolidated Metropolitan Statistical Area (CMSA), as well as the number employed per 100,000 people.

[Total for all of the U.S. was 329,892; 132.64 per 100,000 persons]

MSA/CMSA	Total Employees	Employees per 100,000 pop.
Abilene, TX MSA	162	135.39
Albany, GA MSA	81	71.96
Albany – Schenectady – Troy, NY MSA	1322	151.21
Albuquerque, NM MSA	793	165.01
Alexandria, LA MSA	184	139.86
Allentown – Bethlehem – Easton, PA – NJ MSA	1004	146.21
Altoona, PA MSA	195	149.38
Amarillo, TX MSA	271	144.50
Anchorage, AK MSA	400	176.73
Anderson, IN MSA	149	114.03
Anderson, SC MSA	338	232.79
Anniston, AL MSA	82	70.67
Appleton – Oshkosh – Neenah, WI MSA	389	123.44
Asheville, NC MSA	304	173.89
Athens, GA MSA	228	145.90
Atlanta, GA MSA	3863	136.33
Atlantic City, NJ MSA	356	111.45
Augusta, GA – SC MSA	812	204.63
Austin, TX MSA	755	96.60
Bakersfield, CA MSA	411	75.62
Baltimore, MD MSA	4898	205.61
Bangor, ME MSA	213	240.01
Baton Rouge, LA MSA	574	108.66
Battle Creek, MI MSA	154	113.25
Beaumont – Port Arthur, TX MSA	389	107.69
Bellingham, WA MSA	94	73.56
Benton Harbor, MI MSA	172	106.58
Billings, MT MSA	156	137.54
Biloxi – Gulfport, MS MSA	272	137.98
Binghamton, NY MSA	281	106.24
Birmingham, AL MSA	1875	206.54
Bismarck, ND MSA	255	304.18
Bloomington, IN MSA	122	111.95
Bloomington – Normal, IL MSA	121	93.67
Boise City, ID MSA	260	126.35
Boston – Lawrence – Salem, MA – NH CMSA	7687	184.27
Bradenton, FL MSA	251	118.56

[Continued]

★ 705 ★

Clinical Laboratory Technologists and Technicians
[Continued]

MSA/CMSA	Total Employees	Employees per 100,000 pop.
Bremerton, WA MSA	180	94.87
Brownsville – Harlingen, TX MSA	215	82.65
Bryan – College Station, TX MSA	96	78.78
Buffalo – Niagara Falls, NY CMSA	1895	159.34
Burlington, NC MSA	391	361.32
Burlington, VT MSA	208	158.25
Canton, OH MSA	586	148.69
Casper, WY MSA	94	153.53
Cedar Rapids, IA MSA	221	130.95
Champaign – Urbana – Rantoul, IL MSA	207	119.64
Charleston, SC MSA	825	162.76
Charleston, WV MSA	402	160.51
Charlotte – Gastonia – Rock Hill, NC – SC MSA	1297	111.61
Charlottesville, VA MSA	497	379.08
Chattanooga, TN – GA MSA	446	102.95
Cheyenne, WY MSA	79	108.01
Chicago – Gary – Lake County, IL – IN – WI CMSA	12380	153.49
Chico, CA MSA	224	123.00
Cincinnati – Hamilton, OH – KY – IN CMSA	2774	159.05
Clarksville – Hopkinsville, TN – KY MSA	172	101.51
Cleveland – Akron – Lorain, OH CMSA	4509	163.38
Colorado Springs, CO MSA	518	130.47
Columbia, MO MSA	466	414.67
Columbia, SC MSA	719	158.60
Columbus, GA – AL MSA	340	139.88
Columbus, OH MSA	2012	146.07
Corpus Christi, TX MSA	381	108.89
Cumberland, MD – WV MSA	187	183.98
Dallas – Fort Worth, TX CMSA	4542	116.90
Danville, VA MSA	103	94.75
Davenport – Rock Island – Moline, IA – IL MSA	439	125.12
Dayton – Springfield, OH MSA	1611	169.35
Daytona Beach, FL MSA	340	91.72
Decatur, AL MSA	95	72.21
Decatur, IL MSA	171	145.90
Denver – Boulder, CO CMSA	2686	145.32
Des Moines, IA MSA	721	183.49
Detroit – Ann Arbor, MI CMSA	7183	153.97
Dothan, AL MSA	145	110.72
Dubuque, IA MSA	100	115.74
Duluth, MN – WI MSA	478	199.19
Eau Claire, WI MSA	174	126.51
El Paso, TX MSA	657	111.05
Elkhart – Goshen, IN MSA	82	52.50
Elmira, NY MSA	125	131.31
Enid, OK MSA	83	146.29

[Continued]

★ 705 ★

Clinical Laboratory Technologists and Technicians
[Continued]

MSA/CMSA	Total Employees	Employees per 100,000 pop.
Erie, PA MSA	433	157.13
Eugene – Springfield, OR MSA	357	126.19
Evansville, IN – KY MSA	419	150.18
Fargo – Moorhead, ND – MN MSA	266	173.52
Fayetteville, NC MSA	443	161.35
Fayetteville – Springdale, AR MSA	112	98.76
Fitchburg – Leominster, MA MSA	106	103.12
Flint, MI MSA	579	134.51
Florence, AL MSA	159	121.07
Florence, SC MSA	180	157.42
Fort Collins – Loveland, CO MSA	258	138.61
Fort Myers – Cape Coral, FL MSA	379	113.10
Fort Pierce, FL MSA	344	137.01
Fort Smith, AR – OK MSA	205	116.54
Fort Walton Beach, FL MSA	224	155.80
Fort Wayne, IN MSA	556	152.83
Fresno, CA MSA	726	108.77
Gadsden, AL MSA	96	96.15
Gainesville, FL MSA	599	293.47
Glens Falls, NY MSA	189	159.44
Grand Forks, ND MSA	108	152.79
Grand Rapids, MI MSA	934	135.68
Great Falls, MT MSA	101	130.00
Greeley, CO MSA	154	116.83
Green Bay, WI MSA	166	85.31
Greensboro – Winston-Salem – High Point, NC MSA	1371	145.53
Greenville – Spartanburg, SC MSA	784	122.34
Hagerstown, MD MSA	180	148.28
Harrisburg – Lebanon – Carlisle, PA MSA	886	150.68
Hartford – New Britain – Middletown, CT CMSA	1502	138.33
Hickory – Morganton, NC MSA	381	171.85
Honolulu, HI MSA	1137	135.97
Houma – Thibodaux, LA MSA	211	115.40
Houston – Galveston – Brazoria, TX CMSA	5550	149.55
Huntington – Ashland, WV – KY – OH MSA	372	119.03
Huntsville, AL MSA	324	135.61
Indianapolis, IN MSA	2050	164.02
Iowa City, IA MSA	434	451.52
Jackson, MI MSA	182	121.53
Jackson, MS MSA	920	232.68
Jackson, TN MSA	147	188.51
Jacksonville, FL MSA	1364	150.43
Jacksonville, NC MSA	102	68.07
Jamestown – Dunkirk, NY	135	95.14
Janesville – Beloit, WI MSA	151	108.24
Johnson City – Kingsport – Bristol, TN – VA MSA	666	152.74

[Continued]

★ 705 ★

Clinical Laboratory Technologists and Technicians
[Continued]

MSA/CMSA	Total Employees	Employees per 100,000 pop.
Johnstown, PA MSA	356	147.57
Joplin, MO MSA	210	155.66
Kalamazoo, MI MSA	440	196.95
Kankakee, IL MSA	424	440.50
Kansas City, MO – KS MSA	2612	166.76
Killeen – Temple, TX MSA	492	192.71
Knoxville, TN MSA	939	155.25
Kokomo, IN MSA	85	87.68
La Crosse, WI MSA	239	244.12
Lafayette, LA MSA	265	126.95
Lafayette – West Lafayette, IN MSA	173	132.47
Lake Charles, LA MSA	228	135.61
Lakeland – Winter Haven, FL MSA	459	113.23
Lancaster, PA MSA	336	79.47
Lansing – East Lansing, MI MSA	726	167.79
Laredo, TX MSA	67	50.29
Las Cruces, NM MSA	119	87.82
Las Vegas, NV MSA	874	117.88
Lawrence, KS MSA	120	146.70
Lawton, OK MSA	143	128.27
Lewiston – Auburn, ME MSA	162	183.80
Lexington-Fayette, KY MSA	850	243.95
Lima, OH MSA	165	106.91
Lincoln, NE MSA	415	194.25
Little Rock – North Little Rock, AR MSA	893	174.03
Longview – Marshall, TX MSA	129	79.42
Los Angeles – Anaheim – Riverside, CA CMSA	15629	107.55
Louisville, KY – IN MSA	1658	174.04
Lubbock, TX MSA	448	201.23
Lynchburg, VA MSA	138	97.05
Macon – Warner Robins, GA MSA	441	156.88
Madison, WI MSA	979	266.70
Manchester, NH MSA	218	147.49
Mansfield, OH MSA	88	69.77
McAllen – Edinburg – Mission, TX MSA	144	37.54
Medford, OR MSA	154	105.20
Melbourne – Titusville – Palm Bay, FL MSA	534	133.84
Memphis, TN – AR – MS MSA	2011	204.84
Merced, CA MSA	91	51.01
Miami – Fort Lauderdale, FL CMSA	5010	156.93
Midland, TX MSA	57	53.47
Milwaukee – Racine, WI CMSA	2739	170.42
Minneapolis – St. Paul, MN – WI MSA	3816	154.86
Mobile, AL MSA	720	150.97
Modesto, CA MSA	356	96.08
Monroe, LA MSA	310	218.02

[Continued]

★ 705 ★

Clinical Laboratory Technologists and Technicians
[Continued]

MSA/CMSA	Total Employees	Employees per 100,000 pop.
Montgomery, AL MSA	412	140.85
Muncie, IN MSA	187	156.28
Muskegon, MI MSA	192	120.77
Naples, FL MSA	194	127.55
Nashville, TN MSA	1902	193.09
New Bedford, MA MSA	269	153.15
New Haven – Meriden, CT MSA	843	159.00
New London – Norwich, CT – RI MSA	290	108.69
New Orleans, LA MSA	2154	173.88
New York – Northern New Jersey – Long Island, NY – NJ – CT CMSA	24130	133.41
Norfolk – Virginia Beach – Newport News, VA MSA	1593	114.10
Ocala, FL MSA	176	90.33
Odessa, TX MSA	160	134.53
Oklahoma City, OK MSA	1716	178.97
Olympia, WA MSA	179	111.02
Omaha, NE – IA MSA	1339	216.57
Orlando, FL MSA	1063	99.09
Owensboro, KY MSA	116	133.04
Panama City, FL MSA	142	111.82
Parkersburg – Marietta, WV – OH MSA	190	127.37
Pascagoula, MS MSA	161	139.70
Pensacola, FL MSA	496	144.02
Peoria, IL MSA	439	129.43
Philadelphia – Wilmington – Trenton, PA – NJ – DE – MD CMSA	10435	176.88
Phoenix, AZ MSA	2685	126.53
Pine Bluff, AR MSA	145	169.62
Pittsburgh – Beaver Valley, PA CMSA	3838	171.13
Pittsfield, MA MSA	128	161.51
Portland, ME MSA	549	255.02
Portland – Vancouver, OR – WA CMSA	2033	137.56
Portsmouth – Dover – Rochester, NH – ME MSA	213	95.27
Poughkeepsie, NY MSA	226	87.10
Providence – Pawtucket – Fall River, RI – MA CMSA	1889	165.48
Provo – Orem, UT MSA	277	105.09
Pueblo, CO MSA	176	143.03
Raleigh – Durham, NC MSA	1889	256.84
Rapid City, SD MSA	155	190.55
Reading, PA MSA	448	133.13
Redding, CA MSA	184	125.14
Reno, NV MSA	529	207.72
Richland – Kennewick – Pasco, WA MSA	153	101.98
Richmond – Petersburg, VA MSA	1655	191.19
Roanoke, VA MSA	265	118.05
Rochester, MN MSA	847	795.53
Rochester, NY MSA	1575	157.12
Rockford, IL MSA	343	120.89

[Continued]

★ 705 ★

Clinical Laboratory Technologists and Technicians
[Continued]

MSA/CMSA	Total Employees	Employees per 100,000 pop.
Sacramento, CA MSA	1838	124.10
Saginaw – Bay City – Midland, MI MSA	638	159.77
St. Cloud, MN MSA	240	125.71
St. Joseph, MO MSA	106	127.58
St. Louis, MO – IL MSA	4449	182.03
Salem, OR MSA	245	88.12
Salinas – Seaside – Monterey, CA MSA	246	69.17
Salt Lake City – Ogden, UT MSA	1677	156.40
San Angelo, TX MSA	201	204.15
San Antonio, TX MSA	2209	169.65
San Diego, CA MSA	3483	139.43
San Francisco – Oakland – San Jose, CA CMSA	8104	129.60
Santa Barbara – Santa Maria – Lompoc, CA MSA	389	105.25
Santa Fe, NM MSA	143	122.18
Sarasota, FL MSA	305	109.80
Savannah, GA MSA	393	161.98
Scranton – Wilkes-Barre, PA MSA	1113	151.60
Seattle – Tacoma, WA CMSA	3977	155.40
Sharon, PA MSA	190	157.02
Sheboygan, WI MSA	91	87.60
Sherman – Denison, TX MSA	161	169.44
Shreveport, LA MSA	511	152.84
Sioux City, IA – NE MSA	211	183.45
Sioux Falls, SD MSA	301	243.12
South Bend – Mishawaka, IN MSA	371	150.17
Spokane, WA MSA	645	178.49
Springfield, IL MSA	392	206.81
Springfield, MO MSA	545	226.52
Springfield, MA MSA	666	125.77
State College, PA MSA	131	105.83
Steubenville – Weirton, OH – WV MSA	162	113.67
Stockton, CA MSA	432	89.88
Syracuse, NY MSA	1008	152.76
Tallahassee, FL MSA	348	148.97
Tampa – St. Petersburg – Clearwater, FL MSA	2980	144.10
Terre Haute, IN MSA	154	117.73
Texarkana, TX – Texarkana, AR MSA	169	140.68
Toledo, OH MSA	1093	177.98
Topeka, KS MSA	318	197.54
Tucson, AZ MSA	888	133.16
Tulsa, OK MSA	907	127.93
Tuscaloosa, AL MSA	162	107.63
Tyler, TX MSA	257	169.85
Utica – Rome, NY MSA	336	106.12
Victoria, TX MSA	79	106.24
Visalia – Tulare – Porterville, CA MSA	212	67.97

[Continued]

★ 705 ★

Clinical Laboratory Technologists and Technicians
[Continued]

MSA/CMSA	Total Employees	Employees per 100,000 pop.
Waco, TX MSA	278	146.99
Washington, DC – MD – VA MSA	5937	151.32
Waterbury, CT MSA	395	178.23
Waterloo – Cedar Falls, IA MSA	160	109.13
Wausau, WI MSA	200	173.31
West Palm Beach – Boca Raton – Delray Beach, FL MSA	986	114.18
Wheeling, WV – OH MSA	238	149.40
Wichita, KS MSA	910	187.52
Wichita Falls, TX MSA	135	110.31
Williamsport, PA MSA	137	115.41
Wilmington, NC MSA	158	131.36
Worcester, MA MSA	800	183.11
Yakima, WA MSA	129	68.32
York, PA MSA	501	119.90
Youngstown – Warren, OH MSA	783	158.95
Yuba City, CA MSA	134	109.26
Yuma, AZ MSA	56	52.39

Source: Census of Population and Housing, 1990: Equal Employment Opportunity (EEO) File on CD-ROM [machine-readable datafiles]. Prepared by the Bureau of the Census. Washington, DC: The Bureau, 1992.

★ 706 ★

Employment

Dental Assistants

The table below presents the number of civilians 16 years old or older who reported working as dental assistants during the 1990 Census. Data are provided by total number employed in each Metropolitan Statistical Area (MSA) or Consolidated Metropolitan Statistical Area (CMSA), as well as the number employed per 100,000 people.

[Total for all of the U.S. was 179,287; 72.09 per 100,000 persons]

MSA/CMSA	Total Employees	Employees per 100,000 pop.
Abilene, TX MSA	52	43.46
Albany, GA MSA	64	56.86
Albany – Schenectady – Troy, NY MSA	456	52.16
Albuquerque, NM MSA	466	96.97
Alexandria, LA MSA	88	66.89
Allentown – Bethlehem – Easton, PA – NJ MSA	559	81.41
Altoona, PA MSA	97	74.31
Amarillo, TX MSA	80	42.66
Anchorage, AK MSA	249	110.01
Anderson, IN MSA	58	44.39
Anderson, SC MSA	148	101.93
Anniston, AL MSA	67	57.74

[Continued]

★ 706 ★

Dental Assistants
[Continued]

MSA/CMSA	Total Employees	Employees per 100,000 pop.
Appleton–Oshkosh–Neenah, WI MSA	290	92.03
Asheville, NC MSA	92	52.63
Athens, GA MSA	65	41.60
Atlanta, GA MSA	1714	60.49
Atlantic City, NJ MSA	160	50.09
Augusta, GA–SC MSA	441	111.14
Austin, TX MSA	419	53.61
Bakersfield, CA MSA	459	84.46
Baltimore, MD MSA	1645	69.05
Bangor, ME MSA	65	73.24
Baton Rouge, LA MSA	336	63.60
Battle Creek, MI MSA	146	107.37
Beaumont–Port Arthur, TX MSA	213	58.97
Bellingham, WA MSA	107	83.74
Benton Harbor, MI MSA	106	65.68
Billings, MT MSA	95	83.76
Biloxi–Gulfport, MS MSA	119	60.37
Binghamton, NY MSA	149	56.33
Birmingham, AL MSA	642	70.72
Bismarck, ND MSA	74	88.27
Bloomington, IN MSA	94	86.26
Bloomington–Normal, IL MSA	73	56.51
Boise City, ID MSA	183	88.93
Boston–Lawrence–Salem, MA–NH CMSA	3524	84.48
Bradenton, FL MSA	209	98.72
Bremerton, WA MSA	248	130.71
Brownsville–Harlingen, TX MSA	95	36.52
Bryan–College Station, TX MSA	42	34.47
Buffalo–Niagara Falls, NY CMSA	808	67.94
Burlington, NC MSA	96	88.71
Burlington, VT MSA	81	61.63
Canton, OH MSA	339	86.02
Casper, WY MSA	40	65.33
Cedar Rapids, IA MSA	158	93.62
Champaign–Urbana–Rantoul, IL MSA	70	40.46
Charleston, SC MSA	325	64.12
Charleston, WV MSA	112	44.72
Charlotte–Gastonia–Rock Hill, NC–SC MSA	643	55.33
Charlottesville, VA MSA	88	67.12
Chattanooga, TN–GA MSA	315	72.71
Cheyenne, WY MSA	70	95.70
Chicago–Gary–Lake County, IL–IN–WI CMSA	6321	78.37
Chico, CA MSA	174	95.54
Cincinnati–Hamilton, OH–KY–IN CMSA	1255	71.96
Clarksville–Hopkinsville, TN–KY MSA	125	73.77
Cleveland–Akron–Lorain, OH CMSA	2138	77.47

[Continued]

★ 706 ★

Dental Assistants
[Continued]

MSA/CMSA	Total Employees	Employees per 100,000 pop.
Colorado Springs, CO MSA	387	97.48
Columbia, MO MSA	52	46.27
Columbia, SC MSA	300	66.18
Columbus, GA–AL MSA	143	58.83
Columbus, OH MSA	914	66.36
Corpus Christi, TX MSA	233	66.59
Cumberland, MD–WV MSA	36	35.42
Dallas–Fort Worth, TX CMSA	2618	67.38
Danville, VA MSA	96	88.31
Davenport–Rock Island–Moline, IA–IL MSA	284	80.94
Dayton–Springfield, OH MSA	624	65.60
Daytona Beach, FL MSA	258	69.60
Decatur, AL MSA	52	39.53
Decatur, IL MSA	42	35.83
Denver–Boulder, CO CMSA	1758	95.11
Des Moines, IA MSA	266	67.70
Detroit–Ann Arbor, MI CMSA	4033	86.45
Dothan, AL MSA	107	81.70
Dubuque, IA MSA	131	151.62
Duluth, MN–WI MSA	169	70.43
Eau Claire, WI MSA	119	86.52
El Paso, TX MSA	283	47.84
Elkhart–Goshen, IN MSA	65	41.61
Elmira, NY MSA	51	53.57
Enid, OK MSA	15	26.44
Erie, PA MSA	300	108.86
Eugene–Springfield, OR MSA	185	65.39
Evansville, IN–KY MSA	138	49.46
Fargo–Moorhead, ND–MN MSA	135	88.06
Fayetteville, NC MSA	238	86.68
Fayetteville–Springdale, AR MSA	103	90.82
Fitchburg–Leominster, MA MSA	91	88.52
Flint, MI MSA	337	78.29
Florence, AL MSA	99	75.38
Florence, SC MSA	127	111.07
Fort Collins–Loveland, CO MSA	147	78.97
Fort Myers–Cape Coral, FL MSA	214	63.86
Fort Pierce, FL MSA	159	63.33
Fort Smith, AR–OK MSA	92	52.30
Fort Walton Beach, FL MSA	71	49.38
Fort Wayne, IN MSA	308	84.66
Fresno, CA MSA	394	59.03
Gadsden, AL MSA	45	45.07
Gainesville, FL MSA	108	52.91
Glens Falls, NY MSA	11	9.28
Grand Forks, ND MSA	58	82.06

[Continued]

★ 706 ★

Dental Assistants
[Continued]

MSA/CMSA	Total Employees	Employees per 100,000 pop.
Grand Rapids, MI MSA	537	78.01
Great Falls, MT MSA	99	127.43
Greeley, CO MSA	100	75.86
Green Bay, WI MSA	138	70.92
Greensboro – Winston-Salem – High Point, NC MSA	592	62.84
Greenville – Spartanburg, SC MSA	341	53.21
Hagerstown, MD MSA	94	77.43
Harrisburg – Lebanon – Carlisle, PA MSA	369	62.76
Hartford – New Britain – Middletown, CT CMSA	919	84.64
Hickory – Morganton, NC MSA	155	69.91
Honolulu, HI MSA	770	92.08
Houma – Thibodaux, LA MSA	104	56.88
Houston – Galveston – Brazoria, TX CMSA	2363	63.67
Huntington – Ashland, WV – KY – OH MSA	121	38.72
Huntsville, AL MSA	113	47.30
Indianapolis, IN MSA	839	67.13
Iowa City, IA MSA	127	132.13
Jackson, MI MSA	84	56.09
Jackson, MS MSA	325	82.20
Jackson, TN MSA	27	34.62
Jacksonville, FL MSA	598	65.95
Jacksonville, NC MSA	84	56.06
Jamestown – Dunkirk, NY	66	46.51
Janesville – Beloit, WI MSA	89	63.79
Johnson City – Kingsport – Bristol, TN – VA MSA	389	89.21
Johnstown, PA MSA	141	58.45
Joplin, MO MSA	139	103.03
Kalamazoo, MI MSA	203	90.86
Kankakee, IL MSA	58	60.26
Kansas City, MO – KS MSA	1211	77.32
Killeen – Temple, TX MSA	216	84.61
Knoxville, TN MSA	425	70.27
Kokomo, IN MSA	112	115.53
La Crosse, WI MSA	166	169.55
Lafayette, LA MSA	86	41.20
Lafayette – West Lafayette, IN MSA	44	33.69
Lake Charles, LA MSA	113	67.21
Lakeland – Winter Haven, FL MSA	238	58.71
Lancaster, PA MSA	326	77.10
Lansing – East Lansing, MI MSA	394	91.06
Laredo, TX MSA	7	5.25
Las Cruces, NM MSA	82	60.51
Las Vegas, NV MSA	498	67.16
Lawrence, KS MSA	70	85.58
Lawton, OK MSA	74	66.38
Lewiston – Auburn, ME MSA	64	72.61

[Continued]

★ 706 ★

Dental Assistants
[Continued]

MSA/CMSA	Total Employees	Employees per 100,000 pop.
Lexington-Fayette, KY MSA	232	66.58
Lima, OH MSA	34	22.03
Lincoln, NE MSA	185	86.59
Little Rock-North Little Rock, AR MSA	443	86.34
Longview-Marshall, TX MSA	95	58.49
Los Angeles-Anaheim-Riverside, CA CMSA	11513	79.23
Louisville, KY-IN MSA	580	60.88
Lubbock, TX MSA	110	49.41
Lynchburg, VA MSA	140	98.45
Macon-Warner Robins, GA MSA	126	44.82
Madison, WI MSA	223	60.75
Manchester, NH MSA	162	109.60
Mansfield, OH MSA	82	65.01
McAllen-Edinburg-Mission, TX MSA	129	33.63
Medford, OR MSA	193	131.84
Melbourne-Titusville-Palm Bay, FL MSA	353	88.48
Memphis, TN-AR-MS MSA	527	53.68
Merced, CA MSA	121	67.82
Miami-Fort Lauderdale, FL CMSA	1977	61.92
Midland, TX MSA	31	29.08
Milwaukee-Racine, WI CMSA	1409	87.67
Minneapolis-St. Paul, MN-WI MSA	2179	88.43
Mobile, AL MSA	183	38.37
Modesto, CA MSA	335	90.41
Monroe, LA MSA	40	28.13
Montgomery, AL MSA	145	49.57
Muncie, IN MSA	76	63.51
Muskegon, MI MSA	92	57.87
Naples, FL MSA	93	61.14
Nashville, TN MSA	832	84.46
New Bedford, MA MSA	122	69.46
New Haven-Meriden, CT MSA	543	102.42
New London-Norwich, CT-RI MSA	244	91.45
New Orleans, LA MSA	671	54.16
New York-Northern New Jersey-Long Island, NY-NJ-CT CMSA	15901	87.91
Norfolk-Virginia Beach-Newport News, VA MSA	1083	77.57
Ocala, FL MSA	148	75.96
Odessa, TX MSA	55	46.24
Oklahoma City, OK MSA	676	70.50
Olympia, WA MSA	134	83.11
Omaha, NE-IA MSA	441	71.33
Orlando, FL MSA	613	57.14
Owensboro, KY MSA	73	83.73
Panama City, FL MSA	86	67.72
Parkersburg-Marietta, WV-OH MSA	98	65.70
Pascagoula, MS MSA	76	65.95

[Continued]

★ 706 ★

Dental Assistants
[Continued]

MSA/CMSA	Total Employees	Employees per 100,000 pop.
Pensacola, FL MSA	355	103.08
Peoria, IL MSA	247	72.82
Philadelphia – Wilmington – Trenton, PA – NJ – DE – MD CMSA	4403	74.64
Phoenix, AZ MSA	1486	70.02
Pine Bluff, AR MSA	36	42.11
Pittsburgh – Beaver Valley, PA CMSA	1504	67.06
Pittsfield, MA MSA	37	46.69
Portland, ME MSA	121	56.21
Portland – Vancouver, OR – WA CMSA	1538	104.07
Portsmouth – Dover – Rochester, NH – ME MSA	133	59.49
Poughkeepsie, NY MSA	227	87.49
Providence – Pawtucket – Fall River, RI – MA CMSA	821	71.92
Provo – Orem, UT MSA	238	90.29
Pueblo, CO MSA	96	78.02
Raleigh – Durham, NC MSA	525	71.38
Rapid City, SD MSA	88	108.18
Reading, PA MSA	244	72.51
Redding, CA MSA	139	94.53
Reno, NV MSA	315	123.69
Richland – Kennewick – Pasco, WA MSA	102	67.99
Richmond – Petersburg, VA MSA	529	61.11
Roanoke, VA MSA	159	70.83
Rochester, MN MSA	108	101.44
Rochester, NY MSA	762	76.02
Rockford, IL MSA	176	62.03
Sacramento, CA MSA	1449	97.83
Saginaw – Bay City – Midland, MI MSA	402	100.67
St. Cloud, MN MSA	159	83.28
St. Joseph, MO MSA	63	75.83
St. Louis, MO – IL MSA	1854	75.86
Salem, OR MSA	277	99.63
Salinas – Seaside – Monterey, CA MSA	338	95.03
Salt Lake City – Ogden, UT MSA	1013	94.48
San Angelo, TX MSA	66	67.03
San Antonio, TX MSA	1015	77.95
San Diego, CA MSA	2187	87.55
San Francisco – Oakland – San Jose, CA CMSA	5682	90.86
Santa Barbara – Santa Maria – Lompoc, CA MSA	335	90.64
Santa Fe, NM MSA	74	63.22
Sarasota, FL MSA	134	48.24
Savannah, GA MSA	137	56.47
Scranton – Wilkes-Barre, PA MSA	459	62.52
Seattle – Tacoma, WA CMSA	2577	100.70
Sharon, PA MSA	83	68.59
Sheboygan, WI MSA	80	77.01
Sherman – Denison, TX MSA	21	22.10

[Continued]

★ 706 ★

Dental Assistants
[Continued]

MSA/CMSA	Total Employees	Employees per 100,000 pop.
Shreveport, LA MSA	223	66.70
Sioux City, IA – NE MSA	57	49.56
Sioux Falls, SD MSA	107	86.42
South Bend – Mishawaka, IN MSA	132	53.43
Spokane, WA MSA	385	106.54
Springfield, IL MSA	96	50.65
Springfield, MO MSA	226	93.93
Springfield, MA MSA	462	87.25
State College, PA MSA	71	57.36
Steubenville – Weirton, OH – WV MSA	132	92.62
Stockton, CA MSA	377	78.44
Syracuse, NY MSA	439	66.53
Tallahassee, FL MSA	94	40.24
Tampa – St. Petersburg – Clearwater, FL MSA	1327	64.17
Terre Haute, IN MSA	62	47.40
Texarkana, TX – Texarkana, AR MSA	66	54.94
Toledo, OH MSA	383	62.36
Topeka, KS MSA	98	60.88
Tucson, AZ MSA	552	82.77
Tulsa, OK MSA	602	84.91
Tuscaloosa, AL MSA	84	55.81
Tyler, TX MSA	48	31.72
Utica – Rome, NY MSA	214	67.59
Victoria, TX MSA	88	118.34
Visalia – Tulare – Porterville, CA MSA	210	67.32
Waco, TX MSA	95	50.23
Washington, DC – MD – VA MSA	2649	67.51
Waterbury, CT MSA	113	50.99
Waterloo – Cedar Falls, IA MSA	101	68.89
Wausau, WI MSA	96	83.19
West Palm Beach – Boca Raton – Delray Beach, FL MSA	705	81.64
Wheeling, WV – OH MSA	58	36.41
Wichita, KS MSA	326	67.18
Wichita Falls, TX MSA	95	77.63
Williamsport, PA MSA	72	60.65
Wilmington, NC MSA	84	69.83
Worcester, MA MSA	334	76.45
Yakima, WA MSA	117	61.96
York, PA MSA	377	90.22
Youngstown – Warren, OH MSA	271	55.01
Yuba City, CA MSA	76	61.97
Yuma, AZ MSA	7	6.55

Source: Census of Population and Housing, 1990: Equal Employment Opportunity (EEO) File on CD-ROM [machine-readable datafiles]. Prepared by the Bureau of the Census. Washington, DC: The Bureau, 1992.

★ 707 ★
Employment

Dental Hygienists

The table below presents the number of civilians 16 years old or older who reported working as dental hygienists during the 1990 Census. Data are provided by total number employed in each Metropolitan Statistical Area (MSA) or Consolidated Metropolitan Statistical Area (CMSA), as well as the number employed per 100,000 people.

[Total for all of the U.S. was 72,394; 29.11 per 100,000 persons]

MSA/CMSA	Total Employees	Employees per 100,000 pop.
Abilene, TX MSA	54	45.13
Albany, GA MSA	23	20.43
Albany–Schenectady–Troy, NY MSA	498	56.96
Albuquerque, NM MSA	175	36.41
Alexandria, LA MSA	13	9.88
Allentown–Bethlehem–Easton, PA–NJ MSA	242	35.24
Altoona, PA MSA	20	15.32
Amarillo, TX MSA	54	28.79
Anchorage, AK MSA	95	41.97
Anderson, IN MSA	36	27.55
Anderson, SC MSA	7	4.82
Anniston, AL MSA	42	36.20
Appleton–Oshkosh–Neenah, WI MSA	134	42.52
Asheville, NC MSA	54	30.89
Athens, GA MSA	56	35.84
Atlanta, GA MSA	1155	40.76
Atlantic City, NJ MSA	149	46.65
Augusta, GA–SC MSA	134	33.77
Austin, TX MSA	257	32.88
Bakersfield, CA MSA	68	12.51
Baltimore, MD MSA	687	28.01
Bangor, ME MSA	56	63.10
Baton Rouge, LA MSA	73	13.82
Battle Creek, MI MSA	87	63.98
Beaumont–Port Arthur, TX MSA	88	24.36
Bellingham, WA MSA	44	34.43
Benton Harbor, MI MSA	32	19.83
Billings, MT MSA	19	16.75
Biloxi–Gulfport, MS MSA	35	17.76
Binghamton, NY MSA	184	69.57
Birmingham, AL MSA	283	31.17
Bismarck, ND MSA	38	45.33
Bloomington, IN MSA	25	22.94
Bloomington–Normal, IL MSA	48	37.16
Boise City, ID MSA	107	52.00
Boston–Lawrence–Salem, MA–NH CMSA	1914	45.88
Bradenton, FL MSA	101	47.71
Bremerton, WA MSA	41	21.61
Brownsville–Harlingen, TX MSA	11	4.23
Bryan–College Station, TX MSA	18	14.77
Buffalo–Niagara Falls, NY CMSA	650	54.65
Burlington, NC MSA	63	58.22

[Continued]

★ 707 ★

Dental Hygienists
[Continued]

MSA/CMSA	Total Employees	Employees per 100,000 pop.
Burlington, VT MSA	105	79.88
Canton, OH MSA	27	6.85
Casper, WY MSA	12	19.60
Cedar Rapids, IA MSA	69	40.88
Champaign–Urbana–Rantoul, IL MSA	66	38.14
Charleston, SC MSA	167	32.95
Charleston, WV MSA	89	35.54
Charlotte–Gastonia–Rock Hill, NC–SC MSA	291	25.04
Charlottesville, VA MSA	23	17.54
Chattanooga, TN–GA MSA	187	43.17
Cheyenne, WY MSA	9	12.30
Chicago–Gary–Lake County, IL–IN–WI CMSA	2308	28.62
Chico, CA MSA	38	20.87
Cincinnati–Hamilton, OH–KY–IN CMSA	585	33.54
Clarksville–Hopkinsville, TN–KY MSA	49	28.92
Cleveland–Akron–Lorain, OH CMSA	782	28.34
Colorado Springs, CO MSA	98	24.68
Columbia, MO MSA	21	18.69
Columbia, SC MSA	145	31.99
Columbus, GA–AL MSA	50	20.57
Columbus, OH MSA	537	38.99
Corpus Christi, TX MSA	65	18.58
Cumberland, MD–WV MSA	44	43.29
Dallas–Fort Worth, TX CMSA	1062	27.33
Danville, VA MSA	12	11.04
Davenport–Rock Island–Moline, IA–IL MSA	90	25.65
Dayton–Springfield, OH MSA	323	33.95
Daytona Beach, FL MSA	106	28.59
Decatur, AL MSA	65	49.41
Decatur, IL MSA	35	29.86
Denver–Boulder, CO CMSA	690	37.33
Des Moines, IA MSA	159	40.47
Detroit–Ann Arbor, MI CMSA	2020	43.30
Dothan, AL MSA	46	35.12
Dubuque, IA MSA	18	20.83
Duluth, MN–WI MSA	96	40.00
Eau Claire, WI MSA	44	31.99
El Paso, TX MSA	99	16.73
Elkhart–Goshen, IN MSA	36	23.05
Elmira, NY MSA	51	53.57
Erie, PA MSA	70	25.40
Eugene–Springfield, OR MSA	118	41.71
Evansville, IN–KY MSA	86	30.83
Fargo–Moorhead, ND–MN MSA	93	60.67
Fayetteville, NC MSA	95	34.60
Fayetteville–Springdale, AR MSA	43	37.92

[Continued]

★ 707 ★

Dental Hygienists
[Continued]

MSA/CMSA	Total Employees	Employees per 100,000 pop.
Fitchburg – Leominster, MA MSA	45	43.78
Flint, MI MSA	236	54.83
Florence, AL MSA	24	18.27
Florence, SC MSA	47	41.10
Fort Collins – Loveland, CO MSA	85	45.67
Fort Myers – Cape Coral, FL MSA	131	39.09
Fort Pierce, FL MSA	93	37.04
Fort Smith, AR – OK MSA	64	36.38
Fort Walton Beach, FL MSA	55	38.25
Fort Wayne, IN MSA	165	45.35
Fresno, CA MSA	145	21.72
Gadsden, AL MSA	46	46.07
Gainesville, FL MSA	146	71.53
Glens Falls, NY MSA	33	27.84
Grand Forks, ND MSA	32	45.27
Grand Rapids, MI MSA	439	63.77
Great Falls, MT MSA	6	7.72
Greeley, CO MSA	38	28.83
Green Bay, WI MSA	71	36.49
Greensboro – Winston-Salem – High Point, NC MSA	471	50.00
Greenville – Spartanburg, SC MSA	158	24.65
Hagerstown, MD MSA	39	32.13
Harrisburg – Lebanon – Carlisle, PA MSA	182	30.95
Hartford – New Britain – Middletown, CT CMSA	364	33.52
Hickory – Morganton, NC MSA	65	29.32
Honolulu, HI MSA	189	22.60
Houma – Thibodaux, LA MSA	21	11.49
Houston – Galveston – Brazoria, TX CMSA	819	22.07
Huntington – Ashland, WV – KY – OH MSA	72	23.04
Huntsville, AL MSA	123	51.48
Indianapolis, IN MSA	375	30.00
Iowa City, IA MSA	36	37.45
Jackson, MI MSA	43	28.71
Jackson, MS MSA	160	40.47
Jackson, TN MSA	17	21.80
Jacksonville, FL MSA	286	31.54
Jacksonville, NC MSA	57	38.04
Jamestown – Dunkirk, NY	25	17.62
Janesville – Beloit, WI MSA	58	41.57
Johnson City – Kingsport – Bristol, TN – VA MSA	107	24.54
Johnstown, PA MSA	35	14.51
Joplin, MO MSA	19	14.08
Kalamazoo, MI MSA	126	56.40
Kansas City, MO – KS MSA	465	29.69
Killeen – Temple, TX MSA	98	38.39
Knoxville, TN MSA	292	48.28

[Continued]

★ 707 ★

Dental Hygienists
[Continued]

MSA/CMSA	Total Employees	Employees per 100,000 pop.
Kokomo, IN MSA	18	18.57
La Crosse, WI MSA	30	30.64
Lafayette, LA MSA	44	21.08
Lafayette – West Lafayette, IN MSA	65	49.77
Lake Charles, LA MSA	10	5.95
Lakeland – Winter Haven, FL MSA	73	18.01
Lancaster, PA MSA	140	33.11
Lansing – East Lansing, MI MSA	286	66.10
Laredo, TX MSA	6	4.50
Las Cruces, NM MSA	20	14.76
Las Vegas, NV MSA	246	33.18
Lawrence, KS MSA	16	19.56
Lawton, OK MSA	12	10.76
Lewiston – Auburn, ME MSA	33	37.44
Lexington-Fayette, KY MSA	92	26.40
Lima, OH MSA	54	34.99
Lincoln, NE MSA	56	26.21
Little Rock – North Little Rock, AR MSA	185	36.05
Longview – Marshall, TX MSA	82	50.48
Los Angeles – Anaheim – Riverside, CA CMSA	2997	20.62
Louisville, KY – IN MSA	180	18.89
Lubbock, TX MSA	20	8.98
Lynchburg, VA MSA	28	19.69
Macon – Warner Robins, GA MSA	146	51.94
Madison, WI MSA	255	69.47
Manchester, NH MSA	39	26.39
Mansfield, OH MSA	43	34.09
McAllen – Edinburg – Mission, TX MSA	13	3.39
Medford, OR MSA	44	30.06
Melbourne – Titusville – Palm Bay, FL MSA	125	31.33
Memphis, TN – AR – MS MSA	232	23.63
Merced, CA MSA	22	12.33
Miami – Fort Lauderdale, FL CMSA	1213	37.99
Midland, TX MSA	45	42.21
Milwaukee – Racine, WI CMSA	610	37.95
Minneapolis – St. Paul, MN – WI MSA	1414	57.38
Mobile, AL MSA	111	23.27
Modesto, CA MSA	116	31.31
Monroe, LA MSA	23	16.18
Montgomery, AL MSA	65	22.22
Muncie, IN MSA	27	22.56
Muskegon, MI MSA	58	36.48
Naples, FL MSA	42	27.61
Nashville, TN MSA	348	35.33
New Bedford, MA MSA	44	25.05
New Haven – Meriden, CT MSA	275	51.87

[Continued]

★ 707 ★

Dental Hygienists
[Continued]

MSA/CMSA	Total Employees	Employees per 100,000 pop.
New London – Norwich, CT – RI MSA	117	43.85
New Orleans, LA MSA	274	22.12
New York – Northern New Jersey – Long Island, NY – NJ – CT CMSA	5288	29.24
Norfolk – Virginia Beach – Newport News, VA MSA	323	23.14
Ocala, FL MSA	22	11.29
Oklahoma City, OK MSA	249	25.97
Olympia, WA MSA	81	50.24
Omaha, NE – IA MSA	129	20.86
Orlando, FL MSA	265	24.70
Owensboro, KY MSA	13	14.91
Panama City, FL MSA	38	29.92
Parkersburg – Marietta, WV – OH MSA	43	28.83
Pascagoula, MS MSA	28	24.30
Pensacola, FL MSA	127	36.88
Peoria, IL MSA	157	46.29
Philadelphia – Wilmington – Trenton, PA – NJ – DE – MD CMSA	1672	28.34
Phoenix, AZ MSA	737	34.73
Pine Bluff, AR MSA	5	5.85
Pittsburgh – Beaver Valley, PA CMSA	521	23.23
Pittsfield, MA MSA	26	32.81
Portland, ME MSA	123	57.13
Portland – Vancouver, OR – WA CMSA	828	56.03
Portsmouth – Dover – Rochester, NH – ME MSA	167	74.69
Poughkeepsie, NY MSA	94	36.23
Providence – Pawtucket – Fall River, RI – MA CMSA	406	35.57
Provo – Orem, UT MSA	47	17.83
Pueblo, CO MSA	20	16.25
Raleigh – Durham, NC MSA	238	32.36
Rapid City, SD MSA	29	35.65
Reading, PA MSA	76	22.58
Redding, CA MSA	44	29.92
Reno, NV MSA	105	41.23
Richland – Kennewick – Pasco, WA MSA	38	25.33
Richmond – Petersburg, VA MSA	200	23.10
Roanoke, VA MSA	67	29.85
Rochester, MN MSA	27	25.36
Rochester, NY MSA	541	53.97
Rockford, IL MSA	81	28.55
Sacramento, CA MSA	510	34.43
Saginaw – Bay City – Midland, MI MSA	168	42.07
St. Cloud, MN MSA	89	46.62
St. Louis, MO – IL MSA	499	20.42
Salem, OR MSA	126	45.32
Salinas – Seaside – Monterey, CA MSA	134	37.68
Salt Lake City – Ogden, UT MSA	195	18.19
San Angelo, TX MSA	11	11.17

[Continued]

★ 707 ★

Dental Hygienists
[Continued]

MSA/CMSA	Total Employees	Employees per 100,000 pop.
San Antonio, TX MSA	294	22.58
San Diego, CA MSA	608	24.34
San Francisco – Oakland – San Jose, CA CMSA	2693	43.07
Santa Barbara – Santa Maria – Lompoc, CA MSA	141	38.15
Santa Fe, NM MSA	21	17.94
Sarasota, FL MSA	145	52.20
Savannah, GA MSA	112	46.16
Scranton – Wilkes-Barre, PA MSA	198	26.97
Seattle – Tacoma, WA CMSA	1254	49.00
Sharon, PA MSA	13	10.74
Sheboygan, WI MSA	35	33.69
Sherman – Denison, TX MSA	21	22.10
Shreveport, LA MSA	83	24.82
Sioux City, IA – NE MSA	18	15.65
Sioux Falls, SD MSA	39	31.50
South Bend – Mishawaka, IN MSA	90	36.43
Spokane, WA MSA	133	36.80
Springfield, IL MSA	52	27.43
Springfield, MO MSA	73	30.34
Springfield, MA MSA	292	55.14
State College, PA MSA	29	23.43
Steubenville – Weirton, OH – WV MSA	55	38.59
Stockton, CA MSA	79	16.44
Syracuse, NY MSA	360	54.56
Tallahassee, FL MSA	84	35.96
Tampa – St. Petersburg – Clearwater, FL MSA	451	21.81
Terre Haute, IN MSA	22	16.82
Texarkana, TX – Texarkana, AR MSA	10	8.32
Toledo, OH MSA	342	55.69
Topeka, KS MSA	49	30.44
Tucson, AZ MSA	202	30.29
Tulsa, OK MSA	221	31.17
Tuscaloosa, AL MSA	16	10.63
Tyler, TX MSA	72	47.58
Utica – Rome, NY MSA	73	23.06
Victoria, TX MSA	15	20.17
Visalia – Tulare – Porterville, CA MSA	13	4.17
Waco, TX MSA	33	17.45
Washington, DC – MD – VA MSA	1262	32.16
Waterbury, CT MSA	115	51.89
Waterloo – Cedar Falls, IA MSA	30	20.46
Wausau, WI MSA	92	79.72
West Palm Beach – Boca Raton – Delray Beach, FL MSA	276	31.96
Wheeling, WV – OH MSA	82	51.47
Wichita, KS MSA	123	25.35
Wichita Falls, TX MSA	53	43.31

[Continued]

★ 707 ★

Dental Hygienists
[Continued]

MSA/CMSA	Total Employees	Employees per 100,000 pop.
Williamsport, PA MSA	24	20.22
Wilmington, NC MSA	68	56.53
Worcester, MA MSA	151	34.56
Yaklma, WA MSA	57	30.19
York, PA MSA	148	35.42
Youngstown – Warren, OH MSA	96	19.49
Yuba City, CA MSA	10	8.15
Yuma, AZ MSA	16	14.97

Source: Census of Population and Housing, 1990; Equal Employment Opportunity (EEO) File on CD ROM [machine-readable datafiles]. Prepared by the Bureau of the Census. Washington, DC: The Bureau, 1992.

★ 708 ★

Employment

Dental Laboratory and Medical Appliance Technicians

The table below presents the number of civilians 16 years old or older who reported working as dental laboratory and medical appliance technicians during the 1990 Census. Data are provided by total number employed in each Metropolitan Statistical Area (MSA) or Consolidated Metropolitan Statistical Area (CMSA), as well as the number employed per 100,000 people.

[Total for all of the U.S. was 56,964; 22.90 per 100,000 persons]

MSA/CMSA	Total Employees	Employees per 100,000 pop.
Abilene, TX MSA	11	9.19
Albany, GA MSA	34	30.21
Albany – Schenectady – Troy, NY MSA	189	21.62
Albuquerque, NM MSA	139	28.92
Alexandria, LA MSA	33	25.08
Allentown – Bethlehem – Easton, PA – NJ MSA	114	16.60
Altoona, PA MSA	13	9.96
Amarillo, TX MSA	73	38.92
Anchorage, AK MSA	90	39.76
Anderson, IN MSA	32	24.49
Appleton – Oshkosh – Neenah, WI MSA	68	21.58
Asheville, NC MSA	49	28.03
Athens, GA MSA	59	37.76
Atlanta, GA MSA	798	28.16
Atlantic City, NJ MSA	69	21.60
Augusta, GA – SC MSA	173	43.60
Austin, TX MSA	100	12.79
Bakersfield, CA MSA	78	14.35
Baltimore, MD MSA	567	23.80
Bangor, ME MSA	34	38.31
Baton Rouge, LA MSA	74	14.01

[Continued]

★ 708 ★

Dental Laboratory and Medical Appliance Technicians
[Continued]

MSA/CMSA	Total Employees	Employees per 100,000 pop.
Battle Creek, MI MSA	49	36.03
Beaumont – Port Arthur, TX MSA	58	16.06
Bellingham, WA MSA	30	23.48
Benton Harbor, MI MSA	54	33.46
Billings, MT MSA	20	17.63
Biloxi – Gulfport, MS MSA	71	36.02
Binghamton, NY MSA	49	18.53
Birmingham, AL MSA	152	16.74
Bismarck, ND MSA	35	41.75
Bloomington – Normal, IL MSA	8	6.19
Boise City, ID MSA	54	26.24
Boston – Lawrence – Salem, MA – NH CMSA	717	17.19
Bradenton, FL MSA	61	28.81
Bremerton, WA MSA	78	41.11
Brownsville – Harlingen, TX MSA	23	8.84
Bryan – College Station, TX MSA	14	11.49
Buffalo – Niagara Falls, NY CMSA	273	22.95
Burlington, NC MSA	85	78.55
Burlington, VT MSA	44	33.48
Canton, OH MSA	15	3.81
Casper, WY MSA	14	22.87
Cedar Rapids, IA MSA	55	32.59
Champaign – Urbana – Rantoul, IL MSA	18	10.40
Charleston, SC MSA	135	26.63
Charleston, WV MSA	23	9.18
Charlotte – Gastonia – Rock Hill, NC – SC MSA	254	21.86
Charlottesville, VA MSA	46	35.09
Chattanooga, TN – GA MSA	79	18.24
Cheyenne, WY MSA	12	16.41
Chicago – Gary – Lake County, IL – IN – WI CMSA	2041	25.30
Chico, CA MSA	23	12.63
Cincinnati – Hamilton, OH – KY – IN CMSA	333	19.09
Clarksville – Hopkinsville, TN – KY MSA	47	27.74
Cleveland – Akron – Lorain, OH CMSA	544	19.71
Colorado Springs, CO MSA	108	27.20
Columbia, MO MSA	13	11.57
Columbia, SC MSA	74	16.32
Columbus, GA – AL MSA	93	38.26
Columbus, OH MSA	272	19.75
Corpus Christi, TX MSA	51	14.58
Cumberland, MD – WV MSA	10	9.84
Dallas – Fort Worth, TX CMSA	944	24.30
Davenport – Rock Island – Moline, IA – IL MSA	112	31.92
Dayton – Springfield, OH MSA	219	23.02
Daytona Beach, FL MSA	88	23.74
Decatur, AL MSA	33	25.08

[Continued]

★ 708 ★

Dental Laboratory and Medical Appliance Technicians

[Continued]

MSA/CMSA	Total Employees	Employees per 100,000 pop.
Decatur, IL MSA	12	10.24
Denver–Boulder, CO CMSA	613	33.17
Des Moines, IA MSA	54	13.74
Detroit–Ann Arbor, MI CMSA	1330	28.51
Dothan, AL MSA	46	35.12
Dubuque, IA MSA	27	31.25
Duluth, MN–WI MSA	52	21.67
Eau Claire, WI MSA	72	52.35
El Paso, TX MSA	84	14.20
Elkhart–Goshen, IN MSA	22	14.08
Enid, OK MSA	35	61.69
Erie, PA MSA	133	48.26
Eugene–Springfield, OR MSA	62	21.91
Evansville, IN–KY MSA	50	17.92
Fargo–Moorhead, ND–MN MSA	95	61.97
Fayetteville, NC MSA	75	27.32
Fayetteville–Springdale, AR MSA	27	23.81
Fitchburg–Leominster, MA MSA	36	35.02
Flint, MI MSA	82	19.05
Florence, AL MSA	22	16.75
Florence, SC MSA	31	27.11
Fort Collins–Loveland, CO MSA	68	36.53
Fort Myers–Cape Coral, FL MSA	114	34.02
Fort Pierce, FL MSA	66	26.29
Fort Smith, AR–OK MSA	84	47.75
Fort Walton Beach, FL MSA	55	38.25
Fort Wayne, IN MSA	119	32.71
Fresno, CA MSA	157	23.52
Gadsden, AL MSA	6	6.01
Gainesville, FL MSA	63	30.87
Glens Falls, NY MSA	27	22.78
Grand Forks, ND MSA	18	25.47
Grand Rapids, MI MSA	95	13.80
Great Falls, MT MSA	5	6.44
Greeley, CO MSA	11	8.34
Green Bay, WI MSA	103	52.93
Greensboro–Winston-Salem–High Point, NC MSA	184	19.53
Greenville–Spartanburg, SC MSA	119	18.57
Hagerstown, MD MSA	6	4.94
Harrisburg–Lebanon–Carlisle, PA MSA	187	31.80
Hartford–New Britain–Middletown, CT CMSA	292	26.89
Hickory–Morganton, NC MSA	45	20.30
Honolulu, HI MSA	220	26.31
Houma–Thibodaux, LA MSA	38	20.78
Houston–Galveston–Brazoria, TX CMSA	690	18.59
Huntington–Ashland, WV–KY–OH MSA	37	11.84

[Continued]

★ 708 ★

Dental Laboratory and Medical Appliance Technicians
[Continued]

MSA/CMSA	Total Employees	Employees per 100,000 pop.
Huntsville, AL MSA	97	40.60
Indianapolis, IN MSA	380	30.40
Iowa City, IA MSA	42	43.70
Jackson, MI MSA	36	24.04
Jackson, MS MSA	137	34.65
Jackson, TN MSA	8	10.26
Jacksonville, FL MSA	212	23.38
Jacksonville, NC MSA	36	24.03
Jamestown – Dunkirk, NY	14	9.87
Johnson City – Kingsport – Bristol, TN – VA MSA	106	24.31
Johnstown, PA MSA	21	8.70
Joplin, MO MSA	25	18.53
Kalamazoo, MI MSA	40	17.90
Kankakee, IL MSA	13	13.51
Kansas City, MO – KS MSA	540	34.48
Killeen – Temple, TX MSA	74	28.99
Knoxville, TN MSA	94	15.54
Kokomo, IN MSA	36	37.13
La Crosse, WI MSA	26	26.56
Lafayette, LA MSA	41	19.64
Lafayette – West Lafayette, IN MSA	33	25.27
Lake Charles, LA MSA	19	11.30
Lakeland – Winter Haven, FL MSA	79	19.49
Lancaster, PA MSA	88	20.81
Lansing – East Lansing, MI MSA	144	33.28
Laredo, TX MSA	8	6.00
Las Cruces, NM MSA	3	2.21
Las Vegas, NV MSA	245	33.04
Lawrence, KS MSA	5	6.11
Lawton, OK MSA	9	8.07
Lewiston – Auburn, ME MSA	12	13.61
Lexington-Fayette, KY MSA	109	31.28
Lima, OH MSA	10	6.48
Lincoln, NE MSA	76	35.57
Little Rock – North Little Rock, AR MSA	126	24.56
Longview – Marshall, TX MSA	18	11.08
Los Angeles – Anaheim – Riverside, CA CMSA	4384	30.17
Louisville, KY – IN MSA	195	20.47
Lubbock, TX MSA	47	21.11
Lynchburg, VA MSA	2	1.41
Macon – Warner Robins, GA MSA	48	17.08
Madison, WI MSA	117	31.87
Manchester, NH MSA	77	52.09
Mansfield, OH MSA	10	7.93
McAllen – Edinburg – Mission, TX MSA	55	14.34
Medford, OR MSA	70	47.82

[Continued]

★ 708 ★

Dental Laboratory and Medical Appliance Technicians
[Continued]

MSA/CMSA	Total Employees	Employees per 100,000 pop.
Melbourne – Titusville – Palm Bay, FL MSA	83	20.80
Memphis, TN – AR – MS MSA	238	24.24
Merced, CA MSA	9	5.04
Miami – Fort Lauderdale, FL CMSA	1118	35.02
Midland, TX MSA	9	8.44
Milwaukee – Racine, WI CMSA	524	32.60
Minneapolis – St. Paul, MN – WI MSA	990	40.18
Mobile, AL MSA	57	11.95
Modesto, CA MSA	97	26.18
Montgomery, AL MSA	81	27.69
Muncie, IN MSA	19	15.88
Muskegon, MI MSA	25	15.72
Naples, FL MSA	45	29.59
Nashville, TN MSA	182	18.48
New Bedford, MA MSA	21	11.96
New Haven – Meriden, CT MSA	139	26.22
New London – Norwich, CT – RI MSA	48	17.99
New Orleans, LA MSA	422	34.06
New York – Northern New Jersey – Long Island, NY – NJ – CT CMSA	5129	28.36
Norfolk – Virginia Beach – Newport News, VA MSA	278	19.91
Ocala, FL MSA	22	11.29
Odessa, TX MSA	10	8.41
Oklahoma City, OK MSA	197	20.55
Olympia, WA MSA	57	35.35
Omaha, NE – IA MSA	139	22.48
Orlando, FL MSA	222	20.69
Owensboro, KY MSA	7	8.03
Panama City, FL MSA	26	20.47
Parkersburg – Marietta, WV – OH MSA	14	9.39
Pascagoula, MS MSA	9	7.81
Pensacola, FL MSA	72	20.91
Peoria, IL MSA	134	39.51
Philadelphia – Wilmington – Trenton, PA – NJ – DE – MD CMSA	1522	25.80
Phoenix, AZ MSA	612	28.84
Pine Bluff, AR MSA	39	45.62
Pittsburgh – Beaver Valley, PA CMSA	352	15.69
Pittsfield, MA MSA	12	15.14
Portland, ME MSA	59	27.41
Portland – Vancouver, OR – WA CMSA	461	31.19
Portsmouth – Dover – Rochester, NH – ME MSA	11	4.92
Poughkeepsie, NY MSA	60	23.12
Providence – Pawtucket – Fall River, RI – MA CMSA	248	21.73
Provo – Orem, UT MSA	23	8.73
Pueblo, CO MSA	46	37.38
Raleigh – Durham, NC MSA	248	33.72
Rapid City, SD MSA	58	71.30

[Continued]

★ 708 ★

Dental Laboratory and Medical Appliance Technicians
[Continued]

MSA/CMSA	Total Employees	Employees per 100,000 pop.
Reading, PA MSA	59	17.53
Redding, CA MSA	24	16.32
Reno, NV MSA	111	43.59
Richmond – Petersburg, VA MSA	112	12.94
Roanoke, VA MSA	19	8.46
Rochester, MN MSA	132	123.98
Rochester, NY MSA	223	22.25
Rockford, IL MSA	78	27.49
Sacramento, CA MSA	452	30.52
Saginaw – Bay City – Midland, MI MSA	99	24.79
St. Cloud, MN MSA	56	29.33
St. Joseph, MO MSA	6	7.22
St. Louis, MO – IL MSA	821	33.59
Salem, OR MSA	36	12.95
Salinas – Seaside – Monterey, CA MSA	70	19.68
Salt Lake City – Ogden, UT MSA	289	26.95
San Angelo, TX MSA	29	29.45
San Antonio, TX MSA	448	34.41
San Diego, CA MSA	721	28.86
San Francisco – Oakland – San Jose, CA CMSA	1977	31.62
Santa Barbara – Santa Maria – Lompoc, CA MSA	134	36.25
Santa Fe, NM MSA	44	37.59
Sarasota, FL MSA	78	28.08
Savannah, GA MSA	50	20.61
Scranton – Wilkes-Barre, PA MSA	133	18.12
Seattle – Tacoma, WA CMSA	837	32.71
Sharon, PA MSA	29	23.97
Sheboygan, WI MSA	37	35.62
Sherman – Denison, TX MSA	27	28.41
Shreveport, LA MSA	212	63.41
Sioux City, IA – NE MSA	25	21.74
Sioux Falls, SD MSA	20	16.15
South Bend – Mishawaka, IN MSA	74	29.95
Spokane, WA MSA	143	39.57
Springfield, IL MSA	60	31.65
Springfield, MO MSA	68	28.26
Springfield, MA MSA	98	18.51
State College, PA MSA	18	14.54
Stockton, CA MSA	72	14.98
Syracuse, NY MSA	100	15.15
Tallahassee, FL MSA	37	15.84
Tampa – St. Petersburg – Clearwater, FL MSA	607	29.35
Terre Haute, IN MSA	55	42.05
Toledo, OH MSA	137	22.31
Topeka, KS MSA	67	41.62
Tucson, AZ MSA	163	24.44

[Continued]

★ 708 ★

Dental Laboratory and Medical Appliance Technicians
[Continued]

MSA/CMSA	Total Employees	Employees per 100,000 pop.
Tulsa, OK MSA	160	22.57
Tuscaloosa, AL MSA	56	37.20
Tyler, TX MSA	14	9.25
Utica–Rome, NY MSA	123	38.85
Victoria, TX MSA	7	9.41
Visalia–Tulare–Porterville, CA MSA	43	13.79
Waco, TX MSA	6	3.17
Washington, DC–MD–VA MSA	941	23.98
Waterbury, CT MSA	39	17.60
Waterloo–Cedar Falls, IA MSA	21	14.32
Wausau, WI MSA	10	8.67
West Palm Beach–Boca Raton–Delray Beach, FL MSA	239	27.68
Wheeling, WV–OH MSA	15	9.42
Wichita, KS MSA	245	50.49
Wichita Falls, TX MSA	15	12.26
Williamsport, PA MSA	11	9.27
Wilmington, NC MSA	34	28.27
Worcester, MA MSA	76	17.40
Yakima, WA MSA	52	27.54
York, PA MSA	85	20.34
Youngstown–Warren, OH MSA	53	10.76
Yuba City, CA MSA	37	30.17
Yuma, AZ MSA	4	3.74

Source: Census of Population and Housing, 1990: Equal Employment Opportunity (EEO) File on CD-ROM [machine-readable datafiles]. Prepared by the Bureau of the Census. Washington, DC: The Bureau, 1992.

★ 709 ★

Employment

Dentists

The table below presents the number of civilians 16 years old or older who reported working as dentists during the 1990 Census. Data are provided by total number employed in each Metropolitan Statistical Area (MSA) or Consolidated Metropolitan Statistical Area (CMSA), as well as the number employed per 100,000 people.

[Total for all of the U.S. was 155,529; 62.53 per 100,000 persons]

MSA/CMSA	Total Employees	Employees per 100,000 pop.
Abilene, TX MSA	51	42.62
Albany, GA MSA	58	51.53
Albany–Schenectady–Troy, NY MSA	505	57.76
Albuquerque, NM MSA	372	77.41
Alexandria, LA MSA	83	63.09
Allentown–Bethlehem–Easton, PA–NJ MSA	433	63.06

[Continued]

★ 709 ★

Dentists
[Continued]

MSA/CMSA	Total Employees	Employees per 100,000 pop.
Altoona, PA MSA	57	43.66
Amarillo, TX MSA	131	69.85
Anchorage, AK MSA	209	92.34
Anderson, IN MSA	69	52.81
Anderson, SC MSA	22	15.15
Anniston, AL MSA	47	40.51
Appleton – Oshkosh – Neenah, WI MSA	231	73.31
Asheville, NC MSA	73	41.76
Athens, GA MSA	88	56.31
Atlanta, GA MSA	1802	63.60
Atlantic City, NJ MSA	168	52.60
Augusta, GA – SC MSA	267	67.29
Austin, TX MSA	460	58.86
Bakersfield, CA MSA	205	37.72
Baltimore, MD MSA	1653	69.39
Bangor, ME MSA	40	45.07
Baton Rouge, LA MSA	369	69.85
Battle Creek, MI MSA	61	44.86
Beaumont – Port Arthur, TX MSA	131	36.27
Bellingham, WA MSA	82	64.17
Benton Harbor, MI MSA	71	44.00
Billings, MT MSA	58	51.14
Biloxi – Gulfport, MS MSA	91	46.16
Binghamton, NY MSA	133	50.28
Birmingham, AL MSA	543	59.81
Bismarck, ND MSA	45	53.68
Bloomington, IN MSA	75	68.82
Bloomington – Normal, IL MSA	65	50.32
Boise City, ID MSA	129	62.69
Boston – Lawrence – Salem, MA – NH CMSA	3470	83.18
Bradenton, FL MSA	85	40.15
Bremerton, WA MSA	159	83.80
Brownsville – Harlingen, TX MSA	53	20.38
Bryan – College Station, TX MSA	59	48.42
Buffalo – Niagara Falls, NY CMSA	790	66.43
Burlington, NC MSA	85	78.55
Burlington, VT MSA	124	94.34
Canton, OH MSA	241	61.15
Casper, WY MSA	56	91.46
Cedar Rapids, IA MSA	107	63.40
Champaign – Urbana – Rantoul, IL MSA	80	46.24
Charleston, SC MSA	303	59.78
Charleston, WV MSA	120	47.91
Charlotte – Gastonia – Rock Hill, NC – SC MSA	445	38.29
Charlottesville, VA MSA	70	53.39
Chattanooga, TN – GA MSA	273	63.02

[Continued]

★ 709 ★

Dentists
[Continued]

MSA/CMSA	Total Employees	Employees per 100,000 pop.
Cheyenne, WY MSA	35	47.85
Chicago – Gary – Lake County, IL – IN – WI CMSA	5923	73.44
Chico, CA MSA	140	76.87
Cincinnati – Hamilton, OH – KY – IN CMSA	1069	61.29
Clarksville – Hopkinsville, TN – KY MSA	103	60.79
Cleveland – Akron – Lorain, OH CMSA	1845	66.85
Colorado Springs, CO MSA	315	79.34
Columbia, MO MSA	72	64.07
Columbia, SC MSA	323	71.25
Columbus, GA – AL MSA	04	34.56
Columbus, OH MSA	1010	73.33
Corpus Christi, TX MSA	180	51.44
Cumberland, MD – WV MSA	70	68.87
Dallas – Fort Worth, TX CMSA	2505	64.47
Danville, VA MSA	21	19.32
Davenport – Rock Island – Moline, IA – IL MSA	185	52.73
Dayton – Springfield, OH MSA	492	51.72
Daytona Beach, FL MSA	193	52.06
Decatur, AL MSA	74	56.25
Decatur, IL MSA	52	44.37
Denver – Boulder, CO CMSA	1504	81.37
Des Moines, IA MSA	197	50.14
Detroit – Ann Arbor, MI CMSA	3430	73.52
Dothan, AL MSA	24	18.33
Dubuque, IA MSA	57	65.97
Duluth, MN – WI MSA	150	62.51
Eau Claire, WI MSA	92	66.89
El Paso, TX MSA	232	39.22
Elkhart – Goshen, IN MSA	56	35.85
Elmira, NY MSA	38	39.92
Enid, OK MSA	37	65.22
Erie, PA MSA	201	72.94
Eugene – Springfield, OR MSA	159	56.20
Evansville, IN – KY MSA	170	60.93
Fargo – Moorhead, ND – MN MSA	90	58.71
Fayetteville, NC MSA	117	42.61
Fayetteville – Springdale, AR MSA	67	59.08
Fitchburg – Leominster, MA MSA	43	41.83
Flint, MI MSA	261	60.63
Florence, AL MSA	47	35.79
Florence, SC MSA	52	45.48
Fort Collins – Loveland, CO MSA	170	91.33
Fort Myers – Cape Coral, FL MSA	173	51.62
Fort Pierce, FL MSA	145	57.75
Fort Smith, AR – OK MSA	121	68.78
Fort Walton Beach, FL MSA	75	52.16

[Continued]

★ 709 ★

Dentists
[Continued]

MSA/CMSA	Total Employees	Employees per 100,000 pop.
Fort Wayne, IN MSA	150	41.23
Fresno, CA MSA	349	52.29
Gadsden, AL MSA	26	26.04
Gainesville, FL MSA	204	99.95
Glens Falls, NY MSA	40	33.74
Grand Forks, ND MSA	55	77.81
Grand Rapids, MI MSA	400	58.11
Great Falls, MT MSA	60	77.23
Greeley, CO MSA	57	43.24
Green Bay, WI MSA	121	62.18
Greensboro – Winston-Salem – High Point, NC MSA	506	53.71
Greenville – Spartanburg, SC MSA	209	32.61
Hagerstown, MD MSA	78	64.25
Harrisburg – Lebanon – Carlisle, PA MSA	316	53.74
Hartford – New Britain – Middletown, CT CMSA	1034	95.23
Hickory – Morganton, NC MSA	34	15.34
Honolulu, HI MSA	769	91.96
Houma – Thibodaux, LA MSA	115	62.90
Houston – Galveston – Brazoria, TX CMSA	2207	59.47
Huntington – Ashland, WV – KY – OH MSA	187	59.83
Huntsville, AL MSA	134	56.09
Indianapolis, IN MSA	811	64.89
Iowa City, IA MSA	149	155.02
Jackson, MI MSA	95	63.44
Jackson, MS MSA	497	125.70
Jackson, TN MSA	53	67.96
Jacksonville, FL MSA	516	56.91
Jacksonville, NC MSA	29	19.35
Jamestown – Dunkirk, NY	69	48.63
Janesville – Beloit, WI MSA	45	32.26
Johnson City – Kingsport – Bristol, TN – VA MSA	259	59.40
Johnstown, PA MSA	65	26.94
Joplin, MO MSA	68	50.40
Kalamazoo, MI MSA	176	78.78
Kankakee, IL MSA	49	50.91
Kansas City, MO – KS MSA	1351	86.26
Killeen – Temple, TX MSA	107	41.91
Knoxville, TN MSA	370	61.18
Kokomo, IN MSA	19	19.60
La Crosse, WI MSA	120	122.57
Lafayette, LA MSA	130	62.28
Lafayette – West Lafayette, IN MSA	48	36.75
Lake Charles, LA MSA	124	73.75
Lakeland – Winter Haven, FL MSA	83	20.47
Lancaster, PA MSA	218	51.56
Lansing – East Lansing, MI MSA	286	66.10

[Continued]

★ 709 ★

Dentists
[Continued]

MSA/CMSA	Total Employees	Employees per 100,000 pop.
Laredo, TX MSA	37	27.77
Las Cruces, NM MSA	27	19.92
Las Vegas, NV MSA	312	42.08
Lawrence, KS MSA	63	77.02
Lawton, OK MSA	68	60.99
Lewiston – Auburn, ME MSA	39	44.25
Lexington-Fayette, KY MSA	237	68.02
Lima, OH MSA	48	31.10
Lincoln, NE MSA	143	66.93
Little Rock – North Little Rock, AR MSA	300	58.47
Longview – Marshall, TX MSA	127	78.19
Los Angeles – Anaheim – Riverside, CA CMSA	10022	68.97
Louisville, KY – IN MSA	650	68.23
Lubbock, TX MSA	118	53.00
Lynchburg, VA MSA	48	33.76
Macon – Warner Robins, GA MSA	194	69.01
Madison, WI MSA	262	71.37
Manchester, NH MSA	94	63.60
Mansfield, OH MSA	79	62.63
McAllen – Edinburg – Mission, TX MSA	102	26.59
Medford, OR MSA	149	101.78
Melbourne – Titusville – Palm Bay, FL MSA	255	63.91
Memphis, TN – AR – MS MSA	690	70.28
Merced, CA MSA	73	40.92
Miami – Fort Lauderdale, FL CMSA	2121	66.44
Midland, TX MSA	68	63.78
Milwaukee – Racine, WI CMSA	1169	72.74
Minneapolis – St. Paul, MN – WI MSA	1955	79.34
Mobile, AL MSA	260	54.52
Modesto, CA MSA	156	42.10
Monroe, LA MSA	93	65.40
Montgomery, AL MSA	130	44.44
Muncie, IN MSA	29	24.24
Muskegon, MI MSA	37	23.27
Naples, FL MSA	41	26.96
Nashville, TN MSA	612	62.13
New Bedford, MA MSA	95	54.09
New Haven – Meriden, CT MSA	402	75.82
New London – Norwich, CT – RI MSA	200	74.96
New Orleans, LA MSA	820	66.19
New York – Northern New Jersey – Long Island, NY – NJ – CT CMSA	17057	94.30
Norfolk – Virginia Beach – Newport News, VA MSA	665	47.63
Ocala, FL MSA	62	31.82
Odessa, TX MSA	27	22.70
Oklahoma City, OK MSA	674	70.29
Olympia, WA MSA	162	100.47

[Continued]

★ 709 ★

Dentists
[Continued]

MSA/CMSA	Total Employees	Employees per 100,000 pop.
Omaha, NE – IA MSA	458	74.08
Orlando, FL MSA	465	43.35
Owensboro, KY MSA	58	66.52
Panama City, FL MSA	53	41.73
Parkersburg – Marietta, WV – OH MSA	80	53.63
Pascagoula, MS MSA	51	44.25
Pensacola, FL MSA	124	36.00
Peoria, IL MSA	174	51.30
Philadelphia – Wilmington – Trenton, PA – NJ – DE – MD CMSA	4094	69.40
Phoenix, AZ MSA	1236	58.24
Pine Bluff, AR MSA	13	15.21
Pittsburgh – Beaver Valley, PA CMSA	1914	85.34
Pittsfield, MA MSA	49	61.83
Portland, ME MSA	206	95.69
Portland – Vancouver, OR – WA CMSA	1136	76.87
Portsmouth – Dover – Rochester, NH – ME MSA	174	77.83
Poughkeepsie, NY MSA	250	96.35
Providence – Pawtucket – Fall River, RI – MA CMSA	723	63.34
Provo – Orem, UT MSA	122	46.28
Pueblo, CO MSA	73	59.33
Raleigh – Durham, NC MSA	479	65.13
Rapid City, SD MSA	96	118.02
Reading, PA MSA	124	36.85
Redding, CA MSA	70	47.61
Reno, NV MSA	200	78.53
Richland – Kennewick – Pasco, WA MSA	47	31.33
Richmond – Petersburg, VA MSA	655	75.67
Roanoke, VA MSA	153	68.16
Rochester, MN MSA	127	119.28
Rochester, NY MSA	806	80.41
Rockford, IL MSA	188	66.26
Sacramento, CA MSA	1165	78.66
Saginaw – Bay City – Midland, MI MSA	214	53.59
St. Cloud, MN MSA	124	64.95
St. Joseph, MO MSA	50	60.18
St. Louis, MO – IL MSA	1453	59.45
Salem, OR MSA	207	74.45
Salinas – Seaside – Monterey, CA MSA	252	70.85
Salt Lake City – Ogden, UT MSA	701	65.38
San Angelo, TX MSA	28	28.44
San Antonio, TX MSA	934	71.73
San Diego, CA MSA	1622	64.93
San Francisco – Oakland – San Jose, CA CMSA	5946	95.09
Santa Barbara – Santa Maria – Lompoc, CA MSA	265	71.70
Santa Fe, NM MSA	100	85.44
Sarasota, FL MSA	225	81.00

[Continued]

★ 709 ★

Dentists
[Continued]

MSA/CMSA	Total Employees	Employees per 100,000 pop.
Savannah, GA MSA	148	61.00
Scranton–Wilkes-Barre, PA MSA	408	55.57
Seattle–Tacoma, WA CMSA	2146	83.86
Sharon, PA MSA	92	76.03
Sheboygan, WI MSA	65	62.57
Sherman–Denison, TX MSA	42	44.20
Shreveport, LA MSA	211	63.11
Sioux City, IA–NE MSA	51	44.34
Sioux Falls, SD MSA	70	56.54
South Bend–Mishawaka, IN MSA	166	67.19
Spokane, WA MSA	184	50.92
Springfield, IL MSA	142	74.91
Springfield, MO MSA	113	46.97
Springfield, MA MSA	346	65.34
State College, PA MSA	54	43.62
Steubenville–Weirton, OH–WV MSA	64	44.91
Stockton, CA MSA	300	62.42
Syracuse, NY MSA	421	63.80
Tallahassee, FL MSA	118	50.51
Tampa–St. Petersburg–Clearwater, FL MSA	1001	48.41
Terre Haute, IN MSA	79	60.39
Texarkana, TX Texarkana, AR MSA	63	52.44
Toledo, OH MSA	340	55.36
Topeka, KS MSA	136	84.48
Tucson, AZ MSA	476	71.38
Tulsa, OK MSA	490	69.12
Tuscaloosa, AL MSA	53	35.21
Tyler, TX MSA	122	80.63
Utica–Rome, NY MSA	168	53.06
Victoria, TX MSA	6	8.07
Visalia–Tulare–Porterville, CA MSA	128	41.04
Waco, TX MSA	93	49.17
Washington, DC–MD–VA MSA	3248	82.78
Waterbury, CT MSA	119	53.69
Waterloo–Cedar Falls, IA MSA	74	50.47
Wausau, WI MSA	70	60.66
West Palm Beach–Boca Raton–Delray Beach, FL MSA	804	93.11
Wheeling, WV–OH MSA	69	43.31
Wichita, KS MSA	153	31.53
Wichita Falls, TX MSA	87	71.09
Williamsport, PA MSA	60	50.54
Wilmington, NC MSA	60	49.88
Worcester, MA MSA	213	48.75
Yakima, WA MSA	148	78.38
York, PA MSA	165	39.49
Youngstown–Warren, OH MSA	306	62.12

[Continued]

★ 709 ★

Dentists

[Continued]

MSA/CMSA	Total Employees	Employees per 100,000 pop.
Yuba City, CA MSA	112	91.32
Yuma, AZ MSA	61	57.07

Source: Census of Population and Housing, 1990: Equal Employment Opportunity (EEO) File on CD-ROM [machine-readable datafiles]. Prepared by the Bureau of the Census. Washington, DC: The Bureau, 1992.

★ 710 ★

Employment

Dietitians

The table below presents the number of civilians 16 years old or older who reported working as dietitians during the 1990 Census. Data are provided by total number employed in each Metropolitan Statistical Area (MSA) or Consolidated Metropolitan Statistical Area (CMSA), as well as the number employed per 100,000 people.

[Total for all of the U.S. was 90,223; 36.28 per 100,000 persons]

MSA/CMSA	Total Employees	Employees per 100,000 pop.
Abilene, TX MSA	30	25.07
Albany, GA MSA	86	76.40
Albany–Schenectady–Troy, NY MSA	406	46.44
Albuquerque, NM MSA	222	46.19
Alexandria, LA MSA	69	52.45
Allentown–Bethlehem–Easton, PA–NJ MSA	183	26.65
Altoona, PA MSA	37	28.34
Amarillo, TX MSA	116	61.85
Anchorage, AK MSA	85	37.55
Anderson, IN MSA	41	31.38
Anderson, SC MSA	71	48.90
Anniston, AL MSA	40	34.47
Appleton–Oshkosh–Neenah, WI MSA	60	19.04
Asheville, NC MSA	39	22.31
Athens, GA MSA	69	44.16
Atlanta, GA MSA	1025	36.17
Atlantic City, NJ MSA	129	40.39
Augusta, GA–SC MSA	194	48.89
Austin, TX MSA	208	26.61
Bakersfield, CA MSA	101	18.58
Baltimore, MD MSA	1024	42.99
Bangor, ME MSA	56	63.10
Baton Rouge, LA MSA	143	27.07
Battle Creek, MI MSA	30	22.06
Beaumont–Port Arthur, TX MSA	119	32.94
Bellingham, WA MSA	42	32.87
Benton Harbor, MI MSA	65	40.28

[Continued]

★ 710 ★

Dietitians
[Continued]

MSA/CMSA	Total Employees	Employees per 100,000 pop.
Billings, MT MSA	16	14.11
Biloxi – Gulfport, MS MSA	106	53.77
Binghamton, NY MSA	105	39.70
Birmingham, AL MSA	374	41.20
Bismarck, ND MSA	81	96.62
Bloomington, IN MSA	50	45.88
Bloomington – Normal, IL MSA	39	30.19
Boise City, ID MSA	79	38.39
Boston – Lawrence – Salem, MA – NH CMSA	2154	51.63
Bradenton, FL MSA	57	26.92
Bremerton, WA MSA	64	33.73
Brownsville – Harlingen, TX MSA	60	23.07
Bryan – College Station, TX MSA	34	27.90
Buffalo – Niagara Falls, NY CMSA	739	62.14
Burlington, NC MSA	52	48.05
Burlington, VT MSA	48	36.52
Canton, OH MSA	107	27.15
Casper, WY MSA	36	58.80
Cedar Rapids, IA MSA	104	61.62
Champaign – Urbana – Rantoul, IL MSA	122	70.51
Charleston, SC MSA	170	33.54
Charleston, WV MSA	118	47.11
Charlotte – Gastonia – Rock Hill, NC – SC MSA	397	34.16
Charlottesville, VA MSA	106	80.85
Chattanooga, TN – GA MSA	120	27.70
Cheyenne, WY MSA	22	30.08
Chicago – Gary – Lake County, IL – IN – WI CMSA	2882	35.70
Chico, CA MSA	65	35.69
Cincinnati – Hamilton, OH – KY – IN CMSA	774	44.38
Clarksville – Hopkinsville, TN – KY MSA	63	37.18
Cleveland – Akron – Lorain, OH CMSA	1157	41.92
Colorado Springs, CO MSA	164	41.31
Columbia, MO MSA	90	80.09
Columbia, SC MSA	302	66.62
Columbus, GA – AL MSA	102	41.96
Columbus, OH MSA	726	52.71
Corpus Christi, TX MSA	111	31.72
Cumberland, MD – WV MSA	35	34.43
Dallas – Fort Worth, TX CMSA	1432	36.86
Danville, VA MSA	28	25.76
Davenport – Rock Island – Moline, IA – IL MSA	160	45.60
Dayton – Springfield, OH MSA	631	66.33
Daytona Beach, FL MSA	128	34.53
Decatur, AL MSA	59	44.85
Decatur, IL MSA	34	29.01
Denver – Boulder, CO CMSA	582	31.49

[Continued]

★ 710 ★

Dietitians
[Continued]

MSA/CMSA	Total Employees	Employees per 100,000 pop.
Des Moines, IA MSA	166	42.25
Detroit – Ann Arbor, MI CMSA	1814	38.88
Dothan, AL MSA	33	25.20
Dubuque, IA MSA	32	37.04
Duluth, MN – WI MSA	139	57.92
Eau Claire, WI MSA	74	53.80
El Paso, TX MSA	120	20.28
Elkhart – Goshen, IN MSA	36	23.05
Elmira, NY MSA	59	61.98
Enid, OK MSA	10	17.63
Erie, PA MSA	73	26.49
Eugene – Springfield, OR MSA	82	28.98
Evansville, IN – KY MSA	84	30.11
Fargo – Moorhead, ND – MN MSA	70	45.66
Fayetteville, NC MSA	99	36.06
Fayetteville – Springdale, AR MSA	26	22.93
Fitchburg – Leominster, MA MSA	46	44.75
Flint, MI MSA	98	22.77
Florence, AL MSA	33	25.13
Florence, SC MSA	37	32.36
Fort Collins – Loveland, CO MSA	82	44.05
Fort Myers – Cape Coral, FL MSA	99	29.54
Fort Pierce, FL MSA	49	19.52
Fort Smith, AR – OK MSA	57	32.40
Fort Walton Beach, FL MSA	38	26.43
Fort Wayne, IN MSA	138	37.93
Fresno, CA MSA	271	40.60
Gadsden, AL MSA	21	21.03
Gainesville, FL MSA	135	66.14
Glens Falls, NY MSA	33	27.84
Grand Forks, ND MSA	32	45.27
Grand Rapids, MI MSA	185	26.87
Great Falls, MT MSA	15	19.31
Greeley, CO MSA	40	30.34
Green Bay, WI MSA	70	35.97
Greensboro – Winston-Salem – High Point, NC MSA	345	36.62
Greenville – Spartanburg, SC MSA	251	39.17
Hagerstown, MD MSA	73	60.14
Harrisburg – Lebanon – Carlisle, PA MSA	162	27.55
Hartford – New Britain – Middletown, CT CMSA	430	39.60
Hickory – Morganton, NC MSA	73	32.93
Honolulu, HI MSA	218	26.07
Houma – Thibodaux, LA MSA	52	28.44
Houston – Galveston – Brazoria, TX CMSA	1181	31.82
Huntington – Ashland, WV – KY – OH MSA	115	36.80
Huntsville, AL MSA	91	38.09

[Continued]

★ 710 ★

Dietitians
[Continued]

MSA/CMSA	Total Employees	Employees per 100,000 pop.
Indianapolis, IN MSA	611	48.89
Iowa City, IA MSA	122	126.93
Jackson, MI MSA	23	15.36
Jackson, MS MSA	166	41.98
Jackson, TN MSA	37	47.45
Jacksonville, FL MSA	261	28.78
Jacksonville, NC MSA	17	11.35
Jamestown – Dunkirk, NY	97	68.36
Janesville – Beloit, WI MSA	36	25.80
Johnson City – Kingsport – Bristol, TN – VA MSA	152	34.86
Johnstown, PA MSA	113	46.84
Joplin, MO MSA	74	54.85
Kalamazoo, MI MSA	77	34.47
Kankakee, IL MSA	28	29.09
Kansas City, MO – KS MSA	649	41.44
Killeen – Temple, TX MSA	109	42.69
Knoxville, TN MSA	191	31.58
Kokomo, IN MSA	80	82.52
La Crosse, WI MSA	69	70.48
Lafayette, LA MSA	78	37.37
Lafayette – West Lafayette, IN MSA	84	64.32
Lake Charles, LA MSA	24	14.27
Lakeland – Winter Haven, FL MSA	116	28.61
Lancaster, PA MSA	56	13.24
Lansing – East Lansing, MI MSA	159	36.75
Laredo, TX MSA	7	5.25
Las Cruces, NM MSA	12	8.86
Las Vegas, NV MSA	203	27.38
Lawrence, KS MSA	19	23.23
Lawton, OK MSA	11	9.87
Lewiston – Auburn, ME MSA	27	30.63
Lexington-Fayette, KY MSA	197	56.54
Lima, OH MSA	66	42.76
Lincoln, NE MSA	71	33.23
Little Rock – North Little Rock, AR MSA	270	52.62
Longview – Marshall, TX MSA	47	28.94
Los Angeles – Anaheim – Riverside, CA CMSA	4208	28.96
Louisville, KY – IN MSA	354	37.16
Lubbock, TX MSA	90	40.42
Lynchburg, VA MSA	25	17.58
Macon – Warner Robins, GA MSA	141	50.16
Madison, WI MSA	240	65.38
Manchester, NH MSA	45	30.44
Mansfield, OH MSA	34	26.95
McAllen – Edinburg – Mission, TX MSA	76	19.82
Medford, OR MSA	38	25.96

[Continued]

★ 710 ★

Dietitians
[Continued]

MSA/CMSA	Total Employees	Employees per 100,000 pop.
Melbourne – Titusville – Palm Bay, FL MSA	72	18.05
Memphis, TN – AR – MS MSA	446	45.43
Merced, CA MSA	36	20.18
Miami – Fort Lauderdale, FL CMSA	1070	33.52
Midland, TX MSA	19	17.82
Milwaukee – Racine, WI CMSA	677	42.12
Minneapolis – St. Paul, MN – WI MSA	942	38.23
Mobile, AL MSA	152	31.87
Modesto, CA MSA	93	25.10
Monroe, LA MSA	79	55.56
Montgomery, AL MSA	81	27.69
Muncie, IN MSA	54	45.13
Muskegon, MI MSA	70	44.03
Naples, FL MSA	35	23.01
Nashville, TN MSA	498	50.56
New Bedford, MA MSA	89	50.67
New Haven – Meriden, CT MSA	260	49.04
New London – Norwich, CT – RI MSA	88	32.98
New Orleans, LA MSA	452	36.49
New York – Northern New Jersey – Long Island, NY – NJ – CT CMSA	7325	40.50
Norfolk – Virginia Beach – Newport News, VA MSA	407	29.15
Ocala, FL MSA	41	21.04
Odessa, TX MSA	24	20.18
Oklahoma City, OK MSA	358	37.34
Olympia, WA MSA	34	21.09
Omaha, NE – IA MSA	258	41.73
Orlando, FL MSA	410	38.22
Owensboro, KY MSA	32	36.70
Panama City, FL MSA	67	52.76
Parkersburg – Marietta, WV – OH MSA	49	32.85
Pascagoula, MS MSA	29	25.16
Pensacola, FL MSA	107	31.07
Peoria, IL MSA	159	46.88
Philadelphia – Wilmington – Trenton, PA – NJ – DE – MD CMSA	2407	40.80
Phoenix, AZ MSA	437	20.59
Pine Bluff, AR MSA	44	51.47
Pittsburgh – Beaver Valley, PA CMSA	884	39.42
Pittsfield, MA MSA	31	39.12
Portland, ME MSA	97	45.06
Portland – Vancouver, OR – WA CMSA	437	29.57
Portsmouth – Dover – Rochester, NH – ME MSA	130	58.15
Poughkeepsie, NY MSA	99	38.16
Providence – Pawtucket – Fall River, RI – MA CMSA	435	38.11
Provo – Orem, UT MSA	75	28.45
Pueblo, CO MSA	39	31.69
Raleigh – Durham, NC MSA	443	60.23

[Continued]

★ 710 ★

Dietitians
[Continued]

MSA/CMSA	Total Employees	Employees per 100,000 pop.
Rapid City, SD MSA	70	86.06
Reading, PA MSA	76	22.58
Redding, CA MSA	17	11.56
Reno, NV MSA	57	22.38
Richland–Kennewick–Pasco, WA MSA	49	32.66
Richmond–Petersburg, VA MSA	450	51.98
Roanoke, VA MSA	84	37.42
Rochester, MN MSA	112	105.19
Rochester, NY MSA	413	41.20
Rockford, IL MSA	92	32.43
Sacramento, CA MSA	483	32.61
Saginaw–Bay City–Midland, MI MSA	190	47.58
St. Cloud, MN MSA	54	28.28
St. Joseph, MO MSA	23	27.68
St. Louis, MO–IL MSA	1142	46.72
Salem, OR MSA	95	34.17
Salinas–Seaside–Monterey, CA MSA	45	12.65
Salt Lake City–Ogden, UT MSA	487	45.42
San Angelo, TX MSA	25	25.39
San Antonio, TX MSA	428	32.87
San Diego, CA MSA	649	25.98
San Francisco–Oakland–San Jose, CA CMSA	2157	34.49
Santa Barbara–Santa Maria–Lompoc, CA MSA	130	35.17
Santa Fe, NM MSA	69	58.95
Sarasota, FL MSA	64	23.04
Savannah, GA MSA	86	35.45
Scranton–Wilkes-Barre, PA MSA	304	41.41
Seattle–Tacoma, WA CMSA	1079	42.16
Sharon, PA MSA	61	50.41
Sheboygan, WI MSA	34	32.73
Sherman–Denison, TX MSA	6	6.31
Shreveport, LA MSA	157	46.96
Sioux City, IA–NE MSA	30	26.08
Sioux Falls, SD MSA	53	42.81
South Bend–Mishawaka, IN MSA	119	48.17
Spokane, WA MSA	161	44.55
Springfield, IL MSA	65	34.29
Springfield, MO MSA	83	34.50
Springfield, MA MSA	149	28.14
State College, PA MSA	44	35.55
Steubenville–Weirton, OH–WV MSA	31	21.75
Stockton, CA MSA	90	18.73
Syracuse, NY MSA	375	56.83
Tallahassee, FL MSA	91	38.96
Tampa–St. Petersburg–Clearwater, FL MSA	688	33.27
Terre Haute, IN MSA	94	71.86

[Continued]

★ 710 ★

Dietitians
[Continued]

MSA/CMSA	Total Employees	Employees per 100,000 pop.
Texarkana, TX – Texarkana, AR MSA	57	47.45
Toledo, OH MSA	235	38.27
Topeka, KS MSA	134	83.24
Tucson, AZ MSA	213	31.94
Tulsa, OK MSA	236	33.29
Tuscaloosa, AL MSA	154	102.31
Tyler, TX MSA	28	18.51
Utica – Rome, NY MSA	177	55.90
Victoria, TX MSA	18	24.21
Visalia – Tulare – Porterville, CA MSA	60	19.24
Waco, TX MSA	87	46.00
Washington, DC – MD – VA MSA	1694	43.17
Waterbury, CT MSA	51	23.01
Waterloo – Cedar Falls, IA MSA	27	18.42
Wausau, WI MSA	71	61.53
West Palm Beach – Boca Raton – Delray Beach, FL MSA	282	32.66
Wheeling, WV – OH MSA	79	49.59
Wichita, KS MSA	182	37.50
Wichita Falls, TX MSA	59	48.21
Williamsport, PA MSA	28	23.59
Wilmington, NC MSA	84	69.83
Worcester, MA MSA	177	40.51
Yakima, WA MSA	62	32.83
York, PA MSA	120	28.72
Youngstown – Warren, OH MSA	281	57.04
Yuba City, CA MSA	41	33.43
Yuma, AZ MSA	7	6.55

Source: Census of Population and Housing, 1990: Equal Employment Opportunity (EEO) File on CD-ROM [machine-readable datafiles]. Prepared by the Bureau of the Census. Washington, DC: The Bureau, 1992.

★ 711 ★

Employment

Health Aides, Except Nursing

The table below presents the number of civilians 16 years old or older who reported working as health aides, except nursing, during the 1990 Census. Data are provided by total number employed in each Metropolitan Statistical Area (MSA) or Consolidated Metropolitan Statistical Area (CMSA), as well as the number employed per 100,000 people.

[Total for all of the U.S. was 222,977; 89.65 per 100,000 persons]

MSA/CMSA	Total Employees	Employees per 100,000 pop.
Abilene, TX MSA	127	106.14
Albany, GA MSA	31	27.54
Albany – Schenectady – Troy, NY MSA	1287	147.20
Albuquerque, NM MSA	417	86.77
Alexandria, LA MSA	65	49.41
Allentown – Bethlehem – Easton, PA – NJ MSA	760	110.68
Altoona, PA MSA	263	201.47
Amarillo, TX MSA	212	113.04
Anchorage, AK MSA	103	45.51
Anderson, IN MSA	129	98.72
Anderson, SC MSA	66	45.46
Anniston, AL MSA	34	29.30
Appleton – Oshkosh – Neenah, WI MSA	315	99.96
Asheville, NC MSA	262	149.87
Athens, GA MSA	124	79.35
Atlanta, GA MSA	1865	65.82
Atlantic City, NJ MSA	351	109.89
Augusta, GA – SC MSA	444	111.89
Austin, TX MSA	590	75.49
Bakersfield, CA MSA	266	48.94
Baltimore, MD MSA	2895	121.53
Bangor, ME MSA	168	189.31
Baton Rouge, LA MSA	363	68.72
Battle Creek, MI MSA	191	140.46
Beaumont – Port Arthur, TX MSA	222	61.46
Bellingham, WA MSA	125	97.82
Benton Harbor, MI MSA	142	87.99
Billings, MT MSA	79	69.65
Biloxi – Gulfport, MS MSA	93	47.18
Binghamton, NY MSA	617	233.27
Birmingham, AL MSA	939	103.44
Bismarck, ND MSA	233	277.94
Bloomington, IN MSA	31	28.45
Bloomington – Normal, IL MSA	167	129.28
Boise City, ID MSA	234	113.72
Boston – Lawrence – Salem, MA – NH CMSA	4644	111.32
Bradenton, FL MSA	152	71.80
Bremerton, WA MSA	124	65.36
Brownsville – Harlingen, TX MSA	147	56.51
Bryan – College Station, TX MSA	101	82.88
Buffalo – Niagara Falls, NY CMSA	2167	182.21
Burlington, NC MSA	98	90.56

[Continued]

★ 711 ★

Health Aides, Except Nursing
[Continued]

MSA/CMSA	Total Employees	Employees per 100,000 pop.
Burlington, VT MSA	114	86.73
Canton, OH MSA	321	81.45
Casper, WY MSA	61	99.63
Cedar Rapids, IA MSA	115	68.14
Champaign – Urbana – Rantoul, IL MSA	98	56.64
Charleston, SC MSA	314	61.95
Charleston, WV MSA	216	86.24
Charlotte – Gastonia – Rock Hill, NC – SC MSA	778	66.95
Charlottesville, VA MSA	160	122.04
Chattanooga, TN – GA MSA	318	73.41
Cheyenne, WY MSA	64	87.50
Chicago – Gary – Lake County, IL – IN – WI CMSA	5571	69.07
Chico, CA MSA	101	55.46
Cincinnati – Hamilton, OH – KY – IN CMSA	1654	94.83
Clarksville – Hopkinsville, TN – KY MSA	83	48.99
Cleveland – Akron – Lorain, OH CMSA	3046	110.37
Colorado Springs, CO MSA	250	62.97
Columbia, MO MSA	210	186.87
Columbia, SC MSA	442	97.50
Columbus, GA – AL MSA	127	52.25
Columbus, OH MSA	1298	94.23
Corpus Christi, TX MSA	284	81.17
Cumberland, MD – WV MSA	140	137.74
Dallas – Fort Worth, TX CMSA	2266	58.32
Danville, VA MSA	59	54.27
Davenport – Rock Island – Moline, IA – IL MSA	454	129.40
Dayton – Springfield, OH MSA	983	103.34
Daytona Beach, FL MSA	348	93.87
Decatur, AL MSA	67	50.93
Decatur, IL MSA	171	145.90
Denver – Boulder, CO CMSA	1365	73.85
Des Moines, IA MSA	325	82.71
Detroit – Ann Arbor, MI CMSA	5335	114.36
Dothan, AL MSA	146	111.48
Dubuque, IA MSA	167	193.28
Duluth, MN – WI MSA	296	123.35
Eau Claire, WI MSA	281	204.30
El Paso, TX MSA	282	47.67
Elkhart – Goshen, IN MSA	82	52.50
Elmira, NY MSA	105	110.30
Enid, OK MSA	116	204.46
Erie, PA MSA	341	123.74
Eugene – Springfield, OR MSA	198	69.99
Evansville, IN – KY MSA	326	116.85
Fargo – Moorhead, ND – MN MSA	270	176.13
Fayetteville, NC MSA	147	53.54

[Continued]

★ 711 ★

Health Aides, Except Nursing
[Continued]

MSA/CMSA	Total Employees	Employees per 100,000 pop.
Fayetteville – Springdale, AR MSA	84	74.07
Fitchburg – Leominster, MA MSA	78	75.88
Flint, MI MSA	545	126.61
Florence, AL MSA	94	71.58
Florence, SC MSA	60	52.47
Fort Collins – Loveland, CO MSA	96	51.58
Fort Myers – Cape Coral, FL MSA	209	62.37
Fort Pierce, FL MSA	108	43.02
Fort Smith, AR – OK MSA	91	51.73
Fort Walton Beach, FL MSA	81	56.34
Fort Wayne, IN MSA	233	64.04
Fresno, CA MSA	597	89.44
Gadsden, AL MSA	93	93.15
Gainesville, FL MSA	353	172.95
Glens Falls, NY MSA	156	131.60
Grand Forks, ND MSA	60	84.89
Grand Rapids, MI MSA	671	97.47
Great Falls, MT MSA	65	83.66
Greeley, CO MSA	63	47.79
Green Bay, WI MSA	234	120.25
Greensboro – Winston-Salem – High Point, NC MSA	819	86.93
Greenville – Spartanburg, SC MSA	263	41.04
Hagerstown, MD MSA	176	144.98
Harrisburg – Lebanon – Carlisle, PA MSA	729	123.98
Hartford – New Britain – Middletown, CT CMSA	1403	129.21
Hickory – Morganton, NC MSA	304	137.12
Honolulu, HI MSA	517	61.83
Houma – Thibodaux, LA MSA	189	103.37
Houston – Galveston – Brazoria, TX CMSA	2977	80.22
Huntington – Ashland, WV – KY – OH MSA	253	80.95
Huntsville, AL MSA	168	70.32
Indianapolis, IN MSA	1151	92.09
Iowa City, IA MSA	237	246.57
Jackson, MI MSA	99	66.11
Jackson, MS MSA	265	67.02
Jackson, TN MSA	60	76.94
Jacksonville, FL MSA	611	67.39
Jacksonville, NC MSA	60	40.04
Jamestown – Dunkirk, NY	284	200.15
Janesville – Beloit, WI MSA	148	106.09
Johnson City – Kingsport – Bristol, TN – VA MSA	496	113.75
Johnstown, PA MSA	397	164.56
Joplin, MO MSA	130	96.36
Kalamazoo, MI MSA	219	98.03
Kankakee, IL MSA	139	144.41
Kansas City, MO – KS MSA	1160	74.06

[Continued]

★ 711 ★

Health Aides, Except Nursing
[Continued]

MSA/CMSA	Total Employees	Employees per 100,000 pop.
Killeen–Temple, TX MSA	220	86.17
Knoxville, TN MSA	535	88.46
Kokomo, IN MSA	69	71.17
La Crosse, WI MSA	171	174.66
Lafayette, LA MSA	128	61.32
Lafayette–West Lafayette, IN MSA	52	39.82
Lake Charles, LA MSA	174	103.49
Lakeland–Winter Haven, FL MSA	323	79.68
Lancaster, PA MSA	390	92.24
Lansing–East Lansing, MI MSA	306	70.72
Laredo, TX MSA	62	46.53
Las Cruces, NM MSA	78	57.56
Las Vegas, NV MSA	370	49.90
Lawrence, KS MSA	85	103.91
Lawton, OK MSA	53	47.54
Lewiston–Auburn, ME MSA	102	115.72
Lexington-Fayette, KY MSA	482	138.34
Lima, OH MSA	155	100.43
Lincoln, NE MSA	231	108.13
Little Rock–North Little Rock, AR MSA	495	96.47
Longview–Marshall, TX MSA	133	81.88
Los Angeles–Anaheim–Riverside, CA CMSA	8840	60.83
Louisville, KY–IN MSA	1190	124.91
Lubbock, TX MSA	272	122.17
Lynchburg, VA MSA	215	151.20
Macon–Warner Robins, GA MSA	304	108.15
Madison, WI MSA	422	114.96
Manchester, NH MSA	117	79.16
Mansfield, OH MSA	87	68.97
McAllen–Edinburg–Mission, TX MSA	132	34.42
Medford, OR MSA	139	94.95
Melbourne–Titusville–Palm Bay, FL MSA	255	63.91
Memphis, TN–AR–MS MSA	922	93.91
Merced, CA MSA	107	59.98
Miami–Fort Lauderdale, FL CMSA	2405	75.33
Midland, TX MSA	124	116.31
Milwaukee–Racine, WI CMSA	2154	134.02
Minneapolis–St. Paul, MN–WI MSA	3289	133.48
Mobile, AL MSA	383	80.31
Modesto, CA MSA	302	81.51
Monroe, LA MSA	143	100.57
Montgomery, AL MSA	213	72.82
Muncie, IN MSA	98	81.90
Muskegon, MI MSA	192	120.77
Naples, FL MSA	123	80.87
Nashville, TN MSA	744	75.53

[Continued]

★ 711 ★

Health Aides, Except Nursing
[Continued]

MSA/CMSA	Total Employees	Employees per 100,000 pop.
New Bedford, MA MSA	252	143.47
New Haven – Meriden, CT MSA	552	104.12
New London – Norwich, CT – RI MSA	250	93.70
New Orleans, LA MSA	1027	82.90
New York – Northern New Jersey – Long Island, NY – NJ – CT CMSA	19875	109.88
Norfolk – Virginia Beach – Newport News, VA MSA	787	56.37
Ocala, FL MSA	123	63.13
Odessa, TX MSA	69	58.02
Oklahoma City, OK MSA	870	90.73
Olympia, WA MSA	120	74.42
Omaha, NE – IA MSA	475	76.83
Orlando, FL MSA	670	62.46
Owensboro, KY MSA	61	69.96
Panama City, FL MSA	137	107.88
Parkersburg – Marietta, WV – OH MSA	117	78.43
Pascagoula, MS MSA	64	55.53
Pensacola, FL MSA	256	74.33
Peoria, IL MSA	418	123.24
Philadelphia – Wilmington – Trenton, PA – NJ – DE – MD CMSA	6436	109.10
Phoenix, AZ MSA	1303	61.40
Pine Bluff, AR MSA	73	85.39
Pittsburgh – Beaver Valley, PA CMSA	2629	117.22
Pittsfield, MA MSA	94	118.61
Portland, ME MSA	191	88.72
Portland – Vancouver, OR – WA CMSA	950	64.28
Portsmouth – Dover – Rochester, NH – ME MSA	260	116.29
Poughkeepsie, NY MSA	966	372.31
Providence – Pawtucket – Fall River, RI – MA CMSA	1586	138.94
Provo – Orem, UT MSA	166	62.98
Pueblo, CO MSA	185	150.34
Raleigh – Durham, NC MSA	580	78.86
Rapid City, SD MSA	76	93.43
Reading, PA MSA	303	90.04
Redding, CA MSA	157	106.78
Reno, NV MSA	185	72.64
Richland – Kennewick – Pasco, WA MSA	50	33.33
Richmond – Petersburg, VA MSA	788	91.03
Roanoke, VA MSA	243	108.25
Rochester, MN MSA	291	273.32
Rochester, NY MSA	1213	121.01
Rockford, IL MSA	314	110.67
Sacramento, CA MSA	1053	71.10
Saginaw – Bay City – Midland, MI MSA	328	82.14
St. Cloud, MN MSA	282	147.71
St. Joseph, MO MSA	105	126.38
St. Louis, MO – IL MSA	3213	131.46

[Continued]

★ 711 ★

Health Aides, Except Nursing

[Continued]

MSA/CMSA	Total Employees	Employees per 100,000 pop.
Salem, OR MSA	209	75.17
Salinas – Seaside – Monterey, CA MSA	210	59.05
Salt Lake City – Ogden, UT MSA	581	54.19
San Angelo, TX MSA	77	78.21
San Antonio, TX MSA	843	64.74
San Diego, CA MSA	1464	58.61
San Francisco – Oakland – San Jose, CA CMSA	3679	58.83
Santa Barbara – Santa Maria – Lompoc, CA MSA	296	80.08
Santa Fe, NM MSA	76	64.93
Sarasota, FL MSA	316	113.76
Savannah, GA MSA	231	95.21
Scranton – Wilkes-Barre, PA MSA	819	111.55
Seattle – Tacoma, WA CMSA	2027	79.21
Sharon, PA MSA	140	115.70
Sheboygan, WI MSA	137	131.89
Sherman – Denison, TX MSA	94	98.93
Shreveport, LA MSA	283	84.64
Sioux City, IA – NE MSA	216	187.80
Sioux Falls, SD MSA	141	113.89
South Bend – Mishawaka, IN MSA	179	72.45
Spokane, WA MSA	357	98.79
Springfield, IL MSA	163	85.99
Springfield, MO MSA	232	96.43
Springfield, MA MSA	673	127.10
State College, PA MSA	112	90.48
Steubenville – Weirton, OH – WV MSA	130	91.21
Stockton, CA MSA	386	80.31
Syracuse, NY MSA	664	100.63
Tallahassee, FL MSA	154	65.93
Tampa – St. Petersburg – Clearwater, FL MSA	1830	88.49
Terre Haute, IN MSA	146	111.61
Texarkana, TX – Texarkana, AR MSA	122	101.55
Toledo, OH MSA	816	132.87
Topeka, KS MSA	314	195.06
Tucson, AZ MSA	474	71.08
Tulsa, OK MSA	615	86.75
Tuscaloosa, AL MSA	148	98.32
Tyler, TX MSA	110	72.70
Utica – Rome, NY MSA	630	198.97
Victoria, TX MSA	59	79.34
Visalia – Tulare – Porterville, CA MSA	127	40.72
Waco, TX MSA	146	77.20
Washington, DC – MD – VA MSA	2582	65.81
Waterbury, CT MSA	327	147.54
Waterloo – Cedar Falls, IA MSA	161	109.81
Wausau, WI MSA	137	118.72

[Continued]

★ 711 ★

Health Aides, Except Nursing
[Continued]

MSA/CMSA	Total Employees	Employees per 100,000 pop.
West Palm Beach – Boca Raton – Delray Beach, FL MSA	629	72.84
Wheeling, WV – OH MSA	235	147.52
Wichita, KS MSA	393	80.99
Wichita Falls, TX MSA	97	79.26
Williamsport, PA MSA	172	144.89
Wilmington, NC MSA	59	49.05
Worcester, MA MSA	579	132.52
Yakima, WA MSA	131	69.38
York, PA MSA	359	85.92
Youngstown – Warren, OH MSA	571	115.91
Yuba City, CA MSA	92	75.01
Yuma, AZ MSA	43	40.23

Source: Census of Population and Housing, 1990; Equal Employment Opportunity (EEO) File on CD-ROM [machine readable datafiles]. Prepared by the Bureau of the Census. Washington, DC: The Bureau, 1992.

★ 712 ★

Employment

Health Diagnosing Practitioners

The table below presents the number of civilians 16 years old or older who reported working as health diagnosing practitioners not included in other tabulations during the 1990 Census; for example, chiropractors. Data are provided by total number employed in each Metropolitan Statistical Area (MSA) or Consolidated Metropolitan Statistical Area (CMSA), as well as the number employed per 100,000 people.

[Total for all of the U.S. was 47,114; 18.94 per 100,000 persons]

MSA/CMSA	Total Employees	Employees per 100,000 pop.
Abilene, TX MSA	10	8.36
Albany, GA MSA	6	5.33
Albany – Schenectady – Troy, NY MSA	79	9.04
Albuquerque, NM MSA	140	29.13
Alexandria, LA MSA	4	3.04
Allentown – Bethlehem – Easton, PA – NJ MSA	152	22.14
Altoona, PA MSA	35	26.81
Amarillo, TX MSA	52	27.73
Anchorage, AK MSA	44	19.44
Anderson, IN MSA	14	10.71
Anderson, SC MSA	23	15.84
Anniston, AL MSA	8	6.89
Appleton – Oshkosh – Neenah, WI MSA	90	28.56
Asheville, NC MSA	24	13.73
Athens, GA MSA	8	5.12
Atlanta, GA MSA	802	28.30
Atlantic City, NJ MSA	70	21.91

[Continued]

★ 712 ★

Health Diagnosing Practitioners
[Continued]

MSA/CMSA	Total Employees	Employees per 100,000 pop.
Augusta, GA – SC MSA	49	12.35
Austin, TX MSA	210	26.87
Bakersfield, CA MSA	119	21.90
Baltimore, MD MSA	181	7.60
Bangor, ME MSA	34	38.31
Baton Rouge, LA MSA	84	15.90
Battle Creek, MI MSA	5	3.68
Beaumont – Port Arthur, TX MSA	61	16.89
Bellingham, WA MSA	68	53.22
Benton Harbor, MI MSA	34	21.07
Billings, MT MSA	6	5.29
Biloxi – Gulfport, MS MSA	21	10.65
Binghamton, NY MSA	14	5.29
Birmingham, AL MSA	31	3.41
Bismarck, ND MSA	24	28.63
Bloomington, IN MSA	41	37.62
Bloomington – Normal, IL MSA	3	2.32
Boise City, ID MSA	31	15.07
Boston – Lawrence – Salem, MA – NH CMSA	756	18.12
Bradenton, FL MSA	38	17.95
Bremerton, WA MSA	51	26.88
Brownsville – Harlingen, TX MSA	14	5.38
Bryan – College Station, TX MSA	22	18.05
Buffalo – Niagara Falls, NY CMSA	196	16.48
Burlington, NC MSA	14	12.94
Burlington, VT MSA	32	24.35
Canton, OH MSA	61	15.48
Casper, WY MSA	21	34.30
Cedar Rapids, IA MSA	31	18.37
Champaign – Urbana – Rantoul, IL MSA	23	13.29
Charleston, SC MSA	97	19.14
Charleston, WV MSA	28	11.18
Charlotte – Gastonia – Rock Hill, NC – SC MSA	172	14.80
Charlottesville, VA MSA	8	6.10
Chattanooga, TN – GA MSA	25	5.77
Chicago – Gary – Lake County, IL – IN – WI CMSA	1095	13.58
Chico, CA MSA	55	30.20
Cincinnati – Hamilton, OH – KY – IN CMSA	237	13.59
Clarksville – Hopkinsville, TN – KY MSA	21	12.39
Cleveland – Akron – Lorain, OH CMSA	178	6.45
Colorado Springs, CO MSA	167	42.06
Columbia, MO MSA	22	19.58
Columbia, SC MSA	26	5.74
Columbus, GA – AL MSA	31	12.75
Columbus, OH MSA	207	15.03
Corpus Christi, TX MSA	17	4.86

[Continued]

★ 712 ★

Health Diagnosing Practitioners
[Continued]

MSA/CMSA	Total Employees	Employees per 100,000 pop.
Cumberland, MD – WV MSA	23	22.63
Dallas – Fort Worth, TX CMSA	454	11.68
Danville, VA MSA	14	12.88
Davenport – Rock Island – Moline, IA – IL MSA	154	43.89
Dayton – Springfield, OH MSA	153	16.08
Daytona Beach, FL MSA	74	19.96
Decatur, AL MSA	26	19.76
Decatur, IL MSA	31	26.45
Denver – Boulder, CO CMSA	562	30.41
Des Moines, IA MSA	81	20.61
Detroit – Ann Arbor, MI CMSA	750	16.08
Dothan, AL MSA	28	21.38
Dubuque, IA MSA	6	6.94
Duluth, MN – WI MSA	81	33.75
Eau Claire, WI MSA	33	23.99
El Paso, TX MSA	34	5.75
Elkhart Goshen, IN MSA	36	23.05
Elmira, NY MSA	6	6.30
Enid, OK MSA	16	28.20
Erie, PA MSA	47	17.06
Eugene – Springfield, OR MSA	70	24.74
Evansville, IN – KY MSA	51	18.28
Fargo – Moorhead, ND – MN MSA	33	21.53
Fayetteville, NC MSA	17	6.19
Fayetteville – Springdale, AR MSA	5	4.41
Fitchburg – Leominster, MA MSA	5	4.86
Flint, MI MSA	84	19.51
Florence, AL MSA	8	6.09
Florence, SC MSA	7	6.12
Fort Collins – Loveland, CO MSA	88	47.28
Fort Myers – Cape Coral, FL MSA	108	32.23
Fort Pierce, FL MSA	76	30.27
Fort Smith, AR – OK MSA	22	12.51
Fort Walton Beach, FL MSA	9	6.26
Fort Wayne, IN MSA	48	13.19
Fresno, CA MSA	206	30.86
Gadsden, AL MSA	8	8.01
Gainesville, FL MSA	22	10.78
Glens Falls, NY MSA	12	10.12
Grand Forks, ND MSA	7	9.90
Grand Rapids, MI MSA	50	7.26
Great Falls, MT MSA	7	9.01
Greeley, CO MSA	47	35.65
Green Bay, WI MSA	43	22.10
Greensboro – Winston-Salem – High Point, NC MSA	107	11.36
Greenville – Spartanburg, SC MSA	127	19.82

[Continued]

★ 712 ★

Health Diagnosing Practitioners
[Continued]

MSA/CMSA	Total Employees	Employees per 100,000 pop.
Hagerstown, MD MSA	17	14.00
Harrisburg – Lebanon – Carlisle, PA MSA	152	25.85
Hartford – New Britain – Middletown, CT CMSA	103	9.49
Hickory – Morganton, NC MSA	28	12.63
Honolulu, HI MSA	162	19.37
Houma – Thibodaux, LA MSA	32	17.50
Houston – Galveston – Brazoria, TX CMSA	608	16.38
Huntington – Ashland, WV – KY – OH MSA	84	26.88
Huntsville, AL MSA	25	10.46
Indianapolis, IN MSA	174	13.92
Iowa City, IA MSA	14	14.57
Jackson, MI MSA	19	12.69
Jackson, MS MSA	54	13.66
Jackson, TN MSA	7	8.98
Jacksonville, FL MSA	110	12.13
Jamestown – Dunkirk, NY	14	9.87
Janesville – Beloit, WI MSA	12	8.60
Johnson City – Kingsport – Bristol, TN – VA MSA	22	5.05
Johnstown, PA MSA	36	14.92
Joplin, MO MSA	26	19.27
Kalamazoo, MI MSA	15	6.71
Kankakee, IL MSA	15	15.58
Kansas City, MO – KS MSA	394	25.16
Killeen – Temple, TX MSA	50	19.58
Knoxville, TN MSA	64	10.58
Kokomo, IN MSA	6	6.19
La Crosse, WI MSA	37	37.79
Lafayette, LA MSA	9	4.31
Lafayette – West Lafayette, IN MSA	46	35.22
Lake Charles, LA MSA	38	22.60
Lakeland – Winter Haven, FL MSA	63	15.54
Lancaster, PA MSA	130	30.75
Lansing – East Lansing, MI MSA	45	10.40
Laredo, TX MSA	7	5.25
Las Cruces, NM MSA	23	16.97
Las Vegas, NV MSA	119	16.05
Lawton, OK MSA	13	11.66
Lewiston – Auburn, ME MSA	21	23.83
Lexington-Fayette, KY MSA	78	22.39
Lima, OH MSA	49	31.75
Lincoln, NE MSA	27	12.64
Little Rock – North Little Rock, AR MSA	132	25.73
Longview – Marshall, TX MSA	26	16.01
Los Angeles – Anaheim – Riverside, CA CMSA	4056	27.91
Louisville, KY – IN MSA	176	18.47
Lubbock, TX MSA	12	5.39

[Continued]

★ 712 ★

Health Diagnosing Practitioners
[Continued]

MSA/CMSA	Total Employees	Employees per 100,000 pop.
Lynchburg, VA MSA	19	13.36
Macon – Warner Robins, GA MSA	21	7.47
Madison, WI MSA	72	19.61
Manchester, NH MSA	15	10.15
Mansfield, OH MSA	5	3.96
McAllen – Edinburg – Mission, TX MSA	16	4.17
Medford, OR MSA	21	14.35
Melbourne – Titusville – Palm Bay, FL MSA	65	16.29
Memphis, TN – AR – MS MSA	50	5.09
Merced, CA MSA	4	2.24
Miami – Fort Lauderdale, FL CMSA	547	17.13
Midland, TX MSA	14	13.13
Milwaukee – Racine, WI CMSA	360	22.40
Minneapolis – St. Paul, MN – WI MSA	784	31.82
Mobile, AL MSA	68	14.26
Modesto, CA MSA	142	38.32
Monroe, LA MSA	34	23.91
Montgomery, AL MSA	50	17.09
Muncie, IN MSA	8	6.69
Muskegon, MI MSA	14	8.81
Naples, FL MSA	16	10.52
Nashville, TN MSA	173	17.56
New Bedford, MA MSA	28	15.94
New Haven – Meriden, CT MSA	104	19.62
New London – Norwich, CT – RI MSA	36	13.49
New Orleans, LA MSA	151	12.19
New York – Northern New Jersey – Long Island, NY – NJ – CT CMSA	4477	24.75
Norfolk – Virginia Beach – Newport News, VA MSA	93	6.66
Ocala, FL MSA	42	21.56
Odessa, TX MSA	25	21.02
Oklahoma City, OK MSA	118	12.31
Olympia, WA MSA	49	30.39
Omaha, NE – IA MSA	53	8.57
Orlando, FL MSA	225	20.97
Owensboro, KY MSA	12	13.76
Panama City, FL MSA	25	19.69
Parkersburg – Marietta, WV – OH MSA	11	7.37
Pascagoula, MS MSA	18	15.62
Pensacola, FL MSA	63	18.29
Peoria, IL MSA	56	16.51
Philadelphia – Wilmington – Trenton, PA – NJ – DE – MD CMSA	1060	17.97
Phoenix, AZ MSA	585	27.57
Pine Bluff, AR MSA	13	15.21
Pittsburgh – Beaver Valley, PA CMSA	528	23.54
Pittsfield, MA MSA	35	44.16
Portland, ME MSA	25	11.61

[Continued]

★ 712 ★

Health Diagnosing Practitioners
[Continued]

MSA/CMSA	Total Employees	Employees per 100,000 pop.
Portland – Vancouver, OR – WA CMSA	515	34.85
Portsmouth – Dover – Rochester, NH – ME MSA	36	16.10
Poughkeepsie, NY MSA	84	32.37
Providence – Pawtucket – Fall River, RI – MA CMSA	76	6.66
Provo – Orem, UT MSA	49	18.59
Pueblo, CO MSA	29	23.57
Raleigh – Durham, NC MSA	138	18.76
Rapid City, SD MSA	19	23.36
Reading, PA MSA	76	22.58
Redding, CA MSA	68	46.25
Reno, NV MSA	110	43.19
Richland – Kennewick – Pasco, WA MSA	45	29.99
Richmond – Petersburg, VA MSA	39	4.51
Roanoke, VA MSA	15	6.68
Rochester, MN MSA	23	21.60
Rochester, NY MSA	91	9.08
Rockford, IL MSA	44	15.51
Sacramento, CA MSA	440	29.71
Saginaw – Bay City – Midland, MI MSA	32	8.01
St. Cloud, MN MSA	81	42.43
St. Joseph, MO MSA	14	16.85
St. Louis, MO – IL MSA	474	19.39
Salem, OR MSA	85	30.57
Salinas – Seaside – Monterey, CA MSA	88	24.74
Salt Lake City – Ogden, UT MSA	190	17.72
San Angelo, TX MSA	7	7.11
San Antonio, TX MSA	208	15.97
San Diego, CA MSA	854	34.19
San Francisco – Oakland – San Jose, CA CMSA	2692	43.05
Santa Barbara – Santa Maria – Lompoc, CA MSA	240	64.93
Santa Fe, NM MSA	92	78.60
Sarasota, FL MSA	66	23.76
Savannah, GA MSA	13	5.36
Scranton – Wilkes-Barre, PA MSA	128	17.43
Seattle – Tacoma, WA CMSA	576	22.51
Sharon, PA MSA	23	19.01
Sheboygan, WI MSA	21	20.22
Sherman – Denison, TX MSA	15	15.79
Shreveport, LA MSA	43	12.86
Sioux City, IA – NE MSA	28	24.34
Sioux Falls, SD MSA	22	17.77
South Bend – Mishawaka, IN MSA	8	3.24
Spokane, WA MSA	139	38.47
Springfield, IL MSA	21	11.08
Springfield, MO MSA	47	19.54
Springfield, MA MSA	148	27.95

[Continued]

★ 712 ★

Health Diagnosing Practitioners

[Continued]

MSA/CMSA	Total Employees	Employees per 100,000 pop.
State College, PA MSA	49	39.58
Steubenville – Weirton, OH – WV MSA	4	2.81
Stockton, CA MSA	137	28.50
Syracuse, NY MSA	55	8.34
Tallahassee, FL MSA	42	17.98
Tampa – St. Petersburg – Clearwater, FL MSA	562	27.18
Terre Haute, IN MSA	12	9.17
Texarkana, TX – Texarkana, AR MSA	37	30.80
Toledo, OH MSA	102	16.61
Topeka, KS MSA	35	21.74
Tucson, AZ MSA	210	31.49
Tulsa, OK MSA	221	31.17
Tuscaloosa, AL MSA	24	15.94
Tyler, TX MSA	17	11.24
Utica – Rome, NY MSA	13	4.11
Victoria, TX MSA	11	14.79
Visalia – Tulare – Porterville, CA MSA	70	22.44
Waco, TX MSA	2	1.06
Washington, DC – MD – VA MSA	326	8.31
Waterbury, CT MSA	33	14.89
Waterloo – Cedar Falls, IA MSA	44	30.01
Wausau, WI MSA	10	8.67
West Palm Beach – Boca Raton – Delray Beach, FL MSA	238	27.56
Wheeling, WV – OH MSA	16	10.04
Wichita, KS MSA	109	22.46
Wichita Falls, TX MSA	6	4.90
Williamsport, PA MSA	30	25.27
Wilmington, NC MSA	11	9.15
Worcester, MA MSA	37	8.47
Yakima, WA MSA	22	11.65
York, PA MSA	53	12.68
Youngstown – Warren, OH MSA	56	11.37
Yuba City, CA MSA	45	36.69
Yuma, AZ MSA	28	26.19

Source: *Census of Population and Housing, 1990: Equal Employment Opportunity (EEO) File on CD-ROM* [machine-readable datafiles]. Prepared by the Bureau of the Census. Washington, DC: The Bureau, 1992.

★ 713 ★

Employment

Health Insurance Industry Employment: 1987-1994

Data covers employees on payroll only and does not include agents not directly employed by insurers.

[In billions of dollars, except as noted]

Year	Employment
1987	202.1
1988	216.5
1989	228.1
1990	241.6
1991	258.7
1992	268.3
1993[1]	270.3
1994[2]	273.0
Percent change	
1988-1989	5.4
1989-1990	5.9
1990-1991	7.1
1991-1992	3.7
1992-1993	0.7
1993-1994	1.0

Source: U.S. Department of Commerce. *U.S. Industrial Outlook, 1994: Forecasts for Selected Manufacturing and Service Industries.* Lanham, MD: Bernan Press, 1994, p. 48-1. Estimates and forecasts by the U.S. Department of Commerce, International Trade Administration. Primary sources: American Council of Life Insurance; U.S. Department of Labor, Bureau of Labor Statistics. *Notes:* 1. Estimate. 2. Forecast.

★ 714 ★

Employment

Health Record Technologists and Technicians

The table below presents the number of civilians 16 years old or older who reported working as health record technologists and technicians during the 1990 Census. Data are provided by total number employed in each Metropolitan Statistical Area (MSA) or Consolidated Metropolitan Statistical Area (CMSA), as well as the number employed per 100,000 people.

[Total for all of the U.S. was 55,764; 22.42 per 100,000 persons]

MSA/CMSA	Total Employees	Employees per 100,000 pop.
Abilene, TX MSA	32	26.74
Albany, GA MSA	25	22.21
Albany–Schenectady–Troy, NY MSA	180	20.59
Albuquerque, NM MSA	192	39.95
Alexandria, LA MSA	79	60.05

[Continued]

★ 714 ★

Health Record Technologists and Technicians
[Continued]

MSA/CMSA	Total Employees	Employees per 100,000 pop.
Allentown – Bethlehem – Easton, PA – NJ MSA	85	12.38
Altoona, PA MSA	23	17.62
Amarillo, TX MSA	94	50.12
Anchorage, AK MSA	43	19.00
Anderson, IN MSA	30	22.96
Anderson, SC MSA	63	43.39
Anniston, AL MSA	12	10.34
Appleton – Oshkosh – Neenah, WI MSA	41	13.01
Asheville, NC MSA	56	32.03
Athens, GA MSA	28	17.92
Atlanta, GA MSA	624	22.02
Atlantic City, NJ MSA	32	10.02
Augusta, GA – SC MSA	106	26.71
Austin, TX MSA	214	27.38
Bakersfield, CA MSA	78	14.35
Baltimore, MD MSA	561	23.55
Bangor, ME MSA	15	16.90
Baton Rouge, LA MSA	165	31.23
Battle Creek, MI MSA	8	5.88
Beaumont – Port Arthur, TX MSA	36	9.97
Bellingham, WA MSA	26	20.35
Benton Harbor, MI MSA	27	16.73
Billings, MT MSA	33	29.10
Biloxi – Gulfport, MS MSA	85	43.12
Binghamton, NY MSA	81	30.62
Birmingham, AL MSA	358	39.44
Bismarck, ND MSA	34	40.56
Bloomington – Normal, IL MSA	28	21.68
Boise City, ID MSA	53	25.76
Boston – Lawrence – Salem, MA – NH CMSA	951	22.80
Bradenton, FL MSA	8	3.78
Bremerton, WA MSA	68	35.84
Brownsville – Harlingen, TX MSA	92	35.37
Bryan – College Station, TX MSA	33	27.08
Buffalo – Niagara Falls, NY CMSA	305	25.65
Burlington, NC MSA	7	6.47
Burlington, VT MSA	19	14.46
Canton, OH MSA	110	27.91
Casper, WY MSA	21	34.30
Cedar Rapids, IA MSA	13	7.70
Champaign – Urbana – Rantoul, IL MSA	17	9.83
Charleston, SC MSA	75	14.80
Charleston, WV MSA	21	8.38
Charlotte – Gastonia – Rock Hill, NC – SC MSA	181	15.58
Charlottesville, VA MSA	20	15.25
Chattanooga, TN – GA MSA	151	34.86

[Continued]

★714★

Health Record Technologists and Technicians
[Continued]

MSA/CMSA	Total Employees	Employees per 100,000 pop.
Cheyenne, WY MSA	26	35.55
Chicago – Gary – Lake County, IL – IN – WI CMSA	1934	23.98
Chico, CA MSA	33	18.12
Cincinnati – Hamilton, OH – KY – IN CMSA	433	24.83
Clarksville – Hopkinsville, TN – KY MSA	53	31.28
Cleveland – Akron – Lorain, OH CMSA	543	19.68
Colorado Springs, CO MSA	122	30.73
Columbia, MO MSA	39	34.70
Columbia, SC MSA	112	24.71
Columbus, GA – AL MSA	69	28.39
Columbus, OH MSA	284	20.62
Corpus Christi, TX MSA	76	21.72
Cumberland, MD – WV MSA	25	24.60
Dallas – Fort Worth, TX CMSA	794	20.44
Danville, VA MSA	17	15.64
Davenport – Rock Island – Moline, IA – IL MSA	43	12.26
Dayton – Springfield, OH MSA	273	28.70
Daytona Beach, FL MSA	132	35.61
Decatur, AL MSA	23	17.48
Decatur, IL MSA	6	5.12
Denver – Boulder, CO CMSA	435	23.53
Des Moines, IA MSA	82	20.87
Detroit – Ann Arbor, MI CMSA	1264	27.09
Dothan, AL MSA	15	11.45
Dubuque, IA MSA	17	19.68
Duluth, MN – WI MSA	124	51.67
Eau Claire, WI MSA	49	35.63
El Paso, TX MSA	111	18.76
Elkhart – Goshen, IN MSA	15	9.60
Elmira, NY MSA	51	53.57
Enid, OK MSA	8	14.10
Erie, PA MSA	56	20.32
Eugene – Springfield, OR MSA	99	34.99
Evansville, IN – KY MSA	43	15.41
Fargo – Moorhead, ND – MN MSA	92	60.01
Fayetteville, NC MSA	30	10.93
Fayetteville – Springdale, AR MSA	36	31.74
Fitchburg – Leominster, MA MSA	14	13.62
Flint, MI MSA	93	21.60
Florence, AL MSA	31	23.61
Florence, SC MSA	40	34.98
Fort Collins – Loveland, CO MSA	52	27.94
Fort Myers – Cape Coral, FL MSA	69	20.59
Fort Pierce, FL MSA	24	9.56
Fort Smith, AR – OK MSA	32	18.19
Fort Walton Beach, FL MSA	6	4.17

[Continued]

★714★

Health Record Technologists and Technicians

[Continued]

MSA/CMSA	Total Employees	Employees per 100,000 pop.
Fort Wayne, IN MSA	48	13.19
Fresno, CA MSA	109	16.33
Gadsden, AL MSA	50	50.08
Gainesville, FL MSA	53	25.97
Glens Falls, NY MSA	10	8.44
Grand Forks, ND MSA	18	25.47
Grand Rapids, MI MSA	146	21.21
Great Falls, MT MSA	40	51.49
Greeley, CO MSA	34	25.79
Green Bay, WI MSA	46	23.64
Greensboro – Winston-Salem – High Point, NC MSA	257	27.28
Greenville – Spartanburg, SC MSA	94	14.67
Hagerstown, MD MSA	6	4.94
Harrisburg – Lebanon – Carlisle, PA MSA	125	21.26
Hartford – New Britain – Middletown, CT CMSA	178	16.39
Hickory – Morganton, NC MSA	51	23.00
Honolulu, HI MSA	145	17.34
Houma – Thibodaux, LA MSA	8	4.38
Houston – Galveston – Brazoria, TX CMSA	784	21.13
Huntington – Ashland, WV – KY – OH MSA	89	28.48
Huntsville, AL MSA	13	5.44
Indianapolis, IN MSA	284	22.72
Iowa City, IA MSA	66	68.66
Jackson, MI MSA	31	20.70
Jackson, MS MSA	225	56.90
Jackson, TN MSA	45	57.71
Jacksonville, FL MSA	262	28.90
Jacksonville, NC MSA	32	21.36
Jamestown – Dunkirk, NY	16	11.28
Janesville – Beloit, WI MSA	50	35.84
Johnson City – Kingsport – Bristol, TN – VA MSA	75	17.20
Johnstown, PA MSA	12	4.97
Joplin, MO MSA	26	19.27
Kalamazoo, MI MSA	46	20.59
Kankakee, IL MSA	13	13.51
Kansas City, MO – KS MSA	472	30.14
Killeen – Temple, TX MSA	109	42.69
Knoxville, TN MSA	109	18.02
Kokomo, IN MSA	22	22.69
La Crosse, WI MSA	67	68.43
Lafayette, LA MSA	35	16.77
Lafayette – West Lafayette, IN MSA	34	26.03
Lake Charles, LA MSA	25	14.87
Lakeland – Winter Haven, FL MSA	57	14.06
Lancaster, PA MSA	60	14.19
Lansing – East Lansing, MI MSA	79	18.26

[Continued]

★714★

Health Record Technologists and Technicians
[Continued]

MSA/CMSA	Total Employees	Employees per 100,000 pop.
Laredo, TX MSA	5	3.75
Las Cruces, NM MSA	7	5.17
Las Vegas, NV MSA	140	18.88
Lawrence, KS MSA	35	42.79
Lawton, OK MSA	27	24.22
Lewiston–Auburn, ME MSA	42	47.65
Lexington-Fayette, KY MSA	86	24.68
Lima, OH MSA	29	18.79
Lincoln, NE MSA	19	8.89
Little Rock–North Little Rock, AR MSA	143	27.87
Longview–Marshall, TX MSA	12	7.39
Los Angeles–Anaheim–Riverside, CA CMSA	3157	21.73
Louisville, KY–IN MSA	335	35.16
Lubbock, TX MSA	89	39.98
Lynchburg, VA MSA	24	16.88
Macon–Warner Robins, GA MSA	69	24.55
Madison, WI MSA	186	50.67
Manchester, NH MSA	24	16.24
Mansfield, OH MSA	7	5.55
McAllen–Edinburg–Mission, TX MSA	72	18.77
Medford, OR MSA	23	15.71
Melbourne–Titusville–Palm Bay, FL MSA	59	14.79
Memphis, TN–AR–MS MSA	173	17.62
Merced, CA MSA	39	21.86
Miami–Fort Lauderdale, FL CMSA	719	22.52
Midland, TX MSA	28	26.26
Milwaukee–Racine, WI CMSA	537	33.41
Minneapolis–St. Paul, MN–WI MSA	859	34.86
Mobile, AL MSA	94	19.71
Modesto, CA MSA	100	26.99
Monroe, LA MSA	36	25.32
Montgomery, AL MSA	82	28.03
Muncie, IN MSA	9	7.52
Muskegon, MI MSA	19	11.95
Naples, FL MSA	22	14.46
Nashville, TN MSA	229	23.25
New Bedford, MA MSA	17	9.68
New Haven–Meriden, CT MSA	58	10.94
New London–Norwich, CT–RI MSA	53	19.86
New Orleans, LA MSA	245	19.78
New York–Northern New Jersey–Long Island, NY–NJ–CT CMSA	3141	17.37
Norfolk–Virginia Beach–Newport News, VA MSA	328	23.49
Ocala, FL MSA	40	20.53
Odessa, TX MSA	21	17.66
Oklahoma City, OK MSA	287	29.93
Olympia, WA MSA	51	31.63

[Continued]

★ 714 ★

Health Record Technologists and Technicians
[Continued]

MSA/CMSA	Total Employees	Employees per 100,000 pop.
Omaha, NE – IA MSA	136	22.00
Orlando, FL MSA	233	21.72
Owensboro, KY MSA	11	12.62
Panama City, FL MSA	34	26.77
Parkersburg – Marietta, WV – OH MSA	46	30.84
Pascagoula, MS MSA	67	58.14
Pensacola, FL MSA	87	25.26
Peoria, IL MSA	43	12.68
Philadelphia – Wilmington – Trenton, PA – NJ – DE – MD CMSA	1400	23.73
Phoenlx, AZ MSA	525	24.74
Pine Bluff, AR MSA	14	16.38
Pittsburgh – Beaver Valley, PA CMSA	517	23.05
Pittsfield, MA MSA	5	6.31
Portland, ME MSA	5	2.32
Portland – Vancouver, OR – WA CMSA	381	25.78
Portsmouth – Dover – Rochester, NH – ME MSA	34	15.21
Poughkeepsie, NY MSA	36	13.87
Providence – Pawtucket – Fall River, RI – MA CMSA	250	21.90
Provo – Orem, UT MSA	36	13.66
Pueblo, CO MSA	29	23.57
Raleigh – Durham, NC MSA	301	40.93
Rapid City, SD MSA	45	55.32
Reading, PA MSA	66	19.61
Redding, CA MSA	9	6.12
Reno, NV MSA	54	21.20
Richland – Kennewick – Pasco, WA MSA	4	2.67
Richmond – Petersburg, VA MSA	200	23.10
Roanoke, VA MSA	58	25.84
Rochester, MN MSA	98	92.04
Rochester, NY MSA	184	18.36
Rockford, IL MSA	44	15.51
Sacramento, CA MSA	243	16.41
Saginaw – Bay City – Midland, MI MSA	60	15.03
St. Cloud, MN MSA	96	50.28
St. Joseph, MO MSA	25	30.09
St. Louis, MO – IL MSA	777	31.79
Salem, OR MSA	104	37.41
Salinas – Seaside – Monterey, CA MSA	105	29.52
Salt Lake City – Ogden, UT MSA	225	20.98
San Angelo, TX MSA	57	57.89
San Antonio, TX MSA	364	27.95
San Diego, CA MSA	711	28.46
San Francisco – Oakland – San Jose, CA CMSA	1365	21.83
Santa Barbara – Santa Maria – Lompoc, CA MSA	84	22.73
Santa Fe, NM MSA	49	41.86
Sarasota, FL MSA	48	17.28

[Continued]

★714★

Health Record Technologists and Technicians

[Continued]

MSA/CMSA	Total Employees	Employees per 100,000 pop.
Savannah, GA MSA	73	30.09
Scranton–Wilkes-Barre, PA MSA	179	24.38
Seattle–Tacoma, WA CMSA	798	31.18
Sharon, PA MSA	15	12.40
Sheboygan, WI MSA	21	20.22
Sherman–Denison, TX MSA	20	21.05
Shreveport, LA MSA	104	31.11
Sioux City, IA–NE MSA	14	12.17
Sioux Falls, SD MSA	61	49.27
South Bend–Mishawaka, IN MSA	35	14.17
Spokane, WA MSA	84	23.25
Springfield, IL MSA	87	45.90
Springfield, MO MSA	66	27.43
Springfield, MA MSA	124	23.42
State College, PA MSA	12	9.69
Steubenville–Weirton, OH–WV MSA	10	7.02
Stockton, CA MSA	88	18.31
Syracuse, NY MSA	140	21.22
Tallahassee, FL MSA	30	12.84
Tampa–St. Petersburg–Clearwater, FL MSA	639	30.90
Terre Haute, IN MSA	56	42.81
Texarkana, TX–Texarkana, AR MSA	42	34.96
Toledo, OH MSA	187	30.45
Topeka, KS MSA	48	29.82
Tucson, AZ MSA	418	62.68
Tulsa, OK MSA	124	17.49
Tuscaloosa, AL MSA	10	6.64
Tyler, TX MSA	27	17.84
Utica–Rome, NY MSA	130	41.06
Victoria, TX MSA	30	40.34
Visalia–Tulare–Porterville, CA MSA	44	14.11
Waco, TX MSA	103	54.46
Washington, DC–MD–VA MSA	963	24.54
Waterbury, CT MSA	76	34.29
Waterloo–Cedar Falls, IA MSA	43	29.33
Wausau, WI MSA	31	26.86
West Palm Beach–Boca Raton–Delray Beach, FL MSA	173	20.03
Wheeling, WV–OH MSA	44	27.62
Wichita, KS MSA	155	31.94
Wichita Falls, TX MSA	19	15.53
Williamsport, PA MSA	4	3.37
Wilmington, NC MSA	34	28.27
Worcester, MA MSA	124	28.38
Yakima, WA MSA	88	46.60
York, PA MSA	74	17.71
Youngstown–Warren, OH MSA	127	25.78

[Continued]

★ 714 ★

Health Record Technologists and Technicians
[Continued]

MSA/CMSA	Total Employees	Employees per 100,000 pop.
Yuba City, CA MSA	33	26.91
Yuma, AZ MSA	23	21.52

Source: Census of Population and Housing, 1990: Equal Employment Opportunity (EEO) File on CD-ROM [machine-readable datafiles]. Prepared by the Bureau of the Census. Washington, DC: The Bureau, 1992.

★ 715 ★

Employment

Health Specialties Teachers

The table below presents the number of civilians 16 years old or older who reported working as health specialties teachers during the 1990 Census. Data are provided by total number employed in each Metropolitan Statistical Area (MSA) or Consolidated Metropolitan Statistical Area (CMSA), as well as the number employed per 100,000 people.

[Total for all of the U.S. was 15,711; 6.32 per 100,000 persons]

MSA/CMSA	Total Employees	Employees per 100,000 pop.
Albany, GA MSA	15	13.33
Albany–Schenectady–Troy, NY MSA	71	8.12
Albuquerque, NM MSA	36	7.49
Allentown–Bethlehem–Easton, PA–NJ MSA	10	1.46
Amarillo, TX MSA	24	12.80
Anchorage, AK MSA	22	9.72
Anderson, SC MSA	7	4.82
Anniston, AL MSA	21	18.10
Appleton–Oshkosh–Neenah, WI MSA	39	12.38
Asheville, NC MSA	10	5.72
Athens, GA MSA	84	53.75
Atlanta, GA MSA	70	2.47
Atlantic City, NJ MSA	20	6.26
Augusta, GA–SC MSA	72	18.14
Austin, TX MSA	85	10.88
Bakersfield, CA MSA	6	1.10
Baltimore, MD MSA	175	7.35
Bangor, ME MSA	34	38.31
Baton Rouge, LA MSA	22	4.16
Battle Creek, MI MSA	16	11.77
Beaumont–Port Arthur, TX MSA	64	17.72
Benton Harbor, MI MSA	14	8.68
Biloxi–Gulfport, MS MSA	32	16.23
Binghamton, NY MSA	51	19.28
Birmingham, AL MSA	119	13.11
Bismarck, ND MSA	17	20.28
Bloomington, IN MSA	17	15.60

[Continued]

★ 715 ★

Health Specialties Teachers
[Continued]

MSA/CMSA	Total Employees	Employees per 100,000 pop.
Boise City, ID MSA	14	6.80
Boston–Lawrence–Salem, MA–NH CMSA	274	6.57
Bryan–College Station, TX MSA	62	50.88
Buffalo–Niagara Falls, NY CMSA	98	8.24
Burlington, VT MSA	38	28.91
Casper, WY MSA	15	24.50
Cedar Rapids, IA MSA	13	7.70
Champaign–Urbana–Rantoul, IL MSA	13	7.51
Charleston, SC MSA	63	12.43
Charleston, WV MSA	9	3.59
Charlotte–Gastonia–Rock Hill, NC–SC MSA	89	7.66
Charlottesville, VA MSA	22	16.78
Chattanooga, TN–GA MSA	36	8.31
Chicago–Gary–Lake County, IL–IN–WI CMSA	491	6.09
Chico, CA MSA	30	16.47
Cincinnati–Hamilton, OH–KY–IN CMSA	63	3.61
Clarksville–Hopkinsville, TN–KY MSA	8	4.72
Cleveland–Akron–Lorain, OH CMSA	129	4.67
Colorado Springs, CO MSA	15	3.78
Columbia, MO MSA	28	24.92
Columbia, SC MSA	67	14.78
Columbus, GA–AL MSA	23	9.46
Columbus, OH MSA	164	11.91
Corpus Christi, TX MSA	27	7.72
Cumberland, MD–WV MSA	13	12.79
Dallas–Fort Worth, TX CMSA	195	5.02
Davenport–Rock Island–Moline, IA–IL MSA	61	17.39
Dayton–Springfield, OH MSA	70	7.36
Daytona Beach, FL MSA	6	1.62
Decatur, IL MSA	2	1.71
Denver–Boulder, CO CMSA	124	6.71
Des Moines, IA MSA	25	6.36
Detroit–Ann Arbor, MI CMSA	212	4.54
Dothan, AL MSA	22	16.80
Dubuque, IA MSA	4	4.63
Duluth, MN–WI MSA	33	13.75
Eau Claire, WI MSA	40	29.08
El Paso, TX MSA	24	4.06
Elkhart–Goshen, IN MSA	15	9.60
Elmira, NY MSA	19	19.96
Enid, OK MSA	15	26.44
Erie, PA MSA	28	10.16
Eugene–Springfield, OR MSA	32	11.31
Evansville, IN–KY MSA	30	10.75
Fargo–Moorhead, ND–MN MSA	14	9.13
Fayetteville, NC MSA	15	5.46

[Continued]

★ 715 ★

Health Specialties Teachers

[Continued]

MSA/CMSA	Total Employees	Employees per 100,000 pop.
Fayetteville – Springdale, AR MSA	15	13.23
Fitchburg – Leominster, MA MSA	5	4.86
Flint, MI MSA	23	5.34
Florence, AL MSA	19	14.47
Florence, SC MSA	23	20.11
Fort Collins – Loveland, CO MSA	23	12.36
Fort Smith, AR – OK MSA	14	7.96
Fort Wayne, IN MSA	14	3.85
Fresno, CA MSA	32	4.79
Gadsden, AL MSA	6	6.01
Gainesville, FL MSA	88	43.11
Grand Forks, ND MSA	29	41.03
Grand Rapids, MI MSA	20	2.91
Great Falls, MT MSA	7	9.01
Greeley, CO MSA	3	2.28
Green Bay, WI MSA	4	2.06
Greensboro – Winston-Salem – High Point, NC MSA	83	8.81
Greenville – Spartanburg, SC MSA	60	9.36
Harrisburg – Lebanon – Carlisle, PA MSA	25	4.25
Hartford – New Britain – Middletown, CT CMSA	62	5.71
Hickory – Morganton, NC MSA	8	3.61
Honolulu, HI MSA	36	4.31
Houma – Thibodaux, LA MSA	7	3.83
Houston – Galveston – Brazoria, TX CMSA	208	5.60
Huntington – Ashland, WV – KY – OH MSA	16	5.12
Huntsville, AL MSA	10	4.19
Indianapolis, IN MSA	160	12.80
Iowa City, IA MSA	75	78.03
Jackson, MS MSA	67	16.95
Jackson, TN MSA	7	8.98
Jacksonville, FL MSA	68	7.50
Jacksonville, NC MSA	17	11.35
Janesville – Beloit, WI MSA	6	4.30
Johnson City – Kingsport – Bristol, TN – VA MSA	7	1.61
Johnstown, PA MSA	8	3.32
Joplin, MO MSA	2	1.48
Kalamazoo, MI MSA	19	8.50
Kankakee, IL MSA	18	18.70
Kansas City, MO – KS MSA	161	10.28
Killeen – Temple, TX MSA	12	4.70
Knoxville, TN MSA	76	12.57
Kokomo, IN MSA	5	5.16
La Crosse, WI MSA	9	9.19
Lafayette, LA MSA	12	5.75
Lafayette – West Lafayette, IN MSA	44	33.69
Lake Charles, LA MSA	7	4.16

[Continued]

★ 715 ★

Health Specialties Teachers
[Continued]

MSA/CMSA	Total Employees	Employees per 100,000 pop.
Lakeland – Winter Haven, FL MSA	19	4.69
Lancaster, PA MSA	6	1.42
Lansing – East Lansing, MI MSA	61	14.10
Las Cruces, NM MSA	10	7.38
Las Vegas, NV MSA	19	2.56
Lawrence, KS MSA	7	8.56
Lawton, OK MSA	6	5.38
Lewiston – Auburn, ME MSA	12	13.61
Lexington-Fayette, KY MSA	82	23.53
Lima, OH MSA	16	10.37
Lincoln, NE MSA	31	14.51
Little Rock – North Little Rock, AR MSA	51	9.94
Longview – Marshall, TX MSA	6	3.69
Los Angeles – Anaheim – Riverside, CA CMSA	356	2.45
Louisville, KY – IN MSA	77	8.08
Lubbock, TX MSA	5	2.25
Lynchburg, VA MSA	12	8.44
Macon – Warner Robins, GA MSA	16	5.69
Madison, WI MSA	47	12.80
Manchester, NH MSA	17	11.50
Mansfield, OH MSA	14	11.10
McAllen – Edinburg – Mission, TX MSA	9	2.35
Medford, OR MSA	15	10.25
Melbourne – Titusville – Palm Bay, FL MSA	15	3.76
Memphis, TN – AR – MS MSA	114	11.61
Miami – Fort Lauderdale, FL CMSA	140	4.39
Milwaukee – Racine, WI CMSA	178	11.08
Minneapolis – St. Paul, MN – WI MSA	197	7.99
Mobile, AL MSA	33	6.92
Modesto, CA MSA	15	4.05
Monroe, LA MSA	38	26.72
Muncie, IN MSA	5	4.18
Muskegon, MI MSA	6	3.77
Nashville, TN MSA	54	5.48
New Haven – Meriden, CT MSA	48	9.05
New London – Norwich, CT – RI MSA	30	11.24
New Orleans, LA MSA	157	12.67
New York – Northern New Jersey – Long Island, NY – NJ – CT CMSA	889	4.92
Norfolk – Virginia Beach – Newport News, VA MSA	73	5.23
Ocala, FL MSA	6	3.08
Oklahoma City, OK MSA	83	8.66
Omaha, NE – IA MSA	48	7.76
Orlando, FL MSA	34	3.17
Panama City, FL MSA	7	5.51
Parkersburg – Marietta, WV – OH MSA	13	8.71
Pascagoula, MS MSA	6	5.21

[Continued]

★ 715 ★

Health Specialties Teachers
[Continued]

MSA/CMSA	Total Employees	Employees per 100,000 pop.
Pensacola, FL MSA	22	6.39
Peoria, IL MSA	32	9.43
Philadelphia – Wilmington – Trenton, PA – NJ – DE – MD CMSA	355	6.02
Phoenix, AZ MSA	140	6.60
Pine Bluff, AR MSA	5	5.85
Pittsburgh – Beaver Valley, PA CMSA	227	10.12
Pittsfield, MA MSA	9	11.36
Portland, ME MSA	7	3.25
Portland – Vancouver, OR – WA CMSA	119	8.05
Portsmouth – Dover – Rochester, NH – ME MSA	9	4.03
Poughkeepsie, NY MSA	22	8.48
Providence – Pawtucket – Fall River, RI – MA CMSA	71	6.22
Provo – Orem, UT MSA	75	28.45
Raleigh – Durham, NC MSA	249	33.86
Reading, PA MSA	8	2.38
Reno, NV MSA	18	7.07
Richland – Kennewick – Pasco, WA MSA	8	5.33
Richmond – Petersburg, VA MSA	55	6.35
Rochester, MN MSA	4	3.76
Rochester, NY MSA	77	7.68
Sacramento, CA MSA	73	4.93
Saginaw – Bay City – Midland, MI MSA	8	2.00
St. Louis, MO – IL MSA	229	9.37
Salem, OR MSA	14	5.04
Salinas – Seaside – Monterey, CA MSA	29	8.15
Salt Lake City – Ogden, UT MSA	56	5.22
San Antonio, TX MSA	106	8.14
San Diego, CA MSA	101	4.04
San Francisco – Oakland – San Jose, CA CMSA	373	5.96
Santa Barbara – Santa Maria – Lompoc, CA MSA	22	5.95
Santa Fe, NM MSA	11	9.40
Sarasota, FL MSA	7	2.52
Scranton – Wilkes-Barre, PA MSA	32	4.36
Seattle – Tacoma, WA CMSA	146	5.70
Sharon, PA MSA	4	3.31
Sheboygan, WI MSA	7	6.74
Sherman – Denison, TX MSA	5	5.26
Shreveport, LA MSA	34	10.17
Sioux City, IA – NE MSA	38	33.04
Sioux Falls, SD MSA	9	7.27
South Bend – Mishawaka, IN MSA	25	10.12
Spokane, WA MSA	15	4.15
Springfield, IL MSA	6	3.17
Springfield, MA MSA	23	4.34
State College, PA MSA	21	16.96
Stockton, CA MSA	7	1.46

[Continued]

★ 715 ★

Health Specialties Teachers
[Continued]

MSA/CMSA	Total Employees	Employees per 100,000 pop.
Syracuse, NY MSA	50	7.58
Tallahassee, FL MSA	73	31.25
Tampa – St. Petersburg – Clearwater, FL MSA	96	4.64
Terre Haute, IN MSA	17	13.00
Toledo, OH MSA	22	3.58
Tucson, AZ MSA	116	17.39
Tulsa, OK MSA	25	3.53
Tuscaloosa, AL MSA	23	15.28
Tyler, TX MSA	29	19.17
Utica – Rome, NY MSA	9	2.84
Visalia – Tulare – Porterville, CA MSA	8	2.56
Waco, TX MSA	35	18.51
Washington, DC – MD – VA MSA	169	4.31
Waterloo – Cedar Falls, IA MSA	20	13.64
Wausau, WI MSA	6	5.20
West Palm Beach – Boca Raton – Delray Beach, FL MSA	53	6.14
Wheeling, WV – OH MSA	14	8.79
Wichita, KS MSA	27	5.56
Wichita Falls, TX MSA	5	4.09
Williamsport, PA MSA	5	4.21
Wilmington, NC MSA	5	4.16
Worcester, MA MSA	29	6.64
Yakima, WA MSA	6	3.18
York, PA MSA	16	3.83
Youngstown – Warren, OH MSA	20	4.06
Yuba City, CA MSA	12	9.78
Yuma, AZ MSA	7	6.55

Source: Census of Population and Housing, 1990: Equal Employment Opportunity (EEO) File on CD-ROM [machine-readable datafiles]. Prepared by the Bureau of the Census. Washington, DC: The Bureau, 1992.

★ 716 ★

Employment

Health Technologists and Technicians

The table below presents the number of civilians 16 years old or older who reported working as health technologists and technicians not tabulated elsewhere during the 1990 Census; for example, dispensing opticians, EEG technologists, EKG technologists, emergency medical technicians, nuclear medicine technologists, or surgical technicians. Data are provided by total number employed in each Metropolitan Statistical Area (MSA) or Consolidated Metropolitan Statistical Area (CMSA), as well as the number employed per 100,000 people.

[Total for all of the U.S. was 411,191; 165.33 per 100,000 persons]

MSA/CMSA	Total Employees	Employees per 100,000 pop.
Abilene, TX MSA	201	167.98
Albany, GA MSA	159	141.26
Albany–Schenectady–Troy, NY MSA	1473	168.48
Albuquerque, NM MSA	737	153.36
Alexandria, LA MSA	272	206.76
Allentown–Bethlehem–Easton, PA–NJ MSA	1082	157.57
Altoona, PA MSA	252	193.04
Amarillo, TX MSA	317	169.02
Anchorage, AK MSA	411	181.59
Anderson, IN MSA	178	136.22
Anderson, SC MSA	316	217.64
Anniston, AL MSA	153	131.86
Appleton–Oshkosh–Neenah, WI MSA	438	138.38
Asheville, NC MSA	323	184.76
Athens, GA MSA	366	234.21
Atlanta, GA MSA	4847	171.06
Atlantic City, NJ MSA	436	136.50
Augusta, GA–SC MSA	976	245.96
Austin, TX MSA	1283	164.16
Bakersfield, CA MSA	883	125.07
Baltimore, MD MSA	5219	219.09
Bangor, ME MSA	191	215.22
Baton Rouge, LA MSA	610	115.47
Battle Creek, MI MSA	219	161.05
Beaumont–Port Arthur, TX MSA	700	193.78
Bellingham, WA MSA	104	81.39
Benton Harbor, MI MSA	253	156.77
Billings, MT MSA	269	237.17
Biloxi–Gulfport, MS MSA	325	164.87
Binghamton, NY MSA	406	153.50
Birmingham, AL MSA	1778	195.86
Bismarck, ND MSA	130	155.07
Bloomington, IN MSA	230	211.05
Bloomington–Normal, IL MSA	150	116.12
Boise City, ID MSA	375	182.24
Boston–Lawrence–Salem, MA–NH CMSA	7652	183.43
Bradenton, FL MSA	364	171.94
Bremerton, WA MSA	301	158.65
Brownsville–Harlingen, TX MSA	266	102.26
Bryan–College Station, TX MSA	264	216.64

[Continued]

★ 716 ★

Health Technologists and Technicians
[Continued]

MSA/CMSA	Total Employees	Employees per 100,000 pop.
Buffalo – Niagara Falls, NY CMSA	2042	171.70
Burlington, NC MSA	95	87.79
Burlington, VT MSA	171	130.10
Canton, OH MSA	795	201.72
Casper, WY MSA	61	99.63
Cedar Rapids, IA MSA	243	143.99
Champaign – Urbana – Rantoul, IL MSA	326	188.41
Charleston, SC MSA	683	134.75
Charleston, WV MSA	672	268.31
Charlotte – Gastonia – Rock Hill, NC – SC MSA	1768	152.14
Charlottesville, VA MSA	310	236.45
Chattanooga, TN – GA MSA	746	172.20
Cheyenne, WY MSA	63	86.13
Chicago – Gary – Lake County, IL – IN – WI CMSA	13602	168.64
Chico, CA MSA	409	224.58
Cincinnati – Hamilton, OH – KY – IN CMSA	3415	195.80
Clarksville – Hopkinsville, TN – KY MSA	217	128.07
Cleveland – Akron – Lorain, OH CMSA	5410	196.03
Colorado Springs, CO MSA	659	165.99
Columbia, MO MSA	435	387.08
Columbia, SC MSA	865	190.81
Columbus, GA – AL MSA	463	190.48
Columbus, OH MSA	2869	208.29
Corpus Christi, TX MSA	553	158.05
Cumberland, MD – WV MSA	214	210.54
Dallas – Fort Worth, TX CMSA	5281	135.92
Danville, VA MSA	111	102.11
Davenport – Rock Island – Moline, IA – IL MSA	543	154.76
Dayton – Springfield, OH MSA	1869	196.47
Daytona Beach, FL MSA	809	218.23
Decatur, AL MSA	150	114.02
Decatur, IL MSA	278	237.19
Denver – Boulder, CO CMSA	3383	183.03
Des Moines, IA MSA	886	225.49
Detroit – Ann Arbor, MI CMSA	10872	233.04
Dothan, AL MSA	221	168.75
Dubuque, IA MSA	153	177.08
Duluth, MN – WI MSA	319	132.93
Eau Claire, WI MSA	161	117.05
El Paso, TX MSA	988	167.00
Elkhart – Goshen, IN MSA	197	126.12
Elmlra, NY MSA	86	90.34
Enid, OK MSA	102	179.78
Erie, PA MSA	426	154.59
Eugene – Springfield, OR MSA	396	139.97
Evansville, IN – KY MSA	620	222.23

[Continued]

★716★

Health Technologists and Technicians
[Continued]

MSA/CMSA	Total Employees	Employees per 100,000 pop.
Fargo–Moorhead, ND–MN MSA	207	135.03
Fayetteville, NC MSA	409	148.96
Fayetteville–Springdale, AR MSA	123	108.46
Fitchburg–Leominster, MA MSA	113	109.93
Flint, MI MSA	898	208.61
Florence, AL MSA	158	120.31
Florence, SC MSA	264	230.88
Fort Collins–Loveland, CO MSA	274	147.20
Fort Myers–Cape Coral, FL MSA	687	205.01
Fort Pierce, FL MSA	398	158.52
Fort Smith, AR–OK MSA	267	151.78
Fort Walton Beach, FL MSA	263	182.92
Fort Wayne, IN MSA	590	162.17
Fresno, CA MSA	1083	162.25
Gadsden, AL MSA	175	175.28
Gainesville, FL MSA	533	261.13
Glens Falls, NY MSA	151	127.38
Grand Forks, ND MSA	70	99.03
Grand Rapids, MI MSA	982	142.65
Great Falls, MT MSA	101	130.00
Greeley, CO MSA	170	128.96
Green Bay, WI MSA	377	193.74
Greensboro–Winston-Salem–High Point, NC MSA	1610	170.90
Greenville–Spartanburg, SC MSA	898	140.12
Hagerstown, MD MSA	105	86.50
Harrisburg–Lebanon–Carlisle, PA MSA	1257	213.78
Hartford–New Britain–Middletown, CT CMSA	1802	165.95
Hickory–Morganton, NC MSA	535	241.32
Honolulu, HI MSA	1345	160.84
Houma–Thibodaux, LA MSA	197	107.74
Houston–Galveston–Brazoria, TX CMSA	6580	177.31
Huntington–Ashland, WV–KY–OH MSA	691	221.10
Huntsville, AL MSA	412	172.45
Indianapolis, IN MSA	2978	238.27
Iowa City, IA MSA	513	533.71
Jackson, MI MSA	266	177.62
Jackson, MS MSA	820	207.39
Jackson, TN MSA	216	276.99
Jacksonville, FL MSA	1804	198.96
Jacksonville, NC MSA	230	153.50
Jamestown–Dunkirk, NY	127	89.50
Janesville–Beloit, WI MSA	169	121.14
Johnson City–Kingsport–Bristol, TN–VA MSA	870	199.52
Johnstown, PA MSA	496	205.60
Joplin, MO MSA	209	154.92
Kalamazoo, MI MSA	645	288.71

[Continued]

★ 716 ★

Health Technologists and Technicians
[Continued]

MSA/CMSA	Total Employees	Employees per 100,000 pop.
Kankakee, IL MSA	360	374.01
Kansas City, MO – KS MSA	3002	191.66
Killeen – Temple, TX MSA	287	112.42
Knoxville, TN MSA	1322	218.58
Kokomo, IN MSA	161	166.07
La Crosse, WI MSA	173	176.70
Lafayette, LA MSA	336	160.97
Lafayette – West Lafayette, IN MSA	481	368.31
Lake Charles, LA MSA	121	71.97
Lakeland – Winter Haven, FL MSA	651	160.59
Lancaster, PA MSA	563	133.15
Lansing – East Lansing, MI MSA	948	219.10
Laredo, TX MSA	140	105.07
Las Cruces, NM MSA	211	155.71
Las Vegas, NV MSA	1236	166.70
Lawrence, KS MSA	178	217.61
Lawton, OK MSA	220	197.33
Lewiston – Auburn, ME MSA	75	85.09
Lexington-Fayette, KY MSA	821	235.63
Lima, OH MSA	192	124.40
Lincoln, NE MSA	472	220.93
Little Rock – North Little Rock, AR MSA	858	167.21
Longview – Marshall, TX MSA	238	146.52
Los Angeles – Anaheim – Riverside, CA CMSA	23606	162.45
Louisville, KY – IN MSA	2713	284.78
Lubbock, TX MSA	466	209.31
Lynchburg, VA MSA	156	109.71
Macon – Warner Robins, GA MSA	398	141.59
Madison, WI MSA	950	258.80
Manchester, NH MSA	244	165.08
Mansfield, OH MSA	153	121.30
McAllen – Edinburg – Mission, TX MSA	329	85.78
Medford, OR MSA	180	122.96
Melbourne – Titusville – Palm Bay, FL MSA	726	181.96
Memphis, TN – AR – MS MSA	2260	230.20
Merced, CA MSA	231	129.48
Miami – Fort Lauderdale, FL CMSA	7391	231.51
Midland, TX MSA	139	130.38
Milwaukee – Racine, WI CMSA	3255	202.53
Minneapolis – St. Paul, MN – WI MSA	4176	169.47
Mobile, AL MSA	788	165.23
Modesto, CA MSA	578	156.00
Monroe, LA MSA	213	149.80
Montgomery, AL MSA	542	185.29
Muncie, IN MSA	249	208.09
Muskegon, MI MSA	193	121.40

[Continued]

★716★

Health Technologists and Technicians
[Continued]

MSA/CMSA	Total Employees	Employees per 100,000 pop.
Naples, FL MSA	188	123.60
Nashville, TN MSA	1918	194.72
New Bedford, MA MSA	209	118.99
New Haven – Meriden, CT MSA	1148	216.53
New London – Norwich, CT – RI MSA	512	191.89
New Orleans, LA MSA	2291	184.93
New York – Northern New Jersey – Long Island, NY – NJ – CT CMSA	26587	146.99
Norfolk – Virginia Beach – Newport News, VA MSA	2685	192.32
Ocala, FL MSA	338	173.48
Odessa, TX MSA	109	91.65
Oklahoma City, OK MSA	2064	215.26
Olympia, WA MSA	338	209.63
Omaha, NE – IA MSA	1296	209.62
Orlando, FL MSA	1659	154.65
Owensboro, KY MSA	187	214.48
Panama City, FL MSA	171	134.65
Parkersburg – Marietta, WV – OH MSA	168	112.62
Pascagoula, MS MSA	198	171.81
Pensacola, FL MSA	609	176.83
Peoria, IL MSA	691	203.73
Philadelphia – Wilmington – Trenton, PA – NJ – DE – MD CMSA	11388	193.04
Phoenix, AZ MSA	3912	184.35
Pine Bluff, AR MSA	119	139.20
Pittsburgh – Beaver Valley, PA CMSA	5541	247.06
Pittsfield, MA MSA	159	200.63
Portland, ME MSA	386	179.30
Portland – Vancouver, OR – WA CMSA	2365	160.02
Portsmouth – Dover – Rochester, NH – ME MSA	318	142.23
Poughkeepsie, NY MSA	380	146.46
Providence – Pawtucket – Fall River, RI – MA CMSA	1951	170.91
Provo – Orem, UT MSA	415	157.44
Pueblo, CO MSA	218	177.16
Raleigh – Durham, NC MSA	1888	256.70
Rapid City, SD MSA	140	172.11
Reading, PA MSA	388	115.30
Redding, CA MSA	211	143.50
Reno, NV MSA	409	160.60
Richland – Kennewick – Pasco, WA MSA	161	107.31
Richmond – Petersburg, VA MSA	1383	159.77
Roanoke, VA MSA	365	162.60
Rochester, MN MSA	616	578.57
Rochester, NY MSA	1655	165.10
Rockford, IL MSA	387	136.40
Sacramento, CA MSA	2889	195.06
Saginaw – Bay City – Midland, MI MSA	889	222.63
St. Cloud, MN MSA	243	127.28

[Continued]

★716★

Health Technologists and Technicians
[Continued]

MSA/CMSA	Total Employees	Employees per 100,000 pop.
St. Joseph, MO MSA	137	164.90
St. Louis, MO–IL MSA	5458	223.31
Salem, OR MSA	468	168.33
Salinas–Seaside–Monterey, CA MSA	490	137.77
Salt Lake City–Ogden, UT MSA	1944	181.30
San Angelo, TX MSA	148	150.32
San Antonio, TX MSA	2780	213.50
San Diego, CA MSA	4714	188.71
San Francisco–Oakland–San Jose, CA CMSA	10838	173.32
Santa Barbara–Santa Maria–Lompoc, CA MSA	631	170.72
Santa Fe, NM MSA	229	195.65
Sarasota, FL MSA	520	187.20
Savannah, GA MSA	563	232.05
Scranton–Wilkes-Barre, PA MSA	910	123.95
Seattle–Tacoma, WA CMSA	4354	170.13
Sharon, PA MSA	146	120.66
Sheboygan, WI MSA	203	195.42
Sherman–Denison, TX MSA	182	191.54
Shreveport, LA MSA	504	150.74
Sioux City, IA–NE MSA	235	204.32
Sioux Falls, SD MSA	285	230.19
South Bend–Mishawaka, IN MSA	436	176.48
Spokane, WA MSA	648	179.32
Springfield, IL MSA	319	168.29
Springfield, MO MSA	599	248.97
Springfield, MA MSA	797	150.51
State College, PA MSA	92	74.32
Steubenville–Weirton, OH–WV MSA	204	143.13
Stockton, CA MSA	644	133.99
Syracuse, NY MSA	1075	162.91
Tallahassee, FL MSA	407	174.23
Tampa–St. Petersburg–Clearwater, FL MSA	4274	206.68
Terre Haute, IN MSA	189	144.48
Texarkana, TX–Texarkana, AR MSA	167	139.01
Toledo, OH MSA	1252	203.87
Topeka, KS MSA	324	201.27
Tucson, AZ MSA	1257	188.49
Tulsa, OK MSA	1309	184.64
Tuscaloosa, AL MSA	292	193.99
Tyler, TX MSA	232	153.33
Utica–Rome, NY MSA	408	128.86
Victoria, TX MSA	154	207.10
Visalia–Tulare–Porterville, CA MSA	461	147.79
Waco, TX MSA	231	122.14
Washington, DC–MD–VA MSA	7174	182.84
Waterbury, CT MSA	281	126.79

[Continued]

★ 716 ★

Health Technologists and Technicians
[Continued]

MSA/CMSA	Total Employees	Employees per 100,000 pop.
Waterloo–Cedar Falls, IA MSA	195	133.01
Wausau, WI MSA	245	212.31
West Palm Beach–Boca Raton–Delray Beach, FL MSA	1449	167.80
Wheeling, WV–OH MSA	323	202.76
Wichita, KS MSA	940	193.71
Wichita Falls, TX MSA	155	126.66
Williamsport, PA MSA	135	113.72
Wilmington, NC MSA	220	182.90
Worcester, MA MSA	885	202.56
Yakima, WA MSA	149	78.91
York, PA MSA	624	149.34
Youngstown–Warren, OH MSA	1063	215.79
Yuba City, CA MSA	202	164.71
Yuma, AZ MSA	81	75.78

Source: Census of Population and Housing, 1990: Equal Employment Opportunity (EEO) File on CD-ROM [machine-readable datafiles]. Prepared by the Bureau of the Census. Washington, DC: The Bureau, 1992.

★ 717 ★

Employment

Insurance Industry Employment

The insurance industry employs nearly 3 million. The table below presents the number of people working in each segment of the industry.

[In dollars]

Industry segment	Number
Life and health (direct)	896,000
Agencies, brokers, and service (direct)	827,000
Property and casualty (direct)	536,000
Life and health (Indirect)	289,000
Agencies, brokers, and service (indirect)	215,000
Property and casualty (indirect)	161,000

Source: Health Insurance Association of America (HIAA). *Source Book of Health Insurance Data, 1993.* Washington, DC: Health Insurance Association of America, 1994, p. 9. Used with permission of HIAA. Primary source: Alliance of American Insurers.

★ 718 ★

Employment

Licensed Practical Nurses

The table below presents the number of civilians 16 years old or older who reported working as licensed practical nurses during the 1990 Census. Data are provided by total number employed in each Metropolitan Statistical Area (MSA) or Consolidated Metropolitan Statistical Area (CMSA), as well as the number employed per 100,000 people.

[Total for all of the U.S. was 429,473; 172.68 per 100,000 persons]

MSA/CMSA	Total Employees	Employees per 100,000 pop.
Abilene, TX MSA	395	330.12
Albany, GA MSA	249	221.21
Albany – Schenectady – Troy, NY MSA	2055	235.04
Albuquerque, NM MSA	629	130.88
Alexandria, LA MSA	506	384.63
Allentown – Bethlehem – Easton, PA – NJ MSA	1409	205.19
Altoona, PA MSA	465	356.21
Amarillo, TX MSA	439	234.07
Anchorage, AK MSA	175	77.32
Anderson, IN MSA	286	218.87
Anderson, SC MSA	276	190.09
Anniston, AL MSA	281	242.17
Appleton – Oshkosh – Neenah, WI MSA	666	211.35
Asheville, NC MSA	412	235.67
Athens, GA MSA	248	158.70
Atlanta, GA MSA	3444	121.55
Atlantic City, NJ MSA	599	187.53
Augusta, GA – SC MSA	1306	329.13
Austin, TX MSA	966	123.60
Bakersfield, CA MSA	589	108.38
Baltimore, MD MSA	3970	166.65
Bangor, ME MSA	252	283.96
Baton Rouge, LA MSA	740	140.08
Battle Creek, MI MSA	268	197.08
Beaumont – Port Arthur, TX MSA	940	260.22
Bellingham, WA MSA	143	111.91
Benton Harbor, MI MSA	225	139.42
Billings, MT MSA	255	224.83
Biloxi – Gulfport, MS MSA	406	205.96
Binghamton, NY MSA	530	200.38
Birmingham, AL MSA	2179	240.03
Bismarck, ND MSA	242	288.68
Bloomington, IN MSA	179	164.25
Bloomington – Normal, IL MSA	160	123.86
Boise City, ID MSA	280	136.07
Boston – Lawrence – Salem, MA – NH CMSA	6288	150.73
Bradenton, FL MSA	554	261.68
Bremerton, WA MSA	322	169.71
Brownsville – Harlingen, TX MSA	552	212.21
Bryan – College Station, TX MSA	214	175.61
Buffalo – Niagara Falls, NY CMSA	2836	238.46
Burlington, NC MSA	114	105.35

[Continued]

★718★

Licensed Practical Nurses
[Continued]

MSA/CMSA	Total Employees	Employees per 100,000 pop.
Burlington, VT MSA	253	192.48
Canton, OH MSA	1127	285.96
Casper, WY MSA	87	142.10
Cedar Rapids, IA MSA	209	123.84
Champaign – Urbana – Rantoul, IL MSA	213	123.10
Charleston, SC MSA	1294	255.29
Charleston, WV MSA	560	223.59
Charlotte – Gastonia – Rock Hill, NC – SC MSA	1389	119.53
Charlottesville, VA MSA	281	214.33
Chattanooga, TN – GA MSA	667	153.97
Cheyenne, WY MSA	52	71.09
Chicago – Gary – Lake County, IL – IN – WI CMSA	8506	105.46
Chico, CA MSA	359	197.12
Cincinnati – Hamilton, OH – KY – IN CMSA	3827	219.42
Clarksville – Hopkinsville, TN – KY MSA	431	254.37
Cleveland – Akron – Lorain, OH CMSA	6488	235.09
Colorado Springs, CO MSA	360	90.68
Columbia, MO MSA	421	374.63
Columbia, SC MSA	1204	265.59
Columbus, GA – AL MSA	492	202.41
Columbus, OH MSA	1830	132.86
Corpus Christi, TX MSA	691	197.49
Cumberland, MD – WV MSA	151	148.56
Dallas – Fort Worth, TX CMSA	4800	123.54
Danville, VA MSA	270	248.36
Davenport – Rock Island Moline, IA – IL MSA	373	106.31
Dayton – Springfield, OH MSA	1637	172.09
Daytona Beach, FL MSA	571	154.03
Decatur, AL MSA	230	174.83
Decatur, IL MSA	498	424.89
Denver – Boulder, CO CMSA	2016	109.07
Des Moines, IA MSA	580	147.61
Detroit – Ann Arbor, MI CMSA	7226	154.89
Dothan, AL MSA	273	208.45
Dubuque, IA MSA	194	224.53
Duluth, MN – WI MSA	757	315.45
Eau Claire, WI MSA	301	218.84
El Paso, TX MSA	526	88.91
Elkhart – Goshen, IN MSA	118	75.55
Elmira, NY MSA	283	297.28
Enid, OK MSA	141	248.52
Erie, PA MSA	501	181.80
Eugene – Springfield, OR MSA	269	95.08
Evansville, IN – KY MSA	727	260.58
Fargo – Moorhead, ND – MN MSA	429	279.85
Fayetteville, NC MSA	450	163.90

[Continued]

★ 718 ★

Licensed Practical Nurses
[Continued]

MSA/CMSA	Total Employees	Employees per 100,000 pop.
Fayetteville – Springdale, AR MSA	212	186.93
Fitchburg – Leominster, MA MSA	182	177.05
Flint, MI MSA	677	157.27
Florence, AL MSA	418	318.29
Florence, SC MSA	237	207.27
Fort Collins – Loveland, CO MSA	256	137.53
Fort Myers – Cape Coral, FL MSA	562	167.70
Fort Pierce, FL MSA	557	221.85
Fort Smith, AR – OK MSA	540	306.97
Fort Walton Beach, FL MSA	177	123.11
Fort Wayne, IN MSA	629	172.89
Fresno, CA MSA	979	146.67
Gadsden, AL MSA	174	174.28
Gainesville, FL MSA	382	187.15
Glens Falls, NY MSA	305	257.30
Grand Forks, ND MSA	126	178.26
Grand Rapids, MI MSA	1472	213.83
Great Falls, MT MSA	191	245.85
Greeley, CO MSA	98	74.34
Green Bay, WI MSA	366	188.08
Greensboro – Winston-Salem – High Point, NC MSA	1543	163.78
Greenville – Spartanburg, SC MSA	1006	156.98
Hagerstown, MD MSA	190	156.52
Harrisburg – Lebanon – Carlisle, PA MSA	1368	232.66
Hartford – New Britain – Middletown, CT CMSA	1905	175.44
Hickory – Morganton, NC MSA	314	141.63
Honolulu, HI MSA	1042	124.61
Houma – Thibodaux, LA MSA	281	153.68
Houston – Galveston – Brazoria, TX CMSA	5481	147.69
Huntington – Ashland, WV – KY – OH MSA	738	236.14
Huntsville, AL MSA	292	122.22
Indianapolis, IN MSA	2559	204.75
Iowa City, IA MSA	266	276.74
Jackson, MI MSA	362	241.73
Jackson, MS MSA	1137	287.56
Jackson, TN MSA	227	291.09
Jacksonville, FL MSA	1239	136.65
Jacksonville, NC MSA	202	134.81
Jamestown – Dunkirk, NY	385	271.33
Janesville – Beloit, WI MSA	197	141.21
Johnson City – Kingsport – Bristol, TN – VA MSA	1254	287.58
Johnstown, PA MSA	847	351.09
Joplin, MO MSA	366	271.29
Kalamazoo, MI MSA	553	247.53
Kankakee, IL MSA	231	239.99
Kansas City, MO – KS MSA	2639	168.49

[Continued]

★ 718 ★

Licensed Practical Nurses
[Continued]

MSA/CMSA	Total Employees	Employees per 100,000 pop.
Killeen – Temple, TX MSA	600	235.02
Knoxville, TN MSA	1286	212.63
Kokomo, IN MSA	149	153.69
La Crosse, WI MSA	165	168.53
Lafayette, LA MSA	448	214.62
Lafayette – West Lafayette, IN MSA	228	174.58
Lake Charles, LA MSA	515	306.30
Lakeland – Winter Haven, FL MSA	767	189.20
Lancaster, PA MSA	1015	240.05
Lansing – East Lansing, MI MSA	563	130.12
Laredo, TX MSA	288	216.15
Las Cruces, NM MSA	193	142.42
Las Vegas, NV MSA	768	103.58
Lawrence, KS MSA	39	47.68
Lawton, OK MSA	308	276.27
Lewiston – Auburn, ME MSA	280	317.67
Lexington-Fayette, KY MSA	713	204.63
Lima, OH MSA	272	176.23
Lincoln, NE MSA	507	237.31
Little Rock – North Little Rock, AR MSA	1881	366.58
Longview – Marshall, TX MSA	345	212.40
Los Angeles – Anaheim – Riverside, CA CMSA	15872	109.22
Louisville, KY – IN MSA	1425	149.58
Lubbock, TX MSA	849	381.34
Lynchburg, VA MSA	248	174.40
Macon – Warner Robins, GA MSA	580	206.33
Madison, WI MSA	554	150.92
Manchester, NH MSA	191	129.22
Mansfield, OH MSA	221	175.21
McAllen – Edinburg – Mission, TX MSA	657	171.30
Medford, OR MSA	117	79.92
Melbourne – Titusville – Palm Bay, FL MSA	503	126.07
Memphis, TN – AR – MS MSA	2023	206.06
Merced, CA MSA	201	112.67
Miami – Fort Lauderdale, FL CMSA	4532	141.95
Midland, TX MSA	144	135.07
Milwaukee – Racine, WI CMSA	2998	186.54
Minneapolis – St. Paul, MN – WI MSA	4402	178.64
Mobile, AL MSA	1167	244.69
Modesto, CA MSA	446	120.37
Monroe, LA MSA	449	315.77
Montgomery, AL MSA	677	231.44
Muncie, IN MSA	205	171.32
Muskegon, MI MSA	397	249.71
Naples, FL MSA	269	176.86
Nashville, TN MSA	2498	253.60

[Continued]

★ 718 ★

Licensed Practical Nurses
[Continued]

MSA/CMSA	Total Employees	Employees per 100,000 pop.
New Bedford, MA MSA	277	157.71
New Haven – Meriden, CT MSA	936	176.54
New London – Norwlch, CT – RI MSA	608	227.87
New Orleans, LA MSA	2306	186.15
New York – Northern New Jersey – Long Island, NY – NJ – CT CMSA	22459	124.17
Norfolk – Virginia Beach – Newport News, VA MSA	2588	185.37
Ocala, FL MSA	211	108.30
Odessa, TX MSA	121	101.74
Oklahoma City, OK MSA	1868	194.82
Olympia, WA MSA	309	191.64
Omaha, NE – IA MSA	988	159.80
Orlando, FL MSA	1813	169.01
Owensboro, KY MSA	218	250.03
Panama City, FL MSA	243	191.35
Parkersburg – Marietta, WV – OH MSA	449	301.00
Pascagoula, MS MSA	194	168.34
Pensacola, FL MSA	861	250.00
Peoria, IL MSA	704	207.56
Philadelphia – Wilmington – Trenton, PA – NJ – DE – MD CMSA	9616	163.00
Phoenix, AZ MSA	2303	108.52
Pine Bluff, AR MSA	235	274.90
Pittsburgh – Beaver Valley, PA CMSA	3893	173.58
Pittsfield, MA MSA	228	287.70
Portland, ME MSA	415	192.77
Portland – Vancouver, OR – WA CMSA	1204	81.47
Portsmouth – Dover – Rochester, NH – ME MSA	438	195.90
Poughkeepsie, NY MSA	401	154.55
Providence – Pawtucket – Fall River, RI – MA CMSA	2202	192.90
Provo – Orem, UT MSA	513	194.62
Pueblo, CO MSA	219	177.97
Raleigh – Durham, NC MSA	1190	161.80
Rapid City, SD MSA	103	126.62
Reading, PA MSA	826	245.45
Redding, CA MSA	129	87.73
Reno, NV MSA	321	126.05
Richland – Kennewick – Pasco, WA MSA	208	138.64
Richmond – Petersburg, VA MSA	2077	239.94
Roanoke, VA MSA	672	299.36
Rochester, MN MSA	668	627.41
Rochester, NY MSA	1886	188.15
Rockford, IL MSA	541	190.68
Sacramento, CA MSA	1752	118.29
Saginaw – Bay City – Midland, MI MSA	898	224.88
St. Cloud, MN MSA	553	289.65
St. Joseph, MO MSA	178	214.24
St. Louis, MO – IL MSA	4464	182.64

[Continued]

★ 718 ★

Licensed Practical Nurses
[Continued]

MSA/CMSA	Total Employees	Employees per 100,000 pop.
Salem, OR MSA	375	134.88
Salinas – Seaside – Monterey, CA MSA	235	66.07
Salt Lake City – Ogden, UT MSA	1033	96.34
San Angelo, TX MSA	309	313.84
San Antonio, TX MSA	3277	251.67
San Diego, CA MSA	2999	120.06
San Francisco – Oakland – San Jose, CA CMSA	6431	102.84
Santa Barbara – Santa Maria – Lompoc, CA MSA	315	85.23
Santa Fe, NM MSA	135	115.34
Sarasota, FL MSA	801	288.36
Savannah, GA MSA	629	259.25
Scranton – Wilkes-Barre, PA MSA	2026	275.96
Seattle – Tacoma, WA CMSA	3086	120.59
Sharon, PA MSA	272	224.79
Sheboygan, WI MSA	252	242.59
Sherman – Denison, TX MSA	175	184.17
Shreveport, LA MSA	928	277.56
Sioux City, IA – NE MSA	189	164.32
Sioux Falls, SD MSA	419	338.42
South Bend – Mishawaka, IN MSA	327	132.36
Spokane, WA MSA	758	209.76
Springfield, IL MSA	584	308.10
Springfield, MO MSA	692	287.62
Springfield, MA MSA	1152	217.56
State College, PA MSA	285	230.24
Steubenville – Weirton, OH – WV MSA	236	165.59
Stockton, CA MSA	475	90.03
Syracuse, NY MSA	1557	235.96
Tallahassee, FL MSA	492	210.62
Tampa – St. Petersburg – Clearwater, FL MSA	4702	227.37
Terre Haute, IN MSA	316	241.57
Texarkana, TX – Texarkana, AR MSA	360	299.67
Toledo, OH MSA	1537	250.27
Topeka, KS MSA	526	326.76
Tucson, AZ MSA	977	146.50
Tulsa, OK MSA	1143	161.22
Tuscaloosa, AL MSA	699	464.38
Tyler, TX MSA	346	228.67
Utica – Rome, NY MSA	1127	355.93
Victoria, TX MSA	258	346.96
Visalia – Tulare – Porterville, CA MSA	432	138.50
Waco, TX MSA	350	185.06
Washington, DC – MD – VA MSA	3682	93.84
Waterbury, CT MSA	641	289.22
Waterloo – Cedar Falls, IA MSA	323	220.31
Wausau, WI MSA	127	110.05

[Continued]

★ 718 ★

Licensed Practical Nurses
[Continued]

MSA/CMSA	Total Employees	Employees per 100,000 pop.
West Palm Beach – Boca Raton – Delray Beach, FL MSA	1117	129.35
Wheeling, WV – OH MSA	522	327.68
Wichita, KS MSA	852	175.57
Wichita Falls, TX MSA	641	523.79
Williamsport, PA MSA	325	273.78
Wilmington, NC MSA	292	242.76
Worcester, MA MSA	844	193.18
Yakima, WA MSA	288	152.52
York, PA MSA	1063	254.40
Youngstown – Warren, OH MSA	1621	329.06
Yuba City, CA MSA	173	141.06
Yuma, AZ MSA	136	127.23

Source: Census of Population and Housing, 1990: Equal Employment Opportunity (EEO) File on CD-ROM [machine-readable datafiles]. Prepared by the Bureau of the Census. Washington, DC: The Bureau, 1992.

★ 719 ★

Employment

Medical Science Teachers

The table below presents the number of civilians 16 years old or older who reported working as medical science teachers during the 1990 Census. Data are provided by total number employed in each Metropolitan Statistical Area (MSA) or Consolidated Metropolitan Statistical Area (CMSA), as well as the number employed per 100,000 people.

[Total for all of the U.S. was 2,743; 1.10 per 100,000 persons]

MSA/CMSA	Total Employees	Employees per 100,000 pop.
Albany, GA MSA	7	6.22
Albany – Schenectady – Troy, NY MSA	5	0.57
Albuquerque, NM MSA	16	3.33
Allentown – Bethlehem – Easton, PA – NJ MSA	5	0.73
Anniston, AL MSA	7	6.03
Appleton – Oshkosh – Neenah, WI MSA	5	1.59
Atlanta, GA MSA	5	0.18
Augusta, GA – SC MSA	24	6.05
Baltimore, MD MSA	35	1.47
Bangor, ME MSA	2	2.25
Beaumont – Port Arthur, TX MSA	9	2.49
Binghamton, NY MSA	8	3.02
Birmingham, AL MSA	50	5.51
Bloomington, IN MSA	4	3.67
Boston – Lawrence – Salem, MA – NH CMSA	33	0.79
Brownsville – Harlingen, TX MSA	3	1.15
Buffalo – Niagara Falls, NY CMSA	17	1.43

[Continued]

★ 719 ★

Medical Science Teachers
[Continued]

MSA/CMSA	Total Employees	Employees per 100,000 pop.
Champaign – Urbana – Rantoul, IL MSA	15	8.67
Charleston, SC MSA	44	8.68
Charlotte – Gastonia – Rock Hill, NC – SC MSA	16	1.38
Charlottesville, VA MSA	16	12.20
Chattanooga, TN – GA MSA	7	1.62
Chicago – Gary – Lake County, IL – IN – WI CMSA	130	1.61
Cincinnati – Hamilton, OH – KY – IN CMSA	16	0.92
Cleveland – Akron – Lorain, OH CMSA	33	1.20
Columbia, MO MSA	7	6.23
Columbia, SC MSA	53	11.69
Columbus, OH MSA	12	0.87
Dallas – Fort Worth, TX CMSA	82	2.11
Davenport – Rock Island – Moline, IA – IL MSA	5	1.43
Des Moines, IA MSA	14	3.56
Detroit – Ann Arbor, MI CMSA	49	1.05
Duluth, MN – WI MSA	7	2.92
Fresno, CA MSA	6	0.90
Gainesville, FL MSA	8	3.92
Grand Forks, ND MSA	8	11.32
Greensboro – Winston-Salem – High Point, NC MSA	30	3.18
Harrisburg – Lebanon – Carlisle, PA MSA	15	2.55
Hartford – New Britain – Middletown, CT CMSA	6	0.55
Honolulu, HI MSA	40	4.78
Houston – Galveston – Brazoria, TX CMSA	112	3.02
Indianapolis, IN MSA	38	3.04
Iowa City, IA MSA	10	10.40
Jackson, MS MSA	16	4.05
Jacksonville, FL MSA	12	1.32
Johnson City – Kingsport – Bristol, TN – VA MSA	13	2.98
Kalamazoo, MI MSA	12	5.37
Lansing – East Lansing, MI MSA	20	4.62
Lexington-Fayette, KY MSA	6	1.72
Little Rock – North Little Rock, AR MSA	12	2.34
Los Angeles – Anaheim – Riverside, CA CMSA	122	0.84
Louisville, KY – IN MSA	15	1.57
Madison, WI MSA	17	4.63
McAllen – Edinburg – Mission, TX MSA	10	2.61
Memphis, TN – AR – MS MSA	31	3.16
Miami – Fort Lauderdale, FL CMSA	22	0.69
Milwaukee – Racine, WI CMSA	7	0.44
Minneapolis – St. Paul, MN – WI MSA	5	0.20
Mobile, AL MSA	26	5.45
Nashville, TN MSA	5	0.51
New Haven – Meriden, CT MSA	31	5.85
New Orleans, LA MSA	76	6.13
New York – Northern New Jersey – Long Island, NY – NJ – CT CMSA	275	1.52

[Continued]

★ 719 ★

Medical Science Teachers
[Continued]

MSA/CMSA	Total Employees	Employees per 100,000 pop.
Norfolk – Virginia Beach – Newport News, VA MSA	7	0.50
Oklahoma City, OK MSA	11	1.15
Omaha, NE – IA MSA	19	3.07
Pensacola, FL MSA	8	2.32
Peoria, IL MSA	7	2.06
Philadelphia – Wilmington – Trenton, PA – NJ – DE – MD CMSA	67	1.14
Pittsburgh – Beaver Valley, PA CMSA	36	1.61
Portland – Vancouver, OR – WA CMSA	27	1.83
Raleigh – Durham, NC MSA	51	6.93
Richmond – Petersburg, VA MSA	32	3.70
Rochester, NY MSA	14	1.40
Sacramento, CA MSA	22	1.49
St. Louis, MO – IL MSA	46	1.88
Salt Lake City – Ogden, UT MSA	14	1.31
San Antonio, TX MSA	25	1.92
San Diego, CA MSA	39	1.56
San Francisco – Oakland – San Jose, CA CMSA	53	0.85
Scranton – Wilkes-Barre, PA MSA	15	2.04
Seattle – Tacoma, WA CMSA	34	1.33
Sioux City, IA – NE MSA	6	5.22
Springfield, IL MSA	26	13.72
Syracuse, NY MSA	31	4.70
Tampa – St. Petersburg – Clearwater, FL MSA	18	0.87
Toledo, OH MSA	6	0.98
Tucson, AZ MSA	6	0.90
Tulsa, OK MSA	21	2.96
Washington, DC – MD – VA MSA	66	1.68
Wichita, KS MSA	16	3.30
Worcester, MA MSA	23	5.26

Source: Census of Population and Housing, 1990: Equal Employment Opportunity (EEO) File on CD-ROM [machine-readable datafiles]. Prepared by the Bureau of the Census. Washington, DC: The Bureau, 1992.

★ 720 ★

Employment

Medical Scientists

The table below presents the number of civilians 16 years old or older who reported working as medical scientists during the 1990 Census. Data are provided by total number employed in each Metropolitan Statistical Area (MSA) or Consolidated Metropolitan Statistical Area (CMSA), as well as the number employed per 100,000 people.

[Total for all of the U.S. was 27,519; 11.06 per 100,000 persons]

MSA/CMSA	Total Employees	Employees per 100,000 pop.
Albany, GA MSA	6	5.33
Albany–Schenectady–Troy, NY MSA	148	16.93
Albuquerque, NM MSA	168	34.96
Alexandria, LA MSA	8	6.08
Allentown–Bethlehem–Easton, PA–NJ MSA	21	3.06
Amarillo, TX MSA	18	9.60
Anchorage, AK MSA	49	21.65
Appleton–Oshkosh–Neenah, WI MSA	4	1.27
Asheville, NC MSA	12	6.86
Athens, GA MSA	15	9.60
Atlanta, GA MSA	603	21.28
Atlantic City, NJ MSA	7	2.19
Augusta, GA–SC MSA	85	21.42
Austin, TX MSA	101	12.92
Bakersfield, CA MSA	20	3.68
Baltimore, MD MSA	565	23.72
Baton Rouge, LA MSA	52	9.84
Battle Creek, MI MSA	6	4.41
Beaumont–Port Arthur, TX MSA	7	1.94
Billings, MT MSA	6	5.29
Binghamton, NY MSA	12	4.54
Birmingham, AL MSA	203	22.36
Bismarck, ND MSA	14	16.70
Bloomington–Normal, IL MSA	2	1.55
Boise City, ID MSA	33	16.04
Boston–Lawrence–Salem, MA–NH CMSA	977	23.42
Bremerton, WA MSA	11	5.80
Brownsville–Harlingen, TX MSA	8	3.08
Bryan–College Station, TX MSA	13	10.67
Buffalo–Niagara Falls, NY CMSA	173	14.55
Burlington, NC MSA	27	24.95
Burlington, VT MSA	30	22.82
Canton, OH MSA	33	8.37
Casper, WY MSA	2	3.27
Cedar Rapids, IA MSA	12	7.11
Champaign–Urbana–Rantoul, IL MSA	24	13.87
Charleston, SC MSA	110	21.70
Charleston, WV MSA	36	14.37
Charlotte–Gastonia–Rock Hill, NC–SC MSA	23	1.98
Charlottesville, VA MSA	194	147.97
Chattanooga, TN–GA MSA	7	1.62
Chicago–Gary–Lake County, IL–IN–WI CMSA	732	9.08

[Continued]

★ 720 ★

Medical Scientists
[Continued]

MSA/CMSA	Total Employees	Employees per 100,000 pop.
Chico, CA MSA	1	0.55
Cincinnati – Hamilton, OH – KY – IN CMSA	249	14.28
Cleveland – Akron – Lorain, OH CMSA	209	7.57
Colorado Springs, CO MSA	23	5.79
Columbia, MO MSA	93	82.76
Columbia, SC MSA	27	5.96
Columbus, GA – AL MSA	6	2.47
Columbus, OH MSA	190	13.79
Dallas – Fort Worth, TX CMSA	340	8.75
Danville, VA MSA	7	6.44
Dayton – Springfield, OH MSA	43	4.52
Daytona Beach, FL MSA	9	2.43
Denver – Boulder, CO CMSA	523	28.30
Des Moines, IA MSA	17	4.33
Detroit – Ann Arbor, MI CMSA	413	8.85
Dubuque, IA MSA	7	8.10
Duluth, MN – WI MSA	7	2.92
El Paso, TX MSA	31	5.24
Elkhart – Goshen, IN MSA	17	10.88
Erie, PA MSA	12	4.35
Evansville, IN – KY MSA	15	5.38
Fargo – Moorhead, ND – MN MSA	18	11.74
Fayetteville, NC MSA	9	3.28
Fayetteville – Springdale, AR MSA	15	13.23
Fitchburg – Leominster, MA MSA	17	16.54
Flint, MI MSA	18	4.18
Florence, AL MSA	12	9.14
Florence, SC MSA	2	1.75
Fort Collins – Loveland, CO MSA	42	22.56
Fort Myers – Cape Coral, FL MSA	6	1.79
Fort Pierce, FL MSA	10	3.98
Fort Smith, AR – OK MSA	10	5.68
Fort Walton Beach, FL MSA	7	4.87
Fresno, CA MSA	45	6.74
Gainesville, FL MSA	58	28.42
Grand Forks, ND MSA	5	7.07
Grand Rapids, MI MSA	8	1.16
Great Falls, MT MSA	4	5.15
Green Bay, WI MSA	2	1.03
Greensboro – Winston-Salem – High Point, NC MSA	148	15.71
Greenville – Spartanburg, SC MSA	15	2.34
Harrisburg – Lebanon – Carlisle, PA MSA	58	9.86
Hartford – New Britain – Middletown, CT CMSA	209	19.25
Honolulu, HI MSA	71	8.49
Houston – Galveston – Brazoria, TX CMSA	888	23.93
Huntington – Ashland, WV – KY – OH MSA	11	3.52

[Continued]

★ 720 ★

Medical Scientists
[Continued]

MSA/CMSA	Total Employees	Employees per 100,000 pop.
Huntsville, AL MSA	7	2.93
Indianapolis, IN MSA	206	16.48
Iowa City, IA MSA	68	70.75
Jackson, MS MSA	69	17.45
Jackson, TN MSA	10	12.82
Jacksonville, FL MSA	33	3.64
Jacksonville, NC MSA	7	4.67
Jamestown–Dunkirk, NY	8	5.64
Johnson City–Kingsport–Bristol, TN–VA MSA	61	13.99
Joplin, MO MSA	6	4.45
Kalamazoo, MI MSA	111	49.68
Kansas City, MO–KS MSA	188	12.00
Knoxville, TN MSA	33	5.46
Lafayette, LA MSA	7	3.35
Lakeland–Winter Haven, FL MSA	24	5.92
Lancaster, PA MSA	11	2.60
Lansing–East Lansing, MI MSA	63	14.56
Las Cruces, NM MSA	5	3.69
Las Vegas, NV MSA	32	1.32
Lawrence, KS MSA	13	15.89
Lawton, OK MSA	17	15.25
Lexington-Fayette, KY MSA	142	40.75
Lima, OH MSA	6	3.89
Lincoln, NE MSA	20	9.36
Little Rock–North Little Rock, AR MSA	121	23.58
Los Angeles–Anaheim–Riverside, CA CMSA	1604	11.04
Louisville, KY–IN MSA	57	5.98
Lubbock, TX MSA	8	3.59
Macon–Warner Robins, GA MSA	9	3.20
Madison, WI MSA	160	43.59
Mansfield, OH MSA	7	5.55
Melbourne–Titusville–Palm Bay, FL MSA	4	1.00
Memphis, TN–AR–MS MSA	233	23.73
Merced, CA MSA	10	5.61
Miami–Fort Lauderdale, FL CMSA	259	8.11
Milwaukee–Racine, WI CMSA	88	5.48
Minneapolis–St. Paul, MN–WI MSA	487	19.76
Mobile, AL MSA	21	4.40
Modesto, CA MSA	8	2.16
Monroe, LA MSA	16	11.25
Montgomery, AL MSA	5	1.71
Muncie, IN MSA	7	5.85
Nashville, TN MSA	251	25.48
New Haven–Meriden, CT MSA	163	30.74
New London–Norwich, CT–RI MSA	128	47.97
New Orleans, LA MSA	172	13.88

[Continued]

★ 720 ★

Medical Scientists
[Continued]

MSA/CMSA	Total Employees	Employees per 100,000 pop.
New York–Northern New Jersey–Long Island, NY–NJ–CT CMSA	2151	11.89
Norfolk–Virginia Beach–Newport News, VA MSA	45	3.22
Oklahoma City, OK MSA	122	12.72
Olympia, WA MSA	33	20.47
Omaha, NE–IA MSA	72	11.65
Orlando, FL MSA	42	3.92
Owensboro, KY MSA	7	8.03
Parkersburg–Marietta, WV–OH MSA	2	1.34
Pascagoula, MS MSA	9	7.81
Pensacola, FL MSA	10	2.90
Peoria, IL MSA	8	2.36
Philadelphia–Wilmington–Trenton, PA–NJ–DE–MD CMSA	1254	21.26
Phoenix, AZ MSA	126	5.94
Pittsburgh–Beaver Valley, PA CMSA	220	9.81
Pittsfield, MA MSA	21	26.50
Portland, ME MSA	10	4.65
Portland–Vancouver, OR–WA CMSA	290	19.62
Poughkeepsie, NY MSA	27	10.41
Providence–Pawtucket–Fall River, RI–MA CMSA	104	9.11
Provo–Orem, UT MSA	21	7.97
Raleigh–Durham, NC MSA	912	124.00
Reading, PA MSA	3	0.89
Redding, CA MSA	6	4.08
Reno, NV MSA	26	10.21
Richland–Kennewick–Pasco, WA MSA	24	16.00
Richmond–Petersburg, VA MSA	160	18.48
Roanoke, VA MSA	14	6.24
Rochester, MN MSA	149	139.95
Rochester, NY MSA	121	12.07
Sacramento, CA MSA	271	18.30
Saginaw–Bay City–Midland, MI MSA	47	11.77
St. Cloud, MN MSA	2	1.05
St. Louis, MO–IL MSA	372	15.22
Salinas–Seaside–Monterey, CA MSA	11	3.09
Salt Lake City–Ogden, UT MSA	244	22.76
San Antonio, TX MSA	161	12.36
San Diego, CA MSA	646	25.86
San Francisco–Oakland–San Jose, CA CMSA	1429	22.85
Santa Barbara–Santa Maria–Lompoc, CA MSA	40	10.82
Santa Fe, NM MSA	42	35.88
Savannah, GA MSA	12	4.95
Scranton–Wilkes-Barre, PA MSA	15	2.04
Seattle–Tacoma, WA CMSA	626	24.46
Sheboygan, WI MSA	15	14.44
Shreveport, LA MSA	80	23.93
Sioux City, IA–NE MSA	10	8.69

[Continued]

★ 720 ★

Medical Scientists
[Continued]

MSA/CMSA	Total Employees	Employees per 100,000 pop.
Sioux Falls, SD MSA	5	4.04
South Bend – Mishawaka, IN MSA	13	5.26
Spokane, WA MSA	18	4.98
Springfield, IL MSA	41	21.63
Springfield, MO MSA	7	2.91
Springfield, MA MSA	15	2.83
State College, PA MSA	8	6.46
Syracuse, NY MSA	98	14.85
Tallahassee, FL MSA	20	8.56
Tampa – St. Petersburg – Clearwater, FL MSA	95	4.59
Terre Haute, IN MSA	5	3.82
Toledo, OH MSA	64	10.42
Topeka, KS MSA	28	17.39
Tucson, AZ MSA	197	29.54
Tulsa, OK MSA	12	1.69
Tuscaloosa, AL MSA	8	5.31
Tyler, TX MSA	24	15.86
Victoria, TX MSA	6	8.07
Visalia – Tulare – Porterville, CA MSA	8	2.56
Washington, DC – MD – VA MSA	1891	48.20
Waterbury, CT MSA	5	2.26
West Palm Beach – Boca Raton – Delray Beach, FL MSA	19	2.20
Wichita, KS MSA	28	5.77
Worcester, MA MSA	91	20.83
York, PA MSA	6	1.44
Yuma, AZ MSA	5	4.68

Source: Census of Population and Housing, 1990: Equal Employment Opportunity (EEO) File on CD-ROM [machine-readable datafiles]. Prepared by the Bureau of the Census. Washington, DC: The Bureau, 1992.

★ 721 ★

Employment

Medicine and Health Managers

The table below presents the number of civilians 16 years old or older who reported working as medicine and health managers during the 1990 Census. Data are provided by total number employed in each Metropolitan Statistical Area (MSA) or Consolidated Metropolitan Statistical Area (CMSA), as well as the number employed per 100,000 people.

[Total for all of the U.S. was 233,621; 93.93 per 100,000 persons]

MSA/CMSA	Total Employees	Employees per 100,000 pop.
Abilene, TX MSA	102	85.25
Albany, GA MSA	172	152.81
Albany–Schenectady–Troy, NY MSA	1184	135.42
Albuquerque, NM MSA	534	111.12
Alexandria, LA MSA	161	122.38
Allentown–Bethlehem–Easton, PA–NJ MSA	533	77.62
Altoona, PA MSA	90	68.94
Amarillo, TX MSA	131	69.85
Anchorage, AK MSA	220	97.20
Anderson, IN MSA	70	53.57
Anderson, SC MSA	149	102.62
Anniston, AL MSA	53	45.68
Appleton–Oshkosh–Neenah, WI MSA	243	77.11
Asheville, NC MSA	251	143.58
Athens, GA MSA	123	78.71
Atlanta, GA MSA	2564	90.49
Atlantic City, NJ MSA	285	89.23
Augusta, GA–SC MSA	527	132.81
Austin, TX MSA	729	93.27
Bakersfield, CA MSA	268	49.31
Baltimore, MD MSA	2962	124.34
Bangor, ME MSA	96	108.18
Baton Rouge, LA MSA	336	63.60
Battle Creek, MI MSA	166	122.07
Beaumont–Port Arthur, TX MSA	174	48.17
Bellingham, WA MSA	109	85.30
Benton Harbor, MI MSA	99	61.35
Billings, MT MSA	153	134.90
Biloxi–Gulfport, MS MSA	163	82.69
Binghamton, NY MSA	216	81.66
Birmingham, AL MSA	997	109.82
Bismarck, ND MSA	96	114.52
Bloomington, IN MSA	99	90.84
Bloomington–Normal, IL MSA	65	50.32
Boise City, ID MSA	243	118.09
Boston–Lawrence–Salem, MA–NH CMSA	5818	139.47
Bradenton, FL MSA	123	58.10
Bremerton, WA MSA	134	70.63
Brownsville–Harlingen, TX MSA	189	72.66
Bryan–College Station, TX MSA	91	74.67
Buffalo–Niagara Falls, NY CMSA	1121	94.26
Burlington, NC MSA	147	135.84

[Continued]

★ 721 ★

Medicine and Health Managers
[Continued]

MSA/CMSA	Total Employees	Employees per 100,000 pop.
Burlington, VT MSA	162	123.25
Canton, OH MSA	276	70.03
Casper, WY MSA	41	66.97
Cedar Rapids, IA MSA	96	56.88
Champaign – Urbana – Rantoul, IL MSA	128	73.98
Charleston, SC MSA	500	98.64
Charleston, WV MSA	237	94.63
Charlotte – Gastonia – Rock Hill, NC – SC MSA	973	83.73
Charlottesville, VA MSA	250	190.68
Chattanooga, TN – GA MSA	392	90.49
Cheyenne, WY MSA	62	84.77
Chicago – Gary – Lake County, IL – IN – WI CMSA	7871	97.59
Chico, CA MSA	155	85.11
Cincinnati – Hamilton, OH – KY – IN CMSA	1694	97.13
Clarksville – Hopkinsville, TN – KY MSA	146	86.17
Cleveland – Akron – Lorain, OH CMSA	2632	95.37
Colorado Springs, CO MSA	377	94.96
Columbia, MO MSA	222	197.55
Columbia, SC MSA	425	93.75
Columbus, GA – AL MSA	178	73.23
Columbus, OH MSA	1326	96.27
Corpus Christi, TX MSA	254	72.59
Cumberland, MD – WV MSA	71	69.85
Dallas – Fort Worth, TX CMSA	3665	94.33
Danville, VA MSA	61	56.11
Davenport – Rock Island – Moline, IA – IL MSA	252	71.82
Dayton – Springfield, OH MSA	978	102.81
Daytona Beach, FL MSA	336	90.64
Decatur, AL MSA	174	132.26
Decatur, IL MSA	40	34.13
Denver – Boulder, CO CMSA	1903	102.96
Des Moines, IA MSA	406	103.33
Detroit – Ann Arbor, MI CMSA	4708	100.92
Dothan, AL MSA	117	89.34
Dubuque, IA MSA	64	74.07
Duluth, MN – WI MSA	265	110.43
Eau Claire, WI MSA	125	90.88
El Paso, TX MSA	379	64.06
Elkhart – Goshen, IN MSA	66	42.25
Elmira, NY MSA	56	58.83
Enid, OK MSA	55	96.94
Erie, PA MSA	347	125.92
Eugene – Springfield, OR MSA	244	86.25
Evansville, IN – KY MSA	237	84.95
Fargo – Moorhead, ND – MN MSA	221	144.17
Fayetteville, NC MSA	197	71.75

[Continued]

★ 721 ★

Medicine and Health Managers
[Continued]

MSA/CMSA	Total Employees	Employees per 100,000 pop.
Fayetteville – Springdale, AR MSA	107	94.35
Fitchburg – Leominster, MA MSA	126	122.57
Flint, MI MSA	350	81.31
Florence, AL MSA	83	63.20
Florence, SC MSA	113	98.82
Fort Collins – Loveland, CO MSA	207	111.21
Fort Myers – Cape Coral, FL MSA	299	89.22
Fort Pierce, FL MSA	143	56.96
Fort Smith, AR – OK MSA	195	110.85
Fort Walton Beach, FL MSA	145	100.85
Fort Wayne, IN MSA	453	124.52
Fresno, CA MSA	521	78.05
Gadsden, AL MSA	108	108.17
Gainesville, FL MSA	401	196.46
Glens Falls, NY MSA	106	89.42
Grand Forks, ND MSA	21	29.71
Grand Rapids, MI MSA	508	73.79
Great Falls, MT MSA	88	113.27
Greeley, CO MSA	70	53.10
Green Bay, WI MSA	100	51.39
Greensboro – Winston-Salem – High Point, NC MSA	964	102.33
Greenville – Spartanburg, SC MSA	375	58.52
Hagerstown, MD MSA	107	88.14
Harrisburg – Lebanon – Carlisle, PA MSA	524	89.12
Hartford – New Britain – Middletown, CT CMSA	1390	128.01
Hickory – Morganton, NC MSA	158	71.27
Honolulu, HI MSA	745	89.09
Houma – Thibodaux, LA MSA	61	33.36
Houston – Galveston – Brazoria, TX CMSA	3606	97.17
Huntington – Ashland, WV – KY – OH MSA	245	78.39
Huntsville, AL MSA	132	55.25
Indianapolis, IN MSA	1617	129.38
Iowa City, IA MSA	139	144.61
Jackson, MI MSA	143	95.49
Jackson, MS MSA	442	111.79
Jackson, TN MSA	59	75.66
Jacksonville, FL MSA	1018	112.27
Jacksonville, NC MSA	45	30.03
Jamestown – Dunkirk, NY	108	76.11
Janesville – Beloit, WI MSA	115	82.43
Johnson City – Kingsport – Bristol, TN – VA MSA	460	105.49
Johnstown, PA MSA	141	58.45
Joplin, MO MSA	127	94.14
Kalamazoo, MI MSA	208	93.10
Kankakee, IL MSA	79	82.07
Kansas City, MO – KS MSA	1760	112.37

[Continued]

★ 721 ★

Medicine and Health Managers
[Continued]

MSA/CMSA	Total Employees	Employees per 100,000 pop.
Killeen – Temple, TX MSA	226	88.52
Knoxville, TN MSA	497	82.17
Kokomo, IN MSA	55	56.73
La Crosse, WI MSA	108	110.31
Lafayette, LA MSA	127	60.84
Lafayette – West Lafayette, IN MSA	69	52.83
Lake Charles, LA MSA	105	62.45
Lakeland – Winter Haven, FL MSA	236	58.22
Lancaster, PA MSA	328	77.57
Lansing – East Lansing, MI MSA	413	95.45
Laredo, TX MSA	50	37.53
Las Cruces, NM MSA	78	57.56
Las Vegas, NV MSA	469	63.25
Lawrence, KS MSA	45	55.01
Lawton, OK MSA	76	68.17
Lewiston – Auburn, ME MSA	73	82.82
Lexington-Fayette, KY MSA	402	138.31
Lima, OH MSA	156	101.08
Lincoln, NE MSA	344	161.02
Little Rock – North Little Rock, AR MSA	729	142.07
Longview – Marshall, TX MSA	86	52.95
Los Angeles – Anaheim – Riverside, CA CMSA	14175	97.55
Louisville, KY – IN MSA	798	83.77
Lubbock, TX MSA	346	155.41
Lynchburg, VA MSA	153	107.60
Macon – Warner Robins, GA MSA	323	114.90
Madison, WI MSA	424	115.50
Manchester, NH MSA	102	69.01
Mansfield, OH MSA	122	96.72
McAllen – Edinburg – Mission, TX MSA	108	28.16
Medford, OR MSA	130	88.80
Melbourne – Titusville – Palm Bay, FL MSA	299	74.94
Memphis, TN – AR – MS MSA	1108	112.86
Merced, CA MSA	123	68.95
Miami – Fort Lauderdale, FL CMSA	3404	106.62
Midland, TX MSA	76	71.29
Milwaukee – Racine, WI CMSA	1500	93.33
Minneapolis – St. Paul, MN – WI MSA	2742	111.28
Mobile, AL MSA	526	110.29
Modesto, CA MSA	275	74.22
Monroe, LA MSA	97	68.22
Montgomery, AL MSA	377	128.88
Muncie, IN MSA	89	74.38
Muskegon, MI MSA	75	47.17
Naples, FL MSA	67	44.05
Nashville, TN MSA	1241	125.99

[Continued]

★ 721 ★

Medicine and Health Managers
[Continued]

MSA/CMSA	Total Employees	Employees per 100,000 pop.
New Bedford, MA MSA	139	79.14
New Haven – Meriden, CT MSA	764	144.10
New London – Norwich, CT – RI MSA	251	94.07
New Orleans, LA MSA	1281	103.41
New York – Northern New Jersey – Long Island, NY – NJ – CT CMSA	18555	102.59
Norfolk – Virginia Beach – Newport News, VA MSA	1147	82.16
Ocala, FL MSA	166	85.20
Odessa, TX MSA	68	57.17
Oklahoma City, OK MSA	974	101.58
Olympia, WA MSA	188	116.60
Omaha, NE – IA MSA	756	122.28
Orlando, FL MSA	849	79.14
Owensboro, KY MSA	97	111.25
Panama City, FL MSA	98	77.17
Parkersburg – Marietta, WV – OH MSA	143	95.86
Pascagoula, MS MSA	95	82.43
Pensacola, FL MSA	323	93.78
Peoria, IL MSA	370	109.09
Philadelphia – Wilmington – Trenton, PA – NJ – DE – MD CMSA	7022	119.03
Phoenix, AZ MSA	2176	102.54
Pine Bluff, AR MSA	75	87.73
Pittsburgh – Beaver Valley, PA CMSA	2460	109.68
Pittsfield, MA MSA	70	88.33
Portland, ME MSA	338	157.00
Portland – Vancouver, OR – WA CMSA	1610	108.94
Portsmouth – Dover – Rochester, NH – ME MSA	158	70.67
Poughkeepsie, NY MSA	311	119.86
Providence – Pawtucket – Fall River, RI – MA CMSA	1048	91.81
Provo – Orem, UT MSA	151	57.29
Pueblo, CO MSA	90	73.14
Raleigh – Durham, NC MSA	1239	168.46
Rapid City, SD MSA	79	97.12
Reading, PA MSA	224	66.56
Redding, CA MSA	103	70.05
Reno, NV MSA	312	122.51
Richland – Kennewick – Pasco, WA MSA	83	55.32
Richmond – Petersburg, VA MSA	1025	118.41
Roanoke, VA MSA	227	101.12
Rochester, MN MSA	238	223.54
Rochester, NY MSA	820	81.80
Rockford, IL MSA	253	89.17
Sacramento, CA MSA	1417	95.67
Saginaw – Bay City – Midland, MI MSA	237	59.35
St. Cloud, MN MSA	117	61.28
St. Joseph, MO MSA	85	102.31
St. Louis, MO – IL MSA	2107	86.21

[Continued]

★ 721 ★

Medicine and Health Managers
[Continued]

MSA/CMSA	Total Employees	Employees per 100,000 pop.
Salem, OR MSA	281	101.07
Salinas – Seaside – Monterey, CA MSA	144	40.49
Salt Lake City – Ogden, UT MSA	968	90.28
San Angelo, TX MSA	78	79.22
San Antonio, TX MSA	1188	91.24
San Diego, CA MSA	2357	94.35
San Francisco – Oakland – San Jose, CA CMSA	6785	108.50
Santa Barbara – Santa Maria – Lompoc, CA MSA	367	99.29
Santa Fe, NM MSA	195	166.61
Sarasota, FL MSA	189	68.04
Savannah, GA MSA	204	84.08
Scranton – Wilkes-Barre, PA MSA	665	90.58
Seattle – Tacoma, WA CMSA	3060	119.57
Sharon, PA MSA	109	90.08
Sheboygan, WI MSA	45	43.32
Sherman – Denison, TX MSA	114	119.97
Shreveport, LA MSA	424	126.82
Sioux City, IA – NE MSA	119	103.46
Sioux Falls, SD MSA	175	141.35
South Bend – Mishawaka, IN MSA	297	120.22
Spokane, WA MSA	407	112.63
Springfield, IL MSA	260	137.17
Springfield, MO MSA	206	85.62
Springfield, MA MSA	580	109.53
State College, PA MSA	72	58.16
Steubenville – Weirton, OH – WV MSA	128	89.81
Stockton, CA MSA	395	82.18
Syracuse, NY MSA	634	96.08
Tallahassee, FL MSA	321	137.42
Tampa – St. Petersburg – Clearwater, FL MSA	2681	129.64
Terre Haute, IN MSA	152	116.20
Texarkana, TX – Texarkana, AR MSA	79	65.76
Toledo, OH MSA	797	129.78
Topeka, KS MSA	192	119.27
Tucson, AZ MSA	817	122.51
Tulsa, OK MSA	653	92.11
Tuscaloosa, AL MSA	160	106.30
Tyler, TX MSA	139	91.86
Utica – Rome, NY MSA	325	102.64
Victoria, TX MSA	92	123.72
Visalia – Tulare – Porterville, CA MSA	185	59.31
Waco, TX MSA	221	116.86
Washington, DC – MD – VA MSA	4720	120.30
Waterbury, CT MSA	264	119.12
Waterloo – Cedar Falls, IA MSA	124	84.58
Wausau, WI MSA	117	101.39

[Continued]

★ 721 ★

Medicine and Health Managers
[Continued]

MSA/CMSA	Total Employees	Employees per 100,000 pop.
West Palm Beach – Boca Raton – Delray Beach, FL MSA	906	104.92
Wheeling, WV – OH MSA	184	115.50
Wichita, KS MSA	558	114.99
Wichita Falls, TX MSA	169	138.10
Williamsport, PA MSA	113	95.19
Wilmington, NC MSA	137	113.90
Worcester, MA MSA	517	118.33
Yakima, WA MSA	183	96.92
York, PA MSA	330	78.98
Youngstown – Warren, OH MSA	428	86.88
Yuba City, CA MSA	86	70.12
Yuma, AZ MSA	78	72.97

Source: Census of Population and Housing, 1990: Equal Employment Opportunity (EEO) File on CD-ROM [machine-readable datafiles]. Prepared by the Bureau of the Census. Washington, DC: The Bureau, 1992.

★ 722 ★

Employment

Nursing Aides, Orderlies, and Attendants

The table below presents the number of civilians 16 years old or older who reported working as nursing aides, orderlies, and attendants during the 1990 Census. Data are provided by total number employed in each Metropolitan Statistical Area (MSA) or Consolidated Metropolitan Statistical Area (CMSA), as well as the number employed per 100,000 people.

[Total for all of the U.S. was 1,859,694; 747.74 per 100,000 persons]

MSA/CMSA	Total Employees	Employees per 100,000 pop.
Abilene, TX MSA	1342	1121.56
Albany, GA MSA	766	680.52
Albany – Schenectady – Troy, NY MSA	7744	885.73
Albuquerque, NM MSA	2506	521.46
Alexandria, LA MSA	1969	1496.70
Allentown – Bethlehem – Easton, PA – NJ MSA	5647	822.35
Altoona, PA MSA	1294	991.25
Amarillo, TX MSA	1381	736.35
Anchorage, AK MSA	1032	455.96
Anderson, IN MSA	1180	903.05
Anderson, SC MSA	932	641.89
Anniston, AL MSA	719	619.65
Appleton – Oshkosh – Neenah, WI MSA	2107	668.63
Asheville, NC MSA	1352	773.36
Athens, GA MSA	888	568.26
Atlanta, GA MSA	12920	455.97
Atlantic City, NJ MSA	2370	741.98

[Continued]

★ 722 ★

Nursing Aides, Orderlies, and Attendants
[Continued]

MSA/CMSA	Total Employees	Employees per 100,000 pop.
Augusta, GA – SC MSA	3405	858.10
Austin, TX MSA	5231	669.29
Bakersfield, CA MSA	2461	452.83
Baltimore, MD MSA	17239	723.67
Bangor, ME MSA	810	912.73
Baton Rouge, LA MSA	3520	666.33
Battle Creek, MI MSA	1286	945.71
Beaumont – Port Arthur, TX MSA	3757	1040.07
Bellingham, WA MSA	839	656.60
Benton Harbor, MI MSA	1036	641.97
Billings, MT MSA	803	707.99
Biloxi – Gulfport, MS MSA	1393	706.66
Binghamton, NY MSA	2504	946.70
Birmingham, AL MSA	6822	751.48
Bismarck, ND MSA	894	1066.43
Bloomington, IN MSA	590	541.39
Bloomington – Normal, IL MSA	797	616.97
Boise City, ID MSA	1111	539.91
Boston – Lawrence – Salem, MA – NH CMSA	34968	838.23
Bradenton, FL MSA	1647	777.96
Bremerton, WA MSA	1298	684.13
Brownsville – Harlingen, TX MSA	1690	649.70
Bryan – College Station, TX MSA	501	411.12
Buffalo – Niagara Falls, NY CMSA	12773	1074.00
Burlington, NC MSA	636	587.73
Burlington, VT MSA	639	486.16
Canton, OH MSA	3541	898.49
Casper, WY MSA	240	391.99
Cedar Rapids, IA MSA	916	542.76
Champaign – Urbana – Rantoul, IL MSA	854	493.57
Charleston, SC MSA	3108	613.17
Charleston, WV MSA	1451	579.35
Charlotte – Gastonia – Rock Hill, NC – SC MSA	6699	576.46
Charlottesville, VA MSA	1082	825.28
Chattanooga, TN – GA MSA	2942	679.12
Cheyenne, WY MSA	382	522.27
Chicago – Gary – Lake County, IL – IN – WI CMSA	43965	545.09
Chico, CA MSA	1582	868.66
Cincinnati – Hamilton, OH – KY – IN CMSA	11595	664.80
Clarksville – Hopkinsville, TN – KY MSA	1107	653.33
Cleveland – Akron – Lorain, OH CMSA	20180	731.21
Colorado Springs, CO MSA	2010	506.28
Columbia, MO MSA	882	784.84
Columbia, SC MSA	3755	828.31
Columbus, GA – AL MSA	1926	792.36
Columbus, OH MSA	9116	661.82

[Continued]

★ 722 ★

Nursing Aides, Orderlies, and Attendants
[Continued]

MSA/CMSA	Total Employees	Employees per 100,000 pop.
Corpus Christi, TX MSA	2701	771.95
Cumberland, MD – WV MSA	1173	1154.04
Dallas – Fort Worth, TX CMSA	20764	534.41
Danville, VA MSA	999	918.95
Davenport – Rock Island – Moline, IA – IL MSA	2693	767.54
Dayton – Springfield, OH MSA	7500	788.42
Daytona Beach, FL MSA	2709	730.76
Decatur, AL MSA	991	753.29
Decatur, IL MSA	1123	958.14
Denver – Boulder, CO CMSA	9140	494.50
Des Moines, IA MSA	2985	759.68
Detroit – Ann Arbor, MI CMSA	31681	679.09
Dothan, AL MSA	855	652.85
Dubuque, IA MSA	909	1052.05
Duluth, MN – WI MSA	2766	1152.64
Eau Claire, WI MSA	1772	1288.32
El Paso, TX MSA	2875	485.96
Elkhart – Goshen, IN MSA	780	499.37
Elmira, NY MSA	1106	1161.83
Enid, OK MSA	750	1321.94
Erie, PA MSA	2334	846.97
Eugene – Springfield, OR MSA	2026	716.12
Evansville, IN – KY MSA	2686	962.76
Fargo – Moorhead, ND – MN MSA	1511	985.67
Fayetteville, NC MSA	1412	514.27
Fayetteville – Springdale, AR MSA	783	690.42
Fitchburg – Leominster, MA MSA	1039	1010.73
Flint, MI MSA	3050	708.55
Florence, AL MSA	940	715.77
Florence, SC MSA	1119	978.63
Fort Collins – Loveland, CO MSA	1016	545.84
Fort Myers – Cape Coral, FL MSA	2210	659.48
Fort Pierce, FL MSA	1593	634.48
Fort Smith, AR – OK MSA	1503	854.41
Fort Walton Beach, FL MSA	686	477.13
Fort Wayne, IN MSA	2815	773.75
Fresno, CA MSA	4656	697.54
Gadsden, AL MSA	888	889.42
Gainesville, FL MSA	1590	778.99
Glens Falls, NY MSA	1001	844.45
Grand Forks, ND MSA	579	819.15
Grand Rapids, MI MSA	4925	715.43
Great Falls, MT MSA	681	876.55
Greeley, CO MSA	810	614.47
Green Bay, WI MSA	1345	691.18
Greensboro – Winston-Salem – High Point, NC MSA	6333	672.23

[Continued]

★ 722 ★

Nursing Aides, Orderlies, and Attendants

[Continued]

MSA/CMSA	Total Employees	Employees per 100,000 pop.
Greenville – Spartanburg, SC MSA	3317	517.58
Hagerstown, MD MSA	1167	961.34
Harrisburg – Lebanon – Carlisle, PA MSA	4826	820.77
Hartford – New Britain – Middletown, CT CMSA	9983	919.38
Hickory – Morganton, NC MSA	1531	690.57
Honolulu, HI MSA	3743	447.60
Houma – Thibodaux, LA MSA	1078	589.58
Houston – Galveston – Brazoria, TX CMSA	20983	565.42
Huntington – Ashland, WV – KY – OH MSA	2151	688.26
Huntsville, AL MSA	1222	511.49
Indianapolis, IN MSA	8196	655.77
Iowa City, IA MSA	1129	1174.59
Jackson, MI MSA	1176	785.28
Jackson, MS MSA	3575	904.16
Jackson, TN MSA	756	969.45
Jacksonville, FL MSA	5192	572.61
Jacksonville, NC MSA	926	618.00
Jamestown – Dunkirk, NY	1960	1381.30
Janesville – Beloit, WI MSA	1446	1036.48
Johnson City – Kingsport – Bristol, TN – VA MSA	3215	737.31
Johnstown, PA MSA	2682	1111.72
Joplin, MO MSA	934	692.31
Kalamazoo, MI MSA	1905	852.69
Kankakee, IL MSA	906	941.25
Kansas City, MO – KS MSA	10575	675.17
Killeen – Temple, TX MSA	2081	815.12
Knoxville, TN MSA	3747	619.53
Kokomo, IN MSA	865	892.25
La Crosse, WI MSA	1008	1029.58
Lafayette, LA MSA	1278	612.24
Lafayette – West Lafayette, IN MSA	813	622.52
Lake Charles, LA MSA	1398	831.48
Lakeland – Winter Haven, FL MSA	2436	600.91
Lancaster, PA MSA	3365	795.84
Lansing – East Lansing, MI MSA	2459	568.33
Laredo, TX MSA	864	648.46
Las Cruces, NM MSA	649	478.93
Las Vegas, NV MSA	2376	320.45
Lawrence, KS MSA	418	511.01
Lawton, OK MSA	826	740.90
Lewiston – Auburn, ME MSA	988	1120.93
Lexington-Fayette, KY MSA	2242	643.46
Lima, OH MSA	1363	883.12
Lincoln, NE MSA	1548	724.58
Little Rock – North Little Rock, AR MSA	4489	874.85
Longview – Marshall, TX MSA	1730	1065.07

[Continued]

★ 722 ★

Nursing Aides, Orderlies, and Attendants
[Continued]

MSA/CMSA	Total Employees	Employees per 100,000 pop.
Los Angeles – Anaheim – Riverside, CA CMSA	73157	503.44
Louisville, KY – IN MSA	7405	777.30
Lubbock, TX MSA	2378	1068.11
Lynchburg, VA MSA	2159	1518.29
Macon – Warner Robins, GA MSA	2329	828.52
Madison, WI MSA	3063	834.41
Manchester, NH MSA	969	655.58
Mansfield, OH MSA	869	688.93
McAllen – Edinburg – Mission, TX MSA	1884	491.21
Medford, OR MSA	798	545.12
Melbourne – Titusville – Palm Bay, FL MSA	1910	478.72
Memphis, TN – AR – MS MSA	7241	737.56
Merced, CA MSA	955	535.30
Miami – Fort Lauderdale, FL CMSA	23608	739.46
Midland, TX MSA	634	594.69
Milwaukee – Racine, WI CMSA	13118	816.21
Minneapolis – St. Paul, MN – WI MSA	17794	722.12
Mobile, AL MSA	3653	765.95
Modesto, CA MSA	2148	579.72
Monroe, LA MSA	1267	891.05
Montgomery, AL MSA	2045	699.10
Muncie, IN MSA	1036	865.79
Muskegon, MI MSA	1418	891.92
Naples, FL MSA	798	524.66
Nashville, TN MSA	5997	608.82
New Bedford, MA MSA	1887	1074.35
New Haven – Meriden, CT MSA	4934	930.63
New London – Norwich, CT – RI MSA	2862	1072.64
New Orleans, LA MSA	8677	700.43
New York – Northern New Jersey – Long Island, NY – NJ – CT CMSA	181173	1001.66
Norfolk – Virginia Beach – Newport News, VA MSA	8596	615.71
Ocala, FL MSA	1251	642.09
Odessa, TX MSA	707	594.45
Oklahoma City, OK MSA	7396	771.35
Olympia, WA MSA	804	498.64
Omaha, NE – IA MSA	4081	660.08
Orlando, FL MSA	5583	520.44
Owensboro, KY MSA	775	888.87
Panama City, FL MSA	690	543.33
Parkersburg – Marietta, WV – OH MSA	1102	738.76
Pascagoula, MS MSA	542	470.31
Pensacola, FL MSA	2270	659.11
Peoria, IL MSA	2739	807.55
Philadelphia – Wilmington – Trenton, PA – NJ – DE – MD CMSA	43855	743.39
Phoenix, AZ MSA	11016	519.11
Pine Bluff, AR MSA	774	905.40

[Continued]

★ 722 ★

Nursing Aides, Orderlies, and Attendants

[Continued]

MSA/CMSA	Total Employees	Employees per 100,000 pop.
Pittsburgh – Beaver Valley, PA CMSA	18505	825.09
Pittsfield, MA MSA	856	1080.13
Portland, ME MSA	1510	701.41
Portland – Vancouver, OR – WA CMSA	9022	610.46
Portsmouth – Dover – Rochester, NH – ME MSA	1346	602.03
Poughkeepsie, NY MSA	2347	904.56
Providence – Pawtucket – Fall River, RI – MA CMSA	11574	1013.92
Provo – Orem, UT MSA	1297	492.05
Pueblo, CO MSA	1226	996.33
Raleigh – Durham, NC MSA	4750	645.84
Rapid City, SD MSA	312	383.56
Reading, PA MSA	2470	733.98
Redding, CA MSA	1170	795.72
Reno, NV MSA	1103	433.11
Richland – Kennewick – Pasco, WA MSA	545	363.25
Richmond – Petersburg, VA MSA	7295	842.73
Roanoke, VA MSA	2143	954.66
Rochester, MN MSA	1223	1148.68
Rochester, NY MSA	9118	909.61
Rockford, IL MSA	2038	718.32
Sacramento, CA MSA	7917	534.53
Saginaw – Bay City – Midland, MI MSA	3050	763.80
St. Cloud, MN MSA	1600	838.04
St. Joseph, MO MSA	891	1072.42
St. Louis, MO – IL MSA	18788	768.71
Salem, OR MSA	3526	1268.24
Salinas – Seaside – Monterey, CA MSA	1876	527.19
Salt Lake City – Ogden, UT MSA	4147	386.77
San Angelo, TX MSA	1335	1355.91
San Antonio, TX MSA	9592	736.66
San Diego, CA MSA	13287	531.90
San Francisco – Oakland – San Jose, CA CMSA	34278	548.16
Santa Barbara – Santa Maria – Lompoc, CA MSA	2032	549.77
Santa Fe, NM MSA	592	505.80
Sarasota, FL MSA	2476	891.37
Savannah, GA MSA	2007	827.21
Scranton – Wilkes-Barre, PA MSA	6540	890.80
Seattle – Tacoma, WA CMSA	15546	607.46
Sharon, PA MSA	1424	1176.83
Sheboygan, WI MSA	896	862.56
Sherman – Denison, TX MSA	997	1049.24
Shreveport, LA MSA	3470	1037.86
Sioux City, IA – NE MSA	1085	943.33
Sioux Falls, SD MSA	971	784.27
South Bend – Mishawaka, IN MSA	1634	661.40
Spokane, WA MSA	3137	868.10

[Continued]

★ 722 ★

Nursing Aides, Orderlies, and Attendants
[Continued]

MSA/CMSA	Total Employees	Employees per 100,000 pop.
Springfield, IL MSA	1612	850.44
Springfield, MO MSA	2167	900.69
Springfield, MA MSA	6268	1183.72
State College, PA MSA	547	441.89
Steubenville – Weirton, OH – WV MSA	1238	868.63
Stockton, CA MSA	3167	658.93
Syracuse, NY MSA	5136	778.34
Tallahassee, FL MSA	1681	719.61
Tampa – St. Petersburg – Clearwater, FL MSA	14117	682.65
Terre Haute, IN MSA	1045	798.86
Texarkana, TX – Texarkana, AR MSA	1203	1001.40
Toledo, OH MSA	5099	830.28
Topeka, KS MSA	1806	1121.91
Tucson, AZ MSA	4772	715.57
Tulsa, OK MSA	6091	859.15
Tuscaloosa, AL MSA	2274	1510.74
Tyler, TX MSA	1535	1014.48
Utica – Rome, NY MSA	3990	1260.13
Victoria, TX MSA	574	771.91
Visalia – Tulare – Porterville, CA MSA	2905	931.33
Waco, TX MSA	1823	963.92
Washington, DC – MD – VA MSA	19945	508.34
Waterbury, CT MSA	3031	1367.60
Waterloo – Cedar Falls, IA MSA	1303	888.75
Wausau, WI MSA	829	718.37
West Palm Beach – Boca Raton – Delray Beach, FL MSA	5584	646.66
Wheeling, WV – OH MSA	1647	1033.89
Wichita, KS MSA	3163	651.80
Wichita Falls, TX MSA	1571	1283.73
Williamsport, PA MSA	1050	884.51
Wilmington, NC MSA	769	639.32
Worcester, MA MSA	4727	1081.93
Yakima, WA MSA	1355	717.60
York, PA MSA	2874	687.81
Youngstown – Warren, OH MSA	4181	848.73
Yuba City, CA MSA	660	538.15
Yuma, AZ MSA	500	467.75

Source: Census of Population and Housing, 1990: Equal Employment Opportunity (EEO) File on CD-ROM [machine-readable datafiles]. Prepared by the Bureau of the Census. Washington, DC: The Bureau, 1992.

★ 723 ★

Employment

Nursing Services Demand: 1990 to 2020

This table shows the increasing number of full-time equivalent nursing personnel needed to meet U.S. demand for nursing services through the year 2020. The increasing need for nursing personnel for older Americans contributes to a greater need for service to the overall population.

Year	Demand for full-time equivalent nurses for older Americans					All settings for all ages	Percent of total demand attributed to older Americans
	All hospitals	Nursing homes	Home health	Other	All settings		
RNs							
1990	420,600	94,900	29,600	38,900	584,000	1,476,000	39.6
1995	469,300	119,800	32,600	42,900	665,000	1,610,000	41.3
2000	510,100	147,900	35,300	45,800	739,000	1,736,000	42.6
2005	556,400	174,700	37,300	48,900	817,000	1,854,000	44.1
2010	609,200	201,900	39,200	54,100	904,000	1,964,000	46.0
2015	681,300	209,600	41,300	62,000	994,000	2,052,000	48.4
2020	783,900	223,900	45,800	72,200	1,126,000	2,155,000	52.3
LP/VNs							
1990	98,100	112,100	2,300	19,500	232,000	476,000	48.7
1995	97,400	126,700	2,500	20,900	248,000	490,000	50.6
2000	93,400	141,200	2,700	21,600	259,000	500,000	51.8
2005	89,900	154,100	2,900	22,500	269,000	513,000	52.4
2010	88,500	166,900	3,000	24,300	283,000	527,000	53.7
2015	90,200	164,800	3,200	27,100	285,000	529,000	53.9
2020	101,100	167,300	3,500	30,800	303,000	538,000	56.3
Aldes							
1990	159,100	421,900	16,400	-	597,000	860,000	69.4
1995	173,000	483,200	19,100	-	675,000	942,000	71.7
2000	183,400	545,500	21,700	-	751,000	1,023,000	73.4
2005	193,100	602,200	23,900	-	819,000	1,097,000	74.7
2010	207,100	658,500	26,000	-	892,000	1,168,000	76.4
2015	227,700	655,500	28,100	-	911,000	1,178,000	77.3
2020	257,000	671,100	32,000	-	960,000	1,211,000	79.3

Source: U.S. House of Representatives. *Shortage of Health Care Professions Caring for the Elderly: Recommendations for Change.* 102d Cong., 2nd sess., December 1992. Comm. Pub. No. 102-915. Washington, DC: U.S. Government Printing Office, 1993, pp. 40-41. Primary source: Projections prepared by Division of Nursing, Bureau of Health Professions, Health Resources and Services Administration, U.S. Department of Health and Human Services, 1992. *Notes:* RN stands for registered nurse; LPN stands for licensed practical nurse; VN stands for vocational nurse.

★724★

Employment

Occupational Therapists

The table below presents the number of civilians 16 years old or older who reported working as occupational therapists during the 1990 Census. Data are provided by total number employed in each Metropolitan Statistical Area (MSA) or Consolidated Metropolitan Statistical Area (CMSA), as well as the number employed per 100,000 people.

[Total for all of the U.S. was 37,895; 15.24 per 100,000 persons]

MSA/CMSA	Total Employees	Employees per 100,000 pop.
Abilene, TX MSA	35	29.25
Albany, GA MSA	5	4.44
Albany–Schenectady–Troy, NY MSA	163	18.64
Albuquerque, NM MSA	190	39.54
Alexandria, LA MSA	71	53.97
Allentown–Bethlehem–Easton, PA–NJ MSA	219	31.89
Altoona, PA MSA	20	15.32
Amarillo, TX MSA	40	21.33
Anchorage, AK MSA	31	13.70
Anderson, SC MSA	38	26.17
Appleton–Oshkosh–Neenah, WI MSA	59	18.72
Asheville, NC MSA	66	37.75
Athens, GA MSA	37	23.68
Atlanta, GA MSA	331	11.68
Atlantic City, NJ MSA	83	25.98
Augusta, GA–SC MSA	94	23.69
Austin, TX MSA	181	23.16
Bakersfield, CA MSA	32	5.89
Baltimore, MD MSA	532	22.33
Bangor, ME MSA	33	37.19
Baton Rouge, LA MSA	62	11.74
Battle Creek, MI MSA	44	32.36
Beaumont–Port Arthur, TX MSA	7	1.94
Bellingham, WA MSA	25	19.56
Benton Harbor, MI MSA	17	10.53
Billings, MT MSA	33	29.10
Biloxi–Gulfport, MS MSA	11	5.58
Binghamton, NY MSA	24	9.07
Birmingham, AL MSA	243	26.77
Bismarck, ND MSA	17	20.28
Bloomington, IN MSA	7	6.42
Bloomington–Normal, IL MSA	21	16.26
Boise City, ID MSA	22	10.69
Boston–Lawrence–Salem, MA–NH CMSA	1357	32.53
Bradenton, FL MSA	12	5.67
Bremerton, WA MSA	33	17.39
Brownsville–Harlingen, TX MSA	5	1.92
Bryan–College Station, TX MSA	13	10.67
Buffalo–Niagara Falls, NY CMSA	462	38.85
Burlington, VT MSA	17	12.93
Canton, OH MSA	106	26.90
Casper, WY MSA	15	24.50

[Continued]

★ 724 ★

Occupational Therapists
[Continued]

MSA/CMSA	Total Employees	Employees per 100,000 pop.
Cedar Rapids, IA MSA	54	32.00
Champaign–Urbana–Rantoul, IL MSA	43	24.85
Charleston, SC MSA	43	8.48
Charleston, WV MSA	14	5.59
Charlotte–Gastonia–Rock Hill, NC–SC MSA	75	6.45
Charlottesville, VA MSA	61	46.53
Chattanooga, TN–GA MSA	48	11.08
Cheyenne, WY MSA	28	38.28
Chicago–Gary–Lake County, IL–IN–WI CMSA	1371	17.00
Chico, CA MSA	35	19.22
Cincinnati–Hamilton, OH–KY–IN CMSA	221	12.67
Clarksville–Hopkinsville, TN–KY MSA	11	6.49
Cleveland–Akron–Lorain, OH CMSA	469	16.99
Colorado Springs, CO MSA	128	32.24
Columbia, MO MSA	20	17.80
Columbia, SC MSA	38	8.38
Columbus, GA–AL MSA	44	18.10
Columbus, OH MSA	366	26.57
Corpus Christi, TX MSA	23	6.57
Dallas–Fort Worth, TX CMSA	579	14.90
Davenport–Rock Island–Moline, IA–IL MSA	47	13.40
Dayton–Springfield, OH MSA	174	18.29
Daytona Beach, FL MSA	19	5.13
Decatur, AL MSA	3	2.28
Decatur, IL MSA	7	5.97
Denver–Boulder, CO CMSA	554	29.97
Des Moines, IA MSA	67	17.05
Detroit–Ann Arbor, MI CMSA	948	20.32
Dothan, AL MSA	12	9.16
Dubuque, IA MSA	31	35.88
Duluth, MN–WI MSA	75	31.25
Eau Claire, WI MSA	44	31.99
El Paso, TX MSA	60	10.14
Elmira, NY MSA	42	44.12
Enid, OK MSA	44	77.55
Erie, PA MSA	61	22.14
Eugene–Springfield, OR MSA	49	17.32
Evansville, IN–KY MSA	18	6.45
Fargo–Moorhead, ND–MN MSA	29	18.92
Fayetteville, NC MSA	53	19.30
Fayetteville–Springdale, AR MSA	8	7.05
Fitchburg–Leominster, MA MSA	14	13.62
Flint, MI MSA	70	16.26
Florence, AL MSA	8	6.09
Florence, SC MSA	18	15.74
Fort Collins–Loveland, CO MSA	72	38.68

[Continued]

★ 724 ★

Occupational Therapists
[Continued]

MSA/CMSA	Total Employees	Employees per 100,000 pop.
Fort Myers – Cape Coral, FL MSA	44	13.13
Fort Pierce, FL MSA	13	5.18
Fort Smith, AR – OK MSA	6	3.41
Fort Walton Beach, FL MSA	28	19.47
Fort Wayne, IN MSA	81	22.26
Fresno, CA MSA	37	5.54
Gadsden, AL MSA	16	16.03
Gainesville, FL MSA	26	12.74
Glens Falls, NY MSA	19	16.03
Grand Forks, ND MSA	29	41.03
Grand Rapids, MI MSA	299	43.43
Great Falls, MT MSA	12	15.45
Greeley, CO MSA	2	1.52
Green Bay, WI MSA	61	31.35
Greensboro – Winston-Salem – High Point, NC MSA	143	15.18
Greenville – Spartanburg, SC MSA	50	7.80
Hagerstown, MD MSA	22	18.12
Harrisburg – Lebanon – Carlisle, PA MSA	53	9.01
Hartford – New Britain – Middletown, CT CMSA	277	25.51
Hickory – Morganton, NC MSA	22	9.92
Honolulu, HI MSA	189	22.60
Houston – Galveston – Brazoria, TX CMSA	606	16.33
Huntington – Ashland, WV – KY – OH MSA	22	7.04
Huntsville, AL MSA	45	18.84
Indianapolis, IN MSA	250	20.00
Iowa City, IA MSA	41	42.66
Jackson, MI MSA	8	5.34
Jackson, MS MSA	50	12.65
Jacksonville, FL MSA	105	11.58
Jacksonville, NC MSA	29	19.35
Jamestown – Dunkirk, NY	3	2.11
Janesville – Beloit, WI MSA	43	30.82
Johnson City – Kingsport – Bristol, TN – VA MSA	30	6.88
Johnstown, PA MSA	74	30.67
Kalamazoo, MI MSA	115	51.47
Kankakee, IL MSA	22	22.86
Kansas City, MO – KS MSA	426	27.20
Killeen – Temple, TX MSA	26	10.18
Knoxville, TN MSA	91	15.05
Kokomo, IN MSA	13	13.41
La Crosse, WI MSA	53	54.13
Lafayette, LA MSA	6	2.87
Lafayette – West Lafayette, IN MSA	22	16.85
Lakeland – Winter Haven, FL MSA	23	5.67
Lancaster, PA MSA	103	24.36
Lansing – East Lansing, MI MSA	60	13.87

[Continued]

★ 724 ★

Occupational Therapists

[Continued]

MSA/CMSA	Total Employees	Employees per 100,000 pop.
Las Cruces, NM MSA	14	10.33
Las Vegas, NV MSA	56	7.55
Lawrence, KS MSA	22	26.90
Lawton, OK MSA	7	6.28
Lewiston – Auburn, ME MSA	7	7.94
Lexington-Fayette, KY MSA	36	10.33
Lincoln, NE MSA	54	25.28
Little Rock – North Little Rock, AR MSA	133	25.92
Longview – Marshall, TX MSA	11	6.77
Los Angeles – Anaheim – Riverside, CA CMSA	1663	11.44
Louisville, KY – IN MSA	82	8.61
Lubbock, TX MSA	24	10.78
Lynchburg, VA MSA	11	7.74
Macon – Warner Robins, GA MSA	24	8.54
Madison, WI MSA	119	32.42
Manchester, NH MSA	36	24.36
Mansfield, OH MSA	6	4.76
McAllen – Edinburg – Mission, TX MSA	12	3.13
Medford, OR MSA	16	10.93
Melbourne – Titusville – Palm Bay, FL MSA	20	5.01
Memphis, TN – AR – MS MSA	72	7.33
Merced, CA MSA	9	5.04
Miami – Fort Lauderdale, FL CMSA	490	15.35
Milwaukee – Racine, WI CMSA	854	53.14
Minneapolis – St. Paul, MN – WI MSA	964	39.12
Mobile, AL MSA	58	12.16
Modesto, CA MSA	68	18.35
Monroe, LA MSA	37	26.02
Montgomery, AL MSA	30	10.26
Muskegon, MI MSA	19	11.95
Naples, FL MSA	19	12.49
Nashville, TN MSA	160	16.24
New Bedford, MA MSA	22	12.53
New Haven – Meriden, CT MSA	145	27.35
New London – Norwich, CT – RI MSA	13	4.87
New Orleans, LA MSA	186	15.01
New York – Northern New Jersey – Long Island, NY – NJ – CT CMSA	3575	19.77
Norfolk – Virginia Beach – Newport News, VA MSA	132	9.45
Ocala, FL MSA	8	4.11
Oklahoma City, OK MSA	110	11.47
Olympia, WA MSA	32	19.85
Omaha, NE – IA MSA	87	14.07
Orlando, FL MSA	177	16.50
Pensacola, FL MSA	26	7.55
Peoria, IL MSA	35	10.32
Philadelphia – Wilmington – Trenton, PA – NJ – DE – MD CMSA	1141	19.34

[Continued]

★ 724 ★

Occupational Therapists
[Continued]

MSA/CMSA	Total Employees	Employees per 100,000 pop.
Phoenix, AZ MSA	348	16.40
Pine Bluff, AR MSA	8	9.36
Pittsburgh – Beaver Valley, PA CMSA	469	20.91
Pittsfield, MA MSA	8	10.09
Portland, ME MSA	42	19.51
Portland – Vancouver, OR – WA CMSA	265	17.93
Portsmouth – Dover – Rochester, NH – ME MSA	118	52.78
Poughkeepsie, NY MSA	48	18.50
Providence – Pawtucket – Fall River, RI – MA CMSA	193	16.91
Provo – Orem, UT MSA	6	2.28
Pueblo, CO MSA	9	7.31
Raleigh – Durham, NC MSA	152	20.67
Reading, PA MSA	34	10.10
Redding, CA MSA	14	9.52
Reno, NV MSA	84	32.98
Richmond – Petersburg, VA MSA	183	21.14
Roanoke, VA MSA	51	22.72
Rochester, MN MSA	54	50.72
Rochester, NY MSA	189	18.85
Rockford, IL MSA	36	12.69
Sacramento, CA MSA	155	10.47
Saginaw – Bay City – Midland, MI MSA	82	20.53
St. Cloud, MN MSA	59	30.90
St. Joseph, MO MSA	12	14.44
St. Louis, MO – IL MSA	449	18.37
Salem, OR MSA	48	17.26
Salinas – Seaside – Monterey, CA MSA	35	9.84
Salt Lake City – Ogden, UT MSA	69	6.44
San Angelo, TX MSA	18	18.28
San Antonio, TX MSA	211	16.20
San Diego, CA MSA	349	13.97
San Francisco – Oakland – San Jose, CA CMSA	1186	18.97
Santa Barbara – Santa Maria – Lompoc, CA MSA	82	22.19
Santa Fe, NM MSA	19	16.23
Sarasota, FL MSA	27	9.72
Savannah, GA MSA	23	9.48
Scranton – Wilkes-Barre, PA MSA	90	12.26
Seattle – Tacoma, WA CMSA	696	27.20
Sheboygan, WI MSA	6	5.78
Sherman – Denison, TX MSA	18	18.94
Shreveport, LA MSA	43	12.86
Sioux Falls, SD MSA	36	29.08
South Bend – Mishawaka, IN MSA	37	14.98
Spokane, WA MSA	127	35.14
Springfield, IL MSA	37	19.52
Springfield, MO MSA	29	12.05

[Continued]

★ 724 ★

Occupational Therapists
[Continued]

MSA/CMSA	Total Employees	Employees per 100,000 pop.
Springfield, MA MSA	73	13.79
State College, PA MSA	18	14.54
Stockton, CA MSA	34	7.07
Syracuse, NY MSA	174	26.37
Tallahassee, FL MSA	10	4.28
Tampa–St. Petersburg–Clearwater, FL MSA	177	8.56
Texarkana, TX–Texarkana, AR MSA	14	11.65
Toledo, OH MSA	165	26.87
Topeka, KS MSA	49	30.44
Tucson, AZ MSA	108	16.19
Tulsa, OK MSA	121	17.07
Tuscaloosa, AL MSA	21	13.95
Tyler, TX MSA	13	8.59
Utica–Rome, NY MSA	109	34.42
Visalia–Tulare–Porterville, CA MSA	10	3.21
Waco, TX MSA	24	12.69
Washington, DC–MD–VA MSA	607	15.47
Waterbury, CT MSA	29	13.08
Wausau, WI MSA	36	31.20
West Palm Beach–Boca Raton–Delray Beach, FL MSA	83	9.61
Wheeling, WV–OH MSA	19	11.93
Wichita, KS MSA	60	12.36
Wichita Falls, TX MSA	26	21.25
Williamsport, PA MSA	4	3.37
Wilmington, NC MSA	4	3.33
Worcester, MA MSA	118	27.01
Yakima, WA MSA	57	30.19
York, PA MSA	37	8.85
Youngstown–Warren, OH MSA	58	11.77

Source: Census of Population and Housing, 1990: Equal Employment Opportunity (EEO) File on CD-ROM [machine-readable datafiles]. Prepared by the Bureau of the Census. Washington, DC: The Bureau, 1992.

★ 725 ★

Employment

Optical Goods Workers

The table below presents the number of civilians 16 years old or older who reported working as optical goods workers during the 1990 Census; for example, ophthalmic laboratory technicians. Data are provided by total number employed in each Metropolitan Statistical Area (MSA) or Consolidated Metropolitan Statistical Area (CMSA), as well as the number employed per 100,000 people.

[Total for all of the U.S. was 74,907; 30.12 per 100,000 persons]

MSA/CMSA	Total Employees	Employees per 100,000 pop.
Abilene, TX MSA	29	24.24
Albany, GA MSA	53	47.09
Albany – Schenectady – Troy, NY MSA	257	29.39
Albuquerque, NM MSA	297	61.80
Alexandria, LA MSA	15	11.40
Allentown – Bethlehem – Easton, PA – NJ MSA	240	34.95
Altoona, PA MSA	25	19.15
Amarillo, TX MSA	118	62.92
Anchorage, AK MSA	37	16.35
Anderson, IN MSA	28	21.43
Anderson, SC MSA	45	30.99
Anniston, AL MSA	76	65.50
Appleton – Oshkosh – Neenah, WI MSA	109	34.59
Asheville, NC MSA	30	17.16
Athens, GA MSA	68	43.52
Atlanta, GA MSA	1024	36.14
Atlantic City, NJ MSA	48	15.03
Augusta, GA – SC MSA	86	21.67
Austin, TX MSA	233	29.81
Bakersfield, CA MSA	116	21.34
Baltimore, MD MSA	753	31.61
Bangor, ME MSA	26	29.30
Baton Rouge, LA MSA	145	27.45
Battle Creek, MI MSA	35	25.74
Beaumont – Port Arthur, TX MSA	149	41.25
Bellingham, WA MSA	50	39.13
Benton Harbor, MI MSA	80	49.57
Billings, MT MSA	72	63.48
Biloxi – Gulfport, MS MSA	80	40.58
Binghamton, NY MSA	60	22.68
Birmingham, AL MSA	188	20.71
Bismarck, ND MSA	67	79.92
Bloomington, IN MSA	16	14.68
Bloomington – Normal, IL MSA	46	35.61
Boise City, ID MSA	89	43.25
Boston – Lawrence – Salem, MA – NH CMSA	1216	29.15
Bradenton, FL MSA	179	84.55
Bremerton, WA MSA	98	51.65
Brownsville – Harlingen, TX MSA	74	28.45
Bryan – College Station, TX MSA	23	18.87
Buffalo – Niagara Falls, NY CMSA	608	51.12
Burlington, NC MSA	56	51.75

[Continued]

★ 725 ★

Optical Goods Workers
[Continued]

MSA/CMSA	Total Employees	Employees per 100,000 pop.
Burlington, VT MSA	57	43.37
Canton, OH MSA	138	35.02
Casper, WY MSA	34	55.53
Cedar Rapids, IA MSA	31	18.37
Champaign – Urbana – Rantoul, IL MSA	79	45.66
Charleston, SC MSA	194	38.27
Charleston, WV MSA	69	27.55
Charlotte – Gastonia – Rock Hill, NC – SC MSA	353	30.38
Charlottesville, VA MSA	54	41.19
Chattanooga, TN – GA MSA	106	24.47
Cheyenne, WY MSA	36	49.22
Chicago – Gary – Lake County, IL – IN – WI CMSA	2388	29.61
Chico, CA MSA	88	48.32
Cincinnati – Hamilton, OH – KY – IN CMSA	742	42.54
Clarksville – Hopkinsville, TN – KY MSA	32	18.89
Cleveland – Akron – Lorain, OH CMSA	1140	41.31
Colorado Springs, CO MSA	166	41.81
Columbia, MO MSA	33	29.36
Columbia, SC MSA	158	34.85
Columbus, GA – AL MSA	54	22.22
Columbus, OH MSA	369	26.79
Corpus Christi, TX MSA	93	26.58
Cumberland, MD WV MSA	9	8.85
Dallas – Fort Worth, TX CMSA	1495	38.48
Danville, VA MSA	16	14.72
Davenport – Rock Island – Moline, IA – IL MSA	100	47.31
Dayton – Springfield, OH MSA	306	32.17
Daytona Beach, FL MSA	162	43.70
Decatur, AL MSA	68	51.69
Decatur, IL MSA	80	68.26
Denver – Boulder, CO CMSA	794	42.96
Des Moines, IA MSA	132	33.59
Detroit – Ann Arbor, MI CMSA	1637	35.09
Dothan, AL MSA	50	38.18
Dubuque, IA MSA	29	33.56
Duluth, MN – WI MSA	100	41.67
Eau Claire, WI MSA	56	40.71
El Paso, TX MSA	147	24.85
Elkhart – Goshen, IN MSA	26	16.65
Elmira, NY MSA	39	40.97
Enid, OK MSA	16	28.20
Erie, PA MSA	105	38.10
Eugene – Springfield, OR MSA	50	17.67
Evansville, IN – KY MSA	84	30.11
Fargo – Moorhead, ND – MN MSA	103	67.19
Fayetteville, NC MSA	62	22.58

[Continued]

★ 725 ★

Optical Goods Workers
[Continued]

MSA/CMSA	Total Employees	Employees per 100,000 pop.
Fayetteville – Springdale, AR MSA	40	35.27
Fitchburg – Leominster, MA MSA	23	22.37
Flint, MI MSA	169	39.26
Florence, AL MSA	25	19.04
Florence, SC MSA	43	37.61
Fort Collins – Loveland, CO MSA	48	25.79
Fort Myers – Cape Coral, FL MSA	90	26.86
Fort Pierce, FL MSA	102	40.63
Fort Smith, AR – OK MSA	52	29.56
Fort Walton Beach, FL MSA	23	16.00
Fort Wayne, IN MSA	128	35.18
Fresno, CA MSA	136	20.37
Gadsden, AL MSA	38	38.06
Gainesville, FL MSA	55	26.95
Glens Falls, NY MSA	112	94.48
Grand Forks, ND MSA	43	60.84
Grand Rapids, MI MSA	250	36.32
Great Falls, MT MSA	43	55.35
Greeley, CO MSA	29	22.00
Green Bay, WI MSA	144	74.00
Greensboro – Winston-Salem – High Point, NC MSA	334	35.45
Greenville – Spartanburg, SC MSA	213	33.24
Hagerstown, MD MSA	28	23.07
Harrisburg – Lebanon – Carlisle, PA MSA	179	30.44
Hartford – New Britain – Middletown, CT CMSA	348	32.05
Hickory – Morganton, NC MSA	40	18.04
Honolulu, HI MSA	228	27.27
Houma – Thibodaux, LA MSA	35	19.14
Houston – Galveston – Brazoria, TX CMSA	1065	28.70
Huntington – Ashland, WV – KY – OH MSA	94	30.08
Huntsville, AL MSA	48	20.09
Indianapolis, IN MSA	391	31.28
Iowa City, IA MSA	38	39.53
Jackson, MI MSA	50	33.39
Jackson, MS MSA	113	28.58
Jackson, TN MSA	80	102.59
Jacksonville, FL MSA	539	59.44
Jacksonville, NC MSA	28	18.69
Jamestown – Dunkirk, NY	10	7.05
Janesville – Beloit, WI MSA	57	40.86
Johnson City – Kingsport – Bristol, TN – VA MSA	114	26.14
Johnstown, PA MSA	38	15.75
Joplin, MO MSA	69	51.15
Kalamazoo, MI MSA	67	29.99
Kansas City, MO – KS MSA	428	27.33
Killeen – Temple, TX MSA	50	19.58

[Continued]

★ 725 ★

Optical Goods Workers
[Continued]

MSA/CMSA	Total Employees	Employees per 100,000 pop.
Knoxville, TN MSA	150	24.80
Kokomo, IN MSA	43	44.35
La Crosse, WI MSA	30	30.64
Lafayette, LA MSA	87	41.68
Lafayette – West Lafayette, IN MSA	86	65.85
Lake Charles, LA MSA	83	49.37
Lakeland – Winter Haven, FL MSA	164	40.46
Lancaster, PA MSA	102	24.12
Lansing – East Lansing, MI MSA	142	32.82
Las Cruces, NM MSA	47	34.68
Las Vegas, NV MSA	168	22.66
Lawrence, KS MSA	7	8.56
Lawton, OK MSA	48	43.05
Lewiston – Auburn, ME MSA	28	31.77
Lexington-Fayette, KY MSA	130	37.31
Lima, OH MSA	32	20.73
Lincoln, NE MSA	62	29.02
Little Rock – North Little Rock, AR MSA	160	31.18
Longview – Marshall, TX MSA	23	14.16
Los Angeles – Anaheim – Riverside, CA CMSA	4549	31.30
Louisville, KY – IN MSA	305	32.02
Lubbock, TX MSA	108	48.61
Lynchburg, VA MSA	76	53.45
Macon – Warner Robins, GA MSA	72	25.61
Madison, WI MSA	125	34.05
Manchester, NH MSA	71	48.03
Mansfield, OH MSA	45	35.68
McAllen – Edinburg – Mission, TX MSA	51	13.30
Medford, OR MSA	14	9.56
Melbourne – Titusville – Palm Bay, FL MSA	152	38.10
Memphis, TN – AR – MS MSA	289	29.44
Merced, CA MSA	16	8.97
Miami – Fort Lauderdale, FL CMSA	1496	46.86
Midland, TX MSA	32	30.02
Milwaukee – Racine, WI CMSA	471	29.31
Minneapolis – St. Paul, MN – WI MSA	1197	48.58
Mobile, AL MSA	163	34.18
Modesto, CA MSA	101	27.26
Monroe, LA MSA	13	9.14
Montgomery, AL MSA	76	25.98
Muncie, IN MSA	31	25.91
Muskegon, MI MSA	56	35.22
Naples, FL MSA	54	35.50
Nashville, TN MSA	290	29.44
New Bedford, MA MSA	51	29.04
New Haven – Meriden, CT MSA	136	25.65

[Continued]

★ 725 ★

Optical Goods Workers
[Continued]

MSA/CMSA	Total Employees	Employees per 100,000 pop.
New London – Norwich, CT – RI MSA	33	12.37
New Orleans, LA MSA	330	26.64
New York – Northern New Jersey – Long Island, NY – NJ – CT CMSA	4560	25.21
Norfolk – Virginia Beach – Newport News, VA MSA	509	36.46
Ocala, FL MSA	51	26.18
Odessa, TX MSA	67	56.33
Oklahoma City, OK MSA	271	28.26
Olympia, WA MSA	31	19.23
Omaha, NE – IA MSA	320	51.76
Orlando, FL MSA	305	28.43
Owensboro, KY MSA	8	9.18
Panama City, FL MSA	60	47.25
Parkersburg – Marietta, WV – OH MSA	62	41.56
Pascagoula, MS MSA	49	42.52
Pensacola, FL MSA	84	24.39
Peoria, IL MSA	116	34.20
Philadelphia – Wilmington – Trenton, PA – NJ – DE – MD CMSA	1526	25.87
Phoenix, AZ MSA	885	41.70
Pine Bluff, AR MSA	38	44.45
Pittsburgh – Beaver Valley, PA CMSA	758	33.80
Pittsfield, MA MSA	33	41.64
Portland, ME MSA	91	42.27
Portland – Vancouver, OR – WA CMSA	682	46.15
Portsmouth – Dover – Rochester, NH – ME MSA	47	21.02
Poughkeepsie, NY MSA	28	10.79
Providence – Pawtucket – Fall River, RI – MA CMSA	383	33.55
Provo – Orem, UT MSA	66	25.04
Pueblo, CO MSA	53	43.07
Raleigh – Durham, NC MSA	258	35.08
Rapid City, SD MSA	23	28.28
Reading, PA MSA	161	47.84
Redding, CA MSA	45	30.60
Reno, NV MSA	95	37.30
Richland – Kennewick – Pasco, WA MSA	28	18.66
Richmond – Petersburg, VA MSA	450	51.98
Roanoke, VA MSA	135	60.14
Rochester, MN MSA	54	50.72
Rochester, NY MSA	1019	101.66
Rockford, IL MSA	90	31.72
Sacramento, CA MSA	480	32.41
Saginaw – Bay City – Midland, MI MSA	120	30.05
St. Cloud, MN MSA	433	226.80
St. Joseph, MO MSA	32	38.52
St. Louis, MO – IL MSA	782	32.00
Salem, OR MSA	63	22.66
Salinas – Seaside – Monterey, CA MSA	25	7.03

[Continued]

★ 725 ★

Optical Goods Workers

[Continued]

MSA/CMSA	Total Employees	Employees per 100,000 pop.
Salt Lake City – Ogden, UT MSA	335	31.24
San Angelo, TX MSA	32	32.50
San Antonio, TX MSA	304	23.35
San Diego, CA MSA	1146	45.88
San Francisco – Oakland – San Jose, CA CMSA	1798	28.75
Santa Barbara – Santa Maria – Lompoc, CA MSA	107	28.95
Santa Fe, NM MSA	16	13.67
Sarasota, FL MSA	131	47.16
Savannah, GA MSA	60	24.73
Scranton – Wilkes-Barre, PA MSA	291	39.64
Seattle – Tacoma, WA CMSA	926	36.18
Sharon, PA MSA	25	20.66
Sheboygan, WI MSA	43	41.40
Sherman – Denison, TX MSA	15	15.79
Shreveport, LA MSA	137	40.98
Sioux City, IA – NE MSA	90	78.25
Sioux Falls, SD MSA	54	43.62
South Bend – Mishawaka, IN MSA	85	34.41
Spokane, WA MSA	91	25.18
Springfield, IL MSA	60	31.65
Springfield, MO MSA	101	41.98
Springfield, MA MSA	173	32.67
State College, PA MSA	30	24.24
Steubenville – Weirton, OH – WV MSA	30	21.05
Stockton, CA MSA	106	22.05
Syracuse, NY MSA	176	26.67
Tallahassee, FL MSA	50	21.40
Tampa – St. Petersburg – Clearwater, FL MSA	1197	57.88
Terre Haute, IN MSA	71	54.28
Texarkana, TX – Texarkana, AR MSA	44	36.63
Toledo, OH MSA	176	28.66
Topeka, KS MSA	92	57.15
Tucson, AZ MSA	305	45.74
Tulsa, OK MSA	268	37.80
Tuscaloosa, AL MSA	70	46.50
Tyler, TX MSA	77	50.89
Utica – Rome, NY MSA	59	18.63
Victoria, TX MSA	27	36.31
Visalia – Tulare – Porterville, CA MSA	23	7.37
Waco, TX MSA	81	42.83
Washington, DC – MD – VA MSA	937	23.88
Waterbury, CT MSA	29	13.08
Waterloo – Cedar Falls, IA MSA	44	30.01
Wausau, WI MSA	32	27.73
West Palm Beach – Boca Raton – Delray Beach, FL MSA	267	30.92
Wheeling, WV – OH MSA	82	51.47

[Continued]

★ 725 ★

Optical Goods Workers
[Continued]

MSA/CMSA	Total Employees	Employees per 100,000 pop.
Wichita, KS MSA	155	31.94
Wichita Falls, TX MSA	15	12.26
Williamsport, PA MSA	39	32.85
Wilmington, NC MSA	42	34.92
Worcester, MA MSA	287	65.69
Yakima, WA MSA	34	18.01
York, PA MSA	135	32.31
Youngstown–Warren, OH MSA	177	35.93
Yuba City, CA MSA	14	11.42
Yuma, AZ MSA	24	22.45

Source: Census of Population and Housing, 1990: Equal Employment Opportunity (EEO) File on CD-ROM [machine-readable datafiles]. Prepared by the Bureau of the Census. Washington, DC: The Bureau, 1992.

★ 726 ★

Employment

Optometrists

The table below presents the number of civilians 16 years old or older who reported working as optometrists during the 1990 Census. Data are provided by total number employed in each Metropolitan Statistical Area (MSA) or Consolidated Metropolitan Statistical Area (CMSA), as well as the number employed per 100,000 people.

[Total for all of the U.S. was 27,515; 11.06 per 100,000 persons]

MSA/CMSA	Total Employees	Employees per 100,000 pop.
Albany, GA MSA	17	15.10
Albany–Schenectady–Troy, NY MSA	123	14.07
Albuquerque, NM MSA	68	14.15
Alexandria, LA MSA	40	30.41
Allentown–Bethlehem–Easton, PA–NJ MSA	126	18.35
Amarillo, TX MSA	20	10.66
Anchorage, AK MSA	31	13.70
Anderson, IN MSA	35	26.79
Anderson, SC MSA	27	18.60
Anniston, AL MSA	18	15.51
Appleton–Oshkosh–Neenah, WI MSA	30	9.52
Asheville, NC MSA	51	29.17
Atlanta, GA MSA	201	7.09
Atlantic City, NJ MSA	24	7.51
Augusta, GA–SC MSA	20	5.04
Austin, TX MSA	82	10.49
Bakersfield, CA MSA	64	11.78
Baltimore, MD MSA	268	11.25
Bangor, ME MSA	2	2.25

[Continued]

★ 726 ★

Optometrists
[Continued]

MSA/CMSA	Total Employees	Employees per 100,000 pop.
Baton Rouge, LA MSA	16	3.03
Battle Creek, MI MSA	17	12.50
Beaumont – Port Arthur, TX MSA	37	10.24
Bellingham, WA MSA	7	5.48
Benton Harbor, MI MSA	39	24.17
Billings, MT MSA	47	41.44
Biloxi – Gulfport, MS MSA	11	5.58
Binghamton, NY MSA	33	12.48
Birmingham, AL MSA	156	17.18
Bismarck, ND MSA	23	27.44
Bloomington, IN MSA	26	23.86
Bloomington – Normal, IL MSA	10	7.74
Boise City, ID MSA	53	25.76
Boston – Lawrence – Salem, MA – NH CMSA	517	12.39
Bradenton, FL MSA	17	8.03
Bremerton, WA MSA	24	12.65
Brownsville – Harlingen, TX MSA	14	5.38
Buffalo – Niagara Falls, NY CMSA	148	12.44
Burlington, NC MSA	33	30.50
Burlington, VT MSA	29	22.06
Canton, OH MSA	92	23.34
Casper, WY MSA	14	22.87
Cedar Rapids, IA MSA	25	14.81
Champaign – Urbana – Rantoul, IL MSA	20	11.56
Charleston, SC MSA	25	4.93
Charleston, WV MSA	55	21.96
Charlotte – Gastonia – Rock Hill, NC – SC MSA	93	8.00
Charlottesville, VA MSA	17	12.97
Chattanooga, TN – GA MSA	33	7.62
Cheyenne, WY MSA	6	8.20
Chicago – Gary – Lake County, IL – IN – WI CMSA	1037	12.86
Chico, CA MSA	21	11.53
Cincinnati – Hamilton, OH – KY – IN CMSA	167	9.58
Clarksville – Hopkinsville, TN – KY MSA	34	20.07
Cleveland – Akron – Lorain, OH CMSA	350	12.68
Colorado Springs, CO MSA	27	6.80
Columbia, SC MSA	79	17.43
Columbus, GA – AL MSA	17	6.99
Columbus, OH MSA	183	13.29
Corpus Christi, TX MSA	17	4.86
Cumberland, MD – WV MSA	8	7.87
Dallas – Fort Worth, TX CMSA	348	8.96
Danville, VA MSA	24	22.08
Davenport – Rock Island – Moline, IA – IL MSA	27	7.70
Dayton – Springfield, OH MSA	108	11.35
Daytona Beach, FL MSA	23	6.20

[Continued]

★ 726 ★

Optometrists
[Continued]

MSA/CMSA	Total Employees	Employees per 100,000 pop.
Decatur, AL MSA	24	18.24
Decatur, IL MSA	20	17.06
Denver–Boulder, CO CMSA	263	14.23
Des Moines, IA MSA	55	14.00
Detroit–Ann Arbor, MI CMSA	445	9.54
Dothan, AL MSA	15	11.45
Dubuque, IA MSA	14	16.20
Duluth, MN–WI MSA	13	5.42
Eau Claire, WI MSA	17	12.36
El Paso, TX MSA	15	2.54
Elkhart–Goshen, IN MSA	62	39.69
Elmira, NY MSA	17	17.86
Enid, OK MSA	10	17.63
Erie, PA MSA	30	10.89
Eugene–Springfield, OR MSA	40	14.14
Evansville, IN–KY MSA	41	14.70
Fargo–Moorhead, ND–MN MSA	5	3.26
Fayetteville, NC MSA	9	3.28
Fitchburg–Leominster, MA MSA	38	36.97
Flint, MI MSA	42	9.76
Florence, AL MSA	22	16.75
Fort Collins–Loveland, CO MSA	41	22.03
Fort Myers–Cape Coral, FL MSA	35	10.44
Fort Pierce, FL MSA	17	6.77
Fort Smith, AR–OK MSA	26	14.78
Fort Walton Beach, FL MSA	21	14.61
Fort Wayne, IN MSA	77	21.16
Fresno, CA MSA	80	11.99
Gainesville, FL MSA	26	12.74
Glens Falls, NY MSA	19	16.03
Grand Forks, ND MSA	11	15.56
Grand Rapids, MI MSA	41	5.96
Great Falls, MT MSA	10	12.87
Greeley, CO MSA	12	9.10
Green Bay, WI MSA	30	15.42
Greensboro–Winston-Salem–High Point, NC MSA	65	6.90
Greenville–Spartanburg, SC MSA	69	10.77
Hagerstown, MD MSA	6	4.94
Harrisburg–Lebanon–Carlisle, PA MSA	74	12.59
Hartford–New Britain–Middletown, CT CMSA	117	10.78
Hickory–Morganton, NC MSA	22	9.92
Honolulu, HI MSA	220	26.31
Houma–Thibodaux, LA MSA	18	9.84
Houston–Galveston–Brazoria, TX CMSA	386	10.40
Huntington–Ashland, WV–KY–OH MSA	3	0.96
Huntsville, AL MSA	12	5.02

[Continued]

★ 726 ★

Optometrists
[Continued]

MSA/CMSA	Total Employees	Employees per 100,000 pop.
Indianapolis, IN MSA	202	16.16
Iowa City, IA MSA	12	12.48
Jackson, MI MSA	14	9.35
Jackson, MS MSA	23	5.82
Jackson, TN MSA	10	12.82
Jacksonville, FL MSA	82	9.04
Jacksonville, NC MSA	7	4.67
Jamestown – Dunkirk, NY	22	15.50
Johnson City – Kingsport – Bristol, TN – VA MSA	59	13.53
Johnstown, PA MSA	32	13.26
Joplin, MO MSA	1	0.74
Kalamazoo, MI MSA	21	9.40
Kansas City, MO – KS MSA	142	9.07
Killeen – Temple, TX MSA	22	8.62
Knoxville, TN MSA	100	16.53
Kokomo, IN MSA	17	17.54
La Crosse, WI MSA	13	13.28
Lafayette, LA MSA	11	5.27
Lafayette – West Lafayette, IN MSA	10	9.05
Lake Charles, LA MSA	23	13.68
Lakeland – Winter Haven, FL MSA	54	13.32
Lancaster, PA MSA	39	9.22
Lansing – East Lansing, MI MSA	56	12.94
Las Cruces, NM MSA	18	13.28
Las Vegas, NV MSA	76	10.25
Lawrence, KS MSA	9	11.00
Lewiston – Auburn, ME MSA	6	6.81
Lexington-Fayette, KY MSA	44	12.63
Lima, OH MSA	5	3.24
Lincoln, NE MSA	17	7.96
Little Rock – North Little Rock, AR MSA	77	15.01
Longview – Marshall, TX MSA	9	5.54
Los Angeles – Anaheim – Riverside, CA CMSA	1733	11.93
Louisville, KY – IN MSA	88	9.24
Lubbock, TX MSA	12	5.39
Lynchburg, VA MSA	13	9.14
Macon – Warner Robins, GA MSA	8	2.85
Madison, WI MSA	63	17.16
Manchester, NH MSA	16	10.82
Mansfield, OH MSA	25	19.82
McAllen – Edinburg – Mission, TX MSA	20	5.21
Medford, OR MSA	23	15.71
Melbourne – Titusville – Palm Bay, FL MSA	21	5.26
Memphis, TN – AR – MS MSA	106	10.80
Merced, CA MSA	52	29.15
Miami – Fort Lauderdale, FL CMSA	342	10.71

[Continued]

717

★ 726 ★

Optometrists
[Continued]

MSA/CMSA	Total Employees	Employees per 100,000 pop.
Midland, TX MSA	6	5.63
Milwaukee – Racine, WI CMSA	137	8.52
Minneapolis – St. Paul, MN – WI MSA	243	9.86
Mobile, AL MSA	34	7.13
Modesto, CA MSA	31	8.37
Monroe, LA MSA	12	8.44
Montgomery, AL MSA	25	8.55
Muskegon, MI MSA	7	4.40
Naples, FL MSA	29	19.07
Nashville, TN MSA	107	10.86
New Bedford, MA MSA	16	9.11
New Haven – Meriden, CT MSA	51	9.62
New London – Norwich, CT – RI MSA	21	7.87
New Orleans, LA MSA	108	8.72
New York – Northern New Jersey – Long Island, NY – NJ – CT CMSA	1953	10.80
Norfolk – Virginia Beach – Newport News, VA MSA	117	8.38
Odessa, TX MSA	20	16.82
Oklahoma City, OK MSA	157	16.37
Olympia, WA MSA	24	14.88
Omaha, NE – IA MSA	48	7.76
Orlando, FL MSA	121	11.28
Owensboro, KY MSA	7	8.03
Panama City, FL MSA	10	7.87
Parkersburg – Marietta, WV – OH MSA	26	17.43
Pensacola, FL MSA	6	1.74
Peoria, IL MSA	27	7.96
Philadelphia – Wilmington – Trenton, PA – NJ – DE – MD CMSA	666	11.29
Phoenix, AZ MSA	228	10.74
Pittsburgh – Beaver Valley, PA CMSA	363	16.19
Portland, ME MSA	43	19.97
Portland – Vancouver, OR – WA CMSA	242	16.37
Portsmouth – Dover – Rochester, NH – ME MSA	18	8.05
Poughkeepsie, NY MSA	42	16.19
Providence – Pawtucket – Fall River, RI – MA CMSA	128	11.21
Provo – Orem, UT MSA	7	2.66
Pueblo, CO MSA	6	4.88
Raleigh – Durham, NC MSA	96	13.05
Rapid City, SD MSA	14	17.21
Reading, PA MSA	44	13.07
Redding, CA MSA	19	12.92
Reno, NV MSA	45	17.67
Richland – Kennewick – Pasco, WA MSA	9	6.00
Richmond – Petersburg, VA MSA	55	6.35
Roanoke, VA MSA	22	9.80
Rochester, MN MSA	2	1.88
Rochester, NY MSA	70	6.98

[Continued]

★ 726 ★

Optometrists
[Continued]

MSA/CMSA	Total Employees	Employees per 100,000 pop.
Rockford, IL MSA	52	18.33
Sacramento, CA MSA	278	18.77
Saginaw – Bay City – Midland, MI MSA	48	12.02
St. Cloud, MN MSA	23	12.05
St. Joseph, MO MSA	27	32.50
St. Louis, MO – IL MSA	284	11.62
Salem, OR MSA	37	13.31
Salinas – Seaside – Monterey, CA MSA	51	14.34
Salt Lake City – Ogden, UT MSA	99	9.23
San Angelo, TX MSA	15	15.23
San Antonio, TX MSA	140	10.75
San Diego, CA MSA	379	15.17
San Francisco – Oakland – San Jose, CA CMSA	1000	15.99
Santa Barbara – Santa Maria – Lompoc, CA MSA	32	8.66
Santa Fe, NM MSA	6	5.13
Sarasota, FL MSA	57	20.52
Savannah, GA MSA	18	7.42
Scranton – Wilkes-Barre, PA MSA	82	11.17
Seattle – Tacoma, WA CMSA	253	9.89
Sharon, PA MSA	20	16.53
Sheboygan, WI MSA	8	7.70
Shreveport, LA MSA	4	1.20
Sioux City, IA – NE MSA	32	27.82
South Bend – Mishawaka, IN MSA	28	11.33
Spokane, WA MSA	58	16.05
Springfield, IL MSA	8	4.22
Springfield, MO MSA	33	13.72
Springfield, MA MSA	25	4.72
State College, PA MSA	13	10.50
Stockton, CA MSA	41	8.53
Syracuse, NY MSA	43	6.52
Tallahassee, FL MSA	19	8.13
Tampa – St. Petersburg – Clearwater, FL MSA	95	4.59
Terre Haute, IN MSA	13	9.94
Texarkana, TX – Texarkana, AR MSA	7	5.83
Toledo, OH MSA	68	11.07
Topeka, KS MSA	13	8.08
Tucson, AZ MSA	43	6.45
Tulsa, OK MSA	78	11.00
Tyler, TX MSA	5	3.30
Utica – Rome, NY MSA	33	10.42
Victoria, TX MSA	21	28.24
Visalia – Tulare – Porterville, CA MSA	61	19.56
Waco, TX MSA	50	26.44
Washington, DC – MD – VA MSA	390	9.94
Waterbury, CT MSA	22	9.93

[Continued]

★ 726 ★

Optometrists
[Continued]

MSA/CMSA	Total Employees	Employees per 100,000 pop.
Waterloo – Cedar Falls, IA MSA	9	6.14
Wausau, WI MSA	11	9.53
West Palm Beach – Boca Raton – Delray Beach, FL MSA	133	15.40
Wheeling, WV – OH MSA	37	23.23
Wichita, KS MSA	81	16.69
Wichita Falls, TX MSA	33	26.97
Williamsport, PA MSA	4	3.37
Worcester, MA MSA	68	15.56
Yakima, WA MSA	15	7.94
York, PA MSA	26	6.22
Youngstown – Warren, OH MSA	64	12.99
Yuba City, CA MSA	17	13.86
Yuma, AZ MSA	5	4.68

Source: Census of Population and Housing, 1990: Equal Employment Opportunity (EEO) File on CD-ROM [machine-readable datafiles]. Prepared by the Bureau of the Census. Washington, DC: The Bureau, 1992.

★ 727 ★

Employment

Pharmacists

The table below presents the number of civilians 16 years old or older who reported working as pharmacists during the 1990 Census. Data are provided by total number employed in each Metropolitan Statistical Area (MSA) or Consolidated Metropolitan Statistical Area (CMSA), as well as the number employed per 100,000 people.

[Total for all of the U.S. was 181,798; 73.10 per 100,000 persons]

MSA/CMSA	Total Employees	Employees per 100,000 pop.
Abilene, TX MSA	74	61.84
Albany, GA MSA	57	50.64
Albany – Schenectady – Troy, NY MSA	992	113.46
Albuquerque, NM MSA	571	118.82
Alexandria, LA MSA	102	77.53
Allentown – Bethlehem – Easton, PA – NJ MSA	485	70.63
Altoona, PA MSA	100	76.60
Amarillo, TX MSA	193	102.91
Anchorage, AK MSA	150	66.27
Anderson, IN MSA	60	45.92
Anderson, SC MSA	95	65.43
Anniston, AL MSA	69	59.47
Appleton – Oshkosh – Neenah, WI MSA	187	59.34
Asheville, NC MSA	196	112.11
Athens, GA MSA	205	131.19
Atlanta, GA MSA	2348	82.87

[Continued]

★ 727 ★

Pharmacists
[Continued]

MSA/CMSA	Total Employees	Employees per 100,000 pop.
Atlantic City, NJ MSA	240	75.14
Augusta, GA – SC MSA	411	103.58
Austin, TX MSA	650	83.17
Bakersfield, CA MSA	286	52.62
Baltimore, MD MSA	1684	70.69
Bangor, ME MSA	36	40.57
Baton Rouge, LA MSA	431	81.59
Battle Creek, MI MSA	62	45.59
Beaumont – Port Arthur, TX MSA	322	89.14
Bellingham, WA MSA	76	59.48
Benton Harbor, MI MSA	119	73.74
Billings, MT MSA	92	81.12
Biloxi – Gulfport, MS MSA	107	54.28
Binghamton, NY MSA	204	77.13
Birmingham, AL MSA	908	100.02
Bismarck, ND MSA	78	93.04
Bloomington, IN MSA	116	106.44
Bloomington – Normal, IL MSA	92	71.22
Boise City, ID MSA	148	71.92
Boston – Lawrence – Salem, MA – NH CMSA	3404	81.60
Bradenton, FL MSA	174	82.19
Bremerton, WA MSA	126	66.41
Brownsville – Harlingen, TX MSA	152	58.43
Bryan – College Station, TX MSA	31	25.44
Buffalo – Niagara Falls, NY CMSA	1156	97.20
Burlington, NC MSA	76	70.23
Burlington, VT MSA	121	92.06
Canton, OH MSA	182	46.18
Casper, WY MSA	57	93.10
Cedar Rapids, IA MSA	108	63.99
Champaign – Urbana – Rantoul, IL MSA	119	68.78
Charleston, SC MSA	501	98.84
Charleston, WV MSA	202	80.65
Charlotte – Gastonia – Rock Hill, NC – SC MSA	839	72.20
Charlottesville, VA MSA	135	102.97
Chattanooga, TN – GA MSA	340	78.48
Cheyenne, WY MSA	41	56.06
Chicago – Gary – Lake County, IL – IN – WI CMSA	5990	74.27
Chico, CA MSA	112	61.50
Cincinnati – Hamilton, OH – KY – IN CMSA	1811	103.83
Clarksville – Hopkinsville, TN – KY MSA	46	27.15
Cleveland – Akron – Lorain, OH CMSA	1937	70.19
Colorado Springs, CO MSA	274	69.02
Columbia, MO MSA	99	88.09
Columbia, SC MSA	503	110.96
Columbus, GA – AL MSA	107	44.02

[Continued]

★ 727 ★

Pharmacists
[Continued]

MSA/CMSA	Total Employees	Employees per 100,000 pop.
Columbus, OH MSA	1539	111.73
Corpus Christi, TX MSA	195	55.73
Cumberland, MD – WV MSA	57	56.08
Dallas – Fort Worth, TX CMSA	2735	70.39
Danville, VA MSA	93	85.55
Davenport – Rock Island – Moline, IA – IL MSA	218	62.13
Dayton – Springfield, OH MSA	709	74.53
Daytona Beach, FL MSA	202	54.49
Decatur, AL MSA	67	50.93
Decatur, IL MSA	103	87.88
Denver – Boulder, CO CMSA	1247	67.47
Des Moines, IA MSA	458	116.56
Detroit – Ann Arbor, MI CMSA	3451	73.97
Dothan, AL MSA	81	61.85
Dubuque, IA MSA	32	37.04
Duluth, MN – WI MSA	163	67.92
Eau Claire, WI MSA	100	72.70
El Paso, TX MSA	419	70.82
Elkhart – Goshen, IN MSA	76	48.66
Elmira, NY MSA	157	164.92
Enid, OK MSA	64	112.81
Erie, PA MSA	152	55.16
Eugene – Springfield, OR MSA	161	56.91
Evansville, IN – KY MSA	207	74.20
Fargo – Moorhead, ND – MN MSA	203	132.42
Fayetteville, NC MSA	140	50.99
Fayetteville – Springdale, AR MSA	109	96.11
Fitchburg – Leominster, MA MSA	87	84.63
Flint, MI MSA	310	72.02
Florence, AL MSA	107	81.48
Florence, SC MSA	145	126.81
Fort Collins – Loveland, CO MSA	167	89.72
Fort Myers – Cape Coral, FL MSA	297	88.63
Fort Pierce, FL MSA	165	65.72
Fort Smith, AR – OK MSA	126	71.63
Fort Walton Beach, FL MSA	87	60.51
Fort Wayne, IN MSA	371	101.98
Fresno, CA MSA	583	87.34
Gadsden, AL MSA	74	74.12
Gainesville, FL MSA	284	139.14
Glens Falls, NY MSA	112	94.48
Grand Forks, ND MSA	19	26.88
Grand Rapids, MI MSA	562	81.64
Great Falls, MT MSA	51	65.64
Greeley, CO MSA	70	53.10
Green Bay, WI MSA	101	51.90

[Continued]

★ 727 ★

Pharmacists

[Continued]

MSA/CMSA	Total Employees	Employees per 100,000 pop.
Greensboro – Winston-Salem – High Point, NC MSA	707	75.05
Greenville – Spartanburg, SC MSA	560	87.38
Hagerstown, MD MSA	91	74.96
Harrisburg – Lebanon – Carlisle, PA MSA	401	68.20
Hartford – New Britain – Middletown, CT CMSA	862	79.39
Hickory – Morganton, NC MSA	197	88.86
Honolulu, HI MSA	364	43.53
Houma – Thibodaux, LA MSA	90	49.22
Houston – Galveston – Brazoria, TX CMSA	2800	75.45
Huntington – Ashland, WV – KY – OH MSA	287	91.83
Huntsville, AL MSA	82	34.32
Indianapolis, IN MSA	1254	100.33
Iowa City, IA MSA	202	210.16
Jackson, MI MSA	104	69.45
Jackson, MS MSA	486	122.91
Jackson, TN MSA	114	146.19
Jacksonville, FL MSA	535	59.00
Jacksonville, NC MSA	59	39.38
Jamestown – Dunkirk, NY	112	78.93
Janesville – Beloit, WI MSA	80	57.34
Johnson City – Kingsport – Bristol, TN – VA MSA	361	82.79
Johnstown, PA MSA	172	71.30
Joplin, MO MSA	46	34.10
Kalamazoo, MI MSA	277	123.99
Kankakee, IL MSA	86	89.35
Kansas City, MO – KS MSA	1534	97.94
Killeen – Temple, TX MSA	139	54.45
Knoxville, TN MSA	562	92.92
Kokomo, IN MSA	83	85.61
La Crosse, WI MSA	73	74.56
Lafayette, LA MSA	143	68.51
Lafayette – West Lafayette, IN MSA	176	134.76
Lake Charles, LA MSA	122	72.56
Lakeland – Winter Haven, FL MSA	221	54.52
Lancaster, PA MSA	217	51.32
Lansing – East Lansing, MI MSA	231	53.39
Laredo, TX MSA	81	60.79
Las Cruces, NM MSA	51	37.64
Las Vegas, NV MSA	403	54.35
Lawrence, KS MSA	122	149.15
Lawton, OK MSA	123	110.33
Lewiston – Auburn, ME MSA	84	95.30
Lexington-Fayette, KY MSA	521	149.53
Lima, OH MSA	92	59.61
Lincoln, NE MSA	150	70.21
Little Rock – North Little Rock, AR MSA	684	133.30

[Continued]

★ 727 ★

Pharmacists
[Continued]

MSA/CMSA	Total Employees	Employees per 100,000 pop.
Longview – Marshall, TX MSA	171	105.28
Los Angeles – Anaheim – Riverside, CA CMSA	8084	55.63
Louisville, KY – IN MSA	761	79.88
Lubbock, TX MSA	244	109.60
Lynchburg, VA MSA	88	61.89
Macon – Warner Robins, GA MSA	187	66.52
Madison, WI MSA	466	126.95
Manchester, NH MSA	129	87.27
Mansfield, OH MSA	126	99.89
McAllen – Edinburg – Mission, TX MSA	141	36.76
Medford, OR MSA	85	58.06
Melbourne – Titusville – Palm Bay, FL MSA	289	72.44
Memphis, TN – AR – MS MSA	714	72.73
Merced, CA MSA	104	58.29
Miami – Fort Lauderdale, FL CMSA	2515	78.78
Midland, TX MSA	77	72.23
Milwaukee – Racine, WI CMSA	1226	76.28
Minneapolis – St. Paul, MN – WI MSA	1994	80.92
Mobile, AL MSA	344	72.13
Modesto, CA MSA	151	40.75
Monroe, LA MSA	327	229.97
Montgomery, AL MSA	283	96.75
Muncie, IN MSA	61	50.98
Muskegon, MI MSA	65	40.88
Naples, FL MSA	97	63.77
Nashville, TN MSA	866	87.92
New Bedford, MA MSA	154	87.68
New Haven – Meriden, CT MSA	317	59.79
New London – Norwich, CT – RI MSA	213	79.83
New Orleans, LA MSA	967	78.06
New York – Northern New Jersey – Long Island, NY – NJ – CT CMSA	14258	78.83
Norfolk – Virginia Beach – Newport News, VA MSA	885	63.39
Ocala, FL MSA	89	45.68
Odessa, TX MSA	77	64.74
Oklahoma City, OK MSA	861	89.80
Olympia, WA MSA	88	54.58
Omaha, NE – IA MSA	821	132.79
Orlando, FL MSA	552	51.46
Owensboro, KY MSA	129	147.95
Panama City, FL MSA	97	76.38
Parkersburg – Marietta, WV – OH MSA	78	52.29
Pascagoula, MS MSA	60	52.06
Pensacola, FL MSA	246	71.43
Peoria, IL MSA	277	81.67
Philadelphia – Wilmington – Trenton, PA – NJ – DE – MD CMSA	5372	91.06
Phoenix, AZ MSA	1545	72.81

[Continued]

★ 727 ★

Pharmacists
[Continued]

MSA/CMSA	Total Employees	Employees per 100,000 pop.
Pine Bluff, AR MSA	34	39.77
Pittsburgh – Beaver Valley, PA CMSA	2487	110.89
Pittsfield, MA MSA	44	55.52
Portland, ME MSA	145	67.35
Portland – Vancouver, OR – WA CMSA	1048	70.91
Portsmouth – Dover – Rochester, NH – ME MSA	133	59.49
Poughkeepsie, NY MSA	262	100.98
Providence – Pawtucket – Fall River, RI – MA CMSA	944	82.70
Provo – Orem, UT MSA	163	61.84
Pueblo, CO MSA	163	132.47
Raleigh – Durham, NC MSA	832	113.12
Rapid City, SD MSA	68	83.60
Reading, PA MSA	163	48.44
Redding, CA MSA	63	42.85
Reno, NV MSA	206	80.89
Richland – Kennewick – Pasco, WA MSA	136	90.65
Richmond – Petersburg, VA MSA	818	94.50
Roanoke, VA MSA	201	89.54
Rochester, MN MSA	206	193.48
Rochester, NY MSA	710	70.83
Rockford, IL MSA	179	63.09
Sacramento, CA MSA	898	60.63
Saginaw – Bay City – Midland, MI MSA	334	83.64
St. Cloud, MN MSA	87	45.57
St. Joseph, MO MSA	31	37.31
St. Louis, MO – IL MSA	1874	76.67
Salem, OR MSA	261	93.88
Salinas – Seaside – Monterey, CA MSA	158	44.42
Salt Lake City – Ogden, UT MSA	898	83.75
San Angelo, TX MSA	91	92.43
San Antonio, TX MSA	936	71.88
San Diego, CA MSA	1376	55.08
San Francisco – Oakland – San Jose, CA CMSA	4136	66.14
Santa Barbara – Santa Maria – Lompoc, CA MSA	196	53.03
Santa Fe, NM MSA	42	35.88
Sarasota, FL MSA	224	80.64
Savannah, GA MSA	254	104.69
Scranton – Wilkes-Barre, PA MSA	636	86.63
Seattle – Tacoma, WA CMSA	2043	79.83
Sharon, PA MSA	48	39.67
Sheboygan, WI MSA	79	76.05
Sherman – Denison, TX MSA	67	70.51
Shreveport, LA MSA	294	87.93
Sioux City, IA – NE MSA	82	71.29
Sioux Falls, SD MSA	182	147.00
South Bend – Mishawaka, IN MSA	161	65.17

[Continued]

★ 727 ★

Pharmacists
[Continued]

MSA/CMSA	Total Employees	Employees per 100,000 pop.
Spokane, WA MSA	279	77.21
Springfield, IL MSA	237	125.03
Springfield, MO MSA	211	87.70
Springfield, MA MSA	502	94.80
State College, PA MSA	71	57.36
Steubenville–Weirton, OH–WV MSA	136	95.42
Stockton, CA MSA	324	67.41
Syracuse, NY MSA	344	52.13
Tallahassee, FL MSA	176	75.34
Tampa–St. Petersburg–Clearwater, FL MSA	1835	88.73
Terre Haute, IN MSA	84	64.21
Texarkana, TX–Texarkana, AR MSA	72	59.93
Toledo, OH MSA	524	85.32
Topeka, KS MSA	138	85.73
Tucson, AZ MSA	656	98.37
Tulsa, OK MSA	621	87.59
Tuscaloosa, AL MSA	216	143.50
Tyler, TX MSA	190	125.57
Utica–Rome, NY MSA	272	85.90
Victoria, TX MSA	70	94.14
Visalia–Tulare–Porterville, CA MSA	141	45.20
Waco, TX MSA	64	33.84
Washington, DC–MD–VA MSA	2299	58.59
Waterbury, CT MSA	274	123.63
Waterloo–Cedar Falls, IA MSA	72	49.11
Wausau, WI MSA	92	79.72
West Palm Beach–Boca Raton–Delray Beach, FL MSA	845	97.86
Wheeling, WV–OH MSA	156	97.93
Wichita, KS MSA	318	65.53
Wichita Falls, TX MSA	86	70.27
Williamsport, PA MSA	69	58.12
Wilmington, NC MSA	136	113.07
Worcester, MA MSA	344	78.74
Yakima, WA MSA	115	60.90
York, PA MSA	276	66.05
Youngstown–Warren, OH MSA	376	76.33
Yuba City, CA MSA	26	21.20
Yuma, AZ MSA	60	56.13

Source: Census of Population and Housing, 1990: Equal Employment Opportunity (EEO) File on CD-ROM [machine-readable datafiles]. Prepared by the Bureau of the Census. Washington, DC: The Bureau, 1992.

★ 728 ★

Employment

Physical Therapists

The table below presents the number of civilians 16 years old or older who reported working as physical therapists during the 1990 Census. Data are provided by total number employed in each Metropolitan Statistical Area (MSA) or Consolidated Metropolitan Statistical Area (CMSA), as well as the number employed per 100,000 people.

[Total for all of the U.S. was 92,022; 37.00 per 100,000 persons]

MSA/CMSA	Total Employees	Employees per 100,000 pop.
Abilene, TX MSA	96	80.23
Albany, GA MSA	33	29.32
Albany–Schenectady–Troy, NY MSA	383	43.81
Albuquerque, NM MSA	331	68.88
Alexandria, LA MSA	44	33.45
Allentown–Bethlehem–Easton, PA–NJ MSA	282	41.07
Altoona, PA MSA	26	19.92
Amarillo, TX MSA	85	45.32
Anchorage, AK MSA	95	41.97
Anderson, IN MSA	27	20.66
Anderson, SC MSA	10	6.89
Anniston, AL MSA	14	12.07
Appleton–Oshkosh–Neenah, WI MSA	163	51.73
Asheville, NC MSA	102	58.35
Athens, GA MSA	63	40.32
Atlanta, GA MSA	1085	38.29
Atlantic City, NJ MSA	148	46.33
Augusta, GA–SC MSA	144	36.29
Austin, TX MSA	496	63.46
Bakersfield, CA MSA	142	20.13
Baltimore, MD MSA	1046	43.91
Bangor, ME MSA	59	66.48
Baton Rouge, LA MSA	186	35.21
Battle Creek, MI MSA	39	28.68
Beaumont–Port Arthur, TX MSA	93	25.75
Bellingham, WA MSA	72	56.35
Benton Harbor, MI MSA	49	30.36
Billings, MT MSA	15	13.23
Biloxi–Gulfport, MS MSA	45	22.83
Binghamton, NY MSA	80	30.25
Birmingham, AL MSA	342	37.67
Bismarck, ND MSA	54	64.42
Bloomington, IN MSA	14	12.85
Bloomington–Normal, IL MSA	29	22.45
Boise City, ID MSA	109	52.97
Boston–Lawrence–Salem, MA–NH CMSA	2632	63.09
Bradenton, FL MSA	66	31.18
Bremerton, WA MSA	77	40.58
Brownsville–Harlingen, TX MSA	48	18.45
Bryan–College Station, TX MSA	22	18.05
Buffalo–Niagara Falls, NY CMSA	562	47.26
Burlington, NC MSA	22	20.33

[Continued]

★ 728 ★

Physical Therapists
[Continued]

MSA/CMSA	Total Employees	Employees per 100,000 pop.
Burlington, VT MSA	104	79.12
Canton, OH MSA	97	24.61
Casper, WY MSA	30	49.00
Cedar Rapids, IA MSA	36	21.33
Champaign – Urbana – Rantoul, IL MSA	69	39.88
Charleston, SC MSA	218	43.01
Charleston, WV MSA	45	17.97
Charlotte – Gastonia – Rock Hill, NC – SC MSA	418	35.97
Charlottesville, VA MSA	76	57.97
Chattanooga, TN – GA MSA	206	47.55
Cheyenne, WY MSA	10	13.67
Chicago – Gary – Lake County, IL – IN – WI CMSA	2899	35.94
Chico, CA MSA	104	57.11
Cincinnati – Hamilton, OH – KY – IN CMSA	561	32.17
Clarksville – Hopkinsville, TN – KY MSA	19	11.21
Cleveland – Akron – Lorain, OH CMSA	992	35.94
Colorado Springs, CO MSA	278	70.02
Columbia, MO MSA	92	81.87
Columbia, SC MSA	163	35.96
Columbus, GA – AL MSA	103	42.37
Columbus, OH MSA	502	36.44
Corpus Christi, TX MSA	175	50.02
Cumberland, MD – WV MSA	32	31.48
Dallas – Fort Worth, TX CMSA	1536	39.53
Danville, VA MSA	16	14.72
Davenport – Rock Island – Moline, IA – IL MSA	112	31.92
Dayton – Springfield, OH MSA	340	35.74
Daytona Beach, FL MSA	87	23.47
Decatur, AL MSA	33	25.08
Decatur, IL MSA	24	20.48
Denver – Boulder, CO CMSA	1281	69.31
Des Moines, IA MSA	133	33.85
Detroit – Ann Arbor, MI CMSA	1639	35.13
Dothan, AL MSA	33	25.20
Dubuque, IA MSA	33	38.19
Duluth, MN – WI MSA	103	42.92
Eau Claire, WI MSA	80	58.16
El Paso, TX MSA	132	22.31
Elkhart – Goshen, IN MSA	36	23.05
Elmira, NY MSA	51	53.57
Enid, OK MSA	34	59.93
Erie, PA MSA	142	51.53
Eugene – Springfield, OR MSA	53	18.73
Evansville, IN – KY MSA	134	48.03
Fargo – Moorhead, ND – MN MSA	73	47.62
Fayetteville, NC MSA	86	31.32

[Continued]

★ 728 ★

Physical Therapists
[Continued]

MSA/CMSA	Total Employees	Employees per 100,000 pop.
Fayetteville – Springdale, AR MSA	31	27.33
Fitchburg – Leominster, MA MSA	23	22.37
Flint, MI MSA	152	35.31
Florence, AL MSA	21	15.99
Florence, SC MSA	44	38.48
Fort Collins – Loveland, CO MSA	132	70.92
Fort Myers – Cape Coral, FL MSA	107	31.93
Fort Pierce, FL MSA	104	41.42
Fort Smith, AR – OK MSA	36	20.46
Fort Walton Beach, FL MSA	53	36.86
Fort Wayne, IN MSA	49	13.47
Fresno, CA MSA	292	43.75
Gadsden, AL MSA	31	31.05
Gainesville, FL MSA	207	101.42
Glens Falls, NY MSA	14	11.81
Grand Forks, ND MSA	78	110.35
Grand Rapids, MI MSA	342	49.68
Great Falls, MT MSA	32	41.19
Greeley, CO MSA	39	29.59
Green Bay, WI MSA	75	38.54
Greensboro – Winston-Salem – High Point, NC MSA	249	26.43
Greenville – Spartanburg, SC MSA	214	33.39
Hagerstown, MD MSA	17	14.00
Harrisburg – Lebanon – Carlisle, PA MSA	248	42.18
Hartford – New Britain – Middletown, CT CMSA	681	62.72
Hickory – Morganton, NC MSA	119	53.68
Honolulu, HI MSA	342	40.90
Houma – Thibodaux, LA MSA	31	16.95
Houston – Galveston – Brazoria, TX CMSA	1337	36.03
Huntington – Ashland, WV – KY – OH MSA	108	34.56
Huntsville, AL MSA	77	32.23
Indianapolis, IN MSA	604	48.33
Iowa City, IA MSA	110	114.44
Jackson, MI MSA	35	23.37
Jackson, MS MSA	62	15.68
Jackson, TN MSA	26	33.34
Jacksonville, FL MSA	282	31.10
Jacksonville, NC MSA	25	16.68
Jamestown – Dunkirk, NY	50	35.24
Janesville – Beloit, WI MSA	32	22.94
Johnson City – Kingsport – Bristol, TN – VA MSA	115	26.37
Johnstown, PA MSA	57	23.63
Joplin, MO MSA	41	30.39
Kalamazoo, MI MSA	82	36.70
Kankakee, IL MSA	33	34.28
Kansas City, MO – KS MSA	670	42.78

[Continued]

★ 728 ★

Physical Therapists
[Continued]

MSA/CMSA	Total Employees	Employees per 100,000 pop.
Killeen–Temple, TX MSA	52	20.37
Knoxville, TN MSA	360	59.52
Kokomo, IN MSA	5	5.16
La Crosse, WI MSA	40	40.86
Lafayette, LA MSA	46	22.04
Lafayette–West Lafayette, IN MSA	29	22.21
Lake Charles, LA MSA	18	10.71
Lakeland–Winter Haven, FL MSA	83	20.47
Lancaster, PA MSA	109	25.78
Lansing–East Lansing, MI MSA	183	42.30
Laredo, TX MSA	21	15.76
Las Cruces, NM MSA	27	19.92
Las Vegas, NV MSA	266	35.88
Lawton, OK MSA	49	43.95
Lewiston–Auburn, ME MSA	19	21.56
Lexington-Fayette, KY MSA	209	59.98
Lima, OH MSA	36	23.33
Lincoln, NE MSA	97	45.40
Little Rock–North Little Rock, AR MSA	222	43.26
Longview–Marshall, TX MSA	21	12.93
Los Angeles–Anaheim–Riverside, CA CMSA	6381	43.91
Louisville, KY–IN MSA	293	30.76
Lubbock, TX MSA	124	55.70
Lynchburg, VA MSA	28	19.69
Macon–Warner Robins, GA MSA	85	30.24
Madison, WI MSA	175	47.67
Manchester, NH MSA	72	48.71
Mansfield, OH MSA	58	45.98
McAllen–Edinburg–Mission, TX MSA	54	14.08
Medford, OR MSA	67	45.77
Melbourne–Titusville–Palm Bay, FL MSA	142	35.59
Memphis, TN–AR–MS MSA	351	35.75
Merced, CA MSA	27	15.13
Miami–Fort Lauderdale, FL CMSA	1245	39.00
Midland, TX MSA	46	43.15
Milwaukee–Racine, WI CMSA	890	55.38
Minneapolis–St. Paul, MN–WI MSA	1212	49.19
Mobile, AL MSA	231	48.44
Modesto, CA MSA	77	20.78
Monroe, LA MSA	16	11.25
Montgomery, AL MSA	79	27.01
Muncie, IN MSA	71	59.34
Muskegon, MI MSA	68	42.77
Naples, FL MSA	22	14.46
Nashville, TN MSA	612	62.13
New Bedford, MA MSA	62	35.30

[Continued]

★ 728 ★

Physical Therapists

[Continued]

MSA/CMSA	Total Employees	Employees per 100,000 pop.
New Haven – Meriden, CT MSA	363	68.47
New London – Norwich, CT – RI MSA	124	46.47
New Orleans, LA MSA	404	32.61
New York – Northern New Jersey – Long Island, NY – NJ – CT CMSA	6901	38.15
Norfolk – Virginia Beach – Newport News, VA MSA	430	30.80
Ocala, FL MSA	33	16.94
Odessa, TX MSA	17	14.29
Oklahoma City, OK MSA	489	51.00
Olympia, WA MSA	57	35.35
Omaha, NE – IA MSA	298	48.20
Orlando, FL MSA	296	27.59
Owensboro, KY MSA	13	14.91
Panama City, FL MSA	26	20.47
Parkersburg – Marietta, WV – OH MSA	52	34.86
Pascagoula, MS MSA	31	26.90
Pensacola, FL MSA	105	30.49
Peoria, IL MSA	88	25.95
Philadelphia – Wilmington – Trenton, PA – NJ – DE – MD CMSA	2774	47.02
Phoenix, AZ MSA	870	41.00
Pine Bluff, AR MSA	7	8.19
Pittsburgh – Beaver Valley, PA CMSA	910	40.57
Pittsfield, MA MSA	48	60.57
Portland, ME MSA	95	44.13
Portland – Vancouver, OR – WA CMSA	749	50.68
Portsmouth – Dover – Rochester, NH – ME MSA	100	44.73
Poughkeepsie, NY MSA	57	21.97
Providence – Pawtucket – Fall River, RI – MA CMSA	418	36.62
Provo – Orem, UT MSA	49	18.59
Pueblo, CO MSA	46	37.38
Raleigh – Durham, NC MSA	431	58.60
Rapid City, SD MSA	32	39.34
Reading, PA MSA	112	33.28
Redding, CA MSA	78	53.05
Reno, NV MSA	141	55.37
Richland – Kennewick – Pasco, WA MSA	36	23.99
Richmond – Petersburg, VA MSA	382	44.13
Roanoke, VA MSA	74	32.97
Rochester, MN MSA	108	101.44
Rochester, NY MSA	300	29.93
Rockford, IL MSA	91	32.07
Sacramento, CA MSA	569	38.42
Saginaw – Bay City – Midland, MI MSA	84	21.04
St. Cloud, MN MSA	92	48.19
St. Joseph, MO MSA	31	37.31
St. Louis, MO – IL MSA	1114	45.58
Salem, OR MSA	103	37.05

[Continued]

★ 728 ★

Physical Therapists
[Continued]

MSA/CMSA	Total Employees	Employees per 100,000 pop.
Salinas – Seaside – Monterey, CA MSA	54	15.18
Salt Lake City – Ogden, UT MSA	383	35.72
San Angelo, TX MSA	26	26.41
San Antonio, TX MSA	469	36.02
San Diego, CA MSA	1030	41.23
San Francisco – Oakland – San Jose, CA CMSA	3105	49.65
Santa Barbara – Santa Maria – Lompoc, CA MSA	251	67.91
Santa Fe, NM MSA	79	67.50
Sarasota, FL MSA	158	56.88
Savannah, GA MSA	40	16.49
Scranton – Wilkes-Barre, PA MSA	258	35.14
Seattle – Tacoma, WA CMSA	1489	58.18
Sharon, PA MSA	32	26.45
Sheboygan, WI MSA	23	22.14
Sherman – Denison, TX MSA	20	21.05
Shreveport, LA MSA	151	45.16
Sioux City, IA – NE MSA	52	45.21
Sioux Falls, SD MSA	55	44.42
South Bend – Mishawaka, IN MSA	139	56.26
Spokane, WA MSA	305	84.40
Springfield, IL MSA	77	40.62
Springfield, MO MSA	80	33.25
Springfield, MA MSA	240	45.32
State College, PA MSA	28	22.62
Steubenville – Weirton, OH – WV MSA	15	10.52
Stockton, CA MSA	125	26.01
Syracuse, NY MSA	201	30.46
Tallahassee, FL MSA	48	20.55
Tampa – St. Petersburg – Clearwater, FL MSA	836	40.43
Terre Haute, IN MSA	19	14.52
Texarkana, TX – Texarkana, AR MSA	38	31.63
Toledo, OH MSA	258	42.01
Topeka, KS MSA	60	37.27
Tucson, AZ MSA	244	36.59
Tulsa, OK MSA	243	34.28
Tuscaloosa, AL MSA	71	47.17
Tyler, TX MSA	95	62.79
Utica – Rome, NY MSA	73	23.06
Victoria, TX MSA	28	37.65
Visalia – Tulare – Porterville, CA MSA	89	28.53
Waco, TX MSA	10	5.29
Washington, DC – MD – VA MSA	1649	42.03
Waterbury, CT MSA	118	53.24
Waterloo – Cedar Falls, IA MSA	40	27.28
Wausau, WI MSA	30	26.00
West Palm Beach – Boca Raton – Delray Beach, FL MSA	412	47.71

[Continued]

★ 728 ★

Physical Therapists
[Continued]

MSA/CMSA	Total Employees	Employees per 100,000 pop.
Wheeling, WV – OH MSA	45	28.25
Wichita, KS MSA	247	50.90
Wichita Falls, TX MSA	54	44.13
Williamsport, PA MSA	38	32.01
Wilmington, NC MSA	54	44.89
Worcester, MA MSA	241	55.16
Yakima, WA MSA	48	25.42
York, PA MSA	86	20.58
Youngstown – Warren, OH MSA	216	43.85
Yuba City, CA MSA	44	35.88
Yuma, AZ MSA	23	21.52

Source: Census of Population and Housing, 1990: Equal Employment Opportunity (EEO) File on CD-ROM [machine-readable datafiles]. Prepared by the Bureau of the Census. Washington, DC: The Bureau, 1992.

★ 729 ★

Employment

Physicians

The table below presents the number of civilians 16 years old or older who reported working as physicians during the 1990 Census. Data are provided by total number employed in each Metropolitan Statistical Area (MSA) or Consolidated Metropolitan Statistical Area (CMSA), as well as the number employod per 100,000 people

[Total for all of the U.S. was 586,715; 235.90 per 100,000 persons]

MSA/CMSA	Total Employees	Employees per 100,000 pop.
Abilene, TX MSA	224	187.20
Albany, GA MSA	192	170.57
Albany – Schenectady – Troy, NY MSA	2563	293.15
Albuquerque, NM MSA	1751	364.35
Alexandria, LA MSA	213	161.91
Allentown – Bethlehem – Easton, PA – NJ MSA	1360	198.05
Altoona, PA MSA	197	150.91
Amarillo, TX MSA	415	221.28
Anchorage, AK MSA	586	258.90
Anderson, IN MSA	127	97.19
Anderson, SC MSA	305	210.06
Anniston, AL MSA	168	144.79
Appleton – Oshkosh – Neenah, WI MSA	554	175.81
Asheville, NC MSA	632	361.51
Athens, GA MSA	171	109.43
Atlanta, GA MSA	6540	230.81
Atlantic City, NJ MSA	555	173.75
Augusta, GA – SC MSA	1695	427.16

[Continued]

★ 729 ★

Physicians
[Continued]

MSA/CMSA	Total Employees	Employees per 100,000 pop.
Austin, TX MSA	1547	197.93
Bakersfield, CA MSA	782	143.89
Baltimore, MD MSA	9216	386.87
Bangor, ME MSA	276	311.00
Baton Rouge, LA MSA	770	145.76
Battle Creek, MI MSA	236	173.55
Beaumont – Port Arthur, TX MSA	520	143.95
Bellingham, WA MSA	238	186.26
Benton Harbor, MI MSA	227	140.66
Billings, MT MSA	232	204.55
Biloxi – Gulfport, MS MSA	403	204.44
Binghamton, NY MSA	616	232.89
Birmingham, AL MSA	2739	301.72
Bismarck, ND MSA	194	231.42
Bloomington, IN MSA	180	165.17
Bloomington – Normal, IL MSA	161	124.63
Boise City, ID MSA	374	181.75
Boston – Lawrence – Salem, MA – NH CMSA	15667	375.56
Bradenton, FL MSA	331	156.35
Bremerton, WA MSA	339	178.67
Brownsville – Harlingen, TX MSA	225	86.50
Bryan – College Station, TX MSA	162	132.94
Buffalo – Niagara Falls, NY CMSA	3297	277.22
Burlington, NC MSA	149	137.69
Burlington, VT MSA	686	521.92
Canton, OH MSA	664	168.48
Casper, WY MSA	175	285.83
Cedar Rapids, IA MSA	309	183.09
Champaign – Urbana – Rantoul, IL MSA	448	258.92
Charleston, SC MSA	1441	284.29
Charleston, WV MSA	648	258.73
Charlotte – Gastonia – Rock Hill, NC – SC MSA	1799	154.81
Charlottesville, VA MSA	984	750.53
Chattanooga, TN – GA MSA	917	211.68
Cheyenne, WY MSA	182	248.83
Chicago – Gary – Lake County, IL – IN – WI CMSA	22529	279.32
Chico, CA MSA	342	187.79
Cincinnati – Hamilton, OH – KY – IN CMSA	4030	231.06
Clarksville – Hopkinsville, TN – KY MSA	134	79.08
Cleveland – Akron – Lorain, OH CMSA	8707	315.49
Colorado Springs, CO MSA	647	162.97
Columbia, MO MSA	670	596.20
Columbia, SC MSA	1256	277.06
Columbus, GA – AL MSA	556	228.74
Columbus, OH MSA	3469	251.85
Corpus Christi, TX MSA	672	192.06

[Continued]

★ 729 ★

Physicians
[Continued]

MSA/CMSA	Total Employees	Employees per 100,000 pop.
Cumberland, MD–WV MSA	263	258.75
Dallas–Fort Worth, TX CMSA	8758	225.41
Danville, VA MSA	147	135.22
Davenport–Rock Island–Moline, IA–IL MSA	561	159.89
Dayton–Springfield, OH MSA	2095	220.23
Daytona Beach, FL MSA	595	160.50
Decatur, AL MSA	137	104.14
Decatur, IL MSA	198	168.93
Denver–Boulder, CO CMSA	5540	299.73
Des Moines, IA MSA	886	225.49
Detroit–Ann Arbor, MI CMSA	13849	296.86
Dothan, AL MSA	246	187.84
Dubuque, IA MSA	114	131.94
Duluth, MN–WI MSA	458	190.86
Eau Claire, WI MSA	201	146.14
El Paso, TX MSA	887	149.93
Elkhart–Goshen, IN MSA	184	117.80
Elmira, NY MSA	268	281.53
Enid, OK MSA	162	285.54
Erie, PA MSA	633	229.70
Eugene–Springfield, OR MSA	515	182.04
Evansville, IN–KY MSA	583	208.97
Fargo–Moorhead, ND–MN MSA	378	246.58
Fayetteville, NC MSA	496	180.65
Fayetteville–Springdale, AR MSA	248	218.68
Fitchburg–Leominster, MA MSA	189	183.86
Flint, MI MSA	851	197.70
Florence, AL MSA	159	121.07
Florence, SC MSA	236	206.39
Fort Collins–Loveland, CO MSA	437	234.77
Fort Myers–Cape Coral, FL MSA	515	153.68
Fort Pierce, FL MSA	328	130.64
Fort Smith, AR–OK MSA	280	159.17
Fort Walton Beach, FL MSA	220	153.02
Fort Wayne, IN MSA	590	162.17
Fresno, CA MSA	1565	234.46
Gadsden, AL MSA	152	152.24
Gainesville, FL MSA	1220	597.71
Glens Falls, NY MSA	252	212.59
Grand Forks, ND MSA	125	176.85
Grand Rapids, MI MSA	1355	196.83
Great Falls, MT MSA	223	287.03
Greeley, CO MSA	173	131.24
Green Bay, WI MSA	349	179.35
Greensboro–Winston-Salem–High Point, NC MSA	2160	229.28
Greenville–Spartanburg, SC MSA	1128	176.01

[Continued]

★ 729 ★

Physicians
[Continued]

MSA/CMSA	Total Employees	Employees per 100,000 pop.
Hagerstown, MD MSA	114	93.91
Harrisburg–Lebanon–Carlisle, PA MSA	1450	246.60
Hartford–New Britain–Middletown, CT CMSA	3509	323.16
Hickory–Morganton, NC MSA	355	160.13
Honolulu, HI MSA	2223	265.84
Houma–Thibodaux, LA MSA	188	102.82
Houston–Galveston–Brazoria, TX CMSA	9477	255.37
Huntington–Ashland, WV–KY–OH MSA	629	201.26
Huntsville, AL MSA	432	180.82
Indianapolis, IN MSA	3802	304.20
Iowa City, IA MSA	1256	1306.71
Jackson, MI MSA	170	113.52
Jackson, MS MSA	1298	328.28
Jackson, TN MSA	182	233.39
Jacksonville, FL MSA	2021	222.89
Jacksonville, NC MSA	117	78.08
Jamestown–Dunkirk, NY	104	73.29
Janesville–Beloit, WI MSA	158	113.25
Johnson City–Kingsport–Bristol, TN–VA MSA	991	227.27
Johnstown, PA MSA	454	188.19
Joplin, MO MSA	187	138.61
Kalamazoo, MI MSA	695	311.09
Kankakee, IL MSA	146	151.68
Kansas City, MO–KS MSA	4481	286.09
Killeen–Temple, TX MSA	734	287.50
Knoxville, TN MSA	1278	211.30
Kokomo, IN MSA	83	85.61
La Crosse, WI MSA	420	428.99
Lafayette, LA MSA	500	239.53
Lafayette–West Lafayette, IN MSA	205	156.97
Lake Charles, LA MSA	250	148.69
Lakeland–Winter Haven, FL MSA	626	154.42
Lancaster, PA MSA	650	153.73
Lansing–East Lansing, MI MSA	1146	264.86
Laredo, TX MSA	107	80.31
Las Cruces, NM MSA	181	133.57
Las Vegas, NV MSA	1008	135.95
Lawrence, KS MSA	100	122.25
Lawton, OK MSA	142	127.37
Lewiston–Auburn, ME MSA	172	195.14
Lexington-Fayette, KY MSA	1266	363.35
Lima, OH MSA	136	88.12
Lincoln, NE MSA	386	180.68
Little Rock–North Little Rock, AR MSA	1667	324.88
Longview–Marshall, TX MSA	178	109.58
Los Angeles–Anaheim–Riverside, CA CMSA	36656	252.25

[Continued]

★ 729 ★

Physicians
[Continued]

MSA/CMSA	Total Employees	Employees per 100,000 pop.
Louisville, KY – IN MSA	2492	261.58
Lubbock, TX MSA	797	357.98
Lynchburg, VA MSA	221	155.42
Macon – Warner Robins, GA MSA	546	194.23
Madison, WI MSA	1557	424.15
Manchester, NH MSA	293	198.23
Mansfield, OH MSA	98	77.69
McAllen – Edinburg – Mission, TX MSA	379	98.82
Medford, OR MSA	300	204.93
Melbourne – Titusville – Palm Bay, FL MSA	683	171.19
Memphis, TN – AR – MS MSA	2809	286.12
Merced, CA MSA	256	143.50
Miami – Fort Lauderdale, FL CMSA	9695	303.67
Midland, TX MSA	161	151.02
Milwaukee – Racine, WI CMSA	4178	259.96
Minneapolis – St. Paul, MN – WI MSA	6204	251.77
Mobile, AL MSA	1049	219.95
Modesto, CA MSA	656	177.05
Monroe, LA MSA	328	230.68
Montgomery, AL MSA	467	159.65
Muncie, IN MSA	195	162.96
Muskegon, MI MSA	238	149.70
Naples, FL MSA	253	166.34
Nashville, TN MSA	2957	300.20
New Bedford, MA MSA	273	155.43
New Haven – Meriden, CT MSA	2816	531.14
New London – Norwich, CT – RI MSA	522	195.64
New Orleans, LA MSA	4068	328.38
New York – Northern New Jersey – Long Island, NY – NJ – CT CMSA	68056	376.27
Norfolk – Virginia Beach – Newport News, VA MSA	2890	207.00
Ocala, FL MSA	358	183.75
Odessa, TX MSA	120	100.90
Oklahoma City, OK MSA	2514	262.19
Olympia, WA MSA	225	139.55
Omaha, NE – IA MSA	1771	286.45
Orlando, FL MSA	2332	217.39
Owensboro, KY MSA	152	174.33
Panama City, FL MSA	278	218.91
Parkersburg – Marietta, WV – OH MSA	226	151.51
Pascagoula, MS MSA	240	208.26
Pensacola, FL MSA	641	186.12
Peoria, IL MSA	746	219.95
Philadelphia – Wilmington – Trenton, PA – NJ – DE – MD CMSA	20639	349.85
Phoenix, AZ MSA	4860	229.02
Pine Bluff, AR MSA	98	114.64
Pittsburgh – Beaver Valley, PA CMSA	6522	290.80

[Continued]

★ 729 ★

Physicians
[Continued]

MSA/CMSA	Total Employees	Employees per 100,000 pop.
Pittsfield, MA MSA	286	360.88
Portland, ME MSA	939	436.17
Portland – Vancouver, OR – WA CMSA	4114	278.37
Portsmouth – Dover – Rochester, NH – ME MSA	419	187.41
Poughkeepsie, NY MSA	632	243.58
Providence – Pawtucket – Fall River, RI – MA CMSA	2804	245.64
Provo – Orem, UT MSA	340	128.99
Pueblo, CO MSA	211	171.47
Raleigh – Durham, NC MSA	3569	485.26
Rapid City, SD MSA	156	191.78
Reading, PA MSA	573	170.27
Redding, CA MSA	253	172.07
Reno, NV MSA	642	252.09
Richland – Kennewick – Pasco, WA MSA	227	151.30
Richmond – Petersburg, VA MSA	2870	331.55
Roanoke, VA MSA	726	323.42
Rochester, MN MSA	1826	1715.04
Rochester, NY MSA	2726	271.94
Rockford, IL MSA	577	203.37
Sacramento, CA MSA	3457	233.41
Saginaw – Bay City – Midland, MI MSA	786	196.83
St. Cloud, MN MSA	259	135.66
St. Joseph, MO MSA	168	202.21
St. Louis, MO – IL MSA	6506	266.19
Salem, OR MSA	471	169.41
Salinas – Seaside – Monterey, CA MSA	599	168.42
Salt Lake City – Ogden, UT MSA	2628	245.10
San Angelo, TX MSA	189	191.96
San Antonio, TX MSA	3939	302.51
San Diego, CA MSA	6526	261.25
San Francisco – Oakland – San Jose, CA CMSA	19971	319.37
Santa Barbara – Santa Maria – Lompoc, CA MSA	992	268.39
Santa Fe, NM MSA	341	291.35
Sarasota, FL MSA	744	267.84
Savannah, GA MSA	501	206.49
Scranton – Wilkes-Barre, PA MSA	1321	179.93
Seattle – Tacoma, WA CMSA	7360	287.59
Sharon, PA MSA	198	163.63
Sheboygan, WI MSA	131	126.11
Sherman – Denison, TX MSA	135	142.07
Shreveport, LA MSA	930	278.16
Sioux City, IA – NE MSA	244	212.14
Sioux Falls, SD MSA	276	222.92
South Bend – Mishawaka, IN MSA	422	170.81
Spokane, WA MSA	852	235.77
Springfield, IL MSA	629	331.84

[Continued]

★ 729 ★

Physicians
[Continued]

MSA/CMSA	Total Employees	Employees per 100,000 pop.
Springfield, MO MSA	682	283.47
Springfield, MA MSA	1071	202.26
State College, PA MSA	162	130.87
Steubenville – Weirton, OH – WV MSA	119	83.50
Stockton, CA MSA	755	157.09
Syracuse, NY MSA	1545	234.14
Tallahassee, FL MSA	664	284.25
Tampa – St. Petersburg – Clearwater, FL MSA	5203	251.60
Terre Haute, IN MSA	212	162.06
Texarkana, TX – Texarkana, AR MSA	224	186.46
Toledo, OH MSA	1826	297.33
Topeka, KS MSA	399	247.86
Tucson, AZ MSA	1997	299.45
Tulsa, OK MSA	1769	249.52
Tuscaloosa, AL MSA	317	210.60
Tyler, TX MSA	428	282.86
Utica – Rome, NY MSA	513	162.02
Victoria, TX MSA	155	208.44
Visalia – Tulare – Porterville, CA MSA	403	129.20
Waco, TX MSA	341	180.31
Washington, DC – MD – VA MSA	14043	357.91
Waterbury, CT MSA	346	156.12
Waterloo – Cedar Falls, IA MSA	260	177.34
Wausau, WI MSA	266	230.50
West Palm Beach – Boca Raton – Delray Beach, FL MSA	1894	219.34
Wheeling, WV – OH MSA	313	196.48
Wichita, KS MSA	1230	253.47
Wichita Falls, TX MSA	227	185.49
Williamsport, PA MSA	210	176.90
Wilmington, NC MSA	274	227.79
Worcester, MA MSA	1349	308.76
Yakima, WA MSA	283	149.88
York, PA MSA	698	167.05
Youngstown – Warren, OH MSA	1101	223.50
Yuba City, CA MSA	156	127.20
Yuma, AZ MSA	143	133.78

Source: Census of Population and Housing, 1990: Equal Employment Opportunity (EEO) File on CD-ROM [machine-readable datafiles]. Prepared by the Bureau of the Census. Washington, DC: The Bureau, 1992.

★ 730 ★

Employment

Physicians' Assistants

The table below presents the number of civilians 16 years old or older who reported working as physicians' assistants during the 1990 Census. Data are provided by total number employed in each Metropolitan Statistical Area (MSA) or Consolidated Metropolitan Statistical Area (CMSA), as well as the number employed per 100,000 people.

[Total for all of the U.S. was 25,569; 10.28 per 100,000 persons]

MSA/CMSA	Total Employees	Employees per 100,000 pop.
Abilene, TX MSA	42	35.10
Albany – Schenectady – Troy, NY MSA	111	12.70
Albuquerque, NM MSA	113	23.51
Alexandria, LA MSA	32	24.32
Allentown – Bethlehem – Easton, PA – NJ MSA	34	4.95
Altoona, PA MSA	10	7.66
Amarillo, TX MSA	44	23.46
Anchorage, AK MSA	32	14.14
Anderson, IN MSA	6	4.59
Anderson, SC MSA	8	5.51
Anniston, AL MSA	33	28.44
Appleton – Oshkosh – Neenah, WI MSA	18	5.71
Asheville, NC MSA	33	18.88
Athens, GA MSA	20	12.80
Atlanta, GA MSA	374	13.20
Atlantic City, NJ MSA	40	12.52
Augusta, GA – SC MSA	80	20.16
Austin, TX MSA	84	10.75
Bakersfield, CA MSA	31	5.70
Baltimore, MD MSA	250	10.49
Bangor, ME MSA	7	7.89
Baton Rouge, LA MSA	98	18.55
Battle Creek, MI MSA	19	13.97
Beaumont – Port Arthur, TX MSA	62	17.16
Bellingham, WA MSA	7	5.48
Benton Harbor, MI MSA	26	16.11
Billings, MT MSA	7	6.17
Binghamton, NY MSA	8	3.02
Birmingham, AL MSA	61	6.72
Bloomington, IN MSA	11	10.09
Boise City, ID MSA	66	32.07
Boston – Lawrence – Salem, MA – NH CMSA	339	8.13
Bradenton, FL MSA	57	26.92
Brownsville – Harlingen, TX MSA	25	9.61
Buffalo – Niagara Falls, NY CMSA	137	11.52
Burlington, VT MSA	34	25.87
Canton, OH MSA	24	6.09
Casper, WY MSA	2	3.27
Cedar Rapids, IA MSA	26	15.41
Champaign – Urbana – Rantoul, IL MSA	27	15.60
Charleston, SC MSA	44	8.68
Charleston, WV MSA	39	15.57

[Continued]

★ 730 ★

Physicians' Assistants
[Continued]

MSA/CMSA	Total Employees	Employees per 100,000 pop.
Charlotte – Gastonia – Rock Hill, NC – SC MSA	141	12.13
Chattanooga, TN – GA MSA	45	10.39
Chicago – Gary – Lake County, IL – IN – WI CMSA	679	8.42
Chico, CA MSA	47	25.81
Cincinnati – Hamilton, OH – KY – IN CMSA	107	6.13
Clarksville – Hopkinsville, TN – KY MSA	12	7.08
Cleveland – Akron – Lorain, OH CMSA	465	16.85
Colorado Springs, CO MSA	56	14.11
Columbia, MO MSA	14	12.46
Columbia, SC MSA	72	15.88
Columbus, GA – AL MSA	37	15.22
Columbus, OH MSA	81	5.88
Corpus Christi, TX MSA	20	5.72
Cumberland, MD – WV MSA	18	17.71
Dallas – Fort Worth, TX CMSA	252	6.49
Danville, VA MSA	10	9.20
Davenport – Rock Island – Moline, IA – IL MSA	15	4.28
Dayton – Springfield, OH MSA	74	7.78
Daytona Beach, FL MSA	9	2.43
Decatur, AL MSA	5	3.80
Denver – Boulder, CO CMSA	206	11.15
Des Moines, IA MSA	23	5.85
Detroit – Ann Arbor, MI CMSA	424	9.09
Dothan, AL MSA	28	21.38
Duluth, MN – WI MSA	33	13.75
Eau Claire. WI MSA	15	10.91
El Paso, TX MSA	34	5.75
Elkhart – Goshen, IN MSA	8	5.12
Enid, OK MSA	18	31.73
Erie, PA MSA	20	7.26
Eugene – Springfield, OR MSA	32	11.31
Evansville, IN – KY MSA	72	25.81
Fargo – Moorhead, ND – MN MSA	30	19.57
Fayetteville, NC MSA	67	24.40
Fayetteville – Springdale, AR MSA	11	9.70
Flint, MI MSA	40	9.29
Florence, AL MSA	2	1.52
Florence, SC MSA	19	16.62
Fort Collins – Loveland, CO MSA	36	19.34
Fort Myers – Cape Coral, FL MSA	43	12.83
Fort Pierce, FL MSA	17	6.77
Fort Smith, AR – OK MSA	7	3.98
Fort Walton Beach, FL MSA	8	5.56
Fort Wayne, IN MSA	37	10.17
Fresno, CA MSA	51	7.64
Gadsden, AL MSA	19	19.03

[Continued]

★ 730 ★

Physicians' Assistants
[Continued]

MSA/CMSA	Total Employees	Employees per 100,000 pop.
Gainesville, FL MSA	18	8.82
Glens Falls, NY MSA	14	11.81
Grand Forks, ND MSA	14	19.81
Grand Rapids, MI MSA	44	6.39
Great Falls, MT MSA	3	3.86
Greeley, CO MSA	24	18.21
Green Bay, WI MSA	27	13.88
Greensboro – Winston-Salem – High Point, NC MSA	136	14.44
Greenville – Spartanburg, SC MSA	68	10.61
Hagerstown, MD MSA	9	7.41
Harrisburg – Lebanon – Carlisle, PA MSA	44	7.48
Hartford – New Britain – Middletown, CT CMSA	152	14.00
Hickory – Morganton, NC MSA	15	6.77
Honolulu, HI MSA	182	21.76
Houma – Thibodaux, LA MSA	13	7.11
Houston – Galveston – Brazoria, TX CMSA	480	12.93
Huntington – Ashland, WV – KY – OH MSA	43	13.76
Huntsville, AL MSA	22	9.21
Indianapolis, IN MSA	207	16.56
Iowa City, IA MSA	13	13.52
Jackson, MI MSA	2	1.34
Jackson, MS MSA	9	2.28
Jackson, TN MSA	9	11.54
Jacksonville, FL MSA	93	10.26
Jacksonville, NC MSA	36	24.03
Janesville – Beloit, WI MSA	6	4.30
Johnson City – Kingsport – Bristol, TN – VA MSA	58	13.30
Johnstown, PA MSA	76	31.50
Joplin, MO MSA	2	1.48
Kalamazoo, MI MSA	36	16.11
Kansas City, MO – KS MSA	215	13.73
Killeen – Temple, TX MSA	30	11.75
Knoxville, TN MSA	48	7.94
Kokomo, IN MSA	16	16.50
La Crosse, WI MSA	21	21.45
Lafayette, LA MSA	17	8.14
Lafayette – West Lafayette, IN MSA	32	24.50
Lake Charles, LA MSA	26	15.46
Lakeland – Winter Haven, FL MSA	43	10.61
Lancaster, PA MSA	66	15.61
Lansing – East Lansing, MI MSA	90	20.80
Laredo, TX MSA	15	11.26
Las Cruces, NM MSA	4	2.95
Las Vegas, NV MSA	72	9.71
Lexington-Fayette, KY MSA	45	12.92
Lima, OH MSA	10	6.48

[Continued]

★ 730 ★

Physicians' Assistants

[Continued]

MSA/CMSA	Total Employees	Employees per 100,000 pop.
Lincoln, NE MSA	25	11.70
Little Rock – North Little Rock, AR MSA	53	10.33
Los Angeles – Anaheim – Riverside, CA CMSA	1351	9.30
Louisville, KY – IN MSA	90	9.45
Lubbock, TX MSA	9	4.04
Lynchburg, VA MSA	5	3.52
Macon – Warner Robins, GA MSA	96	34.15
Madison, WI MSA	17	4.63
McAllen – Edinburg – Mission, TX MSA	9	2.35
Medford, OR MSA	24	16.39
Melbourne – Titusville – Palm Bay, FL MSA	50	12.53
Memphis, TN – AR – MS MSA	116	11.82
Merced, CA MSA	14	7.85
Miami – Fort Lauderdale, FL CMSA	341	10.68
Midland, TX MSA	8	7.50
Milwaukee – Racine, WI CMSA	101	6.28
Minneapolis – St. Paul, MN – WI MSA	329	13.35
Mobile, AL MSA	12	2.52
Modesto, CA MSA	15	4.05
Monroe, LA MSA	16	11.25
Montgomery, AL MSA	69	23.59
Muncie, IN MSA	3	2.51
Muskegon, MI MSA	23	14.47
Naples, FL MSA	32	21.04
Nashville, TN MSA	118	11.98
New Haven – Meriden, CT MSA	124	23.39
New London – Norwich, CT – RI MSA	6	2.25
New Orleans, LA MSA	139	11.22
New York – Northern New Jersey – Long Island, NY – NJ – CT CMSA	2413	13.34
Norfolk – Virginia Beach – Newport News, VA MSA	102	7.31
Ocala, FL MSA	70	35.93
Odessa, TX MSA	8	6.73
Oklahoma City, OK MSA	142	14.81
Olympia, WA MSA	28	17.37
Omaha, NE – IA MSA	99	16.01
Orlando, FL MSA	69	6.43
Panama City, FL MSA	18	14.17
Parkersburg – Marietta, WV – OH MSA	39	26.14
Pascagoula, MS MSA	23	19.96
Pensacola, FL MSA	41	11.90
Peoria, IL MSA	31	9.14
Philadelphia – Wilmington – Trenton, PA – NJ – DE – MD CMSA	827	14.02
Phoenix, AZ MSA	180	8.48
Pittsburgh – Beaver Valley, PA CMSA	388	17.30
Portland, ME MSA	24	11.15
Portland – Vancouver, OR – WA CMSA	162	10.96

[Continued]

★ 730 ★

Physicians' Assistants
[Continued]

MSA/CMSA	Total Employees	Employees per 100,000 pop.
Portsmouth – Dover – Rochester, NH – ME MSA	18	8.05
Poughkeepsie, NY MSA	37	14.26
Providence – Pawtucket – Fall River, RI – MA CMSA	59	5.17
Provo – Orem, UT MSA	24	9.11
Pueblo, CO MSA	17	13.82
Raleigh – Durham, NC MSA	122	16.59
Rapid City, SD MSA	16	19.67
Reading, PA MSA	28	8.32
Reno, NV MSA	25	9.82
Richmond – Petersburg, VA MSA	37	4.27
Roanoke, VA MSA	30	13.36
Rochester, MN MSA	35	32.87
Rochester, NY MSA	42	4.19
Rockford, IL MSA	20	7.05
Sacramento, CA MSA	121	8.17
Saginaw – Bay City – Midland, MI MSA	34	8.51
St. Cloud, MN MSA	15	7.86
St. Joseph, MO MSA	32	38.52
St. Louis, MO – IL MSA	215	8.80
Salem, OR MSA	32	11.51
Salinas – Seaside – Monterey, CA MSA	55	15.46
Salt Lake City – Ogden, UT MSA	34	3.17
San Antonio, TX MSA	96	7.37
San Diego, CA MSA	199	7.97
San Francisco – Oakland – San Jose, CA CMSA	551	8.81
Santa Barbara – Santa Maria – Lompoc, CA MSA	69	18.67
Santa Fe, NM MSA	37	31.61
Sarasota, FL MSA	8	2.88
Savannah, GA MSA	18	7.42
Scranton – Wilkes-Barre, PA MSA	89	12.12
Seattle – Tacoma, WA CMSA	297	11.61
Sharon, PA MSA	4	3.31
Sheboygan, WI MSA	14	13.48
Sherman – Denison, TX MSA	9	9.47
Shreveport, LA MSA	29	8.67
Sioux City, IA – NE MSA	20	17.39
Sioux Falls, SD MSA	14	11.31
South Bend – Mishawaka, IN MSA	6	2.43
Spokane, WA MSA	28	7.75
Springfield, IL MSA	11	5.80
Springfield, MO MSA	96	39.90
Springfield, MA MSA	44	8.31
State College, PA MSA	10	8.08
Steubenville – Weirton, OH – WV MSA	7	4.91
Stockton, CA MSA	56	11.65
Syracuse, NY MSA	45	6.82

[Continued]

★ 730 ★

Physicians' Assistants
[Continued]

MSA/CMSA	Total Employees	Employees per 100,000 pop.
Tallahassee, FL MSA	50	21.40
Tampa – St. Petersburg – Clearwater, FL MSA	267	12.91
Terre Haute, IN MSA	18	13.76
Texarkana, TX – Texarkana, AR MSA	25	20.81
Toledo, OH MSA	63	10.26
Topeka, KS MSA	10	6.21
Tucson, AZ MSA	26	3.90
Tulsa, OK MSA	84	11.85
Tuscaloosa, AL MSA	15	9.97
Tyler, TX MSA	23	15.20
Utica – Rome, NY MSA	17	5.37
Victoria, TX MSA	14	18.83
Visalia – Tulare – Porterville, CA MSA	10	3.21
Waco, TX MSA	12	6.35
Washington, DC – MD – VA MSA	469	11.95
Waterbury, CT MSA	22	9.93
Waterloo – Cedar Falls, IA MSA	16	10.91
Wausau, WI MSA	3	2.60
West Palm Beach – Boca Raton – Delray Beach, FL MSA	52	8.02
Wheeling, WV – OH MSA	15	9.42
Wichita, KS MSA	78	16.07
Wichita Falls, TX MSA	25	20.43
Williamsport, PA MSA	16	13.48
Worcester, MA MSA	27	6.18
York, PA MSA	36	8.62
Youngstown – Warren, OH MSA	41	8.32

Source: Census of Population and Housing, 1990: Equal Employment Opportunity (EEO) File on CD-ROM [machine-readable datafiles]. Prepared by the Bureau of the Census. Washington, DC: The Bureau, 1992.

★ 731 ★
Employment
Podiatrists

The table below presents the number of civilians 16 years old or older who reported working as podiatrists during the 1990 Census. Data are provided by total number employed in each Metropolitan Statistical Area (MSA) or Consolidated Metropolitan Statistical Area (CMSA), as well as the number employed per 100,000 people.

[Total for all of the U.S. was 8,908; 3.58 per 100,000 persons]

MSA/CMSA	Total Employees	Employees per 100,000 pop.
Albany – Schenectady – Troy, NY MSA	38	4.35
Albuquerque, NM MSA	7	1.46
Allentown – Bethlehem – Easton, PA – NJ MSA	26	3.79
Amarillo, TX MSA	6	3.20
Atlanta, GA MSA	54	1.91
Atlantic City, NJ MSA	11	3.44
Augusta, GA – SC MSA	15	3.78
Austin, TX MSA	14	1.79
Baltimore, MD MSA	160	6.72
Baton Rouge, LA MSA	6	1.14
Beaumont – Port Arthur, TX MSA	15	4.15
Bellingham, WA MSA	21	16.43
Benton Harbor, MI MSA	6	3.72
Billings, MT MSA	7	6.17
Binghamton, NY MSA	6	2.27
Birmingham, AL MSA	5	0.55
Bloomington, IN MSA	11	10.09
Bloomington – Normal, IL MSA	7	5.42
Boston – Lawrence – Salem, MA – NH CMSA	262	6.28
Buffalo – Niagara Falls, NY CMSA	67	5.63
Canton, OH MSA	6	1.52
Charlotte – Gastonia – Rock Hill, NC – SC MSA	9	0.77
Charlottesville, VA MSA	21	16.02
Chicago – Gary – Lake County, IL – IN – WI CMSA	503	6.24
Cincinnati – Hamilton, OH – KY – IN CMSA	45	2.58
Cleveland – Akron – Lorain, OH CMSA	213	7.72
Colorado Springs, CO MSA	12	3.02
Columbus, GA – AL MSA	7	2.88
Columbus, OH MSA	65	4.72
Dallas – Fort Worth, TX CMSA	83	2.14
Danville, VA MSA	7	6.44
Davenport – Rock Island – Moline, IA – IL MSA	11	3.14
Dayton – Springfield, OH MSA	21	2.21
Daytona Beach, FL MSA	8	2.16
Decatur, IL MSA	6	5.12
Denver – Boulder, CO CMSA	87	4.71
Des Moines, IA MSA	46	11.71
Detroit – Ann Arbor, MI CMSA	229	4.91
Dothan, AL MSA	8	6.11
El Paso, TX MSA	9	1.52
Elkhart – Goshen, IN MSA	3	1.92
Erie, PA MSA	36	13.06

[Continued]

★ 731 ★

Podiatrists
[Continued]

MSA/CMSA	Total Employees	Employees per 100,000 pop.
Fayetteville, NC MSA	12	4.37
Fitchburg – Leominster, MA MSA	15	14.59
Flint, MI MSA	6	1.39
Fort Collins – Loveland, CO MSA	10	5.37
Fort Myers – Cape Coral, FL MSA	43	12.83
Fort Pierce, FL MSA	18	7.17
Fort Smith, AR – OK MSA	13	7.39
Fort Walton Beach, FL MSA	10	6.96
Fort Wayne, IN MSA	7	1.92
Fresno, CA MSA	26	3.90
Gadsden, AL MSA	6	6.01
Gainesville, FL MSA	9	4.41
Glens Falls, NY MSA	5	4.22
Grand Rapids, MI MSA	13	1.89
Great Falls, MT MSA	7	9.01
Green Bay, WI MSA	8	4.11
Greensboro – Winston-Salem – High Point, NC MSA	14	1.49
Greenville – Spartanburg, SC MSA	5	0.78
Hagerstown, MD MSA	10	8.24
Harrisburg – Lebanon – Carlisle, PA MSA	29	4.93
Hartford – New Britain – Middletown, CT CMSA	40	3.68
Honolulu, HI MSA	9	1.08
Houston – Galveston – Brazoria, TX CMSA	48	1.29
Huntington – Ashland, WV – KY – OH MSA	7	2.24
Indianapolis, IN MSA	28	2.24
Iowa City, IA MSA	2	2.08
Jackson, MS MSA	9	2.28
Jackson, TN MSA	6	7.69
Jacksonville, FL MSA	34	3.75
Jamestown – Dunkirk, NY	31	21.85
Janesville – Beloit, WI MSA	10	7.17
Johnson City – Kingsport – Bristol, TN – VA MSA	25	5.73
Kankakee, IL MSA	6	6.23
Kansas City, MO – KS MSA	20	1.28
Killeen – Temple, TX MSA	4	1.57
Kokomo, IN MSA	7	7.22
Lafayette, LA MSA	6	2.87
Lakeland – Winter Haven, FL MSA	10	2.47
Lancaster, PA MSA	9	2.13
Las Cruces, NM MSA	6	4.43
Las Vegas, NV MSA	4	0.54
Lawrence, KS MSA	10	12.23
Little Rock – North Little Rock, AR MSA	7	1.36
Los Angeles – Anaheim – Riverside, CA CMSA	417	2.87
Louisville, KY – IN MSA	8	0.84
Lubbock, TX MSA	13	5.84

[Continued]

★ 731 ★

Podiatrists
[Continued]

MSA/CMSA	Total Employees	Employees per 100,000 pop.
Lynchburg, VA MSA	5	3.52
Manchester, NH MSA	10	6.77
Memphis, TN – AR – MS MSA	26	2.65
Miami – Fort Lauderdale, FL CMSA	184	5.76
Milwaukee – Racine, WI CMSA	36	2.24
Minneapolis – St. Paul, MN – WI MSA	35	1.42
Mobile, AL MSA	7	1.47
Monroe, LA MSA	7	4.92
Montgomery, AL MSA	10	3.42
Muskegon, MI MSA	7	4.40
Naples, FL MSA	13	8.55
Nashville, TN MSA	27	2.74
New Bedford, MA MSA	21	11.96
New Haven – Meriden, CT MSA	39	7.36
New London – Norwich, CT – RI MSA	5	1.87
New Orleans, LA MSA	25	2.02
New York – Northern New Jersey – Long Island, NY – NJ – CT CMSA	1515	8.38
Norfolk – Virginia Beach – Newport News, VA MSA	16	1.15
Ocala, FL MSA	9	4.62
Odessa, TX MSA	5	4.20
Oklahoma City, OK MSA	14	1.46
Olympia, WA MSA	16	9.92
Omaha, NE – IA MSA	16	2.59
Orlando, FL MSA	25	2.33
Pascagoula, MS MSA	5	4.34
Philadelphia – Wilmington – Trenton, PA – NJ – DE – MD CMSA	608	10.31
Phoenix, AZ MSA	106	5.00
Pine Bluff, AR MSA	7	8.19
Pittsburgh – Beaver Valley, PA CMSA	149	6.64
Portland – Vancouver, OR – WA CMSA	38	2.57
Portsmouth – Dover – Rochester, NH – ME MSA	3	1.34
Poughkeepsie, NY MSA	6	2.31
Providence – Pawtucket – Fall River, RI – MA CMSA	62	5.43
Provo – Orem, UT MSA	16	6.07
Raleigh – Durham, NC MSA	4	0.54
Rapid City, SD MSA	8	9.83
Reading, PA MSA	18	5.35
Reno, NV MSA	8	3.14
Richland – Kennewick – Pasco, WA MSA	8	5.33
Richmond – Petersburg, VA MSA	33	3.81
Roanoke, VA MSA	5	2.23
Rochester, MN MSA	17	15.97
Rochester, NY MSA	22	2.19
Sacramento, CA MSA	34	2.30
Saginaw – Bay City – Midland, MI MSA	19	4.76
St. Cloud, MN MSA	2	1.05

[Continued]

★ 731 ★

Podiatrists
[Continued]

MSA/CMSA	Total Employees	Employees per 100,000 pop.
St. Joseph, MO MSA	6	7.22
St. Louis, MO–IL MSA	76	3.11
Salinas–Seaside–Monterey, CA MSA	17	4.78
Salt Lake City–Ogden, UT MSA	33	3.08
San Angelo, TX MSA	8	8.13
San Antonio, TX MSA	64	4.92
San Diego, CA MSA	73	2.92
San Francisco–Oakland–San Jose, CA CMSA	444	7.10
Santa Fe, NM MSA	7	5.98
Sarasota, FL MSA	31	11.16
Savannah, GA MSA	3	1.24
Scranton–Wilkes-Barre, PA MSA	84	11.44
Seattle–Tacoma, WA CMSA	109	4.26
Sharon, PA MSA	9	7.44
Shreveport, LA MSA	5	1.50
South Bend–Mishawaka, IN MSA	9	3.64
Spokane, WA MSA	17	4.70
Springfield, IL MSA	7	3.69
Springfield, MA MSA	9	1.70
State College, PA MSA	16	12.93
Steubenville–Weirton, OH–WV MSA	9	6.31
Stockton, CA MSA	25	5.20
Syracuse, NY MSA	44	6.67
Tampa–St. Petersburg–Clearwater, FL MSA	96	4.64
Toledo, OH MSA	15	2.44
Topeka, KS MSA	12	7.45
Tucson, AZ MSA	47	7.05
Tulsa, OK MSA	13	1.83
Utica–Rome, NY MSA	27	8.53
Victoria, TX MSA	14	18.83
Visalia–Tulare–Porterville, CA MSA	9	2.89
Waco, TX MSA	6	3.17
Washington, DC–MD–VA MSA	117	2.98
Waterloo–Cedar Falls, IA MSA	7	4.77
West Palm Beach–Boca Raton–Delray Beach, FL MSA	102	11.81
Wheeling, WV–OH MSA	5	3.14
Wichita, KS MSA	3	0.62
Williamsport, PA MSA	5	4.21
Wilmington, NC MSA	6	4.99
Worcester, MA MSA	15	3.43
Yakima, WA MSA	7	3.71
York, PA MSA	38	9.09
Youngstown–Warren, OH MSA	37	7.51
Yuma, AZ MSA	11	10.29

Source: Census of Population and Housing, 1990: Equal Employment Opportunity (EEO) File on CD-ROM [machine-readable datafiles]. Prepared by the Bureau of the Census. Washington, DC: The Bureau, 1992.

★ 732 ★

Employment

Psychologists

The table below presents the number of civilians 16 years old or older who reported working as psychologists during the 1990 Census. Data are provided by total number employed in each Metropolitan Statistical Area (MSA) or Consolidated Metropolitan Statistical Area (CMSA), as well as the number employed per 100,000 people.

[Total for all of the U.S. was 191,962; 77.18 per 100,000 persons]

MSA/CMSA	Total Employees	Employees per 100,000 pop.
Abilene, TX MSA	113	94.44
Albany, GA MSA	16	14.21
Albany–Schenectady–Troy, NY MSA	994	113.69
Albuquerque, NM MSA	706	146.91
Alexandria, LA MSA	40	30.41
Allentown–Bethlehem–Easton, PA–NJ MSA	469	68.30
Altoona, PA MSA	46	35.24
Amarillo, TX MSA	78	41.59
Anchorage, AK MSA	327	144.47
Anderson, IN MSA	71	54.34
Anderson, SC MSA	94	64.74
Anniston, AL MSA	20	17.24
Appleton–Oshkosh–Neenah, WI MSA	165	52.36
Asheville, NC MSA	135	77.22
Athens, GA MSA	143	91.51
Atlanta, GA MSA	2066	72.91
Atlantic City, NJ MSA	159	49.78
Augusta, GA–SC MSA	221	55.69
Austin, TX MSA	764	97.75
Bakersfield, CA MSA	213	39.19
Baltimore, MD MSA	2211	92.81
Bangor, ME MSA	155	174.66
Baton Rouge, LA MSA	305	57.74
Battle Creek, MI MSA	61	44.86
Beaumont–Port Arthur, TX MSA	73	20.21
Bellingham, WA MSA	129	100.95
Benton Harbor, MI MSA	85	52.67
Billings, MT MSA	141	124.32
Biloxi–Gulfport, MS MSA	114	57.83
Binghamton, NY MSA	194	73.35
Birmingham, AL MSA	402	44.28
Bismarck, ND MSA	36	42.94
Bloomington, IN MSA	115	105.53
Bloomington–Normal, IL MSA	137	106.05
Boise City, ID MSA	190	92.33
Boston–Lawrence–Salem, MA–NH CMSA	7316	175.37
Bradenton, FL MSA	79	37.32
Bremerton, WA MSA	112	59.03
Brownsville–Harlingen, TX MSA	18	6.92
Bryan–College Station, TX MSA	147	120.63
Buffalo–Niagara Falls, NY CMSA	940	79.04
Burlington, NC MSA	17	15.71

[Continued]

★ 732 ★

Psychologists
[Continued]

MSA/CMSA	Total Employees	Employees per 100,000 pop.
Burlington, VT MSA	342	260.20
Canton, OH MSA	160	40.60
Casper, WY MSA	64	104.53
Cedar Rapids, IA MSA	76	45.03
Champaign – Urbana – Rantoul, IL MSA	175	101.14
Charleston, SC MSA	354	69.84
Charleston, WV MSA	125	49.91
Charlotte – Gastonia – Rock Hill, NC – SC MSA	621	53.44
Charlottesville, VA MSA	179	136.53
Chattanooga, TN – GA MSA	214	49.40
Cheyenne, WY MSA	52	71.09
Chicago – Gary – Lake County, IL – IN – WI CMSA	6206	76.94
Chico, CA MSA	224	123.00
Cincinnati – Hamilton, OH – KY – IN CMSA	1217	69.78
Clarksville – Hopkinsville, TN – KY MSA	65	38.36
Cleveland – Akron – Lorain, OH CMSA	1677	60.76
Colorado Springs, CO MSA	434	109.32
Columbia, MO MSA	269	239.37
Columbia, SC MSA	523	115.37
Columbus, GA – AL MSA	116	47.72
Columbus, OH MSA	1087	78.92
Corpus Christi, TX MSA	181	51.73
Cumberland, MD – WV MSA	46	45.26
Dallas – Fort Worth, TX CMSA	2442	62.85
Danville, VA MSA	25	23.00
Davenport – Rock Island – Moline, IA – IL MSA	165	47.03
Dayton – Springfield, OH MSA	786	82.63
Daytona Beach, FL MSA	137	36.96
Decatur, AL MSA	49	37.25
Decatur, IL MSA	57	48.63
Denver – Boulder, CO CMSA	2937	158.90
Des Moines, IA MSA	343	87.29
Detroit – Ann Arbor, MI CMSA	3578	76.69
Dothan, AL MSA	46	35.12
Dubuque, IA MSA	62	71.76
Duluth, MN – WI MSA	189	78.76
Eau Claire, WI MSA	123	89.43
El Paso, TX MSA	210	35.50
Elkhart – Goshen, IN MSA	61	39.05
Elmira, NY MSA	73	76.68
Enid, OK MSA	29	51.11
Erie, PA MSA	205	74.39
Eugene – Springfield, OR MSA	270	95.44
Evansville, IN – KY MSA	158	56.63
Fargo – Moorhead, ND – MN MSA	86	56.10
Fayetteville, NC MSA	114	41.52

[Continued]

★ 732 ★

Psychologists
[Continued]

MSA/CMSA	Total Employees	Employees per 100,000 pop.
Fayetteville – Springdale, AR MSA	57	50.26
Fitchburg – Leominster, MA MSA	101	98.25
Flint, MI MSA	188	43.67
Florence, AL MSA	50	38.07
Florence, SC MSA	33	28.86
Fort Collins – Loveland, CO MSA	259	139.15
Fort Myers – Cape Coral, FL MSA	225	67.14
Fort Pierce, FL MSA	144	57.35
Fort Smith, AR – OK MSA	43	24.44
Fort Walton Beach, FL MSA	128	89.03
Fort Wayne, IN MSA	190	52.22
Fresno, CA MSA	502	75.21
Gadsden, AL MSA	20	20.03
Gainesville, FL MSA	347	170.01
Glens Falls, NY MSA	63	53.15
Grand Forks, ND MSA	51	72.15
Grand Rapids, MI MSA	542	78.73
Great Falls, MT MSA	34	43.76
Greeley, CO MSA	66	50.07
Green Bay, WI MSA	142	72.97
Greensboro – Winston-Salem – High Point, NC MSA	567	60.19
Greenville – Spartanburg, SC MSA	318	49.62
Hagerstown, MD MSA	61	50.25
Harrisburg – Lebanon – Carlisle, PA MSA	367	62.42
Hartford – New Britain – Middletown, CT CMSA	1275	117.42
Hickory – Morganton, NC MSA	83	37.44
Honolulu, HI MSA	509	60.87
Houma – Thibodaux, LA MSA	14	7.66
Houston – Galveston – Brazoria, TX CMSA	2516	67.80
Huntington – Ashland, WV – KY – OH MSA	144	46.08
Huntsville, AL MSA	137	57.34
Indianapolis, IN MSA	792	63.37
Iowa City, IA MSA	108	112.36
Jackson, MI MSA	64	42.74
Jackson, MS MSA	256	64.75
Jackson, TN MSA	58	74.38
Jacksonville, FL MSA	594	65.51
Jacksonville, NC MSA	32	21.36
Jamestown – Dunkirk, NY	98	69.07
Janesville – Beloit, WI MSA	81	58.06
Johnson City – Kingsport – Bristol, TN – VA MSA	220	50.45
Johnstown, PA MSA	101	41.87
Joplin, MO MSA	96	71.16
Kalamazoo, MI MSA	291	130.25
Kankakee, IL MSA	48	49.87
Kansas City, MO – KS MSA	1149	73.36

[Continued]

★ 732 ★

Psychologists
[Continued]

MSA/CMSA	Total Employees	Employees per 100,000 pop.
Killeen–Temple, TX MSA	110	43.09
Knoxville, TN MSA	439	72.58
Kokomo, IN MSA	25	25.79
La Crosse, WI MSA	105	107.25
Lafayette, LA MSA	144	68.99
Lafayette–West Lafayette, IN MSA	123	94.18
Lake Charles, LA MSA	85	50.55
Lakeland–Winter Haven, FL MSA	181	44.65
Lancaster, PA MSA	279	65.99
Lansing–East Lansing, MI MSA	375	86.67
Laredo, TX MSA	7	5.25
Las Cruces, NM MSA	76	56.08
Las Vegas, NV MSA	261	35.20
Lawrence, KS MSA	99	121.03
Lawton, OK MSA	63	56.51
Lewiston–Auburn, ME MSA	34	38.57
Lexington-Fayette, KY MSA	318	91.27
Lima, OH MSA	61	39.52
Lincoln, NE MSA	311	145.57
Little Rock–North Little Rock, AR MSA	460	89.65
Longview–Marshall, TX MSA	32	19.70
Los Angeles–Anaheim–Riverside, CA CMSA	13098	90.14
Louisville, KY–IN MSA	630	66.13
Lubbock, TX MSA	150	70.07
Lynchburg, VA MSA	94	66.10
Macon–Warner Robins, GA MSA	115	40.91
Madison, WI MSA	528	143.84
Manchester, NH MSA	101	68.33
Mansfield, OH MSA	35	27.75
McAllen–Edinburg–Mission, TX MSA	98	25.55
Medford, OR MSA	84	57.38
Melbourne–Titusville–Palm Bay, FL MSA	170	42.61
Memphis, TN–AR–MS MSA	597	60.81
Merced, CA MSA	44	24.66
Miami–Fort Lauderdale, FL CMSA	2169	67.94
Midland, TX MSA	78	73.16
Milwaukee–Racine, WI CMSA	1307	81.32
Minneapolis–St. Paul, MN–WI MSA	3072	124.67
Mobile, AL MSA	217	45.50
Modesto, CA MSA	149	40.21
Monroe, LA MSA	50	35.16
Montgomery, AL MSA	140	47.86
Muncie, IN MSA	126	105.30
Muskegon, MI MSA	87	54.72
Naples, FL MSA	92	60.49
Nashville, TN MSA	748	75.94

[Continued]

★ 732 ★

Psychologists
[Continued]

MSA/CMSA	Total Employees	Employees per 100,000 pop.
New Bedford, MA MSA	112	63.77
New Haven – Meriden, CT MSA	922	173.90
New London – Norwich, CT – RI MSA	288	107.94
New Orleans, LA MSA	770	62.16
New York – Northern New Jersey – Long Island, NY – NJ – CT CMSA	22031	121.80
Norfolk – Virginia Beach – Newport News, VA MSA	1272	91.11
Ocala, FL MSA	93	47.73
Odessa, TX MSA	21	17.66
Oklahoma City, OK MSA	640	66.75
Olympia, WA MSA	160	99.23
Omaha, NE – IA MSA	366	59.20
Orlando, FL MSA	679	63.30
Owensboro, KY MSA	38	43.58
Panama City, FL MSA	86	67.72
Parkersburg – Marietta, WV – OH MSA	56	37.54
Pascagoula, MS MSA	54	46.86
Pensacola, FL MSA	384	111.50
Peoria, IL MSA	235	69.29
Philadelphia – Wilmington – Trenton, PA – NJ – DE – MD CMSA	5773	97.86
Phoenix, AZ MSA	1640	77.28
Pine Bluff, AR MSA	35	40.94
Pittsburgh – Beaver Valley, PA CMSA	1710	76.24
Pittsfield, MA MSA	99	124.92
Portland, ME MSA	267	124.02
Portland – Vancouver, OR – WA CMSA	1186	80.25
Portsmouth – Dover – Rochester, NH – ME MSA	326	145.81
Poughkeepsie, NY MSA	414	159.56
Providence – Pawtucket – Fall River, RI – MA CMSA	1189	104.16
Provo – Orem, UT MSA	294	111.54
Pueblo, CO MSA	142	115.40
Raleigh – Durham, NC MSA	978	132.97
Rapid City, SD MSA	19	23.36
Reading, PA MSA	156	46.36
Redding, CA MSA	80	54.41
Reno, NV MSA	261	102.49
Richland – Kennewick – Pasco, WA MSA	101	67.32
Richmond – Petersburg, VA MSA	823	95.07
Roanoke, VA MSA	214	95.33
Rochester, MN MSA	121	113.65
Rochester, NY MSA	1052	104.95
Rockford, IL MSA	131	46.17
Sacramento, CA MSA	1338	90.34
Saginaw – Bay City – Midland, MI MSA	247	61.86
St. Cloud, MN MSA	181	94.80
St. Joseph, MO MSA	52	62.59
St. Louis, MO – IL MSA	1484	60.72

[Continued]

★ 732 ★

Psychologists
[Continued]

MSA/CMSA	Total Employees	Employees per 100,000 pop.
Salem, OR MSA	270	97.11
Salinas – Seaside – Monterey, CA MSA	274	77.04
Salt Lake City – Ogden, UT MSA	694	64.73
San Angelo, TX MSA	76	77.19
San Antonio, TX MSA	834	64.05
San Diego, CA MSA	2765	110.69
San Francisco – Oakland – San Jose, CA CMSA	8905	142.40
Santa Barbara – Santa Maria – Lompoc, CA MSA	489	132.30
Santa Fe, NM MSA	148	126.45
Sarasota, FL MSA	244	87.84
Savannah, GA MSA	81	33.39
Scranton – Wilkes-Barre, PA MSA	437	59.52
Seattle – Tacoma, WA CMSA	2934	114.65
Sharon, PA MSA	52	42.97
Sheboygan, WI MSA	47	45.25
Sherman – Denison, TX MSA	64	67.35
Shreveport, LA MSA	155	46.36
Sioux City, IA – NE MSA	62	53.90
Sioux Falls, SD MSA	155	125.19
South Bend – Mishawaka, IN MSA	116	46.95
Spokane, WA MSA	322	89.11
Springfield, IL MSA	70	36.93
Springfield, MO MSA	163	67.75
Springfield, MA MSA	723	136.54
State College, PA MSA	162	130.87
Steubenville – Weirton, OH – WV MSA	46	32.28
Stockton, CA MSA	306	63.67
Syracuse, NY MSA	760	115.18
Tallahassee, FL MSA	384	164.38
Tampa – St. Petersburg – Clearwater, FL MSA	1545	74.71
Terre Haute, IN MSA	52	39.75
Texarkana, TX – Texarkana, AR MSA	14	11.65
Toledo, OH MSA	290	47.22
Topeka, KS MSA	174	108.09
Tucson, AZ MSA	681	102.12
Tulsa, OK MSA	471	66.44
Tuscaloosa, AL MSA	183	121.58
Tyler, TX MSA	93	61.46
Utica – Rome, NY MSA	201	63.48
Victoria, TX MSA	19	25.55
Visalia – Tulare – Porterville, CA MSA	168	53.86
Waco, TX MSA	157	83.01
Washington, DC – MD – VA MSA	4881	124.40
Waterbury, CT MSA	202	91.14
Waterloo – Cedar Falls, IA MSA	117	79.80
Wausau, WI MSA	48	41.59

[Continued]

★ 732 ★

Psychologists
[Continued]

MSA/CMSA	Total Employees	Employees per 100,000 pop.
West Palm Beach – Boca Raton – Delray Beach, FL MSA	615	71.22
Wheeling, WV – OH MSA	83	52.10
Wichita, KS MSA	290	59.76
Wichita Falls, TX MSA	63	51.48
Williamsport, PA MSA	59	49.70
Wilmington, NC MSA	51	42.40
Worcester, MA MSA	571	130.69
Yakima, WA MSA	134	70.97
York, PA MSA	110	26.33
Youngstown – Warren, OH MSA	178	36.13
Yuba City, CA MSA	74	60.34
Yuma, AZ MSA	10	9.35

Source: Census of Population and Housing, 1990: Equal Employment Opportunity (EEO) File on CD-ROM [machine-readable datafiles]. Prepared by the Bureau of the Census. Washington, DC: The Bureau, 1992.

★ 733 ★

Employment

Psychology Teachers

The table below presents the number of civilians 16 years old or older who reported working as psychology teachers during the 1990 Census. Data are provided by total number employed in each Metropolitan Statistical Area (MSA) or Consolidated Metropolitan Statistical Area (CMSA), as well as the number employed per 100,000 people.

[Total for all of the U.S. was 4,518; 1.82 per 100,000 persons]

MSA/CMSA	Total Employees	Employees per 100,000 pop.
Albany – Schenectady – Troy, NY MSA	27	3.09
Albuquerque, NM MSA	44	9.16
Allentown – Bethlehem – Easton, PA – NJ MSA	7	1.02
Appleton – Oshkosh – Neenah, WI MSA	13	4.13
Athens, GA MSA	33	21.12
Atlanta, GA MSA	38	1.34
Atlantic City, NJ MSA	10	3.13
Augusta, GA – SC MSA	4	1.01
Austin, TX MSA	40	5.12
Bakersfield, CA MSA	7	1.29
Baltimore, MD MSA	58	2.43
Bangor, ME MSA	6	6.76
Baton Rouge, LA MSA	6	1.14
Battle Creek, MI MSA	16	11.77
Binghamton, NY MSA	28	10.59
Birmingham, AL MSA	14	1.54
Bloomington, IN MSA	9	8.26

[Continued]

★ 733 ★

Psychology Teachers
[Continued]

MSA/CMSA	Total Employees	Employees per 100,000 pop.
Bloomington – Normal, IL MSA	19	14.71
Boise City, ID MSA	6	2.92
Boston – Lawrence – Salem, MA – NH CMSA	128	3.07
Brownsville – Harlingen, TX MSA	9	3.46
Bryan – College Station, TX MSA	7	5.74
Buffalo – Niagara Falls, NY CMSA	10	0.84
Burlington, VT MSA	21	15.98
Canton, OH MSA	1	0.25
Champaign – Urbana – Rantoul, IL MSA	25	14.45
Charleston, SC MSA	23	4.54
Charleston, WV MSA	8	3.19
Charlotte – Gastonia – Rock Hill, NC – SC MSA	32	2.75
Charlottesville, VA MSA	6	4.58
Chattanooga, TN – GA MSA	20	4.62
Chicago – Gary – Lake County, IL – IN – WI CMSA	87	1.08
Chico, CA MSA	12	6.59
Cincinnati – Hamilton, OH – KY – IN CMSA	48	2.75
Clarksville – Hopkinsville, TN – KY MSA	6	3.54
Cleveland – Akron – Lorain, OH CMSA	38	1.38
Colorado Springs, CO MSA	8	2.02
Columbia, MO MSA	11	9.79
Columbia, SC MSA	12	2.65
Columbus, OH MSA	20	1.45
Dallas – Fort Worth, TX CMSA	40	1.11
Davenport – Rock Island – Moline, IA – IL MSA	8	2.28
Dayton – Springfield, OH MSA	22	2.31
Decatur, AL MSA	5	3.80
Decatur, IL MSA	7	5.97
Denver – Boulder, CO CMSA	31	1.68
Des Moines, IA MSA	12	3.05
Detroit – Ann Arbor, MI CMSA	36	0.77
Duluth, MN – WI MSA	2	0.83
El Paso, TX MSA	14	2.37
Eugene – Springfield, OR MSA	32	11.31
Evansville, IN – KY MSA	8	2.87
Fayetteville – Springdale, AR MSA	21	18.52
Fort Pierce, FL MSA	10	3.98
Fort Wayne, IN MSA	8	2.20
Gainesville, FL MSA	13	6.37
Greeley, CO MSA	18	13.65
Greensboro – Winston-Salem – High Point, NC MSA	12	1.27
Harrisburg – Lebanon – Carlisle, PA MSA	17	2.89
Houston – Galveston – Brazoria, TX CMSA	42	1.13
Huntington – Ashland, WV – KY – OH MSA	13	4.16
Huntsville, AL MSA	16	6.70
Indianapolis, IN MSA	12	0.96

[Continued]

★ 733 ★

Psychology Teachers
[Continued]

MSA/CMSA	Total Employees	Employees per 100,000 pop.
Iowa City, IA MSA	20	20.81
Jackson, MS MSA	31	7.84
Jamestown–Dunkirk, NY	7	4.93
Janesville–Beloit, WI MSA	14	10.04
Johnson City–Kingsport–Bristol, TN–VA MSA	14	3.21
Joplin, MO MSA	7	5.19
Kalamazoo, MI MSA	6	2.69
Kansas City, MO–KS MSA	15	0.96
Killeen–Temple, TX MSA	9	3.53
La Crosse, WI MSA	5	5.11
Lafayette–West Lafayette, IN MSA	9	6.89
Lakeland–Winter Haven, FL MSA	7	1.73
Lansing–East Lansing, MI MSA	40	9.24
Lawrence, KS MSA	41	50.12
Lawton, OK MSA	11	9.87
Lexington-Fayette, KY MSA	9	2.58
Little Rock–North Little Rock, AR MSA	5	0.97
Los Angeles–Anaheim–Riverside, CA CMSA	181	1.25
Lubbock, TX MSA	47	21.11
Madison, WI MSA	21	5.72
Melbourne–Titusville–Palm Bay, FL MSA	4	1.00
Memphis, TN–AR–MS MSA	16	1.63
Midland, TX MSA	6	5.63
Milwaukee–Racine, WI CMSA	43	2.68
Minneapolis–St. Paul, MN–WI MSA	42	1.70
Montgomery, AL MSA	21	7.18
Muncie, IN MSA	23	19.22
Nashville, TN MSA	22	2.23
New Haven–Meriden, CT MSA	17	3.21
New London–Norwich, CT–RI MSA	9	3.37
New Orleans, LA MSA	36	2.91
New York–Northern New Jersey–Long Island, NY–NJ–CT CMSA	464	2.57
Norfolk–Virginia Beach–Newport News, VA MSA	15	1.07
Odessa, TX MSA	5	4.20
Oklahoma City, OK MSA	16	1.67
Olympia, WA MSA	6	3.72
Omaha, NE–IA MSA	24	3.88
Orlando, FL MSA	7	0.65
Parkersburg–Marietta, WV–OH MSA	7	4.69
Philadelphia–Wilmington–Trenton, PA–NJ–DE–MD CMSA	83	1.41
Phoenix, AZ MSA	17	0.80
Pittsburgh–Beaver Valley, PA CMSA	55	2.45
Portland–Vancouver, OR–WA CMSA	16	1.08
Portsmouth–Dover–Rochester, NH–ME MSA	8	3.58
Provo–Orem, UT MSA	13	4.93
Raleigh–Durham, NC MSA	41	5.57

[Continued]

★ 733 ★

Psychology Teachers

[Continued]

MSA/CMSA	Total Employees	Employees per 100,000 pop.
Reading, PA MSA	2	0.59
Reno, NV MSA	25	9.82
Roanoke, VA MSA	10	4.45
Rochester, MN MSA	6	5.64
Rochester, NY MSA	13	1.30
Rockford, IL MSA	5	1.76
Sacramento, CA MSA	41	2.77
St. Cloud, MN MSA	3	1.57
St. Louis, MO – IL MSA	19	0.78
Salt Lake City – Ogden, UT MSA	14	1.31
San Antonio, TX MSA	35	2.69
San Diego, CA MSA	52	2.08
San Francisco – Oakland – San Jose, CA CMSA	132	2.11
Santa Barbara – Santa Maria – Lompoc, CA MSA	10	2.71
Scranton – Wilkes-Barre, PA MSA	11	1.50
Seattle – Tacoma, WA CMSA	66	2.58
Sioux City, IA – NE MSA	5	4.35
Spokane, WA MSA	6	1.66
Springfield, IL MSA	12	6.33
Springfield, MO MSA	17	7.07
Springfield, MA MSA	30	5.67
Stockton, CA MSA	7	1.46
Syracuse, NY MSA	11	1.67
Tallahassee, FL MSA	25	10.70
Tampa – St. Petersburg – Clearwater, FL MSA	20	0.97
Terre Haute, IN MSA	6	4.59
Toledo, OH MSA	32	5.21
Tucson, AZ MSA	15	2.25
Tulsa, OK MSA	12	1.69
Tuscaloosa, AL MSA	7	4.65
Waco, TX MSA	8	4.23
Washington, DC – MD – VA MSA	44	1.12
Wausau, WI MSA	7	6.07
West Palm Beach – Boca Raton – Delray Beach, FL MSA	20	2.32
Wheeling, WV – OH MSA	6	3.77
Wichita, KS MSA	16	3.30
Wilmington, NC MSA	5	4.16
Worcester, MA MSA	5	1.14
Yakima, WA MSA	16	8.47
York, PA MSA	15	3.59
Yuba City, CA MSA	5	4.08

Source: Census of Population and Housing, 1990: Equal Employment Opportunity (EEO) File on CD-ROM [machine-readable datafiles]. Prepared by the Bureau of the Census. Washington, DC: The Bureau, 1992.

★ 734 ★

Employment

Radiologic Technicians

The table below presents the number of civilians 16 years old or older who reported working as radiologic technicians during the 1990 Census. Data are provided by total number employed in each Metropolitan Statistical Area (MSA) or Consolidated Metropolitan Statistical Area (CMSA), as well as the number employed per 100,000 people.

[Total for all of the U.S. was 130,383; 52.42 per 100,000 persons]

MSA/CMSA	Total Employees	Employees per 100,000 pop.
Abilene, TX MSA	44	36.77
Albany, GA MSA	81	71.96
Albany – Schenectady – Troy, NY MSA	472	53.99
Albuquerque, NM MSA	310	64.51
Alexandria, LA MSA	67	50.93
Allentown – Bethlehem – Easton, PA – NJ MSA	389	56.65
Altoona, PA MSA	61	46.73
Amarillo, TX MSA	108	57.59
Anchorage, AK MSA	117	51.69
Anderson, IN MSA	84	64.28
Anderson, SC MSA	123	84.71
Anniston, AL MSA	54	46.54
Appleton – Oshkosh – Neenah, WI MSA	147	46.65
Asheville, NC MSA	94	53.77
Athens, GA MSA	37	23.68
Atlanta, GA MSA	1511	53.33
Atlantic City, NJ MSA	142	44.46
Augusta, GA – SC MSA	214	53.93
Austin, TX MSA	298	38.13
Bakersfield, CA MSA	363	66.79
Baltimore, MD MSA	1453	60.99
Bangor, ME MSA	78	87.89
Baton Rouge, LA MSA	322	60.95
Battle Creek, MI MSA	84	61.77
Beaumont – Port Arthur, TX MSA	295	81.67
Bellingham, WA MSA	44	34.43
Benton Harbor, MI MSA	87	53.91
Billings, MT MSA	91	80.23
Biloxi – Gulfport, MS MSA	82	41.60
Binghamton, NY MSA	92	34.78
Birmingham, AL MSA	643	70.83
Bismarck, ND MSA	81	96.62
Bloomington, IN MSA	50	45.88
Bloomington – Normal, IL MSA	43	33.29
Boise City, ID MSA	135	65.61
Boston – Lawrence – Salem, MA – NH CMSA	2728	65.39
Bradenton, FL MSA	128	60.46
Bremerton, WA MSA	119	62.72
Brownsville – Harlingen, TX MSA	81	31.14
Bryan – College Station, TX MSA	79	64.83
Buffalo – Niagara Falls, NY CMSA	726	61.04
Burlington, NC MSA	50	46.21

[Continued]

★ 734 ★

Radiologic Technicians
[Continued]

MSA/CMSA	Total Employees	Employees per 100,000 pop.
Burlington, VT MSA	52	39.56
Canton, OH MSA	354	89.82
Casper, WY MSA	10	16.33
Cedar Rapids, IA MSA	96	56.88
Champaign–Urbana–Rantoul, IL MSA	144	83.22
Charleston, SC MSA	300	59.19
Charleston, WV MSA	161	64.28
Charlotte–Gastonia–Rock Hill, NC–SC MSA	597	51.37
Charlottesville, VA MSA	150	114.41
Chattanooga, TN–GA MSA	420	96.95
Cheyenne, WY MSA	36	49.22
Chicago–Gary–Lake County, IL–IN–WI CMSA	4049	50.20
Chico, CA MSA	115	63.15
Cincinnati–Hamilton, OH–KY–IN CMSA	1087	62.32
Clarksville–Hopkinsville, TN–KY MSA	89	52.53
Cleveland–Akron–Lorain, OH CMSA	1855	67.21
Colorado Springs, CO MSA	140	35.26
Columbia, MO MSA	147	130.81
Columbia, SC MSA	202	44.56
Columbus, GA–AL MSA	124	51.01
Columbus, OH MSA	855	62.07
Corpus Christi, TX MSA	217	62.02
Cumberland, MD–WV MSA	57	56.08
Dallas–Fort Worth, TX CMSA	1516	39.02
Danville, VA MSA	60	55.19
Davenport–Rock Island–Moline, IA–IL MSA	246	70.11
Dayton–Springfield, OH MSA	507	53.30
Daytona Beach, FL MSA	184	49.63
Decatur, AL MSA	75	57.01
Decatur, IL MSA	72	61.43
Denver–Boulder, CO CMSA	926	50.10
Des Moines, IA MSA	235	59.81
Detroit–Ann Arbor, MI CMSA	2792	59.85
Dothan, AL MSA	108	82.47
Dubuque, IA MSA	91	105.32
Duluth, MN–WI MSA	210	87.51
Eau Claire, WI MSA	118	85.79
El Paso, TX MSA	185	31.27
Elkhart–Goshen, IN MSA	30	19.21
Elmira, NY MSA	93	97.69
Enid, OK MSA	20	35.25
Erie, PA MSA	163	59.15
Eugene–Springfield, OR MSA	150	53.02
Evansville, IN–KY MSA	222	79.57
Fargo–Moorhead, ND–MN MSA	105	68.49
Fayetteville, NC MSA	160	58.27

[Continued]

★ 734 ★

Radiologic Technicians
[Continued]

MSA/CMSA	Total Employees	Employees per 100,000 pop.
Fayetteville–Springdale, AR MSA	61	53.79
Fitchburg–Leominster, MA MSA	41	39.88
Flint, MI MSA	352	81.77
Florence, AL MSA	62	47.21
Florence, SC MSA	88	76.96
Fort Collins–Loveland, CO MSA	76	40.83
Fort Myers–Cape Coral, FL MSA	142	42.37
Fort Pierce, FL MSA	94	37.44
Fort Smith, AR–OK MSA	106	60.26
Fort Walton Beach, FL MSA	96	66.77
Fort Wayne, IN MSA	257	70.64
Fresno, CA MSA	359	53.78
Gadsden, AL MSA	66	66.11
Gainesville, FL MSA	192	94.07
Glens Falls, NY MSA	52	43.87
Grand Forks, ND MSA	23	32.54
Grand Rapids, MI MSA	275	39.95
Great Falls, MT MSA	97	124.85
Greeley, CO MSA	74	56.14
Green Bay, WI MSA	81	41.63
Greensboro–Winston-Salem–High Point, NC MSA	522	55.41
Greenville–Spartanburg, SC MSA	398	62.10
Hagerstown, MD MSA	44	36.25
Harrisburg–Lebanon–Carlisle, PA MSA	379	64.46
Hartford–New Britain–Middletown, CT CMSA	663	61.06
Hickory–Morganton, NC MSA	158	71.27
Honolulu, HI MSA	266	31.81
Houma–Thibodaux, LA MSA	104	56.88
Houston–Galveston–Brazoria, TX CMSA	1729	46.59
Huntington–Ashland, WV–KY–OH MSA	263	84.15
Huntsville, AL MSA	134	56.09
Indianapolis, IN MSA	937	74.97
Iowa City, IA MSA	132	137.33
Jackson, MI MSA	53	35.39
Jackson, MS MSA	251	63.48
Jackson, TN MSA	44	56.42
Jacksonville, FL MSA	587	64.74
Jacksonville, NC MSA	27	18.02
Jamestown–Dunkirk, NY	51	35.94
Janesville–Beloit, WI MSA	73	52.33
Johnson City–Kingsport–Bristol, TN–VA MSA	238	54.58
Johnstown, PA MSA	177	73.37
Joplin, MO MSA	52	38.54
Kalamazoo, MI MSA	109	48.79
Kankakee, IL MSA	58	60.26
Kansas City, MO–KS MSA	947	60.46

[Continued]

★ 734 ★

Radiologic Technicians
[Continued]

MSA/CMSA	Total Employees	Employees per 100,000 pop.
Killeen – Temple, TX MSA	131	51.31
Knoxville, TN MSA	377	62.33
Kokomo, IN MSA	17	17.54
La Crosse, WI MSA	84	85.80
Lafayette, LA MSA	166	79.52
Lafayette – West Lafayette, IN MSA	35	26.80
Lake Charles, LA MSA	124	73.75
Lakeland – Winter Haven, FL MSA	140	34.54
Lancaster, PA MSA	177	41.86
Lansing – East Lansing, MI MSA	278	64.25
Laredo, TX MSA	27	20.26
Las Cruces, NM MSA	53	39.11
Las Vegas, NV MSA	299	40.33
Lawrence, KS MSA	8	9.78
Lawton, OK MSA	88	78.93
Lewiston – Auburn, ME MSA	56	63.53
Lexington-Fayette, KY MSA	225	64.58
Lima, OH MSA	115	74.51
Lincoln, NE MSA	155	72.55
Little Rock – North Little Rock, AR MSA	260	50.67
Longview – Marshall, TX MSA	107	65.87
Los Angeles – Anaheim – Riverside, CA CMSA	7188	49.46
Louisville, KY – IN MSA	669	70.22
Lubbock, TX MSA	120	53.90
Lynchburg, VA MSA	110	77.36
Macon – Warner Robins, GA MSA	177	62.97
Madison, WI MSA	288	78.46
Manchester, NH MSA	60	40.59
Mansfield, OH MSA	52	41.23
McAllen – Edinburg – Mission, TX MSA	74	19.29
Medford, OR MSA	63	43.04
Melbourne – Titusville – Palm Bay, FL MSA	221	55.39
Memphis, TN – AR – MS MSA	689	70.18
Merced, CA MSA	82	45.96
Miami – Fort Lauderdale, FL CMSA	2083	65.25
Midland, TX MSA	27	25.33
Milwaukee – Racine, WI CMSA	1086	67.57
Minneapolis – St. Paul, MN – WI MSA	1181	47.93
Mobile, AL MSA	250	52.42
Modesto, CA MSA	165	44.53
Monroe, LA MSA	128	90.02
Montgomery, AL MSA	146	49.91
Muncie, IN MSA	69	57.66
Muskegon, MI MSA	77	48.43
Naples, FL MSA	60	39.45
Nashville, TN MSA	628	63.75

[Continued]

★ 734 ★

Radiologic Technicians
[Continued]

MSA/CMSA	Total Employees	Employees per 100,000 pop.
New Bedford, MA MSA	57	32.45
New Haven–Meriden, CT MSA	446	84.12
New London–Norwich, CT–RI MSA	195	73.08
New Orleans, LA MSA	802	64.74
New York–Northern New Jersey–Long Island, NY–NJ–CT CMSA	8347	46.15
Norfolk–Virginia Beach–Newport News, VA MSA	914	65.47
Ocala, FL MSA	149	76.48
Odessa, TX MSA	92	77.35
Oklahoma City, OK MSA	641	66.85
Olympia, WA MSA	80	49.62
Omaha, NE–IA MSA	354	57.26
Orlando, FL MSA	488	45.49
Owensboro, KY MSA	74	84.87
Panama City, FL MSA	71	55.91
Parkersburg–Marietta, WV–OH MSA	142	95.19
Pascagoula, MS MSA	154	133.63
Pensacola, FL MSA	265	76.94
Peoria, IL MSA	262	77.25
Philadelphia–Wilmington–Trenton, PA–NJ–DE–MD CMSA	3936	66.72
Phoenix, AZ MSA	1246	58.72
Pine Bluff, AR MSA	44	51.47
Pittsburgh–Beaver Valley, PA CMSA	1636	72.94
Pittsfield, MA MSA	43	54.26
Portland, ME MSA	131	60.85
Portland–Vancouver, OR–WA CMSA	853	57.72
Portsmouth–Dover–Rochester, NH–ME MSA	88	39.36
Poughkeepsie, NY MSA	121	46.63
Providence–Pawtucket–Fall River, RI–MA CMSA	757	66.32
Provo–Orem, UT MSA	145	55.01
Pueblo, CO MSA	87	70.70
Raleigh–Durham, NC MSA	446	60.64
Rapid City, SD MSA	50	61.47
Reading, PA MSA	148	43.98
Redding, CA MSA	55	37.41
Reno, NV MSA	147	57.72
Richland–Kennewick–Pasco, WA MSA	103	68.65
Richmond–Petersburg, VA MSA	485	56.03
Roanoke, VA MSA	247	110.03
Rochester, MN MSA	283	265.80
Rochester, NY MSA	506	50.48
Rockford, IL MSA	236	83.18
Sacramento, CA MSA	588	39.70
Saginaw–Bay City–Midland, MI MSA	252	63.11
St. Cloud, MN MSA	104	54.47
St. Joseph, MO MSA	31	37.31
St. Louis, MO–IL MSA	1260	51.55

[Continued]

★ 734 ★

Radiologic Technicians
[Continued]

MSA/CMSA	Total Employees	Employees per 100,000 pop.
Salem, OR MSA	114	41.00
Salinas – Seaside – Monterey, CA MSA	105	29.52
Salt Lake City – Ogden, UT MSA	473	44.11
San Angelo, TX MSA	74	75.16
San Antonio, TX MSA	709	54.45
San Diego, CA MSA	1113	44.56
San Francisco – Oakland – San Jose, CA CMSA	2952	47.21
Santa Barbara – Santa Maria – Lompoc, CA MSA	254	68.72
Santa Fe, NM MSA	32	27.34
Sarasota, FL MSA	186	66.96
Savannah, GA MSA	126	51.93
Scranton – Wilkes-Barre, PA MSA	560	76.28
Seattle – Tacoma, WA CMSA	1277	49.90
Sharon, PA MSA	121	100.00
Sheboygan, WI MSA	30	28.88
Sherman – Denison, TX MSA	64	67.35
Shreveport, LA MSA	187	55.93
Sioux City, IA – NE MSA	61	53.04
Sioux Falls, SD MSA	139	112.27
South Bend – Mishawaka, IN MSA	156	63.14
Spokane, WA MSA	288	79.70
Springfield, IL MSA	168	88.63
Springfield, MO MSA	269	111.81
Springfield, MA MSA	355	67.04
State College, PA MSA	22	17.77
Steubenville – Weirton, OH – WV MSA	110	77.18
Stockton, CA MSA	178	37.03
Syracuse, NY MSA	420	63.65
Tallahassee, FL MSA	73	31.25
Tampa – St. Petersburg – Clearwater, FL MSA	1282	61.99
Terre Haute, IN MSA	64	48.93
Texarkana, TX – Texarkana, AR MSA	103	85.74
Toledo, OH MSA	434	70.67
Topeka, KS MSA	101	62.74
Tucson, AZ MSA	429	64.33
Tulsa, OK MSA	395	55.72
Tuscaloosa, AL MSA	53	35.21
Tyler, TX MSA	88	58.16
Utica – Rome, NY MSA	157	49.58
Victoria, TX MSA	54	72.62
Visalia – Tulare – Porterville, CA MSA	85	27.25
Waco, TX MSA	84	44.42
Washington, DC – MD – VA MSA	1580	40.27
Waterbury, CT MSA	189	85.28
Waterloo – Cedar Falls, IA MSA	65	44.34
Wausau, WI MSA	97	84.06

[Continued]

★ 734 ★

Radiologic Technicians
[Continued]

MSA/CMSA	Total Employees	Employees per 100,000 pop.
West Palm Beach – Boca Raton – Delray Beach, FL MSA	423	48.99
Wheeling, WV – OH MSA	107	67.17
Wichita, KS MSA	359	73.98
Wichita Falls, TX MSA	77	62.92
Williamsport, PA MSA	102	85.92
Wilmington, NC MSA	113	93.94
Worcester, MA MSA	321	73.47
Yakima, WA MSA	117	61.96
York, PA MSA	274	65.57
Youngstown – Warren, OH MSA	441	89.52
Yuba City, CA MSA	38	30.98
Yuma, AZ MSA	19	17.77

Source: Census of Population and Housing, 1990: Equal Employment Opportunity (EEO) File on CD-ROM [machine-readable datafiles]. Prepared by the Bureau of the Census. Washington, DC: The Bureau, 1992.

★ 735 ★

Employment

Registered Nurses

The table below presents the number of civilians 16 years old or older who reported working as registered nurses during the 1990 Census. Data are provided by total number employed in each Metropolitan Statistical Area (MSA) or Consolidated Metropolitan Statistical Area (CMSA), as well as the number employed per 100,000 people.

[Total for all of the U.S. was 1,885,129; 757.96 per 100,000 persons]

MSA/CMSA	Total Employees	Employees per 100,000 pop.
Abilene, TX MSA	709	592.54
Albany, GA MSA	695	617.44
Albany – Schenectady – Troy, NY MSA	8865	1013.95
Albuquerque, NM MSA	4043	841.28
Alexandria, LA MSA	1002	761.65
Allentown – Bethlehem – Easton, PA – NJ MSA	6708	976.86
Altoona, PA MSA	1314	1006.57
Amarillo, TX MSA	1497	798.20
Anchorage, AK MSA	1933	854.03
Anderson, IN MSA	988	756.11
Anderson, SC MSA	794	546.85
Anniston, AL MSA	927	798.90
Appleton – Oshkosh – Neenah, WI MSA	2431	771.45
Asheville, NC MSA	1631	932.95
Athens, GA MSA	933	597.06
Atlanta, GA MSA	20779	733.33
Atlantic City, NJ MSA	2717	850.61

[Continued]

★ 735 ★

Registered Nurses
[Continued]

MSA/CMSA	Total Employees	Employees per 100,000 pop.
Augusta, GA – SC MSA	3772	950.58
Austin, TX MSA	4644	594.19
Bakersfield, CA MSA	2202	405.17
Baltimore, MD MSA	22864	959.80
Bangor, ME MSA	1002	1129.08
Baton Rouge, LA MSA	2842	537.99
Battle Creek, MI MSA	1125	827.32
Beaumont – Port Arthur, TX MSA	2315	640.87
Bellingham, WA MSA	735	575.21
Benton Harbor, MI MSA	1364	845.22
Billings, MT MSA	967	852.59
Biloxi – Gulfport, MS MSA	1671	847.69
Binghamton, NY MSA	2423	916.08
Birmingham, AL MSA	8681	956.26
Bismarck, ND MSA	1032	1231.05
Bloomington, IN MSA	679	623.06
Bloomington – Normal, IL MSA	900	696.70
Boise City, ID MSA	1488	723.12
Boston – Lawrence – Salem, MA – NH CMSA	45789	1097.63
Bradenton, FL MSA	1808	854.01
Bremerton, WA MSA	1038	547.09
Brownsville – Harlingen, TX MSA	913	350.99
Bryan – College Station, TX MSA	541	413.91
Buffalo – Niagara Falls, NY CMSA	12242	1029.36
Burlington, NC MSA	644	595.12
Burlington, VT MSA	1278	972.31
Canton, OH MSA	3426	869.31
Casper, WY MSA	579	945.68
Cedar Rapids, IA MSA	1584	938.57
Champaign – Urbana – Rantoul, IL MSA	1494	863.46
Charleston, SC MSA	3875	764.49
Charleston, WV MSA	2069	826.10
Charlotte – Gastonia – Rock Hill, NC – SC MSA	8479	729.63
Charlottesville, VA MSA	1672	1275.29
Chattanooga, TN – GA MSA	3294	760.37
Cheyenne, WY MSA	567	775.20
Chicago – Gary – Lake County, IL – IN – WI CMSA	67351	835.04
Chico, CA MSA	1371	752.80
Cincinnati – Hamilton, OH – KY – IN CMSA	16080	921.95
Clarksville – Hopkinsville, TN – KY MSA	821	484.54
Cleveland – Akron – Lorain, OH CMSA	25497	923.86
Colorado Springs, CO MSA	2759	694.94
Columbia, MO MSA	1844	1640.88
Columbia, SC MSA	4786	1055.74
Columbus, GA – AL MSA	1726	710.08
Columbus, OH MSA	12013	872.14

[Continued]

★ 735 ★

Registered Nurses
[Continued]

MSA/CMSA	Total Employees	Employees per 100,000 pop.
Corpus Christi, TX MSA	2138	611.04
Cumberland, MD – WV MSA	1105	1087.14
Dallas – Fort Worth, TX CMSA	24762	637.31
Danville, VA MSA	708	651.27
Davenport – Rock Island – Moline, IA – IL MSA	2710	772.39
Dayton – Springfield, OH MSA	9585	1007.60
Daytona Beach, FL MSA	3054	823.82
Decatur, AL MSA	812	617.23
Decatur, IL MSA	794	677.44
Denver – Boulder, CO CMSA	15362	831.13
Des Moines, IA MSA	3989	1015.20
Detroit – Ann Arbor, MI CMSA	36224	776.47
Dothan, AL MSA	1026	783.42
Dubuque, IA MSA	953	1102.97
Duluth, MN – WI MSA	2102	875.94
Eau Claire, WI MSA	1164	846.28
El Paso, TX MSA	2931	495.43
Elkhart – Goshen, IN MSA	761	487.20
Elmira, NY MSA	1138	1195.44
Enid, OK MSA	389	685.64
Erie, PA MSA	2747	996.84
Eugene – Springfield, OR MSA	1736	613.62
Evansville, IN – KY MSA	2702	968.49
Fargo – Moorhead, ND – MN MSA	1891	1233.56
Fayetteville, NC MSA	1334	485.86
Fayetteville – Springdale, AR MSA	693	611.06
Fitchburg – Leominster, MA MSA	1155	1123.57
Flint, MI MSA	3457	803.10
Florence, AL MSA	838	638.10
Florence, SC MSA	823	719.76
Fort Collins – Loveland, CO MSA	1287	691.43
Fort Myers – Cape Coral, FL MSA	2823	842.40
Fort Pierce, FL MSA	2096	834.82
Fort Smith, AR – OK MSA	1302	740.15
Fort Walton Beach, FL MSA	854	593.98
Fort Wayne, IN MSA	3637	999.69
Fresno, CA MSA	4231	633.87
Gadsden, AL MSA	774	775.24
Gainesville, FL MSA	2724	1334.57
Glens Falls, NY MSA	1006	848.67
Grand Forks, ND MSA	600	848.86
Grand Rapids, MI MSA	5648	820.45
Great Falls, MT MSA	734	944.77
Greeley, CO MSA	734	556.82
Green Bay, WI MSA	1764	906.50
Greensboro – Winston-Salem – High Point, NC MSA	7699	817.22

[Continued]

★ 735 ★

Registered Nurses
[Continued]

MSA/CMSA	Total Employees	Employees per 100,000 pop.
Greenville – Spartanburg, SC MSA	4072	635.40
Hagerstown, MD MSA	840	691.97
Harrisburg – Lebanon – Carlisle, PA MSA	5385	915.84
Hartford – New Britain – Middletown, CT CMSA	11373	1047.39
Hickory – Morganton, NC MSA	1546	697.34
Honolulu, HI MSA	5718	683.78
Houma – Thibodaux, LA MSA	808	441.91
Houston – Galveston – Brazoria, TX CMSA	25328	682.50
Huntington – Ashland, WV – KY – OH MSA	2401	768.25
Huntsville, AL MSA	1901	029.10
Indianapolis, IN MSA	11864	949.26
Iowa City, IA MSA	2144	2230.57
Jackson, MI MSA	1079	720.51
Jackson, MS MSA	3332	842.70
Jackson, TN MSA	768	984.84
Jacksonville, FL MSA	6356	700.98
Jacksonville, NC MSA	638	425.79
Jamestown – Dunkirk, NY	1106	779.45
Janesville – Beloit, WI MSA	1034	741.17
Johnson City – Kingsport – Bristol, TN – VA MSA	2819	646.49
Johnstown, PA MSA	2315	959.60
Joplin, MO MSA	980	726.41
Kalamazoo, MI MSA	2228	997.27
Kankakee, IL MSA	938	974.49
Kansas City, MO – KS MSA	13272	847.36
Killeen – Temple, TX MSA	1762	690.17
Knoxville, TN MSA	4574	756.26
Kokomo, IN MSA	744	767.44
La Crosse, WI MSA	1109	1132.74
Lafayette, LA MSA	1194	572.00
Lafayette – West Lafayette, IN MSA	990	758.05
Lake Charles, LA MSA	962	572.16
Lakeland – Winter Haven, FL MSA	2336	576.25
Lancaster, PA MSA	3308	782.36
Lansing – East Lansing, MI MSA	3094	715.09
Laredo, TX MSA	364	273.19
Las Cruces, NM MSA	593	437.61
Las Vegas, NV MSA	3957	533.68
Lawrence, KS MSA	488	596.59
Lawton, OK MSA	634	568.68
Lewiston – Auburn, ME MSA	728	825.95
Lexington-Fayette, KY MSA	3504	1005.66
Lima, OH MSA	1292	837.11
Lincoln, NE MSA	2030	950.19
Little Rock – North Little Rock, AR MSA	5199	1013.22
Longview – Marshall, TX MSA	772	475.28

[Continued]

★ 735 ★

Registered Nurses
[Continued]

MSA/CMSA	Total Employees	Employees per 100,000 pop.
Los Angeles – Anaheim – Riverside, CA CMSA	90853	625.21
Louisville, KY – IN MSA	8211	861.90
Lubbock, TX MSA	2050	920.79
Lynchburg, VA MSA	1139	800.99
Macon – Warner Robins, GA MSA	1903	676.98
Madison, WI MSA	4295	1170.03
Manchester, NH MSA	1418	959.35
Mansfield, OH MSA	911	722.23
McAllen – Edinburg – Mission, TX MSA	1233	321.47
Medford, OR MSA	992	677.65
Melbourne – Titusville – Palm Bay, FL MSA	2793	700.04
Memphis, TN – AR – MS MSA	7824	796.95
Merced, CA MSA	893	500.55
Miami – Fort Lauderdale, FL CMSA	23615	739.68
Midland, TX MSA	485	454.92
Milwaukee – Racine, WI CMSA	15128	941.27
Minneapolis – St. Paul, MN – WI MSA	24305	986.35
Mobile, AL MSA	3606	756.10
Modesto, CA MSA	2136	576.48
Monroe, LA MSA	864	607.63
Montgomery, AL MSA	2286	781.49
Muncie, IN MSA	672	561.60
Muskegon, MI MSA	937	589.37
Naples, FL MSA	1014	666.67
Nashville, TN MSA	8668	879.98
New Bedford, MA MSA	1341	763.49
New Haven – Meriden, CT MSA	5352	1009.47
New London – Norwich, CT – RI MSA	2267	849.64
New Orleans, LA MSA	8505	686.54
New York – Northern New Jersey – Long Island, NY – NJ – CT CMSA	154588	854.68
Norfolk – Virginia Beach – Newport News, VA MSA	9643	690.71
Ocala, FL MSA	1318	676.48
Odessa, TX MSA	615	517.09
Oklahoma City, OK MSA	6610	689.38
Olympia, WA MSA	1225	759.75
Omaha, NE – IA MSA	6659	1077.05
Orlando, FL MSA	8163	760.94
Owensboro, KY MSA	699	801.71
Panama City, FL MSA	846	666.17
Parkersburg – Marietta, WV – OH MSA	1247	835.96
Pascagoula, MS MSA	835	724.56
Pensacola, FL MSA	2846	826.35
Peoria, IL MSA	3247	957.33
Philadelphia – Wilmington – Trenton, PA – NJ – DE – MD CMSA	57777	979.38
Phoenix, AZ MSA	17061	803.97
Pine Bluff, AR MSA	457	534.58

[Continued]

★ 735 ★

Registered Nurses
[Continued]

MSA/CMSA	Total Employees	Employees per 100,000 pop.
Pittsburgh – Beaver Valley, PA CMSA	24455	1090.38
Pittsfield, MA MSA	890	1123.03
Portland, ME MSA	2397	1113.43
Portland – Vancouver, OR – WA CMSA	13352	903.45
Portsmouth – Dover – Rochester, NH – ME MSA	1913	855.63
Poughkeepsie, NY MSA	3119	1202.10
Providence – Pawtucket – Fall River, RI – MA CMSA	10537	923.08
Provo – Orem, UT MSA	1466	556.17
Pueblo, CO MSA	1069	868.75
Raleigh – Durham, NC MSA	8688	1181.27
Rapid City, SD MSA	785	965.05
Reading, PA MSA	3207	952.98
Redding, CA MSA	1062	722.27
Reno, NV MSA	1910	750.00
Richland – Kennewick – Pasco, WA MSA	979	652.52
Richmond – Petersburg, VA MSA	7939	917.12
Roanoke, VA MSA	2157	960.90
Rochester, MN MSA	2596	2438.25
Rochester, NY MSA	9523	950.01
Rockford, IL MSA	2319	817.36
Sacramento, CA MSA	10345	698.47
Saginaw – Bay City – Midland, MI MSA	2955	740.01
St. Cloud, MN MSA	1529	800.85
St. Joseph, MO MSA	767	923.17
St. Louis, MO – IL MSA	21966	898.74
Salem, OR MSA	1719	618.29
Salinas – Seaside – Monterey, CA MSA	1833	515.38
Salt Lake City – Ogden, UT MSA	6728	627.48
San Angelo, TX MSA	772	784.09
San Antonio, TX MSA	8607	661.01
San Diego, CA MSA	16984	679.90
San Francisco – Oakland – San Jose, CA CMSA	49907	798.09
Santa Barbara – Santa Maria – Lompoc, CA MSA	2089	565.19
Santa Fe, NM MSA	836	714.27
Sarasota, FL MSA	2516	905.77
Savannah, GA MSA	2153	887.39
Scranton – Wilkes-Barre, PA MSA	7126	970.61
Seattle – Tacoma, WA CMSA	20805	812.96
Sharon, PA MSA	1219	1007.41
Sheboygan, WI MSA	675	649.81
Sherman – Denison, TX MSA	625	657.75
Shreveport, LA MSA	2945	880.84
Sioux City, IA – NE MSA	1276	1109.39
Sioux Falls, SD MSA	1870	1510.39
South Bend – Mishawaka, IN MSA	1852	749.64
Spokane, WA MSA	4140	1145.66

[Continued]

★ 735 ★

Registered Nurses
[Continued]

MSA/CMSA	Total Employees	Employees per 100,000 pop.
Springfield, IL MSA	2124	1120.55
Springfield, MO MSA	2237	929.79
Springfield, MA MSA	5153	973.15
State College, PA MSA	687	554.99
Steubenville–Weirton, OH–WV MSA	1205	845.48
Stockton, CA MSA	2528	525.98
Syracuse, NY MSA	5919	897.00
Tallahassee, FL MSA	1695	725.61
Tampa–St. Petersburg–Clearwater, FL MSA	16745	809.74
Terre Haute, IN MSA	806	616.15
Texarkana, TX–Texarkana, AR MSA	1036	862.38
Toledo, OH MSA	6575	1070.62
Topeka, KS MSA	1805	1121.29
Tucson, AZ MSA	5607	840.78
Tulsa, OK MSA	4827	680.86
Tuscaloosa, AL MSA	1587	1054.33
Tyler, TX MSA	1279	845.29
Utica–Rome, NY MSA	2787	880.20
Victoria, TX MSA	461	619.95
Visalia–Tulare–Porterville, CA MSA	1241	397.86
Waco, TX MSA	1158	612.30
Washington, DC–MD–VA MSA	31739	808.93
Waterbury, CT MSA	2851	1286.38
Waterloo–Cedar Falls, IA MSA	1208	823.95
Wausau, WI MSA	878	760.83
West Palm Beach–Boca Raton–Delray Beach, FL MSA	6738	780.30
Wheeling, WV–OH MSA	1599	1003.76
Wichita, KS MSA	4917	1013.25
Wichita Falls, TX MSA	862	704.37
Williamsport, PA MSA	869	732.04
Wilmington, NC MSA	1369	1138.14
Worcester, MA MSA	5428	1242.38
Yakima, WA MSA	1079	571.43
York, PA MSA	2714	649.52
Youngstown–Warren, OH MSA	4291	871.06
Yuba City, CA MSA	595	485.15
Yuma, AZ MSA	472	441.55

Source: Census of Population and Housing, 1990: Equal Employment Opportunity (EEO) File on CD-ROM [machine-readable datafiles]. Prepared by the Bureau of the Census. Washington, DC: The Bureau, 1992.

★ 736 ★

Employment

Registered Nurses Supply and Demand Projections: 1990-2020

From the source: "These data show that the supply for registered nurses will increase into the middle of the first decade in the next century but will decline thereafter."

Year	DFTERN[1] to provide nursing service to older Americans	Supply of FTE[2] registered nurses	Percent of supply needed to satisfy demand
1990	584,000	1,435,000	40.7
1995	665,000	1,585,000	41.9
2000	739,000	1,647,000	44.9
2005	817,000	1,676,000	48.7
2010	904,000	1,637,000	55.2
2015	994,000	1,623,000	61.2
2020	1,126,000	1,555,000	72.4

Source: U.S. House of Representatives. *Shortage of Health Care Professions Caring for the Elderly: Recommendations for Change.* 102d Cong., 2nd sess., December 1992. Comm. Pub. No. 102-915. Washington, DC: U.S. Government Printing Office, 1993, p. 42. Primary source: Projections prepared by Division of Nursing, Bureau of Health Professions, Health Resources and Services Administration, U.S. Department of Health and Human Services, 1992. *Notes:* 1. DFTERN stands for demand for full-time equivalent registered nurses. 2. FTE stands for full-time equivalent.

★ 737 ★

Employment

Respiratory Therapists

The table below presents the number of civilians 16 years old or older who reported working as respiratory therapists during the 1990 Census. Data are provided by total number employed in each Metropolitan Statistical Area (MSA) or Consolidated Metropolitan Statistical Area (CMSA), as well as the number employed per 100,000 people.

[Total for all of the U.S. was 65,589; 26.37 per 100,000 persons]

MSA/CMSA	Total Employees	Employees per 100,000 pop.
Abilene, TX MSA	56	46.80
Albany, GA MSA	22	19.54
Albany – Schenectady – Troy, NY MSA	183	20.93
Albuquerque, NM MSA	193	40.16
Alexandria, LA MSA	37	28.12
Allentown – Bethlehem – Easton, PA – NJ MSA	98	14.27
Altoona, PA MSA	20	15.32
Amarillo, TX MSA	35	18.66
Anchorage, AK MSA	48	21.21
Anderson, IN MSA	32	24.49

[Continued]

★ 737 ★

Respiratory Therapists
[Continued]

MSA/CMSA	Total Employees	Employees per 100,000 pop.
Anderson, SC MSA	39	26.86
Appleton–Oshkosh–Neenah, WI MSA	73	23.17
Asheville, NC MSA	45	25.74
Athens, GA MSA	20	12.80
Atlanta, GA MSA	1055	37.23
Atlantic City, NJ MSA	51	15.97
Augusta, GA–SC MSA	122	30.75
Austin, TX MSA	204	26.10
Bakersfield, CA MSA	58	10.67
Baltimore, MD MSA	629	26.40
Bangor, ME MSA	44	49.58
Baton Rouge, LA MSA	106	20.07
Battle Creek, MI MSA	35	25.74
Beaumont–Port Arthur, TX MSA	129	35.71
Bellingham, WA MSA	53	41.48
Benton Harbor, MI MSA	32	19.83
Billings, MT MSA	20	17.63
Biloxi–Gulfport, MS MSA	102	51.74
Binghamton, NY MSA	69	26.09
Birmingham, AL MSA	323	35.58
Bismarck, ND MSA	77	91.85
Bloomington, IN MSA	8	7.34
Bloomington–Normal, IL MSA	38	29.42
Boise City, ID MSA	34	16.52
Boston–Lawrence–Salem, MA–NH CMSA	991	23.76
Bradenton, FL MSA	52	24.56
Bremerton, WA MSA	47	24.77
Brownsville–Harlingen, TX MSA	33	12.69
Bryan–College Station, TX MSA	14	11.49
Buffalo–Niagara Falls, NY CMSA	283	23.80
Burlington, NC MSA	18	16.63
Burlington, VT MSA	27	20.54
Canton, OH MSA	114	28.93
Casper, WY MSA	20	32.67
Cedar Rapids, IA MSA	47	27.85
Champaign–Urbana–Rantoul, IL MSA	44	25.43
Charleston, SC MSA	145	28.61
Charleston, WV MSA	71	28.35
Charlotte–Gastonia–Rock Hill, NC–SC MSA	262	22.55
Charlottesville, VA MSA	80	61.02
Chattanooga, TN–GA MSA	146	33.70
Cheyenne, WY MSA	12	16.41
Chicago–Gary–Lake County, IL–IN–WI CMSA	2186	27.10
Chico, CA MSA	117	64.24
Cincinnati–Hamilton, OH–KY–IN CMSA	395	22.65
Clarksville–Hopkinsville, TN–KY MSA	56	33.05

[Continued]

★ 737 ★

Respiratory Therapists
[Continued]

MSA/CMSA	Total Employees	Employees per 100,000 pop.
Cleveland – Akron – Lorain, OH CMSA	887	32.14
Colorado Springs, CO MSA	84	21.16
Columbia, MO MSA	76	67.63
Columbia, SC MSA	194	42.79
Columbus, GA – AL MSA	48	19.75
Columbus, OH MSA	398	28.89
Corpus Christi, TX MSA	82	23.44
Cumberland, MD – WV MSA	32	31.48
Dallas – Fort Worth, TX CMSA	1151	29.62
Davenport – Rock Island – Moline, IA – IL MSA	136	38.76
Dayton – Springfield, OH MSA	478	50.25
Daytona Beach, FL MSA	147	39.65
Decatur, AL MSA	48	36.49
Decatur, IL MSA	45	38.39
Denver – Boulder, CO CMSA	543	29.38
Des Moines, IA MSA	161	40.97
Detroit – Ann Arbor, MI CMSA	1710	36.65
Dothan, AL MSA	68	51.92
Duluth, MN – WI MSA	34	14.17
Eau Claire, WI MSA	50	36.35
El Paso, TX MSA	82	13.86
Elkhart – Goshen, IN MSA	45	28.81
Elmira, NY MSA	12	12.61
Enid, OK MSA	5	8.81
Erie, PA MSA	119	43.18
Eugene – Springfield, OR MSA	68	24.04
Evansville, IN – KY MSA	78	27.96
Fargo – Moorhead, ND – MN MSA	43	28.05
Fayetteville, NC MSA	97	35.33
Fayetteville – Springdale, AR MSA	50	44.09
Fitchburg – Leominster, MA MSA	39	37.94
Flint, MI MSA	151	35.08
Florence, AL MSA	77	58.63
Florence, SC MSA	66	57.72
Fort Collins – Loveland, CO MSA	21	11.28
Fort Myers – Cape Coral, FL MSA	109	32.53
Fort Pierce, FL MSA	74	29.47
Fort Smith, AR – OK MSA	57	32.40
Fort Walton Beach, FL MSA	46	31.99
Fort Wayne, IN MSA	123	33.81
Fresno, CA MSA	178	26.67
Gadsden, AL MSA	16	16.03
Gainesville, FL MSA	102	49.97
Glens Falls, NY MSA	23	19.40
Grand Forks, ND MSA	15	21.22
Grand Rapids, MI MSA	126	18.30

[Continued]

★ 737 ★

Respiratory Therapists
[Continued]

MSA/CMSA	Total Employees	Employees per 100,000 pop.
Great Falls, MT MSA	13	16.73
Greeley, CO MSA	11	8.34
Green Bay, WI MSA	50	25.69
Greensboro – Winston-Salem – High Point, NC MSA	250	26.54
Greenville – Spartanburg, SC MSA	237	36.98
Hagerstown, MD MSA	17	14.00
Harrisburg – Lebanon – Carlisle, PA MSA	121	20.58
Hartford – New Britain – Middletown, CT CMSA	297	27.35
Hickory – Morganton, NC MSA	48	21.65
Honolulu, HI MSA	183	21.88
Houma – Thibodaux, LA MSA	45	24.61
Houston – Galveston – Brazoria, TX CMSA	946	25.49
Huntington – Ashland, WV – KY – OH MSA	133	42.56
Huntsville, AL MSA	34	14.23
Indianapolis, IN MSA	611	48.89
Iowa City, IA MSA	77	80.11
Jackson, MI MSA	22	14.69
Jackson, MS MSA	202	51.09
Jackson, TN MSA	36	46.16
Jacksonville, FL MSA	287	31.65
Jacksonville, NC MSA	27	18.02
Jamestown – Dunkirk, NY	16	11.28
Janesville – Beloit, WI MSA	49	35.12
Johnson City – Kingsport – Bristol, TN – VA MSA	114	26.14
Johnstown, PA MSA	90	37.31
Joplin, MO MSA	35	25.94
Kalamazoo, MI MSA	113	50.58
Kankakee, IL MSA	29	30.13
Kansas City, MO – KS MSA	588	37.54
Killeen – Temple, TX MSA	91	35.64
Knoxville, TN MSA	202	33.40
Kokomo, IN MSA	22	22.69
La Crosse, WI MSA	42	42.90
Lafayette, LA MSA	31	14.85
Lafayette – West Lafayette, IN MSA	32	24.50
Lake Charles, LA MSA	48	28.55
Lakeland – Winter Haven, FL MSA	67	16.53
Lancaster, PA MSA	139	32.87
Lansing – East Lansing, MI MSA	125	28.89
Las Cruces, NM MSA	13	9.59
Las Vegas, NV MSA	139	18.75
Lawrence, KS MSA	14	17.12
Lewiston – Auburn, ME MSA	13	14.75
Lexington-Fayette, KY MSA	133	38.17
Lima, OH MSA	62	40.17
Lincoln, NE MSA	104	48.68

[Continued]

★ 737 ★

Respiratory Therapists
[Continued]

MSA/CMSA	Total Employees	Employees per 100,000 pop.
Little Rock – North Little Rock, AR MSA	284	55.35
Longview – Marshall, TX MSA	47	28.94
Los Angeles – Anaheim – Riverside, CA CMSA	3865	26.60
Louisville, KY – IN MSA	281	29.50
Lubbock, TX MSA	105	47.16
Lynchburg, VA MSA	52	36.57
Macon – Warner Robins, GA MSA	71	25.26
Madison, WI MSA	214	58.30
Manchester, NH MSA	52	35.18
Mansfield, OH MSA	31	24.58
McAllen – Edinburg – Mission, TX MSA	34	8.86
Medford, OR MSA	69	47.13
Melbourne – Titusville – Palm Bay, FL MSA	52	13.03
Memphis, TN – AR – MS MSA	349	35.55
Merced, CA MSA	30	16.82
Miami – Fort Lauderdale, FL CMSA	1445	45.26
Midland, TX MSA	51	47.84
Milwaukee – Racine, WI CMSA	451	28.06
Minneapolis – St. Paul, MN – WI MSA	532	21.59
Mobile, AL MSA	109	22.85
Modesto, CA MSA	97	26.18
Monroe, LA MSA	67	47.12
Montgomery, AL MSA	73	24.96
Muncie, IN MSA	46	38.44
Muskegon, MI MSA	96	60.38
Naples, FL MSA	23	15.12
Nashville, TN MSA	418	42.44
New Bedford, MA MSA	60	34.16
New Haven – Meriden, CT MSA	134	25.27
New London – Norwich, CT – RI MSA	70	26.24
New Orleans, LA MSA	554	44.72
New York – Northern New Jersey – Long Island, NY – NJ – CT CMSA	3060	16.92
Norfolk – Virginia Beach – Newport News, VA MSA	235	16.83
Ocala, FL MSA	30	15.40
Odessa, TX MSA	85	71.47
Oklahoma City, OK MSA	233	24.30
Olympia, WA MSA	13	8.06
Omaha, NE – IA MSA	315	50.95
Orlando, FL MSA	403	37.57
Owensboro, KY MSA	15	17.20
Panama City, FL MSA	38	29.92
Parkersburg – Marietta, WV – OH MSA	33	22.12
Pascagoula, MS MSA	34	29.50
Pensacola, FL MSA	150	43.55
Peoria, IL MSA	114	33.61
Philadelphia – Wilmington – Trenton, PA – NJ – DE – MD CMSA	1491	25.27

[Continued]

★ 737 ★

Respiratory Therapists
[Continued]

MSA/CMSA	Total Employees	Employees per 100,000 pop.
Phoenix, AZ MSA	868	40.90
Pine Bluff, AR MSA	5	5.85
Pittsburgh – Beaver Valley, PA CMSA	682	30.41
Pittsfield, MA MSA	55	69.40
Portland, ME MSA	85	39.48
Portland – Vancouver, OR – WA CMSA	363	24.56
Portsmouth – Dover – Rochester, NH – ME MSA	15	6.71
Poughkeepsie, NY MSA	46	17.73
Providence – Pawtucket – Fall River, RI – MA CMSA	332	29.08
Provo – Orem, UT MSA	50	18.97
Pueblo, CO MSA	88	71.52
Raleigh – Durham, NC MSA	231	31.41
Rapid City, SD MSA	59	72.53
Reading, PA MSA	47	13.97
Redding, CA MSA	93	63.25
Reno, NV MSA	73	28.66
Richland – Kennewick – Pasco, WA MSA	54	35.99
Richmond – Petersburg, VA MSA	223	25.76
Roanoke, VA MSA	91	40.54
Rochester, MN MSA	70	65.75
Rochester, NY MSA	106	10.57
Rockford, IL MSA	140	49.34
Sacramento, CA MSA	382	25.79
Saginaw – Bay City – Midland, MI MSA	137	34.31
St. Cloud, MN MSA	12	6.29
St. Joseph, MO MSA	13	15.65
St. Louis, MO – IL MSA	783	32.04
Salem, OR MSA	60	21.58
Salinas – Seaside – Monterey, CA MSA	59	16.59
Salt Lake City – Ogden, UT MSA	251	23.41
San Angelo, TX MSA	48	48.75
San Antonio, TX MSA	346	26.57
San Diego, CA MSA	750	30.02
San Francisco – Oakland – San Jose, CA CMSA	1444	23.09
Santa Barbara – Santa Maria – Lompoc, CA MSA	65	17.59
Santa Fe, NM MSA	40	34.18
Sarasota, FL MSA	117	42.12
Savannah, GA MSA	164	67.59
Scranton – Wilkes-Barre, PA MSA	156	21.25
Seattle – Tacoma, WA CMSA	577	22.55
Sharon, PA MSA	60	49.59
Sheboygan, WI MSA	4	3.85
Sherman – Denison, TX MSA	30	31.57
Shreveport, LA MSA	161	48.15
Sioux City, IA – NE MSA	53	46.08
Sioux Falls, SD MSA	32	25.85

[Continued]

★ 737 ★

Respiratory Therapists
[Continued]

MSA/CMSA	Total Employees	Employees per 100,000 pop.
South Bend – Mishawaka, IN MSA	66	26.72
Spokane, WA MSA	185	51.19
Springfield, IL MSA	114	60.14
Springfield, MO MSA	128	53.20
Springfield, MA MSA	159	30.03
State College, PA MSA	22	17.77
Steubenville – Weirton, OH – WV MSA	72	50.52
Stockton, CA MSA	68	14.15
Syracuse, NY MSA	208	31.52
Tallahassee, FL MSA	34	14.55
Tampa – St. Petersburg – Clearwater, FL MSA	841	40.67
Terre Haute, IN MSA	30	22.93
Texarkana, TX – Texarkana, AR MSA	42	34.96
Toledo, OH MSA	374	60.90
Topeka, KS MSA	61	37.89
Tucson, AZ MSA	308	46.19
Tulsa, OK MSA	150	21.16
Tuscaloosa, AL MSA	42	27.90
Tyler, TX MSA	173	114.34
Utica – Rome, NY MSA	74	23.37
Victoria, TX MSA	21	28.24
Visalia – Tulare – Porterville, CA MSA	70	22.44
Waco, TX MSA	13	6.87
Washington, DC – MD – VA MSA	050	21.66
Waterbury, CT MSA	159	71.74
Waterloo – Cedar Falls, IA MSA	51	34.70
Wausau, WI MSA	34	29.46
West Palm Beach – Boca Raton – Delray Beach, FL MSA	190	22.00
Wheeling, WV – OH MSA	113	70.93
Wichita, KS MSA	182	37.50
Wichita Falls, TX MSA	9	7.35
Williamsport, PA MSA	34	28.64
Wilmington, NC MSA	35	29.10
Worcester, MA MSA	153	35.02
Yakima, WA MSA	36	19.07
York, PA MSA	150	35.90
Youngstown – Warren, OH MSA	200	40.60
Yuba City, CA MSA	50	40.77
Yuma, AZ MSA	31	29.00

Source: Census of Population and Housing, 1990: Equal Employment Opportunity (EEO) File on CD-ROM [machine-readable datafiles]. Prepared by the Bureau of the Census. Washington, DC: The Bureau, 1992.

★ 738 ★

Employment

Speech Therapists

The table below presents the number of civilians 16 years old or older who reported working as speech therapists during the 1990 Census. Data are provided by total number employed in each Metropolitan Statistical Area (MSA) or Consolidated Metropolitan Statistical Area (CMSA), as well as the number employed per 100,000 people.

[Total for all of the U.S. was 64,713; 26.02 per 100,000 persons]

MSA/CMSA	Total Employees	Employees per 100,000 pop.
Abilene, TX MSA	28	23.40
Albany, GA MSA	22	19.54
Albany–Schenectady–Troy, NY MSA	459	52.50
Albuquerque, NM MSA	305	63.47
Alexandria, LA MSA	40	30.41
Allentown–Bethlehem–Easton, PA–NJ MSA	143	20.82
Altoona, PA MSA	30	22.98
Amarillo, TX MSA	36	19.20
Anchorage, AK MSA	75	33.14
Anderson, IN MSA	18	13.78
Anderson, SC MSA	19	13.09
Anniston, AL MSA	18	15.51
Appleton–Oshkosh–Neenah, WI MSA	110	34.91
Asheville, NC MSA	75	42.90
Athens, GA MSA	38	24.32
Atlanta, GA MSA	605	21.35
Atlantic City, NJ MSA	46	14.40
Augusta, GA–SC MSA	68	17.14
Austin, TX MSA	258	33.01
Bakersfield, CA MSA	117	21.53
Baltimore, MD MSA	730	30.64
Bangor, ME MSA	32	36.06
Baton Rouge, LA MSA	209	39.56
Battle Creek, MI MSA	15	11.03
Beaumont–Port Arthur, TX MSA	85	23.53
Bellingham, WA MSA	37	28.96
Benton Harbor, MI MSA	33	20.45
Billings, MT MSA	74	65.24
Biloxi–Gulfport, MS MSA	94	47.69
Binghamton, NY MSA	73	27.60
Birmingham, AL MSA	211	23.24
Bismarck, ND MSA	39	46.52
Bloomington, IN MSA	41	37.62
Bloomington–Normal, IL MSA	78	60.38
Boise City, ID MSA	77	37.42
Boston–Lawrence–Salem, MA–NH CMSA	1488	35.67
Bradenton, FL MSA	74	34.95
Bremerton, WA MSA	36	18.97
Brownsville–Harlingen, TX MSA	28	10.76
Bryan–College Station, TX MSA	21	17.23
Buffalo–Niagara Falls, NY CMSA	585	49.19
Burlington, NC MSA	32	29.57

[Continued]

★ 738 ★

Speech Therapists
[Continued]

MSA/CMSA	Total Employees	Employees per 100,000 pop.
Burlington, VT MSA	67	50.97
Canton, OH MSA	85	21.57
Casper, WY MSA	22	35.93
Cedar Rapids, IA MSA	109	64.59
Champaign–Urbana–Rantoul, IL MSA	106	61.26
Charleston, SC MSA	136	26.83
Charleston, WV MSA	101	40.33
Charlotte–Gastonia–Rock Hill, NC–SC MSA	300	25.82
Charlottesville, VA MSA	63	48.05
Chattanooga, TN–GA MSA	45	10.39
Cheyenne, WY MSA	13	17.77
Chicago–Gary–Lake County, IL–IN–WI CMSA	2422	30.03
Chico, CA MSA	32	17.57
Cincinnati–Hamilton, OH–KY–IN CMSA	637	36.52
Clarksville–Hopkinsville, TN–KY MSA	32	18.89
Cleveland–Akron–Lorain, OH CMSA	778	28.19
Colorado Springs, CO MSA	93	23.42
Columbia, MO MSA	64	56.95
Columbia, SC MSA	211	46.54
Columbus, GA–AL MSA	57	23.45
Columbus, OH MSA	289	20.98
Corpus Christi, TX MSA	43	12.29
Cumberland, MD–WV MSA	37	36.40
Dallas–Fort Worth, TX CMSA	1012	26.05
Danville, VA MSA	17	15.64
Davenport–Rock Island–Moline, IA–IL MSA	80	22.80
Dayton–Springfield, OH MSA	252	26.49
Daytona Beach, FL MSA	25	6.74
Decatur, AL MSA	9	6.84
Decatur, IL MSA	23	19.62
Denver–Boulder, CO CMSA	646	34.95
Des Moines, IA MSA	98	24.94
Detroit–Ann Arbor, MI CMSA	1063	22.79
Dothan, AL MSA	16	12.22
Dubuque, IA MSA	23	26.62
Duluth, MN–WI MSA	79	32.92
Eau Claire, WI MSA	53	38.53
El Paso, TX MSA	133	22.48
Elkhart–Goshen, IN MSA	25	16.01
Elmira, NY MSA	44	46.22
Enid, OK MSA	11	19.39
Erie, PA MSA	94	34.11
Eugene–Springfield, OR MSA	92	32.52
Evansville, IN–KY MSA	35	12.55
Fargo–Moorhead, ND–MN MSA	66	43.05
Fayetteville, NC MSA	42	15.30

[Continued]

★ 738 ★

Speech Therapists
[Continued]

MSA/CMSA	Total Employees	Employees per 100,000 pop.
Fayetteville – Springdale, AR MSA	49	43.21
Fitchburg – Leominster, MA MSA	31	30.16
Flint, MI MSA	72	16.73
Florence, SC MSA	11	9.62
Fort Collins – Loveland, CO MSA	43	23.10
Fort Myers – Cape Coral, FL MSA	73	21.78
Fort Pierce, FL MSA	12	4.78
Fort Smith, AR – OK MSA	14	7.96
Fort Walton Beach, FL MSA	26	18.08
Fort Wayne, IN MSA	122	33.53
Fresno, CA MSA	175	26.22
Gainesville, FL MSA	97	47.52
Glens Falls, NY MSA	35	29.53
Grand Forks, ND MSA	40	56.59
Grand Rapids, MI MSA	206	29.92
Great Falls, MT MSA	22	28.32
Greeley, CO MSA	24	18.21
Green Bay, WI MSA	84	43.17
Greensboro – Winston-Salem – High Point, NC MSA	192	20.38
Greenville – Spartanburg, SC MSA	148	23.09
Hagerstown, MD MSA	20	16.48
Harrisburg – Lebanon – Carlisle, PA MSA	179	30.44
Hartford – New Britain – Middletown, CT CMSA	342	31.50
Hickory – Morganton, NC MSA	55	24.81
Honolulu, HI MSA	280	33.48
Houma – Thibodaux, LA MSA	52	28.44
Houston – Galveston – Brazoria, TX CMSA	852	22.96
Huntington – Ashland, WV – KY – OH MSA	101	32.32
Huntsville, AL MSA	40	16.74
Indianapolis, IN MSA	424	33.92
Iowa City, IA MSA	42	43.70
Jackson, MI MSA	30	20.03
Jackson, MS MSA	89	22.51
Jackson, TN MSA	36	46.16
Jacksonville, FL MSA	213	23.49
Jacksonville, NC MSA	27	18.02
Jamestown – Dunkirk, NY	83	58.49
Janesville – Beloit, WI MSA	18	12.90
Johnson City – Kingsport – Bristol, TN – VA MSA	79	18.12
Johnstown, PA MSA	113	46.84
Joplin, MO MSA	17	12.60
Kalamazoo, MI MSA	55	24.62
Kankakee, IL MSA	21	21.82
Kansas City, MO – KS MSA	483	30.84
Killeen – Temple, TX MSA	33	12.93
Knoxville, TN MSA	258	42.66

[Continued]

★ 738 ★

Speech Therapists
[Continued]

MSA/CMSA	Total Employees	Employees per 100,000 pop.
Kokomo, IN MSA	13	13.41
La Crosse, WI MSA	32	32.69
Lafayette, LA MSA	80	38.33
Lafayette – West Lafayette, IN MSA	44	33.69
Lake Charles, LA MSA	50	29.74
Lakeland – Winter Haven, FL MSA	39	9.62
Lancaster, PA MSA	137	32.40
Lansing – East Lansing, MI MSA	120	27.73
Las Cruces, NM MSA	58	42.80
Las Vegas, NV MSA	109	14.70
Lawrence, KS MSA	29	35.45
Lawton, OK MSA	21	18.84
Lewiston – Auburn, ME MSA	5	5.67
Lexington-Fayette, KY MSA	147	42.19
Lima, OH MSA	20	12.96
Lincoln, NE MSA	57	26.68
Little Rock – North Little Rock, AR MSA	261	50.87
Longview – Marshall, TX MSA	10	6.16
Los Angeles – Anaheim – Riverside, CA CMSA	2605	17.93
Louisville, KY – IN MSA	250	26.24
Lubbock, TX MSA	90	40.42
Lynchburg, VA MSA	42	29.54
Macon – Warner Robins, GA MSA	102	36.29
Madison, WI MSA	233	63.47
Manchester, NH MSA	46	31.12
Mansfield, OH MSA	40	31.71
McAllen – Edinburg – Mission, TX MSA	54	14.08
Medford, OR MSA	21	14.35
Melbourne – Titusville – Palm Bay, FL MSA	92	23.06
Memphis, TN – AR – MS MSA	267	27.20
Merced, CA MSA	38	21.30
Miami – Fort Lauderdale, FL CMSA	637	19.95
Midland, TX MSA	18	16.88
Milwaukee – Racine, WI CMSA	657	40.88
Minneapolis – St. Paul, MN – WI MSA	893	36.24
Mobile, AL MSA	112	23.48
Modesto, CA MSA	124	33.47
Monroe, LA MSA	49	34.46
Montgomery, AL MSA	41	14.02
Muncie, IN MSA	31	25.91
Muskegon, MI MSA	23	14.47
Naples, FL MSA	34	22.35
Nashville, TN MSA	374	37.97
New Bedford, MA MSA	46	26.19
New Haven – Meriden, CT MSA	262	49.42
New London – Norwich, CT – RI MSA	62	23.24

[Continued]

★ 738 ★

Speech Therapists
[Continued]

MSA/CMSA	Total Employees	Employees per 100,000 pop.
New Orleans, LA MSA	347	28.01
New York – Northern New Jersey – Long Island, NY – NJ – CT CMSA	5616	31.05
Norfolk – Virginia Beach – Newport News, VA MSA	285	20.41
Ocala, FL MSA	23	11.80
Odessa, TX MSA	6	5.04
Oklahoma City, OK MSA	259	27.01
Olympia, WA MSA	58	35.97
Omaha, NE – IA MSA	195	31.54
Orlando, FL MSA	274	25.54
Panama City, FL MSA	23	18.11
Parkersburg – Marietta, WV – OH MSA	47	31.51
Pascagoula, MS MSA	28	24.30
Pensacola, FL MSA	94	27.29
Peoria, IL MSA	176	51.89
Philadelphia – Wilmington – Trenton, PA – NJ – DE – MD CMSA	1918	32.51
Phoenix, AZ MSA	547	25.78
Pine Bluff, AR MSA	37	43.28
Pittsburgh – Beaver Valley, PA CMSA	761	33.93
Pittsfield, MA MSA	39	49.21
Portland, ME MSA	64	29.73
Portland – Vancouver, OR – WA CMSA	362	24.49
Portsmouth – Dover – Rochester, NH – ME MSA	90	40.25
Poughkeepsie, NY MSA	137	52.80
Providence – Pawtucket – Fall River, RI – MA CMSA	284	24.88
Provo – Orem, UT MSA	41	15.55
Pueblo, CO MSA	34	27.63
Raleigh – Durham, NC MSA	206	28.01
Rapid City, SD MSA	47	57.78
Reading, PA MSA	89	26.45
Redding, CA MSA	45	30.60
Reno, NV MSA	97	38.09
Richland – Kennewick – Pasco, WA MSA	26	17.33
Richmond – Petersburg, VA MSA	248	28.65
Roanoke, VA MSA	67	29.85
Rochester, MN MSA	60	56.35
Rochester, NY MSA	417	41.60
Rockford, IL MSA	66	23.26
Sacramento, CA MSA	359	24.24
Saginaw – Bay City – Midland, MI MSA	51	12.77
St. Cloud, MN MSA	48	25.14
St. Joseph, MO MSA	33	39.72
St. Louis, MO – IL MSA	749	30.65
Salem, OR MSA	50	17.98
Salinas – Seaside – Monterey, CA MSA	91	25.59
Salt Lake City – Ogden, UT MSA	385	35.91
San Angelo, TX MSA	27	27.42

[Continued]

★ 738 ★

Speech Therapists
[Continued]

MSA/CMSA	Total Employees	Employees per 100,000 pop.
San Antonio, TX MSA	365	28.03
San Diego, CA MSA	672	26.90
San Francisco – Oakland – San Jose, CA CMSA	1502	24.02
Santa Barbara – Santa Maria – Lompoc, CA MSA	42	11.36
Santa Fe, NM MSA	32	27.34
Sarasota, FL MSA	57	20.52
Savannah, GA MSA	57	23.49
Scranton – Wilkes-Barre, PA MSA	204	27.79
Seattle – Tacoma, WA CMSA	697	27.24
Sharon, PA MSA	34	28.10
Sheboygan, WI MSA	23	22.14
Sherman – Denison, TX MSA	32	33.68
Shreveport, LA MSA	77	23.03
Sioux City, IA – NE MSA	17	14.78
Sioux Falls, SD MSA	48	38.77
South Bend – Mishawaka, IN MSA	70	28.33
Spokane, WA MSA	108	29.89
Springfield, IL MSA	24	12.66
Springfield, MO MSA	91	37.82
Springfield, MA MSA	122	23.04
State College, PA MSA	68	54.93
Steubenville – Weirton, OH – WV MSA	21	14.73
Stockton, CA MSA	90	18.73
Syracuse, NY MSA	214	32.43
Tallahassee, FL MSA	54	23.12
Tampa – St. Petersburg – Clearwater, FL MSA	368	17.80
Terre Haute, IN MSA	43	32.07
Texarkana, TX – Texarkana, AR MSA	53	44.12
Toledo, OH MSA	182	29.64
Topeka, KS MSA	58	36.03
Tucson, AZ MSA	177	26.54
Tulsa, OK MSA	193	27.22
Tuscaloosa, AL MSA	45	29.90
Tyler, TX MSA	39	25.78
Utica – Rome, NY MSA	80	25.27
Victoria, TX MSA	37	49.76
Visalia – Tulare – Porterville, CA MSA	67	21.48
Waco, TX MSA	60	31.73
Washington, DC – MD – VA MSA	1277	32.55
Waterbury, CT MSA	68	30.68
Waterloo – Cedar Falls, IA MSA	42	28.65
Wausau, WI MSA	29	25.13
West Palm Beach – Boca Raton – Delray Beach, FL MSA	225	26.06
Wheeling, WV – OH MSA	41	25.74
Wichita, KS MSA	188	38.74
Wichita Falls, TX MSA	33	26.97

[Continued]

★ 738 ★

Speech Therapists
[Continued]

MSA/CMSA	Total Employees	Employees per 100,000 pop.
Williamsport, PA MSA	52	43.80
Wilmington, NC MSA	33	27.44
Worcester, MA MSA	156	35.71
Yakima, WA MSA	31	16.42
York, PA MSA	75	17.95
Youngstown – Warren, OH MSA	99	20.10
Yuba City, CA MSA	32	26.09
Yuma, AZ MSA	43	40.23

Source: Census of Population and Housing, 1990: Equal Employment Opportunity (EEO) File on CD-ROM [machine-readable datafiles]. Prepared by the Bureau of the Census. Washington, DC: The Bureau, 1992.

★ 739 ★

Employment

Therapists

The table below presents the number of civilians 16 years old or older who reported working as therapists not tabulated elsewhere during the 1990 Census; for example, recreational therapists. Data are provided by total number employed in each Metropolitan Statistical Area (MSA) or Consolidated Metropolitan Statistical Area (CMSA), as well as the number employed per 100,000 people.

[Total for all of the U.S. was 71,402; 28.71 per 100,000 persons]

MSA/CMSA	Total Employees	Employees per 100,000 pop.
Abilene, TX MSA	14	11.70
Albany, GA MSA	31	27.54
Albany – Schenectady – Troy, NY MSA	322	36.83
Albuquerque, NM MSA	237	49.32
Alexandria, LA MSA	83	63.09
Allentown – Bethlehem – Easton, PA – NJ MSA	196	28.54
Altoona, PA MSA	22	16.85
Amarillo, TX MSA	87	46.39
Anchorage, AK MSA	63	27.83
Anderson, IN MSA	21	16.07
Anderson, SC MSA	37	25.48
Anniston, AL MSA	22	18.96
Appleton – Oshkosh – Neenah, WI MSA	96	30.46
Asheville, NC MSA	97	55.49
Athens, GA MSA	27	17.28
Atlanta, GA MSA	829	29.26
Atlantic City, NJ MSA	49	15.34
Augusta, GA – SC MSA	114	28.73
Austin, TX MSA	282	36.08
Bakersfield, CA MSA	77	14.17
Baltimore, MD MSA	694	29.13

[Continued]

★ 739 ★

Therapists
[Continued]

MSA/CMSA	Total Employees	Employees per 100,000 pop.
Bangor, ME MSA	38	42.82
Baton Rouge, LA MSA	53	10.03
Battle Creek, MI MSA	24	17.65
Beaumont – Port Arthur, TX MSA	119	32.94
Bellingham, WA MSA	57	44.61
Benton Harbor, MI MSA	27	16.73
Billings, MT MSA	11	9.70
Biloxi – Gulfport, MS MSA	41	20.80
Binghamton, NY MSA	140	52.93
Birmingham, AL MSA	130	14.32
Bismarck, ND MSA	14	16.70
Bloomington, IN MSA	66	60.56
Bloomington – Normal, IL MSA	52	40.25
Boise City, ID MSA	97	47.14
Boston – Lawrence – Salem, MA – NH CMSA	1911	45.81
Bradenton, FL MSA	37	17.48
Bremerton, WA MSA	11	5.80
Brownsville – Harlingen, TX MSA	28	10.76
Bryan – College Station, TX MSA	15	12.31
Buffalo – Niagara Falls, NY CMSA	346	29.09
Burlington, NC MSA	9	8.32
Burlington, VT MSA	23	17.50
Canton, OH MSA	130	32.99
Casper, WY MSA	5	8.17
Cedar Rapids, IA MSA	50	29.63
Champaign – Urbana – Rantoul, IL MSA	43	24.85
Charleston, SC MSA	102	20.12
Charleston, WV MSA	83	33.14
Charlotte – Gastonia – Rock Hill, NC – SC MSA	173	14.89
Charlottesville, VA MSA	69	52.63
Chattanooga, TN – GA MSA	166	38.32
Cheyenne, WY MSA	13	17.77
Chicago – Gary – Lake County, IL – IN – WI CMSA	2645	32.79
Chico, CA MSA	56	30.75
Cincinnati – Hamilton, OH – KY – IN CMSA	486	27.86
Clarksville – Hopkinsville, TN – KY MSA	31	18.30
Cleveland – Akron – Lorain, OH CMSA	722	26.16
Colorado Springs, CO MSA	145	36.52
Columbia, MO MSA	83	73.86
Columbia, SC MSA	209	46.10
Columbus, GA – AL MSA	62	25.51
Columbus, OH MSA	503	36.52
Corpus Christi, TX MSA	95	27.15
Cumberland, MD – WV MSA	33	32.47
Dallas – Fort Worth, TX CMSA	1276	32.84
Davenport – Rock Island – Moline, IA – IL MSA	72	20.52

[Continued]

★ 739 ★

Therapists
[Continued]

MSA/CMSA	Total Employees	Employees per 100,000 pop.
Dayton – Springfield, OH MSA	507	53.30
Daytona Beach, FL MSA	46	12.41
Decatur, AL MSA	30	22.80
Decatur, IL MSA	24	20.48
Denver – Boulder, CO CMSA	748	40.47
Des Moines, IA MSA	114	29.01
Detroit – Ann Arbor, MI CMSA	1600	34.30
Dothan, AL MSA	36	27.49
Dubuque, IA MSA	13	15.05
Duluth, MN – WI MSA	73	30.42
Eau Claire, WI MSA	96	69.80
El Paso, TX MSA	102	17.24
Elkhart – Goshen, IN MSA	7	4.48
Elmira, NY MSA	32	33.62
Enid, OK MSA	17	29.96
Erie, PA MSA	140	50.80
Eugene – Springfield, OR MSA	39	13.79
Evansville, IN – KY MSA	120	43.01
Fargo – Moorhead, ND – MN MSA	43	28.05
Fayetteville, NC MSA	103	37.51
Fayetteville – Springdale, AR MSA	24	21.16
Fitchburg – Leominster, MA MSA	9	8.76
Flint, MI MSA	162	37.63
Florence, AL MSA	8	6.09
Florence, SC MSA	34	29.73
Fort Collins – Loveland, CO MSA	76	40.83
Fort Myers – Cape Coral, FL MSA	101	30.14
Fort Pierce, FL MSA	33	13.14
Fort Smith, AR – OK MSA	21	11.94
Fort Walton Beach, FL MSA	40	27.82
Fort Wayne, IN MSA	27	7.42
Fresno, CA MSA	211	31.61
Gadsden, AL MSA	14	14.02
Gainesville, FL MSA	108	52.91
Glens Falls, NY MSA	14	11.81
Grand Forks, ND MSA	6	8.49
Grand Rapids, MI MSA	208	30.22
Great Falls, MT MSA	9	11.58
Greeley, CO MSA	51	38.69
Green Bay, WI MSA	39	20.04
Greensboro – Winston-Salem – High Point, NC MSA	211	22.40
Greenville – Spartanburg, SC MSA	112	17.48
Hagerstown, MD MSA	27	22.24
Harrisburg – Lebanon – Carlisle, PA MSA	227	38.61
Hartford – New Britain – Middletown, CT CMSA	409	37.67
Hickory – Morganton, NC MSA	58	26.16

[Continued]

★ 739 ★

Therapists
[Continued]

MSA/CMSA	Total Employees	Employees per 100,000 pop.
Honolulu, HI MSA	232	27.74
Houma – Thibodaux, LA MSA	51	27.89
Houston – Galveston – Brazoria, TX CMSA	834	22.47
Huntington – Ashland, WV – KY – OH MSA	53	16.96
Huntsville, AL MSA	68	28.46
Indianapolis, IN MSA	388	31.04
Iowa City, IA MSA	76	79.07
Jackson, MI MSA	21	14.02
Jackson, MS MSA	87	22.00
Jackson, TN MSA	13	16.67
Jacksonville, FL MSA	159	17.54
Jacksonville, NC MSA	15	10.01
Jamestown – Dunkirk, NY	42	29.60
Janesville – Beloit, WI MSA	39	27.95
Johnson City – Kingsport – Bristol, TN – VA MSA	126	28.90
Johnstown, PA MSA	40	16.58
Joplin, MO MSA	13	9.64
Kalamazoo, MI MSA	163	72.96
Kankakee, IL MSA	37	38.44
Kansas City, MO – KS MSA	426	27.20
Killeen – Temple, TX MSA	62	24.29
Knoxville, TN MSA	177	29.27
Kokomo, IN MSA	11	11.35
La Crosse, WI MSA	38	38.81
Lafayette, LA MSA	29	13.89
Lafayette – West Lafayette, IN MSA	42	32.16
Lake Charles, LA MSA	64	38.06
Lakeland – Winter Haven, FL MSA	120	29.60
Lancaster, PA MSA	193	45.65
Lansing – East Lansing, MI MSA	212	49.00
Laredo, TX MSA	22	16.51
Las Cruces, NM MSA	28	20.66
Las Vegas, NV MSA	163	21.98
Lawrence, KS MSA	35	42.79
Lawton, OK MSA	7	6.28
Lewiston – Auburn, ME MSA	32	36.31
Lexington-Fayette, KY MSA	72	20.66
Lima, OH MSA	27	17.49
Lincoln, NE MSA	66	30.89
Little Rock – North Little Rock, AR MSA	172	33.52
Longview – Marshall, TX MSA	31	19.09
Los Angeles – Anaheim – Riverside, CA CMSA	3538	24.35
Louisville, KY – IN MSA	259	27.19
Lubbock, TX MSA	32	14.37
Lynchburg, VA MSA	64	45.01
Macon – Warner Robins, GA MSA	91	32.37

[Continued]

★ 739 ★

Therapists
[Continued]

MSA/CMSA	Total Employees	Employees per 100,000 pop.
Madison, WI MSA	171	46.58
Manchester, NH MSA	34	23.00
Mansfield, OH MSA	42	33.30
McAllen – Edinburg – Mission, TX MSA	30	7.82
Medford, OR MSA	32	21.86
Melbourne – Titusville – Palm Bay, FL MSA	105	26.32
Memphis, TN – AR – MS MSA	224	22.82
Merced, CA MSA	44	24.66
Miami – Fort Lauderdale, FL CMSA	956	29.94
Midland, TX MSA	22	20.64
Milwaukee – Racine, WI CMSA	593	36.90
Minneapolis – St. Paul, MN – WI MSA	1025	41.60
Mobile, AL MSA	106	22.23
Modesto, CA MSA	75	20.24
Monroe, LA MSA	18	12.66
Montgomery, AL MSA	81	27.69
Muncie, IN MSA	18	15.04
Muskegon, MI MSA	18	11.32
Naples, FL MSA	18	11.83
Nashville, TN MSA	247	25.08
New Bedford, MA MSA	15	8.54
New Haven – Meriden, CT MSA	254	47.91
New London – Norwich, CT – RI MSA	106	39.73
New Orleans, LA MSA	245	19.78
New York – Northern New Jersey – Long Island, NY – NJ – CT CMSA	6671	36.88
Norfolk – Virginia Beach – Newport News, VA MSA	430	30.80
Ocala, FL MSA	56	28.74
Odessa, TX MSA	11	9.25
Oklahoma City, OK MSA	147	15.33
Olympia, WA MSA	70	43.41
Omaha, NE – IA MSA	170	27.50
Orlando, FL MSA	347	32.35
Owensboro, KY MSA	23	26.38
Panama City, FL MSA	9	7.09
Parkersburg – Marietta, WV – OH MSA	61	40.89
Pascagoula, MS MSA	5	4.34
Pensacola, FL MSA	65	18.87
Peoria, IL MSA	98	28.89
Philadelphia – Wilmington – Trenton, PA – NJ – DE – MD CMSA	2187	37.07
Phoenix, AZ MSA	670	31.57
Pine Bluff, AR MSA	15	17.55
Pittsburgh – Beaver Valley, PA CMSA	859	38.30
Pittsfield, MA MSA	36	45.43
Portland, ME MSA	88	40.88
Portland – Vancouver, OR – WA CMSA	512	34.64
Portsmouth – Dover – Rochester, NH – ME MSA	62	27.73

[Continued]

★ 739 ★

Therapists
[Continued]

MSA/CMSA	Total Employees	Employees per 100,000 pop.
Poughkeepsie, NY MSA	242	93.27
Providence – Pawtucket – Fall River, RI – MA CMSA	455	39.86
Provo – Orem, UT MSA	158	59.94
Pueblo, CO MSA	71	57.70
Raleigh – Durham, NC MSA	330	44.87
Rapid City, SD MSA	17	20.90
Reading, PA MSA	134	39.82
Redding, CA MSA	31	21.08
Reno, NV MSA	45	17.67
Richland – Kennewick – Pasco, WA MSA	50	33.33
Richmond – Petersburg, VA MSA	204	23.57
Roanoke, VA MSA	43	19.16
Rochester, MN MSA	41	38.51
Rochester, NY MSA	460	45.89
Rockford, IL MSA	57	20.09
Sacramento, CA MSA	330	22.28
Saginaw – Bay City – Midland, MI MSA	93	23.29
St. Cloud, MN MSA	57	29.86
St. Joseph, MO MSA	67	80.64
St. Louis, MO – IL MSA	685	28.03
Salem, OR MSA	164	58.99
Salinas – Seaside – Monterey, CA MSA	59	16.59
Salt Lake City – Ogden, UT MSA	373	34.79
San Angelo, TX MSA	37	37.58
San Antonio, TX MSA	278	21.35
San Diego, CA MSA	535	21.42
San Francisco – Oakland – San Jose, CA CMSA	2337	37.37
Santa Barbara – Santa Maria – Lompoc, CA MSA	166	44.91
Santa Fe, NM MSA	96	82.02
Sarasota, FL MSA	87	31.32
Savannah, GA MSA	19	7.83
Scranton – Wilkes-Barre, PA MSA	276	37.59
Seattle – Tacoma, WA CMSA	921	35.99
Sharon, PA MSA	26	21.49
Sheboygan, WI MSA	16	15.40
Sherman – Denison, TX MSA	20	21.05
Shreveport, LA MSA	62	18.54
Sioux City, IA – NE MSA	42	36.52
Sioux Falls, SD MSA	28	22.62
South Bend – Mishawaka, IN MSA	65	26.31
Spokane, WA MSA	124	34.31
Springfield, IL MSA	30	15.83
Springfield, MO MSA	59	24.52
Springfield, MA MSA	231	43.62
State College, PA MSA	2	1.62
Steubenville – Weirton, OH – WV MSA	39	27.36

[Continued]

★ 739 ★

Therapists
[Continued]

MSA/CMSA	Total Employees	Employees per 100,000 pop.
Stockton, CA MSA	60	12.48
Syracuse, NY MSA	203	30.76
Tallahassee, FL MSA	74	31.68
Tampa – St. Petersburg – Clearwater, FL MSA	586	28.34
Terre Haute, IN MSA	42	32.11
Texarkana, TX – Texarkana, AR MSA	11	9.16
Toledo, OH MSA	301	49.01
Topeka, KS MSA	95	59.02
Tucson, AZ MSA	240	35.99
Tulsa, OK MSA	210	29.62
Tuscaloosa, AL MSA	89	59.13
Tyler, TX MSA	63	41.64
Utica – Rome, NY MSA	128	40.43
Victoria, TX MSA	8	10.76
Visalia – Tulare – Porterville, CA MSA	83	26.61
Waco, TX MSA	60	31.73
Washington, DC – MD – VA MSA	1305	33.26
Waterbury, CT MSA	138	62.27
Waterloo – Cedar Falls, IA MSA	18	12.28
Wausau, WI MSA	13	11.27
West Palm Beach – Boca Raton – Delray Beach, FL MSA	260	30.11
Wheeling, WV – OH MSA	49	30.76
Wichita, KS MSA	111	22.87
Wichita Falls, TX MSA	54	44.13
Williamsport, PA MSA	13	10.95
Wilmington, NC MSA	25	20.78
Worcester, MA MSA	148	33.87
Yakima, WA MSA	93	49.25
York, PA MSA	121	28.96
Youngstown – Warren, OH MSA	173	35.12
Yuba City, CA MSA	12	9.78
Yuma, AZ MSA	20	18.71

Source: Census of Population and Housing, 1990: Equal Employment Opportunity (EEO) File on CD-ROM [machine-readable datafiles]. Prepared by the Bureau of the Census. Washington, DC: The Bureau, 1992.

★ 740 ★

Employment

Veterinarians

The table below presents the number of civilians 16 years old or older who reported working as veterinarians during the 1990 Census. Data are provided by total number employed in each Metropolitan Statistical Area (MSA) or Consolidated Metropolitan Statistical Area (CMSA), as well as the number employed per 100,000 people.

[Total for all of the U.S. was 48,744; 19.60 per 100,000 persons]

MSA/CMSA	Total Employees	Employees per 100,000 pop.
Abilene, TX MSA	8	6.69
Albany, GA MSA	38	33.76
Albany – Schenectady – Troy, NY MSA	128	14.64
Albuquerque, NM MSA	73	15.19
Alexandria, LA MSA	26	19.76
Allentown – Bethlehem – Easton, PA – NJ MSA	110	16.02
Altoona, PA MSA	11	8.43
Amarillo, TX MSA	42	22.39
Anchorage, AK MSA	35	15.46
Anderson, IN MSA	33	25.25
Anderson, SC MSA	19	13.09
Anniston, AL MSA	9	7.76
Appleton – Oshkosh – Neenah, WI MSA	29	9.20
Asheville, NC MSA	29	16.59
Athens, GA MSA	152	97.27
Atlanta, GA MSA	622	21.95
Atlantic City, NJ MSA	77	24.11
Augusta, GA – SC MSA	20	5.04
Austin, TX MSA	197	25.21
Bakersfield, CA MSA	88	16.19
Baltimore, MD MSA	447	18.76
Bangor, ME MSA	9	10.14
Baton Rouge, LA MSA	175	33.13
Battle Creek, MI MSA	21	15.44
Beaumont – Port Arthur, TX MSA	50	13.84
Bellingham, WA MSA	38	29.74
Benton Harbor, MI MSA	35	21.69
Billings, MT MSA	54	47.61
Biloxi – Gulfport, MS MSA	10	5.07
Binghamton, NY MSA	58	21.93
Birmingham, AL MSA	172	18.95
Bismarck, ND MSA	12	14.31
Bloomington – Normal, IL MSA	12	9.29
Boise City, ID MSA	88	42.77
Boston – Lawrence – Salem, MA – NH CMSA	792	18.99
Bradenton, FL MSA	32	15.12
Bremerton, WA MSA	39	20.56
Brownsville – Harlingen, TX MSA	13	5.00
Bryan – College Station, TX MSA	243	199.41
Buffalo – Niagara Falls, NY CMSA	129	10.85
Burlington, NC MSA	18	16.63
Burlington, VT MSA	37	28.15

[Continued]

★ 740 ★

Veterinarians

[Continued]

MSA/CMSA	Total Employees	Employees per 100,000 pop.
Canton, OH MSA	77	19.54
Casper, WY MSA	2	3.27
Cedar Rapids, IA MSA	5	2.96
Champaign – Urbana – Rantoul, IL MSA	75	43.35
Charleston, SC MSA	67	13.22
Charleston, WV MSA	64	25.55
Charlotte – Gastonia – Rock Hill, NC – SC MSA	219	18.85
Charlottesville, VA MSA	57	43.48
Chattanooga, TN – GA MSA	77	17.77
Cheyenne, WY MSA	12	16.41
Chicago – Gary – Lake County, IL – IN – WI CMSA	955	11.84
Chico, CA MSA	50	27.45
Cincinnati – Hamilton, OH – KY – IN CMSA	350	20.07
Clarksville – Hopkinsville, TN – KY MSA	18	10.62
Cleveland – Akron – Lorain, OH CMSA	405	14.67
Colorado Springs, CO MSA	76	19.14
Columbia, MO MSA	103	91.65
Columbia, SC MSA	57	12.57
Columbus, GA – AL MSA	18	7.41
Columbus, OH MSA	443	32.16
Corpus Christi, TX MSA	57	16.29
Dallas – Fort Worth, TX CMSA	809	20.82
Danville, VA MSA	10	9.20
Davenport – Rock Island – Moline, IA – IL MSA	62	17.67
Dayton – Springfield, OH MSA	165	17.35
Daytona Beach, FL MSA	48	12.95
Decatur, AL MSA	6	4.56
Decatur, IL MSA	26	22.18
Denver – Boulder, CO CMSA	523	28.30
Des Moines, IA MSA	144	36.65
Detroit – Ann Arbor, MI CMSA	711	15.24
Dothan, AL MSA	28	21.38
Dubuque, IA MSA	19	21.99
Duluth, MN – WI MSA	21	8.75
Eau Claire, WI MSA	29	21.08
El Paso, TX MSA	82	13.86
Elkhart – Goshen, IN MSA	53	33.93
Elmira, NY MSA	11	11.56
Enid, OK MSA	28	49.35
Erie, PA MSA	14	5.08
Eugene – Springfield, OR MSA	67	23.68
Evansville, IN – KY MSA	53	19.00
Fargo – Moorhead, ND – MN MSA	43	28.05
Fayetteville, NC MSA	20	7.28
Fayetteville – Springdale, AR MSA	31	27.33
Fitchburg – Leominster, MA MSA	7	6.81

[Continued]

★ 740 ★

Veterinarians
[Continued]

MSA/CMSA	Total Employees	Employees per 100,000 pop.
Flint, MI MSA	39	9.06
Florence, AL MSA	38	28.94
Florence, SC MSA	11	9.62
Fort Collins–Loveland, CO MSA	140	75.21
Fort Myers–Cape Coral, FL MSA	43	12.83
Fort Pierce, FL MSA	30	11.95
Fort Smith, AR–OK MSA	34	19.33
Fort Walton Beach, FL MSA	22	15.30
Fort Wayne, IN MSA	99	27.21
Fresno, CA MSA	105	15.73
Gadsden, AL MSA	6	6.01
Gainesville, FL MSA	173	84.76
Glens Falls, NY MSA	16	13.50
Grand Rapids, MI MSA	88	12.78
Great Falls, MT MSA	28	36.04
Greeley, CO MSA	59	44.76
Green Bay, WI MSA	69	35.46
Greensboro–Winston-Salem–High Point, NC MSA	253	26.86
Greenville–Spartanburg, SC MSA	87	13.58
Hagerstown, MD MSA	31	25.54
Harrisburg–Lebanon–Carlisle, PA MSA	109	18.54
Hartford–New Britain–Middletown, CT CMSA	204	18.79
Hickory–Morganton, NC MSA	22	9.92
Honolulu, HI MSA	123	14.71
Houma–Thibodaux, LA MSA	13	7.11
Houston–Galveston–Brazoria, TX CMSA	806	21.72
Huntington–Ashland, WV–KY–OH MSA	48	15.36
Huntsville, AL MSA	27	11.30
Indianapolis, IN MSA	310	24.80
Iowa City, IA MSA	2	2.08
Jackson, MI MSA	19	12.69
Jackson, MS MSA	97	24.53
Jackson, TN MSA	24	30.78
Jacksonville, FL MSA	185	20.40
Jacksonville, NC MSA	12	8.01
Jamestown–Dunkirk, NY	25	17.62
Janesville–Beloit, WI MSA	46	32.97
Johnson City–Kingsport–Bristol, TN–VA MSA	62	14.22
Johnstown, PA MSA	10	4.15
Joplin, MO MSA	45	33.36
Kalamazoo, MI MSA	46	20.59
Kankakee, IL MSA	4	4.16
Kansas City, MO–KS MSA	445	28.41
Killeen–Temple, TX MSA	37	14.49
Knoxville, TN MSA	161	26.62
Kokomo, IN MSA	12	12.38

[Continued]

★ 740 ★

Veterinarians
[Continued]

MSA/CMSA	Total Employees	Employees per 100,000 pop.
La Crosse, WI MSA	15	15.32
Lafayette, LA MSA	40	19.16
Lafayette – West Lafayette, IN MSA	106	81.17
Lake Charles, LA MSA	35	20.82
Lakeland – Winter Haven, FL MSA	30	7.40
Lancaster, PA MSA	134	31.69
Lansing – East Lansing, MI MSA	206	47.61
Las Cruces, NM MSA	22	16.23
Las Vegas, NV MSA	100	13.49
Lawton, OK MSA	16	14.35
Lewiston – Auburn, ME MSA	12	13.61
Lexington-Fayette, KY MSA	185	53.10
Lima, OH MSA	29	18.79
Lincoln, NE MSA	74	34.64
Little Rock – North Little Rock, AR MSA	140	27.28
Longview – Marshall, TX MSA	27	16.62
Los Angeles – Anaheim – Riverside, CA CMSA	1951	13.43
Louisville, KY – IN MSA	183	19.21
Lubbock, TX MSA	31	13.92
Lynchburg, VA MSA	40	28.13
Macon – Warner Robins, GA MSA	8	2.85
Madison, WI MSA	142	38.68
Manchester, NH MSA	6	4.06
Mansfield, OH MSA	6	4.76
McAllen – Edinburg – Mission, TX MSA	18	4.69
Medford, OR MSA	50	34.16
Melbourne – Titusville – Palm Bay, FL MSA	86	21.56
Memphis, TN – AR – MS MSA	152	15.48
Merced, CA MSA	39	21.86
Miami – Fort Lauderdale, FL CMSA	691	21.64
Milwaukee – Racine, WI CMSA	305	18.98
Minneapolis – St. Paul, MN – WI MSA	669	27.15
Mobile, AL MSA	91	19.08
Modesto, CA MSA	48	12.95
Montgomery, AL MSA	56	19.14
Muncie, IN MSA	24	20.06
Naples, FL MSA	33	21.70
Nashville, TN MSA	185	18.78
New Bedford, MA MSA	11	6.26
New Haven – Meriden, CT MSA	42	7.92
New London – Norwich, CT – RI MSA	48	17.99
New Orleans, LA MSA	265	21.39
New York – Northern New Jersey – Long Island, NY – NJ – CT CMSA	2187	12.09
Norfolk – Virginia Beach – Newport News, VA MSA	233	16.69
Ocala, FL MSA	164	84.17
Odessa, TX MSA	14	11.77

[Continued]

★ 740 ★

Veterinarians
[Continued]

MSA/CMSA	Total Employees	Employees per 100,000 pop.
Oklahoma City, OK MSA	159	16.58
Olympia, WA MSA	49	30.39
Omaha, NE – IA MSA	144	23.29
Orlando, FL MSA	128	11.93
Owensboro, KY MSA	6	6.88
Panama City, FL MSA	32	25.20
Parkersburg – Marietta, WV – OH MSA	12	8.04
Pascagoula, MS MSA	13	11.28
Pensacola, FL MSA	65	18.87
Peoria, IL MSA	50	14.74
Philadelphia – Wilmington – Trenton, PA – NJ – DE – MD CMSA	1308	22.17
Phoenix, AZ MSA	341	16.07
Pine Bluff, AR MSA	8	9.36
Pittsburgh – Beaver Valley, PA CMSA	195	8.69
Pittsfield, MA MSA	2	2.52
Portland, ME MSA	37	17.19
Portland – Vancouver, OR – WA CMSA	357	24.16
Portsmouth – Dover – Rochester, NH – ME MSA	42	18.79
Poughkeepsie, NY MSA	93	35.84
Providence – Pawtucket – Fall River, RI – MA CMSA	178	15.59
Provo – Orem, UT MSA	17	6.45
Pueblo, CO MSA	30	24.38
Raleigh – Durham, NC MSA	314	42.69
Rapid City, SD MSA	19	23.36
Reading, PA MSA	48	14.26
Redding, CA MSA	12	8.16
Reno, NV MSA	110	43.19
Richland – Kennewick – Pasco, WA MSA	6	4.00
Richmond – Petersburg, VA MSA	154	17.79
Roanoke, VA MSA	26	11.58
Rochester, MN MSA	28	26.30
Rochester, NY MSA	227	22.65
Rockford, IL MSA	42	14.80
Sacramento, CA MSA	470	31.73
Saginaw – Bay City – Midland, MI MSA	64	16.03
St. Cloud, MN MSA	65	34.05
St. Louis, MO – IL MSA	497	20.33
Salem, OR MSA	58	20.86
Salinas – Seaside – Monterey, CA MSA	81	22.77
Salt Lake City – Ogden, UT MSA	122	11.38
San Angelo, TX MSA	4	4.06
San Antonio, TX MSA	231	17.74
San Diego, CA MSA	503	20.14
San Francisco – Oakland – San Jose, CA CMSA	1258	20.12
Santa Barbara – Santa Maria – Lompoc, CA MSA	101	27.33
Santa Fe, NM MSA	72	61.52

[Continued]

★ 740 ★

Veterinarians
[Continued]

MSA/CMSA	Total Employees	Employees per 100,000 pop.
Sarasota, FL MSA	92	33.12
Savannah, GA MSA	44	18.14
Scranton – Wilkes-Barre, PA MSA	52	7.08
Seattle – Tacoma, WA CMSA	601	23.48
Sharon, PA MSA	29	23.97
Sheboygan, WI MSA	27	25.99
Sherman – Denison, TX MSA	24	25.26
Shreveport, LA MSA	105	31.41
Sioux City, IA – NE MSA	56	48.69
Sioux Falls, SD MSA	32	25.85
South Bend – Mishawaka, IN MSA	19	7.69
Spokane, WA MSA	65	17.99
Springfield, IL MSA	24	12.66
Springfield, MO MSA	55	22.86
Springfield, MA MSA	66	12.46
State College, PA MSA	22	17.77
Stockton, CA MSA	94	19.56
Syracuse, NY MSA	116	17.58
Tallahassee, FL MSA	47	20.12
Tampa – St. Petersburg – Clearwater, FL MSA	381	18.42
Terre Haute, IN MSA	30	22.93
Texarkana, TX – Texarkana, AR MSA	50	41.62
Toledo, OH MSA	79	12.86
Topeka, KS MSA	13	8.08
Tucson, AZ MSA	142	21.29
Tulsa, OK MSA	156	22.00
Tuscaloosa, AL MSA	48	31.89
Tyler, TX MSA	48	31.72
Utica – Rome, NY MSA	84	26.53
Victoria, TX MSA	5	6.72
Visalia – Tulare – Porterville, CA MSA	48	15.39
Waco, TX MSA	21	11.10
Washington, DC – MD – VA MSA	1085	27.65
Waterbury, CT MSA	18	8.12
Waterloo – Cedar Falls, IA MSA	30	20.46
Wausau, WI MSA	20	17.33
West Palm Beach – Boca Raton – Delray Beach, FL MSA	198	22.93
Wheeling, WV – OH MSA	18	11.30
Wichita, KS MSA	127	26.17
Wichita Falls, TX MSA	25	20.43
Williamsport, PA MSA	3	2.53
Wilmington, NC MSA	51	42.40
Worcester, MA MSA	62	14.19
Yakima, WA MSA	58	30.72
York, PA MSA	48	11.49
Youngstown – Warren, OH MSA	82	16.65

[Continued]

★ 740 ★

Veterinarians
[Continued]

MSA/CMSA	Total Employees	Employees per 100,000 pop.
Yuba City, CA MSA	10	8.15
Yuma, AZ MSA	25	23.39

Source: Census of Population and Housing, 1990: Equal Employment Opportunity (EEO) File on CD-ROM [machine-readable datafiles]. Prepared by the Bureau of the Census. Washington, DC: The Bureau, 1992.

Salaries and Wages: Administration

★ 741 ★

Earnings of Full-time Clerical Workers in Hospitals: 1991

The table shows the number of private hospital workers and their average (mean) hourly earnings.

Occupation[1]	Number of workers	Hourly earnings ($)
Accounting clerks		
I	511	7.12
II	6,104	8.54
III	2,849	10.09
IV	268	11.57
Admitting clerks	26,491	8.02
File clerks		
I	2,694	6.45
II	2,272	8.09
III	103	9.68
General clerks		
I	894	6.53
II	6,713	7.61
III	4,410	8.78
IV	701	9.84
Key entry operators		
I	3,401	7.79
II	1,494	9.40
Medical transcriptionists	16,292	9.45

[Continued]

★ 741 ★

Earnings of Full-time Clerical Workers in Hospitals:
1991
[Continued]

Occupation[1]	Number of workers	Hourly earnings ($)
Messengers	1,317	7.00
Personnel clerks/assistants		
I	301	7.61
II	1,007	9.17
III	774	10.97
IV	129	12.81
Purchasing clerks/assistants		
I	409	7.24
II	999	9.50
III	345	10.93
Secretaries		
I	8,941	8.92
II	10,741	10.57
III	9,107	11.60
IV	2,457	13.79
V	386	15.99
Switchboard operators	9,853	7.95
Typists		
I	1,455	8.47
II	256	8.83
Unit secretaries	59,629	8.19
Word processors		
I	107	8.47
II	210	9.48

Source: U.S. Department of Labor. Bureau of Labor Statistics. *Occupational Wage Survey: Hospitals, January 1991.* Bulletin 2392. Washington, DC: U.S. Government Printing Office, January 1992, pp. 36-40. Source includes results of 1991 White-collar Pay Survey. *Notes:* Because of rounding, sum of individual items may not equal 100. 1. Data for overall occupation may include data for subclassifications not shown separately.

★ 742 ★

Salaries and Wages: Administration

Earnings of Full-time Professional and Administrative Hospital Workers: 1991

The table shows the number of private hospital workers and their average (mean) hourly earnings.

Occupation[1]	Number of workers	Hourly earnings ($)
Accountants		
I	786	11.35
II	2,594	13.41
III	2,143	17.13
IV	961	22.49
V	130	29.28
Attorneys		
III	47	31.05
IV	15	44.68
Auditors		
I	14	10.69
II	27	13.55
III	54	18.69
IV	7	24.11
Buyers		
I	1,231	11.11
II	1,053	14.51
III	131	18.50
Chemists		
III	12	19.84
Chief accountants		
II	35	30.33
III	8	36.70
Computer operators		
I	484	7.60
II	3,281	9.63
III	1,226	11.91
IV	133	14.71
Computer programmers		
I	323	12.12
II	846	13.74
III	966	16.92
IV	244	20.65
Computer systems analysts		
I	1,013	16.50

[Continued]

★ 742 ★

Earnings of Full-time Professional and Administrative Hospital Workers: 1991
[Continued]

Occupation[1]	Number of workers	Hourly earnings ($)
II	1,487	19.86
III	521	23.78
IV	60	26.16
Computer systems analyst supervisors/managers		
I	170	25.53
II	60	29.92
III	6	36.51
Directors of Personnel		
I	287	19.86
II	370	26.98
Drafters		
II	6	10.63
III	21	12.06
IV	29	14.19
Engineers		
II	14	17.71
III	32	20.44
IV	14	25.33
Medical records directors	2,804	18.16
Medical records technicians	12,313	9.70
I	8,917	9.10
II	3,224	11.30
Personnel specialists		
I	215	10.64
II	1,884	13.22
III	2,159	16.62
IV	1,152	21.04
V	81	28.02
Personnel supervisors/managers		
I	243	22.91

[Continued]

★ 742 ★

Earnings of Full-time Professional and Administrative Hospital Workers: 1991
[Continued]

Occupation[1]	Number of workers	Hourly earnings ($)
II	145	28.43
III	27	38.20

Source: U.S. Department of Labor. Bureau of Labor Statistics. *Occupational Wage Survey: Hospitals, January 1991.* Bulletin 2392. Washington, DC: U.S. Government Printing Office, January 1992, pp. 36-40. Source includes results of 1991 White-collar Pay Survey. *Notes:* Because of rounding, sum of individual items may not equal 100. 1. Data for overall occupation may include data for subclassifications not shown separately.

★ 743 ★

Salaries and Wages: Administration

Earnings of Full-time Service Workers in Hospitals: 1991

The table shows the number of private hospital workers and their average (mean) hourly earnings.

Occupation[1]	Number of workers	Hourly earnings ($)
Food service helpers	52,867	6.99
I	39,468	6.72
II	11,626	7.82
Hospital cleaners	92,952	7.14

Source: U.S. Department of Labor. Bureau of Labor Statistics. *Occupational Wage Survey: Hospitals, January 1991.* Bulletin 2392. Washington, DC: U.S. Government Printing Office, January 1992, pp. 36-40. Source includes results of 1991 White-collar Pay Survey. *Notes:* Because of rounding, sum of individual items may not equal 100. 1. Data for overall occupation may include data for subclassifications not shown separately.

Salaries and Wages: Health Care Practitioners

★ 744 ★

Direct Compensation of Health Care Practitioners

Data reflect the median for midlevel practitioner direct compensation. Data are provided by specialty.

[In dollars]

Practitioner	Compensation
Audiologist	37,176
Dietitian/nutritionist	29,762
Midwife	51,411
Nurse anesthetist[1]	77,462
Nurse practitioner	42,500
Optometrist	68,950
Pharmacist	48,695
Physical therapist	47,746
Physician's assistant	43,407
Podiatrist	106,712
Psychologist	60,000
Social worker	39,007
Surgeon's assistant	63,466

Source: Medical Group Management Association. *Physician Compensation and Production Survey: 1993 Report Based on 1992 Data.* Englewood, Colorado: Center for Research in Ambulatory Health Care Administration, September 1993, p. 71. Copyright. Used with permission of the Medical Group Management Association. *Note:* 1. Certified registered.

★ 745 ★

Salaries and Wages: Health Care Practitioners

Earnings of Full-time Health Care Practitioners in Hospital Settings: 1991

The table shows the number of private hospital workers and their average (mean) hourly earnings.

Occupation[1]	Number of workers	Hourly earnings ($)
Medical social workers	11,008	14.73
Medical technologists	42,496	14.71
I	33,213	14.24
II	8,497	16.48
Physical therapists	11,362	17.01

[Continued]

★ 745 ★

Earnings of Full-time Health Care Practitioners in Hospital Settings: 1991
[Continued]

Occupation[1]	Number of workers	Hourly earnings ($)
I	7,938	16.41
II	3,071	18.58

Source: U.S. Department of Labor. Bureau of Labor Statistics. *Occupational Wage Survey: Hospitals, January 1991.* Bulletin 2392. Washington, DC: U.S. Government Printing Office, January 1992, pp. 36-40. Source includes results of 1991 White-collar Pay Survey. *Notes:* Because of rounding, sum of individual items may not equal 100. 1. Data for overall occupation may include data for subclassifications not shown separately.

★ 746 ★

Salaries and Wages: Health Care Practitioners

Earnings of Full-time Technical Support Hospital Workers: 1991

The table shows the number of private hospital workers and their average (mean) hourly earnings.

Occupation[1]	Number of workers	Hourly earnings ($)
Diagnostic medical sonographers	4,686	14.47
I	117	10.70
II	859	13.28
III	3,547	14.74
IV	145	17.72
Electrocardiograph (EKG) technicians	5,751	8.66
I	4,413	8.02
II	1,243	10.58
III	83	13.22
Electroencephalographic (EEG) technicians	2,069	10.70
I	560	8.66
II	1,321	11.10
III	173	13.82
Medical laboratory technicians	13,263	11.33
I	9,132	10.78
II	3,671	12.50
Radiology technicians	33,456	12.75
I	20,428	12.06
II	12,371	13.84

[Continued]

★ 746 ★

Earnings of Full-time Technical Support Hospital Workers: 1991
[Continued]

Occupation[1]	Number of workers	Hourly earnings ($)
Respiratory therapists	26,846	12.60
I	13,294	11.57
II	13,243	13.62
Surgical technicians	17,671	10.03

Source: U.S. Department of Labor. Bureau of Labor Statistics. *Occupational Wage Survey: Hospitals, January 1991.* Bulletin 2392. Washington, DC: U.S. Government Printing Office, January 1992, pp. 36-40. Source includes results of 1991 White-collar Pay Survey. *Notes:* Because of rounding, sum of individual items may not equal 100. 1. Data for overall occupation may include data for subclassifications not shown separately.

★ 747 ★

Salaries and Wages: Health Care Practitioners

Education and Salaries of Selected Health Care Practitioners: 1990

Profession	Years of postsecondary education required	Entry degree	1990 earnings
Audiology[1]	6	M.A./M.S.	$32,000
Clinical psychology[2]	9	Ph.D.	$58,240
Medicine[3]	8[8]	M.D.	$123,802[9]
Nursing[4]	4	B.S.N.	$30,968
Occupational therapy[5]	4	B.A./B.S.	$35,000
Physical therapy[6]	4	B.A./B.S.	$43,281
Psychology[7]	8	Ph.D.	$52,104
Speech-language pathology[1]	6	M.A./M.S.	$30,000

Source: "Compensation and Gender." *ASHA* 36, no. 5 (May 1994), p. 34. *ASHA* is the publication of the American Speech-Language-Hearing Association. *Notes:* CCC-SLP represents Certificate of Clinical Competence—Speech-Language Pathology. CCC-A represents Certificate of Clinical Competence—Audiology. M.A. represents Master of Arts; M.S. represents Master of Science. B.A. represents Bachelor of Arts; B.S. represents Bachelor of Science. B.S.N. represents Bachelor of Science in Nursing. M.D. represents Doctor of Medicine. 1. American Speech-Language-Hearing Association. 1990 Omnibus Survey provided median salary for full-time certified CCC-SLP and CCC-A personnel. 2. American Psychological Association (APA). 1989 APA Salary Survey provided median salary for licensed, doctoral-level clinical psychologists, adjusted 1.04 percent for cost of living. 3. American Medical Association. Center for Health Policy Research (1986). Mean net income for 1986 was adjusted +3.6 percent for inflation. 4. University of Texas Medical Branch at Galveston. *National Survey of Hospital and Medical School Salaries.* Mean 1990 salary of staff nurses. 5. American Occupational Therapy Association. 1990 median salary. 6. American Physical Therapy Association. 1989 mean salary for full-time salaried personnel adjusted +1.04 percent for cost of living. Full-time self-employed physical therapists earned an average of $99,676 in 1989. 7. National Science Foundation Survey (1989). Median 1989 salary for psychologists adjusted 1.04 percent for cost of living. 8. Minimum. 9. 1987 earnings; 1990 data not available.

★ 748 ★

Salaries and Wages: Health Care Practitioners

Emergency Medical Technicians' Salaries: 1991

Data reflect the average annual salaries of emergency medical technicians (EMT) in 1991. Data are provided by employer types.

[In dollars]

Employer	Paramedic	Emergency medical technician-1	Emergency medical technician- basic
Mean[1]	27,320	23,108	21,650
Ambulance services (private)	24,223	19,097	17,227
Fire departments	33,108	32,176	28,029
Hospitals	24,518	18,134	16,401

Source: U.S. Deparment of Labor. *Occupational Outlook Handbook.* 1992-1993 edition. Lincolnwood, IL: VGM Career Horizons, p. 193. Primary source: *Journal of Emergency Medical Services. Note:* 1. All employers.

★ 749 ★

Salaries and Wages: Health Care Practitioners

Veterinary Technicians' Salaries, by Career Path

[In dollars]

Career Path	Salary
Food animal practice[1]	15,000
Government	26,300
Industry	26,100
Mixed animal practice	15,500
Research	26,200
Small animal practice	16,600

[Continued]

★ 749 ★

Veterinary Technicians' Salaries, by Career Path
[Continued]

Career Path	Salary
Specialty practice	19,100
University/college	22,800
Veterinary tech education	24,400
Other	22,200

Source: Decker, Carlene A. "Salaries—The Real Reason for the Shortage: Where Have All the Techs Gone?" *Veterinary Forum* (January 1993), p. 22. Primary source: 1991 national survey of the North American Veterinary Technician Association. *Note:* 1. Includes equine practice.

Salaries and Wages: Health Service Establishments

★ 750 ★

Earnings in Private Health Service Establishments: 1990-1993

Data reflect employment, hours, and earnings in private health service establishments by type. Hospitals, clinics, and other health-related establishments operated by all governments are excluded.

Establishment and measures	Calendar year			1993	
	1990	1991	1992	First quarter	Second quarter
Health services					
Total employment (in thousands)	7,814.3	8,182.9	8,523.3	8,735.7	8,836.4
Nonsupervisory workers					
Employment (in thousands)	6,947.6	7,275.8	7,575.3	7,755.0	7,843.9
Average weekly hours	32.5	32.5	32.8	32.7	32.7
Average hourly earnings (in dollars)	10.40	10.96	11.39	11.68	11.70
Offices and clinics of medical doctors					
Total employment (in thousands)	1,338.2	1,404.5	1,472.7	1,517.6	1,538.1
Nonsupervisory workers					
Employment (in thousands)	1,104.5	1,155.4	1,209.4	1,242.0	1,258.4
Average weekly hours	31.8	31.9	32.1	32.2	32.2
Average hourly earnings (in dollars)	10.58	11.13	11.41	11.72	11.85
Offices and clinics of dentists					
Total employment (in thousands)	512.9	527.6	541.9	552.3	560.0
Nonsupervisory workers					
Employment (in thousands)	449.7	463.5	474.3	483.5	489.8
Average weekly hours	28.4	28.3	28.3	28.1	28.4
Average hourly earnings (in dollars)	10.14	10.62	11.01	11.25	11.34
Nursing and personal care facilities					
Total employment (in thousands)	1,415.4	1,492.6	1,542.7	1,581.9	1,604.6
Nonsupervisory workers					
Employment (in thousands)	1,278.9	1,347.4	1.393.7	1,428.6	1,449.0

[Continued]

★ 750 ★

Earnings in Private Health Service Establishments: 1990-1993

[Continued]

Establishment and measures	Calendar year			1993	
	1990	1991	1992	First quarter	Second quarter
Average weekly hours	32.1	32.1	32.3	32.0	32.2
Average hourly earnings (in dollars)	7.24	7.56	7.85	8.05	8.09
Private hospitals					
Total employment (in thousands)	3,548.7	3,655.1	3,759.8	3,805.5	3,815.4
Nonsupervisory workers					
Employment (in thousands)	3,248.4	3,352.5	3,451.4	3,491.8	3,499.6
Average weekly hours	34.2	34.2	34.4	34.5	34.5
Average hourly earnings (in dollars)	11.79	12.50	13.03	13.38	13.38
All private nonagricultural establishments					
Total employment (in thousands)	91,115	89,854	89,866	89,217	91,297
Nonsupervisory workers					
Employment (in thousands)	73,800	72,650	72,866	72,357	74,316
Average weekly hours	34.5	34.3	34.4	34.0	34.4
Average hourly earnings (in dollars)	10.01	10.32	10.57	10.78	10.79

Source: U.S. Department of Health and Human Services. Health Care Financing Administration (HCFA). *Health Care Financing Review* 15, no. 2 (winter 1993), pp. 213-214. Primary source: U.S. Department of Labor. Bureau of Labor Statistics. *Employment and Earnings.* Monthly reports for January 1990 through September 1993. Washington, DC: U.S. Government Printing Office.

★ 751 ★

Salaries and Wages; Health Service Establishments

Earnings of Part-time Hospital Workers: 1991

The table shows the number of private hospital workers working part-time and their average (mean) hourly earnings. Data are provided for selected occupations.

Occupation	Number of workers	Hourly earnings ($)
Admitting clerks	13,599	7.97
Diagnostic medical sonographers	982	15.18
Electroencephalographic (EEG) technicians	393	11.35
Electrocardiogram (EKG) technicians	2,639	8.92
Food service helpers	35,243	6.56
Licensed practical nurses	36,986	10.70
Medical technologists	15,653	14.84

[Continued]

★ 751 ★

Earnings of Part-time Hospital Workers: 1991
[Continued]

Occupation	Number of workers	Hourly earnings ($)
Nursing assistants	43,930	7.05
Radiology technicians	10,391	12.76
Respiratory therapists	8,391	13.01
Staff nurses[1]	225,193	17.14
I	1,253	15.97
II	215,182	17.08
II (specialists)	6,352	18.04
III	696	20.65
Switchboard operators	7,389	7.69
Unit secretaries	31,226	8.17

Source: U.S. Department of Labor. Bureau of Labor Statistics. *Occupational Wage Survey: Hospitals, January 1991.* Bulletin 2392. Washington, DC: U.S. Government Printing Office, January 1992, pp. 41. Source includes results of 1991 White-collar Pay Survey. *Notes:* Because of rounding, sums of individual items may not equal 100. 1. Data for overall occupation may include data for subclassifications not shown separately.

Salaries and Wages: Managers and Executives

★ 752 ★

Direct Compensation of Health Care Managers

Data reflect medians for direct compensation and total fringe benefits for health services management positions. Data are provided by position title.

[In dollars]

Management position	Compensation	Fringe benefits
Administrator/executive director	63,088	13,950
Assistant administrator	55,000	11,650
Associate administrator/chief operating officer	62,500	15,308
Business office manager	42,000	9,000
Chief financial officer	67,850	12,900
Clinical department manager	46,500	10,938
Controller	50,500	10,080
Director of Human Resources	47,563	10,360
Information systems manager	59,000	11,600

[Continued]

★ 752 ★

Direct Compensation of Health Care Managers
[Continued]

Management position	Compensation	Fringe benefits
Medical director	148,500	21,883
Medical school department/faculty practice plan administrator	56,268	12,250
Office manager	37,440	8,175

Source: Medical Group Management Association. *Membership Compensation Survey: 1993 Report Based on 1993 Data.* Englewood, Colorado: Medical Group Management Association, October 1993, p. 9. Copyright. Used with permission of the Medical Group Management Association. *Notes:* Data from academic practice administrators are excluded for all position categories except "Medical school department/faculty practice plan administrator."

★ 753 ★

Salaries and Wages: Managers and Executives

Hospital Chief Executive Compensation: 1991

Table shows chief executive compensation by hospital ownership type and size. From the source: "Among hospitals that are similar in all respects but ownership, for-profit hospitals tend to pay higher compensation to chief executives than not-for-profit hospitals pay. This fact is not clearly evident in the table ... because the table does not account for other important characteristics (besides size) that vary between for-profit and not-for-profit hospitals" (p. 10).

[In dollars]

Type and size of hospital	Mean	Median	25 percent received more than	25 percent received less than
Not-for-profit				
Small	86,160	65,828	99,542	58,190
Medium	175,631	169,186	212,030	136,152
Large	292,165	271,598	337,789	217,292
For-profit				
Small	72,129	72,518	101,291	45,300
Medium	181,541	157,851	214,993	130,090
Large	1	1	1	1
Government				
Small	55,132	57,190	64,512	47,967
Medium	138,536	129,253	162,937	102,250
Large	240,050	222,551	279,450	164,248

Source: U.S. General Accounting Office. *Hospitals: Chief Executives' Compensation, 1989-1991.* Testimony Before the Subcommittee on Oversight and Investigations, Committee on Energy and Commerce, House of Representatives. Statement of Janet L. Shikles, Assistant Comptroller General, Human Resources Division. GAO/T-HRD-94-70. Washington, DC: U.S. General Accounting Office, 7 December 1992, p. 10. *Notes:* Small hospitals are defined as those having 1 to 100 beds. Medium hospitals are defined as those having 101 to 500 beds. Large hospitals are defined as those having more than 500 beds. 1. Too few cases reported to develop representative figures.

★ 754 ★

Salaries and Wages: Managers and Executives

Hospital Executives' Earnings: 1993

Table reflects the average base salary of hospital executives. Data are for independent hospitals only. Data for chief executive officers (CEOs) are based on surveys of 794 insitutions; data for physician executives are based on surveys of 27 hospitals.

Position	Average base salary ($)	Percent of CEO's salary
Chief of medical affairs	159,300	105
Chief executive officer	151,400	100
Chief operating officer	119,600	79
Chief financial officer	97,700	65
Head of patient care	81,600	54
Head of professional services	81,400	54
Head of human resources	72,800	48
Chief information officer	70,900	47
Head of marketing	57,500	38

Source: "How Hospital Execs Are Faring on Payday." *Medical Economics,* 23 August 1993, p. 18. Primary sources: Hay Management Consultants; *Modern Healthcare* Hospital Compensation Survey. *Notes:* The average base salary for physican executives is higher than the overall survey average for hospital CEOs because data for physician executives came from only 27 institutions with a mean annual revenue of $130 million.

★ 755 ★

Salaries and Wages: Managers and Executives

Salaries of Insurance Company CEOs: 1993

The table below reflects the salaries, bonuses, and stock options of chief executive officers (CEOs) at large insurance carriers. Data are for 1993.

[In dollars]

Company and CEO	Compensation
The Travelers (Sanford Weill)	52,800,000
U.S. Healthcare (Leonard Abramson)	9,820,254
Aetna Life & Casualty (Ronald Compton)	2,340,000
Prudential (Robert C. Winters)	2,299,255
Metropolitan Life (Harry Kamen)	1,161,667
Cigna (W. H. Taylor)	790,000
Blue Cross/Blue Shield (Bernard Tresnowski)	774,000[1]

Source: "Your Insurance Premiums at Work." *Newsweek,* 27 June 1994, p. 8. Primary source: *Hartford Courant;* American Political Network; *Business Week;* CBS. *Note:* 1. 1992 figure.

Salaries and Wages: Nurses

★ 756 ★

Earnings of Full-time Nurses in Hospitals: 1991

The table shows the number of private hospital workers and their average (mean) hourly earnings.

Occupation[1]	Number of workers	Hourly earnings ($)
Nursing supervisors	10,355	21.45
Head nurses	36,262	19.83
Registered nurses	409,681	16.41
Clinical specialists	5,830	21.02
III	5,257	20.84
IV	524	22.98
Nurse anesthetists	3,676	29.19
III	3,676	29.19
Nurse practitioners	1,632	21.36
II	172	17.51
III	1,213	21.52
IV	247	25.00
Staff nurses	396,109	16.20
I	5,504	13.65
II	368,495	16.14
II (specialists)	18,533	17.55
III	3,446	19.10
Licensed practical nurses	94,570	10.21
I	2,321	9.12
II	88,883	10.16
III	3,366	12.21
Nursing assistants	118,493	7.63
I	6,741	5.89
II	98,634	7.59
III	11,714	8.84

Source: U.S. Department of Labor. Bureau of Labor Statistics. *Occupational Wage Survey: Hospitals, January 1991.* Bulletin 2392. Washington, DC: U.S. Government Printing Office, January 1992, pp. 36-40. Source includes results of 1991 White-collar Pay Survey. *Notes:* Because of rounding, sum of individual items may not equal 100. 1. Data for overall occupation may include data for subclassifications not shown separately.

★ 757 ★

Salaries and Wages: Nurses

Nurses' Salaries: 1992

Nurse anesthetist - 68,312

Head nurse - 47,911

Clinical nurse specialist - 45,974

Nurse practitioner - 45,012

Staff nurse - 35,982

Chart shows data from column 1.

	Average 1992 salary	Percent increase
Clinical nurse specialist	45,974	8.8
Head nurse	47,911	5.3
Nurse anesthetist	68,312	8.5
Nurse practitioner	45,012	7.2
Staff nurse	35,982	4.4

Source: "RN Salary Gains: Staff Nurses Get Less, Grow Less." *RN* (May 1993), p. 18. Primary source: University of Texas Medical Branch at Galveston (1993). *National Survey of Hospital and Medical School Salaries, 1992.*

★ 758 ★

Salaries and Wages: Nurses

Nursing Income as Related to Education

[In dollars]

Education	Income[1]
Associate degree	37,182
Diploma	40,247
Baccalaureate degree	40,842
Master's degree/doctorate	46,394

Source: "Nursing Education and Income: Does More Time in the Classroom Mean Higher Pay?" *RN* (December 1993), p. 15. Primary source: *RN* 1993 Salary Survey. Conducted by Medical Economics Research Group (Montvale, NJ). *Notes:* 1. Includes base pay, differentials, and overtime. Figures are medians for nurses working full-time in acute care settings.

Salaries and Wages: Pharmacists and Pharmaceutical Industry

★ 759 ★

Earnings of Full-time Pharmacists and Pharmacy Technicians in Hospitals: 1991

The table shows the number of private hospital workers and their average (mean) hourly earnings.

Occupation[1]	Number of workers	Hourly earnings ($)
Pharmacists	19,445	21.24
I	16,870	20.88
II	2,161	23.98
Pharmacy technicians	16,755	8.45
I	13,570	8.08
II	2,878	10.22

Source: U.S. Department of Labor. Bureau of Labor Statistics. *Occupational Wage Survey: Hospitals, January 1991.* Bulletin 2392. Washington, DC: U.S. Government Printing Office, January 1992, pp. 36-40. Source includes results of 1991 White-collar Pay Survey. *Notes:* Because of rounding, sum of individual items may not equal 100. 1. Data for overall occupation may include data for subclassifications not shown separately

★ 760 ★

Salaries and Wages: Pharmacists and Pharmaceutical Industry

Pharmacists' Salaries: 1990

Table shows the percent distribution of full-time, salaried pharmacists in 1990.

[In dollars]

	Salary
First decile	25,200
First quartile	35,200
Median	41,300
Third quartile	46,700
Ninth decile	52,400

Source: U.S. Deparment of Labor. *Occupational Outlook Handbook.* 1992-1993 edition. Lincolnwood, IL: VGM Career Horizons, 1992, p. 3. Primary source: Bureau of Labor Statistics.

★ 761 ★

Salaries and Wages: Pharmacists and Pharmaceutical Industry

Starting Salaries in the Pharmaceutical Industry

[In dollars]

Position	Salary
Assistant/associate clinical research director	85,000-125,000
Clinical research director	135,000-190,000
Executive director/vice president	235,000-285,000

Source: "Pharmaceutical Industry Starting Salaries." *American Medical News,* 4 October 1993, p. 25. Primary source: Sampson, Neill & Wilkins Inc. *Survey of Physician Salary Ranges Within the Pharmaceutical Industry* (March 1992). *Note:* Does not include bonuses. Some positions guarantee bonuses.

Salaries and Wages: Physicians

★ 762 ★

Average Income of Physicians Compared With Economy Averages: 1978-1990

Year	Mean before-tax annual income[1] of physicians	Average hours worked per year	Per hour	Mean before-tax annual compensation[2] of all employees	Average hours worked per year	Per hour	Ratio of physicians to all employees
1978	64,600	2,696	23.96	15,002	1,863	8.05	3.0
1979	77,400	2,662	29.08	16,262	1,854	8.77	3.3
1980				17,753	1,834	9.68	
1981	89,900	2,645	33.99	19,451	1,832	10.62	3.2
1982	97,700	2,656	36.78	20,890	1,810	11.54	3.2
1983	104,100	2,701	38.54	21,940	1,820	12.06	3.2
1984	108,400	2,708	40.03	22,935	1,828	12.55	3.2
1985	112,200	2,718	41.28	23,866	1,816	13.15	3.1
1986	119,500	2,741	43.60	24,800	1,808	13.72	3.2
1987	132,300	2,746	48.18	25,883	1,809	14.31	3.4
1988	144,700	2,741	52.79	27,176	1,805	15.06	3.5
1989	155,800	2,752	56.61	28,144	1,794	15.66	3.6
1990	164,300	2,752	59.70	29,341	1,794	16.40	3.6

Source: U.S. Department of Labor. Pension and Welfare Benefits Administration. *Trends in Health Benefits.* Washington, DC: U.S. Government Printing Office, 1993, p. 88. Primary source: American Medical Association, and source author's calculations. *Notes:* 1. Income only from physicians' services. 2. Includes wages and salaries, benefits, and employers' contributions for social insurance for all employees in the public and private sectors.

★ 763 ★

Salaries and Wages: Physicians

Income of Self-Employed Physicians: 1990

According to the American Medical Association, in 1990 the average self-employed doctor earned $185,600 after expenses.

Source: "Away From Politics." *International Herald Tribune,* 25 February 1993, p. 3.

★ 764 ★

Salaries and Wages: Physicians

Physicians' Mean Annual Income: 1991

Specialty	Mean annual salary
Family practice	$111,000
Psychiatry	128,000
Internal medicine	150,000
Pathology	198,000
Anesthesiology	221,000
Obstetrics/gynecology	222,000
Radiology	230,000
Surgery	234,000
All	170,000

Source: "Doctors' Income." *Wall Street Journal,* 2 March 1993, p. A20. Primary source: American Medical Association.

★ 765 ★

Salaries and Wages: Physicians

Physicians' Median Incomes: 1992

Data show median income of U.S. physicians.

[In dollars]

	Income
Anesthesiologists	220,000
General/family practice physicians	100,000
Internists	130,000
Obstetricians/gynecologists	190,000
Pathologists	170,000
Pediatricians	112,000
Psychiatrists	120,000

[Continued]

★ 765 ★

Physicians' Median Incomes: 1992
[Continued]

	Income
Radiologists	240,000
Surgeons	207,000

Source: "The Trend in Medicine." Detroit Free Press, 31 March 1994, p. 12A. Primary sources: Association of American Medical Colleges; American Medical Association.

★ 766 ★

Salaries and Wages: Physicians

Salaries of Physicians Employed by HMOs and Hospitals: 1992

According to a survey by the William M. Mercer Co., the average physician employed by a health maintenance organization or hospital received $139,732 in pay and bonuses in 1992.

Source: "Away From Politics." International Herald Tribune, 25 February 1993, p. 3.

Chapter 10
MEDICAL ESTABLISHMENT

The 75 tables in this chapter provide an overview of issues relevant to the medical community. Tables focus on particular areas of the health care universe, notably medical advertising and marketing, medical libraries, and medical publishing. Tables also reflect medical management and administrative concerns; for example, computer applications, fund-raising, medical practice operations, quality programs, hospital ownership and construction, food service, and labor issues, including strikes and layoffs. Special, high-interest aspects of the medical community—medical technology, medical waste, and medical research—also are covered.

Advertising

★ 767 ★

U.S. Food and Drug Administration's Medical Advertising Information Line: January-February 1992

The U.S. Food and Drug Administration (FDA) established its Medical Advertising Information Line in September 1991. The service was instituted so that health care professionals could report inappropriate marketing of drugs and devices. From its establishment through February 21, 1992, the service received more than 1,400 calls. The table below indicates who called the service and for what reason.

	Percent
Callers	
Physicians	29
Pharmacists	18
Dentists	15
Other	38

[Continued]

★ 767 ★

U.S. Food and Drug Administration's Medical Advertising Information Line: January-February 1992

[Continued]

	Percent
Reasons for call	
Information requests	80
Tips	20

Source: "Health Professionals' Line." FDA Consumer (May 1992), p. 3.

★ 768 ★

Advertising

Worldwide Billings of Health Care Advertising Agencies: 1992

Advertising agencies that specialize in health care accounts have been experiencing a growth spurt. According to the source: "Revenues at the top 50 healthcare agencies grew by 14 percent worldwide and 16 percent in the U.S. in 1992.... More than 570 new jobs were added last year at healthcare agencies" (p. 14). The table below reflects worldwide billings for health care ad agencies for 1991 through 1994.

[In million dollars]

Billings	Amount
1991	3.874
1992	4.420
1993[1]	5.127
1994[1]	5.948

Source: Heitzman, Beth. "Finally ... an Ad Sector That's Hiring." ADWEEK, 4 October 1994, p. 14. Primary source: Med Ad News (1991 and 1992 data). Note: 1. Projections compiled by ADWEEK.

Computers

★ 769 ★

Acceptance of Computer-Based Patient Records

The table below shows how soon health information management professionals expect computer-based patient records to be accepted and/or implemented. Data are based on the responses of 1,066 attendees of the American Health Information Management Association's (AHIMA) 1993 national convention.

Time period for acceptance/implementation	Percent of respondents
21st century	11.1
10 years	30.2
7 years	23.1
5 years	27.2
2 years	8.0
Never	0.4

Source: Thierry, Patty. "Survey Shows Optimisim for CPR." *Journal of AHIMA* 64, no. 12 (December 1993), p. 76.

★ 770 ★
Computers

Automation Plans and Critical Paths

Critical paths—monitoring and managing clinical processes—are one method of quality improvement. Figures below represent the findings of a survey inquiring about plans to automate critical paths.

Plans and actions	Percent
Hospitals with plans to automate critical paths	37
Automation actions	
Developed in-house spreadsheet to analyze variances	21
Have automated critical paths/caregivers directly entering data	
into information system	8
Deciding on/developing/implementing automated paths	6
Too soon to say	3
Automation plans	
Would like to automate, but have other information system needs	
and/or priorities	34
None/too soon to say	32
Plan to develop variance analysis/develop outcomes database	
within next 12 months	23

[Continued]

★ 770 ★

Automation Plans and Critical Paths
[Continued]

Plans and actions	Percent
Plan to automate charting based on critical paths within the next 12 months	21

Source: Lumsdon, Kevin, and Mark Hagland. "Mapping Care." *Hospitals & Health Networks,* 20 October 1993, p. 37.

★ 771 ★

Computers

Computers and the Reduction of Health Care Costs

According to researchers at Indiana University, charges to patients treated by doctors who use computers to order drugs and tests are 13 percent lower per hospital admission than charges for patients treated by doctors who use paper. Total charges average $900 less for patients whose doctors use computers compared with those whose doctors using traditional charts. One drawback was noted, however. Doctors using computers spend an average of 5 minutes more per patient to write orders than those doctors using charts.

Source: "Computers Helping Doctors Match Care With Costs Can Lower Bills, Study Says." *Wall Street Journal,* 20 January 1993, p. B6.

★ 772 ★

Computers

Health Insurance Claims Processed Electronically

According to Dr. Louis H. Sullivan, head of the U.S. Department of Health and Human Services during President Bush's administration, a standard claims form and electronic processing of claims could save $2 per claim, or $8 billion annually. The table below compares claims processed traditionally and electronically.

[In percentages]

Method	Amount
Claims processed traditionally	75
Claims processed electronically	25

Source: "Insurers Urged to Process Claims Electronically." *Blues Advantage* 1 (October 1992), p. 10. *Blues Advantage* is a publication of Blue Cross Blue Shield of Michigan.

★ 773 ★

Computers

Obstacles to Computer-Based Patient Records

The data below show responses of 571 health care information management professionals when asked to consider the obstacles to computer-based patient records.

Obstacles	Percent of responses
Hospitals lacking funds	23
Technology lacking	22
Government unable to set reporting standards	20
Clinicians uninterested	13
Hospitals not committed	10
Too many state regulations	9
Hospital politics	4

Source: Bergman, Rhonda. "The Long March Toward Progress; In Pursuit of the Computer-Based Patient Record." *Hospitals* 67, no. 18 (20 September 1993), p. 46. Primary source: 1993 HIMSS/Hewlett-Packard Leadership Survey.

Construction

★ 774 ★

Hospital Construction Plans

According to a survey of hospital executives, construction, expansion, and renovation of facilities continues. The table below identifies the construction plans of the 249 executives surveyed.

Plans	Percent
Expansion/renovation	59
Current construction	37
New/offsite facility	27
Recently completed construction	25
None	13

Source: "Future Plans: Anxious About the Future, Hospitals Step Up Planning." *Hospitals & Health Networks,* 5 October 1993, p. 60. Primary source: TriBrook Group, Inc. (1993).

★ 775 ★

Construction

Value of Construction Contracts and Floor Space of Hospitals: 1976-1993

Covers new structures and additions, and major alterations to existing structures which affect only valuation, since no additional floor area is created by "alteration."

	Nonresidential buildings total	Hospitals
Value (billion dollars)		
1976	31.3	4.5
1977	37.0	4.5
1978	47.4	3.9
1979	53.5	4.8
1980	56.9	5.4
1981	65.5	6.4
1982	64.6	8.0
1983	67.9	8.5
1984	82.1	7.4
1985	92.3	7.8
1986	91.6	7.9
1987	98.8	9.0
1988	97.9	8.2
1989	106.1	8.8
1990	95.5	9.2
1991	86.2	9.6
1992	86.8	10.8
1993	(NA)	(NA)
Floor space (million square feet)		
1976	978	71
1977	1,135	66
1978	1,338	54
1979	1,444	58
1980	1,263	55
1981	1,243	60
1982	1,015	71
1983	1,111	84
1984	1,350	70
1985	1,529	73
1986	1,454	73
1987	1,469	78
1988	1,414	71
1989	1,400	72
1990	1,204	69
1991	981	71

[Continued]

★ 775 ★

Value of Construction Contracts and Floor Space of Hospitals: 1976-1993
[Continued]

	Nonresidential buildings total	Hospitals
1992	937	77
1993	(NA)	(NA)

Source: 1993 Statistical Abstract of the United States on CD-ROM [machine-readable datafiles]. CD-ABSTR-93. Washington, DC: U.S. Department of Commerce, Economics and Statistics Administration, Bureau of the Census, Data User Services Division, 1993. Primary source: Dodge, F. W. *Dodge Construction Potentials.* New York, NY: McGraw-Hill Information Systems Company, National Information Services Division. *Note:* "NA" represents "not applicable."

★ 776 ★

Construction

Value of New Hospital Construction: 1970-1992

In current and constant (1987) dollars. Represents value of construction put in place during year; differs from building permit and construction contract data in timing and coverage. Includes installed cost of normal building service equipment and selected types of industrial production equipment (largely site fabricated). Excludes cost of shipbuilding, land, and most types of machinery and equipment.

[In millions of dollars]

Type of construction	Current dollars						Constant (1987) dollars					1992 (preliminary)
	1970	1980	1985	1990	1991	1992	1970	1980	1985	1990	1991	
Total new construction	100,727	259,746	377,366	442,065	400,955	425,807	309,244	328,435	401,967	397,547	358,549	379,479
Nonresidential buildings	23,008	58,290	103,455	117,971	97,841	85,360	71,796	78,972	111,262	106,067	87,608	75,746
Hospital and institutional	2,555	4,254	6,060	9,450	9,189	10,085	7,976	5,759	6,521	8,494	8,228	8,946
Public construction	27,908	63,646	77,823	107,912	110,249	118,740	84,077	75,790	80,260	97,909	98,967	107,735
Buildings	10,473	20,427	27,861	46,208	50,475	53,085	32,753	27,520	30,000	41,523	45,189	47,106

Source: 1993 Statistical Abstract of the United States on CD-ROM [machine-readable datafiles]. CD-ABSTR-93. Washington, DC: U.S. Department of Commerce, Economics and Statistics Administration, Bureau of the Census, Data User Services Division, 1993. Primary source: U.S. Bureau of the Census. *Current Construction Reports,* Series C30.

Food Service

★ 777 ★

Food Purchases of Largest Health Care Chains: 1992

Data reflect the total facilities, beds, and estimated annual food purchases of the 10 largest health care chains in 1992. Chains are ranked by food purchases.

Organization	Facilities	Beds	Annual food purchases ($MM)
U.S. Veterans Administration	171	64,763	94.80
Beverly Enterprises	882	91,900	90.00
Quorum Group	190	21,819	57.72
Galen Health[1]	77	17,295	45.83
Hillhaven	353	44,067	44.90
Hospital Corporation of America[1]	99	18,299	43.77
Daughters of Charity	58	14,444	41.60
National Medical Enterprises	156	16,903	28.55
Healthtrust[2]	81	9,919	26.29
Manor Care	166	22,663	24.36

Source: "Top Health Care Chains." Restaurants and Institutions (1 March 1994), p. 40. Primary source: *Report on Institutional Food Service* (30 August 1993). *Notes:* 1. Galen Health and Hospital Corporation of America have merged since data was compiled. 2. Healthtrust has annouced plans to merge with Epic Health Care Group.

Grants and Contracts

★ 778 ★

Grants: 1990-1991

Data are reported by subject field and cover grants of $10,000 or more in size. Based on reports of foundations. Grant sample represented a percent of all grant dollars awarded by private, corporate, and community foundations.

Subject field	1990	1991 Number	1991 Percent distribution
Total	57,443	58,218	100.0
Arts and culture	9,053	8,945	15.4
Education	13,319	13,350	22.9
Environment & animals	2,583	3,091	5.3

[Continued]

★ 778 ★

Grants: 1990-1991
[Continued]

Subject field	1990	1991 Number	1991 Percent distribution
Health	7,275	7,473	12.8
Human services	12,360	12,339	21.2
International affairs, development & peace	1,622	1,952	3.4
Public/society benefit	6,649	6,582	11.3
Science and technology	2,074	1,826	3.1
Social sciences	1,049	1,157	2.0
Religion	1,238	1,382	2.4
Other	221	121	0.2

Source: 1993 Statistical Abstract of the United States on CD-ROM [machine-readable datafiles]. CD-ABSTR-93. Washington, DC: U.S. Department of Commerce, Economics and Statistics Administration, Bureau of the Census, Data User Services Division, 1993. Primary source: The Foundation Center. *Foundation Grants Index* (annual). New York, NY. Used with permission of The Foundation Center. *Notes:* Grants may be awarded to multiple types of recipient organizations and would thereby be double-counted.

★ 779 ★

Grants and Contracts

National Heart, Lung, and Blood Institute Research Grants, by Activity: 1991

The table below reflects research grants of the National Heart, Lung, and Blood Institute (NHLBI) for the 1991 fiscal year.

[Costs in thousands of dollars]

	Number of grants obligated	Direct cost	Indirect cost	Total cost	Percent of total NHLBI research grant dollars
Research Project Grants (RPGs)[1]					
Regular Research Grants (R01)	2,027	$281,295	$132,289	$413,584	50.14
Cooperative Agreements (U01)	76	28,771	9,148	37,919	4.60
Program Project Grants (P01)	125	103,944	48,704	152,648	18.51
FIRST Independent Research Support and Transition Award (R29)	355	24,047	12,034	36,081	4.37
Method to Extend Research in Time (MERIT; R37)	152	23,361	12,775	36,136	4.38
Small Business Innovation Research (R43) SBIR Phase I	71	2,936	548	3,484	0.42
Small Business Innovation Research (R44) SBIR Phase II	36	6,269	2,209	8,478	1.03
Subtotal, SBIR	107	9,205	2,757	11,962	1.45
Subtotal, Research Project Grants	2,842	470,623	217,707	688,330	83.44

[Continued]

★ 779 ★

National Heart, Lung, and Blood Institute Research Grants, by Activity: 1991

[Continued]

	Number of grants obligated	Direct cost	Indirect cost	Total cost	Percent of total NHLBI research grant dollars
Research Centers Grants[2]					
Specialized Centers of Research (SCOR; P50)	54	48,827	22,980	71,807	8.71
Enhanced SCOR (P60)	1	2,166	1,001	3,167	0.38
Sickle Cell Centers (P60)	10	13,807	3,393	17,200	2.09
Subtotal, Research Centers Grants	65	64,800	27,374	92,174	11.17
Research Career Programs[3]					
Research Career Development Awards (K04)	65	3,962	317	4,279	0.52
Research Career Awards (RCA; K06)	8	250	20	270	0.03
Preventive Cardiology Academic Awards (PCAA; K07)	23	2,706	215	2,921	0.35
Pulmonary Academic Award (PAA; K07)	20	1,714	137	1,851	0.22
Transfusion Medicine Academic Awards (TMAA; K07)	18	1,540	118	1,658	0.20
Systemic Pulmonary and Vascular Disease Academic Award (SPVDAA; K07)	2	224	18	242	0.03
Clinical Investigator Awards (CIA; K08)	137	9,604	766	10,370	1.26
Physician Scientist Awards (PSA; K11)	82	6,165	486	6,651	0.81
Minority Faculty Development Awards (K14)	18	1,139	87	1,226	0.15
Subtotal, Research Career Programs	373	27,304	2,164	29,468	3.57
Other Research Grants[4]					
Cooperative Clinical Research (R10)	11	929	414	1,343	0.16
Minority Biomedical Research Support (S06, S14)	(28)	1,841	720	2,561	0.31
Small Instrumentation Grant (S15)	104	3,387	0	3,387	0.41
Demonstration and Education Program (R18)	2	998	349	1,347	0.16
Small Research Grants (R03)	16	691	392	1,083	0.13
Other (R09, R25, P09, R13, T15, T09, U09, R55)	43	4,938	260	5,198	0.63
Subtotal, Other Research Grants	176	12,784	2,135	14,919	1.81
Total, NHLBI Research Grants	3,456	575,511	249,380	824,891	100.00

Source: U.S. Department of Health and Human Services. Public Health Service. National Institutes of Health. National Heart, Lung, and Blood Institute (NHLBI). *NHLBI Fact Book, Fiscal Year 1991.* Washington, DC: U.S. Department of Health and Human Services, Public Health Service, National Institutes of Health, National Heart, Lung, and Blood Institute (NHLBI), c. 1992, p. 75. *Notes:* 1. 83.4 percent of total research grants. 2. 11.2 percent of total research grants. 3. 3.6 percent of total research grants. 4. 1.8 percent of total research grants.

★ 780 ★

Grants and Contracts

State Distribution of National Heart, Lung, and Blood Institute Awards: 1991

The table below presents a geographic distribution of awards from the National Heart, Lung, and Blood Institute (NHLBI) for the 1991 fiscal year.

	Totals		Research grants		Research training and development		Contracts	
	Number	Dollars	Number	Dollars	Number	Dollars	Number	Dollars
Alabama	80	16,516,245	68	12,725,040	7	845,864	5	2,945,341
Alaska	1	107,696	1	107,696	-	-	-	-
Arizona	24	5,570,390	21	5,307,186	3	263,204	-	-
Arkansas	4	391,315	2	332,109	1	22,700	1	36,506
California	459	118,204,645	392	102,341,264	46	5,227,260	19	10,636,121
Colorado	52	11,480,780	47	10,406,213	4	905,471	1	169,096
Connecticut	65	11,234,498	54	10,520,713	9	651,605	2	62,180
Delaware	2	186,856	2	186,856	-	-	-	-
District of Columbia	63	12,625,685	50	10,022,785	3	361,162	10	2,241,738
Florida	58	9,238,694	51	8,254,220	3	568,798	4	415,676
Georgia	78	15,233,829	63	13,740,957	8	241,060	7	1,251,812
Hawaii	6	1,612,815	3	213,193	1	108,054	2	1,291,568
Illinois	141	28,297,951	123	25,408,114	12	2,096,210	6	793,627
Indiana	41	6,921,235	36	6,530,169	5	391,066	-	-
Iowa	64	17,190,072	47	15,332,743	17	1,857,329	-	-
Kansas	5	620,116	5	620,116	-	-	-	-
Kentucky	22	3,734,267	21	3,597,132	-	-	1	137,135
Louisiana	32	8,988,818	31	8,863,899	1	124,919	-	-
Maine	3	700,516	3	700,516	-	-	-	-
Maryland	184	60,644,432	136	33,106,911	19	2,258,286	29	25,279,235
Massachusetts	389	114,332,039	337	101,366,252	44	6,292,072	8	6,673,715
Michigan	102	21,308,108	83	17,468,562	12	1,221,154	7	2,618,392
Minnesota	104	38,442,523	79	21,906,311	17	1,386,168	8	15,150,044
Mississippi	18	3,727,385	13	2,368,273	2	182,231	3	1,176,881
Missouri	127	30,481,629	107	27,240,710	13	2,530,436	7	710,483
Nebraska	14	1,713,637	13	1,678,267	1	35,370	-	-
Nevada	10	1,079,395	7	1,005,395	3	74,000	-	-
New Hampshire	12	2,007,795	11	1,779,623	1	228,172	-	-
New Jersey	37	6,029,055	34	5,722,395	1	95,023	2	211,637
New Mexico	23	2,989,787	17	2,392,234	2	55,200	4	542,353
New York	354	83,281,559	304	75,628,876	31	5,078,590	19	4,574,093
North Carolina	195	56,772,686	165	44,189,713	20	2,244,918	10	10,338,055
Ohio	163	41,636,204	143	36,567,431	11	1,883,839	9	3,184,934
Oklahoma	35	5,825,765	30	4,928,815	4	186,272	1	710,678
Oregon	33	6,163,984	27	4,891,326	4	143,940	2	1,128,718
Pennsylvania	259	55,144,655	231	49,978,483	21	2,624,283	7	2,541,889
Rhode Island	23	4,297,376	18	3,847,630	3	192,320	2	257,426
South Carolina	31	4,646,079	29	4,463,585	2	182,494	-	-
South Dakota	3	378,119	3	378,119	-	-	-	-
Tennessee	109	21,528,425	95	19,889,545	9	1,238,736	5	400,144
Texas	228	55,251,625	200	48,137,454	18	1,860,027	10	5,254,144
Utah	63	13,259,402	56	9,641,298	4	388,615	3	3,229,489
Vermont	38	9,819,830	35	9,524,869	3	294,961	-	-
Virginia	65	11,117,459	55	10,057,829	9	838,703	1	220,927

[Continued]

★ 780 ★

State Distribution of National Heart, Lung, and Blood Institute Awards: 1991
[Continued]

	Totals		Research grants		Research training and development		Contracts	
	Number	Dollars	Number	Dollars	Number	Dollars	Number	Dollars
Washington	112	36,847,083	97	33,149,477	11	1,659,001	4	2,038,605
West Virginia	8	850,594	8	850,594	-	-	-	-
Wisconsin	91	15,323,358	83	14,906,366	8	416,992	-	-

Source: U.S. Department of Health and Human Services. Public Health Service. National Institutes of Health. National Heart, Lung, and Blood Institute (NHLBI). *NHLBI Fact Book, Fiscal Year 1991.* Washington, DC: U.S. Department of Health and Human Services, Public Health Service, National Institutes of Health, National Heart, Lung, and Blood Institute (NHLBI), c. 1992, p. 128-148.

★ 781 ★

Grants and Contracts

Value of Grants, by Recipients: 1990-1991

Data are reported by recipient organization and cover grants of $10,000 or more in size. Based on reports of foundations. Grant sample represented a percent of all grant dollars awarded by private, corporate, and community foundations.

	Number of grants		Percent distribution	Dollar value of grants		Percent distribution
	1990	1991	1991	1990	1991	1991
Community improvement organizations	2,630	2,588	4.4	151	151	3.1
Educational institutions	17,766	17,658	30.3	1,733	1,880	38.8
Colleges & universities	10,953	10,686	18.4	1,255	1,340	27.6
Educational support agencies	2,538	2,485	4.3	177	211	4.4
Schools	2,623	2,861	4.9	143	165	3.4
Federated funds	1,961	1,786	3.1	195	185	3.8
Hospitals/medical care facilities	3,050	3,169	5.4	300	345	7.1
Human service agencies	9,689	10,018	17.2	472	485	10.0
International organizations	1,523	1,706	2.9	116	140	2.9
Museums/historical societies	2,832	2,672	4.6	277	319	6.6
Performing arts groups	3,443	3,484	6.0	188	188	3.9

Source: *1993 Statistical Abstract of the United States on CD-ROM* [machine-readable datafiles]. CD-ABSTR-93. Washington, DC: U.S. Department of Commerce, Economics and Statistics Administration, Bureau of the Census, Data User Services Division, 1993. Primary source: The Foundation Center. *Foundation Grants Index* (annual). New York, NY. Used with permission of The Foundation Center. *Notes:* Grants may be awarded to multiple types of recipient organizations and would thereby be double-counted.

★ 782 ★

Grants and Contracts

Value of Grants, by Subject Field: 1990-1991

Data are reported by subject field and cover grants of $10,000 or more in size. Based on reports of foundations. Grant sample represented a percent of all grant dollars awarded by private, corporate, and community foundations.

[In million dollars, except as noted]

	1990	1991	
		Amount	Percent distribution
Total	4,475	4,849	100.0
Arts and culture	639	683	14.1
Education	1,150	1,210	25.0
Environment & animals	208	236	4.9
Health	752	817	16.9
Human services	645	688	14.2
International affairs, development & peace	140	196	4.0
Public/society benefit	491	506	10.4
Science and technology	223	278	5.7
Social sciences	133	133	2.7
Religion	85	98	2.0
Other	7	4	0.1

Source: 1993 Statistical Abstract of the United States on CD-ROM [machine-readable datafiles]. CD-ABSTR-93. Washington, DC: U.S. Department of Commerce, Economics and Statistics Administration, Bureau of the Census, Data User Services Division, 1993. Primary source: The Foundation Center Foundation Grants Index (annual). New York, NY. Used with permission of The Foundation Center. Notes: 1. Grants may be awarded to multiple types of recipient organizations and would thereby be double-counted.

Investment and Ownership

★ 783 ★

Hospital Bondholders

[In percentages]

Bondholders	Percent
Individuals	42
Other	17
Mutual funds	14
Insurance companies	11

[Continued]

★ 783 ★

Hospital Bondholders
[Continued]

Bonholders	Percent
Money markets	8
Banks	8

Source: Winslow, Ron. "Health-Care Reforms Raise Pressure on Hospital Bonds." *Wall Street Journal,* 9 February 1994, p. B4.

★ 784 ★

Investment and Ownership

Hospital Owners: 1992

Data show a percent of total.

Owner	Percent
Free-standing non-profit	44
State and local governments	17
Religous non-profit networks	14
Investors for profit	11
Secular non-profit networks	8
Federal government	6

Source: "State of Emergency." *The Economist,* 23 October 1993, p. 29.

Labor Issues

★ 785 ★

Bloodborne Pathogens Violators

In 1992, the U.S. Occupational Safety and Health Administration (OSHA) began enforcing a bloodborne pathogens standard for medical facilities. That year the agency inspected 1,346 medical facilities such as hospitals and physicians' and dentists' offices. In addition, OSHA received 960 complaints against medical facilities. In 1992, 736 employers were cited as violators. The table below reflects the violators by type of facility.

[In percentages]

Facility	Violators
Hospitals	8
Physicians' offices	4
Dentists' offices	4
Other[1]	84

Source: Voelker, Rebecca. "Bloodborne Standards Reach Beyond Medicine." *American Medical News,* 22-29 March 1993, p. 12. Primary source: American Medical Association. *Notes:* 1. Includes nursing homes, schools, jails, industrial plants, post offices, grocery stores, and police departments.

★ 786 ★

Labor Issues

Employee Benefit Plans in Hospitals With and Without Quality Programs

Data reflect a survey of approximately 2,000 hospitals regarding benefits for their employees. The survey was sponsored by AHA Insurance Resource Inc., the insurance agency of the American Hospital Association, and was conducted by Ernst & Young's actuarial, benefits, and compensation consulting practice. The table below compares the benefits of hospitals with continuous quality improvement (CQI) and total quality management (TQM) programs to those without such efforts.

[In percentages]

Benefits	TQM/CQI hospitals	Non-TQM/CQI hospitals
Flexible benefit programs	64.8	59.4
Employee assistance programs	58.4	51.4
Employee opinion surveys	47.4	35.0
Retirement counseling	36.5	36.7
Long-term care	6.0	5.5

Source: Finnegan, F. Thomas. "Benefit Plans Test Hospitals' Acceptance of Change." *National Underwriter,* 25 October 1993, p. 9.

★ 787 ★

Labor Issues

Employee Benefits for Health Care Employees: 1992

Figures are from the National Association for Health Care Recruitment Survey and reflect the responses of 435 health care facilities.

[In percentages]

Benefit	Employees
Tuition reimbursement	94
Pension plan	92
Dental insurance	89
Pharmacy discount	73
Wellness center	41
Child-care center	40

Source: "How Does Your Hospital Compare?" *Nursing93* (January 1993), p. 8. Springhouse Corporation conducts the survey from which data was taken.

★ 788 ★

Labor Issues

Employee Benefits for Nurses: 1992 and 1993

Figures are from the National Association for Health Care Recruitment Survey and reflect the responses of 402 recruiters.

[In percentages]

Benefit	1993	1992
Tuition reimbursement	94	94
Paid time off for continuing education seminars	83	82
Special orientation for new graduates	78	81
Flexible staffing	82	82
Evening/night shift differential	96	94
Pay differential for weekend shift	65	67
Refresher courses for returning nurses	14	18
Sign-on bonus	16	20
Retention bonus	9	12

Source: "What's Offered?" *Nursing93* (August 1993), p. 8. *Nursing93* and Springhouse Corporation conduct the survey from which data was taken.

★ 789 ★

Labor Issues

Hospital Strikes: 1993

Union employees at 12 hospitals went on strike in the 1993 fiscal year; that is, October 1, 1992, through September 30, 1993.

Hospital (location) and Union	Employees	Number of workers idled	Date strike began	Strike length (days)
Pocono Medical Center (East Stroudsburg, Pennsylvania) Pennsylvania Nurses Association	Nurses	342	10-8-92	21
John F. Kennedy Memorial Hospital (Philadelphia, Pennsylvania) Pennsylvania Nurses Association	Nurses	91	10-26-92	4
Brookdale Hospital Medical Center (New York, New York) National Health and Human Service Employee Union (1199)	Nurses, psychologists	4,000	12-21-92	1
Jamaica Hospital (New York, New York) National Health and Human Service Employees Union (1199)	Nurses	1,600	12-21-92	1
St. John's Episcopal Hospital – South Shore (New York, New York) National Health and Human Service Employees Union (1199)	Nurses	1,400	12-21-92	1
St. John's Queens Hospital (New York, New York) National Health and Human Service Employees Union (1199)	Nurses	200	12-21-92	1
St. Mary's Hospital (New York, New York) National Health and Human Service Employees Union (1199)	Nurses	1,200	12-21-92	1
St. Joseph Medical Center (Joliet, Illinois) Illinois Nurses Association	Nurses	200	1-18-93	63
Kaiser Foundation Hospitals (Los Angeles, California) Service Employees International Union	Non-professionals	12,000	4-1-93	1
Eastern Long Island Hospital (Greenport, New York) National Health and Human Service Employees Union (1199)	All	100	6-29-93	27
Community Memorial Hospital (Hamilton, New York) Service Employees International Union	LPNs, technicians, professionals	100	8-28-93	3
Kadlec Medical Center (Richmond, Washington) Washington State Nurses Association	Nurses	266	9-6-93	39

Source: Burda, David. "Healthcare Picket Lines Increase in '93." *Modern Healthcare,* 17 January 1994, p. 38. Primary source: Federal Mediation and Conciliation Service. *Note:* "LPN" is an abbreviation for "licensed practical nurse."

★ 790 ★

Labor Issues

Insufficient Staffing in Acute Care Hospitals

Figures represent the incidents caused by insufficient staffing in acute care hospitals. Data are provided by frequency and type of incident.

[In percentages]

Incident	Frequency
Medication errors	43
Patient injuries	29
Staff injuries	17
Other	7
Lapses in infection control	4

Source: Sherer, Jill L. "Nurses Call for Regulations on Hospital Staffing Ratios." *Hospitals & Health Networks,* 20 July 1993, p. 56. Primary source: SEIU (1993).

★ 791 ★

Labor Issues

Layoff Targets of Hospital Staffs

The table below presents data from a survey of 1,000 hospitals. Of those polled, 27 percent were cutting staff anywhere from 5 to 14 percent.

Staffing categories	Percent targeted for layoffs
Nonexempt employees	41
Middle managers	32
Nurses	20
Technicians	17
Senior management	15
Therapists	6
Pharmacists	4

Source: "Who's Targeted for Layoffs?" *AJN* (February 1994), p. 76. Primary sources: *Modern Healthcare;* Deloitte & Touche.

Libraries and Information Services

★ 792 ★

Fees for Telephone Hotlines and Other Services for Consumers of Medical Care

The table below lists the cost of special services available to consumers for evaluating the appropriateness of charges for medical care.

SERVICE	COST
Health Care Cost Hotline 900-225-2500	$3.95, first minute.
	$1.95, each additional minute.
Medirisk/Medigard 800-656-3337	$69.00, annual fee for unlimited calls.
Cost Review Services 512-338-9196	$8.00, fee for information on cost of medical care.
	$45.00, fee for consumer advocate activities such as haggling with doctors about fees.

Source: Baird, Jane. "Fiscal Checkups." *Houston Chronicle,* 30 January 1994, STAR edition, Business section, p. 1.

★ 793 ★

Libraries and Information Services

Medical Libraries

The Medical Library Association estimates indicate that there are 33,000 to 36,000 medical and allied scientific libraries.

Source: Medical Library Association. Unpublished data. Chicago, IL (1994).

★ 794 ★

Libraries and Information Services

Medical Library Associations

The table below provides membership and budget information for trade associations of interest to medical librarians and related professionals.

Association	Founding date	Members	Budget
Archivists and Librarians in Health Sciences (ALHHS)[1]	1975	150	$10,000
Association of Academic Health Sciences Library Directors (AAHSLD)	1978	126	NA
Association of Mental Health Librarians (AMHL)	1964	140	<$25,000
Medical Library Association (MLA)	1898	5,000	$1,900,000
Mental Health Librarians Section (MLA-MHLS)	1965	90	<$25,000
Veterinary Medical Libraries Section (VMLS/MLA)	1972	40	<$25,000

Source: Encyclopedia of Associations, 1994. 28th ed. Detroit, MI: Gale Research Inc., 1993, pp. 1096-1097, 1104, 1108. *Notes:* "NA" represents "not available." 1. Formerly Association of Librarians in the History of Health Sciences.

★ 795 ★

Libraries and Information Services

MEDLINE Database

MEDLINE is considered to be the largest medical bibliographic database. It was created and currently is maintained by the U.S. National Library of Medicine. MEDLINE covers in excess of 3,500 clinical and research journals from around the world, dating from 1966 to the present. In total, the database contains more than 7 million references.

Source: Lowe, Henry J., and G. Octo Barnett. "Understanding and Using the Medical Subject Headings (MeSH) Vocabulary to Perform Literature Searches." *Journal of the American Medical Association (JAMA)* 1994, no. 271 (13 April 1994), pp. 1103-1108.

★ 796 ★

Libraries and Information Services

MEDLINE's Top Ten Subheadings

Table shows the subheadings most frequently searched in the MEDLINE database.

Subheading	Number[1]	Percent
Metabolism	373,496	19.0
Pharmacology	285,468	14.5
Physiology	275,155	14.0
Drug effects	271,592	13.8
Etiology	212,736	10.8

[Continued]

★ 796 ★

MEDLINE's Top Ten Subheadings
[Continued]

Subheading	Number[1]	Percent
Pathology	206,308	10.5
Analysis	199,289	10.1
Genetics	188,629	9.6
Methods	176,483	9.0
Diagnosis	166,885	8.5

Source: Pratt, Gregory F. "A Brief Hitchhiker's Guide to MEDLINE." *DATABASE* (February 1994), p. 44. *Note:* 1. Subset used was 1,967,167 recent MEDLINE records.

Licensing

★ 797 ★

Medical Licensing Fees: 1992 and 1993

Figures represent the average cost of licenses to practice medicine. Data are provided for 1992 and 1993.

[In dollars]

Method of licensing	1992	1993
By examination	514	542
By endorsement/reciprocity	269	290
Reregistration	108	117

Source: Oberman, Linda. "Medical Society Fighting Broad Use of Licensing Fees." *American Medical News,* 21 June 1993, p. 6. Primary source: American Medical Association.

★ 798 ★

Licensing

Medical Reregistration Licensing Fees by Location: 1993

Figures represent the cost of licenses to practice medicine in selected states and territories. Data provided are for 1993.

[In dollars]

Location	Fee
Highest fees	
Connecticut	450.00
Texas	292.00
California	250.00
Lowest fees	
Guam	30.00
Indiana	25.00
Puerto RIco	16.66

Source: Oberman, Linda. "Medical Society Fighting Broad Use of Licensing Fees." *American Medical News,* 21 June 1993, p. 6. Primary source: American Medical Association.

Medical Practice Management

★ 799 ★

Hidden Costs of Insurance Claims

Physicians spend an average of $8 for each insurance claim submitted; another $8 is spent for every check written by employers and insurance companies. Investigating the legitimacy of a claim involves additional cost. Thus, up to $25 in administrative costs can be added to a $25 doctor's visit, doubling the cost of medical care.

Source: Goodman, John C., and Gerald L. Musgrave. "How to Solve the Health Care Crisis." *Consumer's Research* 75 (March 1992), pp. 10-14.

★ 800 ★

Medical Practice Management

Locations in Which Physicians Practice Most Economically

Data reflect median professional expenses for each area of the United States.

Location	In dollars	Percent of gross
East	84,870	38.5
New England	77,480	35.7
Mid-East	87,150	40.0
Midwest	91,040	38.1
Great Plains	90,000	37.5
Great Lakes	93,010	40.0
West	93,520	38.5
Far West[1]	89,480	37.5
Rocky Mountain	110,680	42.1
South	102,640	40.0
Mid-South	83,280	37.5
South Atlantic	99,180	40.0
Southwest	115,930	44.4

Source: "Practice Expenses: Doctors Apply the Shears." *Medical Economics,* 25 October 1993, p. 133. *Note:* 1. Includes Alaska and Hawaii.

★ 801 ★

Medical Practice Management

Office and Clinical Supply Expenses, by Specialty

The table below shows the percentage of gross spent for office and clinical supplies. Data are provided by medical specialty.

Specialty	Clinical supplies	Business supplies	All supplies
Allergy and immunology	5.3	2.8	8.1
Cardiology	0.9	1.1	2.0
Cardiovascular surgery	0.7	0.2	0.9
Dermatology	3.6	2.3	5.9
Emergency medicine	0.5	0.3	0.8
Family practice	5.7	2.3	8.0
Gastroenterology	1.5	1.6	3.1
General surgery	1.4	1.3	2.7
Internal medicine	3.2	1.9	5.1
Neurology	1.1	1.7	2.8
Neurosurgery	0.6	1.5	2.1

[Continued]

★ 801 ★

Office and Clinical Supply Expenses, by Specialty
[Continued]

Specialty	Clinical supplies	Business supplies	All supplies
Obstetrics/gynecology	2.4	1.6	4.0
Oncology/hematology	10.6	1.5	12.1
Ophthalmology, dispensing	9.3	1.7	11.0
Ophthalmology, nondispensing	5.7	2.4	8.1
Orthopedic surgery	2.9	1.6	4.5
Otolaryngology	2.3	1.9	4.2
Pediatrics	8.5	2.6	11.1
Plastic surgery	3.2	1.9	5.1
Psychiatry	0.1	1.7	1.8
Radiology	0.7	1.0	1.7
Urology	6.7	1.6	8.3

Source: "Here's What Your Colleagues Are Spending for Supplies." *Medical Economics,* 13 September 1993, p. 56. Primary source: The Society of Medical-Dental Management Consultants. Data apply to practices that use the services of society members. *Notes:* Figures are averages and do not include depreciation on medical and business equipment.

★ 802 ★

Medical Practice Management

Professional Expenses, by Region: 1991

The table below reflects the mean professional expenses for medical practices in 1991. Data are provided by region of the United States.

Expenses	All physicians	Region			
		Northeast	North Central	South	West
In thousands of dollars					
Total	167.5	143.5	160.8	175.8	183.5
Payroll (nonphysician)	62.9	50.2	64.1	68.2	65.8
Office space	37.3	32.0	33.3	38.9	43.5
Medical supplies	18.3	12.2	18.6	20.2	20.8
Medical equipment	9.4	11.3	6.7	9.3	9.9
Liability insurance	15.0	18.5	14.7	12.9	15.1
Other	24.7	19.2	23.4	26.3	28.4
As percent of total expenses[1]					
Payroll (nonphysician)	33.9	30.8	35.4	35.0	33.9
Office space	22.6	25.3	21.4	21.5	22.8
Medical supplies	9.5	7.7	10.2	10.4	9.4
Medical equipment	4.4	4.5	3.7	4.7	4.3

[Continued]

★ 802 ★

Professional Expenses, by Region: 1991
[Continued]

Expenses	All physicians	Region			
		Northeast	North Central	South	West
Liability insurance	13.2	15.4	13.5	12.1	12.7
Other	16.4	16.4	15.8	16.3	16.8

Source: "Where Does Your Money Come From and Where Does It Go?" American Medical News, 2 August 1993, p. 22. Primary source: American Medical Association Center for Health Policy Research. Notes: Percentages were derived by dividing each expense component by total expenses (for each physician in the sample), then taking the average across the whole sample. Percentages will differ from those derived by dividing the mean expense components by mean expenses.

★ 803 ★

Medical Practice Management

Professional Spending, by Specialty: 1992

The table below presents the spending ranges by physicians in professional practice. Data are provided by medical specialty.

[In percentages]

Specialty	Total expenses per doctor											
	$400,000 or more	$300,000-399,999	$250,000-299,999	$200,000-249,999	$150,000-199,999	$125,000-149,999	$100,000-124,999	$80,000-99,999	$60,000-79,999	$40,000-59,999	$20,000-39,999	Less than $20,000
Cardiology	6	4	2	18	10	7	11	5	7	5	6	19
Cardio/thoracic surgery	2	3	1	18	14	3	17	11	5	7	11	8
Family practice	2	1	11	9	9	8	14	11	9	8	8	20
Gastroenterology	4	2	1	9	18	8	22	7	12	9	2	6
General practice	1	1	1	6	7	6	13	6	8	14	14	25
General surgery	1	3	1	10	10	12	14	15	13	10	5	9
Internal medicine	1	1	1	10	10	11	15	13	11	8	8	12
Neurology	1	2	1	9	17	4	18	17	5	8	2	17
Neurosurgery	7	9	2	20	22	9	9	7	7	2	2	4
Obstetrics/gynecology	5	6	4	21	15	10	10	9	3	3	4	10
Orthopedic surgery	10	10	7	15	17	10	4	5	3	4	8	7
Pediatrics	1	1	3	10	9	10	15	6	11	8	5	22
Plastic surgery	10	13	1	18	23	10	10	3	2	5	1	4
Psychiatry	1	1	1	2	2	4	5	1	13	25	32	16
Surgical specialties	6	6	3	16	14	9	10	8	6	6	7	9
All nonsurgical specialties[2]	2	1	1	8	8	7	12	8	9	10	12	22
All doctors	3	3	2	10	10	8	11	8	8	9	10	18

Source: "Practice Expenses: Doctors Apply the Shears." Medical Economics, 25 October 1993, pp. 132-133. Notes: 1. Less than 1 percent. 2. Includes family and general practice.

★ 804 ★

Medical Practice Management

Race/Ethnicity of Patient Populations: 1993-2040

Figures represent projections as to the ethnic mix of physicians' patients.

[In percentages]

Race/ethnicity	1993	2000	2020	2040
African-American	12	12	13	14
Asian-American	3	4	7	9
Hispanic	9	11	16	20
Native American	1	1	1	1
Non-Hispanic White	76	72	64	56

Source: Hearn, Wayne, and Sandra Lee Breisch. "Cultural Competence: Patients Come in Many Stripes, and Understanding This Is Increasingly Important to Delivering Good Care." *American Medical News* 36, no. 40 (25 October 1993), p. 14. Primary source: U.S. Bureau of the Census. *Notes:* Persons of Hispanic origin may be of any race. Figures may total more than 100 percent due to rounding.

Medical Publishing

★ 805 ★

Medical Publishing and Information Needs of Practitioners

In a landmark study, D. G. Covell, G. C. Uman, and P. R. Manning found that 70 percent of a physician's information needs were not addressed in a patient's office visit. Instead of consulting books or paper-based media for the material needed, doctors most often contacted other health care professionals. Despite practitioners' reluctance to consult traditional references, more than 20,000 journals and 17,000 books related to biomedicine are introduced annually.

Source: Lowe, Henry J., and G. Octo Barnett. "Understanding and Using the Medical Subject Headings (MeSH) Vocabulary to Perform Literature Searches." *Journal of the American Medical Association (JAMA)* 1994, no. 271 (13 April 1994), pp. 1103-1108. Primary source: Covell, D. G., G. C. Uman, and P. R. Manning. "Information Needs in Office Practice: Are They Being Met?" *Annals of Internal Medicine* 1985, no. 103, pp. 596-599.

★ 806 ★
Medical Publishing

Reading Level of American Academy of Pediatrics Publications

The mean score of a survey of 396 parents placed their reading level in the seventh/eighth grade range. The table below indicates the reading level of material distributed by the American Academy of Pediatrics.

Publication	Grade level
The Injury Prevention Program (TIPP) pamphlets	
Safe Driving ... A Parental Responsibility	12
The Child as Passenger on an Adult's Bicycle	10
Safe Bicycling Starts Early	11
Choosing the Right Size Bicycle for Your Child	10
Safe Swimming for Your Young Child	11
Protect Your Home Against Fire ... Planning Saves Lives	10
Protect Your Child ... Prevent Poisoning	12
Baby Sitting Reminders	10
Infant Furniture: Cribs	7
Framingham Safety Survey: From 10 to 12 Years	6
Framingham Safety Survey: From 6 to 9 Years	7
Framingham Safety Survey: From 1 to 5 Years (Part 2)	7
Framingham Safety Survey: From 1 to 5 Years (Part 1)	9
Framingham Safety Survey: The First Year of Life	7
Safety for Your Child: 10 Years	8
Safety for Your Child: 8 Years	7
Safety for Your Child: 6 Years	6
Early Childhood Years: Birth to 6 Months	8
Early Childhood Years: 7 to 12 Months	8
Early Childhood Years: 1 to 2 Years	9
Early Childhood Years: 2 to 4 Years	10
Safety for Your Child: 5 Years	7
Safety Tips for Home Playground Equipment	9
Guidelines for Parents	
Child Sexual Abuse: What It Is and How to Prevent It	10
Hepatitis B	13
Healthy Start Food to Grow on Program[1]	
Feeding Kids Right Isn't Always Easy: Tips for Preventing Food Hassles	9
Growing Up Healthy: Fat, Cholesterol and More	9
Right From the Start: ABC's of Good Nutrition for Young Children	8
What's to Eat? Healthy Food for Hungry Children	10
Patient medication instructions	
Codeine	12
Diphenhydramine	10
Acetaminophen	10
Pseudoephedrine	11

[Continued]

★ 806 ★

Reading Level of American Academy of Pediatrics Publications
[Continued]

Publication	Grade level
Other pamphlets	
Newborns: Care of the Uncircumcised Penis	12
Child Care: What's Best for Your Family	10
Television and the Family	13
Guidelines for Your Family's Health Insurance	12
Sex Education: A Bibliography of Educational Material for Children, Adolescents, and Their Families	17
A Guide to Children's Dental Health	10
Sports and Your Child	11
Deciding to Wait: Guidelines for Teens	8
Guidelines for Teens: Acne Treatment and Control	9
Marijuana: Your Child and Drugs	13
Better Health Through Fitness	12
Smoking: Straight Talk for Teens	10
Tobacco Use: A Message to Parents and Teens	9
Choking Prevention and First Aid for Infants and Children	8
Important Information for Teens Who Get Headaches	14
Surviving: Coping With Adolescent Depression and Suicide	11
Teens Who Drink and Drive: Reducing the Death Toll	16
Cocaine: Your Child and Drugs	11
Alcohol: Your Child and Drugs	10
Making the Right Choice: Facts Young People Need to Know About Avoiding Pregnancy	11
Hepatitis B	12
Posters	
Choking/CPR[2]	8
Cards	
Child Vaccination Record Card	12
Books	
Caring for Your Baby and Young Child: Birth to Age 5[3]	12
Caring for Your Adolescent: Ages 12 to 21[3]	15
Magazines	
Healthy Kids: Birth to 3 (spring/summer 1992)	12
Healthy Kids: 4 to 10 (spring/summer 1993)	10

Source: Davis, Terry C., E. J. Mayeaux, Doren Fredrickson, and others. "Reading Ability of Parents Compared With Reading Level of Pediatric Patient Education Materials." *Pediatrics* 1994, no. 93 (March 1994), pp. 460-468. *Notes:* 1. Produced as a cooperative effort by the American Academy of Pediatrics (AAP), the American Dietetic Association (ADA), and the Food Marketing Institute (FMI). 2. CPR stands for cardiopulmonary resuscitation. 3. Published by Bantam Books (New York, NY), 1991.

★ 807 ★

Medical Publishing

Reading Level of Commercial Baby Books

The mean score of a survey of 396 parents placed their reading level in the seventh/eighth grade range. The table below indicates the reading level of mass market publications about baby and child care.

Title (author and publisher)	Publication date	Price	Reading level
Infants and Mothers: Differences in Development (T. B. Brazelton; New York, NY: Bantam)	1983	14.95	11
The Good Housekeeping Illustrated Book of Pregnancy and Baby Care (J. M. Carter, editor; New York, NY: William Morrow)	1990	25.00	11
The Baby Owner's Manual: What to Expect and How to Survive the First Year (E. R. Christophersen; Shawnee Mission, KS: Westport)	1988	7.95	12
What to Expect the First Year (A. Eisenberg, H. E. Murkoff, and S. E. Hathaway; New York, NY: Workman)	1989	12.95	14
What to Expect When You're Expecting (A. Eisenberg and S. E. Hathaway; New York, NY: Workman)	1991	10.95	15
Solve Your Child's Sleep Problems (R. Ferber; New York, NY: Simon & Schuster)	1985	8.95	14
The Essential Partnership: How Parents and Children Can Meet the Emotional Challenges of Infancy and Childhood (S. L. Greenspan; New York, NY: Penguin)	1989	8.95	15
The Mommy Book (K. H. Hull; New York, NY: Harper Collins)	1986	5.99	10
Babyhood: Stage by Stage, From Birth to Age Two (P. Leach; New York, NY: Random House)	1983	12.95	14
Your Baby and Child From Birth to Age Five, 2nd revised edition (P. Leach; New York, NY: Random House)	1989	29.95	11
The Complete Book of Breastfeeding (S. W. Olds; New York, NY: Workman)	1987	7.95	16
Parents' Book for the Toddler Years (A. Popper; New York, NY: Ballantine)	1986	4.95	11
The First Twelve Months of Life (Princeton Center for Infancy and Early Childhood; New York, NY: Putnam)	1982	10.95	11
The Well Pregnancy Book	1986	16.95	16

[Continued]

★ 807 ★

Reading Level of Commercial Baby Books
[Continued]

Title (author and publisher)	Publication date	Price	Reading level
(M. Samuels and N. Samuels; New York, NY: Simon & Schuster)			
The Pregnancy Book for Today's Woman (H. I. Shapiro; New York, NY: Harper & Row)	1983	12.95	19
Dr. Spock's Baby and Child Care, 6th edition (B. Spock and M. Rothenberg; New York, NY: Pocket Books)	1992	6.99	10

Source: Davis, Terry C., E. J. Mayeaux, Doren Fredrickson, and others. "Reading Ability of Parents Compared With Reading Level of Pediatric Patient Education Materials." *Pediatrics* 1994, no. 93 (March 1994), pp. 460-468.

★ 808 ★

Medical Publishing

Reading Level of Selected Centers for Disease Control Immunization Pamphlets

The mean score of a survey of 396 parents placed their reading level in the seventh/eighth grade range. The table below indicates the reading level of material on immunization prepared for parents by the Centers for Disease Control.

Publication	Grade level
Before It's Too Late, Vaccinate: Diphtheria, Tetanus, and Pertussis	11
Before It's Too Late, Vaccinate: Ten Questions and Answers About How to Help Protect Your Child From Getting Deadly Diseases	10
Diphtheria, Tetanus, and Pertussis: What You Need to Know	10
Measles, Mumps, and Rubella: What You Need to Know	12
Polio: What You Need to Know	10

Source: Davis, Terry C., E. J. Mayeaux, Doren Fredrickson, and others. "Reading Ability of Parents Compared With Reading Level of Pediatric Patient Education Materials." *Pediatrics* 1994, no. 93 (March 1994), pp. 460-468.

Medical Publishing: Books

★ 809 ★

American Medical Book Production: 1991-1993

Figures reflect production data for hardcover and trade paperback books in the medicine subject category. Data for 1991 and 1992 are final; data for 1993 are preliminary.

Year	Number
1991	
All hard and paper	3,027
1992	
Hard and trade paper	
Books	2,499
Editions	714
Totals	3,213
All hard and paper	3,234
1993	
Hard and trade paper	2,014
Books	625
Editions	2,639
Totals	2,651
All hard and paper	

Source: Ink, Gary. "Inching Ahead." *Publishers Weekly,* 7 March 1994, p. S28. *Notes:* Figures for mass market paperbound book production are based on entries in R. R. Bowker's *Paperbound Books In Print.* Other figures are from the *Weekly Record (American Book Publishing Record)* database. Figures under "Books" and "Editions" designate new books and new editions.

★ 810 ★

Medical Publishing: Books

Mass Market Medical Paperbacks: 1991-1993

Figures reflect the output of mass market paperback books in the medicine subject category. Data for 1991 and 1992 are final; data for 1993 are preliminary.

Year	Number
1991	32
1992	21
1993	12

Source: Ink, Gary. "Inching Ahead." *Publishers Weekly,* 7 March 1994, p. S30.

★ 811 ★

Medical Publishing: Books

Prices of Medical Books: 1991-1993

The table below reflects the average per-volume prices of hardcover, mass market paperbacks, and trade paperbacks in the medicine subject category. Data for 1991 and 1992 are final; data for 1993 are preliminary.

Type of book	1991 prices	1992 Volumes	1992 $ Total	1992 Prices	1993 Volumes	1993 $ Total	1993 Prices
Hardcover[1]	40.19	1,460	61,075	41.83	1,133	46,483.63	41.02
Mass market paperbacks	5.88	21	189.43	9.02	12	117.76	9.81
Trade paperbacks	24.20	855	22,364	26.16	699	19,784.80	28.30

Source: Ink, Gary. "Inching Ahead." *Publishers Weekly,* 7 March 1994, pp. S30-S31. *Note:* 1. Less than $81.00.

Medical Publishing: Periodicals

★ 812 ★

Medical Periodicals: 1977-1994

The table below lists the numbers, prices, and percent increases for medical periodicals, dating from 1977 through 1994. Index of 100.0 equivalent to average prices for 1977. In 1994, 1 title was dropped, and 1 was added; 73 percent of the titles increased their prices.

Year	Number of titles	Average price	Percent increase	Index
1977	172	51.31	-	100.0
1978	172	57.06	11.2	111.2
1979	172	63.31	11.0	123.4
1980	172	73.37	15.9	143.0
1981	172	86.38	17.7	168.4
1982	172	102.87	19.1	200.5
1983	177	112.72	9.6	219.7
1984	182	125.57	11.4	244.7
1985	182	137.92	9.8	268.8
1986	182	151.77	10.0	295.8
1987	182	169.36	11.6	330.1
1988	182	180.67	6.7	352.1
1989	182	199.22	10.3	388.3
1990	182	217.87	9.4	424.6
1991	182	249.94	14.7	487.1
1992	182	276.01	10.4	537.9

[Continued]

★ 812 ★

Medical Periodicals: 1977-1994

[Continued]

Year	Number of titles	Average price	Percent increase	Index
1993	182	288.38	4.5	562.0
1994	182	321.39	11.5	626.4

Source: Carpenter, Kathryn Hammell, and Adrian W. Alexander. "U.S. Periodical Price Index for 1994." *American Libraries* 25, no. 5 (May 1994), p. 459.

★ 813 ★

Medical Publishing: Periodicals

Percent Changes in Prices of Medical Periodicals: 1992-1994

The table below provides the annual price percent changes and the percent of titles increasing in price for medical periodicals from 1992 through 1994.

Year	Price percent changes	Percent of titles with price increases
1992	+10.4	83
1993	+4.5	72
1994	+11.4	73

Source: Carpenter, Kathryn Hammell, and Adrian W. Alexander. "U.S. Periodical Price Index for 1994." *American Libraries* 25, no. 5 (May 1994), pp. 452- 453.

★ 814 ★

Medical Publishing: Periodicals

Prices of U.S. Medical Periodicals: 1994

The table below provides the average prices of U.S. medical periodicals by Library of Congress classifications. Data are for 1994.

[In dollars]

Subject category	Number of titles			Average price			Percent increase		
	1994	1993	1992	1994	1993	1992	1994-1993	1993-1992	1992-1991
Medicine	263	263	262	190.76	174.84	163.63	9.1	6.9	5.3
Medicine (general)	28	29	26	162.96	150.78	147.36	8.1	2.3	-16.7
Public aspects of medicine	36	36	38	167.60	154.55	137.00	8.4	12.8	10.8
Internal medicine	103	102	101	194.94	176.45	164.63	10.5	7.2	2.9
Surgery	22	22	22	188.82	171.05	154.00	10.4	11.1	13.1

[Continued]

★ 814 ★

Prices of U.S. Medical Periodicals: 1994

[Continued]

Subject category	Number of titles			Average price			Percent increase		
	1994	1993	1992	1994	1993	1992	1994-1993	1993-1992	1992-1991
Therapeutics, pharmacology	18	18	18	193.78	198.06	182.25	-2.2	8.7	12.7
All others	56	56	57	211.63	191.44	184.86	10.5	3.6	13.7

Source: Carpenter, Kathryn Hammell, and Adrian W. Alexander. "U.S. Periodical Price Index for 1994." *American Libraries* 25, no. 5 (May 1994), p. 454.

★ 815 ★

Medical Publishing: Periodicals

Subscription Prices of Periodicals: 1994

The table below provides the average subscription prices of periodicals by subject category. Data are for 1994.

[In dollars]

Subject category	Price
Russian translations	964.13
Chemistry and physics	678.03
Medicine	321.39
Mathematics	271.68
Zoology	243.38
Engineering	195.62
Psychology	171.80
Sociology and anthropology	106.28
Business and economics	88.10
Home economics	82.23
Journalism and communications	80.14
Industrial arts	78.78
Labor and industrial relations	78.42
Law	76.06
Education	74.76
Political science	70.50
Library and information sciences	63.04
Agriculture	57.06
History	44.99
Fine and applied arts	44.92
Philosophy and religion	40.25
Literature and language	39.72
Physical education and recreation	39.47
General interest periodicals	37.39
Children's periodicals	20.43

Source: Carpenter, Kathryn Hammell, and Adrian W. Alexander. "U.S. Periodical Price Index for 1994." *American Libraries* 25, no. 5 (May 1994), p. 450.

Medical Research

★ 816 ★

Federal Funding for Health Research and Development and Percent Distribution According to Agency for Selected Fiscal Years: 1970-1991

Data for this table were compiled by the National Institutes of Health using federal government sources.

Agency	1970[1]	1975[1]	1980	1985	1990	1991[2]
	Amount in millions ($)					
Total	1,667	2,832	4,723	6,791	9,791	10,711
	Percent distribution					
All federal agencies	100.0	100.0	100.0	100.0	100.0	100.0
Department of Health and Human Services	70.6	77.6	78.2	79.7	85.2	86.0
National Institutes of Health	52.4	66.4	67.4	71.1	72.9	72.0
Centers for Disease Control and Prevention	-	1.5	1.8	0.7	1.0	1.1
Other Public Health Service	16.2	8.3	7.9	7.3	10.8	12.3
Other Department of Health and Human Services	2.0	1.3	1.1	0.6	0.5	0.7
Other agencies	29.4	22.4	21.8	18.9	14.8	14.0
Department of Agriculture	3.0	2.2	3.1	2.1	1.1	1.1
Department of Defense	7.5	4.1	4.5	6.5	4.4	3.2
Department of Education[3]	-	-	0.7	0.6	0.6	0.4
Department of Energy[4]	6.3	5.8	4.5	2.6	2.8	3.4
Department of the Interior	0.7	0.3	0.5	0.4	0.4	0.4
Environmental Protection Agency	-	1.3	1.7	0.8	0.3	0.3
International Development Cooperation Agency[5]	0.6	0.2	0.3	0.6	0.2	0.2
National Aeronautics and Space Administration	5.2	2.6	1.5	1.7	1.5	1.5
National Science Foundation	1.7	1.6	1.6	1.3	0.8	0.7
Department of Veterans Affairs	3.5	3.3	2.8	3.3	2.4	2.4
All other departments and agencies	0.9	1.0	0.4	0.4	0.2	0.3

Source: U.S. Department of Health and Human Services. Public Health Service. Centers for Disease Control and Prevention. National Center for Health Statistics. *Health, United States, 1992.* Hyattsville, MD: Public Health Service, 1993, p. 176. Primary sources: 1) U.S. Department of Health and Human Services. Public Health Service. National Institutes of Health (NIH). *NIH Data Book, 1992.* NIH Publication No. 92-1261. Bethesda, MD: U.S. Department of Health and Human Services, Public Health Service, September 1992. 2) U.S. Department of Health and Human Services. Public Health Service. National Institutes of Health. Office of Science Policy and Legislation. Unpublished data. *Notes:* 1. Data for fiscal year ending June 30; all other data for fiscal year ending September 30. 2. Preliminary figures. 3. Office of Handicapped Research, formerly included in "Other Department of Health and Human Services" category. 4. Includes Atomic Energy Commission and Energy Research and Development Administration. 5. Includes Department of State and Agency for International Development.

★ 817 ★

Medical Research

National Expenditures for Total Health Costs, Total R&D, and Health R&D: 1983-1992

This table compares national total health care costs and total national research and development (R&D) expenditures to health-related R&D support.

[In billions of dollars]

National expenditures for:	1983	1984	1985	1986	1987	1988	1989	1990	1991 (estimated)	1992 (estimated)
Total health costs[1]	355.0	387.1	420.3	453.4	492.4	542.1	599.8	668.7	746.0	832.2
Total R&D[2]	89.1	101.1	113.8	119.5	125.4	133.7	140.8	146.2	150.8	157.4
Health R&D	10.8	12.2	13.6	14.9	16.9	19.0	20.9	23.1	25.8	28.7

Source: U.S. Department of Health and Human Services. Public Health Service. National Institutes of Health. *NIH Data Book, 1993: Basic Data Relating to the National Institutes of Health.* Compiled by Office of Science Policy and Technology Transfer, with assistance of National Institutes of Health's Division of Research Grants. NIH Publication No. 93-1261. Bethesda, MD: U.S. Department of Health and Human Services, Public Health Service, National Institutes of Health, September 1993, p. 1. *Notes:* 1. Source of this data is Health Care Financing Administration and Office of Strategic Planning and Evaluation, Office of Science Policy and Technology Transfer (formerly Office of Science Policy and Legislation), National Institutes of Health. 2. Source of this data is National Science Foundation and Office of Strategic Planning and Evaluation, Office of Science Policy and Technology Transfer (formerly Office of Science Policy and Legislation), National Institutes of Health.

★ 818 ★

Medical Research

National Funding for Health Research and Development: 1960-1991

The table below reflects national funding for health-related research and development according to the source of funds for selected years. Data for this table were compiled by the National Institutes of Health using multiple sources. Data include revisions.

Year and period	All funding	Source of funds			
		Federal	State and local	Industry[1]	Private nonprofit organizations
Amount in millions ($)					
1960	886	448	46	253	139
1965	1,890	1,174	90	450	176
1970	2,847	1,667	170	795	215
1971	3,168	1,877	198	860	233
1972	3,536	2,147	228	934	227
1973	3,750	2,225	245	1,048	232
1974	4,443	2,754	254	1,183	252
1975	4,701	2,832	286	1,319	264
1976	5,107	3,059	312	1,469	267
1977	5,568	3,396	338	1,614	220
1978	6,273	3,811	416	1,800	246

[Continued]

★ 818 ★

National Funding for Health Research and Development:
1960-1991
[Continued]

Year and period	All funding	Source of funds			
		Federal	State and local	Industry[1]	Private nonprofit organizations
1979	7,162	4,321	465	2,093	284
1980	7,967	4,723	480	2,459	305
1981	8,738	4,848	564	2,998	328
1982	9,595	4,970	642	3,593	390
1983	10,778	5,399	718	4,205	456
1984	12,159	6,087	800	4,765	507
1985	13,565	6,791	884	5,352	538
1986	14,900	6,895	1,034	6,188	782
1987	16,940	7,847	1,191	7,103	800
1988	19,011	8,425	1,300	8,432	854
1989	20,977	9,163	1,471	9,404	939
1990[2]	23,076	9,791	1,632	10,634	1,020
1991[2]	25,560	10,711	1,702	12,020	1,128

Source: U.S. Department of Health and Human Services. Public Health Service. Centers for Disease Control and Prevention. National Center for Health Statistics. *Health, United States, 1992.* Hyattsville, MD: Public Health Service, 1993, p. 175. Primary sources: 1) U.S. Department of Health and Human Services. Public Health Service. National Institutes of Health. *NIH Data Book, 1992.* NIH Publication No. 92-1261. Bethesda, MD: U.S. Department of Health and Human Services, Public Health Service, September 1992. 2) U.S. Department of Health and Human Services. Public Health Service. National Institutes of Health. Office of Science Policy and Legislation. Selected data. *Notes:* 1. Includes expenditures for drug research. These expenditures are included in the "Drugs and Sundries" component of the Health Care Financing Administration's National Health Expenditure Series, not under "Research." 2. Preliminary figures.

★ 819 ★
Medical Research

Percent Change in National Funding for Health Research and Development: 1960-1991

The table below reflects the average annual percent change in national funding for health-related research and development according to the source of funds for selected years. Data for this table were compiled by the National Institutes of Health using multiple sources. Data include revisions.

Year and period	All funding	Source of funds			
		Federal	State and local	Industry[1]	Private nonprofit organizations
Average annual percent change					
1960-91	11.5	10.8	12.4	13.3	7.0
1960-65	16.4	21.2	14.4	12.2	4.8
1965-70	8.5	7.3	13.6	12.1	4.1
1970-75	10.6	11.2	11.0	10.7	4.2
1970-71	11.3	12.6	16.5	8.2	8.4
1971-72	11.6	14.4	15.2	8.6	-2.6
1972-73	6.1	3.6	7.5	12.2	2.2
1973-74	18.5	23.8	3.7	12.9	8.6
1974-75	5.8	2.8	12.6	11.5	4.8
1975-80	11.1	10.8	10.9	13.3	2.9
1975-76	8.6	8.0	9.1	11.4	1.1
1976-77	9.0	11.0	8.3	9.9	-17.6
1977-78	12.7	12.2	23.1	11.5	11.8
1978-79	14.2	13.4	11.8	16.3	15.4
1979-80	11.2	9.3	3.2	17.5	7.4
1980-85	11.2	7.5	13.0	16.8	12.0
1980-81	9.7	2.6	17.5	21.9	7.5
1981-82	9.8	2.5	13.8	19.8	18.9
1982-83	12.3	8.6	11.8	17.0	16.9
1983-84	12.8	12.7	11.4	13.3	11.2
1984-85	11.6	11.6	10.5	12.3	6.1
1985-90	11.2	7.6	13.0	14.7	13.6
1985-86	9.8	1.5	17.0	15.6	45.4
1986-87	13.7	13.8	15.2	14.8	2.3
1987-88	12.2	7.4	9.2	18.7	6.8
1988-89	10.3	8.8	13.2	11.5	10.0

[Continued]

★ 819 ★

Percent Change in National Funding for Health Research and Development: 1960-1991
[Continued]

Year and period	All funding	Source of funds			
		Federal	State and local	Industry[1]	Private nonprofit organizations
1989-90	10.0	6.9	10.9	13.1	8.6
1990-91	10.8	9.4	4.3	13.0	10.6

Source: U.S. Department of Health and Human Services. Public Health Service. Centers for Disease Control and Prevention. National Center for Health Statistics. *Health, United States, 1992.* Hyattsville, MD: Public Health Service, 1993, p. 175. Primary sources: 1) U.S. Department of Health and Human Services. Public Health Service. National Institutes of Health. *NIH Data Book, 1992.* NIH Publication No. 92-1261. Bethesda, MD: U.S. Department of Health and Human Services, Public Health Service, September 1992. 2) U.S. Department of Health and Human Services. Public Health Service. National Institutes of Health. Office of Science Policy and Legislation. Selected data.

★ 820 ★

Medical Research

U.S. R&D Facilities of Foreign Companies in the Medical Equipment and Biotechnology Industries: 1992

Japan - 17
United Kingdom - 13
Germany - 12
France - 11
Switzerland - 11
Netherlands - 4
Other countries - 4
Sweden - 2

Chart shows data from column 1.

Country	Number of biotechnology facilities	Number of medical equipment facilities
Japan	17	1
United Kingdom	13	-
Germany	12	2
France	11	-
Switzerland	11	-
Netherlands	4	-

[Continued]

★ 820 ★

U.S. R&D Facilities of Foreign Companies in the Medical Equipment and Biotechnology Industries: 1992
[Continued]

Country	Number of biotechnology facilities	Number of medical equipment facilities
Other countries	4	-
Sweden	2	-

Source: U.S. Department of Commerce. Economics and Statistics Administration. Office of the Chief Economist. *Foreign Direct Investment in the United States: An Update.* Washington, DC: U.S. Department of Commerce, Economics and Statistics Administration, Office of the Chief Economist, June 1993, p. 72. Primary source: Compiled by Economics and Statistics Administration (ESA), Office of Business Analysis, from data from the Japan Economic Institute, company officials, company publications, and industry trade journals. *Note:* "R&D" represents "research and development."

Medical Technology

★ 821 ★

Biotech Products Under Development: 1989-1993

The table below presents the number of products under development in the United States from 1989 through 1993.

Products	1989	1990	1991	1993
Clotting factors	2	2	4	1
Colony stimulating factors	7	9	8	6
Dismutases	3	3	1	1
Erythropoeitins	4	5	4	1
Gene therapy	[1]	[1]	[1]	1
Growth factors	2	7	11	9
Human growth hormones	3	5	7	4
Interferons	12	13	16	11
Interleukins	12	14	13	10
Monoclonal antibodies	25	41	58	50
Recombinant soluble CD4s	2	4	2	2
Tissue plasminogen activators	[1]	[1]	4	1
Tumor necrosis factors	4	4	2	3
Vaccines	13	15	18	20
Other	6	4	10	23

Source: "U.S. Maintains Its Lead." *Chemistry and Industry,* 18 October 1993, p. 784. Primary source: U.S. Pharmaceutical Manufacturers Association. *Note:* 1. Category not included in that year's survey.

★ 822 ★

Medical Technology

Biotechnology Patents: 1992

Figures indicate health-related patents issued by the U.S. Patents and Trademark Office in 1992.

Patents	Number
Biotechnology	4,446
Health care-related biotechnology	2,094
Genetic engineering	373
Health care-related genetic engineering	178

Source: "U.S. Maintains Its Lead." *Chemistry and Industry,* 18 October 1993, p. 784. Primary source: U.S. Pharmaceutical Manufacturers Association.

★ 823 ★

Medical Technology

Drug Firms Focus on Biotechnology: 1992

In 1992, biotechnology-related research-and-development expenditures of pharmaceutical companies exceeded those of biotechnology companies, yet drug firms employed almost a third less researchers than biotechnology companies.

Firm	Employment	Research and development spending
Drug companies	11,000	$2.7 billion
Biotechnology companies	15,800	$2.0 billion

Source: "Is Biotech Leadership Changing?" *R&D Magazine* (December 1993), p. 19. Primary source: Institute for Biotechnology Information.

★ 824 ★

Medical Technology

Management Priorities of Biotechnology Companies

Data reflect the survey responses of senior executives from developing biotechnology companies.

Priority	Percent
Strengthening quality efforts	71
Improving time-to-market of products	67
Establishing corporate partnerships	54
Raising capital	50
Improving overall management effectiveness	46

Source: Gupta, Udayan. "Now or Never: Can the Biotech Industry Deliver? For Most Companies, It's Put-up-or-Shut-up Time." *Wall Street Journal,* 20 May 1994, p. R12. Primary source: KPMG Peat Marwick.

★ 825 ★

Medical Technology

Marketing Biotechnology Products

The table below indicates the steps in bringing a biotechnology product to market. In general, this requires 7.5 to 11 years.

[In years]

Step	Time
Determine biology of disease and potential therapeutic impact of compound	2-4
Isolate compound and figure out how to get it to specific sites in the body	1-2
Design system to produce, modify, and purify compound on a commercial scale	1-2
Produce enough of the drug for testing	1
Test in animals for safety and efficacy; design appropriate delivery system for people	1.5-2
Clinical trials	3-5
Manage regulatory process	2-2.5

Source: Gupta, Udayan. "Now or Never: Can the Biotech Industry Deliver? For Most Companies, It's Put-up-or-Shut-up Time." *Wall Street Journal,* 20 May 1994, p. R12. Primary source: McKinsey & Co. *Note:* 1. As needed.

★ 826 ★

Medical Technology

Sources of Capital for Biotechnology: 1989-1993

Data below indicate the amounts sources of capital have raised for biotechnology.

[In million dollars]

Source	1989	1990	1991	1992	1993
Initial public offerings	300	358	1,188	829	527
Secondary public offerings	400	299	2,515	821	931
Venture capital firms	102	124	200	366	411
Private debt	82	424	445	250	455
Shares sold at a discount in private placements	0	0	0	12	413
Other[1]	171	39	74	374	610
Total	1,055	1,244	4,422	2,652	3,347

Source: Gupta, Udayan. "Experience Pays: There's More Money for Biotech Firms, But Start-ups Need Not Apply." *Wall Street Journal,* 20 May 1994, p. R15. Primary source: Ernst & Young. *Notes:* 1. Includes licensing payments and other funding from partnerships with bigger companies.

Medical Waste

★ 827 ★

Medical Waste Treatment Costs

[Values in dollars per pound per hour]

Type of treatment	Operation and maintenance costs	Capital equipment costs
Incineration	0.04	500[1]
Hydropulping	0.06	200
Microwaving	0.15	750
Sterilization	0.07	300
Sterilization/compaction	0.08	400
Sterilization/grinding	0.08	500

Source: Pollution Engineering (September 1990), p. 73. *Note:* 1. Controlled air incinerator.

★ 828 ★

Medical Waste

Offsite Disposal of Medical Waste: 1992-2000

Data include hospital and nonhospital medical waste sent offsite for disposal.

[Tons in thousands]

Year	Hospital waste	Nonhospital waste
1992	215	270
1993	230	290
1994	250	320
1995	270	345
1996	285	365
1997	300	380
1998	315	405
1999	330	420
2000	345	455

Source: Baily, Jeff. "How Two Garbage Giants Fought Over Medical Waste." *Wall Street Journal,* 17 November 1992, p. B6. Primary source: Projections by Arthur D. Little Inc. Magnitudes estimated from published chart.

★ 829 ★

Medical Waste

Recycling Hospital Waste

Type of waste	Total amount of waste		Recycle (percent)	Amount recycled	Percent for disposal	Amount for disposal (pounds)
	Percent	Pounds/day				
Regulated medical waste	9.5	475	-	-	100	475
Aluminum cans	5.0	250	100	250	-	-
Batteries	<1	-	100	all	-	-
Plastics	5.0	250	100	250	-	-
Food waste	30.0	1,500	100	1,500	-	-
			Compost			
Bond Paper	25.0	1,250	-	-	100	1,250
Green bar paper	14.0	700	100	700	-	-
Glass	1.0	50	-	-	100	50
Cardboard	9.5	475	-	-	100	475

Source: Pollution Engineering (September 1990), p. 72.

Philanthropy

★ 830 ★

Community Hospital Gifts

Data reflect sources of community hospital gifts.

Sources	Percent
Individuals	72.6
Corporations	13.8
Foundations	8.7
Other	4.9

Source: "Philanthropy and the '91 Recession." *Volunteer Leader* (fall 1992), p. 11. Primary source: Association for Healthcare Philanthropy (Falls Church, Virginia; 1992).

★ 831 ★

Philanthropy

Corporate Philanthropy: 1970-1991

Data reflect donations by type of beneficiary. Based on a sample of corporations contributing at least $100,000.

[In millions of dollars]

Beneficiary	1975	1980	1985	1990	1991
Total[1]	436.8	994.6	1,694.7	2,051.5	2,245.5
Health and human services[1]	180.0	337.9	494.1	580.2	608.9
Federated drives	104.6	170.7	(NA)	262.6	285.0
Other local health, human services	20.5	41.7	(NA)	(NA)	(NA)
Education[1]	158.4	375.8	650.0	789.2	783.6
Department and research grants[2]	23.8	64.7	(NA)	(NA)	(NA)
Employee matching gifts[2]	14.0	45.4	(NA)	105.0	142.0
Unrestricted operating grants[2]	29.1	56.0	(NA)	(NA)	(NA)
Culture and art	33.0	108.7	187.5	243.6	265.4
Civic, community activities[1]	45.2	116.8	279.5	254.5	253.5
Community improvement	15.2	47.0	(NA)	43.0	(NA)
Environment; ecology	7.5	10.8	(NA)	18.7	22.0

Source: 1993 Statistical Abstract of the United States on CD-ROM [machine-readable datafiles]. CD-ABSTR-93. Washington, DC: U.S. Department of Commerce, Economics and Statistics Administration, Bureau of the Census, Data User Services Division, 1993. Primary source: The Conference Board. *Annual Survey of Corporate Contributions.* New York, NY. Used with permission of the Conference Board. *Notes:* "NA" represents "not available." 1. Includes other beneficiaries not shown separately. 2. Higher education institutions.

★ 832 ★

Philanthropy

Giving, by Source and Use: 1960-1993

[In billions]

Source and use of funds	1960	1970	1980	1990	1991	1992	1993
	Current dollars						
Total	11.05	21.04	48.55	111.89	117.10	121.89	126.22
Sources							
Corporations	0.51	0.82	2.17	5.87	6.00	5.92	5.92
Foundations	0.71	1.90	2.81	7.23	7.72	8.64	9.21
Bequests	0.67	2.13	2.86	7.64	7.78	8.15	8.54
Individuals	9.16	16.19	40.71	91.15	95.60	99.18	102.55
Uses							
Religion	5.01	9.34	22.23	49.79	53.92	54.91	57.15
Education	1.26	2.60	4.96	12.41	13.45	14.29	15.07
Health	0.95	2.40	5.34	9.90	9.68	10.24	10.83
Human Services	1.63	2.92	4.91	11.82	11.11	11.57	12.47
Arts	0.408	0.663	3.15	7.89	8.81	9.32	9.57
Public/society benefit	0.314	0.455	1.46	4.92	4.93	5.05	5.44
Environment/wildlife	-	-	-	2.64	2.93	3.12	3.19
International Affairs	-	-	-	1.50	1.75	1.71	1.86
Unclassified	1.05	2.66	6.50	11.01	10.53	11.67	10.65
	Inflation-adjusted dollars						
Total	61.73	88.06	100.65	127.99	127.30	126.63	126.22
Sources							
Corporations	2.86	3.44	4.50	6.71	6.52	6.15	5.92
Foundations	3.97	7.95	5.83	8.27	8.39	8.98	9.21
Bequests	3.74	8.91	5.93	8.74	8.46	8.46	8.54
Individuals	51.17	67.75	84.39	104.27	103.93	103.04	102.55
Uses							
Religion	27.98	39.09	46.08	56.96	58.62	57.05	57.15
Education	7.04	10.88	10.28	14.20	14.62	14.84	15.07
Health	5.31	10.04	11.07	11.33	10.52	10.64	10.83
Human Services	9.10	12.22	10.18	13.52	12.08	12.02	12.47
Arts	2.28	2.77	6.53	9.03	9.57	9.69	9.57
Public/society benefit	1.75	1.90	3.03	5.63	5.36	5.25	5.44
Environment/wildlife	-	-	-	3.03	3.18	3.24	3.19
International Affairs	-	-	-	1.72	1.90	1.78	1.86
Unclassified	8.27	11.15	13.48	12.59	11.44	12.13	10.65

Source: AAFRC Trust for Philanthropy. *Giving USA 1994.* 39th ed. New York, NY: AAFRC Trust for Philanthropy, 1994, n.p. Used with permission. AAFRC stands for American Association of Fund Raising Counsel.

★ 833 ★

Philanthropy

Sources of Hospital Capital Campaign Funds

Sources	Percent
Individuals	39
Medical staff	16
Foundations	13
Business/corporate foundations	13
Trustees	8
Auxilians	6
Hospital staff	5

Source: "Philanthropy and the '91 Recession." *Volunteer Leader* (fall 1992), p. 11. Primary source: Association for Healthcare Philanthropy (Falls Church, Virginia; 1992).

★ 834 ★

Philanthropy

Top Health-Related Charities

Organization	Public income ($)	Fund-raising support ($)	Fund-raising expense (%)
American Cancer Society	381.95	346.35	16.10
United Cerebral Palsy Association	381.78	47.51	2.35
National Easter Seal Society	313.10	98.94	7.42
American Heart Association	288.49	235.67	13.10
City of Hope	167.46	45.91	3.87
ALSAC – St. Jude Hospital	144.26	90.31	12.50
March of Dimes Foundation	125.36	112.47	15.90
American Lung Association	123.49	95.70	17.40
Muscular Dystrophy Association	110.88	102.94	18.60
National Multiple Sclerosis Association	79.79	72.89	17.70
AmeriCares Foundation	75.82	75.20	1.18
National Mental Health Association	69.60	20.68	1.77

Source: "Top Charities—By Category." *Your Money* (December/January 1994), p. 52.

Total Quality Management

★ 835 ★

Comparison of Cost Savings in Hospitals With and Without Quality Programs

The table below compares hospitals reporting statistically significant, measurable cost savings. Data are for all hospitals, for hospitals with total quality management (TQM) and continuous quality improvement (CQI) programs, and for hospitals without such programs.

[In percentages]

Area of savings	All hospitals	CQI/TQM hospitals	Non-CQI/TQM hospitals
Significantly reduced average length of stay	29.6	32.2	23.8
Departments			
Pharmacy	24.9	26.8	20.7
Laboratory[1]	21.3	23.2	17.2
Patient care units	19.1	21.8	12.9
Billing	18.1	20.1	13.6

Source: "The Quality March: Part Two of a National Survey of Quality Improvement Activities." *Hospitals & Health Networks,* 20 December 1993, p. 42. *Note:* 1. Includes blood bank.

★ 836 ★

Total Quality Management

Cost Savings in Hospitals With Quality Programs

The table below compares cost savings of hospitals with total quality management (TQM) and continuous quality improvement (CQI) programs and hospitals without such programs.

[In percentages]

Amount saved	With CQI/TQM	Without CQI\TQM
No savings yet	57.0	68.8
Less than $100,000	25.6	22.5
More than $100,000	17.4	8.8

Source: "The Quality March: Part Two of a National Survey of Quality Improvement Activities." *Hospitals & Health Networks,* 20 December 1993, p. 42.

★ 837 ★

Total Quality Management

Incentive Programs and Quality Initiatives in Physician Practices

The table below reflects survey responses of physician groups regarding the establishment of incentive programs tied to clinical outcomes or quality initiatives. Data indicate the availability of incentive programs.

[In percentages]

Respondents	Have incentive programs		
	Yes	No	Don't know
Total	11	87	1
By group's size			
14 physicians and under	9	90	1
15-25 physicians	10	88	2
26 or more physicians	14	86	1
By group's region			
South	9	91	0
West	18	80	2
Northeast	9	89	2
Midwest	9	90	1
By group's locale			
Urban	12	86	1
Suburban	11	88	0
Rural	16	83	1

Source: Montegue, Jim. "Outcomes on the Upswing." *Hospitals & Health Networks,* 20 January 1994, p. 56. *Note:* Based on 925 responses.

★ 838 ★

Total Quality Management

Patient Outcome Improvements in Hospitals With and Without Quality Programs

The table below compares hospitals reporting statistically significant improvements in patient outcomes. Data are for all hospitals, for hospitals with total quality management (TQM) and continuous quality improvement (CQI) programs, and for hospitals without such programs.

[In percentages]

Improvements	All hospitals	CQI/TQM hospitals	Non-CQI/TQM hospitals
Reduction in medication errors	40.4	39.3	42.9
Increase in patient satisfaction scores	38.8	40.4	35.3
Reduction in inappropriate use of blood products	37.8	37.8	38.0
Reduction in postoperative infection rates	27.8	28.0	27.4
Reduction in cesarean sections	23.4	25.3	19.3

Source: "The Quality March: Part Two of a National Survey of Quality Improvement Activities." *Hospitals & Health Networks,* 20 December 1993, p. 42.

★ 839 ★

Total Quality Management

Quality Outcomes Databases: Availability

The table below reflects survey responses of physician groups regarding the use of organized clinical outcomes data. Data indicate the availability and perceived value of quality outcomes databases.

[In percentages]

Respondents	Have a database?[1] Yes	No	Description of database[2] Very good	Good	Adequate	Small
Total	35	63	4	15	11	70
By group's size						
14 physicians and under	29	6	8	5	1	9	1	2	6	3
15-25 physicians	32	66		8	21	9	60
26 or more physicians	42	57		2	7	10	80
By group's region						
South	33	62		8	11	8	73
West	39	60		-	20	15	65
Northeast	28	71		12	18	6	64
Midwest	34	65		3	12	9	76
By group's locale						
Urban	39	59		3	15	12	69

[Continued]

★ 839 ★

Quality Outcomes Databases: Availability
[Continued]

Respondents	Have a database?[1]		Description of database[2]			
	Yes	No	Very good	Good	Adequate	Small
Suburban	36	62	8	17	12	64
Rural	28	69	9	-	5	85

Source: Montegue, Jim. "Outcomes on the Upswing." *Hospitals & Health Networks,* 20 January 1994, p. 56. *Notes:* 1. Based on 925 responses. 2. Based on 321 responses.

★ 840 ★

Total Quality Management

Quality Outcomes Databases: Use

The table below reflects survey responses of physician groups regarding the use of organized clinical outcomes data. Data indicate the uses of quality outcomes databases.

[In percentages]

Respondents	Improve patient care	Modify physician behaviors	Obtain managed care contracts	Don't know
Total	85	67	46	6
By group's size				
14 physicians and under	83	55	38	9
15-25 physicians	83	67	45	9
26 or more physicians	86	73	51	3
By group's region				
South	81	62	39	6
West	84	72	45	8
Northeast	91	64	58	6
Midwest	84	65	44	6
By group's locale				
Urban	85	70	49	5
Suburban	89	69	50	4
Rural	78	62	36	11

Source: Montegue, Jim. "Outcomes on the Upswing." *Hospitals & Health Networks,* 20 January 1994, p. 56. *Note:* Based on 321 responses allowed to make multiple affirmative answers.

Chapter 11
POLITICS, OPINION, AND LAW

Tables in this chapter reflect the legal, political, and social climates of modern America. Tables cover such controversial issues as physician-assisted suicide, life support for relatives, and the use of fetal tissue in medical research. Selected legal milestones—notably the $4.25 billion settlement to recipients of breast implants—also are included. Results of polls and surveys show public opinion of the U.S. health care system, and data about state and national health care reform proposals illustrate possible changes for the future.

Attitudes and Opinions: Consumer Issues

★ 841 ★

Behavior of Americans When Dealing With Conflicting Health Information

Data is derived from a 1993 Gallup phone survey asking 1,509 Americans for their reactions to conflicting medical information.

Behavior	Percent
Uses own judgment	56
Seeks doctor's advice	38
Consults books or media	31
Seeks family's or friend's advice	27
Ignores conflicting information	14

Source: "At a Glance: Snapshots of the Workplace Health Industry." *Workplace Health* (September 1993), p. 15. Primary source: *American Medical News*.

★ 842 ★

Attitudes and Opinions: Consumer Issues

Consumer Satisfaction With Health Insurance Coverage

Data show survey responses of 10,000 respondents.

	Percent
Somewhat satisfied	32.0
Neutral; no answer	30.0
Somewhat dissatisfied	12.0
Completely satisfied	11.0
Completely dissatisfied	10.0
No coverage	5.0

Source: Modern Maturity 36, no. 3 (June-July 1993), p. 12.

★ 843 ★

Attitudes and Opinions: Consumer Issues

Consumer Satisfaction With Health Insurance Plans: 1993

From the source: "More than 75 percent of the 5,000 households surveyed ... say they are satisfied with their current plans, while 62 percent would recommend their plans to a friend" (p. 54). The table below shows the ratings of health plans by consumers.

[In percentages]

Item	Satisfied	Dissatisfied	Neutral
Satisfaction with insurance coverage	76	15	9
Satisfaction with insurance by plan type			
HMO/Staff	88	6	6
HMO/IPA	84	10	6
Indemnity	72	18	10
PPO	72	18	10
Satisfaction with range of services by plan type			
HMO/Staff	88	5	7
HMO/IPA	84	9	7
PPO	71	19	10
Indemnity	70	19	11

Source: Cerne, Frank. "Consumers Rate Their Health Plans." *Hospitals & Health Networks,* 5 January 1994, p. 54. Primary source: Sachs Group Inc. *SachsFacts '93.* Evanston, IL: Sachs Group Inc., 1993. *Notes:* HMO is an acronym for Health Maintenance Organization. IPA stands for Independent Practice Association. PPO indicates Preferred Provider Organization.

★ 844 ★

Attitudes and Opinions: Consumer Issues

Consumer Satisfaction With Physician's Ability to Listen

Data in this table represent the results of a national telephone survey conducted in December 1992. A total of 906 adults responded to the question: "My doctor does not spend enough time listening to me about my health. Do you agree or disagree?" According the source: "When Americans are asked to consider how well their doctors listen to them, a slim majority (51 percent) voice satisfaction, while 4 in 10 (42 percent) are less than satisfied. The satisfaction with doctors as listeners increases with age; women over age 64 are the most likely to be pleased." Senior Americans (50 years or older) represented 34 percent of the sample.

[In percentages]

	Agree strongly	Agree somewhat	Disagree somewhat	Disagree strongly	Don't know
Totals	23.0	19.0	22.0	29.0	6.0
Age					
18-29	23.0	21.0	32.0	18.0	6.0
30-39	24.0	17.0	21.0	30.0	7.0
40-49	24.0	21.0	17.0	29.0	6.0
50-64	22.0	21.0	20.0	30.0	5.0
65+	23.0	13.0	17.0	40.0	7.0
Women					
Under 40	24.0	17.0	26.0	27.0	6.0
Over 40	23.0	19.0	15.0	40.0	3.0

Source: Belden & Russonello Research and Communications. *Health and Longevity: Results of a National Survey Conducted for the Alliance for Aging Research.* Washington, DC: Belden & Russonello, December 1992, p. 32. *Note:* Percentages are weighted.

★ 845 ★

Attitudes and Opinions: Consumer Issues

Consumer Satisfaction With Physicians, by Type of Insurance Plan: 1993

Table below reflects data from a survey conducted by Sachs Group Inc. Of those polled, enrollees in IPA health maintenance organizations were the most satisfied with the quality of their doctors.

[In percetnages]

Item	Satisfied	Dissatisfied	Neutral
Quality of physician:			
HMO/IPA	91	4	5
PPO	89	4	7
HMO/Staff	86	6	8

[Continued]

★ 845 ★

Consumer Satisfaction With Physicians, by Type of Insurance Plan: 1993
[Continued]

Item	Satisfied	Dissatisfied	Neutral
Time waiting in physician's office:			
HMO/Staff	67	22	12
HMO/IPA	59	28	13
PPO	53	34	13
Indemnity	48	39	13
Access to out-of-plan physicians:			
PPO	71	18	12
HMO/Staff	42	40	18
HMO/IPA	40	40	20

Source: Cerne, Frank. "Consumers Rate Their Health Plans." *Hospitals & Health Networks,* 5 January 1994, p. 54. Primary source: Sachs Group Inc. *SachsFacts '93.* Evanston, IL: Sachs Group Inc., 1993. *Notes:* HMO is an acronym for Health Maintenance Organization. IPA stands for Independent Practice Association. PPO indicates Preferred Provider Organization.

★ 846 ★

Attitudes and Opinions: Consumer Issues

Health Care Concerns

Data below reflect concerns of survey respondents regarding health care.

Concerns	Percent
Cost	54
Quality	28
Access/availability	13
Other	2
Don't know	2
None	1

Source: "Survey Finds Strong Support for Shared Health Benefits Costs." *Hospitals & Health Networks,* 5 November 1993, p. 46. Primary sources: Employee Benefit Research Institute; *Gallup Report,* 1993.

★ 847 ★

Attitudes and Opinions: Consumer Issues

Health Care Satisfaction

From the source: "A new *Wall Street Journal*/NBC News poll shows that public support for 'the Clinton health plan' is eroding. Yet the same poll, conducted by Republican Robert Teeter and Democrat Peter Hart, shows that backing for the basic provisions in the president's plan is strong. In the poll, 45 percent of Americans now say they oppose the Clinton plan, up from 39 percent in January and 18 percent in September, just after the president outlined the plan in a televised address to Congress. Thirty-seven percent of those surveyed favor the Clinton program, down from 42 percent in January and 51 percent in September. But when read a description of the major provisions of the White House bill—without identifying it—76 percent of the respondents say it has either 'a great deal of appeal' or 'some appeal'" (p. B1).

[In percentages]

Respondents reaction to:	Levels of satisfaction				
	Very satisified	Somewhat satisfied	Somewhat dissatisfied	Very dissatisfied	Not sure
U.S. health care system	11	26	30	30	3
Own medical care and health coverage	40	31	12	16	1

Source: Stout, Hilary. "Many Don't Realize It's Clinton Plan They Like." *Wall Street Journal,* 10 March 1994, p. B1. Primary Source: *Wall Street Journal*/NBC News poll.

Attitudes and Opinions: Costs

★ 848 ★

Consumers' Perceptions of Medical Care Costs

The table below indicates consumer guesses as to the cost of selected medical procedures.

Type of Care	Average National Fee	Low Estimate	High Estimate	Average Estimate
Broken arm	$418	$10	$3,800	$583
Delivery of baby				
Cesarean	2,636	200	70,000	3,661
normal	1,999	45	80,000	2,595
Hysterectomy	2,493	100	45,000	3,048
Mammogram	88	10	4,000	315
Office visit	47	3	200	151
Open-heart surgery	7,280	10	99,000	12,804
Pap smear & exam	105	8	2,000	320
Physical exam	111	8	2,500	270

[Continued]

★ 848 ★

Consumers' Perceptions of Medical Care Costs
[Continued]

Type of Care	Average National Fee	Low Estimate	High Estimate	Average Estimate
Tonsillectomy & adenoidectomy	726	50	12,000	1,437

Source: Ruffenach, Glenn. "Firms Use Financial Incentives to Make Employees Seek Lower Health-Care Fees." *Wall Street Journal,* 9 February 1993, p. B10. Primary source: Medirisk, Inc.

★ 849 ★

Attitudes and Opinions: Costs

Controlling High Health Care Costs

Table below indicates the public's perception regarding ways to control rising health care costs. Respondents were asked to select the statement to which they agreed more. Cutting medical waste, fraud, and high profits was preferred to rationing; that is, limiting the availability of health care.

[In percentages]

Cure	Percent selecting
Cut waste, high profits, fraud	77
Limit health care available[1]	20
Don't know	3

Source: "Bridging the Gap." *Journal of the American Medical Association (JAMA)* 209, no. 19, 19 May 1993, p. 2575. Primary source: Roper Center for Public Opinion Research. *Note:* 1. To average person.

★ 850 ★

Attitudes and Opinions: Costs

Factors Contributing to High Health Care Costs

Data below reflect the public's perception regarding items elevating health care costs. The table shows the percent of respondents indicating that a given item "contributes a great deal" to high health care costs.

Factor	Percent
Malpractice lawsuits	59
Waste and abuse	58
Fraudulent claims	50
Doctors practicing defensive medicine to avoid lawsuits	44
Acquired Immunodeficiency Syndrome (AIDS)	44
New, expensive drugs	43
New technology	39
Urban problems[1]	34
An aging population	29
Expectations of public for the "best" treatment for any condition	25

Source: "Bridging the Gap." *Journal of the American Medical Association (JAMA)* 269, no. 19, 19 May 1993, p. 2575. Primary source: Roper Organization. *Note:* 1. Urban problems include crime, drug abuse, and like concerns.

★ 851 ★

Attitudes and Opinions: Costs

Medical Cost Worries

The table below reflects the feelings of Americans regarding their concerns about money and costs.

[In percentages]

Item	Percent
Medical costs	68
Having enough money for retirement	55
Food costs	36
Education/college costs	34
Housing costs	30
Losing job	29
Clothing costs	26
Family member losing job	24
Caring for aged parents	18
Child care costs	12
None of the above	5

Source: "Money Woes." *Detroit Free Press*, 15 April 1994, p. 3C. Primary source: Americans and Their Money survey.

★ 852 ★

Attitudes and Opinions: Costs

Opinions on Research Spending and Health Care Costs

Data represent the results of a national telephone survey conducted in December 1992. A total of 906 adults responded to the question: "Spending money now on medical research to find cures for major diseases will reduce future health care costs. Do you agree or disagree?" Senior Americans (50 years or older) represented 34 percent of the sample.

[In percentages]

	Agree strongly	Agree somewhat	Disagree somewhat	Disagree strongly	Don't know
Totals	48.0	28.0	11.0	8.0	5.0
Totals collapsed					
Agree	76.0				
Disagree			19.0		
Age					
18-29	48.0	32.0	9.0	5.0	6.0
30-39	53.0	25.0	10.0	10.0	2.0
40-49	53.0	24.0	10.0	12.0	2.0
50-64	50.0	29.0	12.0	6.0	3.0
65+	34.0	28.0	17.0	8.0	13.0
Presidential vote					
Clinton	55.0	21.0	12.0	27.0	5.0
Bush	41.0	34.0	9.0	9.0	5.0
Perot	41.0	32.0	13.0	11.0	4.0

Source: Belden & Russonello Research and Communications. *Health and Longevity: Results of a National Survey Conducted for the Alliance for Aging Research.* Washington, DC: Belden & Russonello, December 1992, p. 28. *Note:* Percentages are weighted.

Attitudes and Opinions: Ethics and Issues

★ 853 ★

Fetal Tissue Use in Medical Research

Data represent the results of a national telephone survey conducted in December 1992. A total of 906 adults responded to the question: "Scientists should be able to use fetal tissue from abortions to find cures for deadly diseases such as Alzheimer's and Parkinson's. Do you agree or disagree?" Senior Americans (50 years or older) represented 34 percent of the sample.

[In percentages]

	Agree strongly	Agree somewhat	Disagree somewhat	Disagree strongly	Don't know
Totals	38.0	25.0	8.0	24.0	5.0
Totals collapsed					
Agree	63.0				
Disagree			32.0		
Education					
High school or less	33.0	23.0	10.0	28.0	7.0
Some college/vocational	37.0	30.0	6.0	23.0	4.0
College degree or more	48.0	24.0	5.0	19.0	4.0
Household occupation					
Professional white-collar	43.0	21.0	9.0	22.0	4.0
Managerial white-collar	44.0	24.0	5.0	23.0	4.0
Blue-collar	33.0	28.0	8.0	25.0	6.0
Household income					
Less than $15,000	26.0	26.0	7.0	33.0	7.0
$15,000-$34,999	35.0	25.0	10.0	24.0	5.0
$35,000-$49,999	45.0	25.0	5.0	20.0	4.0
$50,000 or more	47.0	23.0	6.0	21.0	2.0
Age					
18-29	32.0	33.0	10.0	23.0	2.0
30-39	32.0	23.0	7.0	31.0	7.0
40-49	41.0	29.0	5.0	22.0	4.0
50-64	43.0	20.0	9.0	22.0	6.0
65+	46.0	16.0	7.0	23.0	7.0
Sex					
Male	43.0	26.0	7.0	19.0	4.0
Female	33.0	23.0	8.0	29.0	6.0

Source: Belden & Russonello Research and Communications. *Health and Longevity: Results of a National Survey Conducted for the Alliance for Aging Research.* Washington, DC: Belden & Russonello, December 1992, p. 31. *Note:* Percentages are weighted.

★ 854 ★

Attitudes and Opinions: Ethics and Issues

Opinions on Doctor-Assisted Suicide

Data represent the results of a national telephone survey conducted in December 1992. A total of 906 adults responded to the question: "Doctors should be allowed by law to help their terminally ill patients commit suicide. Do you agree or disagree?" Senior Americans (50 years or older) represented 34 percent of the sample.

[In percentages]

	Agree strongly	Agree somewhat	Disagree somewhat	Disagree strongly	Don't know
Totals	24.0	19.0	12.0	38.0	6.0
Totals collapsed					
Agree	43.0				
Disagree			50.0		
Sex					
Male	26.0	22.0	12.0	35.0	4.0
Female	21.0	17.0	12.0	41.0	8.0
Age					
18-29	20.0	22.0	13.0	44.0	2.0
30-39	23.0	24.0	13.0	34.0	6.0
40-49	28.0	19.0	8.0	38.0	7.0
50-64	25.0	16.0	15.0	37.0	8.0
65+	24.0	14.0	14.0	38.0	9.0
Race					
White	25.0	21.0	13.0	35.0	6.0
African-American	14.0	15.0	8.0	58.0	5.0
Household income					
Less than $15,000	16.0	13.0	11.0	53.0	7.0
$15,000-$34,999	26.0	18.0	12.0	38.0	5.0
$35,000-$49,999	23.0	24.0	13.0	34.0	6.0
$50,000 or more	27.0	25.0	13.0	31.0	4.0
Household occupation					
Professional white-collar	29.0	22.0	11.0	32.0	4.0
Managerial white-collar	24.0	26.0	10.0	32.0	7.0
Blue-collar	20.0	15.0	16.0	43.0	6.0
Household children					
None	26.0	21.0	13.0	32.0	7.0
18 and under	21.0	17.0	12.0	45.0	4.0

Source: Belden & Russonello Research and Communications. *Health and Longevity: Results of a National Survey Conducted for the Alliance for Aging Research.* Washington, DC: Belden & Russonello, December 1992, p. 34. *Note:* Percentages are weighted.

★ 855 ★

Attitudes and Opinions: Ethics and Issues

Opinions on Medical Research and Health Care Reform

Data represent the results of a national telephone survey conducted in December 1992. A total of 906 adults responded to the question: "Any type of health care reform should include more government emphasis on medical research to cure and prevent diseases. Do you agree or disagree?" Senior Americans (50 years or older) represented 34 percent of the sample.

[In percentages]

	Agree strongly	Agree somewhat	Disagree somewhat	Disagree strongly	Don't know
Totals	51.0	31.0	10.0	4.0	3.0
Totals collapsed					
Agree	82.0				
Disagree			14.0		
Age					
18-29	51.0	37.0	10.0	2.0	1.0
30-39	49.0	33.0	11.0	5.0	3.0
40-49	50.0	32.0	10.0	4.0	4.0
50-64	60.0	24.0	10.0	4.0	2.0
65+	49.0	28.0	11.0	6.0	4.0
Presidential vote					
Clinton	59.0	32.0	6.0	2.0	2.0
Bush	37.0	37.0	17.0	7.0	1.0
Perot	38.0	38.0	14.0	5.0	4.0

Source: Belden & Russonello Research and Communications. *Health and Longevity: Results of a National Survey Conducted for the Alliance for Aging Research.* Washington, DC: Belden & Russonello, December 1992, p. 29. *Note:* Percentages are weighted.

★ 856 ★

Attitudes and Opinions: Ethics and Issues

Patient Opinion and Surrogate Decision Making on Life Support

Data reflect the results of 50 hospital patients and their surrogates regarding life support.

Decisions	Percent
Patients desiring life support	35
Patients favoring euthanasia under some circumstances	62
Surrogates correctly guessing patients wishes about life support	59.3

Source: Suhl, Jeremiah, Pamela Simons, Terry Reedy, and Thomas Garrick. "Myth of Substituted Judgment; Surrogate Decision Making Regarding Life Support Is Unreliable." *Archives of Internal Medicine* 1994, no. 154, 10 January 1994, pp. 90-96.

Attitudes and Opinions: Life Expectancy

★ 857 ★

Desire to Be 100 Years Old

Data represent the results of a national telephone survey conducted in December 1992. A total of 906 adults responded to the question: "If it were possible, would you like to live to be 100 years old?" Senior Americans (50 years or older) represented 34 percent of the sample.

[In poroontagoo]

	Yes	No	Don't know
Total	61.0	34.0	5.0
Sex			
Male	65.0	30.0	4.0
Female	57.0	39.0	5.0
Race			
White	58.0	37.0	5.0
African-American	76.0	17.0	7.0
Age			
18-29	65.0	32.0	3.0
30-39	69.0	26.0	4.0
40-49	61.0	64.0	5.0

[Continued]

★ 857 ★

Desire to Be 100 Years Old
[Continued]

	Yes	No	Don't know
50-64	54.0	40.0	6.0
65 +	52.0	43.0	5.0

Source: Belden & Russonello Research and Communications. *Health and Longevity: Results of a National Survey Conducted for the Alliance for Aging Research.* Washington, DC: Belden & Russonello, December 1992, p. 10. *Note:* Percentages are weighted.

★ 858 ★

Attitudes and Opinions: Life Expectancy

Expectations of Longevity, by Educational and Professional Status

Data represent the results of a national telephone survey conducted in December 1992. A total of 906 adults responded to the question: "How old do you expect to live to be? Until what age?" Older Americans (50 years or older) represented 34 percent of the sample.

[In percentages]

	Less than 80	More than 80	Don't know
Total	36.0	49.0	14.0
Education			
High school or less	36.0	45.0	18.0
Some college/vocational	46.0	41.0	12.0
College degree or more	27.0	63.0	10.0
Household occupation			
Professional white collar	28.0	59.0	13.0
Managerial/technical/sales white collar	40.0	51.0	7.0
Blue collar	38.0	42.0	18.0

Source: Belden & Russonello Research and Communications. *Health and Longevity: Results of a National Survey Conducted for the Alliance for Aging Research.* Washington, DC: Belden & Russonello, December 1992, p. 13. *Note:* Percentages are weighted.

★ 859 ★

Attitudes and Opinions: Life Expectancy

Expectations of Longevity, by Respondent Age

Data represent the results of a national telephone survey conducted in December 1992. A total of 906 adults responded to the question: "How old do you expect to live to be? Until what age?" Senior Americans (50 years or older) represented 34 percent of the sample.

[In percentages]

Age	1991[1]	1992
Less than age 70	8.0	9.0
70 to 74	12.0	14.0
75 to 79	13.0	13.0
80 to 84	25.0	24.0
85 to 94	14.0	12.0
90 to 99	11.0	8.0
100 or older	6.0	4.0
Don't know	11.0	14.0
Subtotal: 80 or older	56.0	48.0

Source: Belden & Russonello Research and Communications. *Health and Longevity: Results of a National Survey Conducted for the Alliance for Aging Research.* Washington, DC: Belden & Russonello, December 1992, p. 12. *Notes:* Percentages are weighted. 1. Alliance for Aging Research, National Public Opinion Survey (Belden & Russonello), November 1991.

Attitudes and Opinions: Medical Establishment

★ 860 ★

Hospitals' Lack of Response to Requests for Data

The table below lists the reasons that hospitals are reluctant to respond to requests for health care data.

[Number of hospitals]

Reason	Hospitals
Unable to compile the data	3
Unwilling to share data	2
Concerned about confidentiality	2
Concerned about legal liability	2
Other	1

Source: "At a Glance: Snapshots of the Workplace Health Industry." *Workplace Health* (September 1993), p. 15. Primary sources: Quorum Health Resources; *Business and Health.*

★ 861 ★

Attitudes and Opinions: Medical Establishment

Physicians' Opinions on Their Careers

Data are the responses of 600 physicians to survey questions regarding selected areas of their careers; for example, emotional demands of the job.

	Percent
Doctors whose family lives suffer from the emotional demands of medicine[1]	90
Residents that are clinically depressed	75
Doctors who restrict their emotional involvement with patients	54
Doctors who would encourage their children to go into medicine[2]	25

Source: "Is Your Doctor Spent?" *USA WEEKEND,* 3-5 June 1994, p. 26. Primary source: *Hippocrates.* *Notes:* 1. Ages 30-39. 2. Decreased from 75 percent in 1984.

Attitudes and Opinions: Privacy

★ 862 ★

Automated Health Information and the Right to Privacy

From the source: "Public fear and distrust of technology and bureaucracy ... [are] likely to increase as collection, storage, and dissemination of information becomes even more automated. Health care information is perhaps the most intimate, personal, and sensitive of any information maintained about an individual. As the U.S. health care system grows in size, scope, and integration, the vulnerability of that information will also increase." Data below are the results of a 1993 poll on health information privacy by Harris-Equifax.

Respondents concerned that:	Percent
Privacy was threatened	80
Consumers lost control of circulation of personal information about themselves	80

Source: Gostin, Lawrence O., Joan Turek-Brezina, Madison Powers, and others. "Privacy and Security of Personal Information in a New Health Care System." *Journal of the American Medical Association (JAMA)* 270, 24 November 1993, pp. 2487-2493.

★ 863 ★

Attitudes and Opinions: Privacy

Privacy Protection of Health-Related Information

Figures reflect the opinions of consumers regarding privacy protection. Data are provided by organization.

[In percentages]

Company	Very important	Somewhat important	Not very important	Not at all important
Banks	72	21	3	3
Health insurance companies	71	23	4	2
Hospitals and clinics	71	23	3	2
Credit card companies	67	22	5	6
Life insurance companies	66	26	5	3
Stock brokerage and investment firms	56	28	7	7
Long-distance telephone companies	53	31	9	5
Companies that sell goods by mail	48	29	12	9

Source: "Yet Another Thing for Marketers to Worry About." *ADWEEK,* 11 October 1993, p. 23. Primary source: Louis Harris & Associates.

Attitudes and Opinions: Workplace Issues

★ 864 ★

Employees' Reasons for Choosing Current Medical Plans

The table below indicates importance of certain factors to employees when they selected their health care coverage. Data were gathered by Hewitt Associates, a benefits consulting firm. From the source: The study "found that, among employees, freedom to choose physicians and hospitals ranked as the most important features of medical plans" (p. 66).

Item	Percent
Freedom to choose any physician	47
Freedom to choose any hospital	30
Freedom to keep current physician	25
Lower plan contribution	25
Lower or no deductible	24
Quality of care	24
Preventative services	19
Low out-of-pocket expenses	18
Little or no paperwork	17
Convenience	13
Like the hospital	10

[Continued]

★ 864 ★

Employees' Reasons for Choosing Current Medical Plans
[Continued]

Item	Percent
Efficient claims	5
Other coverage	4

Source: "Key Features of Employee Health Benefits Plans." *Hospitals & Health Networks,* 5 June 1993, p. 66. Primary source: Hewitt Associates' 1993 Perception Index.

★ 865 ★

Attitudes and Opinions: Workplace Issues

Employers as a Source of Health Information

The table below indicates responses to a poll that asked more than 1,000 working Americans how responsible they felt their employers should be to make them better informed about health care.

[Scale of 1 to 5, with 5 being "most responsible"]

Employee characteristics	Rating
Young employees (18-22 years old)	4.2
Low income employees (less than $25,000)	4.0
Education level:	
High school or lower	4.0
College graduate	3.6
Average	3.8

Source: "At a Glance: Snapshots of the Workplace Health Industry." *Workplace Health* (January 1994), p. 15. Primary source: *Employee Benefit News.*

★ 866 ★

Attitudes and Opinions: Workplace Issues

Most Important Human Resources Issues for the 1990s

```
Health care - 15.1
Downsizing/rightsizing - 11.3
Cultural diversity training - 11.0
Teambuilding - 10.6
Total Quality Management
Employee retention - 7.6
Sexual harassment - 6.2
                        Violence in the workplace - 6.0
Career planning - 4.9
                Substance abuse - 4.6
                Preselection assessment - 3.8
            Immigration - 3.0
            Executive coaching - 2.6
        Executive assessment - 1.6
        Transportation planning - 1.6
    Survivor training - 1.4
    Executive intervention - 0.8
```

Data are the findings of a survey of approximately 300 attendees at the Association of Human Resource Professionals' thirty-sixth annual conference. Participants were asked to name the decade's most important human resources issue.

Issue	Percent
Health care	15.1
Downsizing/rightsizing	11.3
Cultural diversity training	11.0
Teambuilding	10.6
Total Quality Management (TQM)	7.9
Employee retention	7.6
Sexual harassment	6.2
Violence in the workplace	6.0
Career planning	4.9
Substance abuse	4.6
Preselection assessment	3.8
Immigration	3.0
Executive coaching	2.6
Executive assessment	1.6
Transportation planning	1.6

[Continued]

★ 866 ★

Most Important Human Resources Issues for the 1990s
[Continued]

Issue	Percent
Survivor training	1.4
Executive intervention	0.8

Source: Flynn, Gillian. "For Your Information." *Personnel Journal* 73, no. 3 (March 1994), p. 12. Primary source: Executive Career Services and the McGuire Group.

Elections: Campaigns

★ 867 ★

Health Care Campaign Contributions: 1990 and 1992

The table below indicates campaign contributions to congressional candidates by segments of the health care industry during 1990 and 1992.

[In millions of dollars]

	1990	1992
Health professionals	7.1	9.7
Insurance	0.9	9.4
Pharmaceuticals	2.3	3.0
Hospitals/nursing homes	1.3	1.5

Source: Hasson, Judi. "Health-care Lobbying Kicks Into High Gear." *USA TODAY,* 13 May 1993, final edition, p. 2A. Primary source: Center for Responsive Politics and preliminary Political Action Committee (PAC) data through November 23, 1992. *Notes:* Data for the insurance segment include health and other kinds of insurance.

★ 868 ★

Elections: Campaigns

Top 20 Congressional Recipients of Health and Insurance Industry Contributions: 1991-1992 and 1993 (Partial)

[In dollars]

Recipients	Party	State	1991-1992	January - July 1993	Total
Sen. Bob Packwood	Republican	Oregon	541,419	3,000	544,419
Rep. Vic Fazio	Democrat	California	424,545	17,450	441,995
Rep. Richard Gephardt	Democrat	Missouri	254,489	71,502	325,991
Sen. Tom Daschle	Democrat	South Dakota	284,783	3,000	287,783

[Continued]

★ 868 ★

Top 20 Congressional Recipients of Health and Insurance Industry
Contributions: 1991-1992 and 1993 (Partial)

[Continued]

Recipients	Party	State	1991-1992	January - July 1993	Total
Sen. Christopher Dodd	Democrat	Connecticut	276,963	10,000	286,963
Rep. Dan Rostenkowski	Democrat	Illinois	226,548	47,000	273,548
Rep. Michael Andrews	Democrat	Texas	246,184	26,925	273,109
Sen. Charles Grassley	Republican	Iowa	271,344	(1,500)	269,844
Sen. Dan Coats	Republican	Indiana	251,903	1,000	252,903
Sen. Christopher Bond	Republican	Missouri	248,674	1,000	249,674
Sen. John McCain	Republican	Arizona	230,783	18,500	249,283
Sen. Bob Dole	Republican	Kansas	245,787	0	245,787
Sen. Arlen Specter	Republican	Pennsylvania	230,862	11,000	241,862
Rep. Pete Stark	Democrat	California	180,251	53,650	233,901
Rep. Scott McInnis	Republican	Colorado	206,610	1,041	207,651
Sen. Don Nickles	Republican	Oklahoma	200,242	0	200,242
Sen. John Breaux	Democrat	Louisiana	201,200	(1,000)	200,200
Sen. Dianne Feinstein	Democrat	California	150,756	35,000	185,756
Rep. Henry Waxman	Democrat	California	181,850	0	181,850
Sen. Kent Conrad	Democrat	North Dakota	102,500	71,000	173,500

Source: "To Give and to Receive." *Wall Street Journal,* 23 September 1993, p. A6. Primary source: Citizen Action analysis of Federal Election Commission records. *Note:* Figures in parentheses reflect returned contributions.

★ 869 ★

Elections: Campaigns

Top 20 Health and Insurance Contributors to Congressional
Campaigns: 1991-1992 and 1993 (Partial)

[In dollars]

Contributors	1991-1992	January - July 1993	Total
American Medical Association	3,960,296	210,018	4,170,314
National Association of Life Underwriters	1,372,600	204,250	1,576,850
American Dental PAC	1,420,958	119,420	1,540,378
American Academy of Ophthalmology	801,527	50,000	851,527
Independent Insurance Agents of America	590,798	138,468	729,266
American Chiropractic Association	642,746	82,930	725,676
American Council of Life Insurance	577,430	123,421	700,851
American Hospital Association	505,888	152,250	658,138
American Family PAC	503,000	111,400	614,400
Podiatry PAC	401,000	118,600	519,600
American Health Care Association	382,019	107,900	489,919
American Optometric Association	398,366	78,100	476,466
Prudential Insurance Company of America	400,835	54,000	454,835
Massachusetts Mutual Life Insurance Co.	282,338	97,050	379,388
Metropolitan Employees' PAC	266,342	68,281	334,623
National Emergency Medicine PAC	330,725	0	330,725

[Continued]

★ 869 ★

Top 20 Health and Insurance Contributors to Congressional Campaigns: 1991-1992 and 1993 (Partial)
[Continued]

Contributors	1991-1992	January - July 1993	Total
National Association of Independent Insurers	240,725	68,000	308,725
American Nurses' Association	306,519	0	306,519
Psychologists for Legislative Action	273,743	26,975	300,718
Northwestern Mutual Life Insurance Co.	240,580	50,700	291,280

Source: "To Give and to Receive." *Wall Street Journal,* 23 September 1993, p. A6. Primary source: Citizen Action analysis of Federal Election Commission records.

Elections: Political Action Committees

★ 870 ★

Leading Health and Insurance PACs: 1993
[Ranked by contributions through May 1993.]

Group	Contributions (dollars)		
	1991	1993	Change
National Association of Life Underwriters	138,250	155,500	17,250
American Medical Association	104,650	148,736	44,086
American Hospital Association[1]	61,350	123,250	61,900
Independent Insurance Agents of America	126,868	105,906	-20,962
Podiatry PAC	82,250	95,500	13,250
American Council of Life Insurance	85,327	87,000	1,673
American Dental PAC	71,325	82,397	11,072
American Health Care Association	52,000	80,700	28,700
American Family PAC	81,500	79,900	-1,600
Massachusetts Mutual Life Insurance Co.	66,800	72,500	5,750
American Chiropractic Association	21,500	63,930	42,430
Metropolitan Employees	66,750	58,500	-8,250
American Optometric Association	49,550	55,200	5,650
American Physical Therapy	37,950	54,300	16,350
Blue Cross and Blue Shield Association	34,650	53,541	18,891
American International Group Employee	24,528	45,700	21,172
Aetna Life and Casualty Co.	32,450	45,300	12,850
American Society of Anesthesiologists	0	45,300	45,300
Cigna Corp.	56,350	38,750	-17,600
Schering-Plough	15,500	37,000	21,500

Source: Priest, Dana. "Health Plan Worries Spur PACs: Industry Group Donations Up 20%." *Washington Post,* 17 July 1993, p. A19. Primary source: Federal Election Commission records compiled by Citizen Action. *Notes:* PAC is an acronym for Political Action Committee. 1. Most recent month for which data is available is April 1993; 1991 figure is also April.

★ 871 ★

Elections: Political Action Committees

Leading Medical Industry PACs: 1981-1992

From the source: "In the 1992 elections, special interest Political Action Committees (PACs) gave $175 million to congressional candidates, investing a record sum in the members elected ... to Congress.... Medical industry PACs invested a total of $75 million in congessional candidates during the past 12 years—a period when health care costs and prescription drug prices more than doubled." The American Medical Association, for example, contributed nearly $15 million, and the Federation of American Health Systems, which represents more than 1,000 for-profit hospitals, contributed $1 million.

[In millions of dollars]

PAC	Contributions
American Medical Association	14.9
National Association of Life Underwriters	6.7
American Dental Association	5.3
American Academy of Ophthalmology	2.6
American Hospital Association	2.2
American Family Corporation	2.1
American Optometric Association	1.7

Source: Common Cause. "Our System of Government Is Under Threat: Special Interest PAC Money in Congressional Elections." Brochure. Washington, DC: Common Cause, n.d. Common Cause is a nonprofit, nonpartisan citizens' lobbying organization with 270,000 members nationwide. *Notes:* Includes medical industry PAC contributions to congressional candidates from January 1, 1981, through December 31, 1992.

★ 872 ★

Elections: Political Action Committees

Medical Industry PAC Contributions to Congressional Candidates: 1981-1992

```
┌─────────────────────────────────────────────────────────┐
│  ┌─────────────────────────────────────────────┐        │
│  │ Health professionals - 35.3                 │        │
│  └─────────────────────────────────────────────┘        │
│  ┌───────────────────────────────────┐                  │
│  │ Insurance - 23.8                  │                  │
│  └───────────────────────────────────┘                  │
│  ┌───────────────────┐                                   │
│  │                   │ Pharmaceuticals - 10.3            │
│  └───────────────────┘                                   │
│  ┌───────────────────┐                                   │
│  │                   │ Hospitals - 7.3                   │
│  └───────────────────┘                                   │
└─────────────────────────────────────────────────────────┘
```

Since January 1, 1981, health and medicine Political Action Committees (PACs) have contributed $75 million to congressional candidates. The health insurance industry alone contributed in excess of $23 million. The table below reflects PAC contributions from selected segments of the health care industry.

[In millions of dollars]

PACs	Contributions
Health professionals	35.3
Insurance	23.8
Pharmaceuticals	10.3
Hospitals	7.3

Source: Common Cause. "Our System of Government Is Under Threat: Special Interest PAC Money in Congressional Elections." Brochure. Washington, DC: Common Cause, n.d. Common Cause is a nonprofit, nonpartisan citizens' lobbying organization with 270,000 members nationwide. *Note:* Includes contributions from January 1, 1981, through December 31, 1992.

Health Care Reform: Bills

★ 873 ★

Health Care Reform Bills: 1994

The table below presents federal cost and financing information for major health care reform proposals.

BILL & SPONSOR	COST	FINANCING
Health Security Act of 1993 (Clinton)	$390 billion in federal funds over 5 years, plus $57.7 billion in deficit reduction.	$124 billion reduction in Medicare; $65 billion reduction in Medicaid; $89 billion from cigarette taxes and assessment on corporate alliances; $40

[Continued]

★ 873 ★

Health Care Reform Bills: 1994
[Continued]

		billion from other federal programs; $71 billion in new tax revenues.
Health Equity and Access Reform Today Act of 1993 (Chafee/Thomas)	$213 billion in low-income subsidies from 1997 to 2005.	$213 billion in 5-year savings from curbing growth of Medicare and Medicaid.
Managed Competition Act of 1993 (Cooper/Breaux)	$25 billion annually, or $125 billion over 5 years.	$40 billion over 5 years from slowing Medicare growth; $16 billion from capping employer tax deduction for health care at lowest cost health plan; 1 percent tax on health plans to fund graduate medical education.
American Health Security Act of 1993 (Wellstone/McDermott)	$370 billion per year in current private spending rechanneled to federal coffers through taxes.	Federal financing through employer payroll tax and sin taxes.
Affordable Health Care Now Act of 1993 (Michel/Lott)	$17 billion over 5 years.	$13 billion in revenues from raising federal retirement age from 55 to 62; $4 billion from phasing out Medicare subsidiaries for beneficiaries earning more than $100,000.
Consumer Choice Health Security Act of 1993 (Nickles/Stearns)	$137 billion to finance tax changes from 1997 to 1999.	$72 billion in Medicaid reductions from 1995 to 1999 by capping federal spending on acute care at CPI plus 1 percent and calculating payments on per-capita basis. Replaces disproportionate share payments with federal grants to states for home health care for low-income individuals; $67 billion in Medicare

[Continued]

★ 873 ★

Health Care Reform Bills: 1994
[Continued]

		reductions from 1995 to 1999.
Comprehensive Family Health Access and Savings Act (Gramm/Santorum)	$144.2 billion for high-risk subsidies, low-income tax credit and health insurance tax deduction 1995 through 1999.	$112.5 billion from capitating Medicaid program and giving states more flexibility to enroll recipients in low-cost plans or provide medical savings accounts and from estimated effects of lower medical inflation and greater consumer choice.

Source: Wagner, Lynn. "Washington Report: Summary of Major Healthcare Reform Bills." *Modern Healthcare,* 31 January 1994, pp. 24-25. *Note:* CPI represents Consumer Price Index.

★ 874 ★

Health Care Reform: Bills

Health Care Reform Bills and Individual Freedom

From the source: "The National Taxpayers Union Foundation, based in Washington, rated eight health plans now under consideration in Congress (identified by the names of their chief sponsors). The first category tallies the frequency of words in each plan that suggest government restriction or punishment. (This matters because the words selected are the ones that send signals to the courts.) The second category estimates the plans' costs. The third counts career limits placed on medical professionals, and the fourth registers price controls" (p. A12).

Health care bills	Sponsors							
	Gramm & Santorum	Nickles & Stearns	Rowland & Bilirakis	Michel & Lott	Chafee & Thomas	Cooper & Breaux	Wellstone & McDermott	Clinton
Word counts								
"Ban"	0	0	0	0	0	0	0	1
"Enforce"	1	10	39	43	37	10	2	83
"Fine"	0	2	3	3	12	0	1	6
"Limit"	19	30	53	48	80	68	33	231
"Obligation"	1	1	7	4	13	6	3	51
"Penalty"	5	9	21	23	64	5	2	111
"Prison"	0	1	3	2	1	0	1	7
"Prohibit"	5	6	6	9	19	6	7	47
"Require"	54	93	244	321	482	151	103	901
"Restrict"	1	9	3	10	19	2	1	35
"Sanction"	0	3	13	4	21	1	8	21
Total	86	164	392	467	748	249	161	1,494
Change in federal spending 1999 (in billion dollars)	-26	-27	-2	-3	30-90	32	702	608
Career limits Racial/ethnic/geographic	0	0	0	0	0	1	0	4

[Continued]

★ 874 ★

Health Care Reform Bills and Individual Freedom

[Continued]

Health care bills	Sponsors							
	Gramm & Santorum	Nickles & Stearns	Rowland & Bilirakis	Michel & Lott	Chafee & Thomas	Cooper & Breaux	Wellstone & McDermott	Clinton
Limits on going into particular specialties	0	0	0	0	0	2	1	2
Price controls	No	No	No	No	No	No	Yes	Yes

Source: "Removing Our Freedom." *Wall Street Journal,* 27 June 1994, p. A12.

Health Care Reform: Costs

★ 875 ★

Annual Medical Bills Under President Clinton's Proposed Health Care Reform Package

The table below illustrates the amount a typical family of four would pay for coverage of their annual medical bills under the system proposed by President Clinton.

[In dollars]

Medical service	Typical family bill	Low-cost option	High-cost option
1 hospital stay	2,000	0	400
Outpatient lab tests	400	0	80
5 prescription drugs	550	25	360
5 adult doctor visits	500	50	100
6 prenatal/well baby-care visits	600	0	0
2 adult dental checkups	200	200	200
2 children's dental checkups	200	20	40
2 children's eye exams	200	20	40
2 pair children's glasses	150	20	30
1 adult eye exam	100	10	20
1 pair adult glasses	100	100	100
Total	5,000	445	1,370
Deductible		0	400
Annual premium	1,296	872	872
Family cost		1,317	2,642

Source: "Comparing Clinton Health Plans." *USA TODAY,* 13 April 1994, p. 2A. Primary sources: 1) White House. 2) *USA TODAY* research.

★ 876 ★

Health Care Reform: Costs

Effect of Health Care Proposals on Receipts

[In billion dollars]

Health care reform proposals	Estimates					
	1994	1995	1996	1997	1998	1999
Health Security Act:						
Increase tax on tobacco products[1]	...	12.0	11.3	11.2	11.1	11.0
Levy assessment on corporate alliance employers[1]	...	...	3.8	5.0	5.1	5.1
Increase deduction for health insurance costs of the self-employed	-0.1	-0.5	-0.6	-0.9	-1.7	-2.5
Limit exclusion of employer-provided health coverage	...	...	...	5.3	8.1	8.7
Provide deduction for qualified long-term care services	...	...	-0.1	-0.2	-0.2	-0.2
Modify tax treatment of long-term care insurance premiums and benefits	...	...	-0.1	-0.2	-0.3	-0.4
Modify tax treatment of accelerated death benefits	[2]	[2]	[2]	[2]	[2]	[2]
Provide tax credit for cost of personal assistance services	...	...	[2]	-0.1	-0.1	-0.1
Provide tax credit for health service providers in shortage areas	...	...	[2]	[2]	[2]	[2]
Increase expensing limit for medical equipment in shortage areas	...	[2]	[2]	[2]	[2]	[2]
Modify self-employment tax treatment of certain S corporation shareholders and partners	...	...	0.2	0.5	0.5	0.5
Modify penalty for failure to report payment to independent contractors	...	0.1	0.1	0.1	0.1	0.1
Modify tax treatment of health care organizations	...	...	...	0.1	0.2	0.2
Relate early retiree health premium discounts to income	...	...	...	[2]	[2]	0.1
Levy assessment on employers to pay for early retirees[1]	...	...	...	...	2.4	4.3
Modify employer contributions to post-retirement medical life and insurance reserves and retiree health accounts	...	[2]	[2]	[2]	[2]	0.1
Recapture Medicare Part B subsidies	...	...	0.2	0.9	0.8	0.9
Extend Medicare coverage to all state and local government employees[1]	...	...	1.6	1.6	1.5	1.5
Levy assessment on premiums for health coverage purchased through regional alliances[1]	...	...	0.5	1.6	4.3	5.5
Effect of employer mandate, cost containment, and subsidies on individual income and payroll taxes	...	...	0.1	0.9	4.4	9.3
Subtotal, Health Security Act[1]	-0.1	11.6	16.9	25.6	36.2	44.0
Other proposals:						
Modify federal pay raise (receipt effect)	...	-0.1	-0.1	-0.2	-0.3	-0.4
Levy surcharge on civil judgments	...	[2]	[2]	[2]	[2]	[2]
Reform PBGC funding (receipt effect)	[2]	0.1	-0.4	-0.4	-0.5	-0.4
Reallocate Old Age Survivors (OASI) and Disability (DI) tax rates	...	...	...	...	...	...
Adjust civil monetary penalties for inflation	...	[2]	[2]	[2]	[2]	[2]
Increase or establish new BATF fees[1]	...	0.1	0.1	[2]	[2]	[2]
Increase or expand fees collected under securities laws	...	0.4	0.4	0.4	0.4	0.4
Levy fees on users of federal fisheries[1]	...	0.1	0.1	0.1	0.1	0.1

[Continued]

★ 876 ★

Effect of Health Care Proposals on Receipts
[Continued]

Health care reform proposals	Estimates					
	1994	1995	1996	1997	1998	1999
Subtotal, other proposals[1]	[2]	0.5	[2]	-0.2	-0.3	-0.2
Total effect of proposals[1]	-0.1	12.2	16.9	25.5	35.9	43.7

Source: Executive Office of the President. Office of Management and Budget. *Budget of the United States Government, Fiscal Year 1995.* Washington, DC: U.S. Government Printing Office, 1994, p. 242. *Notes:* BATF represents Bureau of Alcohol, Tobacco, and Firearms. PBGC stands for Pension Benefit Guaranty Corporation. 1. Net of income offsets. 2. $50 million or less.

★ 877 ★

Health Care Reform: Costs

Effect of President Clinton's Proposed Health Care Reform on Households

The data below reflect the anticipated effects of President Clinton's proposed health care reform plan on household health spending in 1998. Figures have been adjusted for inflation.

[In dollars]

Household income	Out-of-pocket savings	Tax savings	Reduced wages	Total savings	Health spending as a percentage of income
Less than $18,000	595	-	415	180	17%
$18,000-35,000	250	180	430	0	15%
$35,000-50,000	245	265	295	215	14%
$50,000-80,000	235	295	225	305	13%
More than $80,000	225	325	135	415	12%
Total	310	210	300	220	13%

Source: Pearlstein, Steven. "Win Some, Lose Some in Health Care Reform; Billions Will Change Hands, But to Little Net Effect." *Washington Post National Weekly Edition,* 7-13 March 1994, p. 20.

★ 878 ★

Health Care Reform: Costs

Effect of Proposed Health Care Reform on State Subsidies

A study by the Urban Institute analyzed the impact of President Clinton's proposed health care reform package on federal health care money for 27 states. The study concluded that 25 of the states would benefit, and 2 (Louisiana and New Hampshire) would not. The study also found that the proposed plan treated states uniformly, despite protests otherwise from New York's Governor Mario M. Cuomo. The table below presents the amount selected states gain per resident in federal payments under the proposed system.

[In dollars]

State\territory	Gain per resident
New Mexico	246
West Virginia	232
Alabama	212
Virginia	212
Maryland	206
California	117
New York	92
District of Columbia	73

Source: Morgan, Dan. "Health Plan Effects Vary by State; Most Would Get More Federal Money Under Clinton Proposal, Study Says." *Washington Post,* 14 February 1994, final edition, sec. 1, p. A4.

★ 879 ★

Health Care Reform: Costs

Financing the Health Security Act: Sources of Funds

These estimates were calculated using the economic assumptions in the 1995 budget. Estimates released in November 1993 were based on the economic assumptions in the 1993 Midsession Review. The numbers in this table for the years 1994-1999 are drawn from the budget database, except that they include the Vulnerable Population Adjustment and a Medicare adjustment based on more recent data than were available at the time the budget database was completed.

[In billion dollars]

Programs	1995	1996	1997	1998	1999	2000	1995-2000
Medicare	2.1	9.0	14.3	22.1	31.6	39.2	118.3
Part A savings	0.0	3.3	7.0	12.0	16.4	20.4	59.1
Part B savings	1.9	2.4	2.7	5.3	8.7	11.5	32.4
Parts A and B savings	0.2	1.5	2.2	2.6	4.2	5.0	15.8
HI tax extended to all state & local government employees	0.0	1.6	1.6	1.5	1.5	1.5	7.6
Income-related SMI premium with outlay and premium effects	0.0	0.2	0.9	0.7	0.8	1.0	3.6

[Continued]

★ 879 ★

Financing the Health Security Act: Sources of Funds
[Continued]

Programs	1995	1996	1997	1998	1999	2000	1995-2000
Medicaid	.0	0.8	3.5	9.2	20.1	27.1	60.8
Cash-eligible beneficiaries in alliances	0.0	0.3	1.2	3.7	6.6	9.7	21.5
Reduced disproportionate share hospital payments	0.0	1.0	3.7	10.4	15.2	17.4	47.7
Less Supplemental Services for Children	0.0	-0.1	-0.4	-1.1	-1.6	-1.6	-4.8
Payment lag, administrative savings, and other changes	0.0	-0.4	-1.0	-3.8	-0.1	1.6	-3.6
Other federal programs	.0	0.4	1.2	6.9	9.8	10.9	29.2
Veterans Affairs: third-party receipts	0.0	0.6	1.7	4.4	5.8	6.1	18.5
Defense Department health[1]	0.0	0.1	0.2	0.7	0.8	0.8	2.6
Federal employees health benefits	0.0	-0.2	-0.7	1.8	3.2	4.0	8.2
Tobacco tax/corporate assessment	12.0	15.0	16.2	16.2	16.1	16.1	91.6
Tobacco tax	12.0	11.3	11.2	11.1	11.0	10.9	67.4
Corporate assessment	0.0	3.8	5.0	5.1	5.1	5.2	24.2
Other revenue effects	.1	0.8	8.4	20.0	28.8	34.5	92.6
Exclusion of health insurance from cafeteria plans	0.0	0.0	5.3	8.1	8.7	9.3	31.4
Effects of mandate, cost containment, and discounts	0.0	0.1	0.9	4.4	9.3	13.7	28.4
Dedicated revenues for academic health centers	0.0	0.5	1.6	4.3	5.5	5.8	17.7
Assessments on employers for retiree discounts	0.0	0.0	0.0	2.4	4.3	4.7	11.4
Anti-abuse rule – certain S corporation shareholders	0.0	0.2	0.5	0.5	0.5	0.5	2.2
Modify tax treatment of certain health care organizations	0.0	0.0	0.1	0.2	0.2	0.2	0.7
Reporting penalties – Non-corp. ind. contractors	0.1	0.1	0.1	0.1	0.1	0.1	0.5
Modify tax treatment retirement funding accounts	0.0	0.0	0.0	0.0	0.1	0.1	0.3
Recapture retiree discounts high-income recipients	0.0	0.0	0.0	0.0	0.1	0.1	0.2
Incentives for health providers in shortage areas	-0.0	-0.0	-0.0	-0.0	-0.0	-0.0	-0.1
Debt service	.3	0.6	0.5	0.2	0.6	2.0	4.2
TOTAL	14.5	26.7	44.0	74.7	107.0	129.8	396.8

Source: Executive Office of the President. Office of Management and Budget. *Budget of the United States Government, Fiscal Year 1995.* Washington, DC: U.S. Government Printing Office, 1994, p. 189. *Notes:* "HI" denotes "Hospital Insurance." "SMI" stands for "Supplemental Medical Insurance." 1. Under the proposed legislation, the Secretary of Defense is to decide when the military system will be coordinated with national health reform. The table shows the estimated budgetary effects on the Department of Defense if the military system were to be fully coordinated with national health reform by 1998.

★ 880 ★

Health Care Reform: Costs

Financing the Health Security Act: Uses of Funds

These estimates were calculated using the economic assumptions in the 1995 budget. Estimates released in November 1993 were based on the economic assumptions in the 1993 Midsession Review. The numbers in this table for the years 1994-1999 are drawn from the budget database, except that they include the Vulnerable Population Adjustment and a Medicare adjustment based on more recent data than were available at the time the budget database was completed.

[In billion dollars]

Programs	1995	1996	1997	1998	1999	2000	1995-2000
Veterans, public health, and new administration, and other	3.0	5.2	9.6	8.9	10.0	10.3	47.0
Veterans Health Care Investment Fund	1.0	0.6	1.7	0.0	0.0	0.0	3.3
New public health initiatives	0.4	1.1	1.6	1.3	1.2	1.1	6.7
Net new spending on academic health centers and graduate medical education	0.3	1.8	3.8	4.9	6.2	6.5	23.5
Advance practice nurses (Medicare)	0.0	0.2	0.4	0.5	0.6	0.6	2.2
New federal administrative and start-up costs	1.3	0.9	1.2	0.9	0.6	0.6	5.4
Special Supplemental Food Program (WIC)	0.0	0.5	0.6	0.6	0.7	0.7	3.1
Vulnerable Population Adjustment	0.0	0.1	0.3	0.7	0.8	0.8	2.7
Long-term care	.0	5.1	8.8	12.2	16.0	20.1	62.2
Home-based care for the disabled	0.0	6.0	10.2	13.9	18.2	22.8	71.1
Medicaid offset	0.0	-1.5	-2.4	-2.9	-3.5	-4.1	-14.4
Liberalized Medicaid eligibility and personal needs allowance	0.0	0.4	0.5	0.5	0.5	0.5	2.4
Tax incentives for long-term care	0.0	0.2	0.5	0.7	0.8	0.9	3.1
Medicare drug benefit	.0	6.9	14.0	15.0	16.0	17.2	69.1
100% tax deduction for self-employed health insurance	.5	0.6	0.9	1.7	2.5	2.8	8.9
Discounts	.0	5.8	17.5	41.8	44.3	41.8	151.1
Discounts – net of cushion	0.0	4.5	13.6	31.4	31.7	28.8	109.9
Total discounts	0.0	10.2	31.6	82.7	100.0	103.0	327.4
Employers (net of cushion)	0.0	3.0	9.2	23.7	28.4	28.7	93.1
Non-retired households (net of cushion)	0.0	4.4	14.0	36.8	45.0	46.7	146.9
Retirees-low income discounts (net of cushion)	0.0	0.7	2.1	5.5	6.7	7.0	21.9
Retirees-added discounts (net of cushion)	0.0	0.4	1.4	3.7	4.5	4.8	14.8
Out-of-pocket	0.0	0.3	1.0	2.6	2.7	2.8	9.4
Cushion	0.0	1.3	4.0	10.4	12.6	13.0	41.2
Offsets made possible by health reform	.0	-4.4	-14.1	-40.9	-55.7	-61.2	-176.3
Medicaid	0.0	-3.4	-12.1	-34.9	-47.7	-53.2	-151.3
States' required maintenance of effort	0.0	-2.0	-6.4	-18.1	-22.4	-23.4	-72.3
Discontinued Medicaid coverage	0.0	-1.4	-5.7	-16.8	-25.3	-29.8	-79.0
Basic benefits	0.0	-1.3	-5.2	-15.2	-22.9	-26.9	-71.5
Wrap-around benefits	0.0	-0.1	-0.5	-1.6	-2.4	-2.9	-7.5
Medicare offset for employed beneficiaries	0.0	-1.0	-2.0	-6.0	-8.0	-8.0	-25.0
Total spending	.5	23.5	50.9	79.4	88.8	92.1	338.3
Deficit reduction	1.0	3.2	-6.9	-4.8	18.2	37.7	58.5
Total	14.5	26.7	44.0	74.7	107.0	129.8	396.8

Source: Executive Office of the President. Office of Management and Budget. *Budget of the United States Government, Fiscal Year 1995.* Washington, DC: U.S. Government Printing Office, 1994, p. 190.

★ 881 ★

Health Care Reform: Costs

Health Security Act's Projected Federal Spending and Tax Increases

[In billion dollars]

Taxes/spending	1995	1996	1997	1998	1999	2000	Totals
New taxes							
Tobacco/corporate alliance taxes	12.3	14.9	15.8	15.7	15.5	15.3	89.5
Other tax impacts	.1	.1	6.4	14.5	21.6	25.4	68.1
Total new taxes	12.4	15.0	22.2	30.2	37.1	40.7	157.6
New spending	4.1	25.5	48.1	82.0	84.3	88.4	332.4
Spending cuts[1]	(2.8)	(12.6)	(22.5)	(43.8)	(67.4)	(83.7)	(232.6)
Net new spending	1.3	12.9	25.6	38.2	16.9	4.7	99.8
Deficit reduction (or increase)	11.1	2.1	(3.4)	(8.0)	20.2	36.0	57.7

Source: The Promise, the Proposal, the Purse; A Billion Dollars a Day: The Financing Shortfall in President Clinton's Health Care Proposal. Prepared by the Republican staff of the Joint Economic Committee at the request of Congressman Jim Saxton, Joint Economic Committee member. Washington, DC: n.p., January 1994, p. 20. Primary source: U.S. Department of Treasury. "Financing Health Care Reform" (table; 2 November 1993). *Notes:* Totals may not add due to rounding. 1. Includes Debt Service.

Health Care Reform: Public Opinion

★ 882 ★

Indecision on Health Care Reform: 1993

In October 1993 the Kaiser Health Reform Project conducted a survey to determine the reactions of respondents to proposed changes to the U.S. health care system. According to the source, in many instances respondents showed that they "don't know how they feel" about health care proposals.

[In percentages]

Questions	Current system	Clinton plan	GOP[1] proposals	Don't know
Which plan offers the greatest choice of doctors/hospitals?	47	19	9	24
Which plan requires paying the least taxes?	43	13	14	29
Which plan requires the least out-of-pocket payments?	26	36	8	30
Which plan provides the highest quality care?	34	26	8	31
Which plan offers the best benefits/coverage?	26	34	8	31

Source: Wolf, Richard. "Survey Indicates Public Perplexed Over Reform." *USA TODAY*, 20 October 1993, p. 9A. Primary Source: Kaiser Health Reform Project poll, October 1993. *Notes:* Some responses do not total 100 percent due to rounding. 1. GOP is an acronym for the Republican Party.

★ 883 ★

Health Care Reform: Public Opinion

Universal, All-Inclusive Health Care

The table below reflects responses to a *Safety + Health* poll asking: "Do you support universal, all-inclusive health care?"

[In percentages]

Industry	Percent
Total	46.2
Government/Military	55.1
Wholesale Trade	54.5
Services	54.0
Public Administration	50.0
Construction	46.7
Other	46.7
Transportation/Communication/Utilities	46.2
Retail Trade	42.1
Mining	40.0
Agriculture/Forestry/Fishing	36.8
Finance/Insurance/Real Estate	33.3

Source: Safety + Health (December 1993), p. 91.

Health Care Reform: State Initiatives

★ 884 ★

Health Care Reform Initiatives in Selected States

The effects of rising health care costs on state budgets motivated decision makers to begin reform programs. By 1993, 10 percent of the states had health care reform initiatives in place. States with the most far-reaching initiatives include Florida, Hawaii, Minnesota, Oregon, and Washington. Another 22 percent of the states experienced major health care reform activity in 1993. They are Vermont, New York, West Virginia, Pennsylvania, Wisconsin, Maryland, Kentucky, Tennessee, Texas, Montana, and Iowa.

Source: Claiborne, William. "Health Reform Closer to Home: While Washington Debates, Many States Press Ahead." *Washington Post National Weekly Edition,* 6-12 December 1993, p. 32. Primary sources: 1) National Governors' Association. 2) Intergovernmental Health Policy Project at George Washington University.

★ 885 ★

Health Care Reform: State Initiatives

State Health Insurance Reform

As of May 1992, 22 states passed health insurance reforms, and 13 other states were considering health insurance reform measures.

State	Employee group size	Restrict premium increases	Restrict transfer between rate classes	Guarantee policy renewal	Coverage continuity: employer changing carriers or worker changing jobs	Create reinsurance mechanism	Limit rate differentiation	Guarantee availability of coverage	Community rating	Restrict medical underwriting	Expand insurance commissioner's jurisdiction	Require disclosure of renewal and rate practice
Alaska[1]												
Arkansas	1-25	x	x	x			x					x
California[1]												
Colorado	1-25	x		x	x							x
Connecticut	1-25	x		x	x	x	x	x		x		x
Delaware	2-25	x	x	x			x					x
Florida	1-25	x	x	x			x					x
Georgia	1-50						x				x	
Idaho[1]												
Iowa	2-25	x	x	x	x	x[5]	x			x		x
Kansas[2]		x			x		x					x
Kentucky[1]												
Louisiana	1-35	x	x	x			x			x		x
Maine					x[4]					x		
Maryland[1]												
Massachusetts	1-25	x		x	x	x	x	x	x[6]	x		x
Minnesota[1]												
Missouri[1]												
Nebraska	1-25	x	x	x			x					x
New Jersey[1]												
New Mexico	1-25	x	x	x			x					x
New York[1]												
North Carolina	3-25	x	x	x	x	x	x	x		x	x	x
North Dakota	1-25	x	x	x			x					x
Ohio[1]												
Oregon	3-25	x		x	x	x	x	x	x[6]	x		x
Pennsylvania[1]												
Rhode Island					x							
South Carolina	1-25	x	x	x			x					x
South Dakota	1-25	x	x	x			x					x
Tennessee[1]												
Vermont[2]	1-50	x[3]			x	x	x	x	x	x	x	x
Washington[1]												
West Virginia	2-49	x	x	x			x					x
Wisconsin	2-25	x		x			x				x	x

Source: "Recently Passed/Pending State Health Insurance Reforms." *Insurance Review* 52, no. 3 (May 1992), p. 29. Primary sources: Intergovernmental Health Policy Project at George Washington University (Washington, DC); Health Insurance Association of America (Washington, DC). *Notes:* 1. Reform pending. 2. Two states—Kansas and Vermont—have an additional reform category: "Require whole group coverage." In Vermont this includes the limited use of demographic factors. 3. Limit rate increases to 1 in 6 months. 4. Maine's continuity law applies to all groups regardless of size. 5. Commissioner of insurance to adopt rules for risk transfer or sharing. 6. Limited use of demographic factors.

★ 886 ★

Health Care Reform: State Initiatives

State Programs to Increase Employee Insurance Coverage in Small Firms

From the source: "Nationally, a Robert Wood Johnson Foundation study of 11 innovative programs designed to increase coverage among employees of small firms—a large bloc of the uninsured—found that none enrolled more than 17 percent of their target market; most fell short of 10 percent. The study found that most small employers refused to cover their workers even if offered premiums 25 percent to 50 percent below market rates. Researchers projected that no more than 20 percent of the working uninsured, or 4.6 million people, would be covered through a national extension of such voluntary programs" (p. 36). The table below reflects how well state programs cover the uninsured without mandates.

State	Uninsured	Covered by state program
California	4,000,000	40,000
Florida	2,700,000	23,000
Minnesota	350,000	65,000
Washington	550,000	32,000

Source: Meyer, Harris. "Voluntary State Models Net Small Coverage Gains." *American Medical News,* 21 March 1994, pp. 36-37.

★ 887 ★

Health Care Reform: State Initiatives

State Reform Actions: 1993

From the source: "Managed competition proposals topped a mountain of state health reform proposals in 1993, as state leaders sought to get a foothold before federal legislation passed" (p. 7). The table below indicates the number of states with health-reform related laws in place.

Reform measure	Status of legislation	Number of states
Universal insurance coverage	Passed	1[1]
Managed competition	Under consideration	40
	Passed	5[2]
Single-payer bills	Under consideration	5[3]
Employer mandates	Passed	4[4]
Incremental reforms	Under consideration	40

[Continued]

★ 887 ★

State Reform Actions: 1993
[Continued]

Reform measure	Status of legislation	Number of states
Programs for special populations	Created or expanded	8
Private insurance subsidies	Agreed to fund	7
Provider price controls	Passed	4[5]

Source: Sommerville, Janice. "1993 Reform Action: States Roll Out Experiments, Feds Help With Medicaid Waivers." *American Medical News,* 14 March 1994, p. 7. Primary source: Blue Cross and Blue Shield Association. *Notes:* 1. Washington. 2. Arizona, Florida, Minnesota, North Carolina, Washington. 3. Michigan, Montana, New Mexico, North Dakota, Vermont. 4. Implemented in Hawaii; mandate laws passed but not implemented in Massachusetts, Oregon, and Washington. 5. Maryland, Minnesota, Montana, Vermont.

Legislation and Litigation

★ 888 ★

Breast Implant Litigation Settlement

Silicone breast implant recipients filed lawsuits against manufacturers owing to health risks associated with the implants; for example, ruptures, chronic illnesses, and musculoskeletal problems. A settlement of the litigation will cost implant manufacturers $4.25 billion. The table below shows the distribution of these costs.

[In billion dollars]

	Amount
Total compensation to women	3.23
Administration, claims processing, attorney fees	1.02

Source: "Breast Implant Settlement." *Kansas City Star,* 14 May 1994, p. C6.

★ 889 ★

Legislation and Litigation

Compensation From Injury Due to Childhood Vaccination

The average award to children who have suffered neurological damage as a result of adverse reactions to childhood vaccination is $1.1 million (from a federal vaccine injury compensation program). The compensation to families of children who have died as a result of such complications is capped at $250,000.

Source: Neuman, Elena. "Will It Hurt?" *Insight,* 20 April 1992, n.p.

★ 890 ★

Legislation and Litigation

Malpractice Lawsuits: 1987 and 1992

| 1987 - 46 |
| 1992 - 31 |

The table below shows the percent of patients who successfully sued physicians and hospitals for malpractice in 1987 and 1992.

[In percentages]

Year	Percent
1987	46
1992	31

Source: "Fewer Malpractice Wins." *USA TODAY,* 4 April 1994, final edition, p. 1A.

★ 891 ★

Legislation and Litigation

State Laws Regulating Managed Care

[As of June 1993]

Laws	Number of states
Regulation of utilization review (UR) firms	26
Any willing provider	16
Freedom of choice	12
Fair reimbursement	10

[Continued]

★ 891 ★

State Laws Regulating Managed Care
[Continued]

Laws	Number of states
Mandatory assignment	8
Required disclosure	5

Source: Schwartz, Matthew P. "'Any Willing Provider' Laws Draw Fire." *National Underwriter,* 9 August 1993, p. 3. Primary source: Blue Cross and Blue Shield Association (1993).

Malpractice and Abuse

★ 892 ★

Disciplinary Actions Against Doctors

Dr. Hormoz Rassekh reported a 14 percent increase in disciplinary actions directed against physicians within a 4-year period. In 1993, for example, actions were taken against more than 3,000 physicians. Dr. Rassekh is the president of the Federation of State Medical Boards (FSMB), an organization comprised of state and territorial medical licensing boards.

Source: "Doctor Disciplinary Action Hits Record High." *Los Angeles Times,* 13 April 1994, home edition, Part A, p. 8.

★ 893 ★

Malpractice and Abuse

Formal Disciplinary Actions Against Physicians: 1992

In 1992, 3,370 disciplinary actions were taken by state medical boards against physicians, mostly for substance abuse and improper prescriptions. State boards averaged 5 actions for every 1,000 physicians. The table below shows the number of selected disciplinary actions for 1992. Data are provided by state/territory.

State board[1]	Loss or suspension of license	License restriction	Other prejudicial actions	Non-prejudicial actions	Prejudicial actions per 1,000 in-state physicians[1]
Alabama	9	15	2	8	3.67
Alaska	5	1	0	3	5.20
Arizona					
MD	12	23	79	5	15.75
DO	2	5	5	5	17.07

[Continued]

★ 893 ★

Formal Disciplinary Actions Against Physicians: 1992
[Continued]

State board[1]	Loss or suspension of license	License restriction	Other prejudicial actions	Non-prejudicial actions	Prejudicial actions per 1,000 in-state physicians[1]
Arkansas	12	7	2	0	5.11
California					
MD	84	52	8	17	1.89
DO	6	7	0	0	10.33
Colorado	30	30	13	5	7.60
Connecticut	18	8	2	3	3.00
Delaware	1	0	0	0	0.46
District of Columbia	4	2	0	2	1.71
Florida					
MD	88	49	128	29	9.52
DO	5	4	6	3	8.04
Georgia	33	55	43	37	10.13
Guam	0	0	0	0	0
Hawaii					
MD	2	0	4	2	1.69
DO	3	1	0	0	NA
Idaho	4	2	1	0	4.38
Illinois	29	36	33	11	3.64
Indiana	24	32	29	4	8.40
Iowa	23	30	9	9	12.47
Kansas	9	12	11	2	7.02
Kentucky	16	20	15	21	7.15
Louisiana	19	34	3	0	6.63
Maine					
MD	3	1	3	0	3.15
DO	0	0	0	1	NA
Maryland	43	23	21	8	8.30
Massachusetts	17	10	25	4	2.69
Michigan					
MD	22	15	16	10	3.01
DO	10	5	4	1	4.81
Minnesota	19	16	46	13	8.05
Mississippi	13	17	15	7	11.61
Missouri	33	31	12	13	6.99
Montana	6	4	1	0	7.34
Nebraska	3	4	3	0	3.37
Nevada					
MD	6	2	3	2	5.46
DO	0	0	0	0	0
New Hampshire	2	1	0	0	1.20
New Jersey	39	41	62	6	6.19
New Mexico					
MD	4	4	6	1	4.62
DO	0	0	0	0	0

[Continued]

★ 893 ★

Formal Disciplinary Actions Against Physicians: 1992
[Continued]

State board[1]	Loss or suspension of license	License restriction	Other prejudicial actions	Non-prejudicial actions	Prejudicial actions per 1,000 in-state physicians[1]
New York	78	48	23	59	2.93
North Carolina	29	5	16	1	3.85
North Dakota	5	5	8	0	15.28
Ohio	50	55	58	25	8.60
Oklahoma					
MD	36	28	18	12	16.97
DO	3	6	3	2	13.32
Oregon	10	17	10	14	5.23
Pennsylvania					
MD	17	15	10	5	1.11
DO	2	0	1	1	0.56
Puerto Rico	3	2	3	0	1.24
Rhode Island	3	2	9	0	6.37
South Carolina	21	22	13	5	9.51
South Dakota	2	1	1	0	3.87
Tennessee					
MD	8	2	2	1	1.41
DO	0	0	0	0	0
Texas	59	60	39	13	5.49
Utah	2	4	0	4	1.22
Vermont	6	3	2	0	7.87
Virginia	16	17	19	12	3.80
Virgin Islands	0	0	0	0	0
Washington					
MD	31	25	43	5	0.03
DO	1	2	0	0	NA
West Virginia					
MD	24	13	5	6	13.83
DO	0	0	0	0	0
Wisconsin	24	16	33	2	6.97
Wyoming	3	3	4	0	15.34
Total	1,091	950	930	399	5.01

Source: Oberman, Linda. "Kept 'Out of the Loop': Boards Pondering Role Under Reform." *American Medical News,* 10 May 1993, pp. 3, 10. Primary source: Federation of State Medical Boards. *Notes:* MD is the designation for medical doctor. DO indicates doctor of osteopathy. NA stands for "not applicable." 1. States with only one board are either MD or combined. The number of disciplinary actions includes multiple actions against an individual physician.

★ 894 ★

Malpractice and Abuse

Insurance Complaints Improperly Referred for Investigation by Insurance Carriers

[Figures represent number of complaints]

Carrier	Instructed or allowed to settle with provider	Instructed to submit in writing	Not recognized as potential fraud/abuse	Other[1]	Total
Aetna Life and Casualty Co. (AZ)	2	4	0	0	6
Blue Cross and Blue Shield of Florida	1	5	0	1	7
Blue Shield of Massachusetts	1	0	0	0	1
Blue Cross and Blue Shield of Texas	1	0	1	0	2
Transamerica Occidental Life Insurance Co. (CA)	7	5	3	0	15
Total	12	14	4	1	31

Source: U.S. Senate Committee on Aging. *Medicare Fraud and Abuse: A Neglected Emergency? Hearing Before the Special Committee on Aging.* 102d Cong., 1st sess., 2 October 1991. Serial no. 102-13. Washington, DC: U.S. Government Printing Office, 1992, p. 162. *Notes:* 1. The carrier representative instructed the beneficiary to contact another carrier regarding the complaint but failed to give the beneficiary the carrier's address or telephone number.

★ 895 ★

Malpractice and Abuse

Insurance Fraud and Abuse

Data reflect referred cases indicating potential insurance fraud or abuse.

[Figures represent number of complaints]

Carrier	Cases where providers had recent prior substantiated complaints[1]		Cases that strongly suggested fraudulent or abusive behavior	
	Fully investigated	Not fully investigated	Fully investigated	Not fully investigated
Aetna Life and Casualty Co. (AZ)	0	2	0	1
Blue Cross and Blue Shield of Florida	2	1	0	1
Blue Shield of Massachusetts	1	2	0	0
Blue Cross and Blue Shield of Texas	1	1	0	1
Transamerica Occidental Life Insurance Co. (CA)	0	2	0	0
Total	4	8	0	3

Source: U.S. Senate Committee on Aging. *Medicare Fraud and Abuse: A Neglected Emergency? Hearing Before the Special Committee on Aging.* 102d Cong., 1st sess., 2 October 1991. Serial no. 102-13. Washington, DC: U.S. Government Printing Office, 1992, p. 163. *Note:* 1. Two or more similar, substantiated complaints in the past 2 years.

★ 896 ★

Malpractice and Abuse

Insurance Fraud and Health Care Providers

In 1993 the Federal Bureau of Investigation's health fraud statistics indicated more than 1,000 open cases. An industry survey by the Health Insurance Association of America found consumers to be the largest group of perpetrators. Nevertheless, health care providers were twice as likely to engage in fraudulent activities such as waiving co-pays or deductibles, billing for services not rendered, and falsified diagnoses or treatment dates.

Source: McCormick, Brian. "Survey Claims Fraud; Often a Physician's Crime, Data Debated." *American Medical News,* 16 August 1993, p. 8.

★ 897 ★

Malpractice and Abuse

Malpractice Premiums: 1992

[Numbers in thousands, before reinsurance]

State	Total direct premiums	Rank
Alabama	87,241	18
Alaska	13,994	43
Arizona	107,533	13
Arkansas	25,266	34
California	524,769	2
Colorado	31,905	29
Connecticut	105,684	14
Delaware	20,782	37
District of Columbia	49,741	24
Florida	170,549	8
Georgia	145,048	10
Hawaii	15,688	40
Idaho	14,572	42
Illinois	299,548	3
Indiana	34,934	27
Iowa	48,689	25
Kansas	28,346	32
Kentucky	57,633	22
Louisiana	54,218	23
Maine	28,614	31
Maryland	119,599	11
Massachusetts	31,333	30
Michigan	169,302	9
Minnesota	72,689	20
Mississippi	22,583	36
Missouri	107,857	12
Montana	16,852	39
Nebraska	18,976	38

[Continued]

★ 897 ★

Malpractice Premiums: 1992

[Continued]

State	Total direct premiums	Rank
Nevada	28,265	33
New Hampshire	9,806	47
New Jersey	243,429	5
New Mexico	8,631	51
New York	791,599	1
North Carolina	95,034	16
North Dakota	12,964	45
Ohio	245,292	4
Oklahoma	14,968	41
Oregon	47,420	26
Pennsylvania	219,421	6
Rhode Island	9,562	48
South Carolina	9,132	49
South Dakota	10,661	46
Tennessee	87,262	17
Texas	207,996	7
Utah	23,912	35
Vermont	13,122	44
Virginia	80,024	19
Washington	99,712	15
West Virginia	33,187	28
Wisconsin	59,686	21
Wyoming	8,975	50
Total	4,784,005	-

Source: Best's Review 93, no. 8 (December 1992), p. 32.

★ 898 ★

Malpractice and Abuse

Malpractice Premiums of Obstetricians/ Gynecologists and Internists

The table below presents the average annual malpractice insurance premiums for obstetricians/gynecologists and internists. Premiums are for coverage to $200,000 per case and $600,000 per year. Data are provided for selected states.

[In dollars]

State	Obstetrician/ gynecologist	Internist
Florida	116,436	13,862
New York	84,026	15,759
Michigan	79,808	12,913
California	43,868	5,924

[Continued]

★ 898 ★

Malpractice Premiums of Obstetricians/ Gynecologists and Internists
[Continued]

State	Obstetrician/ gynecologist	Internist
Ohio	28,470	9,668
Illinois	27,964	5,832
Indiana	24,615	2,896

Source: Stevens, Carol. "Malpractice Jackpots Will Be Harder to Win." *Detroit News,* 27 March 1994, pp. 1A, 6A. Primary source: Michigan Physicians Mutual Liability Co.

★ 899 ★

Malpractice and Abuse

Malpractice Premiums of Orthopedic Surgeons

The table below reflects the average malpractice premiums of orthopedic surgeons. Data are provided by state.

[In dollars]

State	Premium	Rank
Alabama	12,860	26
Alaska	45,203	5
Arizona	22,307	15
Arkansas	5,388	49
California	35,218	7
Colorado	10,943	31
Connecticut	14,729	22
Delaware	14,079	23
Florida	73,788	2
Georgia	13,360	24
Hawaii	24,500	12
Idaho	10,624	33
Illinois	21,764	16
Indiana	4,350	51
Iowa	9,462	37
Kansas	6,232	47
Kentucky	10,383	35
Louisiana	7,937	42
Maine	10,050	36
Maryland	19,287	18
Massachusetts	36,190	6
Michigan	108,762	1
Minnesota	7,537	44
Mississippi	12,952	25
Missouri	23,395	13
Montana	10,889	32
Nebraska	4,359	50
Nevada	28,739	9

[Continued]

★ 899 ★

Malpractice Premiums of Orthopedic Surgeons
[Continued]

State	Premium	Rank
New Hampshire	11,148	30
New Jersey	22,982	14
New Mexico	30,770	8
New York	65,451	3
North Carolina	7,320	45
North Dakota	12,032	27
Ohio	17,366	21
Oklahoma	18,299	19
Oregon	10,415	34
Pennsylvania	11,904	28
Rhode Island	46,045	4
South Carolina	6,497	46
South Dakota	5,875	48
Tennessee	8,057	41
Texas	24,868	11
Utah	7,597	43
Vermont	8,564	38
Virginia	8,246	39
Washington	18,258	20
Washington, DC	25,023	10
West Virginia	20,502	17
Wisconsin	8,111	40
Wyoming	11,549	29

Source: Frum, David, and Frank Wolfe. "If You Gotta Get Sued, Get Sued in Utah." *Forbes,* 17 January 1994, p. 72. Primary source: Insurance Research Council, St. Paul Fire and Marine. Member companies of the Physician Insurers Association of America. *Forbes.*

★ 900 ★

Malpractice and Abuse

National Practitioner Data Bank Inquiries: 1991-1993

The National Practitioner Data Bank collects malpractice and disciplinary data on physicians. Doctors, hospitals, state licensing boards, and other authorized organizations may access this data.

	Self-queries	Total queries
First year[1]	2,507	781,247
Second year[2]	13,495	839,202
Third year[3]	13,184	612,612
Cumulative	29,186	2,233,061

Source: Oberman, Linda. "Data Bank Access Debate: Doctors May Have to Ante Up For Queries; Consumers Push to See Files." *American Medical News,* 24-31 May 1993, p. 3. *Notes:* Self-queries represent physicians accessing information about themselves. 1. September 1, 1990, to August 31, 1991. 2. September 1, 1991, to August 31, 1992. 3. September 1, 1992, to April 30, 1993. 4. Through April 30, 1993.

Chapter 12
INTERNATIONAL COMPARISONS

This chapter juxtaposes aspects of health care in the United States with those of the world. Tables compare patient care (for example, number of office visits), costs, and the availability of medical technology in America with foreign nations. Countries selected usually are similar to the United States in economic development. Other tables offer a global view of health care by ranking countries in various categories; for example, prevalence of certain diseases such as AIDS or tuberculosis, infant mortality rates, or the number of uninsured citizens. Tables are organized to reflect the topics and coverage of the preceding chapters of the *Statistical Record of Health and Medicine.*

Health Care Establishment: Costs

★ 901 ★

Comparison of U.S. and Canadian Medical Charges for Selected Procedures

[In dollars]

Country	Fees for procedures							
	Intermediate office visit[1]	Follow-up hospital visit	Hernia repair	Coronary artery bypass[2]	Bone marrow transplant	In vitro fertilization	Lithotripsy	Neurosurgery
Canada	25	15	253	1,129	< 80,000	3,000[3]	4,000	10,000
United States	35	53	876	4,791	up to 200,000	6,000[3]	7,000	20,000

Source: "At a Glance: Snapshots of the Workplace Health Industry." *Workplace Health* (October 1993), p. 15. Korcok, Milan. "Ontario Hospitals Are Looking to Woo U.S. Patients." *American Medical News,* 24-31 May 1993, p. 6. Primary sources: Urban Institute; University of Michigan; *Washington Post. Notes:* 1. Established patient. 2. 3 grafts. 3. Per cycle.

★ 902 ★

Health Care Establishment: Costs

Cost of Blood Tests in Developing Countries

The World Health Organization (WHO) estimates that 1 to 5 percent of new HIV infections in developing countries are due to tainted blood transfusions. The average cost to test a sample of donated blood for HIV infection is $1 in these countries, although their average annual health budgets are only $2 to $3 per person. Still, this indicates improvement: Five years ago it cost $30 to test donated blood in a country where the average annual health care spending was only $1 per person.

Source: Kingman, Sharon. "The Cost of Clean Blood." *New Scientist* 136 (September 1992), p. 20.

★ 903 ★

Health Care Establishment: Costs

Doctors' Fees in Germany

The table below indicates fees paid to doctors by the A.O.K. Sickness Fund, a German health insurance plan.

[In dollars]

Type of Service	Average Charge
Consultation	
Office or phone	5.00
Night	12.50
House call	17.80
At night	45.00
Diagnosis of pregnancy	20.00
Attendance at normal birth	93.75
Attendance at breech birth	143.75
Examination of a baby	22.50
Electrocardiogram	15.60
Chest X-ray	28.13

Source: "How Much a Sickness Fund Pays." *New York Times,* 23 January 1993, p. 4. Remarks: Source also includes average costs of German and American health care per person.

★ 904 ★

Health Care Establishment: Costs

Doctors' Office Visit Charges in Mexico

According to a survey of 242 Mexican doctors commissioned by Families USA Foundation, doctors in Mexico charged an average of $25.00 for an office visit. American doctors charged 2 1/2 to 3 times as much for a similar visit.

Source: Hilts, Philip J. "Mexican Health Care Draws Americans." *Detroit Free Press,* 26 November 1992, p. 23A. Remarks: Source also includes the average prices of five drugs in California and Mexico.

Health Care Establishment: Drugs and Medicine

★ 905 ★

Comparison of Drug Prices in Britain and the United States: 1992

Data show wholesale drug prices in the United States and Britain during 1992.

[Prices in dollars]

Drug	Price per dose	
	Britain	United States
Achromycin	0.08	0.03
Amoxil	0.27	0.17
Ativan	0.04	0.52
Dyazide	0.12	0.27
Elavil	0.04	0.28
Hismanal	0.30	1.33
Inderal	0.04	0.37
Lopressor	0.09	0.38
Nordette	0.05	0.84
Premarin	0.09	0.28
Prozac	1.67	1.61
Valium	0.04	0.45
Xanax	0.14	0.52
Zantac	0.78	1.23
Zovirax	1.81	0.69

Source: "Lower Cost of Prescriptions in Britain Brings Calls for Price Controls on Drugs." *Detroit News,* 3 February 1994, p. 6A. Primary source: Associated Press.

★ 906 ★

Health Care Establishment: Drugs and Medicine

Cost of Aspirin in Selected Cities Worldwide

Figures below represent prices for 100 aspirin tablets in major cities of the world.

[In dollars]

City	Cost
Tokyo, Japan	27
Madrid, Spain	9
Copenhagen, Denmark	8
Toronto, Ontario, Canada	5

Source: "USA Snapshots." *USA TODAY,* 17 January 1994, p. 1D. Primary source: Runzheimer International.

★ 907 ★

Health Care Establishment: Drugs and Medicine

International Pharmaceuticals Industry: 1990

Data reflect the number of firms and the percentages of consolidated worldwide sales for the 12 largest companies. Data are provided by home country.

Country	Number of firms	Rank	Percent of sales	Rank
United States	6	1	49	1
Switzerland	3	2	30	2
Germany	1	3	6	4
Sweden	1	3	6	4
United Kingdom	1	3	9	3

Source: Franko, Lawrence G. "Global Corporate Competition II: Is the Large American Firm an Endangered Species?" *Business Horizons* 34, no. 4 (November 1991), p. 15.

★ 908 ★

Health Care Establishment: Drugs and Medicine

Price of Drugs in California and Mexico

[Average price in dollars]

Drug	Strength (mg)	Number of tablets	Average price	
			California	Mexico
Cardizem	60	30	$24.04	$6.12
Ceclor	250	15	35.87	6.87
Mevacor	20	30	67.62	42.08
Prozac	20	14	33.22	23.49
Tagamet	300	100	77.08	19.60
Xanax	.25	90	64.08	NA
Zantac	160	60	92.31	21.91

Source: "Medicines Across the Border." *Detroit Free Press,* 26 November 1992, p. 23A. Primary source: Families USA Foundation. *Note:* NA stands for not available.

★ 909 ★

Health Care Establishment: Drugs and Medicine

Sales of Ulcer Medications in the United States and World: 1993

The table below reflects the sales of prescription ulcer drugs during 1993.

[In billion dollars]

Drug (manufacturer)	U.S. sales	World sales
Zantac (Glaxo)	1.90	3.50
Tagamet (Smith Kline Beecham)	0.65	1.01
Prilosec (Merck)[1]	0.59	1.62
Pepcid (Merck)	0.54	0.74
Axid (Lilly)	0.30	0.40

Source: Freudenheim, Milt. "New Drug Era Begins as Tagamet Patent Ends." *New York Times,* 17 May 1994, p. C4. Primary source: PaineWebber Securities. *Notes:* 1. Outside of the United States, known as Losec and manufactured by Astra.

★ 910 ★

Health Care Establishment: Drugs and Medicine

Spending on Prescription Drugs in Selected Countries

Data present annual per person spending on prescription drugs and medicines.

[In dollars]

Country	Spending per person
United Kingdom	98
Japan	189
United States	210
Canada	241
France	256
Germany	325

Source: "USA Snapshots." *USA TODAY,* 27 September 1993, p. 1B. Primary source: Pharmaceutical Manufacturers Association.

★ 911 ★

Health Care Establishment: Drugs and Medicine

Tranquilizer Use

Table indicates daily users of tranquilizers per 100 people in selected countries.

Country	Users
Canada	0.1
Denmark	11.1
France	4.7
Germany	4.1
Italy	7.4
Japan	3.4
United States	3.3

Source: "Daily Dose: Tranquilizers or TV?" *Health* (January/February 1994), p. 24. Primary sources: World Health Organization; national surveys.

Health Care Establishment: Equipment and Facilities

★ 912 ★

Deaths From Sepsis in European and U.S. Hospitals

Sepsis is infection that occurs when a person's natural defenses to bacteria are activated; for example, after surgery or from feeding tubes. The table below reports annual deaths in hospitals from sepsis in Europe and the United States.

Location	Deaths
Europe	10,000
United States	200,000

Source: Howard, Nigel. "Who Says Hospitals Are Clean? Nearly Half the Patients in Intensive Care Are Given an Infection." *The European,* 13-19 May 1994, p. 22.

★ 913 ★

Health Care Establishment: Equipment and Facilities

Health Technology Equipment and Facilities in Selected Countries

[Technology facilities per million persons]

	United States	Canada	Germany
MRI machines	3.69	0.46	0.94
Open-heart surgery units	3.26	1.23	0.74
Lithotripsy machines	0.94	0.16	0.34

Source: Collins, Sara. "Cutting Edge Cures." *U.S. News & World Report,* 7 June 1993, p. 58. Primary source: *USN&WR*—Basic data: Dale Rublee, American Medical Association, Center for Health Policy Research, Office of Economic Cooperation and Development. *Notes:* Magnetic Resonance Imaging (MRI) machines are diagnostic tools. Lithotripsy machines dissolve kidney stones.

Health Care Establishment: Medical Personnel

★914★

Comparison of Patient/Doctor Ratios in Haiti and the United States

Country	People per doctor
Haiti	7,140
United States	419

Source: "Fleeing Haiti." *Detroit News,* 10 July 1994, p. B1. Primary sources: U.S. Coast Guard, U.S. Atlantic Command, National Oceanic Service, Joint Information Bureau Headquarters in Guantanamo Bay, National Hurricane Center, Gannett News Service, and *Detroit News.*

★915★

Health Care Establishment: Medical Personnel

Doctor Visits in Selected Countries

Japan - 12.8
Germany - 11.5
Canada - 6.6
United States - 5.3

Data show annual doctor visits per capita.

Country	Visits per capita
Canada	6.6
Germany	11.5
Japan	12.8
United States	5.3

Source: "How Do They Pull It Off?" *Health* (July/August 1993), p. 67.

★916★

Health Care Establishment: Medical Personnel

Hospital Personnel in OECD Countries: 1990

Data show the number of hospital staff per occupied bed in selected Organization for Economic Cooperation and Development (OECD) countries. Data are for 1990.

Country	Number
Austria	0.85
Denmark	2.83
France	1.09
Greece	1.48
Japan	0.79
Netherlands	2.13
Portugal	1.90
Switzerland	1.91
Turkey	1.48
United States	3.35

Source: "Health Care: The Issue Is Front and Center." *Public Perspective* (January/February 1993), p. 6. Primary sources: U.S. Bureau of the Census. *Statistical Abstract of the United States, 1992;* Health Care Financing Administration. *Health Care Financing Review* (summer 1992).

Health Care Establishment: Patient Care

★917★

Acute Inpatient Care Admission Rate, by Country: 1990

Country	Percent of population
Austria	20.5
Denmark	20.5
Finland	16.3
France	20.7
Ireland	14.9
Luxembourg	18.4
Netherlands	10.3
Portugal	10.6

[Continued]

★917★

Acute Inpatient Care Admission Rate, by Country: 1990

[Continued]

Country	Percent of population
Sweden	16.3
United States	12.4

Source: U.S. Department of Health and Human Services. Health Care Financing Adminstration (HCFA). *Health Care Financing Review* 13, no. 4 (summer 1992), pp. 30-31. Primary source: Organization for Economic Cooperation and Development (OECD). *OECD Health Data File* (1992).

★918★

Health Care Establishment: Patient Care

Acute Inpatient Medical Care Beds, by Country: 1990

Country	Average daily census
Austria	46,041
Finland	21,659
France	292,852
Luxembourg	2,671
Netherlands	64,580
Portugal	35,922
Sweden	33,503
Switzerland	43,851
Turkey	100,818
United States	929,000

Source: U.S. Department of Health and Human Services. Health Care Financing Adminstration (HCFA). *Health Care Financing Review* 13, no. 4 (summer 1992), p. 43. Primary source: Organization for Economic Cooperation and Development (OECD). *OECD Health Data File* (1992).

★ 919 ★

Health Care Establishment: Patient Care

Inpatient Care, by Country: 1990

Country	Bed days per person
Austria	3.0
Belgium	2.6
Canada	2.0
Denmark	1.7
Finland	4.1
France	2.9
Germany	3.4
Greece	1.1
Ireland	2.8
Italy	1.8
Japan	4.1
Luxembourg	3.7
Netherlands	3.7
New Zealand	2.1
Norway	5.0
Portugal	1.1
Spain	1.1
Sweden	3.5
Switzerland	2.9
Turkey	0.4
United Kingdom	2.0
United States	1.2

Source: U.S. Department of Health and Human Services. Health Care Financing Adminstration (HCFA). *Health Care Financing Review* 13, no. 4 (summer 1992), p. 25. Primary source: Organization for Economic Cooperation and Development (OECD). *OECD Health Data File* (1992).

★ 920 ★

Health Care Establishment: Patient Care

New Oncology Patients

Table reflects the number of new patients seen per year per oncologist. Data provided for selected countries.

Country	Number
Britain	560
France	200
Germany	140
Netherlands	250
Portugal	200

[Continued]

★ 920 ★

New Oncology Patients
[Continued]

Country	Number
Spain	200
United States	200

Source: "Tracking Cancer Treatment in Britain." *New York Time,* 26 June 1994, p. 4Y. Primary sources: Cancer Research Campaign, Britain; National Cancer Institute, United States; World Health Organization; International Agency for Research on Cancer; Royal College of Radiologists, Britain; CIE Monitor-Glaxo. *Note:* Data based on study published in 1991.

Health Care Establishment: Treatment and Procedures

★ 921 ★

Photorefractive Keratectomy Procedures: 1992 and 2000

The table below shows the estimated number of photorefractive keratectomy (PRK) procedures performed in selected countries. PRK is excimer laser surgery that reshapes the cornea of an eye to correct vision.

Country	1992	2000
United States	[1]	3,400,000
Canada	2,100	203,000
Europe	93,000	2,100,000
Asia	16,200	465,000
Other areas	1,600	437,500

Source: Morgan, Babette. "Seeing Is Believing: Outlook Bright for Laser Surgery That Helps Vision." *St. Louis Post-Dispatch,* 30 August 1993, p. 13BP. Estimates from Arthur D. Little Inc. (January 1992). *Note:* 1. Number of procedures limited by U.S. Food and Drug Administration.

★ 922 ★

Health Care Establishment: Treatment and Procedures

Polio Immunization

Table shows the percent of one-year-olds immunized against polio. Data are from 1990 and 1991.

Country	Percent
Sweden	99
Brazil	98
Cuba	97
Mexico	96
United States	95
Honduras	93
Rwanda	83

Source: Edelman, Marian Wright. "Give Children Health Security." *USA TODAY,* 9 December 1993, p. 15A. Primary sources: Children's Defense Fund; U.S. Committee for UNICEF.

Health Expenditures and Funding

★ 923 ★

Government Expenditures for Health, Housing and Social Security, and Education

| United Kingdom - 15.0 |
| France - 15.0 |
| United States - 14.0 |
| New Zealand - 12.7 |
| Brazil - 7.2 |
| Canada - 6.0 |
| Sri Lanka - 5.0 |
| India - 2.0 |
| Sweden - 0.9 |

Chart shows data from column 1.

Data compare the percentage of total government expenditures for health and related social welfare items with expenditures for education.

Country	Percent of total expenditures		
	Health	Housing and Social Security	Education
New Zealand	12.7	33.8	12.5
United States	14.0	29.0	2.0
Sweden	0.9	55.9	8.7
Brazil	7.2	20.1	5.3
Sri Lanka	5.0	15.0	10.0
India	2.0	7.0	3.0
Canada	6.0	37.0	3.0
France	15.0	46.0	7.0
United Kingdom	15.0	35.0	3.0

Source: "Social Standing." *India Today,* 31 January 1994, p. 100. Primary source: Confederation of Indian Industry (1993).

★ 924 ★

Health Expenditures and Funding

Per Capita Health Expenditures for Selected Countries: 1960-1991

Per capita health expenditures for each country have been adjusted to U.S. dollars using gross domestic product purchasing power parities for each year.

[In dollars]

Country	1960	1965	1970	1975	1980	1985	1990	1991[1]
Australia	99	127	207	438	663	998	1,310	1,407
Austria	69	94	163	369	683	984	1,383	1,448
Belgium	55	84	128	303	571	879	1,242	1,377
Canada	109	154	253	435	743	1,244	1,811	1,915
Denmark	70	125	212	340	582	807	1,051	1,151
Finland	57	95	164	305	517	855	1,291	1,426
France	75	124	203	386	698	1,083	1,528	1,650
Germany	98	135	216	458	811	1,175	1,522	1,659
Greece	16	27	58	102	184	282	400	404
Iceland	53	88	137	290	581	889	1,379	1,447
Ireland	38	53	97	231	449	572	748	845
Italy	51	83	153	280	571	814	1,296	1,408
Japan	27	64	127	256	517	792	1,175	1,267
Luxembourg	-	-	154	326	632	930	1,392	1,494
Netherlands	74	106	207	410	696	931	1,286	1,360
New Zealand	94	-	180	364	562	747	995	1,047
Norway	49	77	134	306	549	846	1,193	1,305
Portugal	-	-	46	157	238	398	554	624
Spain	14	38	82	187	325	452	774	848
Sweden	94	151	271	470	855	1,150	1,455	1,443
Switzerland	96	141	268	512	839	1,224	1,640	1,713
Turkey	-	-	-	36	64	66	133	142
United Kingdom	79	102	147	273	458	685	985	1,043
United States	143	204	346	592	1,063	1,711	2,600	2,868

Source: U.S. Department of Health and Human Services. Public Health Service. Centers for Disease Control and Prevention. National Center for Health Statistics. *Health, United States, 1992.* Hyattsville, MD: Public Health Service, 1993, p. 161. Data compiled by the Organization for Economic Cooperation and Development. Primary sources: 1) Schieber, G. J., J. P Poullier, and L. G. Greenwald. "U.S. Health Expenditure Performance: An International Comparison and Data Update." *Health Care Financing Review* 13, no. 4 (September 1992). 2) Office of National Health Statistics. Office of the Actuary. "National Health Expenditures, 1991." *Health Care Financing Review* 14, no. 2 (winter 1993). 3) Unpublished data. *Notes:* Some numbers in this table have been revised and differ from previous editions of *Health, United States.* 1. Preliminary figures.

★ 925 ★

Health Expenditures and Funding

Percentage of Government Medical Care Expenditures on the Elderly Population by Country: 1980-2025

From the source: "With the shift in the age structure of the population, an associated change will take place in the underlying structure of demand for services, creating imbalances between available physical capacity and professional manpower resources and the structure of demand. This change will undoubtedly create short-term transitional adjustment difficulties. For example, the share of government expenditure on medical care consumed by the age group 65 and over will substantially increase. In the Federal Republic of Germany, Italy, and the United Kingdom, it will increase by 7-9 percentage points between 1980 and 2025; in Canada, Japan, and the United States, the increase will be even more dramatic. This increased share will be reflected in a change in the demand for particular services, with obviously increased needs for nursing home facilities and for professionals and paraprofessionals trained in geriatric care. An associated problem will be the need to 'retool' plants and retrain professionals in specialties less in demand."

Country	1980	2000	2010	2025
Canada	33.3	38.0	40.9	53.1
Germany, Fed. Rep. of[1]	33.1	33.6	39.0	42.6
Italy	31.8	36.2	37.4	40.6
Japan	27.4	37.7	43.8	48.3
United Kingdom	42.1	44.1	44.3	49.4
United States	50.0	54.4	55.6	64.6

Source: Heller, Peter S., Richard Hemming, Peter W. Kohnert, and others. *Aging and Social Expenditure in the Major Industrial Countries, 1980-2025.* International Monetary Fund, September 1986, p. 45. *Notes:* Gross Domestic Product excludes expenditure on medical research and education, administration, and capital investment in the medical sector. 1. People included are those over age sixty.

★ 926 ★

Health Expenditures and Funding

Projected Increases in Real Government Expenditures on Medical Care for Selected Countries: 2000 and 2025

Data show increases in expenditures using 1980 as the reference year.

[Index: 1980 = 100]

Country	Year		
	1980	2000	2025
United States	100.0	130.0	180.0
France	100.0	117.0	130.0
West Germany	100.0	104.0	103.0
Italy	100.0	113.0	121.0
United Kingdom	100.0	105.0	115.0

[Continued]

★ 926 ★

Projected Increases in Real Government Expenditures on Medical Care for Selected Countries: 2000 and 2025

[Continued]

Country	Year		
	1980	2000	2025
Canada	100.0	128.0	174.0
Japan	100.0	130.0	147.0

Source: Aging America: Trends and Projections. 1991 ed. Prepared by the U.S. Senate Special Committee on Aging, the American Association of Retired Persons, the Federal Council on the Aging, and the U.S. Administration on Aging. DHHS Publication No. (FCoA) 91-28001. Washington, DC: U.S. Department of Health and Human Services (DHHS), 1991, p. 270. Primary source: Heller, Peter S., Richard Hemming, and Peter W. Kohnert. *Aging and Social Expenditure in the Major Industrial Countries, 1980-2025.* Occasional Paper 47. International Monetary Fund (IMF), September 1986.

★ 927 ★

Health Expenditures and Funding

Total Health Expenditures as a Percent of Gross Domestic Product for Selected Countries: 1960-1991

Country	1960	1965	1970	1975	1980	1985	1990	1991[1]
Australia	4.9	5.1	5.7	7.5	7.3	7.7	8.2	8.6
Austria	4.4	4.7	5.4	7.3	7.9	8.1	8.3	8.4
Belgium	3.4	3.9	4.1	5.9	6.6	7.4	7.6	7.9
Canada	5.5	6.0	7.1	7.2	7.4	8.5	9.5	10.0
Denmark	3.6	4.8	6.1	6.5	6.8	6.3	6.3	6.5
Finland	3.9	4.9	5.7	6.3	6.5	7.2	7.8	8.9
France	4.2	5.2	5.8	7.0	7.6	8.5	8.8	9.1
Germany	4.8	5.1	5.9	8.1	8.4	8.7	8.3	8.5
Greece	2.9	3.1	4.0	4.1	4.3	4.9	5.4	5.2
Iceland	3.5	4.2	5.2	6.2	6.4	7.1	8.3	8.4
Ireland	4.0	4.4	5.6	8.0	9.2	8.2	7.0	7.3
Italy	3.6	4.3	5.2	6.1	6.9	7.0	8.1	8.3
Japan	3.0	4.5	4.6	5.6	6.6	6.5	6.5	6.6
Luxembourg	-	-	4.1	5.6	6.8	6.8	7.2	7.2
Netherlands	3.9	4.4	6.0	7.6	8.0	8.0	8.2	8.3
New Zealand	4.3	-	5.2	6.7	7.2	6.5	7.3	7.6
Norway	3.3	3.9	5.0	6.7	6.6	6.4	7.4	7.6
Portugal	-	-	3.1	6.4	5.9	7.0	6.7	6.8
Spain	1.5	2.5	3.7	4.8	5.6	5.7	6.6	6.7
Sweden	4.7	5.6	7.2	7.9	9.4	8.8	8.6	8.6
Switzerland	3.3	3.8	5.2	7.0	7.3	7.6	7.8	7.9
Turkey	-	-	-	3.5	4.0	2.8	4.0	4.0

[Continued]

★ 927 ★

Total Health Expenditures as a Percent of Gross Domestic Product for Selected Countries: 1960-1991
[Continued]

Country	1960	1965	1970	1975	1980	1985	1990	1991[1]
United Kingdom	3.9	4.1	4.5	5.5	5.8	6.0	6.2	6.6
United States	5.3	5.9	7.4	8.4	9.2	10.5	12.2	13.2

Source: U.S. Department of Health and Human Services. Public Health Service. Centers for Disease Control and Prevention. National Center for Health Statistics. *Health, United States, 1992.* Hyattsville, MD: Public Health Service, 1993, p. 161. Data compiled by the Organization for Economic Cooperation and Development. Primary sources: 1) Schieber, G. J., J. P Poullier, and L. G. Greenwald. "U.S. Health Expenditure Performance: An International Comparison and Data Update." *Health Care Financing Review* 13, no. 4 (September 1992). 2) Office of National Health Statistics. Office of the Actuary. "National Health Expenditures, 1991." *Health Care Financing Review* 14, no. 2 (winter 1993). 3) Unpublished data. *Notes:* Some numbers in this table have been revised and differ from previous editions of *Health, United States.* 1. Preliminary figures.

★ 928 ★

Health Expenditures and Funding

Total Health Expenditures, by Country: 1990
[National currency in millions]

Country	1990 expenditures
Australia	30,974
Austria	150,000
Belgium	482,150
Canada	61,753
Denmark	50,947
Finland	40,979
France	572,900
Germany	195,000
Greece	572,000
Iceland	29,231
Ireland	1,808
Italy	100,860,000
Japan	28,300,000
Luxembourg	21,000
Netherlands	41,499
New Zealand	5,277
Norway	49,255
Portugal	566,000
Spain	3,300,000
Sweden	116,200
Switzerland	24,300
Turkey	11,240,000

[Continued]

★ 928 ★

Total Health Expenditures, by Country: 1990
[Continued]

Country	1990 expenditures
United Kingdom	34,033
United States	666,187

Source: U.S. Department of Health and Human Services. Health Care Financing Adminstration (HCFA). *Health Care Financing Review* 13, no. 4 (summer 1992), p. 19. Primary source: Organization for Economic Cooperation and Development (OECD). *OECD Health Data File* (1992).

Health Status: Babies and Children

★ 929 ★

Abortion Rates

Data indicate the number of abortions per 1,000 women, ages 15 to 44, in selected countries.

Country	Abortion rate
Australia	16.6
Canada	11.2
China	37.5
Cuba	56.5
Germany	8.7
Ireland[1]	5.4
Italy	12.7
Japan	14.5
Lithuania	30.1
South Korea	6.4
Poland	3.6
Romania	172.4
Russia	119.6
Singapore	25.7
United Kingdom	14.8
United States	26.4

Source: "World Abortion Rates." *The Mirror* (Springfield, Missouri), 13 May 1994, p. 10. Primary source: United Nations Department for Economic and Social Information and Policy Analysis (1994). *Notes:* 1. Based on number of abortions obtained by residents of Ireland in England and Wales.

★ 930 ★

Health Status: Babies and Children

Babies Who Die Before Age One in Selected Countries: 1991

Country	Income per capita	Average number of deaths per 1,000 births
Brazil	$2,920	55
Mexico	2,870	30
Russia	3,220	23
China	370	22
United States	22,560	9

Source: "Infant Mortality: How Brazil Compares." *New York Times,* 14 May 1993, p. A8. Primary source: UNICEF; World Bank Atlas.

★ 931 ★

Health Status: Babies and Children

Deaths From Child Abuse Throughout the World: 1985-1990

Data reflect the deaths from child abuse per 100,000 births from 1985 through 1990. Data are provided by country.

Country	Number
Czechoslovakia	10.1
United States	9.8
Soviet Union	8.7
Denmark	8.1
Japan	7.4

Source: Greene, Marilyn "Women Called Key to Helping Third World." *USA TODAY,* 21 June 1994, p. 8A. Primary source: United Nations Children's Fund. *The Progress of Nations, 1994.*

★ 932 ★

Health Status: Babies and Children

Infant Mortality: 1990

Data reflect mortality rates of babies in selected countries. Data are for 1990.

Country	Mortality rate
Japan	4.0
Ireland	5.0
Finland	6.0
Hong Kong	6.0
Netherlands	6.0
Norway	6.0
Singapore	6.0
Sweden	6.0
Australia	7.0
Austria	7.0
Britain	7.0
Canada	7.0
Denmark	7.0
France	7.0
Germany	7.0
Switzerland	7.0
Greece	8.0
Italy	8.0
New Zealand	8.0
South Korea	8.0
Spain	8.0
Belgium	9.0
Israel	9.0
United States	9.0
Cuba	10.0
Czech Republic	11.0
Portugal	11.0
Jamaica	12.0
Slovakia	12.0
Costa Rica	14.0
Kuwait	14.0
Malaysia	14.0
Poland	14.0
Chile	15.0
Hungary	15.0
Sri Lanka	15.0
Bulgaria	16.0
Taiwan	16.6
Colombia	17.0
Lithuania	17.0
Panama	18.0
United Arab Emirates	18.0
Trinidad	19.0
Yugoslavia	19.0
Belarus	20.0

[Continued]

★ 932 ★

Infant Mortality: 1990
[Continued]

Country	Mortality rate
Estonia	20.0
Kazakhstan	20.0
Mauritius	20.0
Uruguay	20.0
Venezuela	20.0
Ukraine	21.0
Argentina	22.0
Latvia	22.0
Romania	23.0
Oman	24.0
Georgia	25.0
Jordan	25.0
North Korea	25.0
Thailand	27.0
Albania	28.0
Mexico	28.0
Paraguay	28.0
Russian Federation	28.0
Armenia	29.0
China	35.0
Vietnam	37.0
Philippines	46.0
Papua New Guinea	54.0
Mongolia	61.0
Indonesia	71.0
India	83.0
Nepal	90.0
Pakistan	95.0
Bangladesh	97.0
Myanmar	117.0

Source: "Healthy Babies." *Asiaweek,* 1 June 1994, p. 16. Primary source: United Nations Children's Fund. Data for Taiwan from Britannica World Data. *Notes:* Infant mortality is death under the age of 1. Mortality rate is the number of babies who die per 1,000 births.

★ 933 ★

Health Status: Babies and Children

Low Birth Weight Infants

Table shows the percent of babies born at low birth weights in selected countries. Data are from 1990 and 1991.

Country	Percent
Spain	4
Bulgaria	6
Costa Rica	6
United States	7
Botswana	8
El Salvador	11
Haiti	15

Source: Edelman, Marian Wright. "Give Children Health Security." *USA TODAY,* 9 December 1993, p. 15A. Primary sources: Children's Defense Fund; U.S. Committee for UNICEF.

Health Status: Death

★ 934 ★

Circulatory System Disease Age-Adjusted Mortality Rates: 1990

Data reflect mortality rates adjusted on the basis of age distribution of the U.S. total population, 1940. Data are for men and women ages 35 through 74.

[Rate per 100,000]

Country	Men	Women
Canada	301.6	128.2
Denmark	408.2	174.6
England and Wales	454.0	198.8
Finland[1]	569.3	200.6
France	214.1	77.3
Germany[1][2]	393.3	160.2
Iceland	303.2	138.8
Japan	205.7	103.6
Netherlands	347.6	131.6
Northern Ireland	551.0	256.1
Norway	422.4	151.9
Scotland	569.1	279.2
Sweden	360.3	140.8

[Continued]

★ 934 ★

Circulatory System Disease Age-Adjusted Mortality Rates: 1990

[Continued]

Country	Men	Women
Switzerland	285.2	103.3
United States	402.8	188.0

Source: Metropolitan Life Insurance Company. "Heart Disease Mortality: International Comparisons." *Statistical Bulletin* 74, no. 4 (October-December 1993), p. 26. *Notes:* 1. 1989 data. 2. Federal Republic of Germany.

★ 935 ★

Health Status: Death

Circulatory System Disease Relative Mortality Rates: 1990

Data reflect mortality rates from diseases of the ciculatory system for men and women ages 35 through 74.

[Percent of U.S. mortality]

Country	Men	Women
Canada	75	68
Denmark	101	93
England and Wales	113	106
Finland	141	107
France	53	41
Germany[1]	98	85
Iceland	75	74
Japan	51	55
Netherlands	86	70
Northern Ireland	137	136
Norway	105	81
Scotland	141	149
Sweden	89	75
Switzerland	71	55
United States	100	100

Source: Metropolitan Life Insurance Company. "Heart Disease Mortality: International Comparisons." *Statistical Bulletin* 74, no. 4 (October-December 1993), pp. 24-25. *Note:* 1. Federal Republic of Germany.

★ 936 ★

Health Status: Death

Death Rates by Selected Causes for Various Countries

Age-standardized death rate per 100,000 population. The standard population for this table is the European standard.

Country	Year	Ischemic heart disease	Cerebro-vascular disease	Cancer Lung, trachea, bronchus	Cancer Stomach	Cancer Female breast	Bronchitis,[1] emphysema, asthma	Chronic liver disease and cirrhosis	Motor vehicle traffic accidents	Suicide and self-inflicted injury
Australia	1988	200.5	77.9	40.4	9.0	29.6	14.6	8.1	17.8	13.3
Austria	1990	151.0	96.9	34.3	17.8	32.1	18.2	25.8	16.8	21.7
Belgium	1986	110.4	83.0	55.5	13.8	38.1	26.3	12.6	19.6	21.0
Bulgaria	1990	230.1	226.2	30.7	22.7	21.1	13.0	16.0	15.5	13.1
Canada	1989	172.2	52.9	54.3	8.6	34.1	8.4	9.4	15.4	13.1
Czechoslovakia	1990	314.4	183.5	53.2	20.1	28.7	21.1	26.1	13.6	18.3
Denmark	1990	211.1	72.5	53.2	8.5	38.5	39.0	13.4	10.9	22.4
England and Wales	1990	210.0	86.1	53.2	12.6	40.7	12.7	5.7	8.9	7.5
Finland	1989	243.2	98.5	33.8	15.5	23.9	17.2	10.0	14.0	27.5
France	1989	64.3	59.2	34.5	9.2	28.1	10.0	18.3	17.3	19.6
Germany[2]	1989	150.3	87.3	35.9	16.3	32.9	22.3	20.1	11.1	14.5
Hungary	1990	240.0	177.4	61.2	24.4	32.3	40.5	50.7	24.4	38.2
Italy	1988	97.4	102.3	44.1	20.5	29.6	23.9	24.9	14.2	7.0
Japan	1990	37.9	90.3	26.8	35.2	8.5	11.0	12.7	11.1	15.4
Netherlands	1989	134.9	67.8	54.6	13.4	39.0	18.2	5.5	8.9	10.0
New Zealand	1987	248.6	88.8	45.5	10.9	40.2	19.8	4.2	22.8	12.6
Norway	1989	186.9	84.2	27.5	12.3	27.3	13.6	5.7	8.5	15.3
Poland	1990	121.0	73.1	51.4	21.2	22.6	25.0	11.4	22.4	13.8
Portugal	1990	85.6	216.6	21.3	27.8	25.7	13.9	24.5	26.9	8.5
Scotland	1990	258.3	112.9	66.9	13.6	37.5	9.9	9.5	9.9	10.1
Spain	1987	75.3	100.2	30.6	17.1	23.2	10.1	20.6	16.6	7.1
Sweden	1988	209.3	69.0	23.9	10.3	26.8	13.1	6.1	8.8	17.8
Switzerland	1990	109.7	57.2	35.1	10.3	35.8	19.9	9.3	12.8	20.1
United States	1988	188.1	53.6	55.4	5.4	32.0	9.1	11.7	18.7	12.2

Source: 1993 Statistical Abstract of the United States on CD-ROM [machine-readable datafiles]. CD-ABSTR-93. Washington, DC: U.S. Department of Commerce, Economics and Statistics Administration, Bureau of the Census, Data User Services Division, 1993. Primary source: World Health Organization. *1991 World Health Statistics* (annual). Geneva, Switzerland *Notes:* 1. Chronic and unspecified. 2. Former West Germany (prior to unification).

Health Status: Diseases

★ 937 ★

AIDS Cases Worldwide: 1993

The World Health Organization counted in excess of 850,000 cases of AIDS at the end of 1993. The table below indicates the percent of reported cases for each area of the world.

Area	Percent of AIDS Cases
Africa	35.5
Asia	0.5
Europe	12.0
North and South America[1]	11.5
United States	40.0
Western Pacific Region	0.5

Source: Anstett, Patricia. "Needle Exchange Slows the Spread of AIDS." *Detroit Free Press,* 18 January 1994, p. 4F. Primary source: World Health Organization *Note:* 1. Excludes United States.

★ 938 ★

Health Status: Diseases

Cholera: 1992

Table offers data for 1992 regarding cholera cases reported to the Pan American Health Organization, Western Hemisphere. Countries are ranked by number of cases.

Country	1992	
	Cases	Deaths
Peru	206,565	709
Ecuador	31,870	208
Brazil	24,039	312
Bolivia	21,324	383
Guatemala	15,178	207
Colombia[1]	15,129	158
El Salvador	8,109	45
Mexico	7,814	99
Nicaragua	3,067	46
Venezuela	2,456	62
Panama	2,416	49
Argentina	553	15
Honduras	384	17
Guyana	290	4
Belize	154	4

[Continued]

★ 938 ★

Cholera: 1992
[Continued]

Country	1992 Cases	Deaths
United States	102	1
Chile	71	1
French Guyana	16	0
Suriname	12	1
Costa Rica	12	0
Canada	0	0

Source: U.S. Department of Health and Human Services. Public Health Service. Centers for Disease Control and Prevention. "Update: Cholera." *Morbidity and Mortality Weekly Report* 42, no. 5, 12 February 1993, p. 90. *Note:* 1. Preliminary data.

★ 939 ★

Health Status: Diseases

HIV Infections, by Continent

Continent	Number
Australia and the Pacific Islands	25,000+
East Asia	25,000+
Europe and the Commonwealth of Independent States	550,000
Latin America and the Caribbean	1.5 million+
North Africa and the Middle East	75,000+
North America	1 million+
South/Southeast Asia	1.5 million
Sub-Saharan Africa	8 million+

Source: "HIV Infections—Continent by Continent." *World Newsmap of the Week* 56, no. 13, 6 December 1993, n.p.

★ 940 ★

Health Status: Diseases

Prevalence of Human Immunodeficiency Virus in Adults Throughout the World: 1993

The table below reflects the estimated distribution of Human Immunodeficiency Virus (HIV) prevalence in adults for late 1993.

[In millions]

Place	Prevalence
Sub-Saharan Africa	7.00+
South Asia	2.00
Southeast Asia	2.00
Latin America	1.00+
Caribbean	1.00+
North America	.80
Western Europe	.40
North Africa	.08
Middle East	.08
Eastern Europe	.05
Central Asia	.05
East Asia and Pacific	.03
Australasia	.02
Global total	11-12

Source: Berkley, Seth, Peter Piot, and Doris Schopper. "AIDS: Invest Now or Pay More Later." *Finance & Development* 31, no. 2 (June 1994), p. 40. Primary source: World Health Organization.

★ 941 ★

Health Status: Diseases

Tuberculosis: 1992

Data reflect tuberculosis case notifications per 100,000 people during 1992 (unless otherwise noted.) Actual incidence may be higher. Data provided for selected countries.

Country	Cases of tuberculosis
Philippines[1]	324.9
Zambia	297.9
Tuvalu	291.7
Botswana[1]	257.1
Peru	234.1
South Africa	203.7
Mauritania	201.4
Lesotho	181.2
India[1]	160.3
Pakistan[1]	160.0

[Continued]

★ 941 ★

Tuberculosis: 1992
[Continued]

Country	Cases of tuberculosis
Wallis[2]	157.1
Haiti[1]	154.7
Vanuatu[1]	152.9
Kiribati	135.1
Afghanistan[1]	130.4
Guinea-Bissau[1]	126.6
Bolivia	126.5
Ethiopia[1]	116.8
Namibia	114.5
Zimbabwe	114.1
Hong Kong	112.7
South Korea	106.6
Solomon Islands	106.4
Tanzania	102.3
New Caledonia	101.7
Mozambique	101.4
Angola	99.7
Sao Tome[3]	99.2
Morocco	96.5
Equatorial Guinea[1]	93.3
Vietnam[1]	87.8
Burundi[1]	86.3
Mongolia	85.0
Iraq[4]	81.2
Yemen	79.0
Romania	77.6
Honduras	76.1
Gabon	74.9
Uganda	74.2
Sudan	73.2
Nicaragua	72.9
Ivory Coast	70.4
Senegal[4]	67.9
Niger[4]	67.3
Macau[1]	66.8
Brunei	66.7
Central African Republic[1]	66.2
Malawi	64.3
Kazakhstan	64.1
Ecuador[1]	63.7
Madagascar	63.4
Singapore	63.4
Papua New Guinea	62.6
St. Lucia	61.9
Cape Verde	60.9
Kenya	57.9

[Continued]

★ 941 ★

Tuberculosis: 1992
[Continued]

Country	Cases of tuberculosis
Seychelles[4]	57.7
Portugal[1]	55.7
Zaire[1]	54.7
Indonesia	51.5
Cambodia	49.1
Nepal[1]	44.8
Japan[1]	40.6
Maldives	40.5
Thailand	38.4
Malaysia	34.4
Fiji[1]	33.7
China[1]	32.1
Bangladesh	25.7
Sri Lanka	22.8
Myanmar	15.6
France	15.3
United States	10.5
New Zealand	9.5
Bhutan	8.7
Laos	8.5
Australia	5.5

Source: "A New TB Threat." Asiaweek, 4 May 1994, p. 24. Primary source: World Health Organization. Notes: 1. 1991 data. 2. Includes Futuna; 1990 data. 3. Includes Principe; 1991 data. 4. 1990 data.

Health Status: Life Expectancy

★ 942 ★

Life Expectancy at Birth for Selected Countries: 1990

From the source: "As of 1990, life expectancy at birth was highest in Japan—79.3 years... Americans born in 1990 could expect to live an average of 75.6 years, which was a lower life expectancy than that of many other developed nations. The nearly four-year difference in life expectancy between the United States and Japan has more to do with infant mortality than aging. At age 65, life expectancy is about the same in the two countries (Japanese men at that age could expect to live about six months longer and Japanese women about six months less than their counterparts in the United States in 1985). However, the infant mortality rate in Japan is about one-half the U.S. rate." Data are provided by sex and differential.

[Numbers in years]

Country	Both sexes	Men	Women	Difference (women minus men)
Canada	77.3	74.0	80.6	6.6
France	77.6	73.4	81.9	8.5
Germany	77.2	73.4	80.6	7.2
Italy	78.0	74.5	81.4	6.9
Japan	79.3	76.4	82.1	5.7
Sweden	77.7	74.7	80.7	6.0
United Kingdom	76.2	73.2	79.2	6.0
United States	75.6	72.1	79.0	6.9

Source: *Aging America: Trends and Projections.* 1991 ed. Prepared by the U.S. Senate Special Committee on Aging, the American Association of Retired Persons, the Federal Council on the Aging, and the U.S. Administration on Aging. DHHS Publication No. (FCoA) 91-28001. Washington, DC: U.S. Department of Health and Human Services (DHHS), 1991, p. 258. Primary source: U.S. Bureau of the Census. International Data Base.

★ 943 ★

Health Status: Life Expectancy

Life Expectancy in Haiti and the United States

Country	Years
Haiti	55.7
United States	75.9

Source: "Fleeing Haiti." *Detroit News,* 10 July 1994, p. B1. Primary sources: U.S. Coast Guard, U.S. Atlantic Command, National Oceanic Service, Joint Information Bureau Headquarters in Guantanamo Bay, National Hurricane Center, Gannett News Service, and *Detroit News.*

★ 944 ★

Health Status: Life Expectancy

Life Expectancy Worldwide: 1955-2000

In 1950 through 1955, life expectancy worldwide was 47.4 years. Life expectancy is predicted to rise to 64.5 years for 1995 through 2000. The lowest life expectancy for men is 39.4 years in Ethiopia and Sierre Leone. The lowest for women is 42 years in Afghanistan. The highest is 81.9 years for women and 75.8 years for men in Japan.

Source: Guinness Book of Records, 1992. New York: Bantam Books, 1992, p. 197.

Lifestyles and Health: Insurance

★ 945 ★

Insurance Coverage in Selected Nations and the United States: 1990

[In percentages]

Insurance coverage	United States	Canada	France	Germany	Netherlands[2]	United Kingdom
Public insurance						
Primary	18	100	100	90[1]	62[3]	100
Supplemental	None	None	None	None	100[4]	None
Private insurance						
Primary	62	None	None	9	37	None
Supplemental	11	00	00	7	13	10
Uninsured	13	None	None	Negligible	Negligible	None

Source: U.S. Department of Labor. Pension and Welfare Benefits Administration. *Trends in Health Benefits.* Washington, DC: U.S. Government Printing Office, 1993, pp. 23-25. *Notes:* 1. Compulsory for 75 percent. 2. Data on the percent of the Netherlands population covered by public and private plans are for 1990. At this writing, the Netherlands is redesigning the relative roles of its public and private insurance systems. 3. Basic coverage. 4. Long-term and chronic medical expenses.

★ 946 ★

Lifestyles and Health: Insurance

Medical Insurance Payments Worldwide

The table below reflects the percentage of health care bills paid by medical insurance in selected countries.

Country	Percent
United Kingdom	93
Japan	87
Canada	82
United States	61

Source: "USA Snapshots." *USA TODAY,* 17 June 1994, p. 1A. Primary source: United Nations.

★ 947 ★

Lifestyles and Health: Insurance

Population Without Health Insurance

Table ranks the percent of population in selected countries without health insurance.

Country	Percent	Rank
United States	14.7	1
Germany	1.0	2
France	0.5	3

Source: White House Domestic Policy Council. *Health Security: The President's Report to the American People.* Washington, DC: The White House, October 1993, p. 11. Primary source: Organization of Economic Cooperation and Development, Department of Health and Human Resources.

Lifestyles and Health: Smoking

★ 948 ★

Death Rate Among Smokers

Worldwide, almost 3 million people die annually from smoking-related causes—an average of 1 death every 10 seconds. This accounts for 1.5 million deaths in the industrialized world. The table below offers data on deaths in selected countries.

Countries	Deaths
Africa	100,000
Latin America	100,000
Asia[1]	200,000
China	300,000
United States of America	400,000
Former Union of Soviet Socialist Republics countries	400,000

Source: Khaltaev, Nikolai. "Inter-Health Fights Life-Style Diseases." *World Health* (May-June 1991), pp. 18-20. *Note:* 1. Excludes China and India.

★ 949 ★

Lifestyles and Health: Smoking

Smokers Worldwide

Table reflects percentage of adult population that smokes.

Country	Men	Women
Australia	30	27
Cambodia[1]	90	3
China	61	7
Hong Kong[2]	29	3
India	40	3
Indonesia	65	5
Japan	61	14
Malaysia	41	5
New Zealand	28	27
Philippines	64	19
Singapore	30	2
South Korea	70	7
Thailand	47	4
United States[3]	28	24
Vietnam	24	1

Source: "The Cigarette's Open Frontier." *New York Times,* 15 May 1994, p. E16. Primary source: World Health Organization. Provisional estimates for 1994. *Notes:* 1. Cambodian government estimate. 2. Figure from Hong Kong government survey, 1990. 3. Figure for 1991 from Centers for Disease Control.

Lifestyles and Health: Suicide and Homicide

★ 950 ★

Suicide Rates for Selected Countries: 1990

Rate per 100,000 population. Includes deaths resulting indirectly from self-inflicted injuries.

Sex and age	United States[1]	Austria	Canada	Denmark	Japan	Poland	United Kingdom[2]
Male							
Total[3]	20.0	34.8	20.4	32.2	20.4	22.0	12.1
15 to 24 years old	22.0	25.0	25.2	14.1	9.2	16.2	11.7
25 to 34 years old	24.4	32.7	29.3	26.7	18.4	30.4	16.0
35 to 44 years old	22.4	37.3	26.3	44.5	21.5	33.0	17.1
45 to 54 years old	22.7	47.7	22.7	53.0	32.0	38.4	16.4
55 to 64 years old	24.8	44.0	22.9	43.7	32.5	36.3	13.3
65 to 74 years old	33.6	66.8	20.8	47.3	36.6	28.0	13.6
75 yrs. old and over	54.5	107.6	32.7	76.7	62.9	27.3	19.4
Female							
Total[3]	4.8	13.4	5.3	16.3	12.4	4.5	3.7
15 to 24 years old	4.2	5.5	5.1	4.0	4.7	2.8	2.0
25 to 34 years old	5.6	8.4	6.5	6.9	9.0	4.3	3.8
35 to 44 years old	6.6	13.9	8.9	18.4	9.2	6.0	4.5
45 to 54 years old	7.4	16.5	7.3	27.3	15.0	7.4	5.1
55 to 64 years old	7.3	20.8	5.5	31.5	17.6	8.7	5.3
65 to 74 years old	5.9	22.0	6.0	30.0	25.3	7.2	6.1
75 yrs. old and over	6.0	35.5	4.2	32.2	48.6	7.4	6.2

Source: 1993 Statistical Abstract of the United States on CD-ROM [machine-readable datafiles]. CD-ABSTR-93. Washington, DC: U.S. Department of Commerce, Economics and Statistics Administration, Bureau of the Census, Data User Services Division, 1993. Primary source: World Health Organization (Geneva, Switzerland). *World Health Statistics Annual;* and unpublished data. *Notes:* 1. Data for 1989. 2. England and Wales only. 3. Includes under 15 years old not shown separately.

★ 951 ★

Lifestyles and Health: Suicide and Homicide

Teen Suicides Throughout the World: 1991

Data reflect the deaths of teenagers 15 to 19 years old from suicide during 1991. Data are provided by country.

[Per 100,000]

Country	Number
New Zealand	15.7
Finland	15.0
Canada	13.5
Norway	13.4
United States	11.1

Source: Greene, Marilyn. "Women Called Key to Helping Third World." *USA TODAY,* 21 June 1994, p. 8A. Primary source: United Nations Children's Fund. *The Progress of Nations, 1994.*

★ 952 ★

Lifestyles and Health: Suicide and Homicide

Youth Homicides Throughout the World: 1991

Data reflect the deaths of teenagers 15 to 19 years old from homicide during 1991. Data are provided by country.

[Per 100,000]

Country	Number
United States	16.9
Russia	10.2
Kazakhstan	7.8
Kyrgyzstan	6.1
Belarus	5.4

Source: Greene, Marilyn. "Women Called Key to Helping Third World." *USA TODAY,* 21 June 1994, p. 8A. Primary source: United Nations Children's Fund. *The Progress of Nations, 1994.*

Medical Establishment: Administration

★ 953 ★

Hospital Billing in Canada and the United States

The average Canadian hospital utilizes 6 employees and spends 8 percent of its health care dollars on billing the single payer and the provincial government and on other administrative tasks. The average hospital in the United States, however, utilizes 50 employees and spends 18 percent of its health care dollars on billing and administration, using $1 million worth of equipment.

Source: Haiven, Judy. "MediScare." *Mother Jones* 16 (March-April 1991), pp. 50-53, 67-69.

★ 954 ★

Medical Establishment: Administration

Time and Cost of Paperwork for Physicians in Canada and the United States

Table shows the average time and the dollar amount spent on paperwork by doctors.

Location	Time	Cost
Canada	30 seconds	$1.00/patient
United States	7 minutes	$7.00/patient

Source: Haiven, Judy. "MediScare." *Mother Jones* 16 (March-April 1991), pp. 50-53, 67-69.

Medical Establishment: Grants and Contracts

★955★

Distribution of National Heart, Lung, and Blood Institute Awards, by Country: 1991

The table below presents a geographic distribution of awards from the National Heart, Lung, and Blood Institute (NHLBI) for the 1991 fiscal year.

	Totals		Research grants		Research training and development		Contracts	
	Number	Dollars	Number	Dollars	Number	Dollars	Number	Dollars
Belgium	1	84,245	-	-	-	-	1	84,245
Canada	21	3,748,999	10	1,546,135	1	36,242	10	2,166,622
China	1	86,438	1	86,438	-	-	-	
Germany[1]	1	68,494	1	68,494	-	-	-	-
Israel	1	69,781	1	69,781	-	-	-	-
Puerto Rico	1	300,119	1	300,119	-	-	-	-
Sweden	2	52,200	-	-	2	52,200	-	-
Switzerland	1	85,000	-	-	-	-	1	85,000
Thailand	2	188,142	2	188,142	-	-	-	-
Trinidad/Tobago	0	4,000	0	4,000	-	-	-	-
United Kingdom	6	517,487	4	351,034	1	19,700	1	146,753
United States	4,031	974,056,530	3,437	822,577,000	305	45,256,505	199	106,222,642

Source: U.S. Department of Health and Human Services. Public Health Service. National Institutes of Health. National Heart, Lung, and Blood Institute (NHLBI). *NHLBI Fact Book, Fiscal Year 1991.* Washington, DC: U.S. Department of Health and Human Services, Public Health Service, National Institutes of Health, National Heart, Lung, and Blood Institute (NHLBI), c. 1992, p. 146-148. *Note:* 1. Federal Republic of Germany.

Medical Establishment: Technology and Research

★ 956 ★

Biotechnology Patent Holders: 1992

Figures indicate the country of origin for holders of health-related biotechnology patents issued by the U.S. Patents and Trademark Office in 1992.

Country	Percent
United States	69
Japan	13
Europe	12

Source: "U.S. Maintains Its Lead." *Chemistry and Industry,* 18 October 1993, p. 784. Primary source: U.S. Pharmaceutical Manufacturers Association.

★ 957 ★

Medical Establishment: Technology and Research

Worldwide Spending on Medical Research

The table below reflects the percentage of a country's gross national product that is devoted to medical research and development.

Country	Percent	Rank
Japan	3.04	1
Germany	2.67	2
United States	1.8	3

Source: De Bakey, Michael E. "Medical Centers of Excellence and Health Reform." *Science* 262, no. 5133, 22 October 1993, p. 523.

Medical Professions

★ 958 ★

Physician Incomes in Selected Countries: 1990

Table shows annual physician net incomes for 1990.

[In dollars]

Country	Average net income
Canada	105,000
Germany	102,000
Japan	80,000
United States	164,000

Source: "How Do They Pull It Off?" Health (July/August 1993), p. 67.

★ 959 ★

Medical Professions

Practicing Physicians, by Country: 1990

Country	Number of active physicians
Austria	16,425
Belgium	34,275
Canada	59,409
Denmark	14,277
Finland	12,091
France	152,096
Japan	203,797
Luxembourg	766
Netherlands	37,461
Norway	13,234
Portugal	28,016
Spain	148,717
Sweden	24,600
Switzerland	20,030
Turkey	50,639
United States	601,100

Source: U.S. Department of Health and Human Services. Health Care Financing Adminstration (HCFA). Health Care Financing Review 13, no. 4 (summer 1992), p. 45. Primary source: Organization for Economic Cooperation and Development (OECD). OECD Health Data File (1992).

Politics, Opinion, and Law

★ 960 ★

Opinions on Health Care Reform in France and the United States

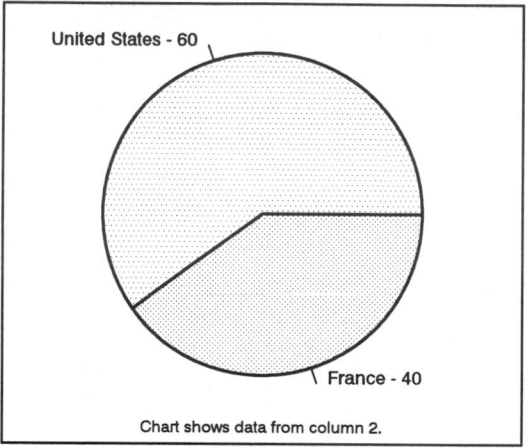

Chart shows data from column 2.

The table below shows the satisfaction ratings of French and American residents with their health care systems, as reported in a 1990 survey.

[In percentages]

Country	Respondents advocating complete system rebuilding	Respondents indicating need for fundamental changes
France	10	40
United States	30	60

Source: Fielding, Jonathan E., and Pierre-Jean Lancry. "Lessons From France—'Vive la Difference': The French Health Care System and U.S. Health System Reform." *Journal of the American Medical Association (JAMA)* 1993, no. 270, 11 August 1993, p. 748-756.

★ 961 ★

Politics, Opinion, and Law

Opinions on Health Care Reform in Selected Countries

Data reflect percent indicating that health care systems in their countries need to be fundamentally changed or rebuilt.

Country	Percent
Canada	43
Germany	48
Japan	53
United States	89

Source: "How Do They Pull It Off?" *Health* (July/August 1993), p. 67.

Sources

"... And So Are Some Other Things: Overall Injuries Seem to Be on the Upswing." *Restaurant Business,* 20 January 1994. Table: 382.

"The 16 Specialties: From AIDS to Urology, 114 Hospitals That Offer Top Care." *U.S. News & World Report,* 18 July 1994. Tables: 197, 198, 199, 200, 201, 202, 203, 204, 205, 206, 207, 208, 209, 210, 211, 212.

"18% Rise in Suicides in the Army Is Found Between 1987 and 1991." *New York Times,* 8 September 1992. Table: 335.

"1991 Service Annual Survey: Business and Selected Professional Services." In CENDATA [online service]. Washington, DC: U.S. Bureau of the Census [issued 26 July 1993]. No. 10.10.4 and No. 10.10.4.4. Table: 575.

"1991 Service Annual Survey: Health Services." In CENDATA [online service]. Washington, DC: U.S. Bureau of the Census [issued 26 July 1993]. No. 10.10.4 and No. 10.10.4.7. Tables: 561, 562, 563, 566, 567, 568, 571, 572, 573, 576, 577, 578, 581, 582, 583, 585, 586, 587, 589, 590, 591, 593, 594, 595, 607, 610, 612, 630, 631, 632, 635, 636, 637, 640, 641, 642, 646, 648, 650, 652, 654, 656, 658.

1993 Statistical Abstract of the United States on CD-ROM [machine-readable datafiles]. CD-ABSTR-93. Washington, DC: U.S. Department of Commerce, Economics and Statistics Administration, Bureau of the Census, Data User Services Division, 1993. Tables: 22, 30, 32, 45, 51, 55, 58, 61, 62, 63, 69, 100, 101, 135, 136, 139, 140, 141, 143, 240, 356, 357, 495, 497, 498, 500, 506, 507, 508, 516, 521, 522, 525, 527, 537, 539, 540, 542, 543, 544, 545, 546, 547, 548, 551, 552, 553, 554, 555, 556, 557, 558, 559, 627, 775, 776, 778, 781, 782, 831, 936, 950.

"Adult Onset of Diabetes." *USA TODAY,* 30 November 1992, final edition. Table: 66.

Aging America: Trends and Projections. 1991 ed. Prepared by the U.S. Senate Special Committee on Aging, the American Association of Retired Persons, the Federal Council on the Aging, and the U.S. Administration on Aging. DHHS Publication No. (FCoA)91-28001. Washington, DC: U.S. Department of Health and Human Services (DHHS), 1991. Tables: 16, 17, 18, 118, 216, 222, 416, 926, 942.

"Alcohol Portrayals and Advertising on Television." *Alcohol Health and Research World* 17, no. 1 (1993). Table: 255.

"Americans Living in Poverty, Lacked Health Insurance." In CENDATA [online service]. Washington, DC: U.S. Bureau of the Census, 1993 [cited 22 November 1993]. No. 5.1. Table: 290.

Anderson, A. C., E. Levine, and B. Stern. "An Estimate of the Need for Environmental Health Academicians in the Workforce." *Public Health Reports* 1990, no. 105 (July/August 1990). Table: 697.

Angier, Natalie. "Early Data Finds Promise in New Cancer Therapy." *New York Times,* 31 July 1992. Table: 57.

Angier, Natalie. "Unusual Therapy Gains Popularity." *New York Times,* 26 January 1993. Table: 254.

"Annual Dues Comparison: Major Medical Associations." *DVM Newsmagazine* (May 1994). Table: 671.

Anstett, Patricia. "Needle Exchange Slows the Spread of AIDS." *Detroit Free Press,* 18 January 1994. Table: 937.

"Appropriateness and the Effect of Guidelines." *Business and Health* 12, no. 3 (Special Report on Guidelines, 1994). Tables: 172, 239.

"At a Glance: Snapshots of the Workplace Health Industry." *Workplace Health* (January 1993). Table: 600.

"At a Glance: Snapshots of the Workplace Health Industry." *Workplace Health* (January 1994). Tables: 132, 865.

"At a Glance: Snapshots of the Workplace Health Industry." *Workplace Health* (July/August 1993). Table: 306.

"At a Glance: Snapshots of the Workplace Health Industry." *Workplace Health* (March 1993). Table: 351.

"At a Glance: Snapshots of the Workplace Health Industry." *Workplace Health* (May 1993). Tables: 253, 326.

"At a Glance: Snapshots of the Workplace Health Industry." *Workplace Health* (October 1993). Table: 901.

"At a Glance: Snapshots of the Workplace Health Industry." *Workplace Health* (September 1993). Tables: 841, 860.

"Away From Politics." *International Herald Tribune,* 19 January 1993. Table: 67.

"Away From Politics." *International Herald Tribune,* 25 February 1993. Tables: 763, 766.

Belden & Russonello Research and Communications. *Health and Longevity: Results of a National Survey Conducted for the Alliance for Aging Research.* Washington, DC: Belden & Russonello, December 1992. Tables: 325, 844, 852, 853, 854, 855, 857, 858, 859.

"Benefits." *Personnel Journal* (November 1993). Table: 345.

Berkley, Seth, Peter Piot, and Doris Schopper. "AIDS: Invest Now or Pay More Later." *Finance & Development* 31, no. 2 (June 1994). Table: 940.

Best's Review 93, no. 8 (December 1992). Table: 897.

"The Big Killers." *Time,* 25 April 1994. Table: 53.

"Big Swing in Plastic Surgeons' Charges." *Medical Economics,* 11 October 1993. Table: 247.

Bio/Technology, 11 March 1993. Table: 185.

"The Bite Is Back." *Chemical Marketing Reporter* 244, no. 6, 9 August 1993. Table: 33.

Boston Globe, 30 May 1993. Table: 597.

"A Breakdown by Race." *U.S. News & World Report,* 13 December 1993. Table: 42.

"Breast Implant Settlement." *Kansas City Star,* 14 May 1994. Table: 888.

"Bridging the Gap." *Journal of the American Medical Association (JAMA)* 269, no. 19, 19 May 1993. Tables: 849, 850.

Brody, Jane E. "Study Documents Lead-Exposure Damage in Middle-Class Children." *New York Times,* 29 October 1992. Table: 26.

Brown, Martin L. "The National Economic Burden of Cancer: An Update." *Journal of the National Cancer Institute* 82, 5 December 1990. Table: 241.

"Brushing Up on Dental Hygiene." *Washington Post,* 11 August 1992, final edition. Table: 36.

"By the Numbers: Why Retiree Medical Benefits Are Changing." *Journal of Accountancy* (September 1993). Table: 368.

"Cancer Risk Lingers After Smokers Quit." *New York Times,* 21 March 1993, late edition (final). Table: 56.

"Cardio/thoracic Surgeons' Latest Fees." *Medical Economics,* 11 October 1993. Table: 242.

Carlson, Eugene. "What Small-Business Owners Face Under Health Plan." *Wall Street Journal,* 28 October 1993. Table: 348.

Carpenter, Kathryn Hammell, and Adrian W. Alexander. "U.S. Periodical Price Index for 1994." *American Libraries* 25, no. 5 (May 1994). Tables: 812, 813.

"Cartilage Transplants in Knees Show Promise." *Wall Street Journal,* 9 June 1993. Table: 244.

Census of Manufactures on CD-ROM, 1987. Geographic Area Series [machine-readable datafiles]. Prepared by U.S. Bureau of the Census. Washington, DC: The Bureau, 1991. Tables: 613, 614, 615, 617, 619, 620, 621, 622, 659, 660, 662, 663.

Census of Population and Housing, 1990: Equal Employment Opportunity (EEO) File on CD-ROM [machine-readable datafiles]. Prepared by the Bureau of the Census. Washington, DC: The Bureau, 1992. Tables: 705, 706, 707, 708, 709, 710, 711, 712, 714, 715, 716, 718, 719, 720, 721, 722, 724, 725, 726, 727, 728, 729, 730, 731, 732, 733, 734, 735, 737, 738, 739, 740.

Census of Population and Housing, 1990: Summary Tape File 3C on CD-ROM [machine-readable datafiles]. Prepared by Bureau of the Census. Washington, DC: The Bureau, 1992. Tables: 372, 373, 375, 376.

Census of Retail Trade on CD-ROM, 1987. Geographic Area Series [machine-readable datafiles]. Prepared by U.S. Bureau of the Census. Washington, DC: The Bureau, 1990. Table: 666.

Census of Service Industries on CD-ROM, 1987. Geographic Area Series [machine-readable datafiles]. Prepared by U.S. Bureau of the Census. Washington, DC: The Bureau, 1990. Tables: 560, 564, 565, 570, 574, 580, 584, 588, 592, 605, 606, 609, 611, 629, 634, 638, 639, 643, 644, 645, 647, 649, 651, 653, 655, 657.

Census of Wholesale Trade on CD-ROM, 1987. Geographic Area Series [machine-readable datafiles]. Prepared by U.S. Bureau of the Census. Washington, DC: The Bureau, 1990. Tables: 667, 669, 670.

Cerne, Frank. "Consumers Rate Their Health Plans." *Hospitals & Health Networks,* 5 January 1994. Tables: 843, 845.

"Child Abuse: Growing Problem in the USA." *USA TODAY,* 7 April 1994, final edition. Table: 214.

"Children Don't Expect a Healthy Future." *Nurse Practitioner* (July/August 1993). Table: 24.

"The Cigarette's Open Frontier." *New York Times,* 15 May 1994. Table: 949.

Claiborne, William. "Health Reform Closer to Home: While Washington Debates, Many States Press Ahead." *Washington Post National Weekly Edition,* 6-12 December 1993. Table: 884.

Colburn, Don. "When Violence Begins at Home." *Washington Post Health,* 15 March 1994. Table: 332.

Collins, Sara. "Cutting Edge Cures." *U.S. News & World Report,* 7 June 1993. Table: 913.

"Combined Annual and Revised Monthly Retail Trade, January 1983 Through December 1992." In CENDATA [online service]. Washington, DC: U.S. Bureau of the Census [issued 16 April 1993]. No. 10.6.1, No. 10.6.2.1., and No. 10.6.2.2. Table: 665.

"Combined Annual and Revised Monthly Wholesale Trade, January 1987 Through December 1993." In CENDATA [online service]. Washington, DC: U.S. Bureau of the Census [issued 1 April 1994]. No. 10.7.1 and No. 10.7.23. Table: 668.

Common Cause. "Our System of Government Is Under Threat: Special Interest PAC Money in Congressional Elections." Brochure. Washington, DC: Common Cause, n.d. Tables: 871, 872.

"Company Health Costs Soar." *USA TODAY,* 27 April 1993. Table: 344.

"Comparing Clinton Health Plans." *USA TODAY,* 13 April 1994. Table: 875.

"Compensation and Gender." *ASHA* 36, no. 5 (May 1994). Table: 747.

"Computers Helping Doctors Match Care With Costs Can Lower Bills, Study Says." *Wall Street Journal,* 20 January 1993. Table: 771.

Condor, Bob. "Have You Juggled Your 8 Glasses Today?" *Chicago Tribune,* 13 February 1994, Zone C. Table: 307.

"Consumer Group Gives Movie Popcorn Two Thumbs Down." *Detroit News,* 26 April 1994. Table: 305.

"The Cost of Losing Weight." *New York Times,* 24 November 1992. Table: 308.

"Costs of Having a Baby." *USA TODAY,* 21 March 1993. Table: 144.

"Costs of Health-care Benefits Rise in 1993." *Personnel Journal* (June 1994). Table: 340.

Crichton, Ginger Munsch. "The Latest High-Tech Instruments Will Make Your Visits With the Dentist Speedier--and More Comfortable." *Dallas Morning News,* 19 April 1993, home final edition. Table: 225.

Culhane, Charles. "Medicare Denial Rates Vary Widely; Carriers Inconsistent in Judging Medical Necessity." *American Medical News,* 18 April 1994. Table: 509.

"Currents." *Hospitals & Health Networks,* 20 January 1994. Table: 295.

"Daily Dose: Tranquilizers or TV?" *Health* (January/February 1994). Table: 911.

Davis, Terry C., E. J. Mayeaux, Doren Fredrickson, and others. "Reading Ability of Parents Compared With Reading Level of Pediatric Patient Education Materials." *Pediatrics* 1994, no. 93 (March 1994). Tables: 806, 807, 808.

Day, Kathleen. "Thinning the Health Care Herd." *Washington Post,* 5 October 1993. Table: 579.

"DC School Foodservice Not Going to Contract." *Food Management* (July 1993). Table: 536.

De Bakey, Michael E. "Medical Centers of Excellence and Health Reform." *Science* 262, no. 5133, 22 October 1993. Table: 957.

De Parle, Jason. "Food Stamp Users up Sharply in Sign of Weak Recovery." *New York Times,* 2 March 1993. Table: 538.

Decker, Carlene A. "Salaries--The Real Reason for the Shortage: Where Have All the Techs Gone?" *Veterinary Forum* (January 1993). Table: 749.

DeLisa, Joel A. "Academic Physiatry: Trends, Opportunities and Challenges." *American Journal of Physical Medicine and Rehabilitation* 72, no. 3 (June 1993). Table: 699.

"Depression Affects Millions." *Business and Health* 12, no. 4. (Supplement A, 1994). Table: 129.

Detroit Free Press, 10 February 1993. Table: 289.

"Doctor Disciplinary Action Hits Record High." *Los Angeles Times,* 13 April 1994, home edition, Part A. Table: 892.

"Doctors' Income." *Wall Street Journal,* 2 March 1993. Table: 764.

Edelman, Marian Wright. "Give Children Health Security." *USA TODAY,* 9 December 1993. Tables: 922, 933.

"Effect of Drug Programs on Total Drug Costs." *National Underwriter,* 26 April 1993. Table: 350.

El-Makkakh, Rif S., and others. "Abuzz Over Bee Keeping." *Science Teacher* 58 (September 1991). Table: 78.

"Employer-Provider Health Care Insurance." *New York Times,* 19 June 1994. Table: 366.

Encyclopedia of Associations, 1994. 28th ed. Detroit, MI: Gale Research Inc., 1993. Table: 794.

"Entitlements for the Retired Take Ever More Money." *New York Times,* 30 August 1992. Tables: 519, 520, 528, 529.

Evans, Roger W. "Organ Procurement Expenditures and the Role of Financial Incentives." *Journal of the American Medical Association (JAMA)* 269, no. 24, 23-30 June 1993. Table: 251.

Executive Office of the President. Office of Management and Budget. *Budget of the United States Government, Fiscal Year 1995.* Washington, DC: U.S. Government Printing Office, 1994. Tables: 876, 879, 880.

"Expected Future Size of the Laboratory Applications Market." *Computers in Healthcare* (September 1993). Table: 608.

"Experts See a Long Battle." *Christian Science Monitor,* 31 July 1992. Table: 50.

Feder, Barnaby J. "Implant Industry Is Facing Cutback by Top Suppliers." *New York Times,* 25 April 1994, late edition. Table: 229.

Ferraiolo, Diane. "General Liability, Medical Malpractice, Surety and Fidelity: 1991." *Best's Review: Property/Casualty Insurance Edition* 93, no. 8 (December 1992). Table: 601.

"Fewer Malpractice Wins." *USA TODAY,* 4 April 1994, final edition. Table: 890.

"Fewest Abortions Since '79." *USA TODAY,* 16 June 1994. Table: 133.

Fielding, Jonathan E., and Pierre-Jean Lancry. "Lessons From France—'Vive la Difference': The French Health Care System and U.S. Health System Reform." *Journal of the American Medical Association (JAMA)* 1993, no. 270, 11 August 19937. Table: 960.

Finnegan, F. Thomas. "Benefit Plans Test Hospitals' Acceptance of Change." *National Underwriter,* 25 October 1993. Table: 786.

"Fleeing Haiti." *Detroit News,* 10 July 1994. Tables: 914, 943.

Flynn, Gillian. "For Your Information." *Personnel Journal* 73, no. 3 (March 1994). Table: 866.

Forrest, Jacqueline Darroch, and Richard R. Fordyce. "Women's Contraceptive Attitudes and Use in 1992." *Family Planning Perspectives* 25, no. 4 (July/August 1993). Table: 138.

Fox, Michael R. "Radiation and Risk: Hanford Workers' Health and the Decline of Scientific Debate." *21st Century Science and Technology* (fall 1993). Table: 72.

Franko, Lawrence G. "Global Corporate Competition II: Is the Large American Firm an Endangered Species?" *Business Horizons* 34, no. 4 (November 1991). Table: 907.

Freudenheim, Milt. "Health Care: A Growing Burden." *New York Times,* 29 January 1991. Table: 341.

Freudenheim, Milt. "Insurers Accused of Discrimination in AIDS Coverage." *New York Times,* 1 June 1993. Table: 49.

Freudenheim, Milt. "New Drug Era Begins as Tagamet Patent Ends." *New York Times,* 17 May 1994. Table: 909.

Freudenheim, Milt. "Retirees Threatened With Loss of Insurance." *New York Times,* 28 June 1992. Table: 365.

Frum, David, and Frank Wolfe. "If You Gotta Get Sued, Get Sued in Utah." *Forbes,* 17 January 1994. Table: 899.

"General Surgeons' Charges for Seven Procedures." *Medical Economics,* 11 October 1993. Table: 248.

Glaser, Martha. "Medicaid Prices Closing in on $20 Per Prescription." *Drug Topics* 136, no. 21, 9 November 1992. Table: 501.

Goodman, John C., and Gerald L. Musgrave. "How to Solve the Health Care Crisis." *Consumer's Research* 75 (March 1992). Table: 799.

Gorov, Lynda. "Nutritionists See Little Good Fortune in Chinese Food." *Boston Globe,* 2 September 1993, city edition. Table: 302.

Gostin, Lawrence O., Joan Turek-Brezina, Madison Powers, and others. "Privacy and Security of Personal Information in a New Health Care System." *Journal of the American Medical Association (JAMA)* 270, 24 November 1993. Table: 862.

Greene, Marilyn. "Women Called Key to Helping Third World." *USA TODAY,* 21 June 1994. Tables: 931, 951, 952.

Guinness Book of Records, 1992. New York: Bantam Books, 1992. Table: 944.

Haiven, Judy. "MediScare." *Mother Jones* 16 (March-April 1991). Tables: 953, 954.

Hall, Mimi. "Study Zeros in on Pregnant Teens, Parents: Both Sides Say New Report Is a Validation of Positions." *USA TODAY,* 20 October 1992, final edition. Table: 134.

Hansen, Mark. "The ADA's Wide Reach: Little League and Health Insurers Among Those Covered by Act." *ABA Journal* (December 1993). Table: 371.

Harvey, S. Marie, and Kathy S. Faber. "Obstacles to Prenatal Care Following Implementation of a Community-Based Program to Reduce Financial Barriers." *Family Planning Perspective* 25, no. 1 (January/February 1993). Table: 147.

Hasson, Judi. "Health-care Lobbying Kicks Into High Gear." *USA TODAY,* 13 May 1993, final edition. Table: 867.

"Health Care Coverage." *San Francisco Examiner,* 28 November 1993. Table: 361.

"Health Care Coverage in the '90s." *Los Angeles Times,* 8 March 1993. Table: 347.

"Health Care Write-Down." *American Medical News,* 1 November 1993. Table: 367.

"Health Care: The Issue Is Front and Center." *Public Perspective* (January/February 1993). Table: 916.

Health Insurance Association of America (HIAA). *Source Book of Health Insurance Data, 1993.* Washington, DC: Health Insurance Association of America, 1994. Tables: 237, 249, 717.

"Health Professionals' Line." *FDA Consumer* (May 1992). Table: 767.

"Healthy Babies." *Asiaweek,* 1 June 1994. Table: 932.

Heitzman, Beth. "Finally ... an Ad Sector That's Hiring." *ADWEEK,* 4 October 1994. Table: 768.

Heller, Peter S., Richard Hemming, Peter W. Kohnert, and others. *Aging and Social Expenditure in the Major Industrial Countries, 1980-2025.* International Monetary Fund, September 1986. Table: 925.

"Hello Boss...." *Detroit Free Press,* 14 March 1993. Table: 385.

"Hidden Factors Boost Annual Cost to $8,000 for Average Household." *Christian Science Monitor,* 18 November 1991. Table: 413.

Hilts, Philip J. "Mexican Health Care Draws Americans." *Detroit Free Press,* 26 November 1992. Table: 904.

"HIV Infections--Continent by Continent." *World Newsmap of the Week* 56, no. 13, 6 December 1993. Table: 939.

"Hospitals Seeing More Outpatients." *Food Management* (July 1993). Table: 232.

"How Dental Fillings Compare." *Consumer Reports* 56 (May 1991). Table: 35.

"How Do They Pull It Off?" *Health* (July/August 1993). Tables: 915, 958, 961.

"How Employers Are Helping Workers Stay Healthy." *Washington Post,* 18 May 1993, final edition. Table: 389.

"How Hospital Execs Are Faring on Payday." *Medical Economics,* 23 August 1993. Table: 754.

"How Much a Sickness Fund Pays." *New York Times,* 23 January 1993. Table: 903.

"How to Lower Blood Pressure." *Consumer Reports* 57 (May 1992). Table: 286.

Howard, Nigel. "Who Says Hospitals Are Clean? Nearly Half the Patients in Intensive Care Are Given an Infection." *The European,* 13-19 May 1994. Table: 912.

"Human Sperm Count Study Shows World-Wide Decline." *Wall Street Journal,* 11 September 1992. Table: 125.

"In the Stores." *Consumer Reports* 57 (August 1992). Table: 79.

"Indemnity Plan Costs vs. Managed-Care Plan Costs in Selected U.S. Cities, 1992." *Modern Healthcare,* 8 March 1993. Table: 347.

"Infant Mortality: How Brazil Compares." *New York Times,* 14 May 1993. Table: 930.

Ink, Gary. "Inching Ahead." *Publishers Weekly,* 7 March 1994. Table: 810.

"Insurers Urged to Process Claims Electronically." *Blues Advantage* 1 (October 1992). Table: 772.

"Is Biotech Leadership Changing?" *R&D Magazine* (December 1993). Table: 823.

"Is Your Doctor Spent?" *USA WEEKEND,* 3-5 June 1994. Table: 861.

Johnson, Julie. "Government Health Spending Soars." *American Medical News,* 10 May 1993. Table: 291.

Johnsson, Julie, and Mike Mitka. "Medicare Efficiency Ratings Are Down in 1992." *American Medical News,* 19 April 1993. Table: 602.

Jonas, Harry S., Sylvia I. Etzel, and Barbara Barzansky. "Educational Programs in U.S. Medical Schools." *Journal of the American Medical Association (JAMA)* 270, no. 9, 1 September 1993. Tables: 691, 692, 695, 700.

"Just the Facts." *Detroit News,* 12 April 1994. Table: 378.

"Key Features of Employee Health Benefits Plans." *Hospitals & Health Networks,* 5 June 1993. Table: 864.

Khaltaev, Nikolai. "Inter-Health Fights Life-Style Diseases." *World Health* (May-June 1991). Table: 948.

"Kids, Shots, and Drug Research: Let's Get Some Answers." *Business Week* 23, 15 February 1992. Table: 213.

Kingman, Sharon. "The Cost of Clean Blood." *New Scientist* 136 (September 1992). Table: 902.

Kirsch, Irwin S., Ann Jungeblut, Lynn Jenkins, and Andrew Kolstad. *Adult Literacy in America: A First Look at the Results of the National Adult Literacy Survey.* Prepared by Educational Testing Service under contract with National Center for Education Statistics. Washington, DC: U.S. Department of Education, Office of Educational Research and Improvement, September 1993. Table: 38.

Korcok, Milan. "Ontario Hospitals Are Looking to Woo U.S. Patients." *American Medical News,* 24-31 May 1993. Table: 901.

Korniewicz, Denise M., Marie Kirwin, Kay Cresci, and others. "In-use Comparison of Latex Gloves in Two High-Risk Units: Surgical Intensive Care and Acquired Immunodificiency Syndrome." *Heart & Lung* 21, no. 1 (January 1992). Table: 230.

Krakower, Jack, and others. "U.S. Medical School Finances." *Journal of the American Medical Association (JAMA)* 270, no. 9, 1 September 1993. Table: 702.

Krakower, Jack, Janice L. Ganem, and Robert L. Beran. "Medical School Financing, 1991-1992: Comparing Seven Different Types of Schools." *Academic Medicine* 69, no. 1 (January 1994). Tables: 689, 696, 701, 703.

Kramer, Larry. "We Have Lost the War Against AIDS." *USA TODAY* (magazine; May 1992). Table: 48.

Laabs, Jennifer J. "Danger at Work: Fatalities and Injuries on the Rise." *Personnel Journal* (February 1994). Table: 380.

Lane, Charlotte Balcomb. "Lamb Gaining Favor in Central Florida." *Orlando Sentinel,* 31 March 1994. Table. 301.

Leary, Warren. "U.S. Panel Backs Testing All Babies to Uncover Hearing Losses Early." *New York Times,* 10 March 1993. Table: 25.

Lee, Jessica, and Mimi Hall. "White House Presses Health-Care Plan." *USA TODAY,* 23 February 1993, final edition. Table: 287.

Levy, Doug. "Mass Ovarian Cancer Testing Impractical." *USA TODAY,* 1 June 1993. Table: 157.

"Lifestyle--Health: The Right Stuff for a Longer Life." *Newsweek* 117, 15 April 1991. Table: 117.

Lillie-Blanton, Marsha, James C. Anthony, and Charles R. Schuster. "Probing the Meaning of Racial/Ethnic Group Comparisons in Crack Cocaine Smoking." *Journal of the American Medical Association (JAMA)* 269, no. 8, 24 February 1993. Table: 264.

"Lines Drawn for Survival of Preemies." *St. Louis Post-Dispatch,* 25 November 1993. Table: 137.

"Lower Cost of Prescriptions in Britain Brings Calls for Price Controls on Drugs." *Detroit News,* 3 February 1994. Table: 905.

Lumsdon, Kevin, and Mark Hagland. "Mapping Care." *Hospitals & Health Networks,* 20 October 1993. Table: 770.

"Managed Care Facts." *Hospitals,* 5 April 1993. Table: 355.

Manufacturing Chemist (December 1992). Table: 664.

Marley, Sara. "Self-Insurance: P/C Self-Insurance Growth Slows, But Efforts to Control Costs Grow." *Business Insurance,* 7 February 1994. Table: 596.

McCormick, Brian. "Survey Claims Fraud; Often a Physician's Crime, Data Debated." *American Medical News,* 16 August 1993. Table: 896.

McCoy, Frank. "Where Does It Hurt?" *Black Enterprise* (May 1994). Table: 293.

McNichol, Tom. "The New Sex Vow: 'I Won't' Until 'I Do.'" *USA WEEKEND,* 25-27 March 1994. Table: 311.

"Median Fees for Neurosurgeons' Services." *Medical Economics,* 11 October 1993. Table: 245.

Medical Group Management Association. *Membership Compensation Survey: 1993 Report Based on 1993 Data.* Englewood, Colorado: Medical Group Management Association, October 1993. Table: 752.

Medical Group Management Association. *Physician Compensation and Production Survey: 1993 Report Based on 1992 Data.* Englewood, Colorado: Center for Research in Ambulatory Health Care Administration, September 1993. Table: 744.

Medical Library Association. Unpublished data. Chicago, IL (1994). Table: 793.

Medicare and Medicaid's 25th Anniversary--Much Promised, Accomplished, and Left Unfinished: A Report Presented by the Chairman of the Select Committee on Aging. Washington, DC: U.S. Government Printing Office, 1990. Table: 504.

"Medicines Across the Border." *Detroit Free Press,* 26 November 1992. Table: 908.

Metropolitan Life Insurance Company. Claims data. Merged and edited by Corporate Health Strategies Inc. Analyses and computations by Metropolitan Life Insurance Company, Safety Education Division. Table: 278.

Metropolitan Life Insurance Company. "Heart Disease Mortality: International Comparisons." *Statistical Bulletin* 74, no. 4 (October-December 1993). Table: 934, 935.

Metropolitan Life Insurance Company. "Selected Behaviors and Perceptions Among U.S. Adults in 1990." *Statistical Bulletin* 74, no. 4 (October-December 1993). Table: 68.

Mide, Susan. "Healing the Hurt of Homeless Kids." *USA TODAY,* 23 November 1992, final edition. Table: 294.

"Mind Over IAQ? Scientists Reseach Mental Aspects of Poor Indoor Air." *Facilities Design and Management* (February 1993). Table: 73.

Modern Maturity 36, no. 3 (June-July 1993). Table: 842.

"Modest Weight Gain Found in Those Who Quit Smoking." *New York Times,* 15 March 1991. Table: 323.

"Monday Tops List for Risk." *Detroit News,* 20 July 1994. Table: 387.

"Money Woes." *Detroit Free Press,* 15 April 1994. Table: 851.

Monroe, Stephen M. "'Provider' Surveys Top Chains." *Provider* (January 1994). Table: 633.

Montegue, Jim. "Outcomes on the Upswing." *Hospitals & Health Networks,* 20 January 1994. Tables: 837, 839, 840.

Moore, Mary Carroll, and Jean Rogers. *Prevention* 43, no. 11 (November 1991). Tables: 299, 300.

"More Doctors Sign Up to Participate in Medicare." *American Medical News,* 23-30 August 1993. Table: 513.

"More Midwives." *Detroit News,* 25 April 1994. Table: 142.

Morgan, Babette. "Seeing Is Believing: Outlook Bright for Laser Surgery That Helps Vision." *St. Louis Post-Dispatch,* 30 August 1993. Table: 921.

Morgan, Dan. "Health Plan Effects Vary by State; Most Would Get More Federal Money Under Clinton Proposal, Study Says." *Washington Post,* 14 February 1994, final edition. Table: 878.

National Economic, Social, and Environmental Data Bank: The Federal Connection [CD-ROM]. Prepared by U.S. Department of Commerce, Economics and Statistics Administration. Washington, DC: U.S. Department of Commerce, Economics and Statistics Administration, Office of Business Analysis, November 1992. Tables: 39, 116, 238.

National Safety Council. *Accident Facts, 1992.* Itasca, IL: National Safety Council, Safety & Health News Center, 1992. Tables: 74, 75.

NEISS Data Highlights 14 (January-December 1990). Tables: 85, 86, 87, 88, 89, 90, 91, 92, 93, 94, 95, 96, 97.

Neuman, Elena. "Will It Hurt?" *Insight,* 20 April 1992. Table: 889.

"A New TB Threat." *Asiaweek,* 4 May 1994. Table: 941.

Newman, Richard J., Doug Podolsky, and Penny Loeb. "Bad Blood." *U.S. News & World Report* 116, no. 25, 27 June 1994. Tables: 159, 160.

"Nursing Education and Income: Does More Time in the Classroom Mean Higher Pay?" *RN* (December 1993). Table: 758.

"Nursing Enrollments Hit All-Time High." *AJN* (January 1994). Table: 704.

Oberman, Linda. "AMA Has Record Membership; Looks to Market Share Gains." *American Medical News,* 22 February 1993. Table: 672.

Oberman, Linda. "Data Bank Access Debate: Doctors May Have to Ante Up For Queries; Consumers Push to See Files." *American Medical News,* 24-31 May 1993. Table: 900.

Oberman, Linda. "Kept 'Out of the Loop': Boards Pondering Role Under Reform." *American Medical News,* 10 May 1993. Table: 893.

Oberman, Linda. "Medical Society Fighting Broad Use of Licensing Fees." *American Medical News,* 21 June 1993. Table: 798.

"Office Furniture Workers Miss Most Workdays." *Wood and Wood Products* (January 1994). Table: 383.

"Outpatient Procedures: New Data Show Services Likely to Shift to Non-hospital Settings." *Hospitals and Health Networks,* 20 July 1993. Table: 233.

Page, Leigh. "U.S. Hounds Student Loan Defaulters." *American Medical News,* 20 September 1990. Table: 690.

Painter, Kim. "'Don't Worry About Women' Was Lesson." *USA TODAY,* 10 February 1993. Table: 154.

Painter, Kim. "Lifestyles Remain a Major Barrier to Condom Use." *USA TODAY,* 7 July 1992, final edition. Table: 312.

Painter, Kim. "U.S. Found Lagging in Fighting STDs." *USA TODAY,* 1 April 1993. Table: 315.

Pearlstein, Steven. "Win Some, Lose Some in Health Care Reform; Billions Will Change Hands, But to Little Net Effect." *Washington Post National Weekly Edition,* 7-13 March 1994. Table: 877.

"Pediatricians' Latest Charges." *Medical Economics,* 11 October 1993. Table: 167.

Peltola, Heikki. "Mumps Vaccination and Meningitis." *Lancet* 341, no. 88511, 17 April 1993. Table: 28.

"Penicillin From a Screen." *Newsweek* 120, 14 September 1992. Table: 174.

Perlmutter, Cathy. *Prevention* 43, no. 11 (November 1991). Table: 296.

Peters, Shannon. "Employers Provide More Parties, Fewer Gym Facilities in 1993." *Personnel Journal* (May 1994). Table: 388.

Peterson, Karen S. "TV Condom Ads May Reach Teens, Panelists Say." *USA TODAY,* 11 January 1994. Table: 316.

"Pharmaceutical Industry Starting Salaries." *American Medical News,* 4 October 1993. Table: 761.

"Physicians' Fees and the Cost of Living." *Medical Economics,* 11 October 1993. Table: 168.

"Practice Expenses: Doctors Apply the Shears." *Medical Economics,* 25 October 1993. Table: 800.

"Price Tag: Psychotherapy." *New York Times,* 4 February 1993, late edition (final). Tables: 126, 127

Priest, Dana. "Health Plan Worries Spur PACs: Industry Group Donations Up 20%." *Washington Post,* 17 July 1993. Table: 870.

"The Prostate Puzzle." *Consumer Reports* 57 (July 1993). Table: 124.

Pryor, David. "Communism Collapses ... But Nothing Changes the Pharmaceutical Industry's Skyrocketing Pricing Practices." *Congressional Record,* 10 September 1991. Table: 175.

"PyMaH Promoting Ease of Use With New Axillary Thermometer." *Health Industry Today* 56, no. 10 (October 1993). Table: 224.

"The Quality March: Part Two of a National Survey of Quality Improvement Activities." *Hospitals & Health Networks,* 20 December 1993. Table: 836.

"The Range of Fees for OBG Services." *Medical Economics,* 11 October 1993. Table: 165.

"Ranks of the Uninsured Increase." *Nation's Business* (May 1994). Table: 363.

"Removing Our Freedom." *Wall Street Journal,* 27 June 1994. Table: 874.

Rice, Dorothy P. "The Economic Cost of Alcohol Abuse and Alcohol Dependence: 1990." *Alcohol Health and Research World* 17, no. 1 (1993). Table: 259.

Richardson, Rod. "Blacks Reluctant to Donate Organs." *Detroit News,* 1 March 1993. Table: 250.

"RN Salary Gains: Staff Nurses Get Less, Grow Less." *RN* (May 1993). Table: 757.

Rose, Robert L. "Retiree Health Coverage Erodes at Small, Midsize Firms." *Wall Street Journal,* 16 April 1993. Table: 370.

Rosenthal, Elisabeth. "Confusion and Error Are Rife in Hospital Billing Practices." *New York Times,* 27 January 1993. Table: 195.

Rosenthal, Elisabeth. "Doctors Weigh the Cost of a Chicken Pox Vaccine." *New York Times,* 7 July 1993, late edition (final). Table: 20.

Ruffenach, Glenn. "Firms Use Financial Incentives to Make Employees Seek Lower Health-Care Fees." *Wall Street Journal,* 9 February 1993. Table: 848.

Safety + Health (December 1993). Table: 883.

"Safety First." *Business Week* 22, 2 November 1992. Table: 381.

Scan/Info 3 (May 1991). Tables: 121, 155.

Schachner, Michael. "Large Companies Still See Self-Funding as Health Care Cure." *Business Insurance,* 7 February 1994. Table: 362.

Schappert, S.M. *National Ambulatory Medical Care Survey: 1991 Summary.* Advance data from Vital and Health Statistics. No. 230. Hyattsville, MD: National Center for Health Statistics, 1993. Table: 166.

Schwartz, Matthew P. "'Any Willing Provider' Laws Draw Fire." *National Underwriter,* 9 August 1993. Table: 891.

"Sex, Lies, and Statistics." *The Economist,* 23 October 1993. Table: 313.

"Shifting Health Traditions." *Miami Herald,* 2 March 1993. Table: 347.

Smothers, Ronald. "150 Miles Away, the Doctor Is Examining Your Tonsils." *New York Times,* 16 September 1992. Table: 196.

"Social Issues at Work." *Training* (October 1993). Table: 390.

"Social Standing." *India Today,* 31 January 1994. Table: 923.

"Something's in the Air." *Small Business Reports* 19, no. 3 (March 1994). Table: 386.

Sorrels, Valarie L. "Nursing Home Fears." *Geriatric Nursing* (September- October 1991). Table: 107.

Spalding, B. J. "106 U.S. Biopharmaceutical Firms Lose $1.1 Billion." *Bio/Technology* 12 (April 1994). Tables: 623, 624.

Springfield News-Leader, 20 March 1993. Table: 14917.

"The State of Affairs in Work Disability." *Small Business Reports* 19, no. 1 (January 1994). Table: 374.

Stevens, Carol. "Malpractice Jackpots Will Be Harder to Win." *Detroit News,* 27 March 1994. Table: 898.

Stevens, Carol. "Who Will Pay Health Bill for Early Retirees?" *Detroit News,* 27 February 1994. Tables: 343, 369.

Stevens, Larry. "House Calls; Financial Aspects for Physicians." *American Medical News* 36, no. 33, 6 September 1993. Tables: 162, 163.

Stipp, David. "Prevention May Be Costlier Than a Cure." *Wall Street Journal,* 6 July 1994. Table: 236.

Stout, Hilary. "Many Don't Realize It's Clinton Plan They Like." *Wall Street Journal,* 10 March 1994. Table: 847.

Suhl, Jeremiah, Pamela Simons, Terry Reedy, and Thomas Garrick. "Myth of Substituted Judgment; Surrogate Decision Making Regarding Life Support Is Unreliable." *Archives of Internal Medicine* 1994, no. 154, 10 January 1994. Table: 856.

"Suicide's Victims." *USA TODAY,* 24 February 1993. Table: 334.

"Survey Finds Strong Support for Shared Health Benefits Costs." *Hospitals & Health Networks,* 5 November 1993. Table: 846.

Thierry, Patty. "Survey Shows Optimisim for CPR." *Journal of AHIMA* 64, no. 12 (December 1993). Table: 769.

Thompson, Roger. "Employers' Costs for Employees Soar; Health Benefits." *Nation's Business* 80, no. 5 (May 1992). Table: 346.

Thompson, Roger. "Small Firms' Stake in Health Reform." *Nation's Business* 81, no. 11 (November 1993). Table: 364.

"The Three Types of Stroke." *FDA Consumer* (June 1994). Table: 59.

"To Give and to Receive." *Wall Street Journal,* 23 September 1993. Tables: 868, 869.

"Top 10 Teen Killers." *Current Health 2* 20, no. 1 (September 1993). Table: 23.

"Top Health Care Chains." *Restaurants and Institutions* (1 March 1994). Table: 777.

Torrey, E. Fuller. "The Mental Health Mess." *National Review* 44, 28 December 1992. Table: 115.

"Toy-related Deaths." *Time,* 13 December 1993. Table: 81.

"Tracking Cancer Treatment in Britain." *New York Time,* 26 June 1994. Table: 920.

"The Trend in Medicine." *Detroit Free Press,* 31 March 1994. Table: 765.

"U.N. Agency on Sex: Pitfalls and Promise." *New York Times,* 25 June 1992. Tables: 145, 314.

"UN Says AIDS Hits Younger Women Harder." *Detroit Free Press,* 29 July 1993. Table: 148.

U.S. Bureau of the Census. *Annual Survey of Manufactures, 1991. Geographic Area Statistics.* M91(AS)-3. Washington, DC: U.S. Government Printing Office, February 1993. Tables: 616, 618, 661.

U.S. Bureau of the Census. *City Government Finances, 1990-1991.* Series GF/91-4. Washington, DC: U.S. Government Printing Office, 1993. Tables: 420, 421, 422, 423, 424, 425, 426, 427, 428, 429, 430, 431, 432, 433, 434, 435, 436, 437, 438, 439, 440, 441, 442, 443, 444, 445, 446, 447, 448, 449, 450, 451, 452, 453, 454, 455, 456, 457, 458, 459, 460, 461, 462, 463, 464, 465, 466, 467, 468, 469, 470, 471, 472, 473, 474.

U.S. Bureau of the Census. *Poverty in the United States: 1991*. Current Population Reports. Series P-60, no. 181. Washington, DC: U.S. Government Printing Office, 1992. Table: 288.

U.S. Congress. Congressional Budget Office (CBO). *Trends in Health Spending: An Update.* A CBO Study. Washington, DC: Congressional Budget Office, June 1993. Table: 417.

U.S. Congress. Office of Technology Assessment. *Does Health Insurance Make a Difference? Background Paper.* OTA-BP-H-99. Washington, DC: U.S. Government Printing Office, September 1992. Tables: 292, 359.

U.S. Congress. Office of Technology Assessment. *Psychiatric Disabilities, Employment, and the Americans With Disabilities Act.* OTA-BP-BBS-124. Washington, DC: U.S. Government Printing Office, March 1994. Table: 130.

U.S. Congress. Office of Technology Assessment. *Who Goes There: Friend or Foe?* OTA-ISC-537. Washington, DC: U.S. Government Printing Office, June 1993. Table: 336.

U.S. Department of Commerce. Economics and Statistics Administration. Bureau of the Census. *Government Finances, 1989-1990: Preliminary Report.* Series GF-90-5P. Washington, DC: U.S. Government Printing Office, September, 1991. Tables: 419, 47719.

U.S. Department of Commerce. Economics and Statistics Administration. Bureau of the Census. *Sixty-five Plus in America.* Prepared by Cynthia M. Taeuber. Washington, DC: U.S. Government Printing Office, 1992. Table: 108.

U.S. Department of Commerce. Economics and Statistics Administration. Office of the Chief Economist. *Foreign Direct Investment in the United States: An Update.* Washington, DC: U.S. Department of Commerce, Economics and Statistics Administration, Office of the Chief Economist, June 1993. Table: 820.

U.S. Department of Commerce. *U.S. Industrial Outlook '92: Business Forecasts for 350 Industries.* Washington, DC: U.S. Government Printing Office, 1992. Table: 192.

U.S. Department of Commerce. *U.S. Industrial Outlook, 1994: Forecasts for Selected Manufacturing and Service Industries.* Lanham, MD: Bernan Press, 1994. Tables: 603, 604, 713.

U.S. Department of Education. Office of Educational Research and Improvement. National Center for Education Statistics. *Digest of Education Statistics, 1992.* Washington, DC: U.S. Government Printing Office, 1992. Tables: 275, 276, 277, 284, 310, 338, 415, 475, 484, 532, 535.

U.S. Department of Health and Human Services. Health Care Financing Administration (HCFA). Bureau of Data Management and Strategy. *1993 HCFA Statistics.* HCFA Pub. No. 03341. Washington, DC: U.S. Department of Health and Human Services, June 1993. Tables: 491, 499, 503.

U.S. Department of Health and Human Services. Health Care Financing Adminstration (HCFA). *Health Care Financing Review* 13, no. 4 (summer 1992). Tables: 917, 918, 919, 928, 959.

U.S. Department of Health and Human Services. Health Care Financing Administration (HCFA). *Health Care Financing Review* 15, no. 2 (winter 1993). Table: 750.

U.S. Department of Health and Human Services. Public Health Service. Alcohol, Drug Abuse, and Mental Health Administration. *National Household Survey on Drug Abuse: Population Estimates, 1991.* Rockville, MD: U.S. Department of Health and Human Services. Public Health Service. Alcohol, Drug Abuse, and Mental Health Administration, n.d. Tables: 258, 260, 261, 262, 263, 265, 266, 267, 268, 269, 270, 271, 272, 273, 274, 319, 320.

U.S. Department of Health and Human Services. Public Health Service. Centers for Disease Control and Prevention. National Center for Health Statistics. *Current Estimates From the National Health Interview Survey, 1991.* Vital and Health Statistics, Series 10: Data From the National Health Survey, no. 184. DHHS publication no. (PHS) 93-1512. Hyattsville, MD: U.S. Department of Health and Human Services, Public Health Service, Centers for Disease Control and Prevention, National Center for Health Statistics, December 1992. Tables: 40-41, 43, 44, 46, 47, 60, 164, 170.

U.S. Department of Health and Human Services. Public Health Service. Centers for Disease Control and Prevention. National Center for Health Statistics. *Health Promotion and Disease Prevention: United States, 1990.* Vital and Health Statistics, Series10, no. 185. Hyattsville, MD: U.S. Department of Health and Human Services, Public Health Service, Centers for Disease Control and Prevention, National Center for Health Statistics, n.d. Tables: 34, 37, 70, 131, 150, 158, 234, 235, 256, 281, 282, 283, 285, 298, 303, 304, 317, 321, 322.

U.S. Department of Health and Human Services. Public Health Service. Centers for Disease Control and Prevention. National Center for Health Statistics. *Health, United States, 1991.* Hyattsville, MD: Public Health Service, 1992. Table: 333.

U.S. Department of Health and Human Services. Public Health Service. Centers for Disease Control and Prevention. National Center for Health Statistics. *Health, United States, 1992.* Hyattsville, MD: Public Health Service, 1993. Tables: 31, 119, 169, 194, 220, 342, 411, 418, 476, 478, 479, 481, 482, 483, 485, 486, 487, 488, 489, 490, 492, 816, 818, 819, 924, 927.

U.S. Department of Health and Human Services. Public Health Service. Centers for Disease Control and Prevention. "Measles Surveillance—United States, 1991." *CDC Surveillance Summaries. Morbidity and Mortality Weekly Report* 41, no. SS-6, 20 November 1992. Table: 27.

U.S. Department of Health and Human Services. Public Health Service. Centers for Disease Control and Prevention. "Notices to Readers." *Morbidity and Mortality Weekly Report* 43, no. 8, 4 March 1994. Table: 214.

U.S. Department of Health and Human Services. Public Health Service. Centers for Disease Control and Prevention. "Summary of Notifiable Diseases: United States, 1992." *Morbidity and Mortality Weekly Report* 41, no. 55, 24 September 1993. Table: 71.

U.S. Department of Health and Human Services. Public Health Service. Centers for Disease Control and Prevention. "Update: Cholera." *Morbidity and Mortality Weekly Report* 42, no. 5, 12 February 1993. Table: 938.

U.S. Department of Health and Human Services. Public Health Service. Health Resources and Services Administration. *Health Status of Minorities and Low-Income Groups.* 3rd ed. Washington, DC: U.S. Government Printing Office, n.d. Tables: 52, 161.

U.S. Department of Health and Human Services. Public Health Service. Health Resources and Services Administration. *On the Status of Health Personnel in the United States: Seventh Report to the President and Congress.* Rockville, MD: U.S. Department of Health and Human Services, Public Health Service, Health Resources and Services Administration, March 1990. Table: 694.

U.S. Department of Health and Human Services. Public Health Service. National Institute on Aging. *Bound for Good Health: A Collection of Age Pages.* Bethesda, MD: National Institute on Aging, c. 1991. Tables: 9, 10, 11, 12, 19, 122, 123, 152, 173, 184.

U.S. Department of Health and Human Services. Public Health Service. National Institute on Aging. *Physical Frailty: A Reducible Barrier to Independence for Older Americans.* Report to Congress. NIH Publication No. 91-397. Bethesda, MD: Department ofHealth and Human Services, Public Health Service, National Institutes of Health (NIH), September 1991. Table: 106.

U.S. Department of Health and Human Services. Public Health Service. National Institutes of Health. National Heart, Lung, and Blood Institute (NHLBI). *NHLBI Fact Book, Fiscal Year 1991.* Washington, DC: U.S. Department of Health and Human Services, Public Health Service, National Institutes of Health, National Heart, Lung, and Blood Institute (NHLBI), c. 1992. Tables: 779, 780, 955.

U.S. Department of Health and Human Services. Public Health Service. National Institutes of Health. National Institute on Alcohol Abuse and Alcoholism. National Institute on Drug Abuse. *State Resource and Services Related to Alcohol and Other Drug Abuse Problems for Fiscal Year 1990.* Rockville, MD: U.S. Department of Health and Human Services. National Institutes of Health. National Institute on Alcohol Abuse and Alcoholism. National Institute on Drug Abuse, n.d. Table: 257.

U.S. Department of Health and Human Services. Public Health Service. National Institutes of Health. *NIH Data Book, 1993: Basic Data Relating to the National Institutes of Health.* Compiled by Office of Science Policy and Technology Transfer, with ass istance of National Institutes of Health's Division of Research Grants. NIH Publication No. 93-1261. Bethesda, MD: U.S. Department of Health and Human Services, Public Health Service, National Institutes of Health, September 1993. Table: 817.

U.S. Department of Health and Human Services. Social Security Administration (SSA). *Annual Statistical Supplement to the "Social Security Bulletin," 1992.* SSA Publication No. 13-11700. Washington, DC: U.S. Department of Health and Human Services, Social Security Administration, Office of Research and Statistics, 1993. Tables: 309, 496, 510, 511, 512, 514, 515, 517, 518, 524, 526, 533, 549.

U.S. Department of Health and Human Services. Social Security Administration (SSA). Office of Research and Statistics. *SSI Recipients by State and County.* Washington, DC: U.S. Department of Health and Human Services, Social Security Administration, Office of Research and Statistics, December 1990. Table: 550.

U.S. Department of Health and Human Services. Social Security Administration (SSA). Office of the Actuary. "Social Security Area Population Projections." Prepared by Alice H. Wade. *Social Security Bulletin* 51, no. 2 (February 1988). Table: 29.

U.S. Department of Health and Human Services. Social Security Administration (SSA). "Social Security Programs in the United States, 1993." *Social Security Bulletin* 4, no. 4 (22 December 1993). Tables: 505, 530.

U.S. Department of Justice. Federal Bureau of Investigation. *Crime in the United States, 1992: Uniform Crime Reports.* Washington, DC: U.S. Government Printing Office, 3 October 1993. Tables: 327, 328, 331.

U.S. Department of Labor. Bureau of Labor Statistics. *Consumer Expenditure Survey, 1990-1991.* Washington, DC: U.S. Government Printing Office, September 1993. Tables: 393, 394, 395, 396, 397, 398, 399, 400, 401, 402, 403, 404, 405, 406, 407, 408, 409, 410, 412.

U.S. Department of Labor. Bureau of Labor Statistics. *Employee Benefits in Medium and Large Private Establishments, 1991.* Bulletin 2422. Washington, DC: U.S. Government Printing Office, May 1993. Table: 360.

U.S. Department of Labor. Bureau of Labor Statistics. *Fatal Workplace Injuries in 1991: A Collection of Data and Analysis.* Report 845. Washington, DC: U.S. Government Printing Office, April 1993. Table: 377.

U.S. Department of Labor. Bureau of Labor Statistics. *Occupational Injuries and Illnesses in the United States by Industry, 1991.* Bulletin 2424. Washington, DC: U.S. Government Printing Office, May 1993. Table: 384.

U.S. Department of Labor. Bureau of Labor Statistics. *Occupational Projections and Training Data: A Statistical and Research Supplement to the 1992-1993 "Occupational Outlook Handbook."* 1992 edition. Bulletin 2401. Washington, DC: U.S. Government Printing Office, May 1992. Tables: 674, 675, 676, 677, 678, 679, 680, 681, 682, 683, 684, 685, 686, 687.

U.S. Department of Labor. Bureau of Labor Statistics. *Occupational Wage Survey: Hospitals, January 1991.* Bulletin 2392. Washington, DC: U.S. Government Printing Office, January 1992. Tables: 741, 742, 743, 745, 746, 751, 756, 759.

U.S. Deparment of Labor. *Occupational Outlook Handbook.* 1992-1993 edition. Lincolnwood, IL: VGM Career Horizons, 1992. Tables: 688, 748, 760.

U.S. Department of Labor. Pension and Welfare Benefits Administration. *Health Benefits and the Workforce.* Washington, DC: U.S. Government Printing Office, 1992. Table: 354.

U.S. Department of Labor. Pension and Welfare Benefits Administration. *Trends in Health Benefits.* Washington, DC: U.S. Government Printing Office, 1993. Tables: 193, 215, 217, 218, 221, 339, 352, 353, 358, 414, 480, 762, 945.

U.S. Department of Transportation. National Highway Traffic Safety Administration. National Center for Statistics and Analysis. *1991 Alcohol Fatal Crash Facts.* Washington, DC: National Center for Statistics and Analysis, Research and Development, c.1991. Tables: 76, 77.

U.S. Department of Transportation. National Highway Traffic Safety Administration. National Center for Statistics and Analysis. *1991 Pedalcyclist Fatal Crash Facts.* Washington, DC: National Center for Statistics and Analysis, Research and Development, c. 1991. Table: 83.

U.S. Department of Transportation. National Highway Traffic Safety Administration. National Center for Statistics and Analysis. *1991 Traffic Fatality Facts.* Washington, DC: National Center for Statistics and Analysis, Research and Development, c. 1991. Tables: 82, 84.

U.S. Department of Veterans Affairs. Veterans Benefits Administration. Regional Office and Insurance Center. *Servicemen's and Veterans' Group Life Insurance Programs: Twenty-seventh Annual Report, Year Ending June 30, 1992*. Supervised by the Secretary of Veterans Affairs. Philadelphia, PA: Veterans Benefits Administration, c. 1992. Tables: 102, 103, 104.

U.S. General Accounting Office. *Diabetes: Status of the Disease Among American Indians, Blacks and Hispanics*. Washington, DC: U.S. General Accounting Office, 1992. Tables: 64, 65.

U.S. General Accounting Office. *Hospitals: Chief Executives' Compensation, 1989-1991*. Testimony Before the Subcommittee on Oversight and Investigations, Committee on Energy and Commerce, House of Representatives. Statement of Janet L. Shikles, Assistant Comptroller General, Human Resources Division. GAO/T-HRD-94-70. Washington, DC: U.S. General Accounting Office, 7 December 1992. Table: 753.

U.S. House Committee on Ways and Means. *Impact of Substance Abuse on State and Local Child Welfare Systems: Hearing*. Prepared by Richard L. Jones of the Child Welfare League of America. 30 April 1991. Washington, DC: U.S. Government Printing Office,1991. Table: 279.

U.S. House Committee on Ways and Means. *Overview of Entitlement Programs, 1993 Green Book: Background Material and Data Programs Within the Jurisdiction of the Committee on Ways and Means*. 103d Cong., 1st sess., 7 July 1993. Washington, DC: U.S. Government Printing Office, 1993. Table: 391.

U.S. House of Representatives. *Shortage of Health Care Professions Caring for the Elderly: Recommendations for Change*. 102d Cong., 2nd sess., December 1992. Comm. Pub. No. 102-915. Washington, DC: U.S. Government Printing Office, 1993. Tables: 698, 723, 736.

U.S. House Subcommittee on Technology, Environment, and Aviation. *Health Care Reform and Its Possible Effects on Innovative Therapies*. Statement presented by Derrel B. De Passe, Vice President, Worldwide Government Relations Varian Associates, Inc.Washington, DC: Federal Document Clearinghouse Congressional Testimony, 2 February 1994. Table: 628.

"U.S. Maintains Its Lead." *Chemistry and Industry*, 18 October 1993. Table: 956.

U.S. Senate Committee on Aging. *Medicare Fraud and Abuse: A Neglected Emergency? Hearing Before the Special Committee on Aging*, 102d Cong., 1st sess., 2 October 1991. Serial no. 102-13. Washington, DC: U.S. Government Printing Office, 1992. Tables: 186, 187, 188, 189, 190, 191, 227, 228, 894, 895.

U.S. Senate Committee on Veterans' Affairs. *Women's Health Progams Act of 1992*. Report to accompany S. 2973. 102d Cong., 2d sess., 17 September 1992. Washington, DC: U.S. Government Printing Office, 1992. Table: 337.

U.S. Senate Special Committee on Aging. *The Effects of Escalating Drug Costs on the Elderly: Hearing Before the Special Committee on Aging*. 102d Cong., 2nd sess., 22 April 1992. Serial no. 102-21. Washington, DC: U.S. Government Printing Office, 1992. Tables: 176, 177, 178, 179, 180, 181, 182, 183, 531.

The Universal Almanac, 1992. Kansas City, MO: Andrews and McMeel, 1991. Table: 153.

"USA Snapshots." *USA TODAY*, 17 January 1994. Table: 906.

"USA Snapshots." *USA TODAY*, 17 June 1994. Table: 946.

"USA Snapshots." *USA TODAY*, 27 September 1993. Table: 910.

"USA Snapshots." *USA TODAY*, 6 October 1993. Table: 252.

Van Nostrand, J. F., S. E. Furner, and R. Suzman, eds. *Health Data on Older Americans: United States, 1992*. Vital and Health Statistics, Series 3: Analytic and Epidemiological Studies, no. 27. DHHS publication no. (PHS) 93-1411. Hyattsville, MD: U.S. Department of Health and Human Services, Public Health Service, Centers for Disease Control and Prevention, National Center for Health Statistics, 1993. Tables: 13, 14, 15, 109, 110, 223.

Viviano, JoAnne. "State Takes Aim at Spouse Abuse." *Sunday Macomb Daily* (Macomb County, Michigan), 3 July 1994. Tables: 329, 330.

Voelker, Rebecca. "Bloodborne Standards Reach Beyond Medicine." *American Medical News*, 22-29 March 1993. Table: 785.

Wagner, Lynn. "AMA Backs Away From Hard Line on Reform." *Modern Healthcare*, 8 March 1993. Table: 673.

Waldholz, Michael. "An Industry in Adolescence; Think of Biotechnology as a Teenager: Lots of Promise, Lots of Headaches." *Wall Street Journal,* 20 May 1994. Tables: 625, 626.

Waldrop, Judith. "Seasons: The Birthday Boost." *American Demographics* 13 (September 1991). Table: 146.

"The War's Toll." *Detroit Free Press,* 3 July 1994. Tables: 54, 120, 151.

Wellness Letter 8, no. 8 (May 1992). Table: 280.

Wellness Letter 9, no. 10 (July 1993). Table: 80.

Wessel, David. "Health Costs to Fall in Some Industries, Increase in Others, New Analysis Shows." *Wall Street Journal,* 9 February 1994. Table: 349.

"What Gastroenterologists Charge for Three Procedures." *Medical Economics,* 11 October 1993. Table: 243.

"What Orthopedic Surgeons Are Charging." *Medical Economics,* 11 October 1993. Table: 246.

"What the Nutritional Information Means." *Orlando Sentinel Tribune,* 22 November 1992. Table: 297.

"Where IMGs Come From." *American Medical News,* 21 February 1994. Table: 693.

"Where Medicaid Dollars Go." *Washington Post National Weekly Edition,* 14-20 February 1994. Table: 494.

"Which Students Smoke Most?" *USA TODAY,* 15 July 1992, final edition. Table: 318.

White House Domestic Policy Council. *Health Security: The President's Report to the American People.* Washington, DC: The White House, October 1993. Table: 947.

"Who Uses Medicare." *USA TODAY,* 10 March 1993, final edition. Table: 502.

"Who's Big in Home Care." *Business Week,* 14 March 1994. Table: 569.

"Will Social Security Be There When You Need It?" *LAN* (August 1992). Table: 523.

Wilson, Virginia. "Policies for Old-Age Care" *Newsweek* 120, 20 April 1992. Table: 219.

Winslow, Ron. "Pap Smears for Some Women Over 65 Are Cost-Effective, Study Says." *Wall Street Journal,* 15 September 1992. Table: 156.

Wojcik, Joanne. "Managed Care Evolving Despite Clinton Proposal to Reform System." *Business Insurance,* 21 December 1993. Tables: 598, 599.

Wolf, Richard. "Survey Indicates Public Perplexed Over Reform." *USA TODAY,* 20 October 1993. Table: 882.

"Work Accidents." *Traffic Safety* (November/December 1993). Table: 379.

"Workers' Compensation Claims." *Occupational Health and Safety* 62, no. 10 (October 1993). Table: 392.

"World Abortion Rates." *The Mirror* (Springfield, Missouri), 13 May 1994. Table: 929.

"Yet Another Thing for Marketers to Worry About." *ADWEEK,* 11 October 1993. Table: 863.

"Your Insurance Premiums at Work." *Newsweek,* 27 June 1994. Table: 755.

Zaldivar, R. A. "High-Tech Love Affair; Lust for Latest Technology Breaking Health Care's Back." *Phoenix Gazette,* 30 July 1993, final edition. Table: 231.

Keyword Index

This index provides access to all subjects, issues, diseases, medical specialties, industries, companies, programs, insurance carriers, associations, schools, educational programs, occupations, personal names, and locations cited in the tables of *SRHM*. Each citation is followed by table and page reference numbers. Page references do not necessarily identify the page on which a table begins. In the cases where tables span two or more pages, references point to the page on which the index term appears, which may be the second or subsequent page of a table. Frequent cross-references have been added to index citations to facilitate the location of related topics and tables.

Abbey Healthcare Group (Costa Mesa, California)
— revenue, p. 495 [569]
Abbot Laboratories
— sales, p. 572 [664]
Abilene, Texas
— city government expenditures, p. 379 [463]
— clinical laboratory technologists and technicians, p. 602 [705]
— dental assistants, p. 608 [706]
— dental hygienists, p. 615 [707]
— dental laboratory technicians, p. 621 [708]
— dentists, p. 627 [709]
— dietitians, p. 634 [710]
— health aides, p. 641 [711]
— health care managers, p. 688 [721]
— health diagnosing practitioners, p. 647 [712]
— health record technologists and technicians, p. 654 [714]
— health technologists and technicians, p. 667 [716]
— licensed practical nurses, p. 674 [718]
— medical appliance technicians, p. 621 [708]
— nursing aides, p. 694 [722]
— occupational therapists, p. 702 [724]
— optical goods workers, p. 708 [725]
— orderlies, p. 694 [722]
— pharmacists, p. 720 [727]
— physical therapists, p. 727 [728]
— physicians, p. 733 [729]
— physicians' assistants, p. 740 [730]
— psychologists, p. 750 [732]
— radiologic technicians, p. 760 [734]
— registered nurses, p. 766 [735]
— respiratory therapists, p. 773 [737]
— speech therapists, p. 780 [738]
— therapists, p. 786 [739]
— veterinarians, p. 793 [740]
Abortion
— number, p. 123 [145]
— opinions, p. 878 [853]

Abortion continued:
— rates, pp. 112, 934 [133, 929]
— teens, p. 113 [134]
Abramson, Leonard
— salary, p. 812 [755]
Abuse *See:* Child abuse; Disciplinary action; Domestic violence
Abused women
— number in shelters, p. 77 [98]
Academic degrees *See:* Degrees
Accident insurance
— net premiums of carriers, p. 515 [597]
Accidental death
 See also: Accidents; Death
— alcohol-related, pp. 65-66 [76 77]
— children, p. 67 [81]
— cost, p. 64 [74]
— military, pp. 82, 84-85 [102-104]
— motor vehicle-related, p. 68 [82]
— number, p. 28 [32]
— older Americans, p. 6 [9]
— pedestrians, p. 69 [84]
— types, p. 64 [75]
— work fatalities, p. 288 [380]
Accidents
 See also: Occupational accidents; Occupational health and safety
— aircraft, p. 288 [380]
— alcohol-related, pp. 65-66 [76-77]
— children, p. 18 [22]
— cost, p. 64 [74]
— deaths, pp. 10-12, 18-19, 28 [14, 22-23, 32]
— electric shock, p. 67 [79]
— falls, p. 288 [380]
— fatal, pp. 64-66, 68-69, 288 [74-77, 82, 84, 380]
— hair dryers, p. 67 [79]
— infant mortality, p. 121 [141]
— lawn mowers, p. 67 [80]
— motor vehicle, pp. 6, 64-66, 68-69, 197, 288-289 [9, 74-77, 82,

Numbers following p. or pp. are page references. Numbers in [ ] are table references.

Numbers following p. or pp. are page references. Numbers in [ ] are table references.

Numbers following p. or pp. are page references. Numbers in [ ] are table references.

Keyword Index

Numbers following p. or pp. are page references. Numbers in [ ] are table references.

Keyword Index

Americans With Disabilities Act continued:
— complaints, p. 278 [371]
AmeriCares Foundation
— fund-raising, p. 865 [834]
— public income, p. 865 [834]
Amgen
— net income, p. 535 [623]
— revenue, p. 536 [624]
Amherst, New York
— city government expenditures, p. 367 [452]
Amoxil
— price, p. 918 [905]
Amphetamines
— prisoners, p. 99 [114]
Amyotrophic lateral sclerosis *See:* Lou Gehrig's disease
Anaheim, California
— city government expenditures, p. 336 [424]
— clinical laboratory technologists and technicians, p. 605 [705]
— dental assistants, p. 612 [706]
— dental hygienists, p. 618 [707]
— dental laboratory technicians, p. 624 [708]
— dentists, p. 631 [709]
— dietitians, p. 637 [710]
— health aides, p. 644 [711]
— health care managers, p. 691 [721]
— health diagnosing practitioners, p. 650 [712]
— health record technologists and technicians, p. 658 [714]
— health specialties teachers, p. 664 [715]
— health technologists and technicians, p. 670 [716]
— licensed practical nurses, p. 677 [718]
— medical appliance technicians, p. 624 [708]
— medical science teachers, p. 681 [719]
— medical scientists, p. 685 [720]
— nursing aides, p. 698 [722]
— occupational therapists, p. 705 [724]
— optical goods workers, p. 711 [725]
— optometrists, p. 717 [726]
— orderlies, p. 698 [722]
— pharmacists, p. 724 [727]
— physical therapists, p. 730 [728]
— physicians, p. 736 [729]
— physicians' assistants, p. 743 [730]
— podiatrists, p. 747 [731]
— psychologists, p. 753 [732]
— psychology teachers, p. 758 [733]
— radiologic technicians, p. 763 [734]
— registered nurses, p. 770 [735]
— respiratory therapists, p. 777 [737]
— speech therapists, p. 783 [738]
— therapists, p. 789 [739]
— veterinarians, p. 796 [740]
Analgesics
— use, pp. 199, 206, 210-211 [261, 271, 276-277]
Anatomy
— medical school faculty, p. 598 [700]
Anchorage, Alaska
— city government expenditures, p. 333 [421]
— clinical laboratory technologists and technicians, p. 602

Anchorage, Alaska continued:
[705]
— consumer expenditures, p. 322 [410]
— dental assistants, p. 608 [706]
— dental hygienists, p. 615 [707]
— dental laboratory technicians, p. 621 [708]
— dentists, p. 628 [709]
— dietitians, p. 634 [710]
— health aides, p. 641 [711]
— health care managers, p. 688 [721]
— health diagnosing practitioners, p. 647 [712]
— health record technologists and technicians, p. 655 [714]
— health specialties teachers, p. 661 [715]
— health technologists and technicians, p. 667 [716]
— licensed practical nurses, p. 674 [718]
— medical appliance technicians, p. 621 [708]
— medical scientists, p. 683 [720]
— nursing aides, p. 694 [722]
— occupational therapists, p. 702 [724]
— optical goods workers, p. 708 [725]
— optometrists, p. 714 [726]
— orderlies, p. 694 [722]
— pharmacists, p. 720 [727]
— physical therapists, p. 727 [728]
— physicians, p. 733 [729]
— physicians' assistants, p. 740 [730]
— psychologists, p. 750 [732]
— radiologic technicians, p. 760 [734]
— registered nurses, p. 766 [735]
— respiratory therapists, p. 773 [737]
— speech therapists, p. 780 [738]
— therapists, p. 786 [739]
— veterinarians, p. 793 [740]
Anderson, Indiana
— clinical laboratory technologists and technicians, p. 602 [705]
— dental assistants, p. 608 [706]
— dental hygienists, p. 615 [707]
— dental laboratory technicians, p. 621 [708]
— dentists, p. 628 [709]
— dietitians, p. 634 [710]
— health aides, p. 641 [711]
— health care managers, p. 688 [721]
— health diagnosing practitioners, p. 647 [712]
— health record technologists and technicians, p. 655 [714]
— health technologists and technicians, p. 667 [716]
— licensed practical nurses, p. 674 [718]
— medical appliance technicians, p. 621 [708]
— nursing aides, p. 694 [722]
— optical goods workers, p. 708 [725]
— optometrists, p. 714 [726]
— orderlies, p. 694 [722]
— pharmacists, p. 720 [727]
— physical therapists, p. 727 [728]
— physicians, p. 733 [729]
— physicians' assistants, p. 740 [730]
— psychologists, p. 750 [732]
— radiologic technicians, p. 760 [734]
— registered nurses, p. 766 [735]
— respiratory therapists, p. 773 [737]

Numbers following p. or pp. are page references. Numbers in [ ] are table references.

Numbers following p. or pp. are page references. Numbers in [ ] are table references.

Numbers following p. or pp. are page references. Numbers in [ ] are table references.

Numbers following p. or pp. are page references. Numbers in [ ] are table references.

Numbers following p. or pp. are page references. Numbers in [ ] are table references.

Numbers following p. or pp. are page references. Numbers in [ ] are table references.

Numbers following p. or pp. are page references. Numbers in [ ] are table references.

Numbers following p. or pp. are page references. Numbers in [ ] are table references.

Numbers following p. or pp. are page references. Numbers in [ ] are table references.

Numbers following p. or pp. are page references. Numbers in [ ] are table references.

991

Numbers following p. or pp. are page references. Numbers in [ ] are table references.

Numbers following p. or pp. are page references. Numbers in [ ] are table references.

Beloit, Wisconsin continued:
— nursing aides, p. 697 [722]
— occupational therapists, p. 704 [724]
— optical goods workers, p. 710 [725]
— orderlies, p. 697 [722]
— pharmacists, p. 723 [727]
— physical therapists, p. 729 [728]
— physicians, p. 736 [729]
— physicians' assistants, p. 742 [730]
— podiatrists, p. 747 [731]
— psychologists, p. 752 [732]
— psychology teachers, p. 758 [733]
— radiologic technicians, p. 762 [734]
— registered nurses, p. 769 [735]
— respiratory therapists, p. 776 [737]
— speech therapists, p. 782 [738]
— therapists, p. 789 [739]
— veterinarians, p. 795 [740]
Benefit payments
— financial statement, p. 450 [527]
Benign lesions
— excision costs, p. 188 [247]
— hospital care, p. 176 [233]
— outpatient services, p. 176 [233]
Benton Harbor, Michigan
— clinical laboratory technologists and technicians, p. 602 [705]
— dental assistants, p. 609 [706]
— dental hygienists, p. 615 [707]
— dental laboratory technicians, p. 622 [708]
— dentists, p. 628 [709]
— dietitians, p. 634 [710]
— health aides, p. 641 [711]
— health care managers, p. 688 [721]
— health diagnosing practitioners, p. 648 [712]
— health record technologists and technicians, p. 655 [714]
— health specialties teachers, p. 661 [715]
— health technologists and technicians, p. 667 [716]
— licensed practical nurses, p. 674 [718]
— medical appliance technicians, p. 622 [708]
— nursing aides, p. 695 [722]
— occupational therapists, p. 702 [724]
— optical goods workers, p. 708 [725]
— optometrists, p. 715 [726]
— orderlies, p. 695 [722]
— pharmacists, p. 721 [727]
— physical therapists, p. 727 [728]
— physicians, p. 734 [729]
— physicians' assistants, p. 740 [730]
— podiatrists, p. 746 [731]
— psychologists, p. 750 [732]
— radiologic technicians, p. 760 [734]
— registered nurses, p. 767 [735]
— respiratory therapists, p. 774 [737]
— speech therapists, p. 780 [738]
— therapists, p. 787 [739]
— veterinarians, p. 793 [740]
Berkeley, California
— city government expenditures, p. 336 [424]

Beta carotene
— sales, p. 235 [306]
Beta-interferon
— sales, p. 149 [185]
Beth Israel Hospital
— geriatrics, p. 157 [200]
Bethlehem, Pennsylvania
— clinical laboratory technologists and technicians, p. 602 [705]
— dental assistants, p. 608 [706]
— dental hygienists, p. 615 [707]
— dental laboratory technicians, p. 621 [708]
— dentists, p. 627 [709]
— dietitians, p. 634 [710]
— health aides, p. 641 [711]
— health care managers, p. 688 [721]
— health diagnosing practitioners, p. 647 [712]
— health record technologists and technicians, p. 655 [714]
— health specialties teachers, p. 661 [715]
— health technologists and technicians, p. 667 [716]
— licensed practical nurses, p. 674 [718]
— medical appliance technicians, p. 621 [708]
— medical science teachers, p. 680 [719]
— medical scientists, p. 683 [720]
— nursing aides, p. 694 [722]
— occupational therapists, p. 702 [724]
— optical goods workers, p. 708 [725]
— optometrists, p. 714 [726]
— orderlies, p. 694 [722]
— pharmacists, p. 720 [727]
— physical therapists, p. 727 [728]
— physicians, p. 733 [729]
— physicians' assistants, p. 740 [730]
— podiatrists, p. 746 [731]
— psychologists, p. 750 [732]
— psychology teachers, p. 756 [733]
— radiologic technicians, p. 760 [734]
— registered nurses, p. 766 [735]
— respiratory therapists, p. 773 [737]
— speech therapists, p. 780 [738]
— therapists, p. 786 [739]
— veterinarians, p. 793 [740]
Beverly Enterprises
— beds, p. 826 [777]
— facilities, p. 826 [777]
Bhutan
— tuberculosis, p. 945 [941]
Bicycles
— accidents, p. 75 [96]
— product-related injuries, p. 75 [96]
Biliary tract X-ray
— men, p. 182 [238]
— women, p. 182 [238]
Bilirakis, Representative Michael
— health care reform, p. 894 [874]
Billings, Montana
— city government expenditures, p. 361 [446]
— clinical laboratory technologists and technicians, p. 602 [705]
— dental assistants, p. 609 [706]
— dental hygienists, p. 615 [707]

Numbers following p. or pp. are page references. Numbers in [ ] are table references.

Keyword Index

Numbers following p. or pp. are page references. Numbers in [ ] are table references.

Numbers following p. or pp. are page references. Numbers in [ ] are table references.

Numbers following p. or pp. are page references. Numbers in [ ] are table references.

Keyword Index

Numbers following p. or pp. are page references. Numbers in [ ] are table references.

Bristol, Virginia continued:
— speech therapists, p. 782 [738]
— therapists, p. 789 [739]
— veterinarians, p. 795 [740]
Bristol-Meyers Squibb Company
— sales, p. 571 [664]
Britain
— infant mortality, p. 936 [932]
— oncology, p. 926 [920]
— physicians' services, p. 926 [920]
Broccoli
— calcium, p. 228 [296]
Brockton, Massachusetts
— city government expenditures, p. 355 [441]
Bronchitis
— acute conditions, p. 40 [43]
— bed days, p. 41 [44]
  chronic conditions, p. 53 [60]
— deaths, p. 940 [936]
— medical attention, p. 43 [46]
— older Americans, p. 12 [15]
— restricted activity, p. 44 [47]
Bronchus cancer
— deaths, p. 940 [936]
Brookdale Hospital Medical Center (New York, New York)
— labor strike, p. 835 [789]
Brookhaven, New York
— city government expenditures, p. 367 [452]
Brownsville, Texas
— city government expenditures, p. 379 [463]
— clinical laboratory technologists and technicians, p. 603 [705]
— dental assistants, p. 609 [706]
— dental hygienists, p. 615 [707]
— dental laboratory technicians, p. 622 [708]
— dentists, p. 628 [709]
— dietitians, p. 635 [710]
— health aides, p. 641 [711]
— health care managers, p. 688 [721]
— health diagnosing practitioners, p. 648 [712]
— health record technologists and technicians, p. 655 [714]
— health technologists and technicians, p. 667 [716]
— licensed practical nurses, p. 674 [718]
— medical appliance technicians, p. 622 [708]
— medical science teachers, p. 680 [719]
— medical scientists, p. 683 [720]
— nursing aides, p. 695 [722]
— occupational therapists, p. 702 [724]
— optical goods workers, p. 708 [725]
— optometrists, p. 715 [726]
— orderlies, p. 695 [722]
— pharmacists, p. 721 [727]
— physical therapists, p. 727 [728]
— physicians, p. 734 [729]
— physicians' assistants, p. 740 [730]
— psychologists, p. 750 [732]
— psychology teachers, p. 757 [733]
— radiologic technicians, p. 760 [734]

Brownsville, Texas continued:
— registered nurses, p. 767 [735]
— respiratory therapists, p. 774 [737]
— speech therapists, p. 780 [738]
— therapists, p. 787 [739]
— veterinarians, p. 793 [740]
Bryan, Texas
— clinical laboratory technologists and technicians, p. 603 [705]
— dental assistants, p. 609 [706]
— dental hygienists, p. 615 [707]
— dental laboratory technicians, p. 622 [708]
— dentists, p. 628 [709]
— dietitians, p. 635 [710]
— health aides, p. 641 [711]
— health care managers, p. 688 [721]
— health diagnosing practitioners, p. 648 [712]
— health record technologists and technicians, p. 655 [714]
— health specialties teachers, p. 662 [715]
— health technologists and technicians, p. 667 [716]
— licensed practical nurses, p. 674 [718]
— medical appliance technicians, p. 622 [708]
— medical scientists, p. 683 [720]
— nursing aides, p. 695 [722]
— occupational therapists, p. 702 [724]
— optical goods workers, p. 708 [725]
— orderlies, p. 695 [722]
— pharmacists, p. 721 [727]
— physical therapists, p. 727 [728]
— physicians, p. 734 [729]
— psychologists, p. 750 [732]
— psychology teachers, p. 757 [733]
— radiologic technicians, p. 760 [734]
— registered nurses, p. 767 [735]
— respiratory therapists, p. 774 [737]
— speech therapists, p. 780 [738]
— therapists, p. 787 [739]
— veterinarians, p. 793 [740]
Buffalo, New York
— city government expenditures, p. 367 [452]
— clinical laboratory technologists and technicians, p. 603 [705]
— consumer expenditures, p. 318 [408]
— dental assistants, p. 609 [706]
— dental hygienists, p. 615 [707]
— dental laboratory technicians, p. 622 [708]
— dentists, p. 628 [709]
— dietitians, p. 635 [710]
— health aides, p. 641 [711]
— health care managers, p. 688 [721]
— health diagnosing practitioners, p. 648 [712]
— health record technologists and technicians, p. 655 [714]
— health specialties teachers, p. 662 [715]
— health technologists and technicians, p. 668 [716]
— licensed practical nurses, p. 674 [718]
— medical appliance technicians, p. 622 [708]
— medical science teachers, p. 680 [719]
— medical scientists, p. 683 [720]
— nursing aides, p. 695 [722]
— occupational therapists, p. 702 [724]
— optical goods workers, p. 708 [725]

Keyword Index

Numbers following p. or pp. are page references. Numbers in [ ] are table references.

Numbers following p. or pp. are page references. Numbers in [ ] are table references.

Keyword Index

Numbers following p. or pp. are page references. Numbers in [ ] are table references.

Numbers following p. or pp. are page references. Numbers in [ ] are table references.

1005

Keyword Index

Numbers following p. or pp. are page references. Numbers in [ ] are table references.

Numbers following p. or pp. are page references. Numbers in [ ] are table references.

Numbers following p. or pp. are page references. Numbers in [ ] are table references.

Numbers following p. or pp. are page references. Numbers in [ ] are table references.

Numbers following p. or pp. are page references. Numbers in [ ] are table references.

Numbers following p. or pp. are page references. Numbers in [ ] are table references.

Numbers following p. or pp. are page references. Numbers in [ ] are table references.

Keyword Index

Numbers following p. or pp. are page references. Numbers in [ ] are table references.

Numbers following p. or pp. are page references. Numbers in [ ] are table references.

1017

Numbers following p. or pp. are page references. Numbers in [ ] are table references.

Keyword Index

Numbers following p. or pp. are page references. Numbers in [ ] are table references.

Numbers following p. or pp. are page references. Numbers in [ ] are table references.

Numbers following p. or pp. are page references. Numbers in [ ] are table references.

Numbers following p. or pp. are page references. Numbers in [ ] are table references.

Numbers following p. or pp. are page references. Numbers in [ ] are table references.

Numbers following p. or pp. are page references. Numbers in [ ] are table references.

Numbers following p. or pp. are page references. Numbers in [ ] are table references.

Numbers following p. or pp. are page references. Numbers in [ ] are table references.

Numbers following p. or pp. are page references. Numbers in [ ] are table references.

Dieting
— persons attempting to lose weight, p. 232 [303]
Dietitians
— employment, p. 634 [710]
— salaries and wages, p. 804 [744]
Diets
— cancer, p. 48 [54]
— deaths, p. 48 [54]
Digestive system conditions
— acute conditions, p. 40 [43]
— bed days, p. 41 [44]
— chronic conditions, p. 52 [60]
— medical attention, p. 43 [46]
— office visits, p. 137 [166]
— restricted activity, p. 44 [47]
Dilation and curettage
— abortion, p. 136 [165]
— cost, p. 136 [165]
— diagnostic, p. 136 [165]
— inappropriate procedures, p. 183 [239]
Dilation and evacuation
— cost, p. 136 [165]
Diphtheria
— cases, p. 61 [71]
— vaccinations, pp. 164-165 [213-214]
Directors of Human Resources
— fringe benefits, p. 810 [752]
— salaries and wages, p. 810 [752]
Directors of Personnel
— earnings, p. 802 [742]
Disabilities
 See also: Work disabilities; specific types (e.g., Paralysis)
— children, p. 20 [25]
  chronic conditions, p. 52 [60]
— cognitive, pp. 93-94 [109-110]
— hearing impairment, pp. 7, 20 [11, 25]
— long-term, p. 478 [552]
— Medicaid, pp. 413, 415 [496-497]
— older Americans, p. 7 [11]
— orthopedic, p. 52 [60]
— physical, p. 89 [106]
— short-term, p. 478 [552]
— social welfare programs, pp. 471 [546-547]
— veterans, p. 487 [559]
— work, pp. 278, 280, 283-284 [372-373, 375-376]
— workers, p. 447 [525]
Disability Insurance
— administrative costs, p. 447 [524]
— financial statement, p. 450 [527]
Discectomy
— cost, p. 187 [245]
Disciplinary action
— National Practitioner Data Bank, p. 915 [900]
— physicians, p. 907 [892]
— state medical boards, pp. 907 [892-893]
Diseases See: Health Status of Americans chapter; specific
  diseases
Dislocations
— acute conditions, p. 40 [43]

Dislocations continued:
— bed days, p. 41 [44]
— medical attention, p. 43 [46]
— restricted activity, p. 44 [47]
Dismutases
— biotechnology products, p. 858 [821]
District of Columbia
— abused women, p. 77 [98]
— accidental death, p. 28 [32]
— accidents, p. 28 [32]
— Aid to Families With Dependent Children, pp. 466, 473 [542, 548]
— alcohol abuse treatment programs, p. 195 [257]
— atherosclerosis, p. 28 [32]
— births, pp. 114-115 [135-136]
— births to teenage mothers, p. 115 [136]
— cancer, p. 28 [32]
— cerebrovascular diseases, p. 28 [32]
— child nutrition programs, p. 457 [535]
— chiropractors' offices and clinics, p. 553 [645]
— chronic obstructive pulmonary diseases, p. 28 [32]
— cirrhosis, p. 28 [32]
— city government expenditures, p. 342 [428]
— deaths, p. 28 [32]
— dental equipment wholesalers, p. 576 [669]
— dental laboratories, pp. 521, 523 [606, 609]
— dental supply wholesalers, p. 576 [669]
— dentists' offices and clinics, pp. 550, 555 [643, 647]
— diabetes, p. 28 [32]
— disciplinary action, p. 908 [893]
— drug and medicine wholesalers, p. 574 [667]
— drug and proprietary retailers, p. 573 [666]
— drug proprietaries wholesalers, p. 574 [667]
— drug stores, p. 573 [666]
— druggists' sundries wholesalers, p. 574 [667]
— end-stage renal disease facilities, p. 438 [517]
— flu, p. 28 [32]
— food stamps, p. 461 [539]
— grants, p. 829 [780]
— Head Start programs, p. 453 [532]
— health care reform, p. 898 [878]
— health practitioners' offices and clinics, p. 563 [655]
— health services, p. 488 [560]
— heart disease, p. 28 [32]
— home health care, pp. 438, 492 [517, 565]
— homeless persons, p. 79 [99]
— hospital charges, p. 429 [511]
— hospital equipment wholesalers, p. 576 [669]
— hospital supply wholesalers, p. 576 [669]
— hospitals, p. 506 [584]
— institutionalized populations, pp. 77, 79, 88, 98 [98-99, 105, 113]
— insurance coverage of residents, p. 227 [295]
— intermediate care facilities, p. 539 [629]
— kidney dialysis centers, p. 496 [570]
— liver disease, p. 28 [32]
— local government expenditures, p. 330 [419]
— low birth weight babies, p. 115 [136]
— malpractice insurance premiums, p. 911 [897]
— Medicaid, p. 412 [495]

Numbers following p. or pp. are page references. Numbers in [ ] are table references.

1029

Numbers following p. or pp. are page references. Numbers in [ ] are table references.

Numbers following p. or pp. are page references. Numbers in [ ] are table references.

Keyword Index

1031

Numbers following p. or pp. are page references. Numbers in [ ] are table references.

1032

Numbers following p. or pp. are page references. Numbers in [ ] are table references.

1033

Keyword Index

Numbers following p. or pp. are page references. Numbers in [ ] are table references.

Keyword Index

Numbers following p. or pp. are page references. Numbers in [ ] are table references.

Numbers following p. or pp. are page references. Numbers in [ ] are table references.

Numbers following p. or pp. are page references. Numbers in [ ] are table references.

Numbers following p. or pp. are page references. Numbers in [ ] are table references.

Numbers following p. or pp. are page references. Numbers in [ ] are table references.

Fall River, Massachusetts continued:
— respiratory therapists, p. 778 [737]
— speech therapists, p. 784 [738]
— therapists, p. 791 [739]
— veterinarians, p. 797 [740]
Falls
— deaths, pp. 67-68 [81]
— work fatalities, p. 288 [380]
Family coverage
— employee benefits, p. 272 [360]
Family medicine
   See also: Family practice
— medical school faculty, pp. 598 [699-700]
Family planning
— Medicaid, p. 415 [497]
Family practice
— associate's degrees, p. 587 [682]
— awards, p. 587 [682]
— bachelor's degrees, p. 587 [682]
— business supply expenditures, p. 841 [801]
— doctoral degrees, p. 587 [682]
— earnings, p. 817 [765]
— first-professional degrees, p. 587 [682]
— geriatrics, p. 597 [698]
— master's degrees, p. 587 [682]
— medical supply expenditures, p. 841 [801]
— physicians, pp. 597, 817 [698, 764]
— professional spending, p. 843 [803]
— salaries and wages, p. 817 [764]
Fans
— product-related injuries, p. 70 [86]
Fargo, North Dakota
— city government expenditures, p. 370 [454]
— clinical laboratory technologists and technicians, p. 604 [705]
— dental assistants, p. 610 [706]
— dental hygienists, p. 616 [707]
— dental laboratory technicians, p. 623 [708]
— dentists, p. 629 [709]
— dietitians, p. 636 [710]
— health aides, p. 642 [711]
— health care managers, p. 689 [721]
— health diagnosing practitioners, p. 649 [712]
— health record technologists and technicians, p. 656 [714]
— health specialties teachers, p. 662 [715]
— health technologists and technicians, p. 669 [716]
— licensed practical nurses, p. 675 [718]
— medical appliance technicians, p. 623 [708]
— medical scientists, p. 684 [720]
— nursing aides, p. 696 [722]
— occupational therapists, p. 703 [724]
— optical goods workers, p. 709 [725]
— optometrists, p. 716 [726]
— orderlies, p. 696 [722]
— pharmacists, p. 722 [727]
— physical therapists, p. 728 [728]
— physicians, p. 735 [729]
— physicians' assistants, p. 741 [730]
— psychologists, p. 751 [732]

Fargo, North Dakota continued:
— radiologic technicians, p. 761 [734]
— registered nurses, p. 768 [735]
— respiratory therapists, p. 775 [737]
— speech therapists, p. 781 [738]
— therapists, p. 788 [739]
— veterinarians, p. 794 [740]
Farming
— group health plans, p. 268 [356]
FAS 106
— effect on leading companies, p. 276 [367]
Fatalities *See:* Accidental death; Accidents; Death;
   Occupational accidents
Fatigue
— stress, p. 249 [326]
Fayetteville, Arkansas
— clinical laboratory technologists and technicians, p. 604 [705]
— dental assistants, p. 610 [706]
— dental hygienists, p. 616 [707]
— dental laboratory technicians, p. 623 [708]
— dentists, p. 629 [709]
— dietitians, p. 636 [710]
— health aides, p. 643 [711]
— health care managers, p. 690 [721]
— health diagnosing practitioners, p. 649 [712]
— health record technologists and technicians, p. 656 [714]
— health specialties teachers, p. 663 [715]
— health technologists and technicians, p. 669 [716]
— licensed practical nurses, p. 676 [718]
— medical appliance technicians, p. 623 [708]
— medical scientists, p. 684 [720]
— nursing aides, p. 696 [722]
— occupational therapists, p. 703 [724]
— optical goods workers, p. 710 [725]
— orderlies, p. 696 [722]
— pharmacists, p. 722 [727]
— physical therapists, p. 729 [728]
— physicians, p. 735 [729]
— physicians' assistants, p. 741 [730]
— psychologists, p. 752 [732]
— psychology teachers, p. 757 [733]
— radiologic technicians, p. 762 [734]
— registered nurses, p. 768 [735]
— respiratory therapists, p. 775 [737]
— speech therapists, p. 782 [738]
— therapists, p. 788 [739]
— veterinarians, p. 794 [740]
Fayetteville, North Carolina
— clinical laboratory technologists and technicians, p. 604 [705]
— dental assistants, p. 610 [706]
— dental hygienists, p. 616 [707]
— dental laboratory technicians, p. 623 [708]
— dentists, p. 629 [709]
— dietitians, p. 636 [710]
— health aides, p. 642 [711]
— health care managers, p. 689 [721]
— health diagnosing practitioners, p. 649 [712]
— health record technologists and technicians, p. 656 [714]
— health specialties teachers, p. 662 [715]

Fayetteville, North Carolina continued:
— health technologists and technicians, p. 669 [716]
— licensed practical nurses, p. 675 [718]
— medical appliance technicians, p. 623 [708]
— medical scientists, p. 684 [720]
— nursing aides, p. 696 [722]
— occupational therapists, p. 703 [724]
— optical goods workers, p. 709 [725]
— optometrists, p. 716 [726]
— orderlies, p. 696 [722]
— pharmacists, p. 722 [727]
— physical therapists, p. 728 [728]
— physicians, p. 735 [729]
— physicians' assistants, p. 741 [730]
— podiatrists, p. 747 [731]
— psychologists, p. 751 [732]
— radiologic technicians, p. 761 [734]
— registered nurses, p. 768 [735]
— respiratory therapists, p. 775 [737]
— speech therapists, p. 781 [738]
— therapists, p. 788 [739]
— veterinarians, p. 794 [740]

Fazio, Representative Vic
— campaign contributions, p. 888 [868]

Fecal-occult blood testing
— cost, p. 185 [241]

Federal government
— child nutrition expenditures, p. 458 [536]
— child nutrition programs, p. 458 [536]
— diabetes, p. 56 [65]
— education expenditures, p. 929 [923]
— expenditures, pp. 326-329, 401-402, 440, 451, 476, 479, 853
    [415-418, 484-485, 519, 528, 551, 553, 816]
— food stamps program, p. 460 [538]
— health care expenditures, p. 929 [923]
— Health Security Act expenditures, p. 901 [881]
— hospital ownership, p. 832 [784]
— housing expenditures, p. 929 [923]
— Medicaid, p. 411 [494]
— pensions, p. 327 [416]
— personal expenditures, p. 408 [492]
— research and development, pp. 854, 856 [818-819]
— Social Security, p. 929 [923]
— social welfare programs, pp. 476, 479 [551, 553]

Federal Republic of Germany *See:* Germany

Federated funds
— grants, p. 830 [781]

Feinstein, Senator Dianne
— campaign contributions, p. 888 [868]

Fences
— accidents, p. 72 [90]
— product-related injuries, p. 72 [90]

Fertility
— men, p. 105 [125]
— rate, p. 118 [139]

Fetal alcohol syndrome
— cost, p. 197 [259]

Fetal tissue
— research, p. 878 [853]

Fever
— acute conditions, p. 41 [43]
— bed days, p. 42 [44]
— medical attention, p. 44 [46]
— restricted activity, p. 45 [47]

Figs
— calcium, p. 228 [296]

Fiji
— tuberculosis, p. 945 [941]

File clerks
— earnings, p. 799 [741]

Finance
— health care plans, p. 267 [355]
— health insurance, p. 273 [361]

Financial Aid for Disadvantaged Health Professions Students
— financial assistance programs, p. 591 [689]

Financial assistance programs
— state funded, p. 591 [689]

Finland
— asthma, p. 940 [936]
— breast cancer, p. 940 [936]
— bronchitis, p. 940 [936]
— bronchus cancer, p. 940 [936]
— cerebrovascular disease, p. 940 [936]
— chronic liver disease, p. 940 [936]
— circulatory system disease mortality rates, pp. 938-939 [934-935]
— cirrhosis, p. 940 [936]
— emphysema, p. 940 [936]
— health care expenditures, pp. 930, 932-933 [924, 927-928]
— hospital care, p. 926 [919]
— infant mortality, p. 936 [932]
— inpatient care, pp. 924-925 [917-918]
— ischemic heart disease, p. 940 [936]
— lung cancer, p. 940 [936]
— physicians, p. 955 [959]
— self-inflicted injuries, p. 940 [936]
— stomach cancer, p. 940 [936]
— suicide, pp. 940, 951 [936, 951]
— trachea cancer, p. 940 [936]
— traffic accidents, p. 940 [936]

Fire departments
— emergency medical technicians, p. 807 [748]
— paramedics, p. 807 [748]

Fireplaces
— product-related injuries, p. 70 [86]

Fireworks
— product-related injuries, p. 74 [94]

First Health Strategies Inc
— claims paid, p. 515 [596]

FIRST Independent Research Support and Transition Award
— costs, p. 827 [779]
— grants, p. 827 [779]

Fishing
— accidents, p. 75 [96]
— group health plans, p. 268 [356]
— product-related injuries, p. 75 [96]

Numbers following p. or pp. are page references. Numbers in [ ] are table references.

Numbers following p. or pp. are page references. Numbers in [ ] are table references.

Keyword Index

Fort Lauderdale, Florida continued:
— orderlies, p. 698 [722]
— pharmacists, p. 724 [727]
— physical therapists, p. 730 [728]
— physicians, p. 737 [729]
— physicians' assistants, p. 743 [730]
— podiatrists, p. 748 [731]
— psychologists, p. 753 [732]
— radiologic technicians, p. 763 [734]
— registered nurses, p. 770 [735]
— respiratory therapists, p. 777 [737]
— speech therapists, p. 783 [738]
— therapists, p. 790 [739]
— veterinarians, p. 796 [740]

Fort Myers, Florida
— clinical laboratory technologists and technicians, p. 604 [705]
— dental assistants, p. 610 [706]
— dental hygienists, p. 617 [707]
— dental laboratory technicians, p. 623 [708]
— dentists, p. 629 [709]
— dietitians, p. 636 [710]
— health aides, p. 643 [711]
— health care managers, p. 690 [721]
— health diagnosing practitioners, p. 649 [712]
— health record technologists and technicians, p. 656 [714]
— health technologists and technicians, p. 669 [716]
— licensed practical nurses, p. 676 [718]
— medical appliance technicians, p. 623 [708]
— medical scientists, p. 684 [720]
— nursing aides, p. 696 [722]
— occupational therapists, p. 704 [724]
— optical goods workers, p. 710 [725]
— optometrists, p. 716 [726]
— orderlies, p. 696 [722]
— pharmacists, p. 722 [727]
— physical therapists, p. 729 [728]
— physicians, p. 735 [729]
— physicians' assistants, p. 741 [730]
— podiatrists, p. 747 [731]
— psychologists, p. 752 [732]
— radiologic technicians, p. 762 [734]
— registered nurses, p. 768 [735]
— respiratory therapists, p. 775 [737]
— speech therapists, p. 782 [738]
— therapists, p. 788 [739]
— veterinarians, p. 795 [740]

Fort Pierce, Florida
— clinical laboratory technologists and technicians, p. 604 [705]
— dental assistants, p. 610 [706]
— dental hygienists, p. 617 [707]
— dental laboratory technicians, p. 623 [708]
— dentists, p. 629 [709]
— dietitians, p. 636 [710]
— health aides, p. 643 [711]
— health care managers, p. 690 [721]
— health diagnosing practitioners, p. 649 [712]
— health record technologists and technicians, p. 656 [714]

Fort Pierce, Florida continued:
— health technologists and technicians, p. 669 [716]
— licensed practical nurses, p. 676 [718]
— medical appliance technicians, p. 623 [708]
— medical scientists, p. 684 [720]
— nursing aides, p. 696 [722]
— occupational therapists, p. 704 [724]
— optical goods workers, p. 710 [725]
— optometrists, p. 716 [726]
— orderlies, p. 696 [722]
— pharmacists, p. 722 [727]
— physical therapists, p. 729 [728]
— physicians, p. 735 [729]
— physicians' assistants, p. 741 [730]
— podiatrists, p. 747 [731]
— psychologists, p. 752 [732]
— psychology teachers, p. 757 [733]
— radiologic technicians, p. 762 [734]
— registered nurses, p. 768 [735]
— respiratory therapists, p. 775 [737]
— speech therapists, p. 782 [738]
— therapists, p. 788 [739]
— veterinarians, p. 795 [740]

Fort Smith, Arkansas
— clinical laboratory technologists and technicians, p. 604 [705]
— dental assistants, p. 610 [706]
— dental hygienists, p. 617 [707]
— dental laboratory technicians, p. 623 [708]
— dentists, p. 629 [709]
— dietitians, p. 636 [710]
— health aides, p. 643 [711]
— health care managers, p. 690 [721]
— health diagnosing practitioners, p. 649 [712]
— health record technologists and technicians, p. 656 [714]
— health specialties teachers, p. 663 [715]
— health technologists and technicians, p. 669 [716]
— licensed practical nurses, p. 676 [718]
— medical appliance technicians, p. 623 [708]
— medical scientists, p. 684 [720]
— nursing aides, p. 696 [722]
— occupational therapists, p. 704 [724]
— optical goods workers, p. 710 [725]
— optometrists, p. 716 [726]
— orderlies, p. 696 [722]
— pharmacists, p. 722 [727]
— physical therapists, p. 729 [728]
— physicians, p. 735 [729]
— physicians' assistants, p. 741 [730]
— podiatrists, p. 747 [731]
— psychologists, p. 752 [732]
— radiologic technicians, p. 762 [734]
— registered nurses, p. 768 [735]
— respiratory therapists, p. 775 [737]
— speech therapists, p. 782 [738]
— therapists, p. 788 [739]
— veterinarians, p. 795 [740]

Fort Walton Beach, Florida
— clinical laboratory technologists and technicians, p. 604 [705]
— dental assistants, p. 610 [706]

Numbers following p. or pp. are page references. Numbers in [ ] are table references.

1046

Numbers following p. or pp. are page references. Numbers in [ ] are table references.

Numbers following p. or pp. are page references. Numbers in [ ] are table references.

Numbers following p. or pp. are page references. Numbers in [ ] are table references.

1049

Keyword Index

Numbers following p. or pp. are page references. Numbers in [ ] are table references.

Keyword Index

Numbers following p. or pp. are page references. Numbers in [ ] are table references.

Numbers following p. or pp. are page references. Numbers in [ ] are table references.

Keyword Index

Numbers following p. or pp. are page references. Numbers in [ ] are table references.

Numbers following p. or pp. are page references. Numbers in [ ] are table references.

Numbers following p. or pp. are page references. Numbers in [ ] are table references.

Hammond, Indiana
— city government expenditures, p. 348 [434]

Hampton, Virginia
— city government expenditures, p. 383 [466]

Hand garden tools
— accidents, p. 76 [97]
— product-related injuries, p. 76 [97]

Handlers
— group health plans, p. 267 [356]

Handrails
— accidents, p. 72 [90]
— product-related injuries, p. 72 [90]

Hansen disease
— cases, p. 61 [71]

Hardening of the arteries
— chronic conditions, p. 53 [60]

Hardware
— product-related injuries, p. 72 [90]

Harlingen, Texas
— clinical laboratory technologists and technicians, p. 603 [705]
— dental assistants, p. 609 [706]
— dental hygienists, p. 615 [707]
— dental laboratory technicians, p. 622 [708]
— dentists, p. 628 [709]
— dietitians, p. 635 [710]
— health aides, p. 641 [711]
— health care managers, p. 688 [721]
— health diagnosing practitioners, p. 648 [712]
— health record technologists and technicians, p. 655 [714]
— health technologists and technicians, p. 667 [716]
— licensed practical nurses, p. 674 [718]
— medical appliance technicians, p. 622 [708]
— medical science teachers, p. 680 [719]
— medical scientists, p. 683 [720]
— nursing aides, p. 695 [722]
— occupational therapists, p. 702 [724]
— optical goods workers, p. 708 [725]
— optometrists, p. 715 [726]
— orderlies, p. 695 [722]
— pharmacists, p. 721 [727]
— physical therapists, p. 727 [728]
— physicians, p. 734 [729]
— physicians' assistants, p. 740 [730]
— psychologists, p. 750 [732]
— psychology teachers, p. 757 [733]
— radiologic technicians, p. 760 [734]
— registered nurses, p. 767 [735]
— respiratory therapists, p. 774 [737]
— speech therapists, p. 780 [738]
— therapists, p. 787 [739]
— veterinarians, p. 793 [740]

Harrington Services Corp
— claims paid, p. 515 [596]

Harrisburg, Pennsylvania
— clinical laboratory technologists and technicians, p. 604 [705]
— dental assistants, p. 611 [706]
— dental hygienists, p. 617 [707]

Harrisburg, Pennsylvania continued:
— dental laboratory technicians, p. 623 [708]
— dentists, p. 630 [709]
— dietitians, p. 636 [710]
— health aides, p. 643 [711]
— health care managers, p. 690 [721]
— health diagnosing practitioners, p. 650 [712]
— health record technologists and technicians, p. 657 [714]
— health specialties teachers, p. 663 [715]
— health technologists and technicians, p. 669 [716]
— licensed practical nurses, p. 676 [718]
— medical appliance technicians, p. 623 [708]
— medical science teachers, p. 681 [719]
— medical scientists, p. 684 [720]
— nursing aides, p. 697 [722]
— occupational therapists, p. 704 [724]
— optical goods workers, p. 710 [725]
— optometrists, p. 716 [726]
— orderlies, p. 697 [722]
— pharmacists, p. 723 [727]
— physical therapists, p. 729 [728]
— physicians, p. 736 [729]
— physicians' assistants, p. 742 [730]
— podiatrists, p. 747 [731]
— psychologists, p. 752 [732]
— psychology teachers, p. 757 [733]
— radiologic technicians, p. 762 [734]
— registered nurses, p. 769 [735]
— respiratory therapists, p. 776 [737]
— speech therapists, p. 782 [738]
— therapists, p. 788 [739]
— veterinarians, p. 795 [740]

Hartford, Connecticut
— city government expenditures, p. 340 [426]
— clinical laboratory technologists and technicians, p. 604 [705]
— dental assistants, p. 611 [706]
— dental hygienists, p. 617 [707]
— dental laboratory technicians, p. 623 [708]
— dentists, p. 630 [709]
— dietitians, p. 636 [710]
— health aides, p. 643 [711]
— health care managers, p. 690 [721]
— health diagnosing practitioners, p. 650 [712]
— health record technologists and technicians, p. 657 [714]
— health specialties teachers, p. 663 [715]
— health technologists and technicians, p. 669 [716]
— inappropriate procedures, p. 142 [172]
— licensed practical nurses, p. 676 [718]
— medical appliance technicians, p. 623 [708]
— medical science teachers, p. 681 [719]
— medical scientists, p. 684 [720]
— nursing aides, p. 697 [722]
— occupational therapists, p. 704 [724]
— optical goods workers, p. 710 [725]
— optometrists, p. 716 [726]
— orderlies, p. 697 [722]
— pharmacists, p. 723 [727]
— physical therapists, p. 729 [728]
— physicians, p. 736 [729]

Numbers following p. or pp. are page references. Numbers in [ ] are table references.

Hartford, Connecticut continued:
— physicians' assistants, p. 742 [730]
— podiatrists, p. 747 [731]
— psychologists, p. 752 [732]
— radiologic technicians, p. 762 [734]
— registered nurses, p. 769 [735]
— respiratory therapists, p. 776 [737]
— speech therapists, p. 782 [738]
— therapists, p. 788 [739]
— veterinarians, p. 795 [740]

Hashish
— use, p. 209 [275]

Hatchets
— accidents, p. 76 [97]
— product-related injuries, p. 76 [97]

Hawaii
— abortion, p. 112 [133]
— abused women, p. 78 [98]
— accidental death, p. 29 [32]
— accidents, p. 29 [32]
— Aid to Families With Dependent Children, pp. 466, 473 [542, 548]
— alcohol abuse treatment programs, p. 195 [257]
— atherosclerosis, p. 29 [32]
— births, pp. 114, 116 [135-136]
— births to teenage mothers, p. 116 [136]
— cancer, p. 29 [32]
— cerebrovascular diseases, p. 29 [32]
— child nutrition programs, p. 457 [535]
— chiropractors' offices and clinics, p. 553 [645]
— chronic obstructive pulmonary diseases, p. 29 [32]
— cirrhosis, p. 29 [32]
— city government expenditures, p. 345 [431]
— deaths, p. 29 [32]
— dental equipment wholesalers, p. 576 [669]
— dental laboratories, pp. 521, 523 [606, 609]
— dental supply wholesalers, p. 576 [669]
— dentists' offices and clinics, pp. 550, 555 [643, 647]
— diabetes, p. 29 [32]
— disciplinary action, p. 908 [893]
— drug and medicine wholesalers, p. 574 [667]
— drug and proprietary retailers, p. 573 [666]
— drug proprietaries wholesalers, p. 574 [667]
— drug stores, p. 573 [666]
— druggists' sundries wholesalers, p. 574 [667]
— end-stage renal disease facilities, p. 439 [517]
— flu, p. 29 [32]
— food stamps, p. 462 [539]
— grants, p. 829 [780]
— Head Start programs, p. 453 [532]
— health care reform, p. 902 [884]
— health practitioners' offices and clinics, p. 563 [655]
— health services, p. 488 [560]
— heart disease, p. 29 [32]
— home health care, pp. 439, 492 [517, 565]
— homeless persons, p. 80 [99]
— hospital charges, p. 430 [511]
— hospital equipment wholesalers, p. 576 [669]
— hospital supply wholesalers, p. 576 [669]

Hawaii continued:
— hospitals, p. 506 [584]
— institutionalized populations, pp. 78, 80, 89, 99 [98-99, 105, 1
— insurance coverage of residents, p. 227 [295]
  intermediate care facilities, p. 539 [629]
— kidney dialysis centers, p. 496 [570]
— liver disease, p. 29 [32]
— local government expenditures, p. 330 [419]
— low birth weight babies, p. 116 [136]
— malpractice insurance premiums, pp. 911, 913 [897, 899]
— Medicaid, p. 413 [495]
— medical and surgical hospitals, p. 503 [580]
— medical doctors' offices and clinics, pp. 551, 557 [644, 649]
— medical equipment rental and leasing, p. 499 [574]
— medical equipment wholesalers, p. 576 [669]
— medical laboratories, pp. 439, 523, 525 [517, 609, 611]
— medical supply wholesalers, p. 576 [669]
— Medicare, pp. 423, 436 [506, 515]
— mental health expenditures, p. 108 [128]
— mental hospitals, p. 509 [588]
— military personnel, p. 89 [105]
— National School Lunch Program, p. 464 [540]
— nursing facilities, p. 543 [634]
— nursing homes, p. 92 [108]
— ophthalmic goods wholesalers, p. 578 [670]
— optometrists' offices and clinics, p. 561 [653]
— osteopaths' offices and clinics, p. 559 [651]
— personal care facilities, p. 543 [634]
— physicians' offices and clinics, pp. 551, 557, 559 [644, 649, 6
— pneumonia, p. 29 [32]
— podiatrists' offices and clinics, p. 565 [657]
— prisoners, p. 99 [113]
— psychiatric hospitals, p. 509 [588]
— skilled nursing care facilities, p. 547 [639]
— skilled nursing facilities, p. 439 [517]
— skilled nursing facility charges, p. 432 [512]
— Social Security, pp. 443, 445 [521-522]
— social welfare, p. 473 [548]
— specialty hospitals, p. 512 [592]
— state government expenditures, p. 393 [477]
— state medical boards, p. 908 [893]
— suicide, p. 29 [32]
— Supplemental Social Income, p. 473 [548]
— Supplementary Social Insurance, pp. 466, 475 [542, 550]
— work disabilities, pp. 279-280, 282-284 [372-376]

Hay fever
— chronic conditions, p. 54 [60]

Hayward, California
— city government expenditures, p. 336 [424]

Hazelnuts
— calcium, p. 228 [296]

Head nurses
— earnings, pp. 813-814 [756-757]

Head of human resources
— earnings, p. 812 [754]

Head of marketing
— earnings, p. 812 [754]

Head of patient care
— earnings, p. 812 [754]

Numbers following p. or pp. are page references. Numbers in [ ] are table references.

Numbers following p. or pp. are page references. Numbers in [ ] are table references.

Keyword Index

Numbers following p. or pp. are page references. Numbers in [ ] are table references.

Numbers following p. or pp. are page references. Numbers in [ ] are table references.

Numbers following p. or pp. are page references. Numbers in [ ] are table references.

Numbers following p. or pp. are page references. Numbers in [ ] are table references.

Numbers following p. or pp. are page references. Numbers in [ ] are table references.

Hospital supply wholesalers continued:
— establishments, p. 576 [669]
— number, p. 576 [669]
Hospitals
  See also: specific types (e.g., Psychiatric hospitals)
— billing practices, pp. 155, 952 [195, 953]
— bloodborne pathogens, p. 833 [785]
— bondholders, p. 831 [783]
— campaign contributions, pp. 888, 892 [867, 872]
— Canada, p. 952 [953]
— capital campaigns, p. 865 [833]
— charges, p. 428 [511]
— charitable contributions, pp. 863, 865 [830, 833]
— city government expenditures, pp. 332-336, 339-355, 357-
    367, 369-379, 381-388, 390-391 [420-471, 473-474]
— construction, pp. 823-825 [774-776]
— continuous quality improvement, p. 833 [786]
— continuous quality management, pp. 866, 868 [835-836, 838]
— emergency medical technicians, p. 807 [748]
— employee benefits, p. 833 [786]
— employment, p. 506 [584]
— establishments, p. 506 [584]
— executive compensation, pp. 811-812 [753-754]
— expenses, pp. 504, 507 [581, 585]
— federal government expenditures, pp. 326, 401 [415, 484]
— grants, p. 830 [781]
— infection control, p. 836 [790]
— labor strikes, p. 835 [789]
— layoffs, p. 836 [791]
— leading providers, p. 502 [579]
— local government expenditures, pp. 389, 392, 401 [472, 475,
    484]
— malpractice lawsuits, p. 906 [890]
— medical waste, p. 862 [829]
— medication errors, p. 836 [790]
— mental health services, p. 82 [101]
— number, p. 506 [584]
— occupational injuries, p. 289 [382]
— OSHA violations, p. 833 [785]
— ownership, p. 832 [784]
— paramedics, p. 807 [748]
— patient injuries, p. 836 [790]
— privacy protection, pp. 883, 885 [860, 863]
— receipts, pp. 505, 508 [582, 586]
— revenue, pp. 505, 508 [583, 587]
— rural, p. 156 [196]
— salaries and wages, pp. 799, 801, 803-805, 809, 813, 815
    [741-743, 745-746, 751, 756, 759]
— staff injuries, p. 836 [790]
— state government expenditures, pp. 392, 401 [475, 484]
— total quality management, pp. 833, 866, 868 [786, 835-836,
    838]
— U.S. Veterans Administration, p. 485 [557]
— urban, p. 156 [196]
Houma, Louisiana
— clinical laboratory technologists and technicians, p. 604
    [705]
— dental assistants, p. 611 [706]
— dental hygienists, p. 617 [707]

Houma, Louisiana continued:
— dental laboratory technicians, p. 623 [708]
— dentists, p. 630 [709]
— dietitians, p. 636 [710]
— health aides, p. 643 [711]
— health care managers, p. 690 [721]
— health diagnosing practitioners, p. 650 [712]
— health record technologists and technicians, p. 657 [714]
— health specialties teachers, p. 663 [715]
— health technologists and technicians, p. 669 [716]
— licensed practical nurses, p. 676 [718]
— medical appliance technicians, p. 623 [708]
— nursing aides, p. 697 [722]
— optical goods workers, p. 710 [725]
— optometrists, p. 716 [726]
— orderlies, p. 697 [722]
— pharmacists, p. 723 [727]
— physical therapists, p. 729 [728]
— physicians, p. 736 [729]
— physicians' assistants, p. 742 [730]
— psychologists, p. 752 [732]
— radiologic technicians, p. 762 [734]
— registered nurses, p. 769 [735]
— respiratory therapists, p. 776 [737]
— speech therapists, p. 782 [738]
— therapists, p. 789 [739]
— veterinarians, p. 795 [740]
House calls
— availability of physicians, p. 134 [163]
— cost, p. 133 [162]
Household chemicals
— product-related injuries, p. 72 [89]
Housewares
— product-related injuries, p. 73 [93]
Housing
— expenditures, p. 481 [555]
— federal government expenditures, pp. 477, 929 [551, 923]
— foreign government expenditures, p. 929 [923]
— local government expenditures, p. 484 [556]
— social welfare programs, pp. 477, 484 [551, 556]
— state government expenditures, p. 484 [556]
Housing benefits
— beneficiaries, p. 470 [545]
— expenditures, p. 467 [543]
Houston, Texas
— city government expenditures, p. 379 [463]
— clinical laboratory technologists and technicians, p. 604 [705]
— consumer expenditures, p. 320 [409]
— dental assistants, p. 611 [706]
— dental hygienists, p. 617 [707]
— dental laboratory technicians, p. 623 [708]
— dentists, p. 630 [709]
— dietitians, p. 636 [710]
— employee sick days, p. 291 [386]
— health aides, p. 643 [711]
— health care managers, p. 690 [721]
— health diagnosing practitioners, p. 650 [712]
— health maintenance organizations, p. 261 [347]
— health record technologists and technicians, p. 657 [714]

Numbers following p. or pp. are page references. Numbers in [ ] are table references.

1065

Keyword Index

Numbers following p. or pp. are page references. Numbers in [ ] are table references.

Numbers following p. or pp. are page references. Numbers in [ ] are table references.

Numbers following p. or pp. are page references. Numbers in [ ] are table references.

Keyword Index

Numbers following p. or pp. are page references. Numbers in [ ] are table references.

1070

Keyword Index

Numbers following p. or pp. are page references. Numbers in [ ] are table references.

Numbers following p. or pp. are page references. Numbers in [ ] are table references.

Keyword Index

1073

Numbers following p. or pp. are page references. Numbers in [ ] are table references.

Numbers following p. or pp. are page references. Numbers in [ ] are table references.

Keyword Index

Numbers following p. or pp. are page references. Numbers in [ ] are table references.

Numbers following p. or pp. are page references. Numbers in [ ] are table references.

Keyword Index

Numbers following p. or pp. are page references. Numbers in [ ] are table references.

Numbers following p. or pp. are page references. Numbers in [ ] are table references.

Numbers following p. or pp. are page references. Numbers in [ ] are table references.

Numbers following p. or pp. are page references. Numbers in [ ] are table references.

1081

Keyword Index

Numbers following p. or pp. are page references. Numbers in [ ] are table references.

Numbers following p. or pp. are page references. Numbers in [ ] are table references.

Keyword Index

Numbers following p. or pp. are page references. Numbers in [ ] are table references.

Numbers following p. or pp. are page references. Numbers in [ ] are table references.

Numbers following p. or pp. are page references. Numbers in [ ] are table references.

Numbers following p. or pp. are page references. Numbers in [ ] are table references.

Numbers following p. or pp. are page references. Numbers in [ ] are table references.

Numbers following p. or pp. are page references. Numbers in [ ] are table references.

Numbers following p. or pp. are page references. Numbers in [ ] are table references.

Numbers following p. or pp. are page references. Numbers in [ ] are table references.

1091

Keyword Index

Numbers following p. or pp. are page references. Numbers in [ ] are table references.

Numbers following p. or pp. are page references. Numbers in [ ] are table references.

Keyword Index

Numbers following p. or pp. are page references. Numbers in [ ] are table references.

Keyword Index

Numbers following p. or pp. are page references. Numbers in [ ] are table references.

Numbers following p. or pp. are page references. Numbers in [ ] are table references.

Keyword Index

Numbers following p. or pp. are page references. Numbers in [ ] are table references.

Numbers following p. or pp. are page references. Numbers in [ ] are table references.

1101

Medical illustrating
— associate's degrees, p. 582 [674]
— awards, p. 582 [674]
— bachelor's degrees, p. 582 [674]
— doctoral degrees, p. 582 [674]
— first-professional degrees, p. 582 [674]
— master's degrees, p. 582 [674]
Medical information
— conflicting, p. 870 [841]
Medical instrument manufacturers
— cost of materials, p. 530 [616]
— electromedical equipment, p. 528 [614]
— employment, pp. 529-530, 533, 538 [615-616, 620, 627]
— end-of-year inventories, p. 530 [616]
— establishments, pp. 529, 533, 538 [615, 620, 627]
— medical instruments, pp. 529, 533 [615, 620]
— medical supplies, p. 529 [615]
— new capital expenditures, p. 530 [616]
— number, pp. 529, 533 [615, 620]
— ophthalmic goods, p. 531 [617]
— optical instruments, p. 532 [619]
— optical lenses, p. 532 [619]
— payroll, p. 530 [616]
— production workers, p. 530 [616]
— salaries and wages, pp. 530, 538 [616, 627]
— surgical appliances, p. 534 [621]
— surgical instruments, p. 533 [620]
— surgical supplies, p. 534 [621]
— value-added by manufacture, p. 530 [616]
— value of shipments, p. 530 [616]
— x-ray apparatus and tubes, p. 535 [622]
Medical instruments
— manufacturers, pp. 529, 533, 538 [615, 620, 627]
Medical laboratories
— employment, pp. 523, 525 [609, 611]
— establishments, pp. 523, 525 [609, 611]
— Medicaid, p. 415 [497]
— Medicare, pp. 433, 437 [514, 517]
— number, pp. 523, 525 [609, 611]
— receipts, pp. 525, 527 [610, 612]
— U.S. Veterans Administration, p. 485 [557]
Medical laboratory degrees
— associate's degrees, p. 586 [681]
— awards, p. 586 [681]
— bachelor's degrees, p. 586 [681]
— doctoral degrees, p. 586 [681]
— first-professional degrees, p. 586 [681]
— master's degrees, p. 586 [681]
Medical laboratory technicians
— earnings, p. 805 [746]
Medical laboratory technologies
— associate's degrees, p. 586 [681]
— awards, p. 586 [681]
— bachelor's degrees, p. 586 [681]
— doctoral degrees, p. 586 [681]
— first-professional degrees, p. 586 [681]
— master's degrees, p. 586 [681]
Medical libraries
— associations, p. 838 [794]

Medical libraries continued:
— number, p. 837 [793]
Medical Library Association
— budget, p. 838 [794]
— members, p. 838 [794]
Medical licenses
— fees, pp. 839-840 [797-798]
Medical malpractice
  See also: Disciplinary action; Fraud; Litigation
— effect on cost of health care, p. 876 [850]
— hospitals, p. 906 [890]
— insurance premiums, pp. 911-913 [897-899]
— lawsuits, pp. 906 [889-890]
— market shares of insurers, p. 517 [601]
— National Practitioner Data Bank, p. 915 [900]
— orthopedic surgeons' insurance premiums, p. 913 [899]
— physicians, p. 906 [890]
Medical office management
— associate's degrees, p. 582 [674]
— awards, p. 582 [674]
— bachelor's degrees, p. 582 [674]
— doctoral degrees, p. 582 [674]
— first-professional degrees, p. 582 [674]
— master's degrees, p. 582 [674]
Medical periodicals
— cost, pp. 850-852 [812-813, 815]
— number, p. 850 [812]
Medical practice management
  See also: Medical administration
— administration, pp. 822, 840 [771, 799]
— computers, p. 822 [771]
— expenditures, p. 842 [802]
— expenses, p. 843 [803]
— patient population, p. 844 [804]
— professional expenses, p. 841 [800]
— supply expenditures, p. 841 [801]
Medical professions
— effect of health care reform, p. 894 [874]
Medical publishing
— books, pp. 849-850 [809-811]
— information needs of practitioners, p. 844 [805]
— periodicals, pp. 850-852 [812-815]
— reading level of material, pp. 845, 847-848 [806-808]
Medical radiation dosimetry
— associate's degrees, p. 584 [678]
— awards, p. 584 [678]
— bachelor's degrees, p. 584 [678]
— doctoral degrees, p. 584 [678]
— first-professional degrees, p. 584 [678]
— master's degrees, p. 584 [678]
Medical record technologists *See:* Health record
  technologists and technicians
Medical records
  See also: Computers
— computer-based patient records, pp. 821, 823 [769, 773]
— computerized, p. 884 [862]
— privacy protection, pp. 883-885 [860, 862-863]
Medical records administration
— associate's degrees, p. 586 [680]

Numbers following p. or pp. are page references. Numbers in [ ] are table references.

Keyword Index

Numbers following p. or pp. are page references. Numbers in [ ] are table references.

Numbers following p. or pp. are page references. Numbers in [ ] are table references.

Numbers following p. or pp. are page references. Numbers in [ ] are table references.

Mental health and human services technology
— associate's degrees, p. 587 [683]
— awards, p. 587 [683]
— bachelor's degrees, p. 587 [683]
— doctoral degrees, p. 587 [683]
— first-professional degrees, p. 587 [683]
— master's degrees, p. 587 [683]
Mental Health Librarians Section
— budget, p. 838 [794]
— members, p. 838 [794]
Mental hospitals
— beds, p. 82 [101]
— employment, p. 509 [588]
— establishments, p. 509 [588]
— expenditures, p. 82 [101]
— Medicaid, p. 415 [497]
— mental health services, p. 82 [101]
— number, pp. 81, 509 [100, 588]
— residents, p. 81 [100]
Mental illness
　See also: Mental health; Mental hospitals; specific
　diseases
— Americans With Disabilities Act, p. 278 [371]
— disorders, pp. 33, 110, 112 [38, 130, 132]
— emotional disorders, p. 110 [131]
— homeless persons, p. 100 [115]
— office visits, p. 137 [166]
— treatment, p. 112 [132]
Mental retardation
— facilities, p. 81 [100]
— nursing home residents, p. 93 [109]
— persons with, p. 33 [38]
— students with, p. 39 [42]
Merced, California
— clinical laboratory technologists and technicians, p. 605 [705]
— dental assistants, p. 612 [706]
— dental hygienists, p. 618 [707]
— dental laboratory technicians, p. 625 [708]
— dentists, p. 631 [709]
— dietitians, p. 638 [710]
— health aides, p. 644 [711]
— health care managers, p. 691 [721]
— health diagnosing practitioners, p. 651 [712]
— health record technologists and technicians, p. 658 [714]
— health technologists and technicians, p. 670 [716]
— licensed practical nurses, p. 677 [718]
— medical appliance technicians, p. 625 [708]
— medical scientists, p. 685 [720]
— nursing aides, p. 698 [722]
— occupational therapists, p. 705 [724]
— optical goods workers, p. 711 [725]
— optometrists, p. 717 [726]
— orderlies, p. 698 [722]
— pharmacists, p. 724 [727]
— physical therapists, p. 730 [728]
— physicians, p. 737 [729]
— physicians' assistants, p. 743 [730]
— psychologists, p. 753 [732]

Merced, California continued:
— radiologic technicians, p. 763 [734]
— registered nurses, p. 770 [735]
— respiratory therapists, p. 777 [737]
— speech therapists, p. 783 [738]
— therapists, p. 790 [739]
— veterinarians, p. 796 [740]
Merck and Company
— Pepcid sales, p. 920 [909]
— Prilosec sales, p. 920 [909]
— sales, p. 571 [664]
Meriden, Connecticut
— clinical laboratory technologists and technicians, p. 606 [705]
— dental assistants, p. 612 [706]
— dental hygienists, p. 618 [707]
— dental laboratory technicians, p. 625 [708]
— dentists, p. 631 [709]
— dietitians, p. 638 [710]
— health aides, p. 645 [711]
— health care managers, p. 692 [721]
— health diagnosing practitioners, p. 651 [712]
— health record technologists and technicians, p. 658 [714]
— health specialties teachers, p. 664 [715]
— health technologists and technicians, p. 671 [716]
— licensed practical nurses, p. 678 [718]
— medical appliance technicians, p. 625 [708]
— medical science teachers, p. 681 [719]
— medical scientists, p. 685 [720]
— nursing aides, p. 698 [722]
— occupational therapists, p. 705 [724]
— optical goods workers, p. 711 [725]
— optometrists, p. 718 [726]
— orderlies, p. 698 [722]
— pharmacists, p. 724 [727]
— physical therapists, p. 731 [728]
— physicians, p. 737 [729]
— physicians' assistants, p. 743 [730]
— podiatrists, p. 748 [731]
— psychologists, p. 754 [732]
— psychology teachers, p. 758 [733]
— radiologic technicians, p. 764 [734]
— registered nurses, p. 770 [735]
— respiratory therapists, p. 777 [737]
— speech therapists, p. 783 [738]
— therapists, p. 790 [739]
— veterinarians, p. 796 [740]
Mesa, Arizona
— city government expenditures, p. 334 [422]
Mesquite, Texas
— city government expenditures, p. 379 [463]
Messengers
— earnings, p. 800 [741]
Methamphetamines
— prisoners, p. 99 [114]
Method to Extend Research in Time
— costs, p. 827 [779]
— grants, p. 827 [779]
Metropolitan Employees
— campaign contributions, p. 890 [870]

Numbers following p. or pp. are page references. Numbers in [ ] are table references.

Numbers following p. or pp. are page references. Numbers in [ ] are table references.

Keyword Index

1107

Numbers following p. or pp. are page references. Numbers in [ ] are table references.

Midland, Michigan continued:
— psychologists, p. 754 [732]
— radiologic technicians, p. 764 [734]
— registered nurses, p. 771 [735]
— respiratory therapists, p. 778 [737]
— speech therapists, p. 784 [738]
— therapists, p. 791 [739]
— veterinarians, p. 797 [740]

Midland, Texas
— city government expenditures, p. 379 [463]
— clinical laboratory technologists and technicians, p. 605 [705]
— dental assistants, p. 612 [706]
— dental hygienists, p. 618 [707]
— dental laboratory technicians, p. 625 [708]
— dentists, p. 631 [709]
— dietitians, p. 638 [710]
— health aides, p. 644 [711]
— health care managers, p. 691 [721]
— health diagnosing practitioners, p. 651 [712]
— health record technologists and technicians, p. 658 [714]
— health technologists and technicians, p. 670 [716]
— licensed practical nurses, p. 677 [718]
— medical appliance technicians, p. 625 [708]
— nursing aides, p. 698 [722]
— optical goods workers, p. 711 [725]
— optometrists, p. 718 [726]
— orderlies, p. 698 [722]
— pharmacists, p. 724 [727]
— physical therapists, p. 730 [728]
— physicians, p. 737 [729]
— physicians' assistants, p. 743 [730]
— psychologists, p. 753 [732]
— psychology teachers, p. 758 [733]
— radiologic technicians, p. 763 [734]
— registered nurses, p. 770 [735]
— respiratory therapists, p. 777 [737]
— speech therapists, p. 783 [738]
— therapists, p. 790 [739]

Midwives
— births attended by, p. 121 [142]
— salaries and wages, p. 804 [744]

Migraine headaches
— chronic conditions, p. 53 [60]

Migrant programs
— Head Start programs, p. 455 [532]

Military personnel
— institutionalized population, p. 87 [105]
— mortality rate, pp. 82, 84-85 [102-104]
— suicide, p. 254 [335]
— veterans' compensation, p. 486 [558]
— veterans' pension benefits, p. 486 [558]

Millwork
— lost workdays due to illness or injury, p. 289 [383]

Milwaukee, Wisconsin
— city government expenditures, p. 386 [469]
— clinical laboratory technologists and technicians, p. 605 [705]
— consumer expenditures, p. 317 [407]

Milwaukee, Wisconsin continued:
— dental assistants, p. 612 [706]
— dental hygienists, p. 618 [707]
— dental laboratory technicians, p. 625 [708]
— dentists, p. 631 [709]
— dietitians, p. 638 [710]
— health aides, p. 644 [711]
— health care managers, p. 691 [721]
— health diagnosing practitioners, p. 651 [712]
— health record technologists and technicians, p. 658 [714]
— health specialties teachers, p. 664 [715]
— health technologists and technicians, p. 670 [716]
— inappropriate procedures, p. 142 [172]
— licensed practical nurses, p. 677 [718]
— medical appliance technicians, p. 625 [708]
— medical science teachers, p. 681 [719]
— medical scientists, p. 685 [720]
— nursing aides, p. 698 [722]
— occupational therapists, p. 705 [724]
— optical goods workers, p. 711 [725]
— optometrists, p. 718 [726]
— orderlies, p. 698 [722]
— pharmacists, p. 724 [727]
— physical therapists, p. 730 [728]
— physicians, p. 737 [729]
— physicians' assistants, p. 743 [730]
— podiatrists, p. 748 [731]
— psychologists, p. 753 [732]
— psychology teachers, p. 758 [733]
— radiologic technicians, p. 763 [734]
— registered nurses, p. 770 [735]
— respiratory therapists, p. 777 [737]
— speech therapists, p. 783 [738]
— therapists, p. 790 [739]
— veterinarians, p. 796 [740]

Minibikes
— product-related injuries, p. 75 [96]

Mining
— health care costs per employee, p. 262 [349]
— work fatalities, p. 287 [379]

Minneapolis, Minnesota
— city government expenditures, p. 358 [443]
— clinical laboratory technologists and technicians, p. 605 [705]
— consumer expenditures, p. 317 [407]
— dental assistants, p. 612 [706]
— dental hygienists, p. 618 [707]
— dental laboratory technicians, p. 625 [708]
— dentists, p. 631 [709]
— dietitians, p. 638 [710]
— employee sick days, p. 291 [386]
— health aides, p. 644 [711]
— health care managers, p. 691 [721]
— health diagnosing practitioners, p. 651 [712]
— health maintenance organizations, p. 261 [347]
— health record technologists and technicians, p. 658 [714]
— health specialties teachers, p. 664 [715]
— health technologists and technicians, p. 670 [716]
— inappropriate procedures, p. 142 [172]
— indemnity plans, p. 261 [347]

Numbers following p. or pp. are page references. Numbers in [ ] are table references.

1109

Numbers following p. or pp. are page references. Numbers in [ ] are table references.

Numbers following p. or pp. are page references. Numbers in [ ] are table references.

Numbers following p. or pp. are page references. Numbers in [ ] are table references.

Keyword Index

Numbers following p. or pp. are page references. Numbers in [ ] are table references.

Numbers following p. or pp. are page references. Numbers in [ ] are table references.

Numbers following p. or pp. are page references. Numbers in [ ] are table references.

Numbers following p. or pp. are page references. Numbers in [ ] are table references.

Mumps
— cases, p. 61 [71]
— epidemics, p. 22 [28]
— vaccinations, pp. 164-165 [213-214]

Muncie, Indiana
— clinical laboratory technologists and technicians, p. 606 [705]
— dental assistants, p. 612 [706]
— dental hygienists, p. 618 [707]
— dental laboratory technicians, p. 625 [708]
— dentists, p. 631 [709]
— dietitians, p. 638 [710]
— health aides, p. 644 [711]
— health care managers, p. 691 [721]
— health diagnosing practitioners, p. 651 [712]
— health record technologists and technicians, p. 658 [714]
— health specialties teachers, p. 664 [715]
— health technologists and technicians, p. 670 [716]
— licensed practical nurses, p. 677 [718]
— medical appliance technicians, p. 625 [708]
— medical scientists, p. 685 [720]
— nursing aides, p. 698 [722]
— optical goods workers, p. 711 [725]
— orderlies, p. 698 [722]
— pharmacists, p. 724 [727]
— physical therapists, p. 730 [728]
— physicians, p. 737 [729]
— physicians' assistants, p. 743 [730]
— psychologists, p. 753 [732]
— psychology teachers, p. 758 [733]
— radiologic technicians, p. 763 [734]
— registered nurses, p. 770 [735]
— respiratory therapists, p. 777 [737]
— speech therapists, p. 783 [738]
— therapists, p. 790 [739]
— veterinarians, p. 796 [740]

Murder
  See also: Homicide
— family, p. 252 [331]
— men, p. 252 [332]
— number, p. 250 [327]
— women, p. 252 [332]
— workplace, p. 287 [378]

Murine typhus fever
— cases, p. 61 [71]

Muscular Dystrophy Association
— fund-raising, p. 865 [834]
— public income, p. 865 [834]

Musculoskeletal conditions
— acute conditions, p. 40 [43]
— bed days, p. 42 [44]
— chronic conditions, p. 52 [60]
— medical attention, p. 43 [46]
— office visits, p. 137 [166]
— restricted activity, p. 45 [47]

Museums/historical societies
— grants, p. 830 [781]

Music therapy
— associate's degrees, p. 590 [687]

Music therapy continued:
— awards, p. 590 [687]
— bachelor's degrees, p. 590 [687]
— doctoral degrees, p. 590 [687]
— first-professional degrees, p. 590 [687]
— master's degrees, p. 590 [687]

Muskegon, Michigan
— clinical laboratory technologists and technicians, p. 606 [705]
— dental assistants, p. 612 [706]
— dental hygienists, p. 618 [707]
— dental laboratory technicians, p. 625 [708]
— dentists, p. 631 [709]
— dietitians, p. 638 [710]
— health aides, p. 644 [711]
— health care managers, p. 691 [721]
— health diagnosing practitioners, p. 651 [712]
— health record technologists and technicians, p. 658 [714]
— health specialties teachers, p. 664 [715]
— health technologists and technicians, p. 670 [716]
— licensed practical nurses, p. 677 [718]
— medical appliance technicians, p. 625 [708]
— nursing aides, p. 698 [722]
— occupational therapists, p. 705 [724]
— optical goods workers, p. 711 [725]
— optometrists, p. 718 [726]
— orderlies, p. 698 [722]
— pharmacists, p. 724 [727]
— physical therapists, p. 730 [728]
— physicians, p. 737 [729]
— physicians' assistants, p. 743 [730]
— podiatrists, p. 748 [731]
— psychologists, p. 753 [732]
— radiologic technicians, p. 763 [734]
— registered nurses, p. 770 [735]
— respiratory therapists, p. 777 [737]
— speech therapists, p. 783 [738]
— therapists, p. 790 [739]

Mustard greens
— calcium, p. 228 [296]

Mutual funds
— hospital bondholders, p. 831 [783]

Mutual of Omaha
— net premiums, p. 515 [597]

Myanmar
— infant mortality, p. 937 [932]
— tuberculosis, p. 945 [941]

Myocardial infarction
— prisoners, p. 97 [112]

Myringotomy
— hospital care, p. 176 [233]
— outpatient services, p. 176 [233]

Nails
— accidents, p. 72 [90]
— product-related injuries, p. 72 [90]

Namibia
— tuberculosis, p. 944 [941]

Naples, Florida
— clinical laboratory technologists and technicians, p. 606 [705]
— dental assistants, p. 612 [706]

Numbers following p. or pp. are page references. Numbers in [ ] are table references.

Numbers following p. or pp. are page references. Numbers in [ ] are table references.

Numbers following p. or pp. are page references. Numbers in [ ] are table references.

Neenah, Wisconsin continued:
— optical goods workers, p. 708 [725]
— optometrists, p. 714 [726]
— orderlies, p. 694 [722]
— pharmacists, p. 720 [727]
— physical therapists, p. 727 [728]
— physicians, p. 733 [729]
— physicians' assistants, p. 740 [730]
— psychologists, p. 750 [732]
— psychology teachers, p. 756 [733]
— radiologic technicians, p. 760 [734]
— registered nurses, p. 766 [735]
— respiratory therapists, p. 774 [737]
— speech therapists, p. 780 [738]
— therapists, p. 786 [739]
— veterinarians, p. 793 [740]
Nepal
— infant mortality, p. 937 [932]
— tuberculosis, p. 945 [941]
Nephritis
— deaths, pp. 10-12, 27, 103 [14, 31, 119]
— men, p. 103 [119]
— older Americans, pp. 10-12 [14]
Nephrosis
— deaths, pp. 10-12, 27, 103 [14, 31, 119]
— men, p. 103 [119]
— older Americans, pp. 10-12 [14]
Nephrotic syndrome
— deaths, pp. 10-12, 27, 103 [14, 31, 119]
— men, p. 103 [119]
— older Americans, pp. 10-12 [14]
Nervous system
— office visits, p. 137 [166]
Netherlands
— asthma, p. 940 [936]
— breast cancer, p. 940 [936]
— bronchitis, p. 940 [936]
— bronchus cancer, p. 940 [936]
— cerebrovascular disease, p. 940 [936]
— chronic liver disease, p. 940 [936]
— circulatory system disease mortality rates, pp. 938-939 [934-935]
— cirrhosis, p. 940 [936]
— emphysema, p. 940 [936]
— health care expenditures, pp. 930, 932-933 [924, 927-928]
— health insurance, p. 947 [945]
— hospital care, p. 926 [919]
— hospital personnel, p. 924 [916]
— infant mortality, p. 936 [932]
— inpatient care, pp. 924-925 [917-918]
— ischemic heart disease, p. 940 [936]
— lung cancer, p. 940 [936]
— oncology, p. 926 [920]
— physicians, p. 955 [959]
— physicians' services, p. 926 [920]
— self-inflicted injuries, p. 940 [936]
— stomach cancer, p. 940 [936]
— suicide, p. 940 [936]
— trachea cancer, p. 940 [936]

Netherlands continued:
— traffic accidents, p. 940 [936]
Neuralgia
— chronic conditions, p. 53 [60]
Neuritis
— chronic conditions, pp. 52-53 [60]
Neurological disorders
— Americans With Disabilities Act, p. 278 [371]
Neurology
— associate's degrees, p. 587 [682]
— awards, p. 587 [682]
— bachelor's degrees, p. 587 [682]
— biomaterials, p. 174 [229]
— business supply expenditures, p. 841 [801]
— doctoral degrees, p. 587 [682]
— first-professional degrees, p. 587 [682]
— geriatrics, p. 597 [698]
— leading hospitals for treatment, p. 160 [204]
— master's degrees, p. 587 [682]
— medical school faculty, pp. 598 [699-700]
— medical supply expenditures, p. 841 [801]
— physicians, p. 597 [698]
— professional spending, p. 843 [803]
Neuroplasty
— cost, p. 187 [245]
Neurosurgery
— business supply expenditures, p. 841 [801]
— cost, p. 916 [901]
— fees, p. 187 [245]
— medical supply expenditures, p. 841 [801]
— professional spending, p. 843 [803]
Neurotic disorders
— older Americans, p. 12 [15]
Nevada
— abortion, p. 112 [133]
— abused women, p. 78 [98]
— accidental death, p. 28 [32]
— accidents, p. 28 [32]
— Aid to Families With Dependent Children, pp. 466, 473 [542, 548]
— alcohol abuse treatment programs, p. 195 [257]
— atherosclerosis, p. 28 [32]
— births, pp. 114, 116 [135-136]
— births to teenage mothers, p. 116 [136]
— cancer, p. 28 [32]
— cerebrovascular diseases, p. 28 [32]
— child nutrition programs, p. 457 [535]
— chiropractors' offices and clinics, p. 553 [645]
— chronic obstructive pulmonary diseases, p. 28 [32]
— cirrhosis, p. 28 [32]
— city government expenditures, p. 363 [448]
— deaths, p. 28 [32]
— dental equipment wholesalers, p. 577 [669]
— dental laboratories, pp. 521, 524 [606, 609]
— dental supply wholesalers, p. 577 [669]
— dentists' offices and clinics, pp. 550, 555 [643, 647]
— diabetes, p. 28 [32]
— disciplinary action, p. 908 [893]
— drug and medicine wholesalers, p. 575 [667]

Numbers following p. or pp. are page references. Numbers in [ ] are table references.

Nevada continued:
— drug and proprietary retailers, p. 573 [666]
— drug proprietaries wholesalers, p. 575 [667]
— drug stores, p. 573 [666]
— druggists' sundries wholesalers, p. 575 [667]
— end-stage renal disease facilities, p. 439 [517]
— flu, p. 28 [32]
— food stamps, p. 462 [539]
— grants, p. 829 [780]
— Head Start programs, p. 454 [532]
— health practitioners' offices and clinics, p. 563 [655]
— health services, p. 489 [560]
— heart disease, p. 28 [32]
— home health care, pp. 439, 493 [517, 565]
— homeless persons, p. 80 [99]
— hospital charges, p. 429 [511]
— hospital equipment wholesalers, p. 577 [669]
— hospital supply wholesalers, p. 577 [669]
— hospitals, p. 506 [584]
— institutionalized populations, pp. 78, 80, 89, 99 [98-99, 105, 113]
— insurance coverage of residents, p. 227 [295]
— intermediate care facilities, p. 540 [629]
— kidney dialysis centers, p. 496 [570]
— liver disease, p. 28 [32]
— local government expenditures, p. 330 [419]
— low birth weight babies, p. 116 [136]
— malpractice insurance premiums, pp. 912-913 [897, 899]
— Medicaid, p. 412 [495]
— medical and surgical hospitals, p. 503 [580]
— medical doctors' offices and clinics, pp. 552, 557 [644, 649]
— medical equipment rental and leasing, p. 499 [574]
— medical equipment wholesalers, p. 577 [669]
— medical instrument manufacturers, p. 530 [616]
— medical laboratories, pp. 439, 524, 526 [517, 609, 611]
— medical supply manufacturers, p. 530 [616]
— medical supply wholesalers, p. 577 [669]
— Medicare, pp. 422, 436 [506, 515]
— mental health expenditures, p. 108 [128]
— mental hospitals, p. 509 [588]
— military personnel, p. 89 [105]
— National School Lunch Program, p. 464 [540]
— nursing facilities, p. 543 [634]
— nursing homes, p. 92 [108]
— ophthalmic goods wholesalers, p. 578 [670]
— optometrists' offices and clinics, p. 561 [653]
— osteopaths' offices and clinics, p. 559 [651]
— personal care facilities, p. 543 [634]
— physicians' offices and clinics, pp. 552, 557, 559 [644, 649, 651]
— pneumonia, p. 28 [32]
— podiatrists' offices and clinics, p. 565 [657]
— prisoners, p. 99 [113]
— psychiatric hospitals, p. 509 [588]
— skilled nursing care facilities, p. 547 [639]
— skilled nursing facilities, p. 439 [517]
— skilled nursing facility charges, p. 432 [512]
— Social Security, pp. 443, 445 [521-522]
— social welfare, p. 473 [548]

Nevada continued:
— specialty hospitals, p. 512 [592]
— state government expenditures, p. 393 [477]
— state medical boards, p. 908 [893]
— suicide, p. 28 [32]
— Supplemental Social Income, p. 473 [548]
— Supplementary Social Insurance, pp. 466, 475 [542, 550]
— work disabilities, pp. 279, 281, 283, 285 [372-373, 375-376]

New Bedford, Massachusetts
— city government expenditures, p. 355 [441]
— clinical laboratory technologists and technicians, p. 606 [705]
— dental assistants, p. 612 [706]
— dental hygienists, p. 618 [707]
— dental laboratory technicians, p. 625 [708]
— dentists, p. 631 [709]
— dietitians, p. 638 [710]
— health aides, p. 645 [711]
— health care managers, p. 692 [721]
— health diagnosing practitioners, p. 651 [712]
— health record technologists and technicians, p. 658 [714]
— health technologists and technicians, p. 671 [716]
— licensed practical nurses, p. 678 [718]
— medical appliance technicians, p. 625 [708]
— nursing aides, p. 698 [722]
— occupational therapists, p. 705 [724]
— optical goods workers, p. 711 [725]
— optometrists, p. 718 [726]
— orderlies, p. 698 [722]
— pharmacists, p. 724 [727]
— physical therapists, p. 730 [728]
— physicians, p. 737 [729]
— podiatrists, p. 748 [731]
— psychologists, p. 754 [732]
— radiologic technicians, p. 764 [734]
— registered nurses, p. 770 [735]
— respiratory therapists, p. 777 [737]
— speech therapists, p. 783 [738]
— therapists, p. 790 [739]
— veterinarians, p. 796 [740]

New Britain, Connecticut
— city government expenditures, p. 340 [426]
— clinical laboratory technologists and technicians, p. 604 [705]
— dental assistants, p. 611 [706]
— dental hygienists, p. 617 [707]
— dental laboratory technicians, p. 623 [708]
— dentists, p. 630 [709]
— dietitians, p. 636 [710]
— health aides, p. 643 [711]
— health care managers, p. 690 [721]
— health diagnosing practitioners, p. 650 [712]
— health record technologists and technicians, p. 657 [714]
— health specialties teachers, p. 663 [715]
— health technologists and technicians, p. 669 [716]
— licensed practical nurses, p. 676 [718]
— medical appliance technicians, p. 623 [708]
— medical science teachers, p. 681 [719]
— medical scientists, p. 684 [720]
— nursing aides, p. 697 [722]
— occupational therapists, p. 704 [724]

Numbers following p. or pp. are page references. Numbers in [ ] are table references.

1121

Keyword Index

Numbers following p. or pp. are page references. Numbers in [ ] are table references.

Keyword Index

Numbers following p. or pp. are page references. Numbers in [ ] are table references.

1123

Numbers following p. or pp. are page references. Numbers in [ ] are table references.

Keyword Index

Numbers following p. or pp. are page references. Numbers in [ ] are table references.

1126

Numbers following p. or pp. are page references. Numbers in [ ] are table references.

Numbers following p. or pp. are page references. Numbers in [ ] are table references.

Numbers following p. or pp. are page references. Numbers in [ ] are table references.

1129

Numbers following p. or pp. are page references. Numbers in [ ] are table references.

Numbers following p. or pp. are page references. Numbers in [ ] are table references.

Numbers following p. or pp. are page references. Numbers in [ ] are table references.

1132

Keyword Index

Numbers following p. or pp. are page references. Numbers in [ ] are table references.

1134

Keyword Index

Numbers following p. or pp. are page references. Numbers in [ ] are table references.

Numbers following p. or pp. are page references. Numbers in [ ] are table references.

Numbers following p. or pp. are page references. Numbers in [ ] are table references.

Keyword Index

Numbers following p. or pp. are page references. Numbers in [ ] are table references.

Numbers following p. or pp. are page references. Numbers in [ ] are table references.

1139

Oregon continued:
— medical doctors' offices and clinics, pp. 552, 557 [644, 649]
— medical equipment rental and leasing, p. 499 [574]
— medical equipment wholesalers, p. 577 [669]
— medical instrument and supply manufacturers, p. 529 [615]
— medical instrument manufacturers, pp. 530, 533 [616, 620]
— medical laboratories, pp. 439, 524, 526 [517, 609, 611]
— medical supply manufacturers, p. 530 [616]
— medical supply wholesalers, p. 577 [669]
— Medicare, pp. 423, 436 [506, 515]
— mental health expenditures, p. 108 [128]
— mental hospitals, p. 509 [588]
— military personnel, p. 89 [105]
— National School Lunch Program, p. 464 [540]
— nursing facilities, p. 543 [634]
— nursing homes, p. 92 [108]
— ophthalmic goods wholesalers, p. 578 [670]
— optical instrument manufacturers, p. 532 [619]
— optical lens manufacturers, p. 532 [619]
— optometrists' offices and clinics, p. 561 [653]
— osteopaths' offices and clinics, p. 559 [651]
— personal care facilities, p. 543 [634]
— personal services, p. 492 [564]
— pharmaceutical preparation manufacturers, p. 571 [663]
— physicians' offices and clinics, pp. 552, 557, 559 [644, 649, 651]
— pneumonia, p. 28 [32]
— podiatrists' offices and clinics, p. 565 [657]
— prisoners, p. 99 [113]
— psychiatric hospitals, p. 509 [588]
— residential care facilities, p. 546 [638]
— skilled nursing care facilities, p. 547 [639]
— skilled nursing facilities, p. 439 [517]
— skilled nursing facility charges, p. 432 [512]
— Social Security, pp. 443, 445 [521-522]
— social welfare, p. 473 [548]
— specialty hospitals, p. 512 [592]
— state government expenditures, p. 394 [477]
— state medical boards, p. 909 [893]
— suicide, p. 28 [32]
— Supplemental Social Income, p. 473 [548]
— Supplementary Social Insurance, pp. 466, 475 [542, 550]
— surgical appliances, p. 534 [621]
— surgical instrument manufacturers, p. 533 [620]
— surgical supplies, p. 534 [621]
— work disabilities, pp. 279, 281-283, 285 [372-376]
Orem, Utah
— clinical laboratory technologists and technicians, p. 606 [705]
— dental assistants, p. 613 [706]
— dental hygienists, p. 619 [707]
— dental laboratory technicians, p. 625 [708]
— dentists, p. 632 [709]
— dietitians, p. 638 [710]
— health aides, p. 645 [711]
— health care managers, p. 692 [721]
— health diagnosing practitioners, p. 652 [712]
— health record technologists and technicians, p. 659 [714]
— health specialties teachers, p. 665 [715]

Orem, Utah continued:
— health technologists and technicians, p. 671 [716]
— licensed practical nurses, p. 678 [718]
— medical appliance technicians, p. 625 [708]
— medical scientists, p. 686 [720]
— nursing aides, p. 699 [722]
— occupational therapists, p. 706 [724]
— optical goods workers, p. 712 [725]
— optometrists, p. 718 [726]
— orderlies, p. 699 [722]
— pharmacists, p. 725 [727]
— physical therapists, p. 731 [728]
— physicians, p. 738 [729]
— physicians' assistants, p. 744 [730]
— podiatrists, p. 748 [731]
— psychologists, p. 754 [732]
— psychology teachers, p. 758 [733]
— radiologic technicians, p. 764 [734]
— registered nurses, p. 771 [735]
— respiratory therapists, p. 778 [737]
— speech therapists, p. 784 [738]
— therapists, p. 791 [739]
— veterinarians, p. 797 [740]
Organ transplants
— bone marrow, p. 916 [901]
— donors, p. 189 [250]
— employee benefits, p. 270 [359]
— heart, pp. 189-190 [250-251]
— heart/lung, pp. 189-190 [250-251]
— kidney, p. 190 [251]
— kindey, p. 189 [250]
— liver, pp. 189-190 [250-251]
— lung, pp. 189-190 [250-251]
— multiple organs, p. 189 [250]
— pancreas, pp. 189-190 [250-251]
Organic brain syndromes
— nursing home residents, pp. 93-94 [109-110]
Organizations
— grants, p. 830 [781]
Orientation programs
— employee benefits, p. 834 [788]
Orlando, Florida
— clinical laboratory technologists and technicians, p. 606 [705]
— dental assistants, p. 612 [706]
— dental hygienists, p. 619 [707]
— dental laboratory technicians, p. 625 [708]
— dentists, p. 632 [709]
— dietitians, p. 638 [710]
— health aides, p. 645 [711]
— health care managers, p. 692 [721]
— health diagnosing practitioners, p. 651 [712]
— health record technologists and technicians, p. 659 [714]
— health specialties teachers, p. 664 [715]
— health technologists and technicians, p. 671 [716]
— licensed practical nurses, p. 678 [718]
— medical appliance technicians, p. 625 [708]
— medical scientists, p. 686 [720]
— nursing aides, p. 698 [722]
— occupational therapists, p. 705 [724]

Numbers following p. or pp. are page references. Numbers in [ ] are table references.

Numbers following p. or pp. are page references. Numbers in [ ] are table references.

Numbers following p. or pp. are page references. Numbers in [ ] are table references.

Numbers following p. or pp. are page references. Numbers in [ ] are table references.

Keyword Index

Numbers following p. or pp. are page references. Numbers in [ ] are table references.

1144

Numbers following p. or pp. are page references. Numbers in [ ] are table references.

Numbers following p. or pp. are page references. Numbers in [ ] are table references.

Numbers following p. or pp. are page references. Numbers in [ ] are table references.

1147

Keyword Index

Numbers following p. or pp. are page references. Numbers in [ ] are table references.

Numbers following p. or pp. are page references. Numbers in [ ] are table references.

Numbers following p. or pp. are page references. Numbers in [ ] are table references.

Pittsfield, Massachusetts continued:
— health aides, p. 645 [711]
— health care managers, p. 692 [721]
— health diagnosing practitioners, p. 651 [712]
— health record technologists and technicians, p. 659 [714]
— health specialties teachers, p. 665 [715]
— health technologists and technicians, p. 671 [716]
— licensed practical nurses, p. 678 [718]
— medical appliance technicians, p. 625 [708]
— medical scientists, p. 686 [720]
— nursing aides, p. 699 [722]
— occupational therapists, p. 706 [724]
— optical goods workers, p. 712 [725]
— orderlies, p. 699 [722]
— pharmacists, p. 725 [727]
— physical therapists, p. 731 [728]
— physicians, p. 738 [729]
— psychologists, p. 754 [732]
— radiologic technicians, p. 764 [734]
— registered nurses, p. 771 [735]
— respiratory therapists, p. 778 [737]
— speech therapists, p. 784 [738]
— therapists, p. 790 [739]
— veterinarians, p. 797 [740]

Placentas
— infant mortality, p. 121 [141]

Plague
— cases, p. 61 [71]

Plano, Texas
— city government expenditures, p. 379 [463]

Plastic products
— accidents, p. 73 [92]
— injuries, p. 73 [92]
— product-related injuries, p. 73 [92]

Plastic surgery
— business supply expenditures, p. 842 [801]
— fees, p. 188 [247]
— medical supply expenditures, p. 842 [801]
— professional spending, p. 843 [803]

Playground equipment
— accidents, p. 75 [96]
— product-related injuries, p. 75 [96]

Pneumonia
— acute conditions, p. 40 [43]
— bed days, p. 41 [44]
— children, p. 18 [22]
— deaths, pp. 10-11, 18-19, 27-28, 42, 103 [14, 22-23, 31-32, 45, 119]
— home health care, p. 153 [190]
— hospital care, p. 8-9 [13]
— infant mortality, p. 121 [141]
— measles, p. 21 [27]
— medical attention, p. 43 [46]
— men, pp. 8-9, 103 [13, 119]
— older Americans, p. 8-11 [13-14]
— restricted activity, p. 44 [47]
— vaccination, p. 179 [236]

Pocono Medical Center (East Stroudsburg, Pennsylvania)
— labor strike, p. 835 [789]

Podiatrists' offices and clinics
— employment, p. 565 [657]
— establishments, p. 565 [657]
— number, p. 565 [657]
— receipts, p. 566 [658]

Podiatry
— associate's degrees, p. 585 [679]
— awards, p. 585 [679]
— bachelor's degrees, p. 585 [679]
— doctoral degrees, p. 585 [679]
— employment, p. 746 [731]
— first-professional degrees, p. 585 [679]
— master's degrees, p. 585 [679]
— salaries and wages, p. 804 [744]
— student loans, p. 592 [690]

Podiatry PAC
— campaign contributions, p. 890 [870]

Point-of-service plans
— cost, p. 260 [345]
— employee enrollment, p. 267 [355]
— market share, p. 517 [600]

Poland
— abortion, p. 934 [929]
— asthma, p. 940 [936]
— breast cancer, p. 940 [936]
— bronchitis, p. 940 [936]
— bronchus cancer, p. 940 [936]
— cerebrovascular disease, p. 940 [936]
— chronic liver disease, p. 940 [936]
— cirrhosis, p. 940 [936]
— emphysema, p. 940 [936]
— infant mortality, p. 936 [932]
— ischemic heart disease, p. 940 [936]
— lung cancer, p. 940 [936]
— self-inflicted injuries, p. 940 [936]
— stomach cancer, p. 940 [936]
— suicide, p. 940 [936]
— trachea cancer, p. 940 [936]
— traffic accidents, p. 940 [936]

Polio
— immunization, p. 928 [922]
— vaccinations, p. 164 [213]

Poliomyelitis
— cases, p. 61 [71]
— vaccinations, p. 165 [214]

Political action committees
— campaign contributions, pp. 889-892 [869-872]

Pollution
— cancer, p. 49 [54]
— deaths, p. 49 [54]

Pomona, California
— city government expenditures, p. 337 [424]

Ponds
— deaths, p. 67 [81]

Pools
— accidents, p. 75 [96]
— deaths, p. 67 [81]

Numbers following p. or pp. are page references. Numbers in [ ] are table references.

1151

Numbers following p. or pp. are page references. Numbers in [ ] are table references.

Numbers following p. or pp. are page references. Numbers in [ ] are table references.

Numbers following p. or pp. are page references. Numbers in [ ] are table references.

Numbers following p. or pp. are page references. Numbers in [ ] are table references.

1155

Keyword Index

Numbers following p. or pp. are page references. Numbers in [ ] are table references.

Numbers following p. or pp. are page references. Numbers in [ ] are table references.

1157

Numbers following p. or pp. are page references. Numbers in [ ] are table references.

Keyword Index

Numbers following p. or pp. are page references. Numbers in [ ] are table references.

Numbers following p. or pp. are page references. Numbers in [ ] are table references.

Keyword Index

1161

Numbers following p. or pp. are page references. Numbers in [ ] are table references.

Keyword Index

Numbers following p. or pp. are page references. Numbers in [ ] are table references.

Numbers following p. or pp. are page references. Numbers in [ ] are table references.

Numbers following p. or pp. are page references. Numbers in [ ] are table references.

Numbers following p. or pp. are page references. Numbers in [ ] are table references.

Keyword Index

Numbers following p. or pp. are page references. Numbers in [ ] are table references.

Numbers following p. or pp. are page references. Numbers in [ ] are table references.

Keyword Index

Salinas, California continued:
— health specialties teachers, p. 665 [715]
— health technologists and technicians, p. 672 [716]
— licensed practical nurses, p. 679 [718]
— medical appliance technicians, p. 626 [708]
— medical scientists, p. 686 [720]
— nursing aides, p. 699 [722]
— occupational therapists, p. 706 [724]
— optical goods workers, p. 712 [725]
— optometrists, p. 719 [726]
— orderlies, p. 699 [722]
— pharmacists, p. 725 [727]
— physical therapists, p. 732 [728]
— physicians, p. 738 [729]
— physicians' assistants, p. 744 [730]
— podiatrists, p. 749 [731]
— psychologists, p. 755 [732]
— radiologic technicians, p. 765 [734]
— registered nurses, p. 771 [735]
— respiratory therapists, p. 778 [737]
— speech therapists, p. 784 [738]
— therapists, p. 791 [739]
— veterinarians, p. 797 [740]

Salmon
— calcium, p. 228 [296]

Salmonellosis
— cases, p. 61 [71]

Salpingo-oophorectomy
— cost, p. 189 [249]

Salt Lake City, Utah
— city government expenditures, p. 381 [464]
— clinical laboratory technologists and technicians, p. 607 [705]
— dental assistants, p. 613 [706]
— dental hygienists, p. 619 [707]
— dental laboratory technicians, p. 626 [708]
— dentists, p. 632 [709]
— dietitians, p. 639 [710]
— health aides, p. 646 [711]
— health care managers, p. 693 [721]
— health diagnosing practitioners, p. 652 [712]
— health record technologists and technicians, p. 659 [714]
— health specialties teachers, p. 665 [715]
— health technologists and technicians, p. 672 [716]
— inappropriate procedures, p. 142 [172]
— licensed practical nurses, p. 679 [718]
— medical appliance technicians, p. 626 [708]
— medical science teachers, p. 682 [719]
— medical scientists, p. 686 [720]
— nursing aides, p. 699 [722]
— occupational therapists, p. 706 [724]
— optical goods workers, p. 713 [725]
— optometrists, p. 719 [726]
— orderlies, p. 699 [722]
— pharmacists, p. 725 [727]
— physical therapists, p. 732 [728]
— physicians, p. 738 [729]
— physicians' assistants, p. 744 [730]
— podiatrists, p. 749 [731]

Salt Lake City, Utah continued:
— psychologists, p. 755 [732]
— psychology teachers, p. 759 [733]
— radiologic technicians, p. 765 [734]
— registered nurses, p. 771 [735]
— respiratory therapists, p. 778 [737]
— speech therapists, p. 784 [738]
— therapists, p. 791 [739]
— veterinarians, p. 797 [740]

San Angelo, Texas
— city government expenditures, p. 379 [463]
— clinical laboratory technologists and technicians, p. 607 [705]
— dental assistants, p. 613 [706]
— dental hygienists, p. 619 [707]
— dental laboratory technicians, p. 626 [708]
— dentists, p. 632 [709]
— dietitians, p. 639 [710]
— health aides, p. 646 [711]
— health care managers, p. 693 [721]
— health diagnosing practitioners, p. 652 [712]
— health record technologists and technicians, p. 659 [714]
— health technologists and technicians, p. 672 [716]
— licensed practical nurses, p. 679 [718]
— medical appliance technicians, p. 626 [708]
— nursing aides, p. 699 [722]
— occupational therapists, p. 706 [724]
— optical goods workers, p. 713 [725]
— optometrists, p. 719 [726]
— orderlies, p. 699 [722]
— pharmacists, p. 725 [727]
— physical therapists, p. 732 [728]
— physicians, p. 738 [729]
— podiatrists, p. 749 [731]
— psychologists, p. 755 [732]
— radiologic technicians, p. 765 [734]
— registered nurses, p. 771 [735]
— respiratory therapists, p. 778 [737]
— speech therapists, p. 784 [738]
— therapists, p. 791 [739]
— veterinarians, p. 797 [740]

San Antonio, Texas
— city government expenditures, p. 379 [463]
— clinical laboratory technologists and technicians, p. 607 [705]
— dental assistants, p. 613 [706]
— dental hygienists, p. 620 [707]
— dental laboratory technicians, p. 626 [708]
— dentists, p. 632 [709]
— dietitians, p. 639 [710]
— health aides, p. 646 [711]
— health care managers, p. 693 [721]
— health diagnosing practitioners, p. 652 [712]
— health record technologists and technicians, p. 659 [714]
— health specialties teachers, p. 665 [715]
— health technologists and technicians, p. 672 [716]
— licensed practical nurses, p. 679 [718]
— medical appliance technicians, p. 626 [708]
— medical science teachers, p. 682 [719]
— medical scientists, p. 686 [720]
— nursing aides, p. 699 [722]

Numbers following p. or pp. are page references. Numbers in [ ] are table references.

1170

Numbers following p. or pp. are page references. Numbers in [ ] are table references.

Santa Maria, California continued:
— health diagnosing practitioners, p. 652 [712]
— health record technologists and technicians, p. 659 [714]
— health specialties teachers, p. 665 [715]
— health technologists and technicians, p. 672 [716]
— licensed practical nurses, p. 679 [718]
— medical appliance technicians, p. 626 [708]
— medical scientists, p. 686 [720]
— nursing aides, p. 699 [722]
— occupational therapists, p. 706 [724]
— optical goods workers, p. 713 [725]
— optometrists, p. 719 [726]
— orderlies, p. 699 [722]
— pharmacists, p. 725 [727]
— physical therapists, p. 732 [728]
— physicians, p. 738 [729]
— physicians' assistants, p. 744 [730]
— psychologists, p. 755 [732]
— psychology teachers, p. 759 [733]
— radiologic technicians, p. 765 [734]
— registered nurses, p. 771 [735]
— respiratory therapists, p. 778 [737]
— speech therapists, p. 785 [738]
— therapists, p. 791 [739]
— veterinarians, p. 797 [740]

Santa Rosa, California
— city government expenditures, p. 337 [424]

Santorum, Representative Rick
— health care reform, p. 894 [874]

Sao Tome
— tuberculosis, p. 944 [941]

Sarasota, Florida
— clinical laboratory technologists and technicians, p. 607 [705]
— dental assistants, p. 613 [706]
— dental hygienists, p. 620 [707]
— dental laboratory technicians, p. 626 [708]
— dentists, p. 632 [709]
— dietitians, p. 639 [710]
— health aides, p. 646 [711]
— health care managers, p. 693 [721]
— health diagnosing practitioners, p. 652 [712]
— health record technologists and technicians, p. 659 [714]
— health specialties teachers, p. 665 [715]
— health technologists and technicians, p. 672 [716]
— licensed practical nurses, p. 679 [718]
— medical appliance technicians, p. 626 [708]
— nursing aides, p. 699 [722]
— occupational therapists, p. 706 [724]
— optical goods workers, p. 713 [725]
— optometrists, p. 719 [726]
— orderlies, p. 699 [722]
— pharmacists, p. 725 [727]
— physical therapists, p. 732 [728]
— physicians, p. 738 [729]
— physicians' assistants, p. 744 [730]
— podiatrists, p. 749 [731]
— psychologists, p. 755 [732]
— radiologic technicians, p. 765 [734]

Sarasota, Florida continued:
— registered nurses, p. 771 [735]
— respiratory therapists, p. 778 [737]
— speech therapists, p. 785 [738]
— therapists, p. 791 [739]
— veterinarians, p. 798 [740]

Sardines
— calcium, p. 228 [296]

Savannah, Georgia
— city government expenditures, p. 344 [430]
— clinical laboratory technologists and technicians, p. 607 [705]
— dental assistants, p. 613 [706]
— dental hygienists, p. 620 [707]
— dental laboratory technicians, p. 626 [708]
— dentists, p. 633 [709]
— dietitians, p. 639 [710]
— health aides, p. 646 [711]
— health care managers, p. 693 [721]
— health diagnosing practitioners, p. 652 [712]
— health record technologists and technicians, p. 660 [714]
— health technologists and technicians, p. 672 [716]
— licensed practical nurses, p. 679 [718]
— medical appliance technicians, p. 626 [708]
— medical scientists, p. 686 [720]
— nursing aides, p. 699 [722]
— occupational therapists, p. 706 [724]
— optical goods workers, p. 713 [725]
— optometrists, p. 719 [726]
— orderlies, p. 699 [722]
— pharmacists, p. 725 [727]
— physical therapists, p. 732 [728]
— physicians, p. 738 [729]
— physicians' assistants, p. 744 [730]
— podiatrists, p. 749 [731]
— psychologists, p. 755 [732]
— radiologic technicians, p. 765 [734]
— registered nurses, p. 771 [735]
— respiratory therapists, p. 778 [737]
— speech therapists, p. 785 [738]
— therapists, p. 791 [739]
— veterinarians, p. 798 [740]

Savings plans
— cost, p. 256 [339]

SBIR Phase I
— costs, p. 827 [779]
— grants, p. 827 [779]

SBIR Phase II
— costs, p. 827 [779]
— grants, p. 827 [779]

Schenectady, New York
— clinical laboratory technologists and technicians, p. 602 [705]
— dental assistants, p. 608 [706]
— dental hygienists, p. 615 [707]
— dental laboratory technicians, p. 621 [708]
— dentists, p. 627 [709]
— dietitians, p. 634 [710]
— health aides, p. 641 [711]
— health care managers, p. 688 [721]
— health diagnosing practitioners, p. 647 [712]

Numbers following p. or pp. are page references. Numbers in [ ] are table references.

1173

Numbers following p. or pp. are page references. Numbers in [ ] are table references.

Keyword Index

Numbers following p. or pp. are page references. Numbers in [ ] are table references.

Numbers following p. or pp. are page references. Numbers in [ ] are table references.

Numbers following p. or pp. are page references. Numbers in [ ] are table references.

Numbers following p. or pp. are page references. Numbers in [ ] are table references.

Numbers following p. or pp. are page references. Numbers in [ ] are table references.

Numbers following p. or pp. are page references. Numbers in [ ] are table references.

Keyword Index

Numbers following p. or pp. are page references. Numbers in [ ] are table references.

Keyword Index

Numbers following p. or pp. are page references. Numbers in [ ] are table references.

Numbers following p. or pp. are page references. Numbers in [ ] are table references.

Keyword Index

Numbers following p. or pp. are page references. Numbers in [ ] are table references.

Keyword Index

Numbers following p. or pp. are page references. Numbers in [ ] are table references.

Numbers following p. or pp. are page references. Numbers in [ ] are table references.

Keyword Index

Numbers following p. or pp. are page references. Numbers in [ ] are table references.

Numbers following p. or pp. are page references. Numbers in [ ] are table references.

1193

Titusville, Florida continued:
— occupational therapists, p. 705 [724]
— optical goods workers, p. 711 [725]
— optometrists, p. 717 [726]
— orderlies, p. 698 [722]
— pharmacists, p. 724 [727]
— physical therapists, p. 730 [728]
— physicians, p. 737 [729]
— physicians' assistants, p. 743 [730]
— psychologists, p. 753 [732]
— psychology teachers, p. 758 [733]
— radiologic technicians, p. 763 [734]
— registered nurses, p. 770 [735]
— respiratory therapists, p. 777 [737]
— speech therapists, p. 783 [738]
— therapists, p. 790 [739]
— veterinarians, p. 796 [740]

Tobacco
— cancer, p. 48 [54]
— chewing, p. 20 [24]
— cigarettes, pp. 244 [318-319]
— deaths, p. 48 [54]
— smokeless, p. 245 [320]

Tobago
— grants, p. 953 [955]

Toboggans
— accidents, p. 75 [96]
— product-related injuries, p. 75 [96]

Toilet safety rails
— rental, p. 172 [226]

Toilets
— product-related injuries, p. 71 [88]

Tokyo, Japan
— cost of aspirin, p. 919 [906]

Toledo, Ohio
— city government expenditures, p. 371 [455]
— clinical laboratory technologists and technicians, p. 607 [705]
— dental assistants, p. 614 [706]
— dental hygienists, p. 620 [707]
— dental laboratory technicians, p. 626 [708]
— dentists, p. 633 [709]
— dietitians, p. 640 [710]
— health aides, p. 646 [711]
— health care managers, p. 693 [721]
— health diagnosing practitioners, p. 653 [712]
— health record technologists and technicians, p. 660 [714]
— health specialties teachers, p. 666 [715]
— health technologists and technicians, p. 672 [716]
— licensed practical nurses, p. 679 [718]
— medical appliance technicians, p. 626 [708]
— medical science teachers, p. 682 [719]
— medical scientists, p. 687 [720]
— nursing aides, p. 700 [722]
— occupational therapists, p. 707 [724]
— optical goods workers, p. 713 [725]
— optometrists, p. 719 [726]
— orderlies, p. 700 [722]
— pharmacists, p. 726 [727]

Toledo, Ohio continued:
— physical therapists, p. 732 [728]
— physicians, p. 739 [729]
— physicians' assistants, p. 745 [730]
— podiatrists, p. 749 [731]
— psychologists, p. 755 [732]
— psychology teachers, p. 759 [733]
— radiologic technicians, p. 765 [734]
— registered nurses, p. 772 [735]
— respiratory therapists, p. 779 [737]
— speech therapists, p. 785 [738]
— therapists, p. 792 [739]
— veterinarians, p. 798 [740]

Tonawanda, New York
— city government expenditures, p. 368 [452]

Tonsillectomy
— hospital care, p. 176 [233]
— outpatient services, p. 176 [233]

Tonsils
— chronic conditions, pp. 52, 54 [60]

Tools
— product-related injuries, pp. 73, 76 [91, 97]

Topeka, Kansas
— city government expenditures, p. 350 [436]
— clinical laboratory technologists and technicians, p. 607 [705]
— dental assistants, p. 614 [706]
— dental hygienists, p. 620 [707]
— dental laboratory technicians, p. 626 [708]
— dentists, p. 633 [709]
— dietitians, p. 640 [710]
— health aides, p. 646 [711]
— health care managers, p. 693 [721]
— health diagnosing practitioners, p. 653 [712]
— health record technologists and technicians, p. 660 [714]
— health technologists and technicians, p. 672 [716]
— licensed practical nurses, p. 679 [718]
— medical appliance technicians, p. 626 [708]
— medical scientists, p. 687 [720]
— nursing aides, p. 700 [722]
— occupational therapists, p. 707 [724]
— optical goods workers, p. 713 [725]
— optometrists, p. 719 [726]
— orderlies, p. 700 [722]
— pharmacists, p. 726 [727]
— physical therapists, p. 732 [728]
— physicians, p. 739 [729]
— physicians' assistants, p. 745 [730]
— podiatrists, p. 749 [731]
— psychologists, p. 755 [732]
— radiologic technicians, p. 765 [734]
— registered nurses, p. 772 [735]
— respiratory therapists, p. 779 [737]
— speech therapists, p. 785 [738]
— therapists, p. 792 [739]
— veterinarians, p. 798 [740]

TOPS (weight loss program)
— cost, p. 236 [308]

Toronto, Ontario, Canada
— cost of aspirin, p. 919 [906]

Numbers following p. or pp. are page references. Numbers in [ ] are table references.

1194

Numbers following p. or pp. are page references. Numbers in [ ] are table references.

Numbers following p. or pp. are page references. Numbers in [ ] are table references.

Numbers following p. or pp. are page references. Numbers in [ ] are table references.

Keyword Index

Numbers following p. or pp. are page references. Numbers in [ ] are table references.

1198

Numbers following p. or pp. are page references. Numbers in [ ] are table references.

Numbers following p. or pp. are page references. Numbers in [ ] are table references.

Numbers following p. or pp. are page references. Numbers in [ ] are table references.

Numbers following p. or pp. are page references. Numbers in [ ] are table references.

1202

Numbers following p. or pp. are page references. Numbers in [ ] are table references.

Numbers following p. or pp. are page references. Numbers in [ ] are table references.

Numbers following p. or pp. are page references. Numbers in [ ] are table references.

Numbers following p. or pp. are page references. Numbers in [ ] are table references.

Keyword Index

Numbers following p. or pp. are page references. Numbers in [ ] are table references.

Numbers following p. or pp. are page references. Numbers in [ ] are table references.

Keyword Index

Numbers following p. or pp. are page references. Numbers in [ ] are table references.

Numbers following p. or pp. are page references. Numbers in [ ] are table references.

Keyword Index

Numbers following p. or pp. are page references. Numbers in [ ] are table references.

Numbers following p. or pp. are page references. Numbers in [ ] are table references.

Keyword Index

Numbers following p. or pp. are page references. Numbers in [ ] are table references.

Numbers following p. or pp. are page references. Numbers in [ ] are table references.

Numbers following p. or pp. are page references. Numbers in [ ] are table references.

Numbers following p. or pp. are page references. Numbers in [ ] are table references.

Keyword Index

Numbers following p. or pp. are page references. Numbers in [ ] are table references.